1 ml. = 17 minims
1 litre = 1 pint 15 fl. oz. approx.

MEASURES OF LENGTH

1 micron	$= \frac{1}{1000}$ millimetre, or 1 micrometre, represented by μ
1 millimetre	= approximately 0·04 inch
1 inch	= „ 2·5 centimetres

PYE'S
SURGICAL HANDICRAFT

PYE'S
SURGICAL HANDICRAFT

EDITED BY

**JAMES KYLE, M.Ch. (Belf.), F.R.C.S. (I.), F.R.C.S. (Eng.),
F.R.C.S. (Edin.)**

Consultant Surgeon, Royal Infirmary, Aberdeen;
Honorary Clinical Senior Lecturer in Surgery, University of Aberdeen

NINETEENTH EDITION

BALTIMORE
THE WILLIAMS AND WILKINS COMPANY
1969

Distribution by Sole Agents:
United States of America: The Williams & Wilkins Company, Baltimore
Canada: The Macmillan Company of Canada Ltd., Toronto

First Edition, September, 1884 *Second Edition, October, 1885* *Third Edition, July, 1891*	WALTER PYE
Fourth Edition, December, 1899	BERTRAM M. H. ROGERS
Fifth Edition, June, 1909 *Sixth Edition, October, 1912* *Seventh Edition, May, 1916* *Eighth Edition, January, 1919* *Reprinted, January, 1924* *Ninth Edition, December, 1924*	W. H. CLAYTON-GREENE
Tenth Edition, January, 1931	H. W. CARSON
Eleventh Edition, December, 1938 *Twelfth Edition, July, 1940* *Thirteenth Edition, September, 1942* *Reprinted, July, 1943* *Fourteenth Edition, September, 1944* *Reprinted, June, 1945* *Fifteenth Edition, February, 1947* *Sixteenth Edition, February, 1950* *Reprinted, February, 1951* *Reprinted, July, 1952* *Seventeenth Edition, September, 1956* *Eighteenth Edition (Vol. I), January, 1962*	HAMILTON BAILEY
(Vol. II), November, 1962 *Vol. I Reprinted, October, 1965*	HAMILTON BAILEY AND JAMES KYLE
Nineteenth Edition, July, 1969	JAMES KYLE

Editors

Spanish Edition in preparation
Portuguese Edition in preparation

SBN 7236 0217 4

PRINTED IN GREAT BRITAIN BY JOHN WRIGHT & SONS LTD.
AT THE STONEBRIDGE PRESS, BRISTOL BS4 5NU

LIST OF CONTRIBUTORS

DAVID ALAN BAILEY, M.A. (Cantab.), M.Chir., F.R.C.S. (Eng.), Consultant Surgeon, University College Hospital, London, and Barnet General Hospital; Formerly Consultant Surgeon, Royal Northern Hospital, London.

Acute Infections of the Hand and Fingers—560.

A. K. BASU, M.S. (Cal.), F.R.C.S. (Eng.), F.A.C.S., F.A.M.S., Director and Director-Professor, Department of Surgery, Institute of Postgraduate Medical Education and Research, and Surgeon Superintendent S.S.K.M. Hospital, Calcutta; Head of the Department of Chest Surgery, University College of Medicine, Calcutta University, Calcutta.

The Management of Cardiac Cases—320.

C. ALLAN BIRCH, M.D. (Liverp.), F.R.C.P. (Lond.), D.C.H., D.P.H., Honorary Consulting Physician, Chase Farm Hospital, Enfield, Middlesex.

Sulphonamide and Antibiotic Therapy—72. The Treatment of Acute Poisoning—84.

WILLIAM BURNETT, Ch.M. (Aberdeen), F.R.C.S. (Eng.), F.R.F.P.S. (Glasg.), F.R.A.C.S., Professor of Surgery, University of Queensland; Senior Surgeon, Royal Brisbane Hospital; Senior Surgeon, Princess Alexandra Hospital; Honorary Consultant Surgeon, Mater Misericordiae Hospital, Brisbane.

The Management of Biliary and Hepatic Cases—358. The Pancreas—382.

LEWIS BURROWS, M.D., F.A.C.S., Assistant Professor of Surgery, Mount Sinai School of Medicine, City University of New York; Assistant Attending in Surgery, Mount Sinai School of Medicine, City University of New York, and Elmhurst City Hospital, Elmhurst, New York; Consultant, Veterans Administration Hospital, Bronx, New York.

Preparation for Operation (jointly)—133.

JOHN BURTON, H.M. Coroner, Greater London.

Certification of Death and Reporting to the Coroner—763.

DAVID S. CHAPMAN, M.D. (Newcastle), M.S. (Durham), F.R.C.S. (Eng.), formerly Professor of Surgery, University of Natal and Head of Division of Surgery, King Edward VIII Hospital, Durban, South Africa.

The Treatment of Wounds—51.

H. S. M. CRABB, M.D.S. (Lond.), Ph.D. (Bristol), F.D.S. R.C.S. (Eng.), Professor of Conservative Dentistry, University of Leeds; Consultant Dental Surgeon, United Leeds Hospitals.

Emergency Dental Treatment—594.

DAVID L. CROSBY, M.B. (Wales), F.R.C.S., Consultant Surgeon, United Cardiff Hospitals, Cardiff.

The Administration of Enemata and Rectal Suppositories (jointly)—404.

HUGH DUDLEY, Ch.M. (Edin.), F.R.C.S. (Edin.), F.R.A.C.S., Foundation Professor of Surgery and Chairman, Department of Surgery, Monash University, Melbourne; Honorary Consultant Surgeon, Alfred Hospital; Consultant Surgeon, Prince Henry's Hospital, Melbourne.

Respiratory Obstruction and Respiratory Insufficiency—11. Shock and Resuscitation—20. Water and Electrolyte Balance and Infusions, Blood Transfusions, and Nutrition (jointly)—32.

H. H. G. EASTCOTT, M.S. (Lond.), F.R.C.S. (Eng.), Consultant Surgeon, St. Mary's Hospital, The Royal Masonic Hospital, King Edward VII Hospital for Officers, and to the Royal Navy.

Peripheral Vascular Surgery—524.

ERIC L. FARQUHARSON, M.D., F.R.C.S. (Edin.), F.R.C.S. (Eng.), Consultant Surgeon, Royal Infirmary, Edinburgh.

Injuries of the Hand and Fingers—545.

J. D. FERGUSSON, M.D. (Cantab.), F.R.C.S. (Eng.), Consultant Surgeon, St. Peter's, St. Paul's, and St. Philip's Hospitals and to the Central Middlesex Hospital; Director of Teaching and Research, Institute of Urology (University of London).

The Upper Urinary Tract (jointly)—436. The Lower Urinary Tract (jointly)—446.

FREDERICK PATRICK FITZGERALD, M.A., M.B., Ch.B. (Dublin), F.R.C.S.I., Consultant Orthopædic Surgeon, Royal Northern Hospital, London; Orthopædic Surgeon, Royal Free Hospital, London.

Plaster-of-Paris Technique—253.

GILBERT FORBES, M.D., B.Sc., F.R.C.S. (Glasg.), F.R.C.S. (Edin.), F.C.Path., Regius Professor of Forensic Medicine, University of Glasgow.

Death Certification in Scotland—769.

A. P. M. FORREST, B.Sc., M.D., Ch.M. (St. Andrews), F.R.C.S. (Edin.), F.R.C.S. (Eng.), F.R.C.S. (Glasg.), Professor of Surgery, Welsh National School of Medicine, and Honorary Consultant Surgeon, United Cardiff Hospitals.

Management of Advanced Carcinoma and Care of the Dying—731.

ALBERT FRANKEL, M.D., F.A.C.S., F.A.C.G., Assistant Professor of Surgery, Mount Sinai School of Medicine, City University of New York; Assistant Attending Surgeon, Mount Sinai School of Medicine, City University of New York, and Elmhurst City Division, New York; Attending Surgeon, Veterans Administration Hospital, Bronx, New York.

Assisting at Operations (jointly)—145.

RICHARD HARRINGTON FRANKLIN, M.B., B.S. (Lond.), F.R.C.S. (Eng.), Senior Lecturer and Surgeon, Royal Postgraduate Medical School, London.

The Management of Œsophageal Cases—316.

LEWIS ALEXANDER GILLANDERS, M.B., Ch.B., F.F.R., D.M.R.D., Consultant-in-Charge, Department of Radiodiagnosis, Aberdeen Royal Infirmary; Clinical Senior Lecturer in Radiology, University of Aberdeen.

The House-surgeon and the Department of Radiodiagnosis—703.

MIRIAM AURELIA GOUGH, S.R.N., Mid. Part I, Sister Tutor's Certificate R.C.N., R.N.T., Diploma in Nursing (Lond.); Principal Nurse Tutor, Royal Infirmary, Cardiff.

B. JOAN HARAM, M.R.C.S. (Eng.), L.R.C.P. (Lond.), F.C.Path., Consultant Pathologist, Elizabeth Garrett Anderson Hospital, London.

D. F. N. HARRISON, M.D., M.S. (Lond.), F.R.C.S. (Eng.), Professor of Laryngology and Otology, University of London; Surgeon to the Royal National Throat, Nose, and Ear Hospital, London.

FRANK DUDLEY HART, M.D. (Edin.), F.R.C.P. (Lond.), Physician, Westminster Hospital, St. Stephen's Hospital, and the Hospital of St. John and St. Elizabeth; Consultant Physician, Chelsea Hospital for Women and Queen Alexandra's Military Hospital, Millbank.

JOSEPH GRAEME HUMBLE, C.V.O., M.R.C.P. (Lond.), F.C.Path., Reader in Hæmatology and Consultant Hæmatologist, Westminster Medical School and Hospital.

ALLAN EUGENE KARK, B.Sc., M.B., B.Ch. (Rand), F.R.C.S. (Eng.), F. W. Sichel, Chairman and Professor, Department of Surgery, Mount Sinai School of Medicine, City University of New York.

JAMES KYLE, M.Ch. (Belf.), F.R.C.S. (I.), F.R.C.S. (Eng.), F.R.C.S. (Edin.), Consultant Surgeon, Royal Infirmary, Aberdeen; Honorary Clinical Senior Lecturer in Surgery, University of Aberdeen.

JOHN G. G. LEDINGHAM, D.M. (Oxon.), M.R.C.P., Consultant Physician, United Oxford Hospitals; Lecturer in Clinical Medicine, University of Oxford.

HUGH EVELYN LOCKHART-MUMMERY, M.D., M.Chir. (Cantab.), F.R.C.S. (Eng.), Consultant Surgeon, St. Thomas's Hospital, and St. Mark's Hospital, London.

The late **WILLIAM DANIEL LOVELOCK-JONES**, B.Sc., M.B., Ch.B. (Wales), F.R.C.S. (Edin.), D.P.H. (Lond.), Medical Director and Consultant Surgeon, General Hospital, Amersham.

JOHN FRANCIS MULLAN, M.B. (Belf.) F.R.C.S., F.A.C.S., Chairman and Professor of the Department of Neurological Surgery, University of Chicago School of Medicine, Chicago.

Head Injuries—269.

The late DONALD C. NORRIS, M.D. (Lond.), F.R.C.S. (Eng.), Barrister-at-Law, The Inner Temple; Chief Medical Officer, Metropolitan Water Board, London; Medical Officer, Bank of England.

Medico-legal Reports—757.

G. B. ONG, O.B.E., F.R.C.S. (Eng.), F.R.C.S. (Edin.), F.A.C.S., F.R.A.C.S., Consultant Surgeon to Hong Kong Government, British Military Hospital, Hong Kong, The Grantham Hospital, Kwong Wah Hospital, Nam Long Hospital; Professor of Surgery, University of Hong Kong.

Principles of Minor Surgery—473.

JOHN A. PALMER, M.D., F.R.C.S. (Can.), F.A.C.S., Surgeon, Toronto General Hospital; Consultant in Head and Neck Surgery, Princess Margaret Hospital, Toronto; Assistant Professor, Department of Surgery, University of Toronto.

The Management of Neck and Face Cases.—286.

BRUCE C. PATON, M.R.C.P. (Edin.), F.R.C.S. (Edin.), Associate Professor of Surgery, Director Halsted Laboratory, University of Colorado Medical Center, Denver, Colorado, U.S.A.; Consultant, Denver General Hospital, Denver Veterans Administration Hospital, Denver, Colorado, U.S.A.

Treatment of Snake-bite—681.

CHARLES EDWARD BERNARD RICKARDS, M.B., Ch.B. (Manch.), F.R.C.O.G., Consultant Gynæcologist, Salford Royal Hospital and Hope Hospital, Salford; Lecturer to the Victoria University of Manchester.

The Management of the Gynæcological Patient—488.

FREDERICK HOWARD ROBARTS, M.B., Ch.B., F.R.C.S. (Edin.), Surgeon-in-Charge, Royal Hospital for Sick Children, Edinburgh; Pædiatric Surgeon, Royal Infirmary of Edinburgh; Senior Lecturer in Pædiatric Surgery, University of Edinburgh.

Surgical Pædiatrics—568.

W. N. ROLLASON, M.B. (Birm.), M.R.C.S., D.A., F.F.A. R.C.S., Consultant in Administrative Charge, Department of Anæsthetics, Royal Infirmary, Aberdeen; Clinical Senior Lecturer in Anæsthetics, University of Aberdeen.

Pre-anæsthetic and Post-anæsthetic Care—101. Anæsthesia, General and Local—108.

Sir T. HOLMES SELLORS, D.M., M.Ch. (Oxon.), F.R.C.P. (Lond.), F.R.C.S. (Eng.), Emeritus Surgeon, Middlesex Hospital; Consulting Surgeon, National Heart, London Chest, and Harefield Hospitals.

The Management of Surgical Thoracic Cases—301.

ALEXANDER BURNS WALLACE, C.B.E., M.Sc. (McGill), M.B., Ch.B. (Edin.), F.R.C.S. (Edin.), Reader in Plastic Surgery, University of Edinburgh; Plastic Surgeon, Royal Hospital for Sick Children, Edinburgh.

The Treatment of Burns and Scalds—90.

SIR REGINALD WATSON-JONES, B.Sc., M.Ch.Orth., F.R.C.S. (Eng.), Extra-Orthopædic Surgeon to H.M. the Queen; Consulting Orthopædic Surgeon to the London Hospital; Honorary Consultant Surgeon to the Robert Jones and Agnes Hunt Orthopædic Hospital, Oswestry; Consultant Orthopædic Surgeon to the Royal Air Force.

J. P. WILLIAMS, M.Chir., F.R.C.S. (Eng.), Senior Lecturer, Institute of Urology, London.

The late FREDERICK ARNOLD WILLIAMSON-NOBLE, B.A., M.B. (Cantab.), F.R.C.S. (Eng.), Consultant Ophthalmic Surgeon, St. Mary's Hospital and the Moorfields Eye Hospital, London.

ACKNOWLEDGEMENTS

For Permission to Republish Illustrations

The Publishers of:—

C. A. BIRCH's *Emergencies in Medical Practice* (Messrs. E. & S. Livingstone, Ltd., Edinburgh) (*Fig.* 48).

H. A. F. DUDLEY's *Principles of General Surgical Management* (Messrs. E. & S. Livingstone, Ltd., Edinburgh) (*Figs.* 41, 43).

E. L. FARQUHARSON's *Textbook of Operative Surgery* (Messrs. E. & S. Livingstone, Ltd., Edinburgh) (*Figs.* 397–402, 407, 408).

W. B. GABRIEL's *Principles and Practice of Rectal Surgery* (Messrs. H. K. Lewis & Co. Ltd., London) (*Figs.* 366, 370, 372).

J. F. MULLAN's *Essentials of Neurosurgery* (Springer Publishing Co. Inc., New York) (*Figs.* 209–211).

The Controller of H.M. Stationery Office:—

Monthly Bulletin of the Ministry of Health and the Public Health Laboratory Service (*Fig.* 524).

The Editor of:—

The Lancet (*Fig.* 413).

For presenting Illustrations

Mr. R. B. CATTELL	Mr. G. L. HOWE
Mr. FOSTER MOORE	Messrs. A. L. LATNER and A. J. SMITH
Mr. GIMBLETT	Dr. P. D. LAWLEY
Mr. F. GLENN	Mr. NUTT
Mr. F. M. HANGER	

For presenting Illustration Blocks of Instruments and Apparatus

Messrs. ALLEN & HANBURYS LTD., London.
Messrs. BURROUGHS, WELLCOME & CO. (THE WELLCOME FOUNDATION LTD.), London.
Messrs. CYPRANE LTD., Keighley.
Messrs. DOWN BROS, and MAYER & PHELPS, London.
Messrs. PARKE, DAVIS & CO. LTD., Hounslow, Middlesex.
Messrs. JOHN WEISS & SON LTD., London.
AIRMED, LTD., London.
THE BRITISH OXYGEN CO. LTD., Brentford.
MEDICAL & INDUSTRIAL EQUIPMENT, LTD., London.

For executing Drawings

Miss BROWN-KELLY	Mr. D. P. HAMMERSLEY
Mr. CHARLES EDWARD CHRYSLER	Miss JILL HASSELL
Mr. TOM FISHER	Mr. R. J. MARSHALL

For verifying Scientific Values

Documenta Geigy, Messrs. Geigy Ltd., Basle and Manchester.

CONTENTS

PREFACE TO NINETEENTH EDITION

THIS Nineteenth Edition of *Pye's Surgical Handicraft* appears only fifteen years before the handbook celebrates its centenary. In 1884, surgery was in its infancy and a laparotomy was regarded as a hazardous undertaking. During the next eighty-five years, developments in all branches of medicine have taken place at an ever-increasing rate, and this was particularly true of surgery.

In order to provide guidance on the practical application of this new knowledge to the surgical patient, inevitably "Pye" steadily grew in size until, in its Eighteenth Edition, it appeared as two volumes. To some extent this format defeated the original intention of providing a compact, easily portable handbook for the senior student, young doctor, and surgical nurse. For this reason the present edition of "Pye" again is being published as a single volume. Some chapters have had to be condensed and amalgamated; a few topics that were not strictly surgical have been omitted. By contrast, and in view of the expansion of medical schools and facilities in Africa, Asia, and Latin America, fuller coverage is given to tropical diseases. The metric system is now used in Britain for prescribing drugs; it has been adopted throughout this edition.

Surgery is an art as well as a science and it is timely to remind the young doctor that while he can cure sometimes, and alleviate frequently, he must at all times be compassionate. A section giving guidance on the difficult art of caring for the dying is included; more can be learned at the bedside from senior members of the surgical team.

The authors of the various chapters are drawn from five continents. The care with which they have prepared their contributions has greatly simplified my task as editor. I am most grateful to them and also to numerous colleagues in Aberdeen for helpful comments and advice. My sincere thanks are due to my secretary, Miss Marilyn Paterson, who has dealt in a most efficient and uncomplaining fashion with the extensive correspondence. For many years Mr. L. G. Owens, of Messrs. John Wright & Sons Ltd., Bristol, has supervised the production of *Pye's Surgical Handicraft*; I am deeply indebted to him for his interest in and assistance with this latest edition.

JAMES KYLE

74 Rubislaw Den North,
Aberdeen.
March, 1969.

INTRODUCTION

By the late HAMILTON BAILEY

(Editor 1938–1961)

Pye's Surgical Handicraft was one of the first medical books published by Messrs. John Wright & Sons Ltd. The First Edition appeared in 1884. When we reflect that only eight books out of every thousand that are published live for twenty years, and that the life of a book on an ever-advancing subject like surgery is very much shorter than the average, it is clear that Mr. Pye put into the hands of the profession a work of exceptional merit.

While still a final-year medical student at St. Bartholomew's Hospital, Walter Pye wrote a series of articles on the development of the kidneys, which attracted much attention, revealing his originality and literary ability. After he qualified in 1876 and had spent a year in resident appointments at his own hospital, he was elected Lecturer on Physiology at St. Mary's Hospital Medical School. It was not long before a vacancy occurred on the surgical staff of St. Mary's Hospital and, although only 24 years of age, Pye was elected. Among other appointments which followed was that of assistant in the Museum of the Royal College of Surgeons, and in the course of these duties Pye had to revise the catalogue of surgical instruments. For this task he enlisted the aid of the senior cutler of the firm of Messrs. Weiss & Sons. There can be little doubt that the combined duties of demonstrating practical surgery at St. Mary's Hospital and working with a practical instrument maker at the Royal College of Surgeons inspired *Surgical Handicraft*. While preparing the third edition, Pye contracted influenza; it is said that the additional strain entailed by bringing the book up to date under adverse conditions led to his breakdown. He went to Cairo to seek health, but on his return it was only too evident that he was suffering from progressive organic nervous disease, from which he died on 2 Sept., 1892, at the age of 39.

WALTER PYE
1853–1892

PYE'S
SURGICAL HANDICRAFT

CHAPTER I

CARDIAC ARREST AND RESUSCITATION

By JAMES KYLE

General Considerations.—Cessation of the heart's action followed by fatal ischæmia of the brain is the sequence of events leading to death in most human beings. In many the heart's failure is the direct result of disease, for which there is at present no known cure. Consequently to interfere in the natural and inexorable progression of events is wrong. To do so is not really prolonging life, only prolonging the act of dying.

But cardiac arrest may occur in subjects believed to be otherwise healthy or in those with an expectation of life of many months. It is these patients who need urgent resuscitation.

There are only *three minutes* in which to restore the circulation to the brain.

The circulation may stop because of ventricular fibrillation (with which there is no effective cardiac output), or because the myocardium ceases to contract or its contraction is so feeble as to be unable to pump blood into the great vessels. Any of these conditions may be referred to as *cardiac arrest*, and the cessation of oxygen transportation by the blood may be called *circulatory arrest*.

Causes of Cardiac Arrest.—

1. Myocardial infarction—often precipitates ventricular fibrillation.
2. Hypoxia. Other factors are usually present.
3. Acid-base upset and hypercapnia.
4. Electrolyte imbalance, e.g., hyperkalæmia gives diastolic arrest or ventricular fibrillation.
5. Drugs, e.g., adrenaline, anæsthetic agents.
6. Cardiac tamponade and disease.
7. Hypothermia and hypotensive anæsthesia—diagnosis may be difficult without monitoring ECG.
8. Fright and viscerocardiac reflexes.
9. Embolism—pulmonary or air embolism (p. 8).
10. Hæmorrhage and shock—from poor venous return.
11. Electrocution.
12. Drowning—salt-water drowning causes hæmoconcentration; fresh-water drowning results in hæmodilution and fatal ionic imbalance.

These possible causes of cardiac arrest should always be in the minds of all members of any surgical team, and early active steps taken to prevent them. Prevention is more effective than treatment.

Confirmation of Circulatory Arrest.—

1. Sudden loss of consciousness.
2. There may be convulsions.
3. Absence of palpable carotid (or femoral) pulse.
4. Cessation of breathing, or irregular gasps.
5. Dilatation of the pupils.

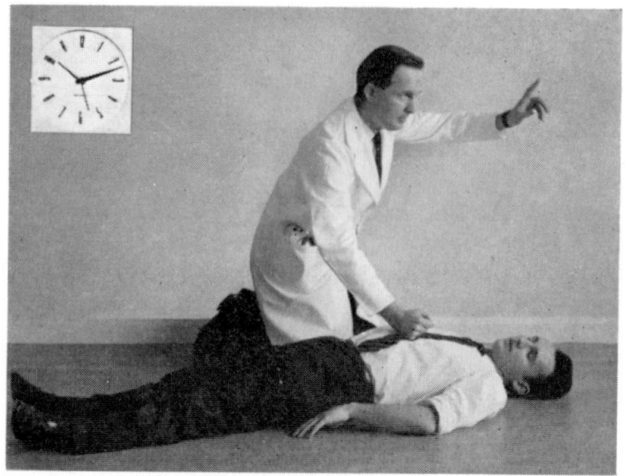

Fig. 1.—(*a*) Lay patient flat; (*b*) Strike the præcordium with the fist; (*c*) Call for assistance; (*d*) Note the time.

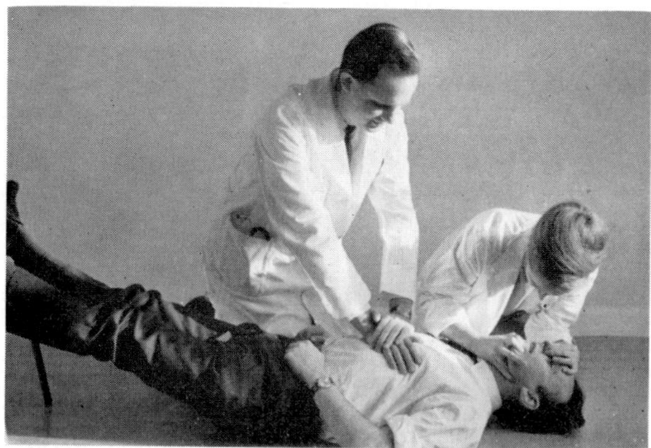

Fig. 2.—(*a*) Elevate legs; (*b*) External cardiac massage—press lower sternum backwards 60 times per minute; (*c*) Mouth-to-mouth respiration—nostrils pinched.

TREATMENT

1. Shout for help, oxygen, and resuscitation equipment.
2. Lay the patient flat.
3. Thump the middle of the sternum once (*Fig.* 1).
4. Note the time.

If the heart does not start beating effectively, then:
 5. Place the patient on the floor or other hard surface.
 6. Raise the legs, e.g., put feet on a chair.
 7. Clear the victim's airway.

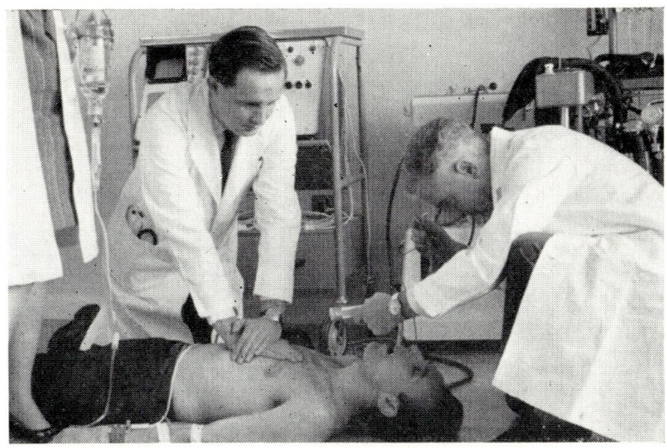

Fig. 3.—(*a*) Intubate the patient and ventilate 8 times per minute with oxygen; (*b*) Continue external massage; (*c*) Connect up cardioscope; (*d*) Set up intravenous infusion of sodium bicarbonate, 8·4 per cent.

 8. Extend the neck and hold chin up.
 9. Inflate lungs once by mouth-to-mouth or mouth-to-nose method or through a Brook airway.
10. Apply external cardiac massage (*Fig.* 2), pressing the lower sternum backwards once per second.
11. Inflate the lungs every eight sternal compressions—use a face-mask and bag, connected to an oxygen cylinder; or Ambu bag (p. 112).
12. Suck out the pharynx to keep airway clear.
13. Call for an anæsthetist.
14. Observe reduction in pupil size as an indication of adequate cerebral perfusion.

These measures provide a temporary oxygen-carrying circulation.

15. Intubate the trachea with a cuffed tube and continue ventilation with oxygen (*Fig.* 3).

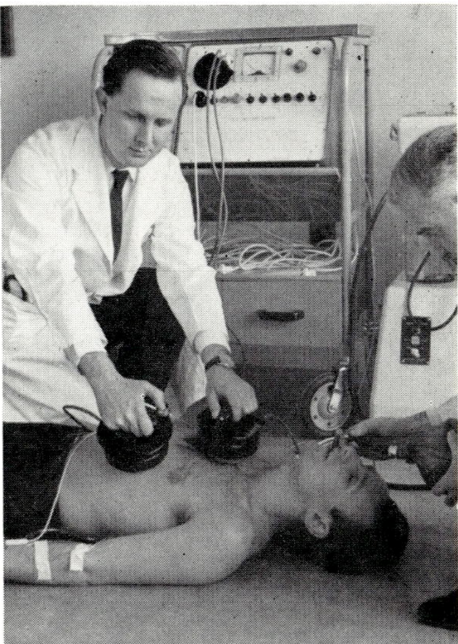

Fig. 4.—Treatment of ventricular fibrillation. (*a*) Place defibrillator electrodes over the præcordium and sternal angle; (*b*) Deliver one or more shocks of 200 joules; (*c*) Continue cardiac massage till normal rhythm returns; (*d*) Continue ventilation.

16. Continue external cardiac massage, lifting hands off the chest between compressions.
17. Set up intravenous infusion and give 50–150 ml. of 8·4 per cent sodium bicarbonate solution.
18. Connect cardioscope or ECG machine to show whether asystole or ventricular fibrillation is present.
19. Treat arrhythmia electrically or with drugs (*see below*).
20. Send an arterial blood sample for analysis of acid-base status.

After spontaneous heart-beat has been restored careful supervision is needed:—

1. Monitor patient's ECG.
2. Record blood-pressure and temperature every 15 minutes.
3. Count respiratory rate; check adequacy of respiration.
4. Check acid-base status several times.
5. Watch urinary output.
6. Be prepared for further episodes of cardiac arrest.

TECHNIQUE OF EXTERNAL CARDIAC MASSAGE

Press with the heel of the hand over the lower third of the patient's sternum. Rest the other hand on top of the first and keep the arms straight. With a sharp jerky movement press vertically backwards once per second, lifting the hands off the chest momentarily between compressions. The aim is to move the sternum backwards 1·5–2 in. (4–5 cm.) with each compression. In an old person one or more ribs are frequently broken, but mechanical damage to the myocardium or liver must be avoided. Only one hand, and much less force, is needed in a young child. Check whether the compressions produce a palpable carotid pulse.

If only one person is present, interrupt cardiac massage every eight strokes to inflate the lungs.

TREATMENT OF VENTRICULAR FIBRILLATION

Apply external defibrillation (*Fig.* 4) (DC countershock—unsynchronized), starting at 200 joules (W seconds) in an adult, 50 joules in a young child. First temporarily disconnect any ECG machine attached to the patient. One 11-cm. electrode is then placed over the apex of the heart, the other over the sternal angle. If the first shock is unsuccessful in stopping fibrillation, increase the current to 300 joules and try again. Further attempts are made after infusing another 100 ml. of 8·4 per cent sodium bicarbonate solution; if this fails, 200 mg. of procaine amide are injected intravenously, and another shock, administered after the drug has reached the heart. Lignocaine in a dose of 1–2 mg. per kg. body-weight may be given in resistant cases.

If fine fibrillation persists on the ECG it may be made coarser by giving 2–5 ml. of 1–10,000 adrenaline hydrochloride intravenously, and then repeating the DC shocks or giving propanolol, 5 mg.

External cardiac massage and ventilation of the lungs are continued between the shocks.

TREATMENT OF ASYSTOLE

Give 2·5 ml. of 1–10,000 adrenaline hydrochloride intravenously and continue external massage. The adrenaline may strengthen the myocardial contraction if and when it is re-established. Should spontaneous beating not recommence in 3–4 minutes, then give 10 ml. of 10 per cent calcium gluconate intravenously. If now the heart-beat starts, but the blood-pressure remains low, inject 100 mg. hydrocortisone intravenously or use pressor drugs, e.g., metaraminol 1–5 mg. intravenously.

Ventricular fibrillation and **asystole** are treated as described above; the electrodes of the defibrillator are applied directly to the front and back of the ventricular mass.

Closure of the chest should be postponed until the pulse-rate and blood-pressure have been stable for at least 15 minutes, but the internal mammary artery must be ligated (or at least clamped) soon after the heart has commenced to beat. Closure of the wound is effected in the following manner. The edges of the pericardium are approximated loosely with widely spaced interrupted sutures of catgut. A narrow stab incision is made in one of the lowest intercostal spaces, as far back as convenient. Through this slit a self-retaining Malecot catheter is drawn, so that the tip projects about 2 in. (5 cm.) into the pleural cavity. The catheter is *not* fixed to the chest wall at this stage.

Employing a large curved needle threaded with two long strands of stout catgut, a series of interrupted stitches is passed through the intercostal space above and out of the intercostal space below, thus encircling the divided ribs. In the absence of a rib-approximator the ribs are forced together by the assistant while the sutures are tied. The muscles and fascia are brought together with interrupted sutures and the skin edges are approximated. The catheter is anchored to the chest wall without transfixing the lumen. The lungs are inflated fully by the anæsthetist, and the tube is clamped with a hæmostat. Later, when the patient has been transferred to his room or ward, the tubing is connected with a water-seal drainage system (p. 310).

AIR EMBOLISM

Air embolism is a rare accident; in most cases air has entered the venous side of the systemic circulation. In the old and frail surprisingly small quantities of air rapidly entering a vein may prove fatal.

Causes of Venous Air Embolism.—The bottle of an intravenous infusion being allowed to run dry is probably the commonest cause of air embolism, but the empty bottle may have been replaced by the time the doctor arrives. Cracks and needle holes in plastic tubing may allow air to be entrained. The application of positive pressure to an intravenous infusion, e.g., with a Higginson's syringe or Martin's pump, is always potentially dangerous; if they are used, supervision must be continuous and uninterrupted. Air may enter a blood donor's vein if the negative pressure in the collecting bottle is faulty. During an operation air may enter the large veins within the skull or neck; induction of a pneumothorax or pneumoperitoneum and vaginal douching may also cause the emergency.

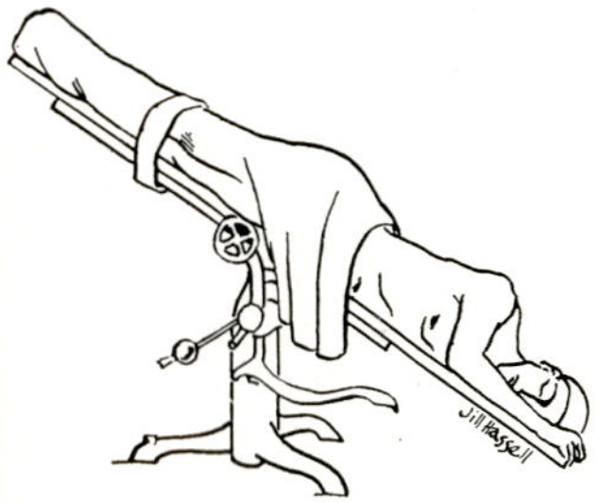

Fig. 7.—The life-saving position in which to place the patient in cases of venous air embolism.

Clinical Manifestations. — Usually the onset is abrupt, with deep inspirations, coughing expirations, cyanosis, then a few gasping breaths, succeeded by unconsciousness and cessation of respiration. The pulse becomes imperceptible, and the blood-pressure falls to an unrecordable level. A stethoscope applied to the præcordium reveals the 'water-wheel' sound—a most unpleasant churning and splashing noise which masks the true heart-sounds. In not a few instances, if the pulps

---

WHEN TO STOP UNSUCCESSFUL RESUSCITATION

Patients have returned to a normal life after an hour of cardiac massage. Recovery is unlikely, however, if spontaneous beating of the heart has not recommenced within 30 minutes of the start of resuscitative efforts. Certainly no junior doctor should cease his efforts in under 30 minutes. The decision to stop is best taken by the anæsthetist and senior clinician together. Frequent repetition of the steps outlined above for the treatment of ventricular fibrillation usually brings success. Asystole carries a worse prognosis. If after giving adrenaline, calcium, and then hydrocortisone there is no sign of electrical activity on the cardioscope, the prognosis is gloomy.

RATIONALE OF BICARBONATE THERAPY

Severe metabolic acidosis follows cardiac arrest and tissue anoxia. The acidosis itself interferes with cardiac conduction and must be rapidly corrected. The 8·4 per cent solution contains 1 mEq. sodium bicarbonate per 1 ml. The number of milliequivalents needed is given by the formula:

$$\frac{M \times t}{10},$$

where $M=$ wt. in kg. and $t=$ duration of arrest in minutes.

Table I.—DRUGS AND SOLUTIONS THAT MAY BE REQUIRED IN THE TREATMENT OF CARDIAC ARREST. THEY SHOULD ALL BE PRESENT ON THE RESUSCITATION TROLLEY

Drugs:—
    Adrenaline injection, B.P., 1–10,000, 1 ml. ampoule × 5
    Ampoules of sterile water, 10 ml. × 10
    Hydrocortisone 100 mg. vials × 2
    Metaraminol, 1 mg./ml., 10 ml. vial × 1
    Noradrenaline injection, 2 ml. ampoules × 4. Dilute to 1–10,000
    Procaine hydrochloride, 1 per cent in 10 ml. ampoules × 2
    Lignocaine hydrochloride, 1 per cent plain, 10 ml. ampoules × 2
    Procaine amide 100 mg./ml., 10 ml. vial × 1
    Calcium gluconate 10 per cent, 10 ml. ampoules × 5
    Propanolol 5 mg., ampoules × 2
    Digoxin 2 mg., ampoules × 2

For Anæsthesia:—
    Thiopentone 0·5 G.
    d-Tubocurarine 15 mg., ampoules × 3
    Atropine 0·6 mg., ampoules × 4
    Neostigmine 0·5 mg., ampoules × 6

Intravenous Fluids:—
    Normal saline
    Dextrose 5 per cent
    Macrodex 6 per cent in saline
    Macrodex 6 per cent in dextrose
    Sodium bicarbonate 8·4 per cent, 250 ml. bottles × 2
    Mannitol 20 per cent, 500 ml. bottle
    Glucose 50 per cent, 50 ml. ampoules × 4

OTHER MEASURES

Periods of anoxia cause cerebral œdema, which may interfere with the circulation to the brain and lead to permanent brain damage; they may also adversely affect renal function. To counteract these tendencies hypothermia and dehydration therapy may be used.

1. *Hypothermia*.—The brain's oxygen requirements decrease sharply as the body temperature is lowered. If consciousness is not regained shortly after the heart is restarted, if there are other neurological changes or hyperpyrexia, then the patient should at once be cooled down 3°–5° C., to 32°–35° C., by placing packs of broken ice around him. Accurate monitoring of the temperature is necessary and smaller doses of drugs are needed by the hypothermic patient.

2. *Dehydration Therapy*.—Urinary output can be increased by giving 500 ml. of 10 per cent mannitol intravenously. This loss of fluid from the body will reduce the tendency to cerebral œdema. Triple-strength plasma will achieve the same objective; it is less popular now. If arrest has lasted more than 10 minutes give 50 ml. of 50 per cent dextrose intravenously.

3. *Plasma Expander*.—If the cardiac arrest was precipitated by hypovolæmia, a plasma expander, e.g., 500 ml. of 6 per cent macrodex, may be infused intravenously.

PLACE OF OPEN (INTERNAL) CARDIAC MASSAGE

This method of massaging the heart will be used when there is a cardiac arrest during an intra-thoracic operation. It is also indicated when there is cardiac tamponade or bilateral pneumothorax.

During external massage it may be noted that the pupils are dilating and the carotid (or femoral) pulse is scarcely palpable, suggesting that compression of the heart's chambers was not being achieved in a really effective manner. In these circumstances internal massage may be resorted to. When cardiac arrest is thought to have been due to massive pulmonary embolus, the chest may be opened and great vessels inspected. In a large hospital, rarely it may be possible to perform pulmonary embolectomy, usually with the help of a by-pass machine.

TECHNIQUE OF INTERNAL (OPEN) CARDIAC MASSAGE

When the thorax is not already open, without counting the ribs, a short, rather deep incision is made in what is believed to be the fourth or fifth left intercostal space. If there is no bleeding, the incision is enlarged so as to divide the intercostal muscles from the lateral border of the sternum to the posterior axillary fold (*Fig.* 5). The pleura is opened. By passing the left hand into the thoracic cavity the palm is insinuated beneath the heart and the intact pericardium, and the heart is compressed against the sternum (*Fig.* 6). Rhythmical compression and complete relaxation (to allow the heart to fill) are continued at the rate of once per second for about 25 seconds. In all probability by this time the wrist will become painful from constriction by the ribs, but sufficient blood to oxygenate the vital centres will have been delivered to enable the next step to be undertaken without endangering the viability of the cerebral cortex.

The hand is withdrawn, the costal cartilages above and below the incision are severed with a knife, and an assistant is instructed to hold the ribs apart or else a rib-spreader is inserted. Following the long axis of the heart, the pericardium is opened widely in front of the phrenic nerve and cardiac massage is commenced.

Three different methods may be used. The most common method is to insert the extended four (index–little) fingers of the right hand behind the ventricles which are then compressed rhythmically against the sternum on the anterior surface of which the thumb or left hand rests (*Fig.* 6). Alternatively, with a large heart, counter-pressure against the fingers and palm of the right hand may be

Macrodex (Pharmacia (Great Britain) Ltd., The Avenue, West Ealing, London, W.13).

provided by those of the surgeon's left hand inserted in front of th[e] With a very small heart it is possible to compress the heart between t[he] fingers and the thenar eminence of the right hand. Compression, whi[ch] to the ventricles only, should be gradual, but pressure exerted mus[t]

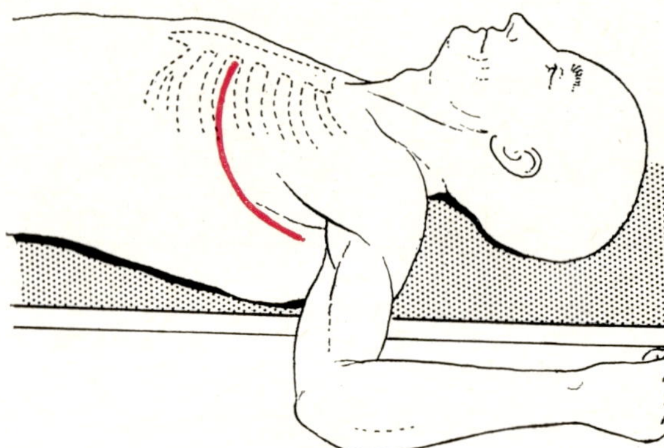

Fig. 5.—Incision for internal cardiac massage. It is made in the 4th or 5th left extends from sternum to posterior axilla.

The finger-tips, and particularly the tip of the thumb, take no part made systole. To ignore this injunction is to run the risk of thrusti[ng] a digit through the wall of the heart. Care must also be exercised the heart or draw it too far over to the left. The blood within t[he]

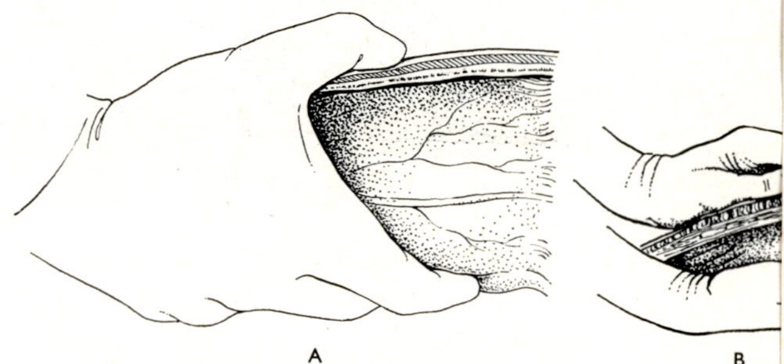

Fig. 6.—Internal cardiac massage. The ventricular mass is compressed a[gainst the] sternum; the fingers must be kept straight. Counter-pressure on the front of th[e heart] is provided either by (A) the thumb or (B) the opposite hand.

having been expelled, relaxation must be abrupt and complete, so the heart to fill to capacity. In this way the heart is squeezed rhythm[ically] times a minute.

Cardiac massage becomes very tiring, and when the operator fe[els] is aching he must take 2 or 3 seconds' rest. This interval allows beats to develop. Artificial ventilation of the lungs must be continued

of the fingers are placed over a jugular vein, bubbles of air can be felt moving beneath. Especially in cases where the patient was in a sitting position, or assumes an upright position after the entry of air into a vein, the state of unconsciousness is preceded by convulsions.

Treatment.—To be successful, immediate action and sustained effort are imperative.

1. Tilt the patient so that the head is low (*Fig.* 7). Large bubbles in the venous system then pass to the veins of the pelvis and the lower extremities, there to be absorbed slowly.

2. Turn the patient on to his left side, i.e., with the right side uppermost. By placing the patient on to the left side, air in the right ventricle rises towards the apex of the heart (*Fig.* 8), breaks the air-lock, and permits the organ to pump whole blood into the pulmonary artery.

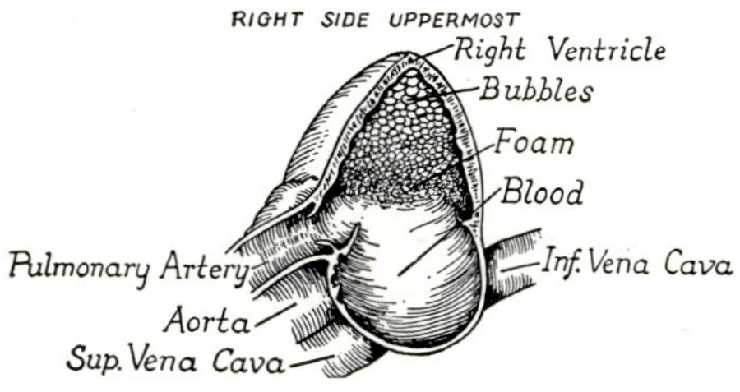

Fig. 8.—With the patient on his left side and tilted head downwards, air in the right side of the heart rises towards the apex.

3. Ventilate the lungs, preferably with pure oxygen, at the earliest possible moment. Even if there is a slight improvement, persevere with postural treatment, if necessary for hours. Success has crowned 8 hours of such treatment.

If these measures do not rapidly bring some evidence of improvement, the patient must be turned on to his back and the heart exposed by an incision through the fifth left interspace (*see Fig.* 5). The right ventricle can then be aspirated under vision, and after discarding froth, the blood is returned to the left ventricle. Massage the heart if necessary, but on no account commence cardiac massage until all the froth has been aspirated.

Arterial Air Embolism.—Air may enter the left side of the heart and the large arteries through the pulmonary veins during thoracic operations or when a pneumothorax is being induced. Rarely a septal defect will permit air on the venous side to pass across to the arterial circulation.

The principal dangers are air either occluding the coronary arteries or passing up to the brain.

Clinical Manifestations.—The onset is more catastrophic than venous air embolism. If the patient is conscious, he feels faint or dizzy. Following these warnings there is loss of consciousness; some regain consciousness but are disorientated. Cyanosis is present almost invariably. Convulsions, localized or generalized, tonic or clonic, often occur. Nearly always the pupils become widely dilated. The patient becomes almost, or completely, pulseless. The 'mill-wheel' murmur is *not* present. As a rule there is slowing of the rate of respiration; sometimes it is of the Cheyne-Stokes variety. Should the patient be so fortunate as to recover from the acute episode, præcordial pain accompanied by considerable dyspnœa lasts for hours, or sometimes days. Various neurological manifestations, including hemiplegia, monoplegia, nystagmus, strabismus, and sometimes blindness, are not infrequent aftermaths.

Pathognomonic Signs: Marbling of the skin of the superior part of the body has often been noted. It is due to embolism of the skin vessels.

Leibermeister's sign: There is pallor of half, or a portion of the tongue, depending upon which lingual artery or portion thereof is blocked. This sign is said to be very constant, but it is often missed because of the anxiety that prevails.

Treatment.—

1. Tilt the patient so that the head is low.

2. Turn him onto his left side; it is more advantageous to turn him still farther—into the half-prone position and hold him there. In this position the openings of the coronary arteries are dependent.

3. Pure oxygen should be administered and artificial ventilation of the lungs carried out.

4. Should these measures fail after 3 minutes' trial, there is only one possible life-saving expedient—that is, to expose the heart (*see Fig*. 5) and aspirate foam from the left ventricle.

CHAPTER II

RESPIRATORY OBSTRUCTION AND RESPIRATORY INSUFFICIENCY

By H. A. F. DUDLEY

HOUSEMEN in surgical units must realize today as never before that next to cardiac arrest (Chapter I) respiratory obstruction and respiratory insufficiency are the two most serious and most common acute disorders they encounter. Although respiratory *obstruction* is not usually difficult to recognize, *insufficiency* may steal upon the clinician unawares so that it is only when some disaster such as cardiac arrest overtakes the patient that it is recognized that for some time gross hypoxia has existed.

RECOGNITION OF RESPIRATORY OBSTRUCTION

The circumstances are of extreme importance. The ill-positioned, unconscious patient, the presence of a space-occupying lesion in the neck or mediastinum, damage either accidental or iatrogenic to the neck or the larynx, the possibility of a foreign body, inflammatory disease of the bronchus—all these must be borne in mind for they set the stage for acute respiratory obstruction even if they do not themselves produce it. Often the last straw is some acute incident which precipitates œdema in, or provokes obturation of, an already narrowed airway. Particularly in the casualty department the houseman must bear in mind that he should do nothing injudicious which, should it prove unsuccessful, will make worse the patient already teetering on the brink of acute respiratory obstruction. Thus, frantic attempts at intubation which produce damage to an already partially obstructed larynx may precipitate fatal, complete œdematous obstruction; or blood entering the trachea from a hasty tracheostomy may make hypoxia worse.

Clinical Features.—Activity of the accessory respiratory muscles and stridor are the two cardinal features of incomplete respiratory obstruction. The first merely signifies respiratory effort and is thus not specific, the latter is the consequence of air rushing through a greatly narrowed passage and is not only specific but is usually a harbinger of early doom unless something is done. Indrawing of the intercostal spaces may or may not be present. Incomplete respiratory obstruction does not necessarily imply respiratory insufficiency, although the one is likely to follow hard upon the other. There is not much difficulty in diagnosing complete obstruction—convulsive respiratory effort, cyanosis, unconsciousness, convulsions, and circulatory arrest are the sequelæ over a period of less than 2 minutes.

RECOGNITION OF RESPIRATORY INSUFFICIENCY

The definition of respiratory insufficiency is biochemical and biophysical—an abnormal state of blood gases. It follows that it has no clear-cut symptoms or physical signs—indeed it represents a final common state that results from a wide variety of causes. In surgical patients the usual but not invariable situations are:—

1. Inadequate mechanical ventilation from either poor movement or ineffective movement of the chest wall.

2. Blocked respiratory passage by retained sputum with subsequent distal absorptive collapse. To this may be added either the ineffective movement of pre-existing lung disease or the consequent effects of œdema in an infected lung in circumstances where massive inappropriate respiratory efforts are being made.

Given the common underlying causes, the houseman's job is to recognize the presence of respiratory insufficiency in individual circumstances. When dyspnœa or cyanosis is present there is little difficulty, but before these have supervened respiratory insufficiency is usually well marked. Thus P_{O_2} may fall from the normal 100 mm. Hg to 60 mm. Hg before saturation is significantly reduced (and cyanosis consequently apparent); a further small fall may precipitate severe desaturation (*see Fig.* 9 for details). This 'slippery slope' of the oxygen dissociation curve should be constantly in the mind's eye of all those dealing with respiratory insufficiency.

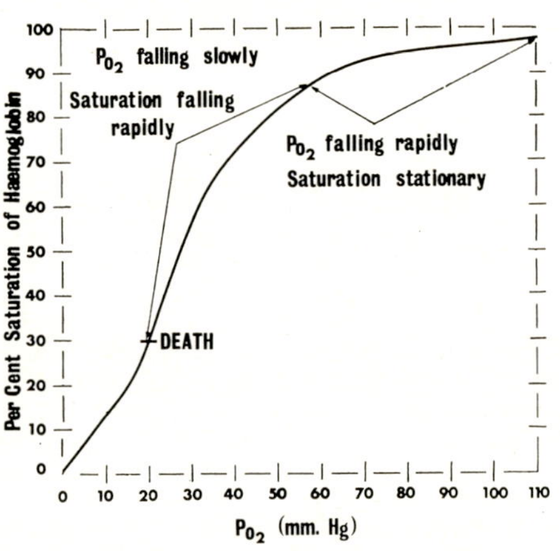

Fig. 9.—The oxygen dissociation curve. Initially P_{O_2} falls rapidly without change in saturation but at a P_{O_2} of approximately 60 mm. Hg, large changes in saturation take place for small changes in P_{O_2}. This is the 'slippery slope'.

In the absence of gross signs, what other guides are present for the clinician? Restlessness and disorientation are two of the most valuable. Although both may have many causes, among the commonest in surgical wards is hypoxia. Sudden changes in mental states should at once raise the question: Is hypoxia present or has hypercarbia developed?

Warning.—It is vital to avoid sedating a restless patient until a diagnosis has been made, for the incautious administration of sedatives to a hypoxic patient is clearly disastrous.

Although *hypercarbia* is mentioned as one manifestation of respiratory insufficiency, it is not commonly encountered as a well-marked syndrome in surgical patients. Consequently, the sweating, vasodilatation, and drowsiness that go with a very high Pco_2 (80–90 mm. Hg) are rarely seen. The explanation is that the surgical patient is not often underventilating in the sense that he has an inadequate stimulus to his respiratory centre or an inadequate mechanical response. Usually he is trying hard to breathe in the face of a situation which involves hypoxia, and because of the free diffusibility of carbon dioxide he may even produce respiratory alkalosis in association with a low Po_2 and clinical deterioration.

AIDS TO THE DIAGNOSIS OF RESPIRATORY INSUFFICIENCY

The final diagnosis rests on proving the definition—abnormality of blood gases—by direct measurement of Po_2 and Pco_2. Both these are now well within the capacity of most hospital biochemical organizations who will provide, in addition, information about hydrogen-ion concentration. To produce such results the laboratory must be provided with an iced, rapidly transported (less than 1 hour old), anaerobically drawn arterial blood sample, although some techniques can make use of capillary blood.

Techniques of Arterial Puncture.—Femoral, brachial, or radial arteries may be used, but the last is to be preferred in that harm is not likely to follow. A short-bevelled 21 S.W.G. needle is attached to a 10-ml. syringe wetted with heparin 1000 U./ml. so that the needle is filled with this solution. The skin is stretched with the thumb and forefinger of the free hand (*Fig.* 10), and the

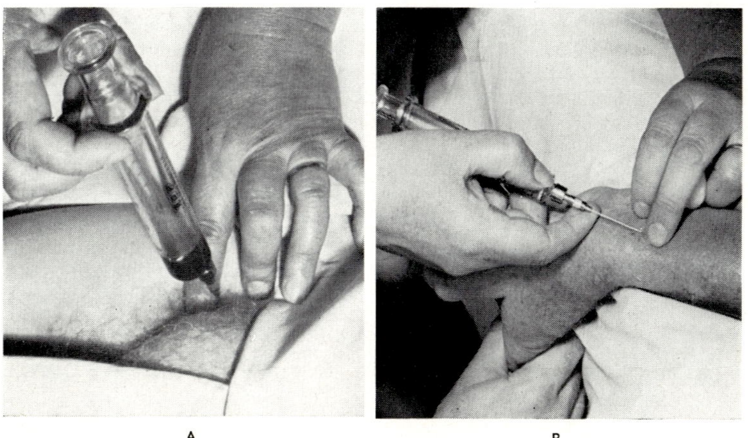

A   B

Fig. 10.—Methods of fixing (A) the femoral and (B) radial arteries for arterial puncture.

artery fixed so that its pulsation can be felt and if possible seen just proximal to the digit of the operator which is pressed against the skin. A quick skin puncture is made at a moderate angle. The needle is then advanced steadily and obliquely into the artery which offers firm resistance. Entry into the lumen of the vessel is signified by a rise of the plunger of the syringe which then fills under arterial pressure alone; failure to detect the added resistance to the arterial wall implies that the needle is lying either to one or other side of the vessel and a fresh puncture should be made. The needle is sharply withdrawn, the syringe capped to avoid aeration of the sample, and firm pressure applied to the puncture site for 3 minutes by the clock. The results should be available within 5 minutes.

In complicated circumstances for repeated sampling a fine cannula should be threaded into the artery and filled with heparin solution 500 U./ml. Needle-cannulæ combinations which have the needle outside the cannula should not be used for this purpose as the needle puncture is not always free from leakage; preferably a cannula is threaded along a guide wire by Seldinger's technique. This manœuvre is so commonly used today for arteriography in X-ray departments that it is usually possible to secure the help of radiologists skilled in percutaneous arterial cannulation should an indwelling conduit be desired. Certainly this is not a procedure for the occasional operator.

ACIDOSIS

Acidosis—a raised blood hydrogen-ion concentration in respiratory insufficiency—is the consequence of:—

1. Underventilation with a rise in P_{CO_2} which in turn displaces the equation

$$CO_2 + H_2O = H_2CO_3 = H^+ \text{ and } HCO_3^-$$

to the right, and

2. The metabolic hydrogen-ion production which is the result of anaerobic metabolism in the hypoxic patient.

Both are of particular importance in that they render the patient more susceptible to acute cardiovascular disturbance such as fibrillation, arrest, and peripheral circulatory failure. The exact dissection of the relative contributions to acidosis of respiratory and metabolic components is a job for the experts, but usually the circumstances will help considerably. When there is evidence of underperfusion, a metabolic acidosis is suspected.

OXYGEN SATURATION MEASUREMENT

When facilities for full blood-gas analysis are not available, saturation measurements are of some use in determining oxygenation. It must be remembered, however, that, as already stated, arterial desaturation is a situation of advanced respiratory failure and requires most urgent and effective management. Absence of desaturation must not lull the houseman into a false sense of security.

PREVENTION AND TREATMENT OF RESPIRATORY OBSTRUCTION

Predisposing factors should be avoided. The unconscious patient is usually at risk (*see* Chapter X) and must be nursed on his side or semi-prone. Where this is impossible (e.g., when other injuries such as fractured femur coexist), prophylactic intubation or tracheostomy should be undertaken (*see below*).

When acute obstruction is diagnosed, an airway must be re-established forthwith. Often this is simple—pulling forward the tongue digitally or with a towel clip (which pierces the tongue without damaging it) and then maintaining forward displacement of the jaw (*Fig.* 11). In the deeply unconscious patient an airway may be inserted, but it is far better to insist that someone is delegated to maintain the jaw forward than to insert an airway casually and hope for the best.

Where simple methods do not suffice and total obstruction is present or impending, it is dramatic but unreliable to undertake emergency tracheostomy. In fact, in a dying patient with respiratory obstruction this may prove the *coup de grâce*, as often an inexperienced surgeon struggles in the acutely congested neck to expose a wind-pipe that is gyrating in the storm of respiratory efforts. Better either:—

1. To intubate the patient, overcoming trismus with a mouth gag. It should be the pride of every house-surgeon to be able to intubate dextrously under direct vision, and the frequency with which endotracheal anæsthesia is used

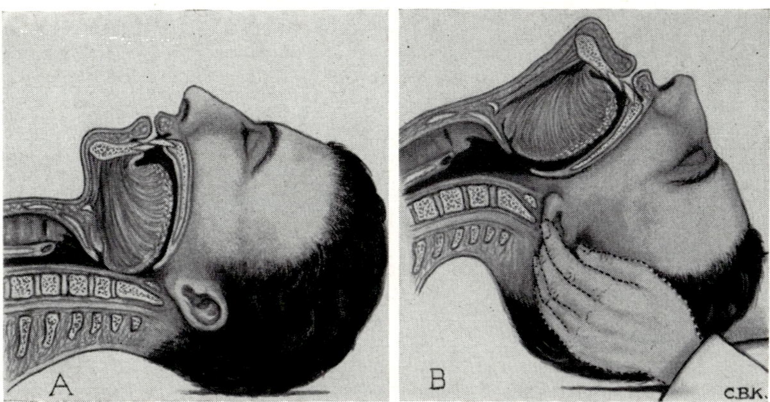

Fig. 11.—Holding the jaw forward to maintain an airway. The same position of head and neck is adopted for bronchoscopy. A shows how the untended jaw permits obstruction of the airway by the tongue. B illustrates (1) the forward displacement of the jaw by pressure at the angle and (2) the extension of the atlanto-occipital joint which permits direct access to the larynx for toilet or bronchoscopy.

provides ample opportunity for him to acquire the technique. Woe betide the ineffective performer who may well worsen a laryngeal œdema and so lessen the chances of survival. If there is any doubt in the mind as to effective intubation it is preferable to:—

2. Plunge a 15-gauge needle through the thyroid membrane. This apparently fine pathway will maintain oxygenation until more effective measures can be set in hand.

Inhalation of Vomitus.—The ill-managed surgical patient or the victim of some acute disaster such as accidental injury or drowning with loss of consciousness may vomit and inhale. Evidence that this has occurred may be provided by the presence of vomitus on the bedclothes or in the hypopharynx, but the absence of such tell-tales are of themselves no indication that the event has not taken place: (1) Because of the tidy habits of nursing staff, or (2) Because the amount of regurgitated material is small. There may, on the one hand, be no overt signs of respiratory problems and, on the other, there may be acute pulmonary œdema. Whenever vomiting has occurred under questionable circumstances, the hypopharynx and larynx should be viewed directly for signs of vomit and the former cleared by suction. If there is obvious respiratory difficulty, urgent bronchoscopy must be done or the trachea intubated so that suction can be applied through the endotracheal tube. While awaiting intubation or bronchoscopy, the patient is laid on his side or face and, if necessary, artificial respiration applied.

Re-establishment of an airway in acute respiratory obstruction from any cause is no guarantee that ventilation will ensue. Not infrequently, either some other respiratory condition is present which interferes with normal gas exchange, or hypoxia has been present for so long that partial or complete respiratory paralysis is already present. It is of the utmost importance to satisfy oneself that breathing is adequate once the airway has been restored.

THERAPEUTIC BRONCHOSCOPY

Therapeutic bronchoscopy is less used than ten years ago and now is more often the province of the anæsthetist than the surgeon. However, the ability expeditiously to pass a bronchoscope should, as with an endotracheal tube, be acquired by all surgeons in training as on occasion it will save lives and, more frequently, if less dramatically, expand a large collapsed area of lung which threatens to delay convalescence.

Indications.—

1. Acute severe pulmonary collapse in the post-operative period which is diagnosed by fever, tachycardia, tracheal deviation, bronchial breathing, and typical radiological apearances.

2. Retained tracheobronchial secretions in a patient too weak to cough where time may be gained to permit elective tracheostomy.

3. Aspiration of vomit, including blood.

Technique.—An adolescent bronchoscope well lubricated with lignocaine (2 per cent jelly) should be used combined with a large-bore sucker. The head is extended to a similar position for that of maintenance of the airway (*see Fig.* 11) and the instrument gently inserted beside the tongue down to the cords. As the patient inspires and the cords open, it is slipped through the cords and down to the carina. (Although uncomfortable, this method is preferable to sousing the cords with local anæsthetic which may then permit inhalation of œsophageal secretions or vomit before the cough reflex is recovered.)

Once the instrument has reached the carina, the patient's head is inclined to either side, so permitting the tip to be slid into each main bronchus. Bronchial toilet is carried out with an œsophageal sucker of large bore and the instrument withdrawn.

This method is not for the tiro. It requires considerable dexterity and sense of timing, but the results are well worth while. A chest film is obtained at the end of the procedure.

EMERGENCY TRACHEOSTOMY (*Fig.* 12)

Very occasionally emergency tracheostomy may be required. The technique used should be the simplest. The head is fully extended on a pillow placed under the shoulders. If necessary 1 per cent procaine is infiltrated in the line of the incision from cricoid to manubrium, but the quantity should be kept at the absolute minimum for tissues much distended by liquid are not easy to dissect. A 6-cm. vertical incision is made exactly in the midline and the dissection carried down to and through the investing fascia. Thereafter blunt dissection spreads the fascia in relation to the thyroid isthmus which can usually be displaced downwards, and by a combination of this and finger palpation the upper ring of the trachea is palpated. The tube is held ready and a horizontal incision made at the level of the second ring. The lower lip of this incision is grasped and the cut converted into a semi-lune on either side. The tracheostomy tube is then slid over the resulting flap into the trachea while an attendant nurse inserts a sterile, soft, plastic catheter to suck out the blood and mucus that

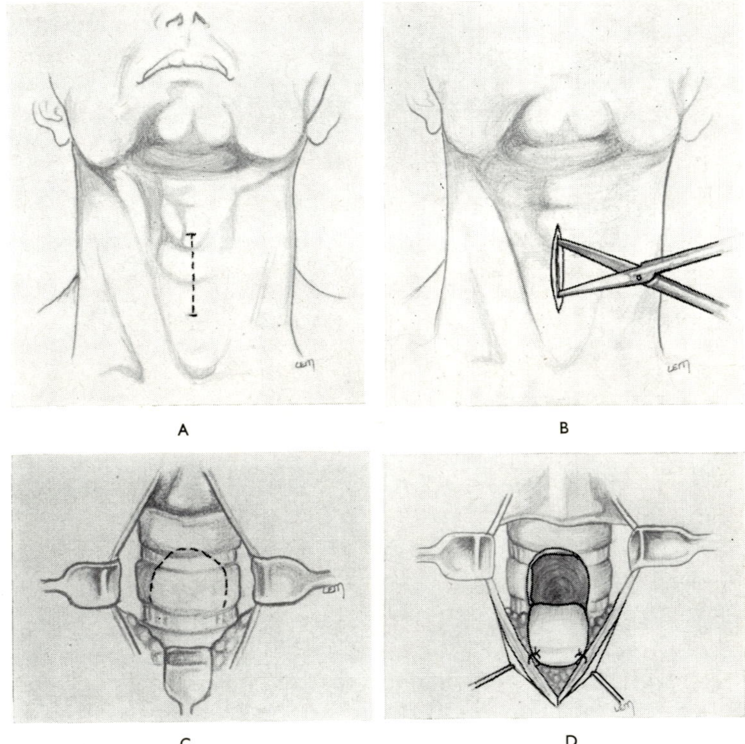

Fig. 12.—The steps in burrowing tracheostomy: **A**, The incision; **B**, Midline separation of pretracheal fascia; **C**, Downward displacement of the thyroid isthmus; **D**, Formation of distal flap of trachea.

inevitably accumulate during the procedure. 'Burrowing' tracheostomy of this type is infinitely to be preferred to formal dissection, particularly in emergency situations.

Choice of Tracheostomy Tubes.—Most institutions have their own favourite tubes. The old-fashioned silver tube lingers on. Its advantages are minimal irritation and a smooth flowing curve which permits it to lie snugly. Its disadvantages are that it does not usually carry a cuff nor is it suited to adaptation to anæsthetic equipment. The best general-purpose tubes are plastic, fitted with a cuff, and designed to match standard fittings (*Fig.* 13).

Management.—The patient is not rendered safe by the relief of respiratory obstruction. Rather he is exposed to new dangers in that the humidifying and filtering mechanism of the nose is by-passed. The house-surgeon must ensure that:—

1. The air or gas mixture supplied is clean. This can be achieved by drawing it from a line or cylinder rather than from the room. When air is entrained by a gas line, it should be filtered.

2. The tracheobronchial tree is kept moist. The simplest way of achieving this is by the regular hourly installation of 2–3 ml. of sodium bicarbonate,

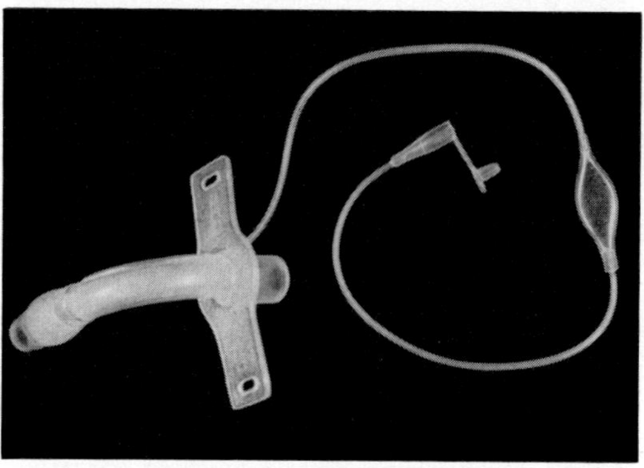

Fig. 13.—A standard cuffed plastic tube for tracheostomy. Anæsthetic connexions can be attached directly.

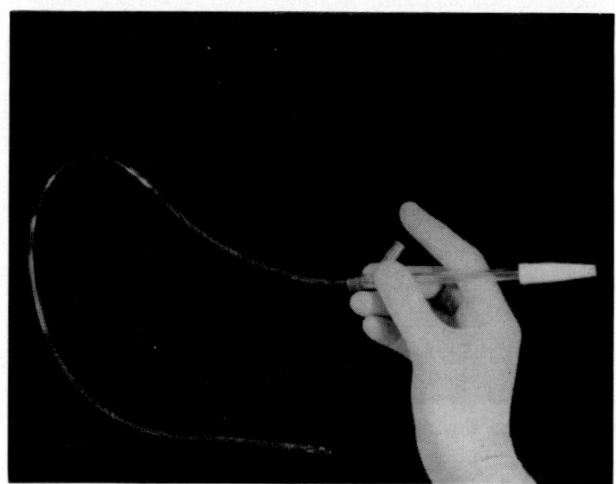

Fig. 14.—A 'Y' catheter for tracheal suction. Negative pressure can be applied at will by a finger over the end of the 'Y'.

1 mEq. per ml. Where equipment is available, all air supplied to the patient should be warmed to body heat and humidified. The gesture of bubbling air through water at room temperature is useless.

3. Careful repeated bacteriological control is kept on the tracheobronchial secretions and therapy promptly instituted as indicated.

Aspiration of Secretions.—Aggressive high-vacuum suction will damage or even strip the mucosa from trachea and bronchi. The technique shown in *Fig.* 14 should be used. The soft, plastic catheter is inserted with the Y-piece open to the atmosphere. With the catheter in situ intermittent suction is applied by placing the thumb over the Y. Negative pressure should not exceed 20 cm. water.

ARTIFICIAL RESPIRATION

Complex methods of external artificial respiration have all been superseded by mouth-to-mouth breathing—Elisha's technique or as it is sometimes dramatically termed 'the kiss of life'. Mouth-to-mouth breathing (including mouth-to-mask and mouth-to-tracheostomy opening) remains the most effective method of performing artificial respiration yet devised; there is evidence that in terms of maximum passive respiratory exchange mouth-to-mouth artificial respiration is superior to all other methods. Furthermore, the method is simple to learn and to carry out; it requires no apparatus; because it is not nearly so tiring as manual methods of artificial respiration, mouth-to-mouth breathing can be continued for more than an hour by most operators; an inadequate jaw-lift can be detected immediately by inability or difficulty in inflating the lungs—in no other method can the operator be sure that he is effecting respiratory exchange.

The unequivocal superiority of mouth-to-mouth over all varieties of manual artificial respiration is so compelling that in all parts of the world it is being adopted as the standard method.

Technique.—Rapidly check that the victim's tongue has not fallen back. Wipe away any vomitus from around the mouth. With one hand lift the lower jaw forwards; with the fingers of the other pinch the nostrils together (*Fig.* 15).

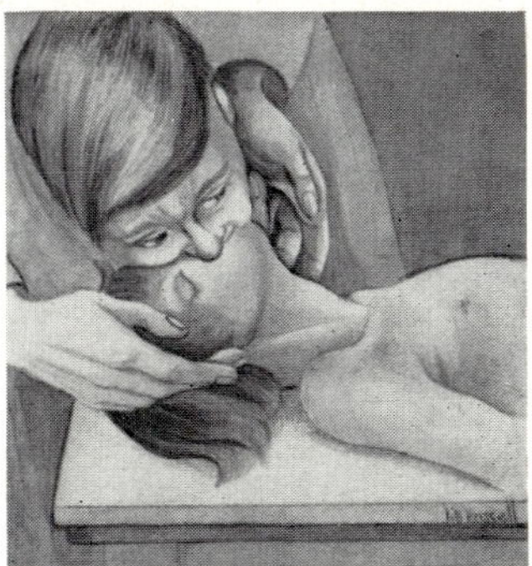

Fig. 15.—Mouth-to-mouth artificial respiration in an adult. Note the position of the left hand of the resuscitator supporting the jaw. His eyes are watching the patient's chest; his right hand should be pinching the nostrils.

After taking a deep breath, place the mouth over the victim's mouth and blow out strongly. Out of the corner of the eye it should be possible to see the patient's chest wall rise as his lungs are inflated. This forced inflation is continued at a rate of 16–20 breaths per minute.

CHAPTER III

SHOCK AND RESUSCITATION

By H. A. F. DUDLEY

'SHOCK' is an imprecise but useful word; it does not describe a physiological entity but rather a clinical appearance. Thus, its use in everyday practice is valuable in conveying information about what a patient looks like but is rarely helpful when it comes to deciding treatment. For, as with any other therapeutic manœuvre, adequate treatment is dependent upon the understanding of mechanisms when these are capable of being elucidated. When summoned to a patient said to be in shock the first question that must be asked is, 'What is the cause?' Only by deciding this can a plan be arrived at.

CAUSES OF SHOCK PICTURE

In dissecting out the major aetiological agents in the causation of a state of shock the first premise is that our use of the term to describe a clinical state of affairs is a shorthand for the appearance of *reduced peripheral blood-flow*. Not only does this affect the easily visible skin and subcutaneous tissues but also the viscera, for example kidney and brain, accounting in this way for the oliguria and disorientation that may accompany a shock state. Most of the clinical manifestations of shock syndromes can be explained by peripheral tissue *hypoxia* based on the low blood-flow. It is the method of production of the reduced perfusion that varies from instance to instance.

The principal aetiological agents responsible for the clinical picture of shock are:—

1. Vasovagal overactivity—fainting.
2. Reduction in circulatory blood-volume.
3. Massive sepsis.
4. Coronary occlusion.
5. Adrenocortical insufficiency.

1. FAINTING AND NEURAL PHENOMENA

In the past it has been customary to include bradycardia, hyperpnœa, and the fainting of emotional stress under the heading of *shock*. Certainly this is so to the layman who habitually describes as 'shocked' anyone who has had a fright. The term 'neurogenic shock' is best not used, although peripheral tissue hypoxia in the brain is characteristic of fainting which has a neurogenic basis. What is important for the houseman to remember is:—

a. Other factors such as blood-loss can, if the patient is upright, lead to the development of the physiological chain of events—adrenaline secretion, muscular vasodilatation, bradycardia, and cerebral hypoxia—which leads to fainting. Thus, fainting may be a component of some particular circumstances of blood-loss; perhaps the most frequently encountered in civilian practice is the patient who has a major gastro-intestinal hæmorrhage and then either defæcates or vomits. The Valsalva effect so produced reduces venous return to the heart and precipitates a faint so that he is picked up from beside the toilet or may sustain a head injury as he falls.

b. If, when a patient faints, he is prevented from falling, the cerebral hypoxia is self-perpetuating and may result in irreversible brain damage and/or a cardiac arrest. Death under light general anæsthesia in the dentist's chair and possibly some fatalities in elderly patients propped upright in bed in hospital may be assigned to this cause.

Management of Fainting.—The patient is placed flat. Unconsciousness is rarely so deep that reflexes are lost but the airway should be assured, if necessary by the use of the semi-prone position. Usually consciousness is soon recovered and there is rarely, if ever, the need to administer vasopressor drugs. Unless the cause is obvious, the patient should be subsequently investigated for precipitating factors such as blood-loss.

2. SHOCK FROM REDUCTION IN CIRCULATORY VOLUME

Three major causes of volume reduction are known—loss of whole blood, loss of plasma as in a burn, and loss of extracellular water. The clinical pictures produced by each have many points of similarity and some points of difference.

Whole blood-loss may be external (which includes by definition the gastro-intestinal tract) or internal into damaged tissues (e.g., a fracture-hæmatoma or an infarcted organ). The effects are the same, although the rate of loss may be slow and progressively reduced into tissues where tension increases gradually.

Plasma loss occurs in burns (p. 92) as a consequence of leakage of protein and exudate through damaged capillaries. Dilute plasma is also lost into an area of inflammation or tissue damage, but the protein content of such loss is rarely important in considering fluid replacement.

Loss of extracellular fluid (ECF) is a consequence of three situations:—

a. Deviation of normal exchange mechanisms. Extracellular fluid is in a constant state of exchange across the gastro-intestinal tract and the nephron. Normally, although large quantities are moved every day in this manner, the net amount of extracellular water that is 'transcellular' (mainly in the lumen of the gut) at any instant is quite small. However, by interfering with reabsorption the extracellular fluid can be continuously drained from its normal site. Such losses occur in vomiting, diarrhœa, fistulæ, and failure of tubular reabsorption of urine. In each instance the fluid lost varies in composition but basically it is rich in sodium ions. Big losses are accompanied by shrinkage of plasma volume and the onset of shock.

b. By increased loss of ECF along a normal pathway. The best single example of this situation is excessive sweating without replacement in a non-acclimatized individual. Sufficient dilute extracellular fluid may be leached out to produce a profound reduction in ECF and a shock state, but this is very rare in temperate climates.

c. The 'third-space phenomenon'. This concept is briefly summarized as follows. The ability of the cell to exclude sodium and so maintain both intracellular integrity and the volume of extracellular fluid is dependent upon active extrusion of the sodium ion by the expenditure of energy; a hypoxic cell is deprived of ability to expend such energy, thus permitting the ingress of sodium and draining such ions out of the extracellular fluid. The effective volume of the ECF is thus reduced and may aggravate the hypoxic insult. Third space must be taken into consideration whenever there has been more than a transient period of markedly reduced tissue perfusion.

PHYSIOLOGICAL ADJUSTMENTS TO LOSS OF CIRCULATORY VOLUME

Two major physiological adjustments occur. First, there is peripheral vaso-constriction which adapts the volume of the vascular tree to the reduced volume of blood it contains (it must be noted that a phrase beloved of many writers on shock—discrepancy between volume of blood and the capacity of the vascular tree—is a physical impossibility). The vasoconstriction is widespread, affecting the capacitance vessels on the venous side of the circulation as well as arterioles. In both instances as the vascular network shrinks the pressure tends to fall, but initially because of increased resistance to flow it is maintained on the arterial side, with or without a mild increase in heart-rate. Measurements of intra-vascular pressure are thus usefully made both on the arterial and venous side of the circulation, particularly the latter (*see* Central Venous Pressure *below*). Secondly, there is, by virtue of the altered pressure relations in the arteriole-capillary-venule loop, an ingress of extracellular water into the circulation producing hæmodilution. Initially, this is quite a rapid progress and after a hæmorrhage of 1·5–2·0 litres three-quarters of the resulting hæmodilution is over in 6–8 hours; this is of importance in the management of patients with suspected continued bleeding into, say, the gastro-intestinal tract. Repeated determinations over some hours indicating a progressively falling hæmoglobin, hæmatocrit, or red-cell count (all rough indications of hæmodilution) are more often than not indications of continued hæmorrhage.

REDUCTION IN CIRCULATING VOLUME: CORRELATION WITH PHYSICAL FINDINGS

Computation of blood-volume deficits is difficult and even direct measurement of blood-volume is only accurate to about 5 per cent (±300 ml. in an average man). No single parameter should be relied on, rather a summation of the following:—

Clinical Status	Vital Signs	Existing Intra-vascular Deficit in Adult
Patient well, not anxious	Pulse, 70–80. B.P., 120 systolic. CVP, 5–10 cm. water. Urine volume at least 40–50 ml. per hour	Less than 70 ml.
Mild anxiety, restlessness, pallor, coldness, possibly sweating. Thirst. Fainting in upright position	Pulse, 90–100. B.P., 90–100 systolic. CVP, 0–5. Urine volume, less than 30 ml. per hour	1–2 litres
Great anxiety, disorientation. Air hunger, icy extremities, fall in body temperature. Severe thirst	Pulse, 130+. B.P., 70 systolic. CVP below atmospheric, −5 cm. water. Urine volume, nil	2–3·5 litres

Points of Differentiation between Whole Blood, Plasma, and ECF Loss			
	Whole Blood	*Plasma*	*ECF*
Hæmatocrit	Normal initially; falls over some hours	Rises	Rises
Skin colour	Pallor	Usually unchanged	Usually unchanged
Tongue	Moist	Moist	Dry

In some circumstances it may be possible to correlate the clinical assessment with measured loss, for example, of blood during the course of an operation or ECF from a fistula. Even if the measurement lacks refinement (as does simple swab weighing), it gives more useful information than an ill-educated guess. Historical evidence may also be useful although lay people and members of the medical and nursing profession all tend to exaggerate visible blood-loss (except surgeons who always underestimate the amount of blood they spill). Finally, semi-objective assessment may be possible by seeing the extent of injury and referring to previously established figures.

When an assessment of whole blood-loss has been made, a decision must be reached on the extent of third-space requirements. When blood-loss exceeds 1 litre, a 2-litre deficit of extracellular fluid should be included for every additional litre of blood-loss.

Metabolic Acidosis in Low Circulating Blood-volume.—When a condition of low flow and hypoxia exists in an actively metabolizing tissue, oxidation is reduced and increased amounts of lactic acid are formed. This leads to the escape of hydrogen ions into the circulation and the development of metabolic acidosis. Increased hydrogen ion concentration depresses myocardial and smooth-muscle contractility, thus interfering with the pumping action of the heart and with the ability of the vascular tree to exert pressure on the contained blood. Metabolic acidosis may complicate the picture of any low blood-volume state and tends to be particularly severe when there is, in addition, a locally compromised area of circulation such as a strangulated loop of gut.

MANAGEMENT OF REDUCED CIRCULATING VOLUME

The object is to restore volume to normal as rapidly as possible taking into consideration losses of ECF in addition to blood or plasma. Restoration is achieved by two means: (1) Stopping the loss, and (2) Replacing that which has occurred. In most, but not all, instances and by the adoption of the techniques to be described it is possible to replace faster than the loss is occurring, but sometimes it may be necessary to establish the conditions under which resuscitation can proceed by taking operative steps to control bleeding. Thus, a furiously bleeding spleen or ruptured ectopic gestation may need to be controlled before blood-volume can be restored. Failure to respond or a response that is temporary indicates a hidden source of bleeding which must be diligently sought for and controlled.

Volume replacement should be undertaken once and for all, either as a preliminary to or after control of loss. It has often been observed that allowing the pendulum to swing from normovolæmia to hypovolæmia by repeatedly allowing losses to occur usually produces a crumbling physiological framework (but *see* Metabolic Acidosis). Accordingly, it is extremely important to have a clear plan outlined by the surgical team, which will allow a smooth progression from resuscitation to operation if this is necessary or from operation to resuscitation if the one must precede the other.

Replacement of Circulating Volume.—The first essential is to withdraw blood for grouping and cross-matching (p. 693). Thereafter the following principles should be observed:—

1. Technique.—A large-bore cannula or needle (No. 14 or bigger) *must* be used. Every house-surgeon seems to have to relearn the lesson that blood-loss from the splenic artery or a ruptured aorta cannot be adequately replaced through a 22-gauge needle. Three alternatives are available:—

a. Insert a standard No. 14 transfusion needle into a forearm vein (*Fig.* 19, p. 37).

b. Use a needle-cannula combination which, if it is plastic, may be inserted at the bend of the elbow.

c. Cut down on the veins of the elbow and insert a large-bore cannula.

These techniques will be found described in detail on pp. 36–41. Without exception the saphenous vein at the ankle should not be used as it is thick-walled and goes into spasm with monotonous regularity. Nor should time be wasted in futile attempts at needling collapsed veins. There are few patients who would not gladly endure a scar on the arm as a means of attaining increased longevity.

2. Initial Infusion.—Even if the cannula is the largest available, blood may initially flow only reluctantly through it. The patient's urgent need is for increased volume which will increase cardiac output and relax vasoconstriction. Thus, it is good practice to administer initially a 'trailer dose' of crystalloid solution and for this purpose the fluid best suited to ECF replacement is ideal. One litre of Ringer-lactate (Hartmann's solution) is rapidly run in over a period of 5–10 minutes. This large infusion will be rapidly dissipated (within an hour or two) into the ECF, but for the moment it expands circulating volume more rapidly than any other technique, particularly because crystalloid fluids flow easily.

3. Later Infusion.—Subsequently blood and other appropriate fluid are transfused plus additional Ringer-lactate to provide for third-space losses (*see above*). Control of rate of transfusion is guided by continued assessment of (i) pulse, (ii) arterial blood-pressure, (iii) central venous pressure, and (iv) urine output. How many of these parameters will be used depends upon the severity and complexity of the situation, but it is a good rule to observe and record too much rather than too little. For this purpose it is essential to have a clear chart and to discipline oneself into meticulous entries at half-hour intervals.

CENTRAL VENOUS PRESSURE (CVP)

For reasons implicit in the outline of the physiology of volume reduction, CVP measured by the insertion of a cannula into the great veins (*see* p. 40) is one of the most reliable guides to the adequacy or inadequacy of fluid replacement. Return of a normal CVP in the presence of presumed normal cardiac function is usually an indication that transfusion has been adequate. Because of peripheral vasoconstriction arterial blood-pressure (but not necessarily peripheral flow) may be normal when the deficit is incompletely replaced. A reduced CVP will reveal this state of affairs and prevent the mistake of proceeding to anæsthetize a patient inadequately replaced when, if anæsthesia is prematurely begun, vasoconstriction is abolished and precipitates a decline in arterial pressure

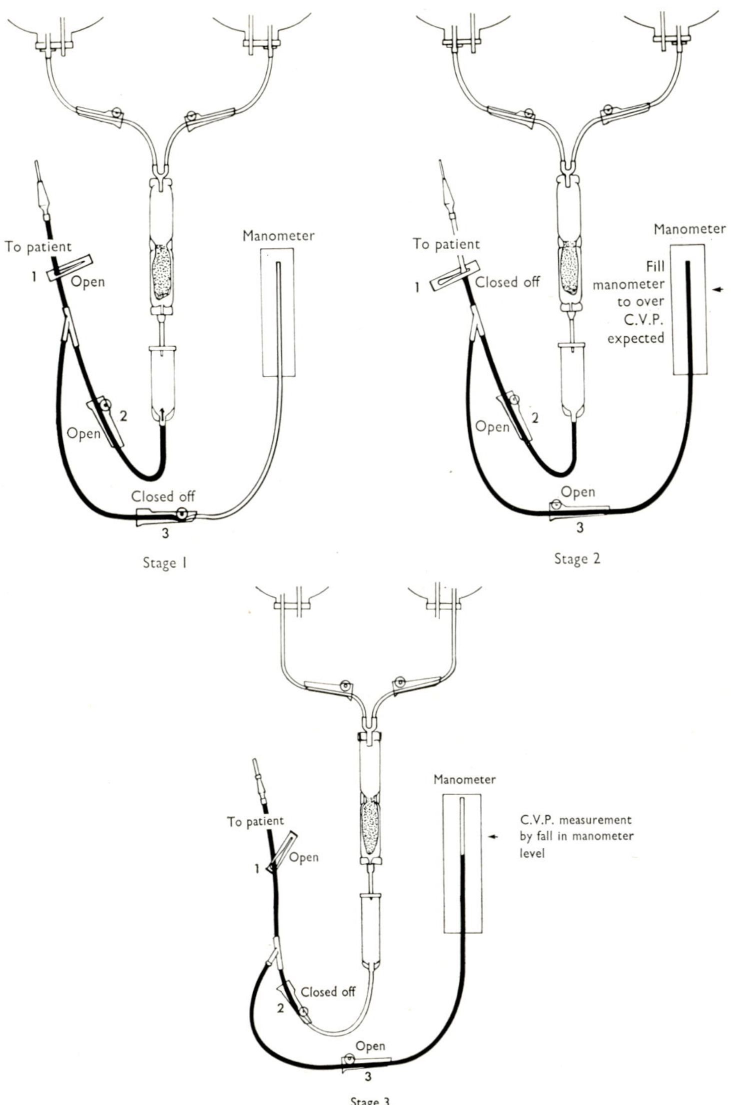

Fig. 16.—Method of connexion of intravenous apparatus to a central venous catheter for the measurement of CVP. Stage 1: the manometer is out of circuit and the drip flows from either bottle. Stage 2: the manometer is filled from the bottle, by clipping off the patient. Stage 3: the manometer fills to the measured CVP by opening clip to patient. The large-bore cannula is inserted into a great vein, e.g., jugular, subclavian, or cephalic, and CVP measured from the patient's mid-axillary line or manubriosternal joint level.

and flow. The measurement of CVP is made after the insertion of a cannula into a great vein (p. 40) and using the apparatus and technique shown in *Fig.* 16.

Urine output is a further satisfactory method of assessing a situation in which loss may be continuous as in a burn or a major operative procedure. A judicious reluctance to insert a urethral catheter in either sex should not be transformed into a doctrinaire refusal to exploit a useful technique which is certain to benefit patient management and, if properly controlled, is devoid of significant risk. In the complicated circumstances of shock when the patient is often restless, when many things may be being done to him and when he may have to be moved from place to place, a No. 14 or No. 16 Foley catheter with a 5-ml. balloon is the most reliable (*see* p. 449).

4. Correction of Acidosis.—When (*a*) acute volume loss has exceeded 2 litres or (*b*) arterial hypotension below 100 mm. Hg systolic has existed for an hour, or (*c*) when response to presumed adequate infusion has been incomplete, metabolic acidosis should be suspected. Confirmation should be sought by arterial blood analysis (*see* p. 13), but if this technique is not immediately available it is better to assume that acidosis is present and to administer sodium bicarbonate, 1 mEq. per ml. in 40-ml. aliquots on the basis of 1 aliquot to each 3 units of blood required. This rule-of-thumb approach is moderately satisfactory but control by *p*H studies is vitally necessary to intelligent therapy.

5. Management of Ancillary Features.—

Pain.—In spite of the experience of World War II and subsequently, there is still a reluctance to use opiate drugs by the only route that will do any good—intravenously. Subcutaneous or intramuscular morphine is too slowly absorbed in the shocked patient to be useful. The best technique is to dilute 15 mg. of morphine in 10 ml. of saline and to inject 1 ml. every 30 seconds until relief is afforded. Precision of this kind is rewarded by the use of a relatively small dose correctly adjusted to the individual patient and sufficiently limited to avoid respiratory depression or masking of physical signs.

Immobilization of Fractures.—This not only limits blood-loss into fracture hæmatomata but also reduces pain. Any major long-bone fracture should be temporarily splinted, pending definitive treatment. Similarly, unnecessary manipulation, transference from bed to stretcher, washing, and fussy documentation should all be avoided. The patient in shock should be got out of it, not subject to catechism or nursing ritual.

Warmth.—The shocked patient complains of *cold* because his metabolic rate falls and/or because he is exposed to a large temperature gradient with the environment. The latter can be corrected by providing a high ambient temperature (21°–24° C., 70°–75° F.), but correction of the former is impossible until increased tissue perfusion raises oxygen consumption. Therefore, external warming is useless and may be harmful if it encourages peripheral vasodilatation.

Oxygen Therapy.—Opinion has ebbed and flowed about the value of oxygen in states of circulating blood-volume reduction. Observation of desaturation of arterial blood and of experimental benefit suggests that it is not to be despised, and an intranasal catheter delivering 4–6 litres a minute should be used until hæmodynamics and urine output have returned to normal.

PLASMA AND PLASMA SUBSTITUTES

When blood has been lost replacement is by lactated Ringer's solution and whole blood. However, in burns and peritonitis plasma or plasma substitutes should be used. **Whole plasma,** usually made from a pool of outdated blood, has enjoyed an unsavoury reputation in the past because of the transmission of infective hepatitis. As now supplied (irradiated or aged), it is probably as safe or safer than whole blood but because the major colloid of plasma is albumin, albumin solutions are satisfactory volume expanders and a good substitute for unrefined plasma. Alternatively, but far less satisfactory, is the use of **dextran**—a long-chain polysaccharide. Although many thousands of units of this substance have been used with success, mystery surrounds its effects on the microcirculation and on blood coaguability. While useful as a stop-gap and in some special circumstances (*see* Low Molecular Weight Dextran, p. 30) its use should be eschewed when adequate albumin, balanced salt solution, and blood are available.

PREPARATION FOR ANÆSTHESIA OF THE PATIENT IN SHOCK

The need to have the patient's blood-volume adequately replaced has already been mentioned. In addition, the stomach must, if possible, be empty. Gastro-intestinal propulsion comes to a halt with a severe injury (and particularly when there is hypotension), so that the important interval is not the time between eating the last meal and the proposed anæsthetic, but the time between eating and injury. If this is less than 3 hours residual gastric contents must be assumed. In some instances an œsophageal tube can be easily passed, but distressing efforts to persuade a patient to swallow a tube should not be persisted with. Further-more, even a stomach tube will not effectively deal with semi-solid or solid gastric content. In such circumstances, it is preferable to practise an anæsthetic induction technique which does not permit regurgitation. Either the cricoid cartilage is firmly pressed directly posteriorly to occlude the œsophagus at its origin, or a No. 16 Foley catheter is passed into the œsophagus and gently inflated until the balloon just grips the œsophageal wall, so obstructing the lumen. Subsequent to the induction of anæsthesia and the passage of an endo-tracheal tube, an œsophageal or stomach tube can safely and easily be inserted to permit gastric aspiration.

SHOCK FROM OTHER CAUSES THAN LOSS OF CIRCULATING VOLUME

Although low blood-volume states are a common situation in hospital practice it is probable that two others are equally if not more so—severe sepsis and coronary occlusion.

3. MASSIVE SEPSIS
(Septic Shock; Bacteriæmia Shock; Bacterial Shock)

Definition.—The term 'massive sepsis' is preferred to septicæmia because the latter is, in fact, a bacteriological diagnosis which may be achieved only in retrospect, if at all. Furthermore, there is some evidence that an acute local process may throw off not so much organisms but products of infection which cause the shock state. The organisms involved are usually intestinal—*Esch. coli, Pseudomonas, Proteus*; the situation may also exist that their multiplication is favoured by some reduction in host resistance, e.g., severe illness, steroids, immuno-suppressive drugs.

It is customary and desirable to distinguish two pathological forms of shock in massive sepsis—instances with and without a focus. In the latter the prognosis is worse than in the former and common portals of entry are the urinary tract, the portal tract, and badly managed intravenous therapy. The pathophysiology of shock with sepsis is incompletely understood, but the current view is that it is predominantly the result of intense arteriolar and possibly venular vasoconstriction, perhaps the consequence of catecholamine and catecholamine-like substances. The arteriolar vasoconstriction reduces or abolishes peripheral blood-flow and the venous effects reduce the blood available for venous return. Thus, cardiac output falls, further aggravating the peripheral hypoxia. There is little evidence of a direct effect of bacterial toxins on the heart nor does selective hepatic vasoconstriction seem to have the same importance in man as it does in the dog and some other species.

Many other factors may contribute to the individual circumstances of a patient who presents with a presumed diagnosis of shock with sepsis. Acute ECF reduction, blood-loss, respiratory insufficiency, metabolic acidosis, and adrenocortical failure (*see* p. 29) may complicate the picture and call for treatment in their own right.

Clinical Features and Diagnosis.—Causes of blood-volume reduction sufficient to account for the profound clinical disturbances are absent, but there may be a history of predisposing drug ingestion or of a febrile illness. In favourable circumstances the diagnosis is made easy by the presence of obvious sepsis or of a portal of entry. On examination, the patient is anxious, cyanosed, has an extremely sluggish capillary return, a cold periphery, and tightly constricted veins. Arterial blood-pressure and CVP are both low.

Although blood-cultures should be taken repeatedly in instances of shock thought to be associated with sepsis they are of more use for retrospective evaluation and the refinement of a chemotherapeutic régime than for urgent diagnosis. By far the most important investigation is a *peripheral blood smear*. With rare exceptions, this will show a leucocytosis and of much greater importance the neutrophils will usually contain toxic granulations and Döhle bodies. Both these are manifestations of severe infection and greatly strengthen the diagnosis.

Management.—The prognosis is poor in septic shock, particularly when there is no obvious focus. The management may be outlined as a series of steps:—

a. Establish a fluid pathway preferably into a great vein so that CVP can be measured.

b. Insert a catheter into the bladder and check hourly urine output.

c. Draw blood for smear and blood-culture.

d. Administer a massive dose of antibiotics chosen with regard to possible aetiology; 10 mega units of penicillin and 2 G. of tetracycline plus 1 G. of kanamycin is a good starting dose to be modified later in the light of bacteriological studies.

e. If CVP is low, replace fluid losses with balanced salt solution.

f. If the patient now comes out of shock, renew the search for a focus and drain it if feasible.

g. If shock persists, it is worth while to give 500 mg. of hydrocortisone on the assumption that adrenocortical insufficiency exists. A non-specific effect of hydrocortisone has been described in some instances but is extremely rare in clinical practice.

If the patient remains in shock after these manœuvres he is almost certainly going to die. It is usual then to administer *vasopressor drugs* such as noradrenaline or metaraminol. These will raise the blood-pressure of virtually any patient unless he is already dead, but they do not result in improved flow and their morale-boosting use is for the benefit of the surgeon, not the patient. It is more rational in septic shock, which is thought to be the consequence of an already overactive vasoconstriction, to attempt to promote blood-flow by inducing vasodilatation. For this purpose drugs such as dibenzaline are now being cautiously employed with as yet equivocal results. Their use should remain restricted to expert teams.

Oxygen therapy and the *relief of anxiety* or *pain* are as much indicated in this form of shock as in any other.

4. CORONARY OCCLUSION

Shock in myocardial infarction is more common in medical than in surgical wards, but it may occasionally complicate a surgical situation. Such association between an operation and a coronary occlusion is much rarer than many surgeons believe, and before assuming that the cause of a post-operative collapse is the consequence of myocardial infarction the houseman must carefully search for other causes and also seek positive confirmation of the diagnosis. Thus, in a recent series of 71 fatalities after gall-bladder surgery—a disease traditionally linked by many with the occurrence of cardiac disorders—not one was found to have been caused by coronary occlusion although many were so diagnosed.

The clinical features are not usually difficult to analyse, although pain may not be so severe. Shock, out of proportion to blood-loss or the extent of other possible precipitating factors, combined with a raised CVP or one that becomes so after the infusion of a small (500-ml.) challenge dose of colloid are the diagnostic features confirmed by progressive ECG signs and ultimately by transaminase determinations. The aim in a surgical setting should be to correct any additional factor which will further embarrass the heart—a full stomach, the pain of an abdominal wound, and the laboured breathing of a post-operative state. Expert cardiological advice should be sought in regard to monitoring, arrhythmias, and the use of cardiac drugs such as digitalis.

5. ADRENOCORTICAL INSUFFICIENCY

This syndrome is rare but perhaps not so rare as it used to be. *De novo* it may occur during the course of severe acute sepsis (e.g., the Waterhouse-Friderichsen syndrome in relation to meningococcal septicæmia) or after a severe head injury, but it is more common to encounter it after steroid drugs have been administered, so suppressing endogenous cortical activity by depressing ACTH production. Thus, it may be seen when surgery is called for in a patient with ulcerative colitis or rheumatoid arthritis. Adrenocortical suppression subsequent to steroid therapy may last up to 2 years, gradually declining in severity; but most instances of acute insufficiency have occurred within 18 months or take place while the patient is on a maintenance dose but is exposed to additional stress, e.g., an operation or infection.

The clinical features are non-specific; the diagnosis is made only by a healthy sense of suspicion and the therapeutic trial of a large (200-mg.) intravenous dose of hydrocortisone. If adrenocortical insufficiency is present the response is dramatic, but it is fair to add that the suspicion is rarely confirmed, some other cause usually being confounded with the diagnosis by hypo-adrenocorticalism.

Prophylaxis is more applicable to this form of shock than any other. Patients who have received steroids in therapeutic doses, within 2 years should be regarded with suspicion if they have to undergo a major surgical procedure, but there is no indication to administer steroids unless they show signs of circulatory failure. Patients actually on therapy should have the operative procedure and post-operative period for the first 4–6 days covered by a dose of 300 mg. daily of hydrocortisone in three divided intramuscular doses of 100 mg. Because of the slow effect of this drug intramuscularly the first dose on the day of operation should be given intravenously. Similarly, patients requiring emergency surgery should receive a large booster dose of 200 mg. intravenously. After the fourth day, and *provided progress is satisfactory*, the dose is halved on successive days until the original maintenance dose is reached.

ADJUVANT MEASURES IN THE MANAGEMENT OF SHOCK

Mannitol.—This carbohydrate is what is known as a disposable solute—that is, once it enters the renal tubule it is not reabsorbed. Consequently it carries with it the water necessary for its excretion and promotes a 'solute diuresis', provided glomerular filtration is adequate. It was introduced in the 1950's as a means of reducing the concentration of tubular urine in circumstances where high concentration of nephrotoxins were considered to be deleterious (e.g., after burns or mismatched transfusion). The more energetic infusion of balanced salt solution and of colloid that characterizes the treatment of shock in the 1960's has rendered mannitol less important as a therapeutic agent. Perhaps its sole use in treatment is in the unexpected circumstances of mismatched transfusion (p. 45) when a large intravascular hæmolysis carries a considerable quantity of hæmoglobin to the nephron under circumstances when glomerular filtration and consequently tubular flow are both reduced. Under such conditions not only should glomerular filtration be increased by rapid infusion of balanced salt solution, but also 50 ml. of 25 per cent mannitol should be *injected*. Maximum solute diuresis is the consequence of the attainment of high plasma concentration and thus there is no place for slow infusion. If a response does not occur, then the renal damage is irreversible by this means and the usual measures must be taken to deal with the problems that ensue (*see* p. 436).

Probably more important than its therapeutic use is the diagnostic administration of mannitol where oliguria or anuria is present. Many patients who have sustained a period of hypotension will be oliguric or effectively anuric. It is of some importance to establish if such oliguria is 'functional' in the sense that it is reversible or if hypoxia in the nephron has passed the stage where rapid recovery may be expected. Under such circumstances the rapid test infusion of 50 ml. of 25 per cent mannitol may establish whether the capability of urine flow exists.

Note.—Such a dose should not be repeated if a diuresis does not result and should not be undertaken in the absence of a catheter which allows the assessment of hourly urine output.

Low Molecular Weight Dextran (LMWD).—The low-cut fractions of dextran have a number of peculiar properties amongst which is an ability to disaggregate clumped erythrocytes. 'Sludging', or aggregation, is thought to be a feature of a number of low-flow states and hypoxia. LMWD has, therefore, been recommended in a wide variety of shocked states. The only relatively unequivocal evidence of its efficiency is in states of local marginal flow such as intestinal or limb ischæmia. Its use should be reserved for such situations, when 1 litre of 5 per cent LMWD in saline may be infused over a period of 1–2 hours.

ANAPHYLACTIC SHOCK

This is a convenient term—although probably a gross oversimplification—for the acute circulatory collapse which is the consequence of hypersensitivity to a drug, toxin, or serum.

The clinical features are acute hypotension, loss of consciousness, patchy mottling of the skin, urticaria, and often, when consciousness is recovered, a persisting sense of anxiety—*the angor animi* of Ryle.

Treatment is expectant and empirical: a massive dose of hydrocortisone intravenously (200–300 mg.) seems to give better results than adrenaline which was for long the main standby. If mismatched transfusion is suspect, 1 litre of balanced salt solution and 50 ml. of 25 per cent mannitol should be infused.

CHAPTER IV

WATER AND ELECTROLYTE BALANCE AND INFUSIONS, BLOOD TRANSFUSION, AND NUTRITION

By H. A. F. DUDLEY and J. KYLE

IN this chapter general principles only will be dealt with. Water and electrolyte balance is one of the fundamental problems in surgical physiology and only diligent observation, wide reading, and hard thinking will enable the house-surgeon to understand the subject. What is written here is but a guide to practical management and not an exhaustive treatise.

NORMAL WATER AND ELECTROLYTE BALANCE

Body water and electrolyte balance are maintained by equating intake to output. Output is determined by environmental circumstances and by the need to excrete waste products. In healthy man a variety of feedback mechanisms adjust intake, e.g., thirst and avidity for salt. In the sick or feeble patient such feedback may be incapable of functioning or may be deprived of expression. It is up to the doctor to anticipate needs by an intelligent appraisal of the physiological status of the patient; for example, renal disease may markedly alter the patient's ability to adjust to changes.

WATER

Body-water content is maintained within narrow limits by the action of the antidiuretic hormone/distal tubule (and collecting-duct) mechanism, reduction of intake leading to increased tubular reabsorption. This mechanism will fail when the collecting duct is damaged or (rarely) when diabetes insipidus exists as in some instances of head injury. In the absence of water intake, body-water losses are those of obligatory urine and transpiration, the latter increased by unfavourable environmental circumstances, e.g., in tropical climates amounting to 2–4 litres per 24 hours.

Features of Acute Water Lack.—These are dryness of mucous membranes, scanty urine with high specific gravity, mental confusion, apathy or irrationality, coma, and ultimately death in hyperpyrexia. There are no circulatory features because the water losses are distributed over the whole body water (approximately 45 litres). Indeed for this reason there may be a deficit of up to 4 litres before there are any clinical manifestations of water lack.

In clinical surgery the two circumstances where water deficiency is seen are: (1) acute upper gastro-intestinal obstruction; and (2) the unconscious or feeble patient who cannot feed himself. Confirmation of the diagnosis is obtained by finding an increased serum-sodium concentration (normal range 130–152 mEq./l.), but by this time the condition is well advanced. The hæmatocrit may be raised— but pre-existing anæmia may lower it.

EXTRACELLULAR FLUID (ECF) VOLUME AND SODIUM

The constancy is a consequence of a balance of ECF volume between absorption and excretion of sodium and water across the gastro-intestinal tract and the nephron. Fine control of sodium excretion is largely the result of changes in the activity of adrenocortical hormones and of the juxtamedullary apparatus. Hyponatræmia, a relative excess of ECF water over sodium, may result from water overloading (particularly by the intravenous route) or from true sodium depletion, common after chronic losses from the alimentary tract. Excessive ADH secretion may follow surgical trauma, certain types of brain injuries and tumours, and liver disease leading to a relative retention of water. In heart failure and hypoproteinæmia, while serum-sodium levels are low there is an increase in total body sodium. Sodium loss in the urine also occurs in Addison's disease, hypopituitarism, and after giving diuretics such as diamox and chlorothiazide. Sometimes it would appear that the 'cell pump' breaks down, allowing larger than normal amounts of sodium to enter the cell, thereby lowering the ECF sodium concentration. Considerable quantities of sodium may be effectively lost in large effusions and exudates.

Clinical Features of ECF Deficit.—The major features of extracellular fluid deficit which produce the clinical picture of 'dehydration'—dry furred tongue, decreased saliva, sunken eyes and cheeks, lax skin, difficulty in speaking and swallowing, and circulatory failure—are the result of loss of normal exchange mechanisms: deviation of gastro-intestinal secretions or failure of reabsorption of sodium and water in the nephron.

The serious features of ECF deficiency are those of circulatory failure, actual or impending. There may be hypotension, tachycardia, inadequate peripheral circulation, and empty veins; weight is lost. The hæmatocrit is raised, but because the loss is usually isotonic or nearly so, there is not much change, if any, in serum-sodium concentration. The diagnosis is made—as always in fluid and electrolyte disorders—by intelligent appreciation of the history and by observations of the clinical features; laboratory tests are less important.

POTASSIUM AND INTRACELLULAR WATER

Intracellular water (ICW) has as its main ion potassium associated with protein and carbohydrate. Major movements of ICW are the result of potassium migration which is mainly the consequence of metabolic events. The normal range of serum potassium is 4·0–5·5 mEq./l.

There can, however, be considerable deficits in body potassium, e.g., after trauma, with little change in serum concentration. Once clinical evidence of hypokalæmia appears, the level is likely to be below 3·5 mEq./l.; more severe degrees are usually accompanied by alkalosis, with a bicarbonate level above 30 mEq./l. In clinical practice loss of potassium is often accompanied by sodium and water losses with acidosis—hence serum-potassium and bicarbonate *concentrations* may appear normal.

Causes of Potassium Loss.—

1. Starvation, when the whole cell matrix is reduced.

2. Lower gastro-intestinal losses, which may contain potassium in concentrations higher than those in the serum.

3. Occasionally significant losses may occur through the kidney, particularly when sodium conservation is maximal; also in the recovery phase of tubular necrosis.

4. Administration or excess secretion of adrenocorticosteroids.

5. Diuretic therapy.

6. Diabetic acidosis.

Clinical Features of Potassium Deficiency.—These are muscular weakness, gastro-intestinal atony, sleepiness, and apathy. In addition, there may be paroxysmal tachycardia, with A–V conduction block. The ECG shows depression of the ST segment, the interval between the Q and the T waves may be lengthened and the latter wave is sometimes inverted (*Fig.* 17 B). All these features can exist when the serum potassium is at the lower limit of normal, for the concentration only falls catastrophically when about one-quarter to one-third of total body potassium is lost. The clinical features of potassium deficiency are exaggerated by alkalosis and by a low concentration of serum sodium and may, for example, be encountered in pyloric stenosis.

Hyperkalæmia.—A rise in serum potassium may result from injudicious administration of potassium salts, or from potassium escaping from cells into the ECF following anoxia or trauma. It is also a feature of uræmia and may be noted after large blood transfusions and in patients with Addison's disease.

Clinically, the main effects of hyperkalæmia are on the conduction system of the heart. This is shown on the ECG: the T wave becomes higher and pointed, then the R wave becomes smaller, the notch of the S wave deeper, so that terminally the trace resembles an electromagnetic sine wave (*Fig.* 17 D). There may be ventricular fibrillation.

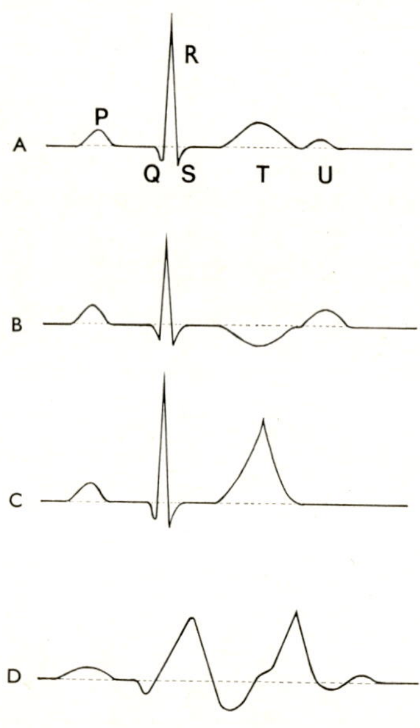

Fig. 17.—Electrocardiograms in: A, Normal subject; B, Hypokalæmia; C, Moderate hyperkalæmia; D, Terminal hyperkalæmia.

PRINCIPLES OF FLUID AND ELECTROLYTE THERAPY

As with shock, diagnosis is of fundamental importance. It is not good enough to say: 'He looks a little dehydrated, let's start on intravenous infusion.' The wisest words in the therapeutics of fluid and electrolyte therapy are those of A. W. Wilkinson: 'The hardest thinking must be done at the bedside.' An intelligent appreciation of the patient's history and a careful physical evaluation, including hæmatocrit, urine volume, and specific gravity, are worth a wealth of laboratory data. Serum and urine electrolytes are useful more for management than for initial therapy.

Once a diagnosis has been arrived at on the basis of history and clinical examination, therapy may commence. The main aims of replacement therapy are to: (1) restore the circulating blood-volumes; (2) ensure an adequate urinary output—1200–1500 ml. per 24 hours for an adult; (3) maintain a normal distribution of electrolytes, especially potassium, between the cells and ECF. Replacement is adjusted to the clinical diagnosis and guided by an assessment of urine output, CVP, skin turgor, and hæmatocrit. The following principles should be observed:—

1. Careful records are essential. Every hospital has its own fluid-balance chart which is always better than anyone else's, but it is essential:—

a. That cumulative totals are available at 24-hour intervals;

b. That the metric system is used.

2. Checks on variable parameters—urine volume, specific gravity, CVP—should be included in the recording chart, preferably at intervals of not more than 4 hours.

3. The patient should be weighed at 24-hour intervals as a cross-check on the fluid-balance chart. This is only needed for infusions being continued beyond 36–48 hours—the majority can be stopped before this.

4. The house-surgeon must make daily checks for evidence of venous distension, pulmonary and dependent œdema, or water intoxication.

If possible, before commencing therapy a **base-line** should be determined, deriving all possible information from the case history, clinical appearance, and measurable parameters outlined above. When on admission there have been fluid and electrolyte losses from the alimentary tract—vomiting or diarrhœa, by aspiration, or from fistulæ—some idea of the order of magnitude of these losses may be obtained from *Table II*, which shows the daily volume and composition of the principal secretions. The volumes of these secretions diminish

Table II.—DAILY VOLUME AND COMPOSITION OF PRINCIPAL ALIMENTARY SECRETIONS

	VOLUME PER 24 HOURS (ml.)	Na (mEq./l.)	K (mEq./l.
Gastric juice	2500	60	10
Succus entericus	3000	130	15
Bile	500	140	5
Pancreatic juice	750	140	5

considerably after a day or two of continuous loss. It is almost impossible to calculate hidden, internal losses of fluid, e.g., into obstructed bowel, pleural effusions, etc., but they should be remembered.

In addition to replacing pre-existing losses, fluid therapy has to provide for the **normal daily output of fluid** in urine (1200–1500 ml.) and by insensible perspiration and respiration (700–1000 ml.). These normal metabolic losses are usually made good by the intravenous administration of 2000 ml. of 5 per cent dextrose and 500 ml. of 0·9 per cent saline. However, in the 24 hours after a major operation the urinary output may be halved, i.e., not more than 1500 ml. of fluid are needed in the first post-operative day. Fever and a high environmental temperature and humidity will increase skin and respiratory fluid losses.

Daily reassessment of the patient's fluid needs is required. **Continuing losses,** e.g., from gastric aspiration or fistulæ, must be replaced. Discontinue infusions as soon as it is safe to do so.

Sodium Administration.—It is rarely necessary to give sodium chloride in a solution stronger than 0·9 per cent (which provides 154 mEq. sodium per litre). Severe salt depletion, actual or relative to water, is the only indication for giving small quantities (up to 500 ml.) of 5 per cent saline.

Potassium Administration.—Potassium chloride should not be given to patients with oliguria, and only with great care to anyone with renal disease. It is always safer to give it by mouth, e.g., in fruit drinks. One gramme of potassium chloride provides 13 mEq. of potassium. If the intravenous route is to be used, 1 C. GKI is added to 500 ml. of 5 per cent dextrose and run in slowly. Do not as a rule give more than 6 G. of KCl per 24 hours, and check the heart's action with repeated electrocardiograms—more valuable than serum concentrations.

Potassium Intoxication.—When there is ECG evidence of cardiac intoxication, give 100 ml. of 50 per cent dextrose plus 10 units insulin intravenously. This may be supplemented by 10 ml. of 10 per cent calcium gluconate and 250 ml. of 1·4 per cent sodium bicarbonate, because hypocalcæmia and hyponatræmia potentiate the toxic effects of hyperkalæmia.

Hyperkalæmia.—Slight to moderate elevations of serum-potassium levels will usually subside once an adequate flow of urine is obtained. If not, the use of ion-exchange resins or dialysis may have to be considered (*see* p. 433).

VENOUS DISTENSION AND CREPITATIONS AT THE BASES OF THE LUNGS

There has been a lot of loose writing on this subject. Venous distension may be obvious as a raised jugular venous pressure (*Fig.* 18) or CVP. It is the consequence of increased blood-volume including increased extracellular volume and may accordingly be seen in plethora from over-transfusion of any colloid or as a consequence of too much salt and water. When sodium chloride or balanced salt solution has been infused in excess, venous distension will be accompanied by transudation into alveoli with crepitations. However, in the early stages of colloid plethora from blood or plasma infusion, crepitations are absent and the only features are tachypnœa and dyspnœa.

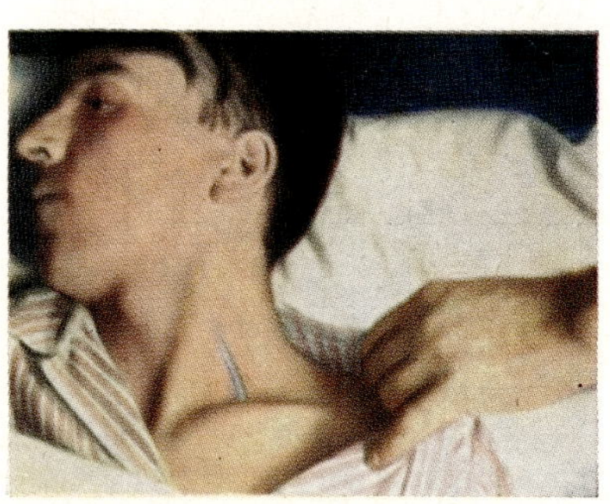

Fig. 18.—Fullness of the external jugular vein in a patient undergoing fluid therapy is indicative that too much fluid has been given.

Infusion of water (as 5 per cent dextrose) does not produce either venous distension or basal crepitations because the water is so rapidly distributed over the large volume of total body water. It follows that crepitations at the bases are heard only when ECF is in excess or there is parenchymal lung disease.

WATER INTOXICATION

The over-infusion of water (usually the consequence of ill-considered therapy in the face of decreased excretory capacity) does not produce signs. Rather there is a group of symptoms—headache, lethargy, muscle cramps, disorientation, convulsions—which is inaccurately if impressively known as 'water intoxication'. The diagnosis is confirmed by finding hyponatræmia and other evidence of hæmodilution.

TECHNIQUES OF INTRAVENOUS THERAPY

Needling.—For the patient in shock, and indeed in any other circumstances, the largest bore needle should be used. Veins suitable for intravenous infusion are shown in *Figs.* 19–21. Anyone who has had a 14- or 15-S.W.G. needle inserted into themselves will understand that a small weal of local anæsthetic is highly desirable. A proximal tourniquet is applied at venous pressure and a 5-minute period allowed to elapse. If distended veins are not then visible it is better to abandon the attempt to needle and make a cut down. Given that

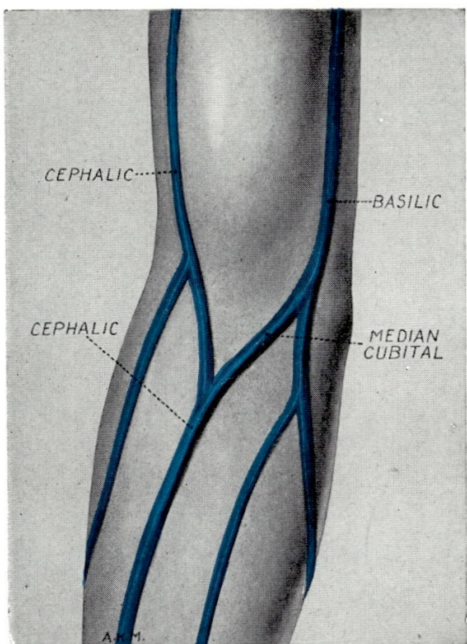

Fig. 19.—The veins of the forearm.

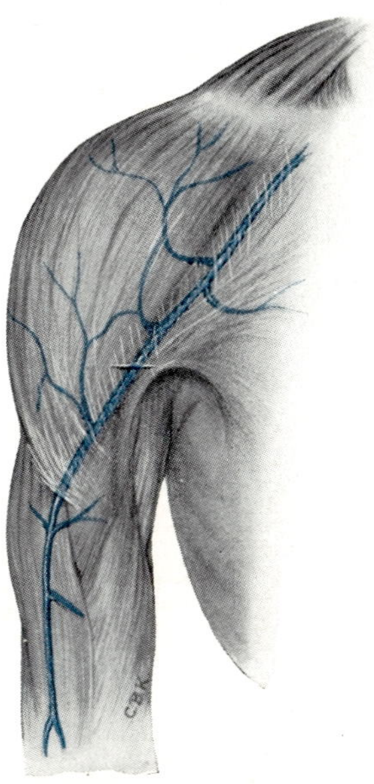

Fig. 20.—The cephalic vein in the delto-pectoral groove has advantages.

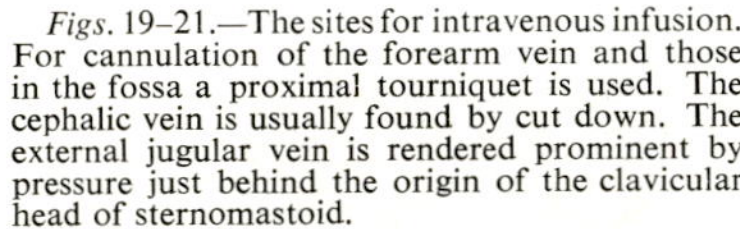

Figs. 19–21.—The sites for intravenous infusion. For cannulation of the forearm vein and those in the fossa a proximal tourniquet is used. The cephalic vein is usually found by cut down. The external jugular vein is rendered prominent by pressure just behind the origin of the clavicular head of sternomastoid.

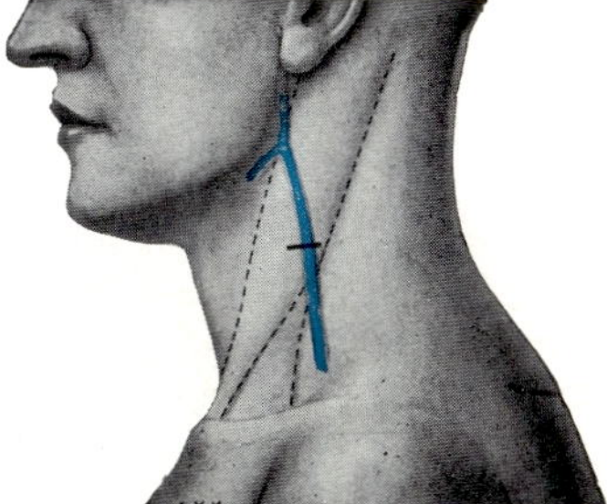

Fig. 21.—The external jugular vein, as it crosses the sternomastoid, can be exposed easily.

veins are visible in forearm or hand, a small blob of 1 per cent procaine or lignocaine is raised *beside* the chosen vein. The needle is then passed through the skin without making any attempt to puncture the vein—the pressure required to penetrate the matted fibre of the dermis is quite different from that necessary

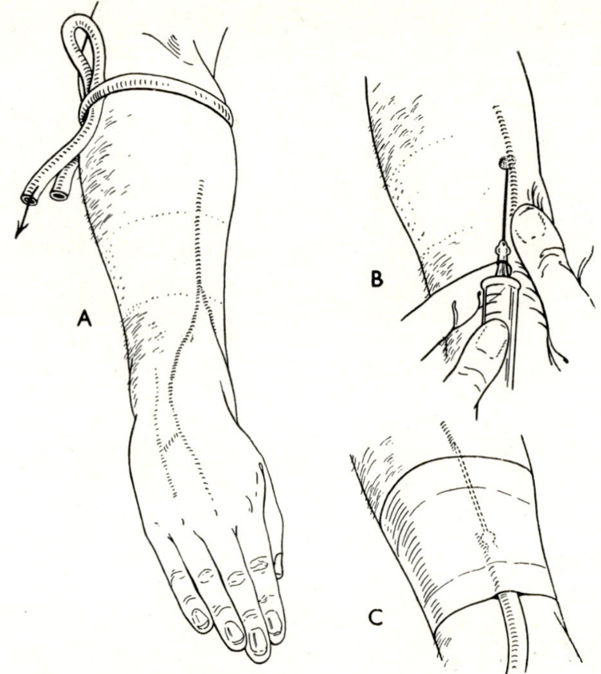

Fig. 22.—Insertion and strapping of needle for intravenous therapy. **A,** Quick release tourniquet; **B,** Insertion of needle through weal of local anæsthetic; **C,** Strapping holding dressing and infusion tubing in position.

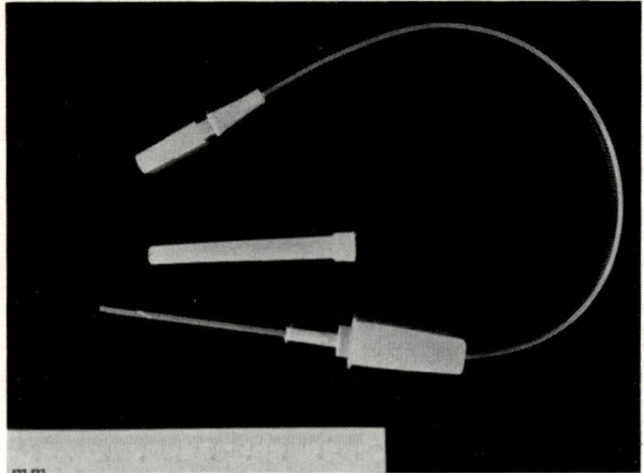

Fig. 23.—An 'Intracath' suitable for peripheral or central venous cannulation: the catheter is internal to the needle.

for penetrating the vein. The point is brought over the vein and deliberate puncture made, the needle being threaded up the vein for at least 2 cm. Reflux of blood confirms the venepuncture, the tourniquet is released, and the infusion apparatus connected. Micropore tape or zinc oxide strapping is used to secure the needle as illustrated in *Fig.* 22.

Needle and Catheter Combinations.—The Intracath, Angiocath, Medicut, or Braunula needle-cannula combinations are inserted by the same techniques (*Fig.* 23). The first can be inserted directly through the weal of local anæsthetic because the needle is outside the cannula, but the 'shoulders' of the cannulæ in the second and third make it necessary to nick the skin at the site of puncture with the No. 16 blade or trocar provided if unnecessary trauma is to be avoided. Thereafter the technique is the same as for needling.

Cutting Down.—The successive steps are illustrated in *Fig.* 24. Notwithstanding the operator's pride, when a cut down is needed the incision should be generous. The insertion of the cannula through the distal flap makes it

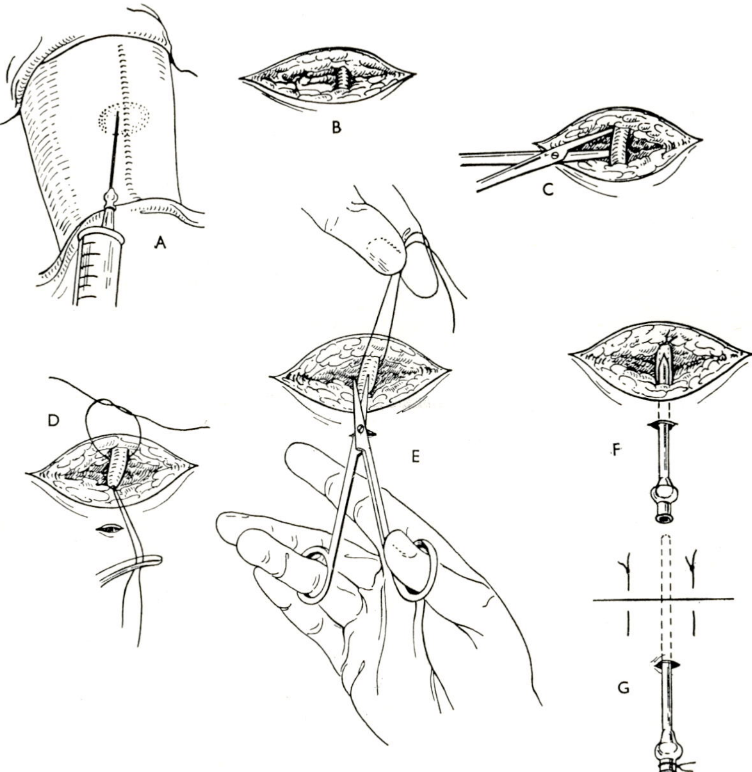

Fig. 24.—Cutting down. Steps in the exposure of a vein and direct insertion of a cannula, which passes separately through the distal skin flap.

Angiocath, Intracath (Bard Davol Ltd., Clacton-on-Sea, Essex).
Braunula (Armour Pharmaceutical Company, Ltd., Eastbourne, and U.S.A.).
Medicut (Argyle Division, Brunswick Corporation, St. Louis, U.S.A.).

3

possible to withdraw it when the infusion is complete without disturbing the original incision.

Cannulæ should be specifically designed for the job and the practice of threading a length of polyethylene tubing on to a needle is deplored. Special cannulæ are available; alternatively, the cannula for an Intracath, or an Angiocath, can be extracted from its pack. The shorter the cannula the better, as increased length increases resistance to flow.

Splinting an Intravenous Infusion Site.—A properly inserted intravenous infusion either by needle or by cannula should not need a splint. In a restless patient it may be necessary to provide a splint to prevent him pulling at the infusion site. Such splintage should be in the position of function.

Puncture of Great Veins.—This is a very useful technique of gaining access to the circulation; venospasm is absent and there is the additional advantage of being able to measure CVP, so useful in the diagnosis and management of shock states (p. 24). There are two techniques of entering the subclavian and one of direct puncture of the innominate from the right side.

Technique of Infraclavicular Puncture.—The subclavian vein is intimately related and attached to the deep aspect of the middle one-third of the clavicle and can be reached by a needle passed backwards and medially from the mid-point of this bone.

The usual technique of infraclavicular puncture is to use an Intracath. After preliminary infiltration of local anæsthetic, a No. 16 scalpel blade is used to make a 3-mm. nick in the skin. A 10-ml. syringe filled with saline is attached to the needle from which the cannula has been withdrawn. The needle is introduced through skin and, with the shaft held almost parallel to the anterior chest wall, is advanced towards the point where the first rib passes under the clavicle—the general direction is towards an area 1–2 cm. above the suprasternal notch.

When the needle point strikes the bone, it is withdrawn 2 cm. and readvanced in the same direction but in a slightly more inferior plane, so that the needle just clears the posterior inferior surface of the clavicle.

A further advance of 2 cm. with suction applied usually results in the syringe rapidly filling with dark red blood which confirms that the puncture is successful. If such does not occur, the needle is withdrawn from under the clavicle and then readvanced in a similar manner but in a slightly more cranial or caudal direction. The syringe is removed, the cannula threaded along the needle and advanced 8–10 cm. Reflux of blood is confirmed and the needle removed along the cannula. It is essential to tape the cannula firmly to the skin of the anterior chest wall.

The supraclavicular route may also be used. The technique is similar, but the site of puncture is the angle between the lateral border of the clavicular head of sternomastoid and the upper border of the clavicle, a point which can best be identified by rotating the head to the opposite side. The direction of the needle is at an angle of 45° to the sagittal plane and 15° forward of the coronal plane.

Routine chest radiography should follow every successful or attempted subclavian vein puncture to guard against the possibility of a pneumothorax going undetected.

Finally, the innominate vein lies behind the right lateral border of the sternum. A needle inserted backwards and medially below the medial third of the clavicle must penetrate the vein and the same routine can then be observed.

Complications.—House-surgeons are advised that puncture of great veins in the thoracocervical region, although a useful procedure, is not to be undertaken lightly. Pneumothorax has been frequently described after infraclavicular puncture, less commonly following supraclavicular. Accurate vein puncture is probably within reach of all, but the technique requires practice and dexterity. An inexperienced house-surgeon should cannulate the external jugular vein or cut down in the cubital fossa and insert a large bore 60-cm. cannula. Threaded proximally this provides a good pathway for intravenous therapy and a measure of venous pressure, which although not 'central' in the strict sense, is often adequate for clinical control.

Whatever the technique adopted, CVP is measured either from mid-axillary line or from manubriosternal junction (*see Fig.* 16, p. 25).

THROMBOPHLEBITIS

Any peripheral intravenous infusion will irritate the vein; the worst offenders are 5 per cent and 10 per cent dextrose, but duration of infusion is more important than the composition of the fluid. The needle or cannula is not of much importance. Pride in the maintenance of an infusion should be tempered by the knowledge that intravenous therapy remains one of the commonest causes of a septicæmia, which may be fatal. The slightest signs of redness, of tenderness, or of systemic infection are an *absolute* indication to remove the infusion and undertake blood-culture. There should be no compromise with this situation else disaster may ensue. For maintenance of intravenous therapy it is better to adopt the technique either of intermittent daily intravenous infusion or of central infusion through a subclavian catheter.

SUPERVISING INTRAVENOUS INFUSIONS

1. There are three main causes of stoppage of an intravenous infusion:-
   a. Damage to the intima by the sharp point of a needle.
   b. Displacement of the needle.
   c. Chemical thrombophlebitis.
Occasionally a minor adjustment of the angle of the needle remedies matters.

2. If some such minor adjustment fails to restart the flow, do not dismantle any part of the apparatus. Rather remove the needle or the cannula and, if necessary, reinsert it into another vein.

3. Never continue an intravenous infusion for more than 24 hours without the sanction of your chief, or the surgical registrar.

4. Check personally the fluid intake and output figures at the end of 24 hours. *Check the balance chart yourself.*

OTHER ROUTES OF FLUID ADMINISTRATION

If it is not possible to give fluids by mouth—always the best way—the intravenous route is the preferred alternative. The amount of fluid infused is known accurately and is effective immediately. However, the method does need both intelligent and continuous supervision by skilled staff.

In places where such staff is not always available it may be safer to use the slower intramuscular route or to resort to the much less predictable practice of rectal infusion. Subcutaneous infusions may be employed in infants (p. 577).

Continuous Intramuscular Infusion.—Perhaps the advantage of this route that transcends all others is that in a hospital without a resident doctor an experienced sister, following telephone instructions, can insert a needle of an infusion apparatus into the muscles of the thigh and administer the stated quantity of fluid herself. Only dextrose and saline solution should be given by this route.

The best site for the injection is the external side of the middle third of the thigh. Billimoria and Dunlop's needle, with its adjustable shield (*Fig.* 25), is

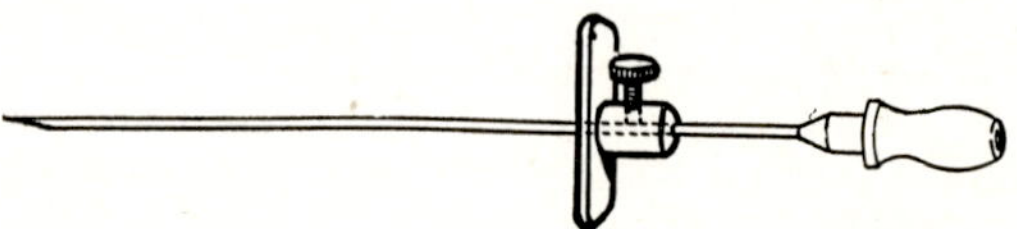

Fig. 25.—Billimoria and Dunlop's needle★ for intramuscular administration of fluid.

an asset. The needle is inserted nearly down to the bone, when the adjustable shield is fixed by turning the screw, making further penetration impossible. It is a good practice to insert the needle through a piece of sterile gauze, which comes to lie between the shield and the skin. Once the needle is in place satisfactorily, it can be kept in position by adhesive plaster placed over the shield. A rate of about 40 drops per minute is suitable for most adults in need of fluid.

Continuous Rectal Infusion.— This method has the advantage of simplicity and requires neither complicated apparatus nor asepsis. Unfortunately, it is not possible to be certain that all fluid run in has been retained, and if retained, that it has been absorbed. The method is not suitable for patients with colonic disease or after colonic surgery. The fluid administered is usually 4 parts of tap water to 1 part of normal saline; about 3·5 litres can be run in during 24 hours at the rate of 40 drops per minute.

Technique.—A preferably unlubricated rectal tube or large Foley bag catheter is inserted 15 cm. into the rectum and secured in position. The flask containing the unsterile solution is suspended 60 cm. above the level of the anus, and connected to the rectal tube or catheter via a drip chamber (*Fig.* 26). The patient may be sedated to reduce the chances of dislodgement.

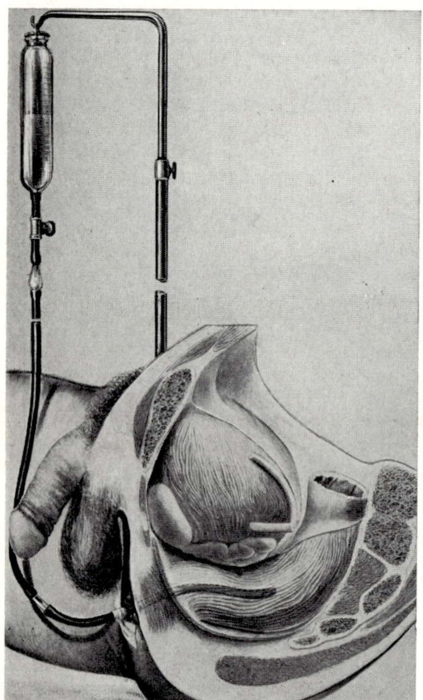

Fig. 26.—The principles of continuous rectal infusion. The outlet of the flask should be 2 ft. (60 cm.) above the level of the anus.

★ Made by C. F. Thackray Ltd., Leeds.

BLOOD TRANSFUSION

Blood transfusion is the best method of treating patients who have suffered a rapid loss of blood or who, more gradually, have become severely anæmic. Blood-transfusion services are in operation in many parts of the world. It is now uncommon not to be able to obtain adequate supplies of blood for transfusion; however, difficulties may arise with rare blood groups. Transfusion services mostly undertake their own blood grouping, but details of cross-matching are given on p. 695 for those for whom such a service is not available.

It is incumbent upon the house-surgeon to:—

1. Order blood in good time by sending a sample for cross-matching, if possible, 24 hours before it is needed.

2. Check *all* the patient's details with those on the bottle of blood supplied.

3. Ensure that there is no avoidable wastage of blood—by ordering too much, or at the wrong time, or storing in the wrong manner.

4. Be familiar with techniques of giving blood, difficulties that may arise, and complications which may follow.

Ordering Blood.—Complete a blood-transfusion request form stating clearly the amount required and the time and date for which the blood is needed.

The request form must give the following details of the patient: (1) Full name; (2) Address; (3) Date of birth; (4) Unit number; (5) History of any previous transfusions and/or pregnancies.

Checking the Compatibility Label.—Before administering the blood supplied the house officer must check the patient's details on the bottle label with those of the intended recipient. *This step must never be omitted.* It is indefensible to proceed if the slightest doubt exists as to whether or not it is the correct blood intended for that particular patient.

Record the serial number and blood group of all blood given in the patient's notes—they will be needed if complications develop.

Verify that the Blood shows No Obvious Sign of Deterioration.—Confirm that the blood is within its expiry date. Hæmolysis due to over-age, infection, or faulty refrigeration may be apparent either as a pinkish discoloration throughout the plasma or as a purplish tinge diffusing upwards from the cell mass. Fat may collect as a whitish layer on the surface and is not a contra-indication to the use of the blood.

Storage.—Blood must be stored in a special refrigerator accurately maintained at 4°–6° C. (38°–42° F.). Transfusion of blood that has been frozen and thawed may cause death. Blood should not be left out of the refrigerator for more than 30 minutes. Reconstituted dried plasma is made up immediately before use.

TECHNIQUE OF ADMINISTRATION

Blood (or plasma) does not need to be heated before use except for exchange transfusions in infants. For the latter type of patient the bottle can be placed in water at a measured temperature not exceeding 40° C. (104° F.).

Giving Sets.—The disposable type of giving set illustrated (*Fig.* 27) is rapidly replacing the old glass-drip-chamber and rubber-tubing sets of former years.

Choice of vein and the mode of entry differ in no respect from those described in connexion with the administration of electrolyte solutions (p. 36). When transfusion is most needed sometimes the veins are collapsed and cannot be entered without cutting down and tying in an intravenous catheter or cannula.

The patient should be watched carefully for the first 30 minutes to ensure a steady flow and to detect any reactions. Check his blood-pressure at least once.

Rate of Transfusion.—A rate of 40 drops per min. is usually adequate if anæmia is being corrected. In severe hypovolæmic shock a faster rate of delivery may be needed. This may necessitate the use of positive pressure with a Martin's pump (*Fig.* 28); blowing into the air inlet tube with a Higginson's syringe is to be deprecated, but direct pressure can be applied to the outside of a plastic pack.

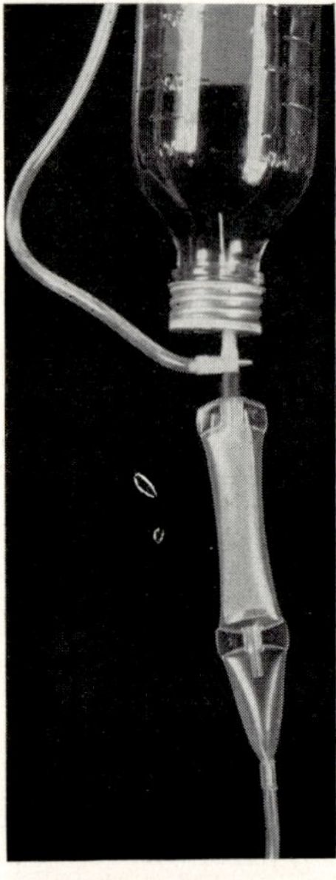

Fig. 27.—The drip-chamber, filter, and laterally-placed air-inlet tube of the Capon Heaton disposable plastic giving set.

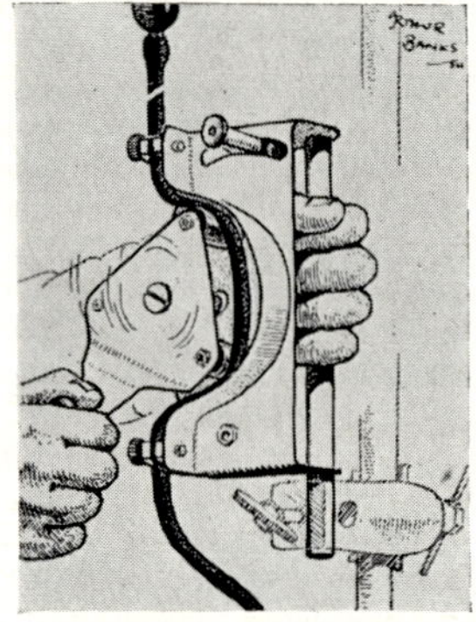

Fig. 28.—Martin's pump in use.

Mechanical Difficulties.—If the blood will not flow properly, check that:—

1. The tourniquet has been removed or that the patient's sleeve is not acting as a tourniquet.

2. There are no acute bends on tubing or intravenous catheter—slight adjustments of the latter or of the position of the patient's arm often improve flow.

3. The air inlet tube is not occluded.

4. There is not an air-lock in the tube—if present disconnect at the catheter end and allow blood and air to run down till all the air is cleared.

5. There is no venospasm—an initial rapid infusion of an electrolyte solution will often overcome this (p. 24).

Obscuration of the Drip Chamber.—If the drip chamber fills up with blood it can be cleared by clamping the tubing, inverting the bottle, and squeezing the plastic chamber to return some blood to the bottle. With a glass chamber a few millilitres of air can be injected into the rubber tubing immediately below it. No injection should be made into plastic tubing. Should clotting occur in a disposable giving set, it must be replaced with another set.

DANGERS OF TRANSFUSION

1. *Circulatory Overloading.*—Watch that the jugular venous pressure (*see Fig.* 18), or CVP, does not rise, especially in the elderly or those with myocardial disease. Venesection may be necessary.

2. *Air Embolism.*—This may result from bottles being allowed to run dry, holes in tubing, or the intravenous catheter being disconnected. (*See* p. 8.)

3. *Transfusion Reactions.*—Minor reactions are not uncommon. The patient may feel warm and have a slight pyrexia. Such mild symptoms usually respond to an antihistamine preparation, e.g., piriton, 1 ml. subcutaneously.

Incompatibility Reactions.—These may be heralded by a feeling of anxiety and constriction across the chest; or they may start suddenly with rigors, acute dyspnœa, and lumbar pain. Symptoms may appear after only a few millilitres of incompatible blood have been run in, or much later. Subsequently jaundice develops; there may be hæmoglobinuria, oliguria, and even anuria.

Treatment.—Stop the transfusion at once. Using a fresh giving set, inject 50 ml. of 25 per cent mannitol or give 5 per cent dextrose or a plasma expander (p. 26). Keep a careful watch on urinary output and serum-urea and potassium levels. If the patient can drink, oral fluids are pushed.

The blood-transfusion service must be told at once of the accident and the remaining blood and the giving set should be returned to them for checking.

Infected Blood.—Transfusion of infected blood quickly produces profound shock with hypotension, cyanosis, rigors, and vomiting.

Treatment.—Stop the transfusion, and replace it with a 5 per cent dextrose infusion containing 500 mg. of a broad-spectrum antibiotic, e.g., tetracycline. Elevation of the foot of the bed and oxygen administration may help. The infected blood is immediately returned to the blood-transfusion service and a sample cultured to detect the organism responsible.

Homologous Serum Jaundice.—This is the one complication which may follow plasma or blood transfusion that is not entirely preventable. Its incidence has now fallen to a fraction of 1 per cent. It may develop in a matter of several weeks or only appear 4–5 months after transfusion. Diagnosis and treatment are as for other forms of hepatitis. All cases of serum hepatitis should be notified to the local blood-transfusion service.

COLLECTING BLOOD

The transfusion service can provide a taking set and a sterile bottle containing anticoagulant, e.g., disodium citrate 2·5 G. and dextrose 3 G. in 120 ml. of pyrogen-free water.

A swab soaked in 0·05 per cent chlorhexidine in 70 per cent alcohol should be placed on the top of the rubber closure and left for 2 minutes. The needle of the air-outlet should be inserted through one of the quadrants marked '1', if the closure conforms to British Standard 2463: 1962. The bottle needle of the taking set should be pushed fully through the other quadrant marked '1'. If the needle of the air-outlet is blocked, e.g., by a plug of rubber, a potentially dangerous situation exists. Blood will flow into the bottle until the pressure of air in the bottle equals the pressure of blood in the vein. If the pressure in the sphygmomanometer is now released, air will pass from the bottle into the vein. A fatal air embolism can result. The tubing should always be clamped before the pressure in the sphygmomanometer is released.

The donor lies with arm abducted. The venous return is occluded with a sphygmomanometer cuff inflated to 40–60 mm. Hg on the upper arm. The skin over a suitable antecubital vein is cleaned with 0·5 per cent chlorhexidine in 70 per cent alcohol. An injection of local anæsthetic is made and the needle is inserted into the vein. When 420 ml. of blood have been collected the tubing is clamped, the sphygmomanometer cuff is removed, a sterile swab placed

Piriton (Allen & Hanburys Ltd., Bethnal Green, London, E.2).

over the skin puncture point and the needle removed. The donor should keep his arm straight, and exert pressure on the swab with the thumb of his other hand for 3 minutes.

Blood may also be collected in a plastic Fenwal bag, the spring balance showing when 300–400 G. have been collected (*Fig.* 29).

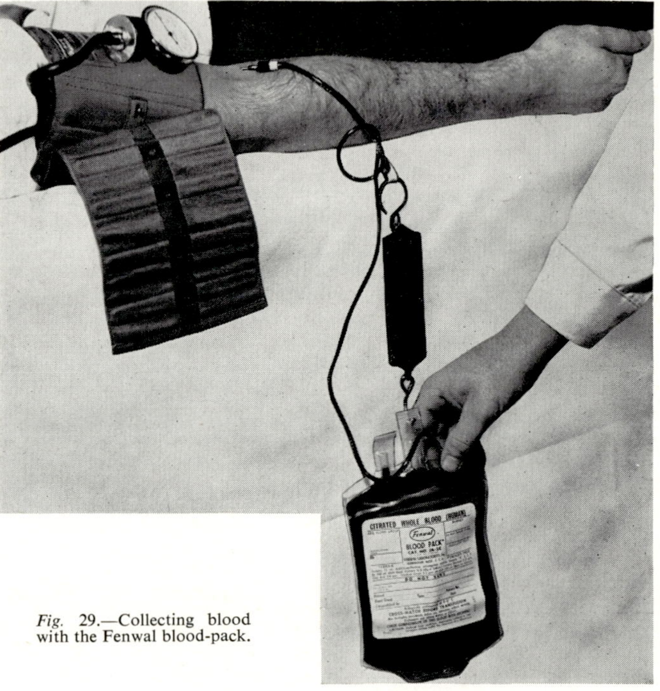

Fig. 29.—Collecting blood with the Fenwal blood-pack.

PACKED RED-CELL TRANSFUSION

Transfusions of concentrated red cells are valuable in elderly anæmic patients. The concentrated cells must be given within 12 hours of their preparation. As a proportion of the serum has been removed, the cell suspension is rather viscous; consequently the largest possible intravenous catheter or needle should be used, and careful supervision is needed.

One bottle (500 ml.) of ordinary blood transfused into an anæmic patient will raise his hæmoglobin by 1 G. per 100 ml. (7 per cent Haldane); one unit of concentrated cells is twice as effective.

EXCHANGE TRANSFUSIONS

(*See* p. 581.)

NUTRITION

Although most house-surgeons have a working knowledge of fluids and electrolyte balance, they often do not realize that a background of understanding

Fenwal bags (Fenwal Laboratories Ltd., Morton Grove, Illinois, U.S.A.).

of nutrition is every bit as important. Many surgical patients come under their care malnourished as a consequence of disease, and many more will, because of complication during their convalescence, become starved or semi-starved. While the direct relationship between malnutrition and complications such as infection and failure of wound healing has yet to be established, there is little doubt that a nutritionally well-cared-for patient will have a smoother convalescence than one who is on the metabolic bread-line.

Basic requirements are shown in the table, which also indicates methods of parenteral supply that will be dealt with below (*Table III*). These are increased by about 15 per cent for a very short time (*circa* 3–4 days) after a major injury,

Table III.—FULL PARENTERAL NUTRITION FOR MAINTENANCE (70-kg. MAN)

SUBSTANCE	AMOUNT	PREPARATION AND VOLUME		CALORIES	WATER CONTENT
Protein	70 G. (1 G. per kg.)	10% protein hydrolysate	700 ml.	200	700 ml.
		or			
		3% synthetic amino-acid mixture	1000 ml.*	120	1000 ml.
Carbohydrate	140 G. (2 G. per kg.)	10% dextrose	1400 ml.	560	1400 ml.
Fat emulsion	140 G. (2 G. per kg.)	20% fat emulsion†	700 ml.	1260	560 ml.
Total	—	—	2800–3100 ml.	2140	3660 ml.

ADDITIONS OR ALTERATIONS TO MAINTENANCE FOR ATTEMPTED REPLETION

Alcohol	70 G. (1 G. per kg.)	Absolute alcohol	88 ml.	Add 490	—
Carbohydrate	280 G. (4 G. per kg.)	20% dextrose	1400 ml.	Add 560	1400 ml.

Lævulose may be substituted for dextrose in this table and further carbohydrate as lævulose or dextrose can be added to bring the total to *circa* 3500 calories a day.

and will remain up for longer periods should infection and other complications supervene. The requirement for total calories rises as much as for protein and there is little evidence to suggest that the interests of the patient are best served by massive protein intakes if these are not balanced by an adequate (40 cal. per G.) non-protein calorie intake. Hence the high-protein diets so beloved of medical and nursing staff are devoid of metabolic meaning although their culinary nature may make them more attractive to the sick patient. Furthermore, greater attention should be directed in surgical nutrition towards regularly supplying the basic needs in the long term than in fretting over the small increase in demand that follows injury and infection. More patients have starved to death at normal or low rates of energy expenditure than have been consumed in the flames of their own excess metabolism.

---

* Trophysan (Sepepharm, Ltd., 15 Hanover Square, London, W.1).
† Intralipid (Paines & Byrne Ltd., Pabyrn Laboratories, Greenford, Middlesex).

INDICATION FOR NUTRITIONAL CONTROL, SUPPLEMENTATION, AND TOTAL PROVISION

Many patients will survive without difficulty a short period of starvation in association with surgical procedures or illnesses and will rapidly regain lost weight when they escape the confines of the hospital. However, for the more seriously ill and those in whom oral intake is restricted for a week or more, supplementation or a complete nutritional takeover by alimentary or parenteral routes is vital. As with fluid and electrolyte balance, the aim should be to prevent and anticipate the development of a gross imbalance and institute intelligent preventive therapy. We do not let patients get thirsty before supplying water; similarly, there is no justification for allowing them to starve for long periods before feeding them. Because nutrition is still not a well-understood subject in a surgical context and because initially changes are undramatic, there is always a tendency to postpone the evil day when something should be done about either finding a pathway into the gastro-intestinal tract or undertaking parenteral nutrition. The tendency to put off until tomorrow what seems capable of being avoided today should be resisted, and a firm cut-off point of no more than 1 week's starvation accepted as the absolute limit. Now that the technique for feeding is so much better developed there is even less excuse for subnutrition in surgical wards.

Indications.—A summary of indications for supplementation or total feeding is as follows:—

1. Pre-operative: the grossly malnourished patient so as to reverse negative nitrogen balance.

2. Post-operative:—

    a. Any patient who comes to surgery in category (1).

    b. Post-operative starvation of more than a week's duration occasioned by complications.

3. The unconscious patient.

4. The feeble patient who is incapable of managing normal dietary manœuvres.

5. Late convalescence after major illnesses (supplementation only).

6. Increased demand from massive injury or sepsis often combined with one or more of the previous factors.

TECHNIQUE OF CALORIE AND NITROGEN SUPPLY

A. By Mouth.—Food is best, but only when it is of the best. Hospital diets are often monotonous and may be unattractive or so different from that to which the patient is accustomed that he will refuse even if basically his appetite is unimpaired. There is also a combination of guilt and denial frequently to be found in nursing staff which leads them to maintain stoutly that the patient is eating adequately of the best food in the world even when he is pecking listlessly at a mess of pottage. The only certain check, and one well worth making, is a rough dietary analysis for 2 days on the fluid-balance chart. Even without recourse to dietetic tables, it is often abundantly clear that the patient is getting around 1000 calories a day instead of the 2500–3000 he may need.

This unsatisfactory situation can be overcome in two ways: when a satisfactory dietetics advice service exists by constructing a reasonable and attractive *personal diet* for the patient; alternatively, either in the absence of such a service or if it proves unable to cope with a recalcitrant or anorectic patient by *supplementary feeding*. There are in turn two methods by which the latter can be undertaken:—

1. *Oral liquid feeds* in the form of milk shakes, egg nogs, or palatable proprietary mixtures. As with ordinary feeding it is useless to leave this form of supplementation as a vague order or encouragement to nurse and patient; if this is done the resulting intake is often derisory. Rather oral supplements should be prescribed on as rigid a schedule as drugs to ensure whatever extra calorie intake is thought desirable. The actual calorie intake should be checked frequently.

2. *Tube Feeding.*—There are situations when the gastro-intestinal tract is normal but the patient is either unable or unwilling to eat. Recourse should then be had without hesitation to supplementary or complete tube feeding. Two techniques are available: a fine (2–3 mm. internal diameter) tube is introduced transnasally (*see* p. 348) and left permanently in situ; alternatively, a larger bore tube (16–18 F) is passed intermittently. In either event food may be given by continuous gravity infusion or intermittently in doses of 200–300 ml. The latter method is quite satisfactory but should not be used if there is the slightest doubt about the ability of the stomach to accept a large quantity of liquid all at once. Sometimes the previous establishment of a gastrostomy (p. 350) or a jejunostomy (for suction or the replacement of fistula losses) allows the use of this for feeding, and in instances where a long period of increased requirement or of difficulty in oral intake (e.g., disintegration of the jaw or mouth, unconsciousness) is anticipated there is a sound case for establishing a gastrostomy for nutritional purposes alone.

Table IV shows four feeds of varying calorie value which will provide a continual spectrum for most surgical circumstances and which are well tolerated.

Table IV.—STANDARD ENTERAL RATIONS

INGREDIENTS	QUANTITY	PROTEIN	FAT	CARBOHYDRATE	CALORIES
Supplement Feed I (high fat, high protein)					
Cows' milk	2000 ml.	68	74	96	1320
50% fat emulsion	100 ml.	—	50	—	450
Lactose	60 G.	—	—	63	240
Water	400 ml.	—	—	—	—
	Total	68	124	159	2010
Full Feed II (high fat, normal protein)					
Cows' milk	1000 ml.	34	37	48	660
50% fat emulsion	270 ml.	—	135	—	1215
Lactose	250 G.	—	—	250	1000
Milk protein	35 G.	35	—	—	140
Water	1700 ml.	—	—	—	—
	Total	69	172	298	3015
Supplement Feed III (high carbohydrate, high protein)					
Complan	200 G.	62	32	88	900
Lactose	150 G.	—	—	150	600
Water	2500 ml.	—	—	—	—
	Total	62	32	238	1500
Full Feed IV (high carbohydrate, high protein)					
Complan	300 G.	93	48	132	1350
Glucose	300 G.	—	—	300	1200
Methyl cellulose	3 G.	—	—	—	—
	Total	93	48	432	2550

Complan (Glaxo Laboratories Ltd., Greenford, Middlesex).

Danger.—The danger of tube feeding by any technique is regurgitation. Constant watchfulness for correct position of the tube (which should be checked before each feed) and a constant clinical assessment of the adequacy of gastro-intestinal function are the house-surgeon's duty. Where doubt as to the position of a tube or the efficiency of gastric emptying is entertained, no hesitation should be had in undertaking a check radiograph, and provided a radio-opaque tube is used its position can be confirmed by a plain film; gastric emptying is ascertained by administering 40 ml. of gastrografin and exposing a flat plate of the abdomen 1 hour later. Three-quarters or more of the contrast medium should be in the small bowel and the head of the meal should have reached the terminal ileum.

B. Parental Nutrition.—Recently it has become possible not only to maintain fluid and electrolyte normality by the intravenous route but also to supply adequate calories and nitrogen. The indications and the rations are the same as for more normal methods of intake and there is nothing to be served by the unbalanced administration of one component of normal diet—man cannot live on nitrogen alone, nor fat alone, nor carbohydrate alone, he needs all three. To these *alcohol* may be added if it is felt useful either for morale or for supplying additional calories. Alcohol provides 7 cal. per ml. and can be metabolized at approximately 8–10 ml. per hour. When it is used, it must not be forgotten that sedation will need to be reduced and that it may have bizarre effects on those unaccustomed to it.

Standard parenteral rations with additional calorie nitrogen supplements are shown in *Table III*. As with other forms of intravenous therapy, the administration may be by intermittent infusion or by central catheter (p. 40). There is less tendency to thrombosis with modern preparations than previously, but prolonged use of the same peripheral vein is to be avoided.

CHAPTER V

THE TREATMENT OF WOUNDS

By D. S. Chapman

A WOUND is the loss of continuity in any tissue caused by violence, which is usually external. Cuts in the skin are known to everyone, but there may be similar and sometimes very extensive wounds of deeper tissues. Thus a fracture is a wound of bone—a simple definition which should make the casualty officer less mesmerized by the radiographic image and more aware of the soft-tissue injury that surrounds the fracture. Sometimes this soft-tissue injury is so great as to determine the life or death of the patient.

DANGERS AND COMPLICATIONS OF WOUNDS

1. Hæmorrhage.—May be external or internal, and in either case may be sufficiently severe as to necessitate blood transfusion. It can be controlled by a firmly applied pressure pad, reinforced if need be by hand pressure and elevation. A tourniquet is seldom necessary.

2. Damage to Important Deeper Structures.—This may not always be apparent and must be looked for. Systematic testing of nerve and tendon function is essential before operation as function cannot be assessed once the part or patient has been anæsthetized.

3. Swelling.—The œdema of trauma commences at the time of wounding and is maximal in 24 hours. Although often minimal, it can cause local tissue hypoxia and pain. Joint stiffness and reduced viability of tissue may result from it; if a limb that is swelling is rigidly encased, e.g., in plaster-of-Paris, ischæmic necrosis may follow. High elevation can prevent or markedly reduce swelling.

4. Infection.—Most wounds are contaminated from the start, but it is only after 6–8 hours that the organisms begin to multiply. Proper wound cleansing and débridement during this interval often prevent clinical infection from developing.

Tetanus and gas gangrene fortunately are rare complications of wounds—*see* p. 67.

FIRST-AID TREATMENT

If the patient is first seen at or near the scene of the accident and his injuries merit his removal to hospital, the attending doctor should apply an emergency dressing, relieve pain, ensure adequate splintage, and send a note with all relevant information to the hospital.

Dressing.—A sterile pressure pad makes an effective dressing. It consists of sterile gauze or lint, on the outer surface of which there are layers of wool to give even pressure over a wide area; the dressing is held in place by a crêpe bandage. Wool should not be placed directly on the surface of a wound. If sterile dressings are not available (most police and road patrol vehicles carry them), then freshly laundered household linen may be used.

Pain.—The psychological response to injury varies greatly, from hysteria, through fatalism, to severe depression. Consequently the assessment of pain can be very difficult. Pain can always be relieved. Minor injuries to limbs and digits may not require any analgesics; for others codeine co. tablets or panadol may suffice. Morphine not only eases pain but lessens anxiety; 10 or 15 mg. may be injected for a major wound, but remember that absorption may be slow in a shocked patient, particularly from the subcutaneous tissues. Both morphine and pethidine (50 mg.) are more rapidly and more certainly effective when given slowly intravenously. Morphine must *not* be given to head injuries.

When pain appears excessive, make sure that bandages are not too tight, that a fracture has not been overlooked, or, later, that there is no infection developing.

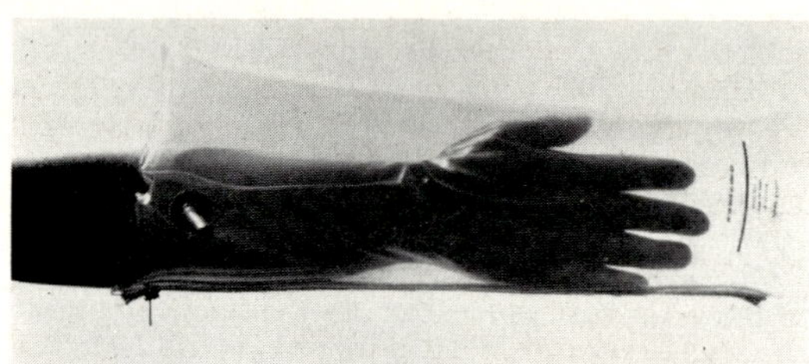

Fig. 30.—Inflatable splint providing rigid and comfortable support for an injured forearm.

Splintage.—Rest for the injured tissues is desirable. Almost all fractures are splinted, but soft tissues also need protection against unnecessary movement. Correct splintage helps relieve pain both before and after operation; elevation reduces swelling.

For the forearm and hand, gutter slabs can be made from plaster-of-Paris. An arm injury can be held efficiently by a sling. For the lower limb the Thomas splint can be used for all injuries (except those of the foot), with the limb secured on the splint by bandaging, plaster-of-Paris (Tobruk plaster), or by traction on the boot. The Tobruk plaster is particularly valuable when a patient must be transported a long distance to a base hospital. Wooden back splints do not stay securely in position for very long.

Recently inflatable plastic bags (*Fig*. 30) of various shapes and sizes to fit a part or the whole of a limb have become available. They are supplied sterile and are easily carried; they should prove a boon in first-aid work. The plastic bag, consisting of two envelopes, is passed directly over the injured part and the outer envelope inflated through a one-way valve, to give even pressure directly on to the skin by the inner lining. This will prevent hæmorrhage, give rigid splintage to any fracture, and provide a sterile dressing.

THE INITIAL ASSESSMENT OF WOUNDS

Adequate treatment is impossible without adequate inspection. Inspection cannot always be completed at the first examination nor is it always wise to try in the casualty department because of the possibility of causing more bleeding, more soiling, and increasing pain. Some wounds can only be fully assessed in the operating theatre.

History.—A full history is required, including the circumstances of wounding, the cause of the injury, the time elapsed, the amount of blood lost, etc. This

Panadol (Bayer Products Co., Surbiton, Surrey).
Inflatable splints (Parke, Davis & Co., Staines Road, Hounslow, Middlesex, and
  Detroit, Michigan, U.S.A.).

information can determine the order of priority in treating multiple injuries and suggest the extent and possibility of contamination of wounds.

Examination.—The casualty doctor wishing to use radiographs will remember the dangers of transporting the patient to another department and the delays that are possible; mostly he should bring the X-ray machine to the seriously injured patient. When examining the wound, the doctor is suitably garbed with gown and sterile mask, and the patient if necessary also wears a mask. The masks can be of the disposable variety. A 'no-touch' technique is used to examine the wound. The full extent, the volume, and depth of injury are ascertained and a decision taken whether the wound is in fact suitable for treatment in that department. The wound is classified (*see below*) and the appropriate treatment policy decided.

With multiple injuries involving more than one body system, several different specialists including an anæsthetist may have to be consulted at an early stage.

CLASSIFICATION OF WOUNDS

Wounds can be broadly considered as *open* or *closed*, the essential difference being that in the open wound there is an access for organisms from the beginning.

The decision to repair any injured structures in an open wound depends entirely on whether it is *tidy* or *untidy*.

OPEN WOUNDS

1. Incised Wound.—This is a wound cleanly cut by a sharp instrument (knife, glass, or razor). This tidy wound has no bruising or crushing of the wound margin; it tends to gape and bleed freely and may be quite large. It might be contaminated and in it important structures may be divided. The damage to all structures is linear, with minimal loss of tissue, and on healing the scar should be linear and the least deforming. If not already infected, the repair of deeper structures can usually be made as a primary procedure.

2. The Puncture (Stab) Wound.—This wound is deeper than it is long, and is caused by such objects as pins, knives, or by a fall on a spike. The entrance wound is often surprisingly small and in fact may be missed. By skin elasticity, for instance, a sword blade 1 in. (2·5 cm.) wide may leave only a $\frac{1}{4}$ in. entrance hole. At any depth, great damage can be done to important deep structures.

External bleeding is usually slight but there may be extensive concealed blood-loss.

3. Perforating and Penetrating Wounds.—These are puncture wounds caused by missiles or other foreign bodies which may lodge in or pass through the tissues. The perforating wound has usually a large ragged exit caused by the foreign body, bone fragments, and other tissues being forced out, and tissues are ploughed up between entrance and exit. The penetrating wound has no exit and the foreign body may be retained far distant from the entrance wound.

4. The Lacerated Wound.—The wounding agent causes tearing, crushing, and forcible disruption of tissues. Not only is there loss of skin continuity but within the zone of violence all the tissues are extensively devitalized by the loss of blood-supply and are liable to infection. This untidy wound may be quite small as when a finger is crushed by a door. The surface wound may be nothing more than a splitting from the pressure, but the deeper structures are torn irregularly, crushed, ragged, and contused. Because of this crushing, bleeding

is often at first slight. For example, when a limb is amputated by a train wheel
the recipient may appear quite well on admission to the hospital. But shock is
usual, by the loss to the body of blood fixed in the crushed tissues. A lacerated
wound is unlikely to heal well.

5. Abrasions and Degloving.—An abrasion is caused by the scraping away
of the superficial layers of the skin; if abraded by a road surface, fragments of
grit are often embedded in it and if left will cause 'tattooing'. Many nerve-
endings are exposed making the wound painful, and it is also prone to infection.
Though the usual violence is shortlived, it might be continued for some time
as when a rope passes rapidly through one's hands and the heat then engendered
causes a *friction burn.*

When deeper pressure is applied in the rubbing, instead of an abrasion a
flap of skin and subcutaneous tissue may be rolled off deeper structures—
degloving (*Fig.* 31). This degloved flap may be devitalized by the pressure, but

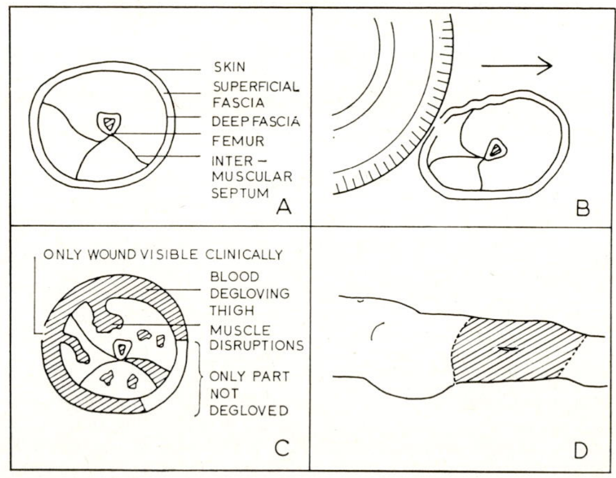

Fig. 31.—Crush injury, with degloving of thigh, by a vehicle's wheel; A, Cross-section
of normal thigh. B, How the limb was rolled and crushed by the wheel. C, Cross-section
to show area of disruption. D, External appearance with small lateral cut but wide area
of crushing and degloving (shaded).

in many cases can and should be saved, as the retention of skin as a dressing
(especially if it is cleansed and sterile), even though dead, is better than no skin
at all.

CLOSED WOUNDS

1. A Contusion.—A contusion is caused by the pressure of a blunt object
(fist, stick, club), by the tearing of tissues, and the forcible angulation of a part
(e.g., a sprain). As a result there is an extravasation into tissues of blood liberated
by the rupture of small vessels. Spreading by continuity in a tissue, the swelling
is augmented by œdema. By definition, the skin is intact but in some cases on
careful inspection it is found split and technically the wound is then open.

If the skin is involved by the contusion the visible bruise is an *ecchymosis.*

Though unattractive, particularly when on the face, and painful at first, even large contusions absorb without aid. The blood cannot in fact be extracted by incision or aspiration.

2. A Hæmatoma.—A hæmatoma is caused by the same type of blunt violence as a contusion but usually larger blood-vessels are ruptured so that blood is poured into a gap between torn tissues or along a fascial plane. The swelling grows rapidly and a large hæmatoma produces shock. A soft-tissue hæmatoma is very often associated with fracture of a large bone. When tightly confined (e.g., subungual) a hæmatoma can be very painful. A knowledge of its natural history is essential in planning treatment. At first the blood is fluid (fluctuant), then it clots (boggy); finally, the hæmatoma is absorbed or becomes infected if the skin is broken or devitalized. If it is very large, serum is absorbed leaving a blood-clot organizing to form a fibrous wall and in this again fluid can collect to form a cyst, a special type being the subdural hæmatoma.

The Crush Injury.—A very heavy object pressing hard against a fixed limb or the trunk creates tremendous changes over large volumes of tissue and can affect them like an 'implosion'—the muscles widely disrupted and bleeding or with large portions dead, tendons and aponeuroses torn from their attachments, large nerves and vessels torn or twisted, yet often without a fracture. When the heavy object also rolls over the fixed part, it rubs the skin virtually off the deeper structures perhaps with only a small break in its continuity (*see Fig*. 31). The 'intact' skin may be considerably bruised, abraded, be obviously dead or it may be degloved. Such an injury, the most serious type of closed injury, may thus present as an apparently minor injury yet the outstanding immediate need is for blood replacement.

The signs and symptoms of the so-called 'crush syndrome' (traumatic anuria, release syndrome) do not appear to be in any way different from those of severe shock (p. 20) as seen with major burns or with irremedial oligæmia from hæmorrhage. In centres aware of the enormous blood-losses possible in soft-tissue injuries caused by crushing, and where blood infusions are given rapidly in adequate amounts, the crush syndrome is not encountered.

A RECORD OF INJURIES

Because of the possibility of litigation and of requiring a record many months later, a pictorial representation—made both at the time of inspection and at operation—is invaluable. This is best made on a prepared chart. Injuries sustained at work or on the roads are very likely to be followed by claims for compensation; detailed records are essential.

THE ASEPTIC TREATMENT OF A LACERATED WOUND

It is expected that the injured person will have arrived with the wound covered, preferably by a sterile pad dressing to prevent infection, to provide compression, to control hæmorrhage and œdema, and to give splintage. A large wound is best left until facilities are available to deal with hæmorrhage should the pad be displaced. Unfortunate subjects quite securely padded have bled to death on removal of the dressing because a doctor feared infection.

The Aim of an Aseptic Technique.—Healing is by an inflammatory response designed to close the breach; the smaller this breach, the more rapid the healing. The aim of surgery is to make all wounds as tidy as possible by removing dead or damaged tissue and by re-alining living tissues neatly together. This is not always possible at operation. As careful a toilet and suture are necessary for small wounds as for those requiring treatment in an operating theatre.

PHASE 1: CLEANSING THE SURROUNDING SKIN

All helpers being gowned, gloved, and masked, the original dressing is removed by sterile forceps and both are discarded into a receiver. While a pad of sterile dry gauze is held on the wound and bulging over its edge, the surrounding skin, if hairy, is shaved and then liberally washed with a bland fluid. Soap and water are satisfactory, but more effective in removing skin fats, grease, and oil debris is a detergent such as 1 per cent cetrimide (cetavlon). An alternative is savlon (0·5 per cent cetrimide with chlorhexidine 0·05 per cent), now with a bactericidal effect. If the wound is very soiled, the wash can be augmented by one of commercial ether which is not harmful. Then follows a similar wash in sterile water or saline. If wounds are multiple or very large, it is advisable after this preliminary wash with packs to repeat it in a more definite way using smaller swabs after having discarded gowns and gloves and starting again. An antiseptic is not used.

If a general anæsthetic is to be employed, this phase is followed immediately by the cleansing of the wound proper. Otherwise, with a sterile pad again applied to the wound, local anæsthetic is injected.

PHASE 2: ANÆSTHESIA

Full anæsthesia of the wounded area is necessary. In many situations circumferential injection of a 1 per cent procaine or lignocaine is satisfactory. Not only the skin, but all the deeper tissues implicated by the wound must be infiltrated; injections must always be made into a site well away from, and towards the wound, viz. ....→ 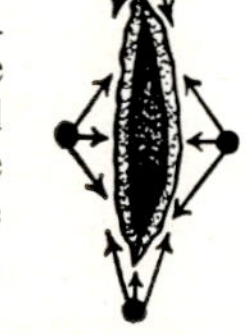 never from the wound peripherally. Vigilance is exercised lest the point of the needle be inserted too far, and so enters lacerated tissues or the cavity of the wound. Should this happen, the needle must be withdrawn at once and a fresh one substituted, otherwise infection may be distributed. When the operator deems it necessary, a general anæsthetic can be given instead.

PHASE 3: CLEANSING OF THE WOUND PROPER

Sterile towels are now applied. The operator is newly gloved and gowned and the dressing over the wound is discarded. Exactly the same order of bland fluid cleansing is used as for the surrounding skin and at the same time obviously loose foreign bodies are extracted by sterile forceps. Following a copious washing with saline, the wound is now ready for the next phase.

PHASE 4: EXPLORATION, IDENTIFICATION, AND EXCISION

Tourniquet or Not?—Where viability is questionable a tourniquet is prohibited. But the identification of damaged structures in a welter of blood is difficult and time-consuming. In such cases it is permissible to at least carry out the exploration and early excision of the wound after exsanguination of the limb using a broad flat Esmarch bandage (*Figs.* 32, 33). But before closure, the tourniquet must be released, the wound allowed to bleed, and hæmostasis secured.

No-touch Technique.—For dealing with small wounds in large numbers, sterile gloves are not always available nor indeed necessary and a no-touch technique can be employed. Even after much practice it requires vigilance for the technique to be employed perfectly. A good method is as depicted in *Fig.* 34, where a sterile towel is laid out and the instruments in use always being laid down with their business ends on this towel while their handles are laid deliberately on an

Cetavlon, Savlon (I.C.I. Ltd., Pharmaceuticals Division, Macclesfield, Cheshire).

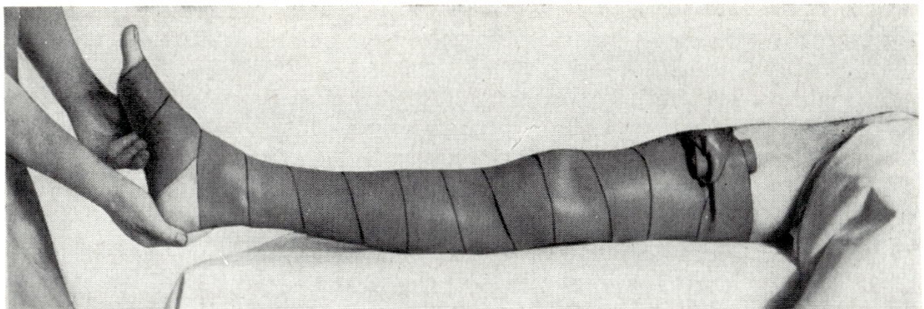

Fig. 32.—Esmarch's bandage applied. Medial view. Note the method of tucking excess bandage

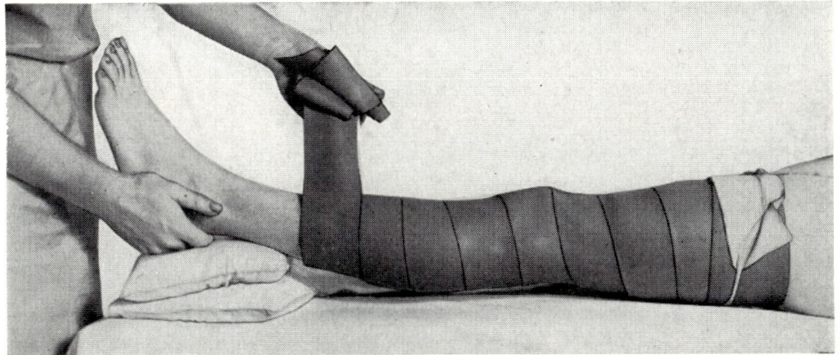

Fig. 33.—Beginning below, the bandage is removed. The major portion of the bandage is unwound. Lateral view.

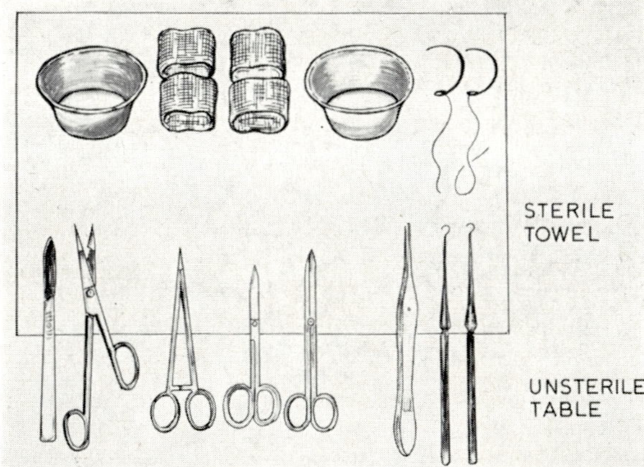

Fig. 34.—No-touch technique. A suitable method for the treatment of small wounds especially when sterile gloves are not available. Only those parts of instruments to touch the wound and all other sterile materials lie on the sterile towel. The handles of instruments lie on an unsterile area. Some of the instruments advised in the text to make up adequate tray sets are depicted.

area left unsterile. At no time will the wound be held by the fingers and gauze for mopping will always be held in forceps as will be other materials employed during the operation.

Instruments.—All instruments and suture materials must be delicate so that further damage is not done. For speed in a busy department and especially for the no-touch technique, trays fully loaded and sterile can be provided and these should include galley pots for local anæsthetic and other fluids, bundles of small gauzes, towels, two pairs of McIndoe's or Gillies's dissecting forceps (one with and one without teeth), suture scissors, scissors with blades curved on the flat, double and single Gillies's skin hooks, also a pair of blunt soft-tissue hooks, and for the quickness of the hand, Gillies's scissors-needle holders. Suitable lengths of fine silk or other non-absorbent material can be threaded on fine curved needles beforehand. Curved needles are essential for reaching the depths of the wound and straight needles should only be employed for the skin.

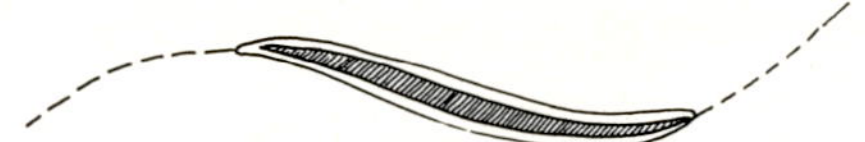

Fig. 35.—A wound which is not straight can be made larger by suitably curved extensions.

Exploration and Identification.—Using the dissecting forceps and skin hooks, the wound is opened and all foreign bodies including grit, hair, and blood-clots are removed. For full exploration it may be advisable to extend a wound in its long axis by making use of skin creases, skin-tension lines, and curves as illustrated in *Fig.* 35.

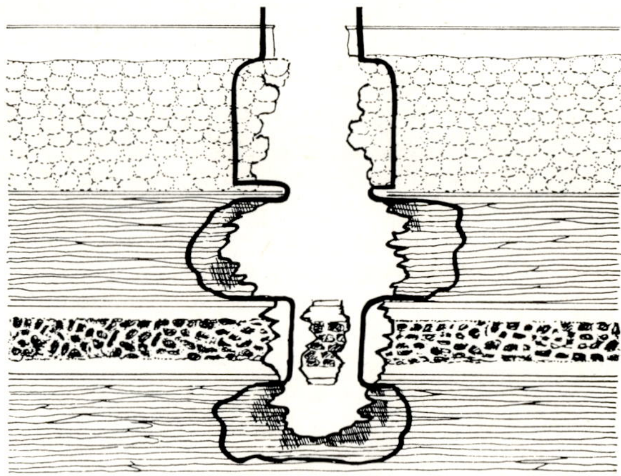

Fig. 36.—To show the extent of excision, layer by layer, necessary in the average lacerated (untidy) wound. Loose bone fragments are removed but normally the bone ends are not touched.

Excision (*Fig.* 36).—Contused or frayed skin edges must be pared but skin must only be grudgingly sacrificed. In excising the skin a tenotomy type of blade (No. 10) can be used to transfix the stretched edge and cut not more than 2 mm. from it.

In general, the walls of the wound are all excised back about 2 mm. All loosened and very bruised tissue is excised; this is best done with a knife rather than by scissors as the latter have some crushing action. Devitalized fat is a good culture medium for infection and should be widely excised when viability is doubtful. Though fasciæ have a poor blood-supply they are valuable in closure, hence only parts which are definitely ragged or bruised should be excised.

Be quite ruthless with damaged muscle; it is fortunate that most muscles act in groups and large parts can be cut out with no great loss of function. Dead muscle of course can bleed (as it does in a butcher's shop), and since it is very variable in appearance—from a dark hæmorrhagic to a dull pale colour—the best criteria that muscle is living are that: (i) it bleeds briskly when it is cut, and (ii) it contracts on grasping with forceps. A full exposure is required.

Detached bone fragments are best removed but those pedicled to periosteum can form a good basis for bone re-formation if they are replaced. As with fasciæ it is difficult to decide on the viability of periosteum and since it is so important in fracture union only that which is completely fragmented should be removed.

Hæmostasis is now effected, but preferably only by forci-pressure, eschewing if possible the use of any ligature material. Small vessels close rapidly without much help and moderate-sized ones by the pressure that will be applied by the dressing. Only the larger ones require ligation, which should be by the finest, 0000 or 00000 size catgut. Non-absorbable ligatures should be avoided.

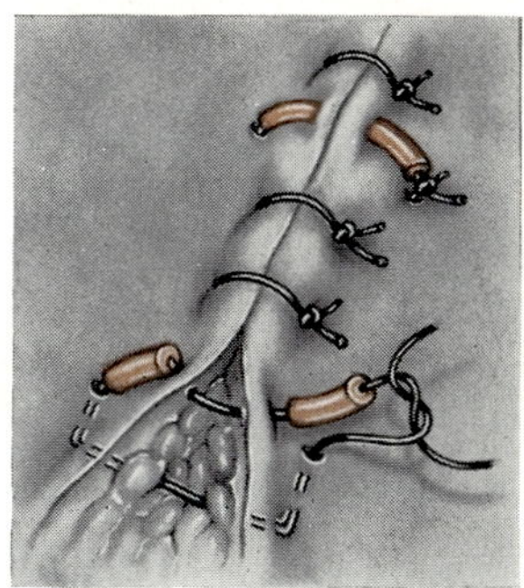

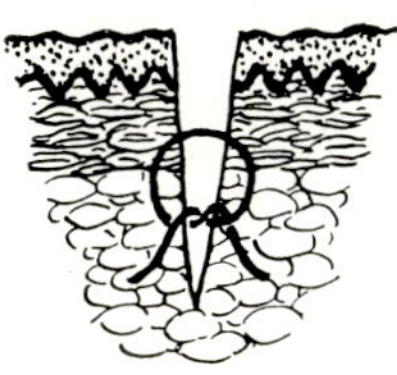

Fig. 37.—Sutures in subcutaneous tissues are inserted so that their knots lie on the deep aspect.

Fig. 38.—Interrupted skin sutures are placed at right-angles to the wound edge and near each other and the skin edge. The vertical mattress sutures evert the skin edges (the rubber tubing is not necessary).

PHASE 5: REPAIR AND CLOSURE OF THE WOUND

The wound is now closed layer by layer as exactly as possible. Repair of large tendons or nerves (*see* p. 551) will depend upon the situation. If not repaired then divided nerve-ends should be united by a single fine unabsorbable stitch through the perineurium, or the ends at least marked. Those tendons not to be repaired are attached to local tissues to prevent retraction. These anchoring stitches should be black for ready localization at a future operation. All findings and procedures are carefully recorded in the operation notes.

Dead space is the biggest problem of all, as collecting blood and serum will invite infection and at least lead to fibrosis which can make a second operation very difficult. Consequently dead space must be obliterated if possible (*Fig.* 37).

Skin edges are apposed exactly by 000 or 0000 non-absorbable sutures placed very close together and as near to the skin edges as possible, so to avoid embarrassing the skin circulation (*Fig.* 38). Not only is perfect apposition so procured but such close suturing encourages the more ready closure of apparently tight wounds. An alternative method to the vertical mattress stitch for securing apposition without inversion is shown in *Fig.* 39. Knots are laid on one side

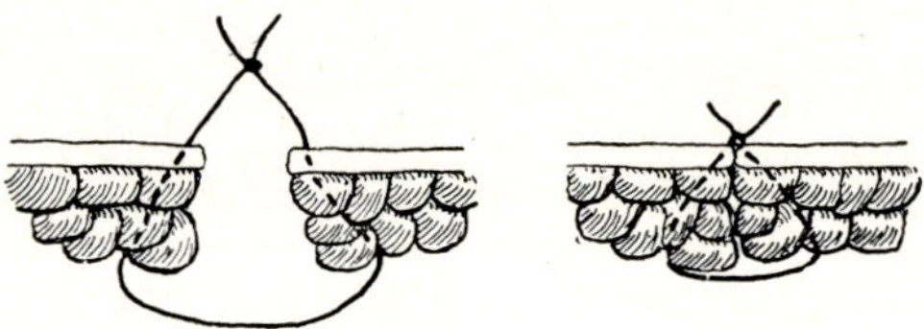

Fig. 39.—A method of inserting ordinary skin stitches so as to avoid any inversion of the skin edges.

of the wound. Where more than one flap abuts, a useful suture to avoid over-crowding of the sutures and necrosis of the corners is the Gillies's angle stitch (*Fig.* 40). Continuous sutures should never be used, for if infection occurs and

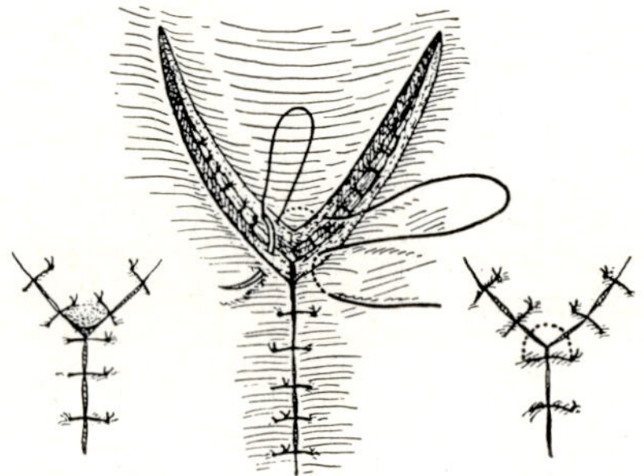

Fig. 40.—Closure of a triangular or Y-shaped wound (centre). If the apex of the top skin triangle is not transfixed with a subcuticular stitch, a gap is liable to remain afterwards (bottom left).

the sutures require removal, the whole wound may gape. For very short wounds, however, particularly when tidy, a refinement is a subcuticular suture (*see Fig.* 322, p. 474).

In general, clips (Michel, van Herff, Kifa) which, to prevent scarring by their points, require removal within 48 hours, should only be considered for the face and neck where the blood-supply is excellent.

In some cases, exact apposition of deeper tissues only (such as the galea aponeurotica for the scalp) may bring the skin edges so exactly together that no skin sutures are needed.

So-called tension sutures are meant to relieve tension and not to cause it, but they are unfortunately usually too tightly applied and certainly worsened when rubber tubing is slotted over them. This only causes more pressure on the skin, with increased probability of infection.

SKIN CLOSURE NOT POSSIBLE

If by the above method of meticulous and admittedly tedious close suturing, wound edges will not meet one another, other methods must be tried. Skin is the perfect dressing for a wound and must be used wherever possible, even at the expense of other parts:—

a. Where skin is more lax, undercutting the skin edges in the plane of subcutaneous fat for some distance around may suffice to allow the skin edges to come together.

b. Relaxing counter-incisions are popular but often lead to other problems of skin loss, they are not easy to plan, and much less necessary than is often thought. Much the best are those made in the form of a V, the apex of this V being furthest from the edge of the original wound, viz.: ....→ 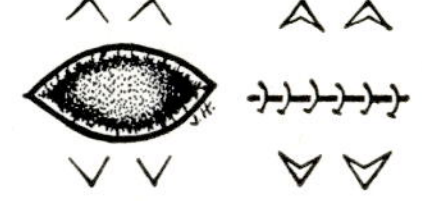 The V's must be made sufficiently far away from the undermined skin edges to be quite certain that the blood-supply of the intervening skin is not jeopardized. After the edges of the original wound have been approximated (and are now found to come together without tension) the somewhat distorted V's can be closed by converting them into Y's.

c. If it is not possible at all to cover the defect in one of these ways even the smallest uninfected wound may be covered by an immediate skin-graft, e.g., using a pedicled skin-flap or by a free partial-thickness graft (Thiersch)—*see* p. 550.

LEAVING THE WOUND OPEN

Most wounds can be closed primarily and drains should be avoided as they invite infection. Exceptions, however, are: (i) those with extensive muscle damage; (ii) where the viability of the tissues left is still suspect; (iii) those grossly infected; (iv) those caused by high velocity projectiles; and (v) when more than 8–12 hours have elapsed since injury. The defect is then loosely packed with strips of a petroleum-jelly dressing or better still one of the newer non-absorbent dressings which allow exudate to escape but do not adhere. Then if the wound presents a healthy appearance in about 4–5 days, *delayed primary suture* is performed by undermining the wound edges, trimming them slightly, and apposing them loosely.

If done later at the end of 7–10 days (*secondary suture*), the method is the same. Both these delayed methods produce third-intention healing as apposed to second-intention healing, when the wound is left open and allowed to heal by granulation tissue.

Special Directions in Respect of Other Types of Wounds commonly encountered.—

Incised Wound.—It is in this, the tidy wound, that primary suture of divided structures, such as digital nerves and tendons, is most often possible. The steps of the operation are the same as given for the lacerated wound except that, no devitalized skin being present, excision of the wound and particularly of the skin edge is not required. In those which are small and not deep, adequate closure can often be obtained by bridge strapping which avoids any surface scar. For this, adhesive plastic tape in strips (steri-strip) can be applied directly to draw the wound edges together.

Steri-strip (Minnesota Mining & Manufacturing Co., London, and St. Paul, U.S.A.).

Puncture wounds are not excised unless as part of the exploration for deeper damage or for removal of devitalized tissue in the path of a foreign body.

Abrasions.—Careful even tedious cleansing is required. Gentle brushing is allowed to remove all the fine pieces of grit; then a petroleum-jelly dressing is applied for comfort.

Facial Wounds.—The skin and soft tissues of the face and neck have so good a blood-supply that despite the frequent bruising and tearing nature of the injuries, much tissue can be left that elsewhere for safety would have had to be removed. Gas gangrene is unknown here. To retain symmetry and mobility of facial expression one must particularly save skin and handle it with great gentleness. While the wound is being cleansed, a gauze pad is held over the eyes by an assistant to prevent irritant fluids from entering. Shaving is carried out widely. After wound cleansing and removal of foreign bodies, wound excision is minimal, only removing tissue which is certainly dead. Hæmostasis is by mosquito forceps pressure and preferably without ligature. Closure of the wound is meticulously exact and in three layers—muscle and fasciæ, then subcutaneous fat, then skin (*Fig.* 41). At all levels the finest suture material (00000) is used, preferably non-absorbable for the deeper layers so as to reduce

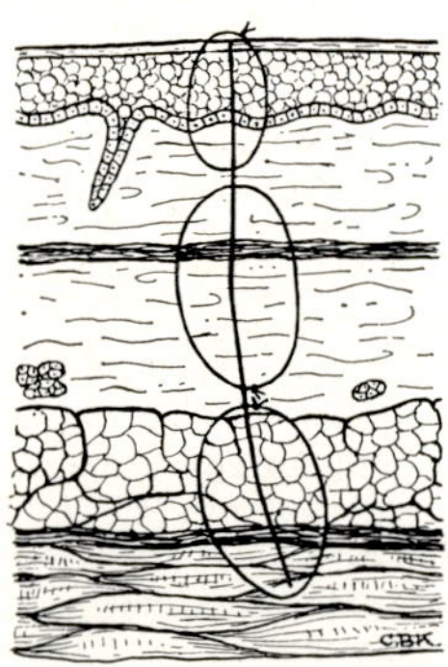

Fig. 41.—Suture of a wound of the face in three layers.

undue tissue reaction. To appose the skin edges, again the finest non-absorbable sutures (preferably on eyeless needles (atraumatic) are applied close together and as near the skin edges as possible; they are tied loosely. No dressing is required, or only a layer of plastic skin. To reduce scarring to a minimum skin sutures are removed within 72 hours.

Contusions and Hæmatomata.—The treatment for these lesions should at first be conservative by relieving pain, gentle firm massage, and by elevation. If a hæmatoma persists or is very painful, fluid blood is aspirated under the most strict aseptic conditions using a wide-bore (No. 15) needle, the puncture hole then sealed by a plastic skin on a pledget of wool (mastisol, collodion, or similar preparation) and a pressure dressing applied. If the swelling is boggy, evacuate old clot through a small incision.

PHASE 6: THE INITIAL DRESSING

If wound edges are perfectly apposed and the part not subsequently disturbed or manipulated, adhesion of wound edges is achieved in some 6 hours and no infection can then enter from without.

Dry skin is more resistant to infection than is moist, and friction adds to the chance of infection. Unless signs of wound distress occur, a dressing should be left alone until the sutures are due to be removed. For a wound of minimal extent, a simple dry dressing is applied and held firmly in place by ventilated strapping (elastic, if required). For small wounds of the face and neck and scalp, which clothing is unlikely to touch, after oozing is controlled, no dressing is required at all. Local antibiotics and antiseptics should not be applied.

When a large wound is likely to ooze despite careful hæmostasis and suturing, a pressure dressing is applied on top of dry gauze. Over the whole of this, to give further mobilization and security, a thin one-layer plaster cast can be used.

Never place wool directly on a wound at any time as it tends to stick and can even become incorporated in the granulation tissue.

A dressing fails if: (i) it is allowed to slip about (it should be fixed by non-elastic strapping to adjacent skin), (ii) it is not sterile, and (iii) it is allowed to become saturated with exudate. In the latter event, the dressing should be removed and replaced by fresh sterile material.

AFTER CARE

Dressings.—Most dressings are left undisturbed until the stitches are removed. The dressing should only be removed earlier if there is: (*a*) hæmatoma formation; (*b*) soaking of the dressing with exudate; (*c*) local pain, tenderness, and discharge, indicating infection; (*d*) unexplained pyrexia.

The dressing of all wounds should be carried out with aseptic precautions in a special room set aside for this purpose, where operating-theatre conditions prevail; sutures are removed there and drains may be shortened, adjusted, or removed.

Movement rapidly disperses fluid and prevents adhesions but has to be balanced against the need for rest, so essential to the repair of soft tissues. They are not so opposite in effect as might be thought and are usually employed together, resting the immediate zone of injury and keeping mobile the parts around, particularly neighbouring joints. The normal fingers of a child can be completely immobilized for a month with a full return of mobility on the day of release, but an old lady similarly confined might have her fingers fixed permanently.

A knowledge of the patient's work and capabilities for adjustment is required so that some form of rehabilitation supervised in the factory or hospital is instituted. Full co-operation must be maintained with the physiotherapist and regular attendance at a clinic is essential.

Recurrent Bleeding.—A well applied pressure dressing prevents all further hæmorrhage except that due to infection. Though the earliest bleeding might be called reactionary and attributed to a rise in blood-pressure when shock is controlled, most early bleeding is in fact due to a badly applied or interfered with dressing.

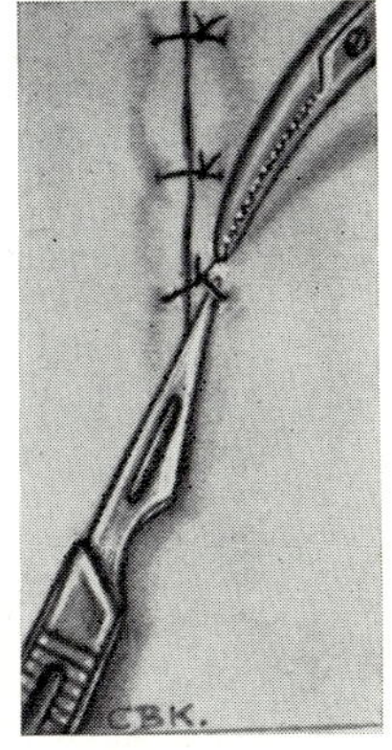

Fig. 42.—Removal of skin sutures. The knot is raised and the stitch severed flush with the skin.

Bleeding due to infection tends to occur any time after the third day and in those wounds where damage has been great (e.g., crushing) and infection likely. Its usually insidious onset by tiny preliminary hæmorrhages must be regarded seriously as a final fatal hæmorrhage from a large vessel may come at any moment. Observing such a case is always trying. Only one attempt to control hæmorrhage by local pressure should be made. Indeed pressure may be difficult to apply as the wound may be macerated, soggy, and already bulging with infected blood-clot. If this fails, wide exploration should be done and amputation may be necessary to save life.

The Removal of Sutures.—After the dressing has been gently lifted from the wound and discarded as described previously, the skin around is cleaned, preferably with ether, so as to keep it dry. Unless removed before their time because of hæmatoma, fever, or local signs of inflammation, skin sutures are usually left from 7 to 10 days; the longer interval is adhered to when the wound overlies large muscle masses where movement is great (e.g., thigh). For the face, neck, and scalp, removal should be at 72 hours.

Technique of Stitch Removal.—To remove a suture, the knot is seized in a hæmostat and sufficient traction exerted to raise the stitch from the skin (*Fig.* 42). Employing a fine pointed scalpel (which is far better than scissors as it causes less pull) the suture is severed *flush with the skin*, and by reason of the tension transmitted by the hæmostat the suture comes away instantly. The importance of the italicized instruction is that no portion that lies above the skin level must enter (and so contaminate) the stitch track. After removal of all sutures, it is usually not necessary at all to cleanse the wound but to leave it entirely dry and apply one of the newer vapour-permeable dressings, as previously described.

THE DRAINAGE OF WOUNDS

Though it is best to dispense with drains particularly when wounds are small, hæmostasis perfect, the wound clean, and where an effective compression dressing has been applied, provision must occasionally be made for the escape of exudates, and this includes blood.

Unless suction can be applied to a drainage-tube, it will only gather fluid from the track it lies in. If allowed to lie over a hollow viscus or vessel its pressure can eventually cause erosion and it should at least be moved (by rotation and shortening) as soon as possible. A track is in fact formed within 48 hours and except where it is needed for the discharge of, for example, pus or urine for a considerable time, a drain should be removed by the end of that period. It is best to place any drain under vision by hand rather than by inserting forceps blindly into the depths. As a general principle the lateral or lower end of a wound is the most suitable place for bringing out a drain.

A small part of the drain should project above the skin level and lie within gauze; depending upon the need, copious amounts of absorbent dressing will be placed over all.

With the popularity now of elastic adhesive strapping and the lessened use of drains even for large wounds, there is an unfortunate tendency to completely cover a dressing, drain and all, by such strapping, thereby encouraging maceration and infection by retained products. One may completely forget that a drain has been enclosed. Though it is permitted for gauze to be sealed over the full length of a wound by strapping, the drain should pass separately into a bulky absorbing dressing held by bandaging or a many-tailed support (for the trunk) (*Fig.* 43).

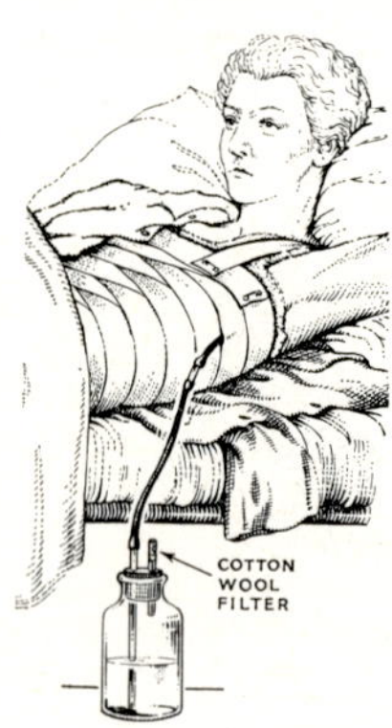

Fig. 43.—Closed drainage after radical mastectomy through a dressing held by a many-tailed bandage. To the air exit tube of the collection bottle can be applied *gentle* suction.

A drain should be secured to the skin by an anchoring suture, either through the edge of its wall, if it is a tube, or completely through it, if made of glove or corrugated rubber. To distinguish this suture from the others, one end should be cut short and the other long and when the loop through the tube is divided for removal of the drain, the remainder of the suture is allowed to stay. For cavity drainage the ruling is that the exit site of drainage should be as dependent as possible and, if necessary, to achieve this, a stab incision will be made separate from the original incision.

The softest, most flexible, and non-irritant materials are used. Latex is less irritant than red rubber and the newer plastics are replacing both. To drain superficial areas a small length of soft rubber tissue (which can be fashioned from an old surgical glove) is best. For deeper wounds and where a thicker discharge is anticipated, one can use a length of corrugated rubber or a tube. A tube conforms well to the shape of a wound and must be firm enough not to kink. Its end should be bevelled and rounded, and to facilitate drainage it should be also fenestrated, the holes made small to prevent either intestine or omentum prolapsing through; and though the calibre should be small enough only for collection purposes, the length must be adequate to reach the depths of a cavity.

The Management of Drainage-tubes.—Supervision of drainage-tube care is an important chore of a house-surgeon. Firstly the drainage should be clearly recorded in the patient's notes: (1) number; (2) locations; (3) type of drains; and equally important is (4) to record their removal.

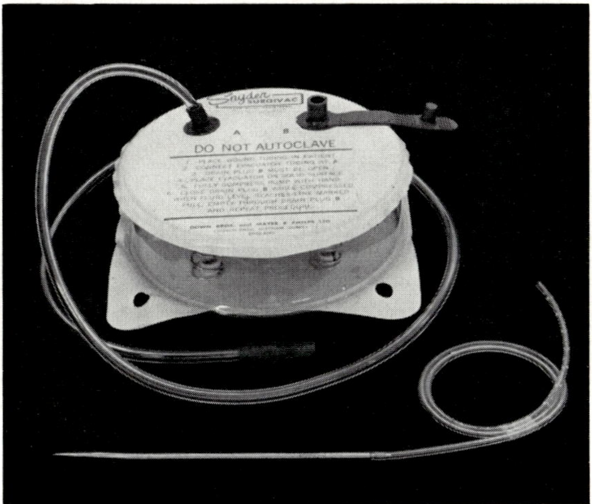

Fig. 44.—Snyder Surgivac suction drainage apparatus.

Unless the outpouring is excessive, a drain inserted to give exit to blood or serum is removed on the second post-operative day, exercising rigorous aseptic precautions. In most cases, in order to attend to a drain, it is unnecessary and most inadvisable to disturb the dressing covering the major part of the wound and only that part of the dressing over the exit of the drain is lifted, following which, all the blood-stained and serum-soaked gauze is removed.

To shorten a tube or other drain, the retaining stitch is severed, and the tube turned in order to loosen it and partially withdrawn without jerking. The greater part of the withdrawn portion is then cut away. The new portion now protruding is transfixed with a sterile safety-pin to prevent the drain disappearing beneath the surface. The pin can be bent to the contour of the part and is held within

Snyder Surgivac apparatus (Down Bros. and Mayer & Phelps Ltd., Mitcham, Surrey, and Zimmer Ltd., Warsaw, Indiana, U.S.A.).

gauze, not to lie on the skin where it might cause pressure necrosis. It is always better to shorten a drain in this way than to remove and replace it by another.

Closed and Suction Drainage.—Where a large cavity remains after a major resection and where there might be an outpouring from cut lymphatics or small blood-vessels frequent changing of dressings is obviated and retrograde infection via the tube prevented by employing closed drainage. *Fig.* 43 illustrates this principle after radical mastectomy. It is better to have already sterilized and available in the theatre the glass connexion and distal tube fixed to the collection bottle. These are attached before the patient leaves the operating theatre. Drainage is then under a water seal to limit infection and can be improved by applying gentle suction on the air outlet tube shown in the figure as 'cotton-wool filter'.

Snyder Surgivac suction drainage bottles and drains are very useful for draining large subcutaneous and intermuscular areas for a few days (*Fig.* 44).

<h3 style="text-align:center">RETAINED EXOGENOUS FOREIGN BODIES</h3>

In most casualty departments, operative search for retained foreign bodies is not fruitful and quite often damaging. The reasons are many—too limited anæsthesia, ignorance of anatomy, a lack of facilities for definite localization, and too restricted an exploration. The smaller the foreign body is, the more difficult it is to find and remove. An operation for one deep in the palm, for example, may cause more harm than a foreign body would do of itself. Metallic and other objects may carry in with them portions of contaminated clothing. Relatively small objects such as needles deep in large muscle masses in the thigh or buttocks should be left there unless infection is associated; pieces of wood and fabric must be removed. It is surprising how large a foreign body can be found deep to a very small entrance wound or scar.

Radiographs.—Where possible three radiographs should be taken at different angles with a skin marker in place and as near to the time of operation as possible. If on radiography the soft-tissue shadows are good, not only metal but wood and glass may also be made visible. Remember that foreign bodies can be moved a great distance by muscle and tendon action from their primary site.

Technique.—A bloodless field should be used wherever possible. For linear bodies, a good method of exploration is to incise at right-angles to the line of the object, and in all cases to use the track or scar as a guide. If the search is prolonged or damage to important structures likely, the operation should be abandoned. It is often better to wait until morning to search for a foreign body than to do so late at night under trying conditions. If there is delay, operation should be preceded by a preliminary course of penicillin and protection given against tetanus.

<h3 style="text-align:center">THE CARE OF INFECTED WOUNDS</h3>

A wound infected from the outset should not be excised (for fear of spreading the infection) and must be treated in the open manner. If a wound becomes infected it must be treated promptly, to let out pus, to remove dead tissue, and to reduce tension that can cause more ischæmia and more necrosis. Infection *per se* is controlled by: (*a*) local mechanical washing, and (*b*) the exhibition of the appropriate antibiotic as shown by bacteriological testing of the pus. However, the main reason for an infection and its persistence is a retained foreign body or necrotic tissue and, in fact, much of what is usually thought to be pus is necrotic tissue, lysed by putrefaction. Attempts to control infection by drugs alone will not then succeed until all dead tissue is removed.

Dead tissue (slough) that is easily visible can be excised without recourse to anæsthesia as it is insensitive. The time-honoured and cheap lavage of such wounds by hydrogen peroxide or surgical hypochlorite solutions (eusol) is not to be lightly discarded in favour of the newer methods of injecting or applying tissue enzymes locally. Since eusol loses its effect on giving off its chlorine within a few minutes of coming into contact with dead tissue, it should not be used as a dressing which will only serve to macerate living tissue. Bathing is done at frequent intervals during the day; between sessions either a bulky dry dressing or an oily one is applied, the latter helping to soften sloughs. Eusol requires to be prepared fresh every day. When the dead tissue is superficial, dry, and well defined it is often quicker to excise and either suture or skin-graft the area.

Enzymatic Débridement.—In the same way as the juice of the paw-paw (papain) can be used by the housewife to tenderize tough meat, so it can also be cheaply used on necrotic wounds. Streptodormase and streptokinase usually in combination as varidase, and either as a surface dressing applied once daily or by injection into a necrotic mass, has been widely used, and it does not seem to be any more effective than the oxidizing or chlorinating compounds.

The newer preparations are pancreatic enzymes, such as tripure novo (which contains trypsin), and other enzymatic compounds such as elase. Debrecin, made from the ficin latex of the fig tree, requires great care in preparation but in favourable cases with soggy sloughs is claimed to give rapid removal (scissors can do this just as well).

Though none of these substances is harmful some are very expensive, and none so far can be said to be dramatic in its action.

Warning.—One should not rely on hot soaks or poultices which make all tissues sodden and lead to slow healing.

TETANUS

Both human and animal fæces contain *Clostridium tetani* which in unfavourable circumstances forms spores. These are plentiful in arable land, in dust, and in plaster, and the spores of some strains are very difficult to destroy, even with prolonged boiling. Vegetative forms develop in an anaerobic environment and release very potent toxins.

Type of Wound.—Deep puncture wounds are those most liable to develop tetanus. But any wound in which there has been contamination of deeper tissues, especially muscle that has been rendered ischæmic, is at risk. The wound need not be large—pricks with the thorns of rose bushes are a well-known cause of tetanus. Wounds occurring on farms, playing fields, and roads, in garages, sewers, and drains are very likely to be contaminated with clostridia.

PREVENTION OF TETANUS

Patients with wounds contaminated by *Cl. tetani* fall into two groups: (1) Those not previously immunized; (2) Those who have had a course of active immunization. Unfortunately, the former group is still much the larger; the hope for the future is that a higher proportion will belong to the immunized group, and this is already true of many children—although neither they nor their parents always know that they have been immunized.

Tetanus can be prevented by: (1) Removing all devitalized tissue and organisms from the wound; (2) Killing any remaining clostridia with antibiotics in patients not already protected; (3) If vegetative clostridia develop, neutralizing the toxin with adequate antitoxin. These methods of prevention are arranged

Varidase (Lederle Laboratories Ltd., Bush House, Aldwych, London, W.C.2).
Elase (Parke, Davis & Co., Staines Road, Hounslow, Middlesex).
Debrecin (Johnson & Johnson Ltd., Slough, Bucks, and New Brunswick, U.S.A.).

in decreasing order of desirability and importance. It is clearly preferable to completely eliminate all clostridia (and the numerous other organisms that accompany them) by very careful wound débridement than it is to try to counteract the toxin released by established tetanus bacilli.

Antibiotics and Antiserum.—Up to 10 per cent of patients exhibit allergic reactions to antitetanic serum (ATS), most of which is produced in horses. Ovine and human antitoxin are made but are scarce and not so readily available in all countries. Further, a second injection of ATS given some time after the first one has very little protective value. In contradistinction to these disadvantages of ATS, fewer patients show any allergic reaction to penicillin, the antibiotic of choice. Tetracycline, erythromycin, and cloxacillin are all effective against *Cl. tetani*. Any one should be given in full doses for at least 5 days, or until the wound is healed.

MANAGEMENT OF POTENTIALLY INFECTED WOUND

First question the patients as to whether or not: (1) They have had a course of tetanus toxoid in the past; (2) They have ever had undesirable reactions to drugs, especially penicillin; (3) Suffer from asthma, hay fever, urticaria, or eczema. If they have not been actively immunized with toxoid, ask if they have ever had an injection of ATS before.

A. Patient not previously Immunized.—

1. If seen within 12 hours.—

a. Careful wound débridement. All foreign material must be removed and all devitalized tissue excised at all levels. Thorough cleansing of the wound with savlon or similar detergent must be carried out. The wound edges must be excised, except in some incised wounds sustained in 'ideal' circumstances. The wound should be closed without tension.

b. Penicillin. For major wounds 1 mega unit intramuscularly every 6 hours for 5 days. For wounds considered less tetanus-prone and in out-patients one injection of a long-acting penicillin preparation, e.g., triplopen, may be substituted.

c. Commence immunization with 0·5 ml. adsorbed toxoid (vaccine) deep subcutaneously or intramuscularly. Further doses are given after 6 weeks, then after 1 year, and booster doses every 5 years.

2. Seen after 12 hours.—As for (1) but, unless patient has had ATS in the past, 1500 units ATS subcutaneously or intramuscularly, observing the precautions outlined below.

B. Previously Immunized Patient.—As (*A*) (1). The antibiotic is not essential but, in heavily contaminated wounds, helps deal with any other organisms present. The booster dose of toxoid provides the main defence against any remaining tetanus bacilli.

PRECAUTIONS WHEN GIVING SERUM

Between 5 and 10 per cent of patients receiving ATS may show reactions to the horse serum. Most of these are *minor reactions* consisting of transient urticaria and skin rashes appearing after a few days. *Serum sickness*, with arthralgia, pyrexia, and œdema, is sometimes seen 5–10 days after injecting ATS. These reactions respond to antihistamines. Fortunately, *anaphylactic shock* is rare; within minutes of giving the injection the patient collapses, with very low blood-pressure and difficulty in breathing. It is treated by immediately injecting 1 ml. of 1–1000 adrenaline intramuscularly, raising the feet, giving oxygen, and setting up an intravenous drip. (*See* Chapter III.)

Triplopen (= benethamine penicillin + procaine penicillin + sodium penicillin G; Glaxo Laboratories Ltd., Greenford, Middlesex).

Procedure for giving Serum.—Always have a 1–1000 solution of adrenaline and a hypodermic syringe ready before giving ATS. Procedure varies with the patient's past history:—

1. No allergic tendencies, no previous ATS injections—give the 1500 units subcutaneously or intramuscularly and keep the patient under observation for 30 minutes.

2. Previous ATS injection—inject 0·2 ml. ATS subcutaneously or intramuscularly. If no adverse reaction after 30 minutes, give the full dose and observe. Repeat doses of equine serum have little protective value—it is better to rely on correct surgical excision, antibiotics, and toxoid.

3. Known general allergic tendencies—make a 1–10 dilution of ATS and give 0·2 ml. subcutaneously. If no reaction in half an hour, give the same dose of undiluted serum subcutaneously, observe for a further 30 minutes, after which the full dose may be given if there are no undesirable side-effects obvious.

4. Previous reaction to serum—use human antitetanic gamma-globulin; a dose of 250 units provides about 4 weeks' protection and is virtually free of side-effects. ATS of ovine origin may also be tried.

Reactions to Tetanus Toxoid.—These are very uncommon. Urticaria, angioneurotic œdema around the lips and eyes, pruritus, and malaise have been described. They respond rapidly to the injection of adrenaline, 1 ml. of 1–1000 solution intramuscularly, or to oral antihistamines, e.g., promethazine (phenergan) 25 mg. t.d.s., or chlorpheniramine (piriton) 8 mg. t.d.s.

TREATMENT OF ESTABLISHED TETANUS

The diagnosis is a clinical one; bacteriological tests are too slow. Many cases are **mild**—the incubation period has been greater than 10 days, there is spasm, some twitching and discomfort in muscles, particularly those of the jaw ('lock-jaw'), face, and spine. In **moderately severe** cases spasm is more widespread and there may be marked risus sardonicus, opisthotonos, and abdominal wall rigidity simulating an acute abdomen. Slight elevation of pulse and of temperature are usual. **Severe** cases of tetanus are not common; the incubation period has only been a few days and the appearance of the first signs is soon followed by generalized convulsions. The management of these severe cases is beyond the scope of this book, except to say that they require urgent tracheostomy, curarization, intermittent positive-pressure ventilation (IPPV), and skilled nursing and anæsthetic supervision, often for weeks, in an intensive therapy unit.

Management of Mild Tetanus.—

1. Antiserum: Observing the precautions outlined above, a 1-ml. test dose is given intramuscularly and, if there is no reaction, 50,000 units ATS are injected slowly intravenously, e.g., through a Gordh needle (p. 126). On each of the following days 25,000 units are given; a similar amount is given weekly if symptoms persist and also to cover any delayed surgical intervention.

2. Sedation: Chlorpromazine 50 mg. every 6 hours or an equivalent dose of barbiturate to keep the patient drowsy.

3. Antibiotics: 2 million units of penicillin intramuscularly every 6 hours; alternatively, tetracycline or cloxacillin. The course is continued for at least 1 week or until the healing of the wound is complete.

4. Tetanus toxoid: A course of active immunization is started, with 0·5 ml. toxoid intramuscularly. Tetanus itself confers little natural immunity.

Phenergan (May & Baker Ltd., Dagenham, Essex).
Piriton (Allen & Hanburys Ltd., Bethnal Green, London, E.2).

5. Operation: Once the patient is saturated with ATS and antibiotics, the wound even if partially healed may be cleansed and properly débrided if this has not already been done.

When there is evidence of laryngeal spasm, a tracheostomy should be performed—always have a tracheostomy set at hand. Certainly in the early stages tetanus patients require continuous supervision by a special nurse, preferably in a quiet room. Watch must be kept on their temperature and urinary output. Later their bowels may require attention and nutritional supplements (p. 46) are usually advisable.

GAS GANGRENE

The clostridia which cause gas gangrene, while found in similar places, are even more widespread than *Cl. tetani*. The three main organisms are *Cl. welchii* (*perfringens*), *Cl. œdematiens*, and *Cl. septicum*; all may be found in hospital wards and operating theatres. Wounds containing clostridia are nearly always contaminated by other organisms as well. The clostridia only develop and release their toxins when the tissue oxygen tension is low, e.g., in dead muscle when arteries have been damaged or in ischæmic limbs.

When crepitation is elicited in the subcutaneous tissues around a wound or incision, the cause is mostly ordinary surgical emphysema, not gas gangrene. The clostridia of gas gangrene may be found in three circumstances:—

1. Wound surface contaminants: Clostridia, particularly *Cl. welchii*, can be obtained from about one-third of wounds sustained out of doors and generally are of no significance.

2. Clostridial cellulitis: Gas is formed in the subcutaneous tissues by the saccharolytic activities of the clostridia, but there is little toxæmia. Proper surgical excision of the wound and the use of an antibiotic are curative.

3. Clostridial necrotizing myositis: Bursting pain develops. Gas issues from the wound; in addition there is a brownish discharge, having a sickly sweet smell. Discoloration and necrosis of muscle proceed quickly, there is profound toxæmia and a hæmolytic type of jaundice. Post-operative necrosing myositis may follow mid-thigh amputation for obliterative arterial disease, the clostridia originating from the patient's own bowel. Gas in the tissues can be demonstrated by radiography.

PREVENTION OF GAS GANGRENE

Nowadays, antiserum is little used in the prevention of gas gangrene in those who have suffered injuries in fields, roads, athletic grounds, etc. Instead reliance is placed on:—

a. Surgical excision—as in tetanus prevention, all ragged edges should be trimmed, foreign bodies removed, and all dead or traumatized tissue excised right down to the bottom of the wound. Only muscle with a good blood-supply is left. There must be no tension in the skin closure—if in doubt, loosely pack the wound wide open. Tourniquets and tight bandages must be avoided.

b. Antibiotics—penicillin 1 million units t.d.s., or equivalent preparations.

TREATMENT OF GAS GANGRENE

All dead muscle and other damaged tissue must be ruthlessly excised, even if the wound has been explored earlier. Full doses of antibiotics are first administered and measures taken to combat shock; blood transfusion is valuable. Polyvalent anti-gas gangrene serum may be given intravenously, observing the precautions given on p. 68 for ATS; 50,000 units are run in slowly in an intravenous infusion. Amputation is rarely necessary in civilian practice; when it is used, the flaps are left open.

Hyperbaric oxygen therapy—soaking the tissues in oxygen at 3 atmospheres' pressure—can produce dramatic results, but the facility is only available in a few special centres.

FACTORS IN THE DELAY OF WOUND HEALING

It will now be evident that many of the factors given below can be eliminated by intelligent treatment and prevention.

No hospital worker has a better opportunity of observing the healing of wounds than the house-surgeon. Delay in healing may be the result of one or more of the following factors:—

1. Hæmorrhage and anæmia—an adequate level of hæmoglobin is required to maintain oxygen transport and so support the increased cellular activity for wound healing.

2. Traumatic œdema—causes reduced tissue oxygenation and viability.

3. Infection—by contamination, and it is greatly increased by tissue necrosis. Always remember the possibility of a retained foreign body.

4. The abuse of topical antibiotics and antiseptics.

5. Nutritional insufficiency.—

a. Protein is required for the growth of capillary endothelium, fibroblasts, and collagen. An adequate intake must be assured, and supplementary feeding (p. 46) may be advisable for very large wounds.

b. Vitamins—an adequate supply of vitamins A and C is desirable. If healing is slow, give 1000 mg. ascorbic acid daily for 3 days, and 100 mg. t.d.s. thereafter. Most vitamin deficiencies are multiple.

If there is a tendency to bleeding from granulation tissue vitamin K should be given, 10 mg. intramuscularly; the patient's blood-clotting mechanism is investigated and the requisite blood samples are withdrawn before giving the vitamin.

6. Other diseases—diabetes is a potent cause for a persistence of infection. Particularly in wounds of the lower limbs in older people, peripheral vascular occlusion often plays a part. The house-surgeon also should be vigilant for the possibility of other diseases which might be attributable for poor wound healing. For instance, pale and soggy granulation tissue, or a wound which shows not one bit of change from the time it was made, might indicate a serious disorder such as leukæmia.

CHAPTER VI

SULPHONAMIDE AND ANTIBIOTIC THERAPY

By C. ALLAN BIRCH

THE SULPHONAMIDES

Mode of Action.—Sulphonamides are similar to *p*-aminosalicylic acid and prevent the utilization of this essential substance by bacteria. They are therefore bacteriostatic but have no bactericidal action. They are antagonized by amino-acids and peptones, and are consequently inactive in the presence of pus. In localized infections they are of little value and they do not neutralize toxins. All sulphonamides (except the insoluble 'gut active' ones) are well absorbed and reach a peak blood level in about 2 hours. Excretion is mainly renal and varies greatly, but is enhanced by an alkaline urine. Sulphonamides form acetylated compounds in the body to varying degrees and these are inert and liable to crystallize out in the urinary tract. The bogy that protein-binding renders sulphonamides inert is not of great importance clinically, but there is a definite interrelationship between the degree of binding and the concentration in the cerebrospinal fluid. Hence, sulphonamides which are long-acting because they are protein-bound are not suitable for treating meningitis.

Resistance.—Sulphonamide-sensitive organisms will be affected, albeit in varying degrees, by any of the sulphonamides and resistant organisms will be resistant to all sulpha drugs.

Indications.—Pyogenic cocci and *Escherichia coli* are generally sensitive to sulphonamides, but the main use of sulphonamides today is against urinary infection, bacillary dysentery, and meningococcal infection—all due to exquisitely sensitive organisms.

Sulphonamides will not interfere with the bactericidal effect of an antibiotic given simultaneously. Indeed, the effect may be enhanced since the antibiotic reduces the number of organisms to a level at which sulphonamides can best act.

As sulphonamides do not vary much in their specificity against particular organisms, the choice is determined mainly by ease of absorption, rate of excretion, and toxic effects.

Dosage.—Most sulphonamides are supplied as 0·5 G. tablets. If they cannot be swallowed, they can be crushed and given through a stomach tube. Broadly speaking, the maximum safe daily dose of 'ordinary' sulphonamides is up to 10 G., and for the smallest infant 2 G. (or 120 mg. per kg. in 24 hours). This rule does not hold for some of the newer sulphonamides and so the manufacturer's literature should be carefully read. Sulphamethoxydiazine (durenate) and other similar compounds are long-acting because they are protein-bound. They are no more effective than the short-acting sulphonamides and carry special risks (*see below*). Sulphamethoxydiazine (durenate) is effective in a dose of 0·5 G. daily after a loading dose of 1 G. It is the least protein-bound of the new long-acting sulphonamides.

Durenate (F.B.A. Pharmaceuticals Ltd., Haywards Heath, Sussex).

Method of Administration.—This is usually by mouth, but sulphadimidine (sulphamezathine) can be injected intravenously and sulphathiazole intramuscularly. For intramuscular injections sulphasomizole (bidizole) is popular since its sodium salt is neutral and so injection is painless. Sulphonamides should never be given intrathecally. With the older sulphonamides, extra fluid was given against the risk of crystalluria, but it is now only necessary to maintain an adequate urinary output (1500 ml. in 24 hours) or less in the case of sulphamethizole (urolucosil). Sulphonamides should not be applied locally to the skin because of the high incidence of sensitivity reactions.

Toxic Effects.—The sulphonamide-protein complex acts as an antigen and may cause a reaction about the ninth day. This usually shows as a recurrence of fever or a rash. Exfoliative dermatitis and polyarteritis nodosa are rare serious effects. Long-acting sulphonamides can cause the Stevens-Johnson syndrome. In the infant, by displacing bilirubin from plasma protein, they may precipitate kernicterus. If sulphonamides are going to be effective, they soon show evidence of this and, to avoid toxic effects, a course of treatment should seldom exceed 7 days.

SOME SULPHONAMIDES

Sulphadimidine (sulphamezathine) probably remains the popular choice for routine use and its 4-hourly dosage produces an effective blood concentration. The sodium salt (1 G. in 3 ml.) can be injected intravenously or intramuscularly.

Sulphacetamide (albucid, cortucid) has the advantage that solutions up to 30 per cent are not very alkaline and so can be used in eye-drops.

Sulphamethizole (urolucosil) is popular for urinary infections. Tablets contain 0·1 G. and a daily dosage of up to 1 G. is sufficient.

Phthalylsulphathiazole is poorly absorbed and so is used for bowel infections. The dose is 10 G. daily.

Sulphamethoxydiazine (durenate) is probably the best of the newer, well-absorbed, but slowly excreted sulphonamides as it is less bound to proteins than its predecessors.

Succinylsulphathiazole is useful for bowel preparation, 10–20 G. daily in divided doses.

THE NITROFURANS

These antibacterial chemicals are unrelated to the sulphonamides and the only member of the group which is commonly used is nitrofurantoin (furadantin). This is a yellow crystalline substance.

Dose.—Furadantin is supplied as 50-mg. tablets—the dose being 5–8 mg. per kg. per 24 hours. Bacteriostatic levels are not attained in the blood but, as 40 per cent of the dose is excreted unchanged in the urine, it is very useful in urinary infections, particularly with *Proteus* and *Pseudomonas* organisms. Furadantin can be administered intravenously in a dose of 7–10 mg. per kg. Fluid intake must be restricted on a low dose, but this is unnecessary with a higher dose.

Contra-indications.—The drug should be avoided if there is renal damage lest high blood levels cause peripheral neuritis. It is best not to give it to children.

The chief side-effect is nausea and this can be minimized by giving the drug with food or magnesium trisilicate or in gelatin capsules.

Sulphamezathine (I.C.I. Ltd., Pharmaceuticals Division, Macclesfield, Cheshire).
Bidizole (May & Baker Ltd., Dagenham, Essex).
Urolucosil (William R. Warner & Co. Ltd., Eastleigh, Hants).
Albucid; Cortucid (British Schering Ltd., Slough, Bucks).
Furadantin (Smith, Kline, & French Laboratories Ltd., Welwyn Garden City, Herts; Norwich Pharmacol Co., U.S.A.).

ANTIBIOTICS
PRACTICAL POINTS AND GENERAL PRINCIPLES OF THERAPY

1. It is best to reserve antibiotics until they are indicated and not to give them for trivial infections. Remember that antibiotics can mask symptoms.

2. Always try to send a specimen for bacteriological examination before starting treatment. Repeat the culture and sensitivity tests in a prolonged case and avoid trying to treat harmless contaminants. Do not rely entirely on the report forms but have personal consultations with the pathologist in a difficult case.

3. Always ask about allergy before starting treatment. Avoid topical applications if possible since they may cause hypersensitivity reactions.

4. If there is no response do not change too quickly to another drug but consider the causes of failure, such as underlying disease, inadequate dosage, and bad drainage.

5. Do not prolong drug treatment unnecessarily.

Mode of Action.—Antibiotics may be bactericidal and bacteriostatic, but the distinction between the modes of actions is not always clear-cut. A bactericidal effect may be vitiated by a small proportion of 'persistent' organisms which survive the drug and cause trouble later. They are unlikely to emerge when the antibacterial effect is rapid. In general, a bactericidal drug is preferable to a bacteriostatic one.

The chief bactericidal antibiotics are: pencillin, cloxacillin (orbenin), carbenicillin (pyopen), streptomycin, polymyxin.

The chief bacteriostatic antibiotics are: tetracycline, chloramphenicol, ampicillin (penbritin).

Antibiotics may be given in combination, but not all combinations are an advantage, some being antagonistic and some synergistic. **Jawetz's law** states that bacteriostatic drugs given together have additive effects, and that bactericidal drugs given together and bactericidal with bacteriostatic drugs may be antagonistic.

PENICILLIN

Benzylpenicillin B.P. (crystalline penicillin G).—This is supplied as a white crystalline powder in rubber-capped vials each containing respectively 100,000, 200,000, 500,000, and 1,000,000 (1 mega) units. Sterile water or physiological saline is injected into the vial and, being very soluble, doses of up to 1 mega unit can be given in 1 or 2 ml. fluid.

Dosage.—This varies from 50,000 units to 1 mega unit or more 12-hourly. Solutions deteriorate on standing but will remain potent for a few hours at room temperature and longer in a refrigerator.

Phenyl mercuric acetate 0·002 per cent may be added to containers holding several intramuscular doses. Such penicillin must never be injected intrathecally. The pain of injection can be greatly reduced by giving it with 1 per cent lignocaine.

Long-acting Penicillin.—Length of action is largely a function of solubility—the less soluble the preparation, the slower the absorption. Hence, all long-acting penicillins are suspensions of solids.

Procaine penicillin injection (B.P.) is an aqueous suspension containing 300,000 units per ml.; 100,000 units of benzylpenicillin per ml. may be added (fortified procaine penicillin injection B.P.). Intravenous injections of procaine penicillin must be avoided as they cause alarming symptoms.

Orbenin, Pyopen, and Penbritin (Beecham Research Laboratories, Brentford, Middlesex).

Benzathine penicillin (*B.P.*) (penidural) contains 300,000 units per ml. Bacteriostatic blood levels are maintained for several days after an intramuscular dose, but its efficacy in acute conditions seems doubtful. There are various proprietary combinations of slow-acting and crystalline penicillin (all-purpose penicillin) intended for the treatment of moderately severe infections by a single injection. The blood concentration of penicillin (however administered) can be increased many times by giving probenecid (benemid) 0·25–0·5 G. 6-hourly (children 0·01–0·025 G. per kg.). It acts by inhibiting penicillin excretion in the renal tubules.

Oral Penicillin.—Manipulation of the penicillanic acid nucleus has produced a series of semi-synthetic penicillins which are either acid- or penicillinase-resistant, or active against a wide range of bacteria.

Phenoxymethyl penicillin (penicillin V) is an example of the group which are acid-resistant. None are very well absorbed. As they are mainly given for mild infections it is difficult to judge their efficacy. They are valuable in the prophylaxis of rheumatic fever but not in gonorrhœa.

Cloxacillin (orbenin) is effective orally against staphylococci which produce penicillinase and so is used in infections resistant to benzylpenicillin. This is its sole indication.

Ampicillin (penbritin) is the so-called broad-spectrum penicillin, being effective against many Gram-positive and Gram-negative bacteria. It is acid-resistant but irregularly absorbed. Its activity is not much reduced by protein-binding. As it is inactivated by penicillinase in the colon it does not cause diarrhœa. It has about the same range as tetracycline, to which it is an alternative, but, in addition, it is bactericidal. The adult dose is 250 to 500 mg. 4-hourly.

Carbenicillin (pyopen) is active against *Pseudomonas pyocyanea* and *Proteus vulgaris*. For mild infections the dose is 1 G. i.m. 6-hourly in adults; for severe infections and septicæmia 12–30 G. may be infused intravenously along with probenecid.

Intrathecal Penicillin.—Penicillin is rarely given intrathecally because other drugs more easily cross the blood–brain barrier. If it is used, 200,000 units should be made up to 10 ml. in physiological saline. No preservative must be present.

Untoward Effects of Penicillin.—Sensitization usually results from previous treatment, but it can arise from inhalations of droplets or drinking milk from cows treated with penicillin. Penicillin may cause immediate anaphylactic shock, usually when injected, or, more often, a delayed reaction with a fever and a rash.

The patient should always be asked about sensitivity and general allergy before penicillin is injected. If there is a history of reaction it is wise to use another antibiotic and to always have adrenaline, aminophylline, and anti-histamines ready in case of need. Sensitivity to one penicillin means sensitivity to all.

ALTERNATIVES TO PENICILLIN

Penicillin—either benzylpenicillin or one of the newer semi-synthetic penicillins, e.g., cloxacillin (orbenin)—and ampicillin (penbritin) are now so effective that they have rendered out of date many of the antistaphylococcal antibiotics of recent years—erythromycin, novobiocin, oleandomycin, vanomycin, etc.—and so these will not be described. But some of the newer antibiotics are useful when penicillin cannot be used, either because the patient is sensitive or the organisms are resistant.

Penidural (John Wyeth & Brother Ltd., Maidenhead, Berks).
Benemid (Merck, Sharp, & Dohme Ltd., Hoddesdon, Herts).

Lincomycin (lincocin).—Its field of usefulness is staphylococcal infections in penicillin-sensitive patients.

Dosage: It is supplied in 500-mg. capsules and 600-mg. ampoules for intravenous and intramuscular use. The daily dose is 2 G.

Fucidin.—This antibiotic, isolated from *Fusidium coccineum*, is very active against Gram-positive and Gram-negative cocci. Pneumococci, streptococci, and *Esch. coli* are resistant. It is well absorbed and slowly excreted, but does not reach the cerebrospinal fluid. Being mainly inactivated in the body, it does not appear in the urine in an active form. Fucidin is a useful addition to the anti-staphylococcal drugs, but resistant strains rapidly emerge. It is said to be able to penetrate pus and necrotic tissue. Fucidin has a close chemical relationship to the corticosteroids but it does not cause any untoward metabolic effects.

Dosage: It is supplied in 250-mg. capsules. The dose is 500 mg. 8-hourly.

Cephalosporins (ceporin).—These are a group of wide-spectrum bactericidal antibiotics extracted from a cephalosporin isolated from a sewage outfall off the coast of Sardinia. In staphylococcal infections their chief virtue is that they are quite unaffected by the penicillinase produced. Against Gram-negative bacilli the spectrum is similar to that of ampicillin. They show cross-resistance with the penicillins, but there is no cross hypersensitivity and so they are useful in patients who are sensitive to penicillin. They have to be given by injection.

Dosage: 250–500 mg. twice a day.

STREPTOMYCIN

This is a bactericidal substance issued as a white freely soluble powder. Its most important use is in tuberculosis. As resistance soon develops it is given with *p*-aminosalicylic 20 G. daily and isoniazid 200 mg. daily in tuberculosis, and with penicillin in other infections. It has to be given by intramuscular injection, as it is not absorbed from the gut, but it may be used in combination with a non-absorbable sulphonamide for bowel infection. When used for urinary infections the urine must be kept alkaline (*p*H 8).

Dosage.—The dose in tuberculosis is 1–2 G. daily in one injection. For other infections the same dose is spread over the day.

Toxic Effects.—Streptomycin causes labyrinthine damage, but if warning signs are heeded and the drug stopped recovery is possible. (Dihydrostreptomycin, while similar therapeutically, causes permanent deafness and should not be used.)

CHLORAMPHENICOL

This synthetic antibiotic is bacteriostatic and effective against a wide range of Gram-positive and Gram-negative organisms. It is very bitter to taste and, for children, the tasteless chloramphenicol palmitate should be used. Chloramphenicol is rapidly absorbed and diffused through the body. It easily passes into the cerebrospinal fluid where it attains a concentration of about half that in the blood. Excretion (partly in an activated form) is by the urine.

Dosage.—It is supplied in 250-mg. capsules for oral use. The daily dose is 50 mg. per kg., reducing to half when the infection responds. For intravenous use, chloramphenicol sodium succinate well diluted with physiological saline should be used—1 G. every 8 hours (children 100 mg. per kg. per day).

Toxic Effects.—There is a definite but slight risk of marrow depression and, although it is a wide-spectrum antibiotic, it is strongly advised that it be reserved solely for typhoid and other salmonella infections and influenzal meningitis.

Lincocin (Upjohn Ltd., Crawley, Sussex).
Fucidin (Leo Laboratories Ltd., Hayes Middlesex).
Ceporin (Glaxo Laboratories Ltd., Greenford, Middlesex).

THE TETRACYCLINES

These are all wide-spectrum bacteriostatic antibiotics with wider indications than for any other antibiotic. There is little to choose between them and they show bacterial cross-resistance. Sufficient remains in the gut for it to have a marked bacteriostatic effect there, often with resulting diarrhœa. Tetracyclines pass into most body spaces but do not readily cross the blood–brain barrier. They attain a higher concentration in the bile than in the blood. Tetracyclines are often used as an alternative to penicillin, but they are less active than penicillin against Gram-positive organisms.

Dosage.—Tetracycline is available in many forms—50- and 250-mg. tablets, and capsules and vials for intramuscular and intravenous use. It is not suitable for intrathecal injection. The average daily adult dose is 1 G. (up to 4 G. for brucellosis). Children should receive 12 mg. per kg. per day.

Demethylchlortetracycline (ledermycin) is just about twice as active against most bacteria as tetracycline and less rapidly excreted. Two oral doses of 150 mg. a day will suffice.

Lymecycline (tetralysal) has activity like tetracycline but with the advantage of great solubility (2·5 G. in 1 ml.), making parenteral administration easier.

The untoward effect of tetracycline is the unopposed growth of resistant organisms resulting in stomatitis, black tongue, proctitis, and staphylococcal diarrhœa

THE POLYMYXINS

Bacillus polymyxa, a soil bacillus, produces several polypeptides of which polymyxin B (aerosporin), colistin sulphonate sodium B.P.—sometimes called polymyxin E—and colistin sulphomethate sodium (colomycin) are commercially available. As they are impure, the dose is stated in units. They are poorly absorbed and so must be injected for systemic infections.

Dosage.—The dose of aerosporin is 250,000 units 4-hourly and of colistin 3–9 million units daily in divided dosage.

Polymyxins are bactericidal and all Gram-negative bacilli (except the *Proteus* species) are highly sensitive. Gram-positive cocci and bacteria are highly resistant. Against *Pseudomonas pyocyanea*, *Hæmophilus influenzæ*, and *Escherichia coli* the polymyxins are more active than against any other bacteria. Organisms do not readily become resistant to polymyxins. With sulphonamides, polymyxins act synergistically. For systemic and urinary infections polymyxins must be injected as they are poorly absorbed from the gut.

Toxic Effect.—Excretion is by the kidneys and overdosage can cause renal damage.

The chief indication for polymyxins is urinary infection by *Pseudomonas pyocyanea*, giving 100,000–500,000 units daily.

Meningitis due to *Pseudomonas* and *Hæmophilus influenzæ* can be treated by colistin intramuscularly (10,000 units per kg. 4-hourly), but as the drug does not pass the blood–brain barrier, intrathecal injections are necessary, giving 500–1000 units per kg. body-weight in one daily injection.

NEOMYCIN

This antibiotic, in the same group as streptomycin, is chiefly used for its action on the bowel, as it is not absorbed. It rapidly suppresses staphylococci, *Proteus*, and coliform organisms, and so is used in the preparation of the bowel for surgery (*see* p. 136).

Ledermycin (Lederle Laboratories, Bush House, Aldwych, London, W.C.2).
Tetralysal (Carlo Erba (U.K.) Ltd., 28 Great Peter Street, London, S.W.1).
Aerosporin (Burroughs, Wellcome & Co., Euston Road, London, N.W.1).
Colomycin (Pharmax Ltd., Crayford, Dartford, Kent).

Another indication is to suppress the intestinal flora in hepatic failure.
Dosage.—1 G. 4-hourly orally.

NYSTATIN

This antifungal antibiotic was discovered in the New York State Department of Health Laboratories. It does not act on bacteria. It is insoluble and so is used as tablets for its effect on the gut or preferably topically in the mouth (100,000 units in 1 dose) for monilial infections (candidiasis) which sometimes complicate the use of wide-spectrum antibiotics in debilitated patients.

Dosage.—500,000 units three times per day.

CHAPTER VII

THE CLINICAL USE OF ANTICOAGULANTS

By F. Dudley Hart and J. G. Humble

THE use and abuse of anticoagulants is a vexed question and opinions are more freely available than facts. They remain, nevertheless, very useful drugs in everyday use in hospitals throughout the world. Heparin is a quick-acting physiological anticoagulant given intravenously; of the oral preparations the choice lies between warfarin sodium (marevan), phenindione (dindevan), nicoumalone (sinthrome), phenprocoumon (marcoumar), ethyl biscoumacetate (tromexan), and cumetharol (dicumoxane). It is common practice to give heparin intravenously or intramuscularly for immediate effect, and at the same time to give an oral preparation for continued therapy.

Indications for Anticoagulant Therapy.—

1. Thrombosis in the veins of a limb (usually a leg) after operation or childbirth.

2. Peripheral arterial embolism and thrombosis.

3. Coronary thrombosis.

4. Cavernous sinus thrombosis.

5. Mesenteric thrombosis.

6. Following certain arterial operations.

Anticoagulants can also be used in a variety of other conditions such as venous thrombosis occurring in certain medical diseases.

Bleeding from the site of operation is unlikely if heparin is commenced after the third post-operative day. Post-partum hæmorrhage also is unlikely if anticoagulant therapy is delayed until the third day after delivery. Unless it is excessive, menstruation is not a contra-indication.

Cautions and Contra-indications.—When the clotting-time has been prolonged artificially a potential bleeding-point is liable to become the site of considerable hæmorrhage. For instance a peptic ulcer, a papilloma of the bladder, renal pelvis, colon, or uterus, or a leaking aneurysm of the circle of Willis, may commence to bleed profusely. When a potential source of hæmorrhage such as one of these is known to be present or is suspected, anticoagulant therapy should be employed only if there is a full appreciation of the liability to, and preparedness for, the onset of considerable hæmorrhage. Because of the danger of cerebral hæmorrhage, anticoagulant therapy is rarely used in cases of cerebral thrombosis. As heparin is largely excreted in the urine, renal insufficiency will lead to its retention in the body, and necessitate drastic reduction in dosage: this applies particularly to elderly patients.

HEPARIN

Heparin is a very satisfactory anticoagulant, as its action is short-lived and cessation of the drug is soon followed by a return of the clotting-time of the blood to normal. Heparin is issued in international units, and although subject

Marevan and Dindevan (Duncan, Flockhart, & Evans Ltd., Birkbeck Street, London, E.2).

Sinthrome and Tromexan (Geigy Pharmaceutical Co. Ltd., Wythenshawe, Manchester, 23).

Marcoumar (Roche Products Ltd., 15 Manchester Square, London, W.1).

Dicumoxane (M.C.P. Pure Drugs Ltd., Alperton, Middlesex).

to some variation, 100 such units are approximately equal to 1 mg. of crystalline heparin. Heparin can be given by intermittent intravenous or intramuscular injection, or by adding it to the contents of a flask of a continuous intravenous drip apparatus.

As active mobility of the patient during administration is highly desirable, intermittent administration of the drug is preferable unless the details specified in the following paragraph are observed meticulously.

Administration.—After a preliminary investigation of the clotting-time of the patient's blood, an indwelling hollow needle with a renewable diaphragm, such as Gordh's needle (*Fig.* 45), is inserted into a suitable vein, and 12,500 international units of heparin are injected intravenously. Thereafter 10,000 units are injected intravenously every 4 hours until the clotting-time, tested not less than 3 hours after the last injection of heparin, is approximately three times its pre-treatment level. Subsequent dosage is such as will maintain that level—probably 10,000 units 4–6-hourly. Regular interspacing of injections is absolutely essential and a dose must never be omitted, day or night. Night dosage is particularly important because it is during the nocturnal hours (because of relative immobility) that further clotting tends to occur. An indwelling needle obviates the discomfort of frequent intravenous injections and subsequent hæmatomata which in a heparinized patient occur so readily at the site of such injections. It also saves the house-surgeon making visits to the bedside at precise intervals, both day and night, for after instructions as to how they are carried out, technically simple injections can be given by the nurse-in-charge. If possible the patient should be ambulatory during the treatment. If this is impracticable, the patient should be as active as is possible in bed, and movements of the legs must be encouraged.

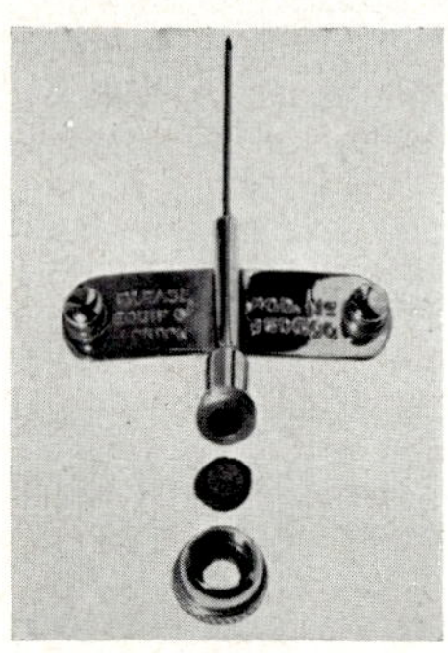

Fig. 45.—Gordh's needle, showing diaphragm and cap.

Should blood transfusion prove necessary, heparin, 3 units per ml., *over and above the dosage otherwise required* is added to the donor blood before the bottle containing the blood is connected to the giving set.

In addition to serving as an anticoagulant, heparin acts also as a vascular antispasmodic. Soon after the commencement of heparin therapy a cold, aching, thrombosed limb will be seen to flush, and the aching lessens or ceases. In some cases generalized flushing of the entire body surface ensues.

Intramuscular injection: Alternatively, heparin can be given in similar dosage 6–8-hourly by intramuscular injection. Once adequate heparinization has been obtained, painful bruising is prone to occur at the site of injections; but in a short course in conjunction with an oral anticoagulant, this disadvantage is insufficient to condemn the method, though in general the intravenous route is greatly to be preferred.

When heparin and an oral anticoagulant are both to be used, the two drugs are started together, intravenous heparin being discontinued after 24–36 hours, oral therapy continuing for the rest of the course (*see below*).

Complications.—These are: (1) hæmatoma; (2) hæmothorax; (3) retroperitoneal or other hæmorrhage; (4) hæmaturia; (5) febrile reactions due to drug impurities; (6) anaphylactic reactions.

Slight hæmaturia, slight epistaxis, and bruising are to be regarded not as untoward manifestations but as signs that the dosage of the anticoagulant therapy is adequate and is achieving the purpose for which the therapy was given. Should more severe or protracted bleeding demand discontinuation of the anticoagulant therapy an intravenous injection of 5–10 ml. of 1 per cent protamine sulphate will help to restore rapidly the normal clotting-time.

ORALLY ADMINISTERED ANTICOAGULANTS

Many oral preparations are now available.

The therapeutic effect of orally administered anticoagulants is not apparent for between 24 and 36 hours. Consequently should a quick effect be required, heparin also must be given to cover this initial period.

Dosage is based on daily prothrombin estimations, and oral anticoagulants should not be used if such estimations cannot be carried out reliably and promptly. The chosen preparation is given usually in the morning and evening, and the daily dosage reduced gradually to that which keeps the blood pro-thrombin level between 20 and 40 per cent of normal. There is considerable variation in the required dosage in different patients, and even in the same patient; occasionally divergence in the rate of absorption, and other factors, make the control more difficult. Care should be taken that other drugs, parti-cularly salicylates, which affect the prothrombin time, are not given in large doses during anticoagulant therapy. Should this be unavoidable, the dose of the oral anticoagulant will probably have to be reduced. The dosage of the oral anticoagulant is maintained until the patient is fully ambulatory: embolic disasters may occur if therapy is discontinued before full mobility has been regained. Today many patients, particularly males under the age of 60 years, are maintained for several weeks or months on oral anticoagulants following coronary thrombosis, in particular diabetics, the sluggish and obese, those with a degree of cardiac decompensation, and those who have had repeated venous or arterial (coronary) thromboses. Subsequently prothrombin estimations are performed every 1–4 weeks during out-patient attendance.

A Combined Course of Anticoagulant Therapy is, usually, somewhat as follows:

	Heparin + Warfarin Sodium	
1st 24 hours	12,500 units I.V. *statim* and 10,000 units 4-hourly	10–20 mg. by mouth 12-hourly
2nd 24 hours	Reduce and discontinue over 4–12 hours only if prothrombin time satisfactory	5–10 mg. by mouth 12-hourly
3rd 24 hours and subse-quently	Nil	According to plasma prothrombin estimations 0–10 mg. 12-hour-ly

The prothrombin time (*Fig.* 46) should be maintained at about 2–3 times the normal, remembering that the normal value varies according to the method used in the determination by the laboratory. For the first few days daily estimations are essential. Should there be reason for suspecting that serious hæmorrhage may occur, more frequent estimations are advisable. In favourable circumstances, when satisfactory control has been obtained, the period between estimations is lengthened gradually. A chart like *Fig.* 46 is valuable.

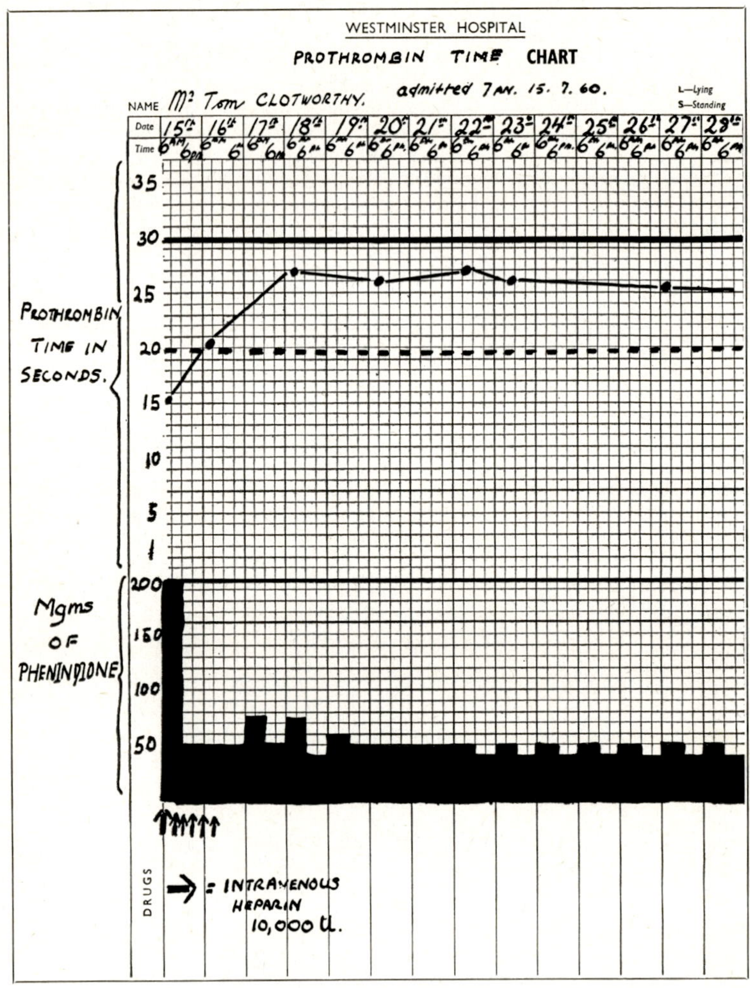

Fig. 46.—Chart of a patient undergoing anticoagulant therapy.

Contra-indications.—Oral anticoagulants must not be given in the presence of liver disease, blood dyscrasia, or nephritis. When the patient is elderly or is suffering from cardiac congestive failure, especial caution should be exercised in the oral administration of anticoagulants, a smaller dose being required.

Complications.—Overdosage can cause any of the manifestations of bleeding set out under 'Heparin'; antidotes are blood transfusion and phytomenadione (vitamin K_1), 5–20 mg. orally or intravenously. Toxic effects due to the drug used, usually phenindione, include skin reactions and, more rarely, renal and hepatic damage.

LOW MOLECULAR WEIGHT DEXTRAN

Low molecular weight dextran (rheomacrodex) helps to prevent the clumping of red blood-corpuscles. It may be given when there is a need both to achieve this effect and for intravenous fluid. A 10 per cent solution is given intravenously in burns, shock, and ileus; the solution is available in 500-ml. bottles.

Rheomacrodex (Pharmacia (Great Britain) Ltd., The Avenue, London, W.13).

CHAPTER VIII

THE TREATMENT OF ACUTE POISONING

By C. ALLAN BIRCH

DIAGNOSIS

THE fact that someone has been poisoned is often obvious from the circumstances. He may, for example, be found in a gas-filled room or with an empty tablet bottle by his side. But the diagnosis may be missed unless the possibility of poisoning crosses the mind of the doctor faced with any patient comatose or severely ill without other obvious cause. Sometimes hypothermia is a striking feature. Poisoning does not produce lateralizing signs, but there are snags, and evidence of 'natural' disease may coexist, as when a hemiplegic patient poisons himself. Diagnosis is urgent and so it usually depends on clinical acumen rather than on special tests. Barbiturate poisoning may resemble insulin coma and when hypoglycæmia is a possibility, particularly if the patient is a diabetic on insulin, it is wise to inject 20 ml. of 50 per cent dextrose (10 G.) intravenously. It will not harm the poisoned patient and if he is in an insulin coma it will bring him round.

WHAT POISON WAS TAKEN?

The answer may be given by the relatives and friends, but it is as well to preserve specimens of blood and urine for examination. Great difficulty may be experienced when more than one substance has been taken, e.g., barbiturates and alcohol. When unidentified tablets are incriminated, help in identification may be obtained from the Poisons Information Centres in London (Guy's Hospital), Edinburgh, Belfast, Cardiff, Leeds, Newcastle, Birmingham, and Suffolk.* However, time should not be lost before starting life-saving measures (*see below*).

FIRST-AID METHODS
A. COAL GAS POISONING

Open doors and windows and drag the victim out by the heels. First ask yourself, however, 'Is it safe to enter?' and, if there is doubt, go in 'roped' so that

---

* London: National Poisons Information Centre, Guy's Hospital, London Bridge—HOP 7600.

Edinburgh: Regional Poisoning Treatment Centre, Royal Infirmary, Edinburgh—FOUntainbridge 2477.

Belfast: Institute of Clinical Science, Grosvenor Road, Belfast 12—Belfast 30503.

Cardiff: Poisons Information Centre, Cardiff Royal Infirmary, Cardiff—Cardiff 33101.

Leeds: Poisons Information Centre, General Infirmary, Leeds—Leeds 30715.

Newcastle: Regional Poison Information Centre, Royal Victoria Infirmary, Newcastle—Newcastle 25131.

Birmingham: The General Hospital, Birmingham—Central 8611.

Brandon, Suffolk: U.S. Poison Control Centre, 48th Tactical Hospital, U.S.A.F., R.A.F., Lakenheath, Brandon, Suffolk—Lakenheath 2371, ext. 4.

you can be dragged out if need be. Keep the head low as coal gas (but not carbon monoxide) is lighter than air. Artificial respiration (*see* p. 19) may be needed.

B. INGESTED POISONS
(Other than Corrosives)

If the patient is conscious, induce vomiting by making him drink a tumblerful of salty water. It may be necessary to stimulate his pharynx with the finger. If he is comatose, empty the stomach with a Senoran's evacuator and keep the contents. Then (or preferably in hospital) proceed to wash out the stomach. As this can be dangerous, if not done properly, the technique is given in detail.

Technique of Gastric Lavage.—The necessary apparatus is as follows:—

1. Stomach tube. This may be the one which fits the Senoran's evacuator. It should be not less than $\frac{1}{2}$ in. (1·25 cm.) in diameter, 60 in. (150 cm.) long, and fairly stiff. A distance of 20 in. (50 cm.) from the tip should be marked by putting a safety-pin through the wall, but not the lumen, of the tube. When passed, the safety-pin should be just inside the lips. It is as well to cut a few side-holes near the end of the tube.

2. A plastic or enamelled funnel.

3. A tongue clip (not the crushing variety).

4. Two mouth gags.

5. Two jugs (1 and 4 pints; 0·5 and 2 litres).

6. A pail.

7. Rubber sheeting or newspapers for the floor.

If the patient is deeply unconscious with impending respiratory failure, a useful preliminary in hospital is to have an anæsthetist pass a cuffed endo-tracheal tube. Failing this, the risk of fluid entering the lungs must be avoided by having the head low. The prone position is best with the head over the end of the table (*Fig.* 47). If an operating table is available the patient may be put in the Trendelenburg position but it is then necessary to draw the tongue forwards with a clip and to remove fluid from the mouth by a sucker. If the patient is not deeply comatose he may struggle, but this is less likely in the prone position. Immobilization by straps may be necessary. The dentures must be removed and the mouth opened by a gag or a boxwood wedge with a central hole (*Fig.* 48). Pass the tube quickly into the stomach. (Only when it is impossible to open the mouth should a nasogastric tube be used. It may then be passed through the nose.) It is as well first to attach the Senoran's evacuator and to empty the stomach. Then replace the evacuator with the funnel and pour in up to a pint of warm water. Lower the funnel over the pail to siphon back the fluid. Bicarbonate solution may be used, but not in barbiturate poison-ing as it increases the solubility. Up to 2 gallons (9 litres) in all may be used, but it is best not to put too much fluid in the stomach at a time lest it forces the pylorus and so defeats the object of the lavage.

Gastric lavage may be omitted if a long time has elapsed since the poison was ingested. The length of time varies with the poison. All the barbiturate ingested will have been absorbed in 4–6 hours and, after that time, lavage is unnecessary. Big doses of aspirin cause gastric stasis and so, in aspirin poisoning, lavage is indicated over a longer period. When there is doubt it is best to wash out the stomach, but always with proper precautions.

The old-fashioned practice of giving a cathartic via the tube, after lavage, is not recommended, for the resulting diarrhœa may complicate the picture by causing loss of fluid. But it is still a good idea, having emptied the stomach, to introduce some universal antidote (powdered activated charcoal 2 parts, magnesium oxide 1 part, and tannic acid 1 part). The dose is a dessertspoonful made into a paste, as it is fluffy. Ordinary charcoal (burnt toast, etc.) is useless.

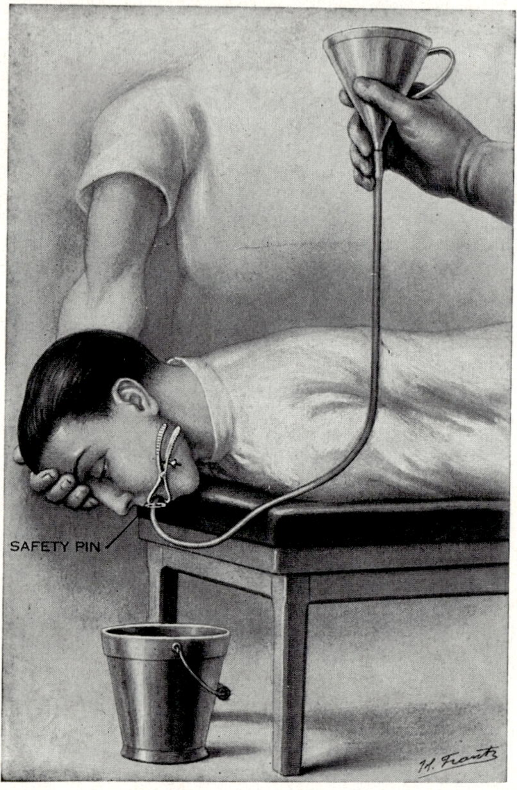

Fig. 47.—Washing out the stomach. For the sake of clarity, the operator's hand holding the tube and the assistant's hand holding the gag are not shown. The head must on no account be raised higher than is shown.

C. CORROSIVE POISONS

Give milk, white of egg, or magnesia, and also pethidine for pain. *Do not attempt gastric lavage.*

TREATMENT

After giving first aid, the basic principles in all poisonings are:—

1. To deal with the process which is endangering life, e.g., dehydration (by intravenous fluid); pain (by pethidine); shock (by noradrenaline drip); restlessness and convulsions (by intramuscular paraldehyde).

2. To eliminate the poison (by forced diuresis, dialysis, exchange transfusions and (for carbon-monoxide poisoning) artificial respiration and hyperbaric oxygen therapy.

General Management of the Patient Comatose from Poison.—The general nursing care is that given to any comatose patient, using the semi-prone position with frequent changes from side to side, maintaining a good airway, guarding against pressure sores, and watching the bladder. Tube feeding is needed if coma is prolonged (p. 49). Catheterization will probably be necessary and a thin, plastic Gibbon catheter should be used. A ripple bed will help to prevent bedsores. Warming should be avoided even though the patient appears shocked.

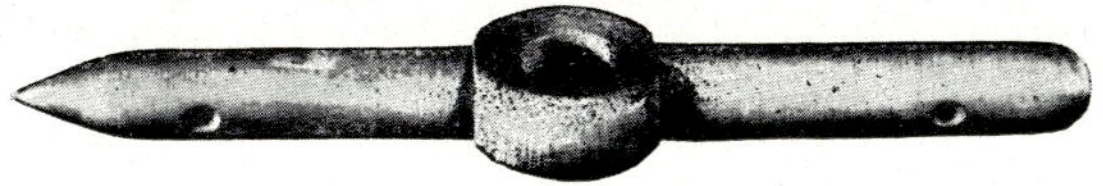

Fig. 48.—Boxwood wedge with central hole to take œsophageal tube.

This is because a lowered temperature depresses metabolism and diminishes the effect of the poison. Bronchoscopy and suction may be needed to maintain an airway and, if insufficient, tracheostomy (*see* p. 16) and intermittent positive-pressure ventilation by breathing machine will be needed. The fluid intake and output must be carefully measured. If it seems probable that material has been aspirated into the lungs, 2–4 mega units of penicillin should be given intramuscularly each day and there is something to be said for giving it routinely to all comatose poisoned patients.

These general measures will often pull the patient through, but the serious effects of some common poisons call for special treatment.

BARBITURATE POISONING

Serious barbiturate poisoning causes circulatory and respiratory depression. If these can be successfully combated and a good urinary output maintained, then recovery is possible, despite prolonged coma. Sometimes an early anoxic phase shows itself disappointingly late as convulsions and death. Analeptics are not needed.

Here we are concerned more with the handicraft of management than with discussions of details of barbiturate excretion. Blood levels are useful guides to progress (send 15 to 20 ml. of heparinized blood). Special methods to get rid of barbiturate are:—

1. The artificial kidney (discuss the case with the doctor in the special unit).
2. Peritoneal dialysis (*see* p. 433).
3. 'Blood lavage'. This is designed to enhance renal excretion of barbiturates by creating an absolute diuresis. Give intravenously a solution containing 15 per cent of urea with 40 mEq./l. sodium lactate and 12 mEq./l. potassium chloride and 200 mEq./l. dextrose. The blood-urea is raised to about 250 mg. per 100 ml. and the drip should be adjusted to keep pace with the urinary flow.

Phenobarbitone is the most slowly excreted barbiturate, but its renal clearance is increased when the urine is alkaline. Bicarbonate should be given intravenously in an amount sufficient to keep the urine alkaline to phenol-red indicator —i.e., to give a definite red colour (*p*H 8·4). Special *p*H indicator papers should be used. The initial dose of bicarbonate should be 230 mg. per kg., given as an injection of sodium bicarbonate (B.P.) 5 per cent.

CARBON MONOXIDE POISONING

Sixty per cent carboxyhæmoglobin (HbCO) is necessary to cause coma in non-anæmic patients, but lower levels may be fatal in the decrepit, the diseased, the drugged, and the drunk—the four D's of carbon monoxide poisoning. Carbon monoxide is eliminated at the rate of 30 to 50 per cent per hour and more rapidly if pure oxygen is breathed. Hence the essentials of treatment are to provide a clear airway and encourage full and deep breathing. A mixture of carbon dioxide and oxygen causes more rapid elimination of carbon monoxide than does oxygen alone, and 5 per cent carbon dioxide in oxygen is officially recommended. (Carbon dioxide is contra-indicated in anoxia and asphyxia from other causes.) Elimination can be more rapidly attained by breathing pure oxygen at 2 atmospheres' pressure in a special chamber.

SALICYLATE POISONING

Salicylates upset acid-base metabolism by a complex mechanism in which overbreathing plays a big part. They are excreted in the urine, partly unaltered and partly conjugated with protein. When the urine is alkaline (pH 7) the excretion of unconjugated salicylate is increased. Hence benefit is obtained from bicarbonate therapy. In severe cases, watch on the acid-base balance, blood gases, and fluid output is essential. Some form of dialysis is often helpful and an exchange transfusion will get rid of the protein-bound fraction.

FERROUS SULPHATE POISONING

Iron tablets are often attractive to children and poisoning by them is a serious emergency. The drug of choice is desferal which forms an iron complex which is rapidly excreted in the urine. Inject 2000 mg. in 8 ml. of water intramuscularly. Wash out the stomach with 1 per cent sodium bicarbonate and give 5000 mg. desferal in 50–100 ml. of water by mouth. Give desferal in physiological saline by intravenous drip at not more than 15 mg. per kg. per hour (maximum dose 30 mg. per kg. in 24 hours).

CYANIDE POISONING

Cyanides are one of the few poisons for which there is a specific antidote. Treatment is aimed at inactivating circulating cyanide by using nitrites to convert hæmoglobin into methæmoglobin which will not combine with cyanide. Give amyl nitrite to breathe (it is useless to try artificial respiration and only by inactivating cyanide can the patient's life be saved). Then give 10 ml. of 3 per cent sodium nitrite intravenously. Follow this by 50 ml. of 25 per cent sodium thiosulphate to form an inactive compound with cyanide. These solutions are supplied in the 'Ampin' emergency kit which is kept in all works using cyanides.

AMPHETAMINE POISONING

Amphetamine and allied drugs stimulate the central nervous system and smooth muscle. Toxic doses cause insomnia, tremors, and a state of euphoria. The pupils are dilated and the mouth dry. Convulsions may occur. Treatment is to control the excitement by barbiturates and to nurse the patient in a quiet, dark room.

Recent ingestion calls for gastric lavage and other general measures.

Desferal (Ciba Laboratories Ltd., Horsham, Sussex).
Ampin Emergency Kit (Cuxson, Gerrard & Co., Oldbury, Birmingham).

ETHYL ALCOHOL POISONING

This produces the familiar picture of severe drunkenness, loss of memory, irregular behaviour, and incoordinated movement going on to coma. It may be complicated by injury and by the effects of other poisons such as barbiturates. Treatment is to use artificial respiration if need be, to prevent aspiration of vomit, and to protect the victim from cold until he becomes sober.

METHYL ALCOHOL POISONING

This results from drinking methylated spirit either neat or as adulterated wine. Mild poisoning may be mistaken for the common 'hangover' of ordinary alcoholism. In more severe cases there is epigastric pain, vomiting, and blindness. Treatment is mainly symptomatic. The eyes should be protected from light. Small amounts of whisky are recommended. This is because ethyl alcohol competes successfully for oxidative enzymes and allows methyl alcohol to be excreted as such. If the arterial blood pH is low, bicarbonate therapy is indicated.

PSYCHIATRIC ASSISTANCE

A brief reminder is added on the medico-legal aspects of poisoning. There is now no legal obligation to report suicidal poisoning, but it is usually wise to bring in a psychiatrist. When poisoning is homicidal a dying declaration may be made or a dying deposition taken.

However, there are many patients, for example, teenagers who have ingested aspirin, who are guilty of self-poisoning (to attract attention) rather than of serious attempts at self-destruction. Both groups should be seen by a psychiatrist before there has been time to fabricate excuses and alibis.

CHAPTER IX

THE TREATMENT OF BURNS AND SCALDS

By A. B. WALLACE

TECHNIQUES in treatment are, and always have been, notoriously diverse, owing in part to variations of the clinical picture and partly to the fact that types of burns vary with forms of employment and industry or existing social habits and conditions.

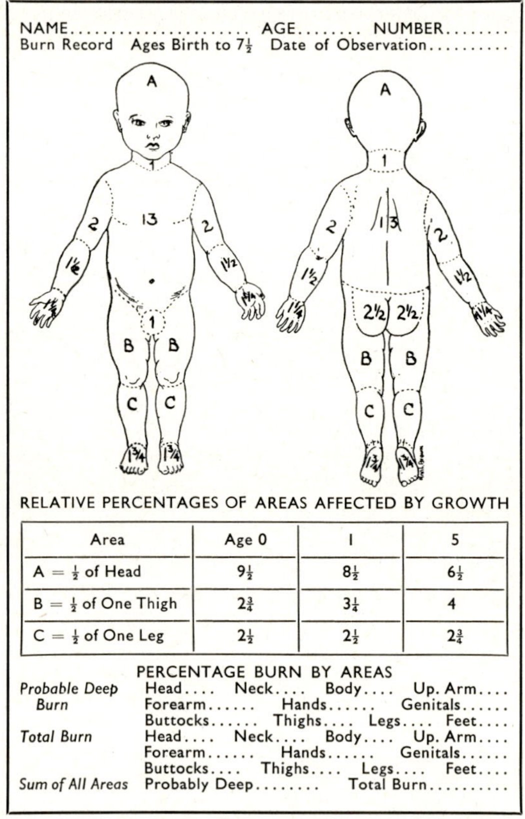

Area	Age 0	1	5
A = ½ of Head	9½	8½	6½
B = ½ of One Thigh	2¾	3¼	4
C = ½ of One Leg	2½	2½	2¾

Fig. 49.—Burn record for children up to 7½ years of age, showing relative percentage of total skin area.

They can differ, therefore, from country to country, from region to region, and even from town to town, and experiences in therapy must of necessity conflict.

Burns commonly affect cutaneous surfaces and from time to time (face burns) the lining of the upper air-passages. They may be extensive, moderate, or slight, and either superficial or deep. In treatment, as in pathology and disturbed physiology, they are best considered as wounds. Wounds can be classified as 'closed' or 'open'; so likewise can burns. Further, wounds cause general reactions; burns lead to various clinical states and treatment demands from the surgeon a considerable knowledge of the reaction of the body to stress.

Burns can kill in many ways, the mortality being highest in the old and the young. Death results most commonly from respiratory complications, cardiac complications, and local or generalized infection.

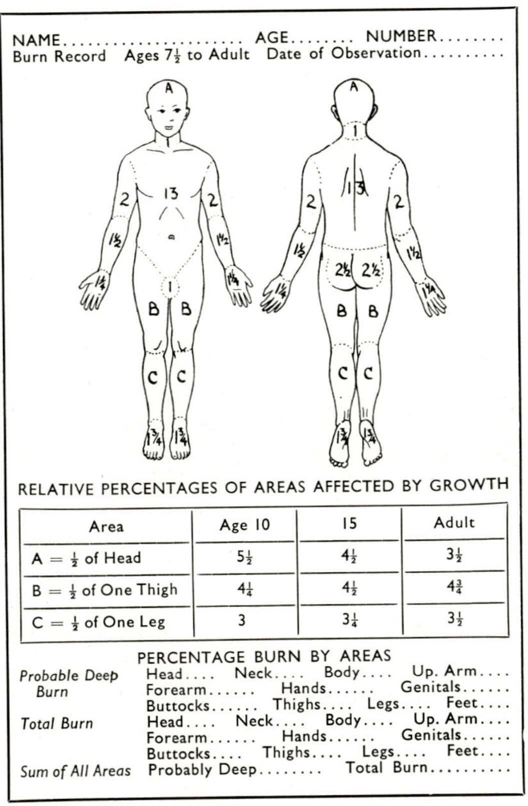

Area	Age 10	15	Adult
A = ½ of Head	5½	4½	3½
B = ½ of One Thigh	4¼	4½	4¾
C = ½ of One Leg	3	3¼	3½

PERCENTAGE BURN BY AREAS

Probable Deep Burn	Head.... Neck.... Body.... Up. Arm....			
	Forearm...... Hands...... Genitals......			
	Buttocks...... Thighs.... Legs.... Feet....			
Total Burn	Head.... Neck.... Body.... Up. Arm....			
	Forearm...... Hands...... Genitals......			
	Buttocks.... Thighs.... Legs.... Feet....			
Sum of All Areas	Probably Deep........ Total Burn..........			

Fig. 50.—Burn record for older children and adults.

The early danger is that of fluid loss. The severity of oligæmic shock is related to the extent of the burn. The later infection is related more to depth than to the surface area. As a guide to treatment, methods of classification both by extent and depth are deemed important.

CLASSIFICATION

Extent.—Tables have been evolved that make estimation of the surface area of burns fairly accurate at any age (*Figs*. 49, 50). A useful though less accurate table is the 'Rule of Nine' (*Fig*. 51).

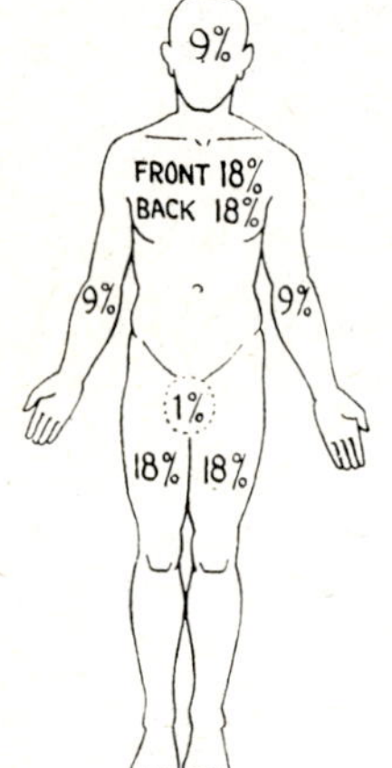

Fig. 51.—The 'Rule of Nine' for calculating burn area as percentage of total skin area.

In general, the estimation of the extent of the surface areas of burns tends to be too high. Areas of erythema are not included in the total.

Depth.—Burns can be superficial or deep. *Superficial* implies involvement of skin, *deep* signifies destruction of skin with possible deeper involvement. The differentiation between a deep and a superficial burn can be difficult. Appearances vary with causal agents, sites affected, and the time that has elapsed since the burning. The light brown tan of a deep flame-burn and the dull white marble-like appearance and firm feel of a deep scald are characteristic, as also are the evident œdema and red blistered surface of the common superficial scald. For many years surgeons have appreciated that the severe continuing pain of the superficial burn is often greater than that of a deep burn.

Loss of sensation to the prick of a sterile needle has been used to distinguish a deep from a superficial burn. It is true that in a deep burn the nerve endings are destroyed and sensation lost, but unfortunately such loss is also present in some superficial burns, particularly the deep dermal burn.

The Deep Dermal Burn.—The slow healing of the deepest superficial burn has led to a subdivision of superficial burns—the deep dermal burn, in which only the deeper dermis, with its few epithelial cells, remains viable. This type of burn results from a relatively long contact with hot fluid, particularly hot fat.

TREATMENT

Fluid Replacement.—The primary aim in the treatment of severe burns is to save life, and this necessitates early restoration of the circulating blood- or plasma-volume and thereafter keeping pace with fluid loss. This is accomplished by the administration of 'replacement fluid'. In addition, every individual requires a daily fluid intake to make up loss from skin, lungs, gut, and kidneys—about 2500 ml. of 'requirement fluid' in an adult.

The fluid lost in a superficial burn contains protein and electrolyte. The loss is greatest in the first 8 hours and continues for 48 hours. In a deep burn, in addition to the aforementioned fluids, there is a considerable loss of erythrocytes, and this loss may amount to almost half the total volume deficit of the first 24 hours. Undoubtedly a severe deep burn leads to an early state of anoxia, and delay in administration of fresh blood can result in irreparable harm.

Further anæmia can develop in the first weeks in deep burns, and continue until the wounds are covered with skin. Delay in administering plasma in superficial burns is likewise unwarrantable. Loss of electrolytes is countered by the administration of plasma.

In general, patients with burns of over 10 per cent surface area have their 'replacement fluids' given intravenously; those with burns of under 10 per cent have their 'replacement fluids' by mouth as orange juice with Hartmann's solution.

The 'requirement fluids' in all patients are given by mouth in non-electrolyte form, e.g., dextrose in water flavoured with orange juice, unless vomiting occurs.

Early indications of the necessity for fluid administration are the development of pallor, thirst, and restlessness, and the urgency for fluid can thus be gauged. A high packed-cell-volume value confirms this need.

The volumes of 'replacement' and 'requirement' fluids to be given depend on the age of the patient and the extent of the burn. Considerable experience is required to estimate these volumes. Tables of normal values of blood-volumes, pressures, output of urine, etc., are valuable.

Tables are useful as guides in assessing a patient's needs or 'budget of fluids'. One of the simplest forms of estimation of 'budget' for the 48-hour period of loss is 3 ml. per kg. per 1 per cent burn, given mainly as plasma. The resuscitation fluid is given at a rate which produces an adequate urinary output (*Table V*). It may be necessary to give the total estimate within the first 12 hours.

Table V.—URINARY OUTPUT

AGE	SATISFACTORY HOURLY URINE OUTPUT
B.–1 yr.	ml. 8–20
1–5	20–25
5–10	25–30
10–14	30–50
14+	50–100

A 'budget' is therefore capable of modification according to the clinical response of the patient. This budget includes the requirement fluid, though there is no danger in giving small quantities at intervals by mouth.

Should intravenous fluid additional to the budget be required this is given at a rate to maintain urinary output. This more energetic approach, with due attention paid to circulatory overloading, reduces the dangers of tissue hypoxia. In deep burns a proportion of the fluid is whole blood. It is important also to administer calcium gluconate intravenously in massive plasma infusions.

There are other methods of calculating the fluids to be administered. The one most popular in the U.S.A. consists of the administration of the following solutions for the first 24-hour period: (1) colloids, 1 ml. per kg. of body-weight for each per cent of body surface burnt; (2) electrolytes (physiological saline solution), 1 ml. per kg. of body-weight for each per cent of body surface burnt; and (3) non-electrolytes, 2000 ml. of 5 per cent dextrose in water (to cover insensible fluid loss and to ensure an adequate output of urine) administered intravenously, or water administered orally. During the second 24-hour period one half of these amounts of colloids and electrolytes are recommended, but the same amount of non-electrolytes as in the first 24 hours.

Progress.—Progress can be assessed by the return of a more normal colour and warmth to the unburned skin and by the lessening of thirst with diminished restlessness, but the most valuable single sign is a satisfactory output of urine. Again a table acts as a guide (*Table V*). The values will be low over the first 12 hours, but thereafter should approximate more and more to the normal. In all extensively burned patients a catheter is passed into the bladder and retained in position. Thus the hourly excretion of urine can be charted. It is important to chart all intake, all output, the temperature, the pulse, and respiration rate.

Other General Measures.—

Sedation.—Rest lowers the oxygen requirement of the tissues and since oligæmic shock causes death by producing tissue anoxia, effective sedation is a logical procedure. It is unwise, however, in a burn of over 10 per cent surface area to administer morphine until after the transfusion or infusion fluids are running. At this time, half the calculated dose can be given intravenously and half subcutaneously.

Oxygen Therapy.—In extensively burnt patients oxygen is of value and is best administered by intranasal catheters at a rate of 3 litres per minute.

Systemic Antibiotic Therapy.—This is of some value and should be given as soon as possible, either intramuscularly, or in the intravenous fluid, in a dosage of 1 mega unit of penicillin in each 24 hours.

Local Treatment.—The local problem in burns is infection, but routine recourse to antibiotics should be avoided. In Burn Units there must be unlimited facilities for the segregation of patients whose wounds become infected. As in all types of wounds, the open burn wound must be closed and the closure maintained. A superficial burn, most commonly caused by hot fluid, can be considered an 'open' wound because the injured surface has lost its protective covering, and so is exposed to infection. The formation of a protective plasma pellicle is to be encouraged in order to close the wound.

A deep burn, caused most commonly by flame, can be considered a 'closed' wound because the covering skin, although coagulated, is present, and this eschar forms a protective covering.

There is general agreement that in any form of wound the perfect dressing to control infection is skin. Next in order of efficacy is the pellicle formed by the clotting of plasma and, third, the eschar covering a deep burn. Each and all of these coverings, if utilized in local care, are of more value than any known form of synthetic dressing.

Though the pellicle and eschar give some protection from infection, they allow considerable loss of fluid by insensible evaporation. It is necessary to allow for this in the daily fluid requirements. At the period of separation of the eschar there is also considerable nitrogen and sodium loss.

The following types of burn require special consideration, for emergency measures are often required.

1. Burns of the Face and Neck with inhalation of steam or hot fumes, which are prone to be followed by œdema of the tracheal mucous membrane, respiratory embarrassment, and even œdema of the lungs.

Encircling Deep Burns of the Neck, which may also lead to constriction of the trachea. Careful watch is kept on the quality and rate of respirations and for evidence of the escape of fine froth from the mouth. If examination of the mucous lining of the pharynx indicates obvious irritative œdema, immediate tracheostomy should be carried out.

2. Deep Burns of the Extremities, in which careful assessment during the first 12 hours reveals inadequacy of the circulation to the fingers and toes. Releasing incisions made through the eschars may preserve the viability of digits and even of hands or feet.

3. Comparatively Small, Deep Burns.—An obviously full-thickness, clearly demarcated burn over an area insufficiently large to cause shock should be excised immediately and covered with a free skin-graft or a flap.

Cleansing: Most burns will not fall into any of these three categories, and the following steps in local care are advised once shock is controlled:—

a. Cleanse the burn and surrounding skin (under strictly aseptic conditions) with 1 per cent cetrimide. A light inhalation anæsthetic may be necessary, but more frequently a small dose of morphine or nepenthe provides adequate sedation.

b. Keep the affected part dry, cool, and, if possible, exposed to light. This encourages a plasma pellicle to form and keeps an eschar firm.

c. Elevate and immobilize the affected part.

The aims are, therefore, to prevent, or at any rate to limit, infection and to avoid further skin damage. The ideal local condition is *dryness* and this is achieved by one of two measures, (*a*) the exposure technique and (*b*) the dressing technique. In each method skilful nursing is essential and poor results follow both exposure neglect and inadequate or soppy dressings, i.e., dressing neglect. The application of antibiotics in any form is not advocated.

Exposure Technique.—The burnt surface is left exposed to the air of the room or ward, the temperature of which must be kept at between 18° and 21°C. (65°–70° F.). A bed cradle, covered with a clean sheet, protects the injured surface and where possible immobilization is accomplished by restraining bands or splints on an extremity or extremities, thereby obviating cracks in the pellicle.

Limbs are positioned to limit œdema. In superficial and deep dermal burns crusts will form within 48 to 60 hours. In superficial burns the crusts separate in 2 weeks; in deep dermal burns in 3–4 weeks.

The exposure technique is not universally applicable, for example in:—

1. Circumferential burns of the trunk and neck—since the undersurface cannot be exposed, and so tends to become moist.

2. Burns of the hand—because (*a*) the digital webs are liable to become moist and (*b*) the position of function should be maintained.

3. Burns that have required releasing incisions.

Dressing Technique.—The burn is covered with non-greasy tulle gras, and over this is placed a dry absorptive dressing. The absorptive material most favoured is Gamgee tissue, sterilized in large rolls and cut to pattern with appropriate large scissors; for instance one piece is fashioned to clothe the posterior part of the trunk and to encircle completely one lower extremity, while a second piece is so cut as to cover the anterior part of the trunk and to encircle the other lower extremity. The dressing must contact the whole burnt area evenly, and should be fixed in position by conforming (e.g., crêpe) bandages. To be effective, the dressings must be constantly absorptive, and if they become moist they must be renewed. Dressings are not infallible, and they can permit infection as readily as they prevent it. *Figs.* 52 and 53 illustrate a burn of the hand in which this method was employed successfully.

Superficial burns, once the crusts have formed and irrespective of the presence or absence of a dressing, are 'closed', and heal by first intention in 3 weeks.

Nursing of Exposed Burns.—Nursing is modified according to the parts involved:—

Face: The patient is nursed on his back. The eyelids, the vestibule of the nose, the lips, and the external auditory canals are smeared lightly with paraffin molle. Any discharge from the eyes, nose, or ears is wiped away.

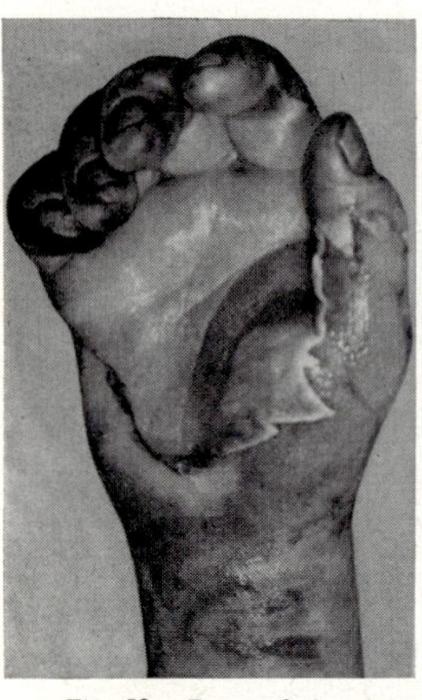
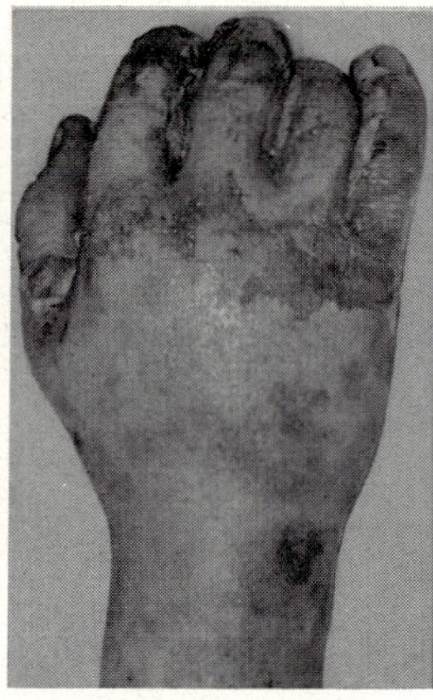
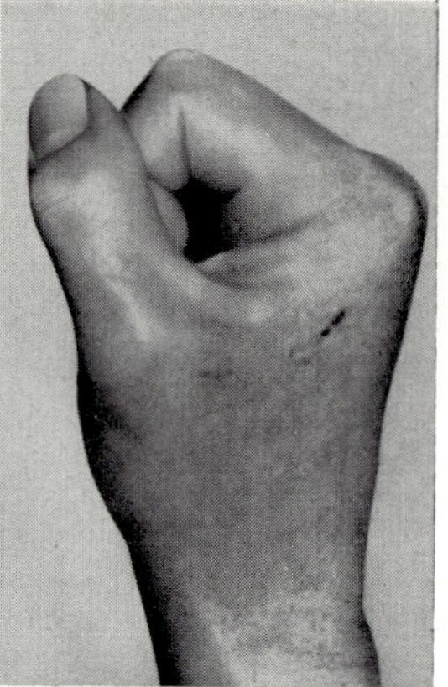

Fig. 52.—Burn of the right hand of a miner treated by absorptive dressings and elevation.

Fig. 53.—Healed within 3 weeks, without grafting.

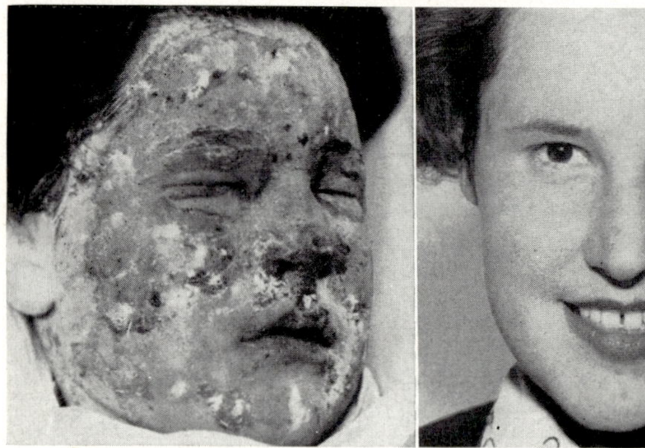
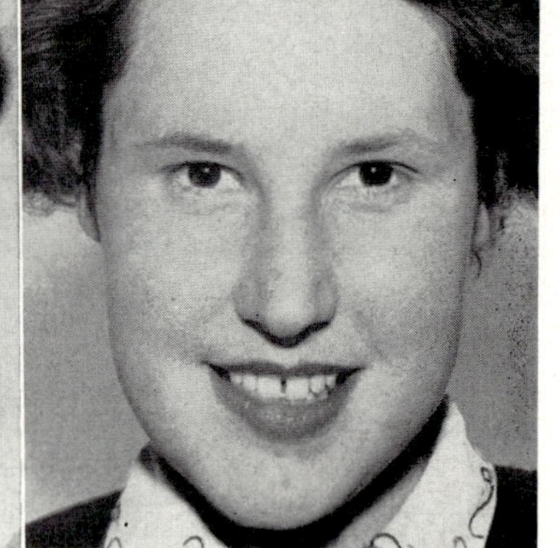

Fig. 54.—Petrol flash burn of face which was treated by exposure. Healed in 3 weeks.

Within about 6 hours the eyelids close from œdema, rendering the patient relatively helpless until the fluid is reabsorbed on the third and fourth days (*Fig.* 54).

Neck: Some hyperextension is required, and it can be secured by placing extra pillows under the shoulders or by lowering the head.

Trunk and Abdomen: When possible the patient lies on the unaffected aspect. When both aspects are involved, a sectional mattress, which allows sections underlying the burnt areas to be removed, is a great advantage. When the burns are superficial, if it is feasible, the patient is allowed up as early as the fourth day.

Buttocks: In children the lower extremities are raised by skin-traction applied via a gallows splint until the buttocks are off the bed. Adults are nursed prone with the legs slightly abducted.

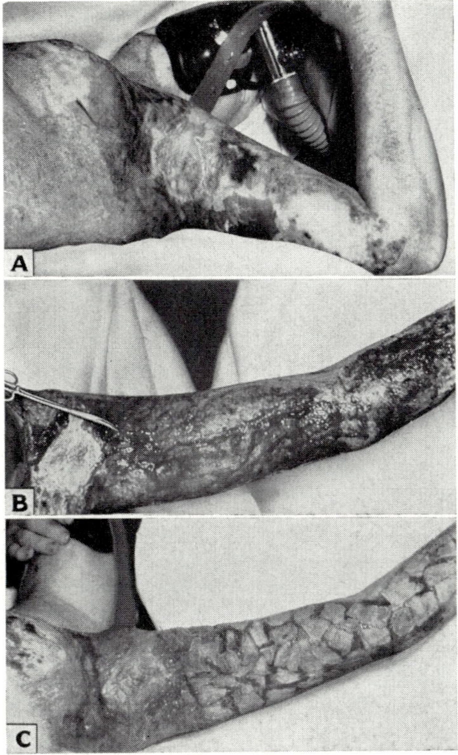

Fig. 55.—A, Flame burn of arm and trunk before being dressed; B, Excision of burn on the ninth day; C, After the application of razor grafts on the fifteenth day.

Lower Extremities: The method of fixation varies according to the distribution of the burns, the choice being between skin-traction, suspension, plaster shells, or simple exposure without splinting. The patient with burns of the *genitalia* is nursed on his back with the legs moderately abducted.

Circumferential burns are notoriously difficult to treat. It is wrong, in the first 12 hours, to cover a circumferential burn, especially of a limb, with dressings. Such a burn should be exposed, the limb elevated, and the distal circulation scrutinized frequently. When deemed necessary, incisions to relieve excessive tension in fingers, hands, forearms, and upper arms often have dramatic results. In such instances, had the limbs been covered, the danger signals would have been obscured and tragedy could not have been averted. In a similar manner, patients with circumferential burns of the neck must be watched for signs of tracheal compression. Tracheostomy or endotracheal intubation may have to be performed urgently.

Deep Burns.—The local control of deep burns is entirely different from that of superficial burns, though the closed wound concept is maintained.

The deep burn dry cover is the original eschar, and a therapeutic dressing, therefore, is often unnecessary. The eschar remains effective for at least 7 to

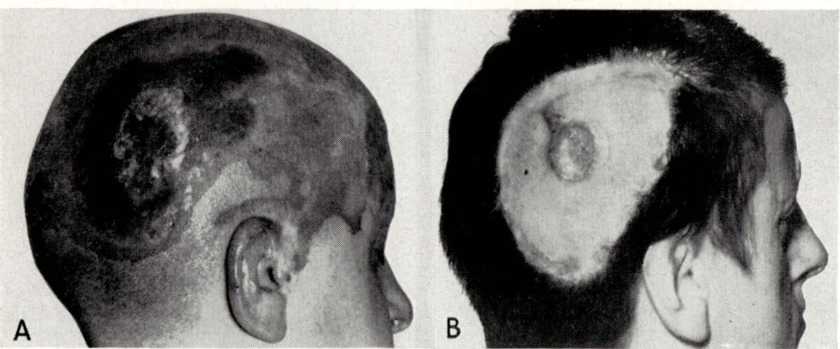

Fig. 56.—A, Fire burn (epileptic), first treated by exposure and on the fourth day by excision and dermatome graft. B, Two months later.

10 days. Because the skin has been destroyed, healing by first intention is impossible, except by surgical aid.

If the eschar is left alone for 14 to 16 days, small areas of moisture will appear, as a rule at the edges, where there is evidence of enzymatic digestion and separation of dead from living tissues. Such areas are liable to become mildly infected. It is essential to interfere before this state occurs because by this time the eschar is no longer a satisfactory dressing and the wound is no longer 'closed' but 'open'. Somewhere between the seventh and tenth days, the surgeon must decide, in every patient with deep burns, the dates of excision of the eschar and the complete covering with skin (*Figs.* 55, 56). The operations should certainly start before the fourteenth day, and before any areas of moisture occur. By so doing, it is possible to obtain healing of a deep burn in stages. The achievement of the highest objective in the treatment of burns, namely skin-grafting followed by prompt healing, is beset with difficulties that include large extent of the burn, insufficiency of suitable skin for grafting, and non-availability of veins for transfusion. Nevertheless an attempt must be made.

In children, following the employment of absorptive dressings, often it is possible to excise some of the eschar about the fourteenth day, and to continue excision of the remainder on two occasions during the next 7 days. Thus, usually complete removal of the eschar is effected by the twenty-first day with a comparatively small total loss of blood. It is most important to excise the deep burn wound when it is dry and it is equally important to cover the area completely with skin. Infection in deep burns is not a natural consequence of the injury, but of inadequate surgery and segregation. At each step the patient is protected with blood transfusion.

Nursing of Burns covered with Absorptive Dressings.—To remain absorptive it is essential that such dressings be surrounded by air. Affected extremities should be elevated; patients with circumferential burns of the trunk are best nursed slung in a hammock of stout open-meshed material, such as nylon— undoubtedly this form of nursing the patient encourages drying. If a hammock is not procurable immediately the customary waterproof or polythene covering of the ordinary mattress must be removed, because it prevents evaporation.

Indications for immediate removal and replacement of the dressings are: (*a*) the dressing becoming moist; (*b*) the dressing becoming loose or displaced; (*c*) unexplained pyrexia or local pain.

If none of these complications arises the dressing over a superficial burn is left in place for 12 days, and that of a deep dermal burn for 2 or 2½ weeks. The dressing covering a deep burn is left in place for 7 to 10 days, when it is removed and a reassessment of the depth and extent of the burn is made, and a plan is formulated for the time of excision of slough and subsequent skin-grafting, as in a deep burn treated by exposure (*see* p. 98).

OTHER ASPECTS OF THE TREATMENT OF BURNS

Toxæmia of Burns.—Undoubtedly the early clinical course of patients with extensive burns does suggest the existence of a burn toxin. In such patients on the third day, with improvement in the peripheral circulation following fluid therapy, there may develop a gradual increasing toxæmia manifested by increasing disorientation, intestinal paresis, and increased pulse- and respiration-rate. This state may be relieved by excision of eschar or the administration of convalescent serum from a burnt patient.

Skin-grafting.—Following complete excision of the eschar, the wound is closed by the application of skin, if possible by autografts. In cases of extensive burns, a skin bank *must* be available, and donors of skin arranged. The operation must be planned carefully and the time for its performance agreed upon, and shaped dressings prepared beforehand. Blood transfusion is the first step. Efficient treatment of one extensively burnt patient demands a surgical team of at least four surgeons, two nurses, and one anæsthetist.

Electrical Burns.—There is both confusion of term and thought in respect of electrical accidents. Death from electric shock is due either to cerebral paralysis or an irreversible ventricular fibrillation. However, in some cases there may result an inhibition of the respiratory and vasomotor centres, with apparent death of the patient. Obviously there is an urgency for the early and continued application of artificial respiration until the breathing is resumed or death is proven.

Following electrical accidents, there may be one of two forms of local lesion. The first is produced by heat either from a flash or by hot elements. The second is the result of the current passing through the body by contact with one or more electrodes.

The first variety most often results in a deep burn requiring excision and grafting; the second variety produces burns of varying degrees of severity which are believed to be due to specific electrical damage of tissue cells. They are manifested by small yellowish areas, or actual charring, surrounded by hyperæmia. The destruction is deep and may involve tendon, muscle, and bone. Progressive œdema ensues, while necrosis of tissue often extends beyond the limits of what was apparent earlier. This may be due to thrombosis of main vessels. Major nerves may be involved and lead to temporary or permanent paralysis. Separation of dead from living tissue is a very slow process, and the residual ulcer is frequently unreceptive to skin-grafts.

In this more severe type of electrical accident, it is unwise to carry out immediate excision, as the full extent of the necrosis is not apparent for at least six to seven days, or even longer. Rigid asepsis must be maintained. Following excision of *all* necrotic tissue, skin-flaps are frequently employed for cover. It is often necessary to sacrifice involved nerves, tendons, muscles, and bone.

Nutrition.—Following injury there is considerable loss of nitrogen; all the problems of its replacement are not yet solved. Further, the basal metabolic rate of severely burnt patients is elevated to levels comparable to those of severe hyperthyroidism. The rise is early and continues until healing. In cases of extensive burns, oral intake for the first two or three days is restricted to fluid requirements. The plan thereafter will depend on the state of the alimentary tract, and it is important to carry out routine abdominal auscultation. If peristaltic sounds are present and flatus has been passed, it is permissible to build up a gradual additional oral intake from the third or fourth day. Average normal intake of specific nutrients may not be enough and higher levels of protein, calories, and vitamins may be necessary. The amount of intake offered will correspond to age, sex, degree of trauma, weight, and previous nutrition. The upper limit of daily intake for an adult will be around 250 grammes of protein and 5000 calories.

To achieve such a high intake, a diet rich in protein (*see* p. 46) could be given, but the appetite is often so poor that it cannot be tolerated, while on operating days, or dressing days, the intake will be negligible.

The second approach is to give a free choice of diet, but add 'supplementary feeds', e.g., concentrated nutrients, which can be incorporated in a fluid formula (*see* p. 49). Examples are whole protein powder, hydrolysed liver powder, and oral fat emulsions. Important points for success are palatability and timing of administration in relation to main feeds, and also small volumes to avoid interference with appetite for the main meals.

With a régime of three supplementary feeds of 450 ml. one can introduce a minimum of 140 G. protein and over 2000 calories, and this, with the ordinary diet, makes the daily total around 200 G. protein and 3500 calories. From time to time there may be anorexia and lack of co-operation. In such cases the use of a nasogastric tube should be considered. This is of special value in children. The newer form of plastic tube is passed readily and causes little irritation. Patients soon become unaware of its presence (p. 348).

In addition to protein, carbohydrates, and fat, vitamins must be administered freely in heavy doses, and also iron. Anabolic steroids may help.

The improved results consequent upon careful nutritional balance in burnt patients are now fully established. Healing is more rapid, skin-grafts are accepted more readily, the resistance of the patient to infection appears to be increased, and blood transfusions are required less frequently.

CHAPTER X

PRE-ANÆSTHETIC AND POST-ANÆSTHETIC CARE

By W. N. ROLLASON

THE ANÆSTHETIC OUT-PATIENT CLINIC

IDEALLY all patients should be seen by the anæsthetist at the time their names are placed on the surgeon's waiting list for operation. In practice the anæsthetic clinic in Britain tends to be restricted to seeing those patients who are (1) having their varicose veins stripped or hernia repaired as out-patients, (2) those to be subjected to special techniques such as controlled hypotension, and (3) those who have systemic disease which is likely to add to the risk of the operation.

In the clinic a full history and examination is undertaken. Any tendency to cough, headache, or vomiting should be noted. Alcohol consumption, smoking habits, and exercise tolerance should be ascertained and the psyche of the patient should be assessed.

It is particularly important to inquire about current and previous drug therapy, e.g., steroids, hypotensive drugs, monoamine oxidase inhibitors, tranquillizers, antibiotics, insulin, anticoagulants, digitalis, and about any drug allergies.

Any particular fears the patient may have, such as claustrophobia associated with the use of a face mask or aichmophobia in relation to an intravenous injection, or the fear of certain techniques such as spinal anæsthesia, should be discussed and resolved. It should rarely be necessary to force an unwelcome technique on a patient.

Where appropriate special investigations are ordered. These include:—

    1. Hæmoglobin.
    2. Urinalysis.
    3. Blood-urea.
    4. Chest radiograph.
    5. Vital capacity.
    6. Peak expiratory flow measurements (p. 165).
    7. An ECG.

ASSESSMENT OF RISK

Patients are placed into one of four grades of risk depending on their physical status.

Grade I.—A normal healthy patient.

Grade II.—A patient with cardiovascular pathology, e.g., hypertension without cardiac failure, *or* respiratory pathology, e.g., mild obstructive airway disease with a vital capacity less than 2 litres and a peak expiratory flow rate less than 200 litres per minute.

Grade III.—A patient with *both* cardiovascular and respiratory pathology, e.g., recently treated cardiac failure and shortness of breath or angina at 50 yards *and* more serious severe obstructive airway disease with a vital capacity less than 1·5 litres and a peak expiratory flow rate of less than 150 litres per minute and not able to work.

Grade IV.—A patient with *both* cardiovascular and respiratory pathology of a *severe* degree, e.g., cor pulmonale, signs of cardiac failure, and an exercise tolerance of not more than 10 yards with effort.

A fifth grade may be added and would include a moribund patient not expected to survive 24 hours with or without an operation.

TREATMENT

Treatment may be instituted as an out-patient and if necessary the patient can be referred to other clinics, e.g., diabetic, dental, cardiological, for advice, so that the patient is in the best possible condition for surgery when he is admitted to hospital. Loose and carious teeth should be removed.

The treatment of anæmia and malnutrition is commenced where necessary.

In cases of obesity the anæsthetist should give the patient a 1000-calorie diet sheet which can be readily understood, and he should be requested to report for a weight check at fortnightly intervals, when encouragement or scolding may be given as appropriate.

Respiratory disease if chronic can be improved. Smoking should be given up for at least 3 weeks prior to the operation. When practicable, operations on patients with chronic bronchitis should be postponed until the better weather. The use of antibiotics, bronchodilators, physiotherapy, and postural drainage should be employed in suitable cases. If post-nasal catarrh and sinus infection are evident the patient should be referred to the E.N.T. department.

For reducing the viscosity of sputum and relieving bronchospasm the following old prescription has been found useful in practice:—

Potassium Iodide	300 mg.
Tinctura Stramonii	1 ml.
Syrupus Tolutanus	4 ml.
Chloroform water	ad 15 ml.

Fifteen ml. of this mixture are given three or four times a day after meals.

PRE-OPERATIVE PREPARATION

The anæsthetist should see the patient a day or two before his operation takes place. The anæsthetic out-patient notes are checked and any change in the patient's condition noted.

Food and drink are withheld for 6 hours preceding operation. Lipstick, nail varnish, and other cosmetics which may mask cyanosis are removed. Dentures, artificial limbs, and artificial eyes should also be taken out.

The patient is asked to pass urine prior to coming to the theatre, and if necessary should be catheterized. The bowel should be empty.

An **identification label** is applied to the wrist and where indicated the side or number of digit to be operated on is marked on the patient's skin with indelible ink.

Consent Form.—The nature of the operation *must* be explained to the patient, and his signature must be obtained for permission to operate and to administer an anæsthetic. No undertaking is given that the operation will be performed by any particular surgeon.

Emergency cases should be delayed, if possible, to allow the stomach to empty, but it must be remembered that the emptying time of the stomach may be delayed for up to 24 hours after accidents, in labour, and in the anxious patient.

Consequently, when immediate operation is essential a wide-bore stomach tube (28–32 F) is passed and aspirated until the stomach is empty. Any dehydration and electrolyte imbalance are corrected by intravenous therapy and blood is cross-matched before the patient comes to theatre in appropriate cases.

PREMEDICATION

This term was introduced in the late 1920's for the administration of drugs to ensure smooth induction and to aid the maintenance of anæsthesia. These drugs are now given for four purposes:—

1. To produce sedation and reduce metabolic rate.
2. To inhibit or modify reflex response from the autonomic nervous system.
3. To prevent post-operative nausea and vomiting.
4. To relieve pre-operative hunger in children.

Premedication should begin the night before operation in the adult and to ensure a good night's sleep a sedative should be given.

Sedative and Analgesic Drugs allay nervousness, reduce the amount of anæsthetic agent required, and reduce post-operative pain, thus preventing restlessness during the recovery period.

Parasympathetic Inhibitors such as atropine and hyoscine are necessary to suppress secretions, especially salivary, tracheobronchial, and gastric, when such agents as ether are employed. They also minimize sweating, thus lessening fluid and heat loss. It has been suggested that vagal inhibition of the heart's action may be a cause of death during anæsthesia, especially with chloroform, during intubation, and after repeated doses of suxamethonium, and that parasympathetic blockade would prevent this. However, in the doses of atropine and scopolamine used the action of the cardiac vagi is not inhibited, but may be modified.

Sympatholytic Drugs such as phentolamine and chlorpromazine may form part of the premedication. The former should be used in a patient with a phæochromocytoma (*see* p. 445), and the latter as an aid in the induction of hypothermia by inhibiting shivering and producing vasodilatation. Patients who have had or who are on steroids should receive an additional dose along with their premedication (*see* p. 445).

Anti-emetics.—Drugs of the phenothiazine group, particularly perphenazine, are powerful anti-emetics and can largely prevent post-operative nausea and vomiting. The dose is 5 mg. pre-operatively by intramuscular injection.

DOSAGE OF PREMEDICATION

In children from 3 to 8 years premedication may be given in the form of a syrup 2 hours prior to induction of anæsthesia. This allays both their hunger and their anxiety, and reduces post-operative restlessness. Trimeprazine (vallergan) forte (6 mg. per ml.) in a dose of 2 mg. per lb. has proved useful for this purpose.

Morphine.—This has been in use as opium for over 2000 years and is probably still unequalled as an analgesic. The standard adult dose is 15 mg., but this should be reduced to 10 mg. in the less robust. Infants under 6 months are very susceptible, and so are the aged, feeble, and debilitated. Children tolerate it well in doses proportional to body-weight. Generally speaking, sedation is unnecessary in children under 2 years of age and, in view of their small tidal volume, respiratory depressants should be avoided. In assessing the dose of a sedative drug it is usually sound to remember that the normal adult dose is

Vallergan (May & Baker Ltd., Dagenham, Essex).

5

based on the 10-stone (70-kg.) man and therefore a child weighing 1 stone may be given 1·5 mg. morphine.

Morphine should be given intramuscularly 1½ hours prior to the induction of anæsthesia so that the peak of respiratory depression has passed.

Morphine plus Atropine.—Morphine may be combined with atropine 0·65 mg. If the atropine sulphate is used this should be given intramuscularly ½ hour before operation, but the longer-acting atropine mucate (hyperduric) may be given with the morphine 1½ hours before operation. Atropine being a respiratory stimulant inhibits the respiratory depressant effects of morphine.

Because morphine and papaveretum (omnopon) may predispose to post-operative vomiting, constipation, and ileus, there is a tendency nowadays to rely on one of the substitutes, particularly pethidine, although omnopon in a dose of 20 mg. remains popular.

Pethidine.*—This was first synthesized in 1939 and pharmacologically is a cross between morphine and atropine. It has a morphine-like action in pain, but is about one-tenth as powerful, 100 mg. being equivalent to about 10 mg. of morphine. Like morphine it may cause hypotension if the head of the patient is raised.

It has a papaverine-like effect on the smooth muscles of the bronchioles, intestines, uterus, and arteries.

On cholinergic nerve-endings its action resembles that of atropine, causing a dry mouth and dilated pupils.

It may release histamine from the tissues and has a quinidine-like effect on the myocardium. The standard adult dose is 100 mg. and should be given intramuscularly 1½ hours before operation. This may be combined with 0·65 mg. of atropine or preferably with 0·4 mg. of hyoscine hydrobromide (scopolamine). In the aged the dose of scopolamine should be reduced to 0·2 mg., as in higher dosage it may cause restlessness and confusion.

Atropine.—This drug has been used in premedication since 1890. The dosage ranges from the small dose of 0·15 mg. in the neonate, where there is virtually no respiratory tract secretion for the first 2 or 3 days of life, to 0·65–1·0 mg. in the adult. The higher dosage is indicated in those with sinus bradycardia and in those undergoing electroplexy, which procedure may produce a bradycardia. If atropine is given in a dose of 0·8 mg. by mouth 1½ hours to 2 hours before operation it acts as well as 0·65 mg. given intramuscularly ½ hour before surgery.

Contra-indication.—In cases of gross tachycardia, e.g., thyrotoxicosis, hyper-pyrexia, or heart disease (particularly mitral stenosis with a fixed output), atropine should be avoided. It should also be avoided in patients who have a phæochromocytoma.

Hyoscine (Scopolamine).—This has been used in premedication since 1900. It is a better drying agent than atropine. It is a mild respiratory stimulant and tachycardia is not often seen. It is a depressant of the central nervous system causing drowsiness, sleep, and amnesia in some patients.

In an adult the combination of scopolamine 0·4 mg. with pethidine 100 mg. or papaveretum 20 mg. forms a useful sedative before operation.

Barbiturates.—The medium-acting barbiturates amylobarbitone (sodium amytal), pentobarbitone (nembutal), quinalbarbitone (seconal), and butobarbitone (soneryl) are useful for sedation for the night before operation (*Table VI*). As these drugs antagonize the convulsant effects of local analgesic drugs they are

---

* Pethidine is known as demerol in the U.S.A.

suitable in the premedication of patients to be operated on under local analgesia. Tuinal is a mixture of quinalbarbitone and amylobarbitone.

There is less hangover with soneryl than with the other barbiturates given in comparable dosage. It acts for 8–10 hours and so is useful for the early morning wakefulness of old age. Soneryl may also be combined with the anti-histaminic

Table VI.—BARBITURATE DRUGS USED FOR PRE-ANÆSTHETIC SEDATION

APPROVED NAME	TRADE NAME	CAPSULE COLOUR	ADULT DOSAGE (mg.)
Amylobarbitone	Sodium amytal	Green	200
Pentobarbitone	Nembutal	Yellow	100–200
Quinalbarbitone	Seconal	Scarlet	100–200
Butobarbitone	Soneryl	White	200

phenergan (promethazine) in the form of sonergan, and this constitutes a useful hypnotic. Each tablet contains 75 mg. butobarbitone and 15 mg. promethazine. The dose is 2 tablets at night time.

Chloral Hydrate.—This is a safe hypnotic, leaves no hangover, and does not produce confusion in the elderly. It is perhaps not used as much as it should be. The hypnotic dose is 1–2 G. It should be well diluted as it can be rather irritating to the alimentary canal. It can also be supplied in tablet form under the names of welldorm (650 mg. dichloralphenazone) and tricloryl (0·5 G. triclofos). The dose is 2 tablets at bedtime. The effect of the drug comes on within an hour and lasts for about 8 hours.

It can also be supplied in the form of a syrup for children and the dose is 0·3 g. per stone (47 mg. per kg.) body-weight.

Paraldehyde.—This is a useful and very safe hypnotic, particularly in the elderly restless patient. The dose is 1–2 drachms (2–4 ml.) orally and the effect comes on in 30 minutes after administration. It does not depress the heart or the respiration, but its stench is its chief disadvantage. In a restless and confused adult 5–10 ml. may be injected intramuscularly. Paraldehyde is self-sterilizing and the dose may be drawn straight from the ampoule.

BASAL NARCOSIS

This is a state produced when premedication is given in doses large enough to cause deep sleep. The patient is put to sleep by a rectal administration in the ward. Medical supervision is essential in case the airway should become obstructed once the patient falls asleep.

Paraldehyde is a safe and efficient basal narcotic. The dose is 4 ml. per stone (6·4 kg.) body-weight up to 40 ml. diluted with olive oil or saline to a 10 per cent solution (approximately 30 ml. of diluent to each 3 ml. of paraldehyde). Paraldehyde should be given ¾–1 hour before operation.

Thiopentone sodium (pentothal) in a dose of 40 mg. per kg. body-weight may also be used. It is diluted with water to make a 5 per cent solution (0·5 G. in 10 ml. water). Sleep occurs in 10–30 minutes.

Either drug is introduced slowly into the rectum by a fine multi-holed catheter whose tip lies about 8 cm. above the anal margin in the adult. The patient should lie on his left side with the buttocks raised by a pillow. This increases

Sodium amytal; Seconal; Tuinal (Eli Lilly & Co. Ltd., Basingstoke, Hants).
Nembutal (Abbott Laboratories Ltd., Queenborough, Kent).
Soneryl; Phenergan; Sonergan (May & Baker, Ltd., Dagenham, Essex).
Pentothal (Abbott Laboratories, Queenborough, Kent).
Tricloryl (Glaxo Laboratories Ltd., Greenford, Middlesex).
Welldorm (Smith & Nephew Pharmaceuticals Ltd., Welwyn Garden City, Herts).

the absorptive area and prevents respiratory obstruction occurring after consciousness has been lost. Careful watching, however, is essential and the patient must not be left unattended.

Tribromethanol (avertin) has been widely used in the past, but its popularity is dwindling, particularly as it is potentially toxic to the liver and kidney.

MODIFICATIONS OF DOSAGE

It is important to remember that the usual adult dose of premedication must be modified in a variety of circumstances.

1. Infants and Children.—Atropine only should be given under the age of 2. Barbiturates should in general be avoided as they predispose to post-operative restlessness. With modern anæsthetic techniques and the correct approach children do well with no premedication at all, but atropine should be given if ether is to be used. Methohexitone (brietal sodium) may be given intramuscularly (6·6 mg. per kg. in a 2 per cent solution) and provides effective basal narcosis in children; it is only given under medical supervision.

2. The Aged.—Owing to the lowered basal metabolic rate and the liability to post-operative pulmonary complications overdosage must be avoided. To prevent confusion the dose of scopolamine should not exceed 0·2 mg.

3. In Shock.—The failure of the peripheral circulation may delay absorption of drugs. Premedication should be given intravenously very slowly and well diluted in these circumstances. Care must be taken to ensure that morphine has not previously been given. In both shock and toxaemia doses of sedative drugs should be halved.

4. In Out-patients.—Here all sedatives must be avoided on account of the risk of subsequent psychological upset and impairment of judgement after leaving hospital. If deemed necessary the normal dose of atropine may be given.

5. In Respiratory Infection.—Here respiratory depressants should be avoided, and in the asthmatic cortisone and aminophylline must be available. Avoid operation if at all possible.

6. In Heart Disease.—In uncompensated heart disease increased sedation is indicated as anxiety and a stormy induction may precipitate acute pulmonary œdema.

7. In Fever.—Owing to the effect of atropine and scopolamine in reducing sweating, and thus heat-loss, these drugs should be used with great caution when the patient is pyrexial. This applies with even greater force in children in whom convulsions may be precipitated more easily than in adults, especially if the work of spontaneous respiration is permitted during anæsthesia.

Induction and maintenance of anæsthesia will be discussed in the next chapter.

POST-OPERATIVE MEDICATION

Object.—The problem here is to eliminate pain, anxiety, and nausea without producing respiratory depression, but no sedative drug should be administered until the patient has regained full consciousness.

Position.—Until consciousness is restored the patient should, where practicable, be nursed in the tonsil position (*Fig.* 57). The foot of the bed should be elevated. In major cases oxygen should be administered for the first 3 post-operative hours, and the blood-pressure and pulse-rate should be frequently checked.

Supervision.—No unconscious patient should ever be left unattended.

Avertin (Bayer Products Co., Surbiton-on-Thames, Surrey).
Brietal sodium (Eli Lilly & Co. Ltd., Basingstoke, Hants).

DRUGS FOR POST-OPERATIVE MEDICATION

Methadone (Physeptone).—This is an analgesic with a similar effect to that of morphine. It can be given by mouth or by injection, and is most useful in the treatment of post-operative pain. Like pethidine it may relieve muscle spasm. It is also useful to relieve the pain associated with paralytic ileus as it does not produce the spastic inactivity of the bowel seen with morphine. The standard adult dose is 10 mg.

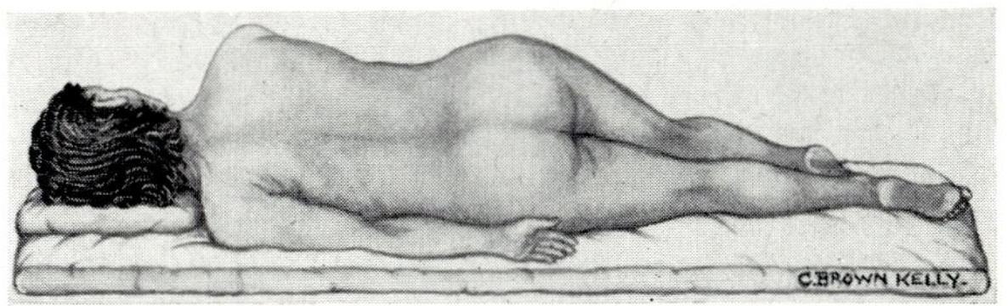

Fig. 57.—Optimum position for a patient while recovering from a general anæsthetic.

Anti-emetics.—It is the author's practice to combine physeptone with 5 mg. perphenazine (fentazin) to also eliminate any tendency to nausea and vomiting.

Other Powerful Analgesics.—Pethidine, morphine, and omnopon may all be used to relieve post-operative pain. Nepenthe (tincture of opium) is given to a child in a dose of 1 drop for each year of age. One drop of nepenthe contains 0·66 mg. morphine.

For minor post-operative discomfort paracetamol (panadol), a derivative of phenacetin, is a useful drug. The dose is 0·5–1·0 G. Disprin and veganin are others, but the latter is constipating. The adult dose for each is 2 tablets 4-hourly if required.

Where there is a combination of discomfort and anxiety 2 tablets of sonalgin (butobarbitone 60 mg., codeine 10 mg., phenacetin 225 mg.) may be useful at bedtime.

For restlessness in the elderly promazine (sparine), chloral, or paraldehyde are useful drugs.

Local Anæsthetic Blocks.—Where pain is prominent, such as after thoracic and upper abdominal surgery, and after hæmorrhoidectomy, epidural and caudal blocks are performed in some units. Alternatively, infiltration of the intercostal nerves and the perianal region with 1 per cent lignocaine in 10 per cent dextran has proved successful and popular in some clinics.

Panadol (Bayer Products Co., Surbiton-on-Thames, Surrey).
Physeptone (Burroughs, Wellcome & Co., Euston Road, London, N.W.1).
Fentazin (Allen & Hanbury, Ltd., London, E.2).
Disprin (Reckitt & Sons Ltd., Hull, Yorks).
Veganin (William R. Warner & Co. Ltd., Eastleigh, Hants).
Sonalgin (May & Baker, Ltd., Dagenham, Essex).
Sparine (John Wyeth & Brother Ltd., Taplow, Maidenhead, Berks).

CHAPTER XI

ANÆSTHESIA, GENERAL AND LOCAL

By W. N. ROLLASON

THE occasional anæsthetist should be able to give an anæsthetic which is simple, safe, and satisfactory, but to do this he must remember to work within the limits of his capability and to refer difficult cases to an experienced colleague. He must keep his head in emergencies and develop that discipline of reaction which will enable him to act unerringly and at speed. He should never sacrifice safety for convenience and he should bear in mind that the administration of anæsthetics can only be learnt in the operating theatre or dental surgery under supervision. All-round confidence, expertise, and appreciation of the broader aspects of the specialty can only be achieved by spending at least 6 months in a teaching department of anæsthetics.

ROUTES OF ADMINISTRATION

Anæsthetics may be introduced into the body by various routes: by absorption from the lungs; by direct injection into a vein; by intramuscular injection; by absorption from the stomach; or by absorption from the rectum. No matter

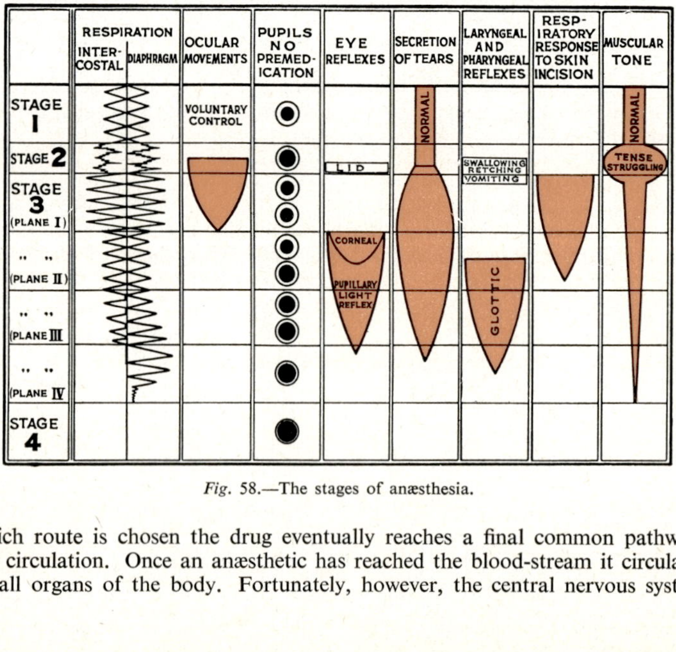

Fig. 58.—The stages of anæsthesia.

which route is chosen the drug eventually reaches a final common pathway, the circulation. Once an anæsthetic has reached the blood-stream it circulates to all organs of the body. Fortunately, however, the central nervous system upon which the drug is required to act receives a greater proportion of the anæsthetic than any other part due to its rich blood-supply. The effect produced can be seen as different layers of the brain are progressively affected by the anæsthetic and forms the basis of the signs and stages of anæsthesia described by Guedel for ether in 1920 (*Fig. 58*).

STAGES AND SIGNS OF ANÆSTHESIA

1st Stage.—This is known as the stage of analgesia or the stage of disorientation. The patient remains conscious but becomes progressively sleepy and analgesic. While providentially the first sense to go is that of smell, it should be remembered that the last sense to disappear is that of hearing and for a time this may become more acute. It is accordingly important to be on guard with one's remarks both during induction and recovery from anæsthesia. At the bottom of this stage the patient passes through a state called *amnalgesia*, where although his eyelash and swallowing reflexes are still present he is unaware of pain, and although he may move when a stimulus is applied, such as the extraction of a tooth, he has no recollection of anything unpleasant. This ultra-light stage of anæsthesia is now widely used in chairside dental anæsthetic practice.

2nd Stage.—This is known as the stage of delirium or excitement or the stage of uninhibited response. The eyelash reflex disappears and the patient becomes quite unconscious. The patient may move, his pupils dilate, the eyeballs rove, and breathing is irregular, but the cough and vomiting reflexes are still present.

3rd Stage.—This is known as the stage of surgical anæsthesia and is characterized by the onset of regular automatic respiration. This stage is divided into four planes:—

First Plane.—In the upper part of this plane the eyelid, swallowing, and vomiting reflexes disappear and at the bottom of this plane the eyeballs become fixed and central.

Second Plane.—In the lower portion of this plane the respiratory response to a skin incision ceases, the pupils are dilated, and the corneal reflex disappears.

Third Plane.—At the onset of this plane a lag develops in the intercostal component of respiration, and at the bottom of this plane intercostal respiration ceases, giving rise to the external paradoxical 'see-saw' pattern of respiration where as the abdomen rises the chest is sucked in. A similar type of respiration may accompany respiratory obstruction or partial curarization.

Fourth Plane.—This plane is characterized by diaphragmatic breathing, widely dilated pupils, absence of the corneal light reflex; the secretion of tears ceases and the laryngeal reflex disappears. At the lower border of this plane diaphragmatic breathing becomes shallow and muscular relaxation is profound.

More recently it has been suggested that the stage of surgical anæsthesia should be divided into only three planes:—
1. Light—until the eyeballs become fixed.
2. Medium—increasing intercostal paralysis.
3. Deep—diaphragmatic respiration.

4th Stage (or the stage of overdosage).—Entry into this stage is characterized by the cessation of respiration, with pallor and cyanosis, and this is quickly followed by cardiac failure and death.

During recovery the same changes take place in the reverse order.

The journey of anæsthesia is accordingly a potentially hazardous one from consciousness towards death, and the safe and reliable anæsthetist ensures that his passenger has a return ticket.

1. ADMINISTRATION OF INHALATION ANÆSTHETICS

The following should be available before induction of anæsthesia: a prop, mouth gag, tongue forceps, pharyngeal airway, nasopharyngeal tube, face-mask, laryngoscope, and endotracheal tubes.

Nowadays inhalation anæsthesia is more often used for *maintaining* anæsthesia as the intravenous, short-acting, barbiturates are usually used for *induction* except in the very young. Moreover, the introduction of curare into clinical practice in 1942 simplified the technique of endotracheal intubation and the maintenance of abdominal relaxation in light planes of anæsthesia, and has tended to replace regional nerve-block techniques in abdominal surgery. Nevertheless, the occasional anæsthetist should be aware of the difficulties he may have to face when administering an inhalational anæsthetic, the most important being respiratory obstruction.

RESPIRATORY OBSTRUCTION

The signs of respiratory obstruction are cyanosis, the use of the accessory muscles of respiration, and external paradoxical respiration—the latter being associated with an indrawing of the upper chest and an outpushing of the abdomen due to strong diaphragmatic action, the lower thoracic region being almost at rest.

Causes of Obstruction.—

1. Obstruction may be caused by the lips in edentulous patients and a Thornton's or London Hospital mouth prop should be inserted (*Fig.* 59).

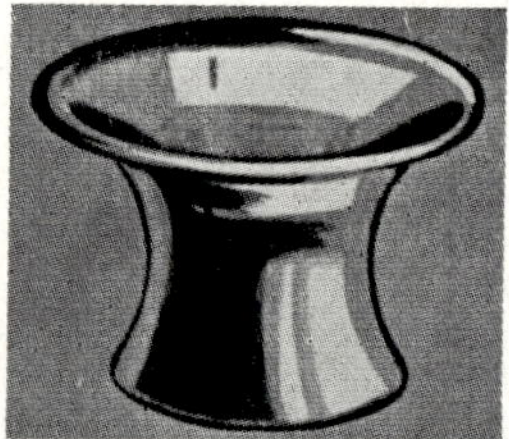

Fig. 59.—London Hospital mouth prop.

2. It may be due to the falling back of the *tongue* and the lower jaw must be pushed forward by pressure behind the angle of the mandible. If this does not relieve the obstruction a well-lubricated nasopharyngeal tube (*Fig.* 60) should

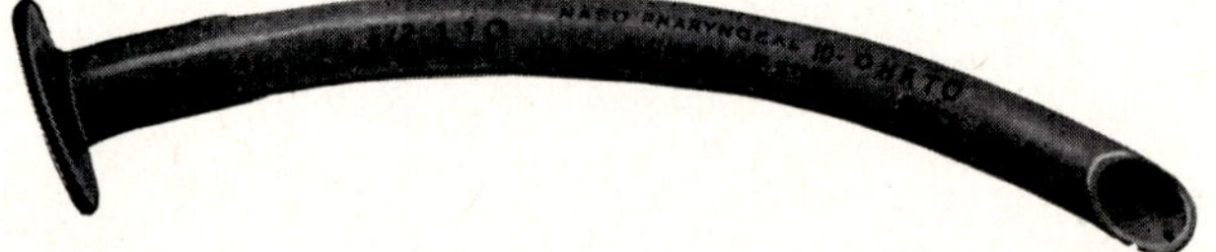

Fig. 60.—Nasopharyngeal tube.

be inserted into the nostril and manipulated so that its distal end lies just beyond the obstruction. It is useful to remember that the distance from the nares to the epiglottis equals that between the nares and the tragus of the ear. With the tube in place and obstruction relieved, anæsthesia is deepened until the jaw relaxes when a pharyngeal airway can be inserted (*Fig.* 61).

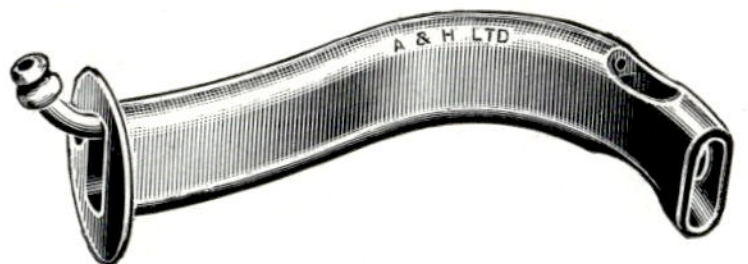

Fig. 61.—Pharyngeal airway.

3. Obstruction above the *glottis* may be due to a foreign body, saliva, vomitus, blood, or œdema. To relieve these cases lower the head of the table, open the jaw using a gag with Ackland's jaws (*Fig.* 62), withdraw the tongue, apply suction,

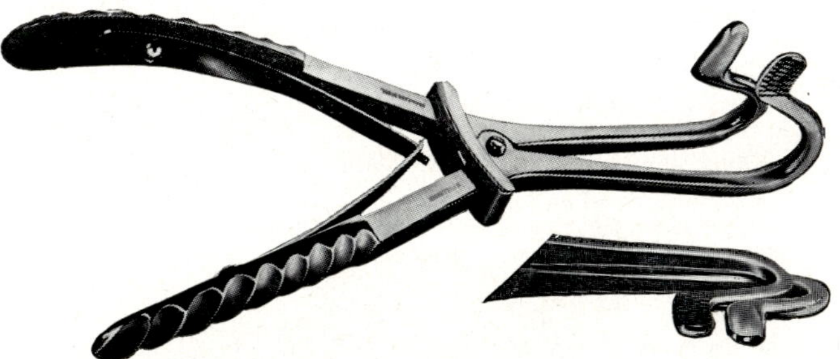

Fig. 62.—Gag with Ackland jaws for opening the mouth. *Inset,* Ackland jaws closed.

and administer oxygen. If unsuccessful, laryngoscopy and intubation may be necessary (*see* p. 120). If an endotracheal tube cannot be inserted, apply pressure to a reservoir bag filled with oxygen after closing the expiratory valve and holding the mask firmly on the face with the jaw well supported

If the patient is *in extremis* a large needle or cricothyrotomy cannula should be inserted through the cricothyroid membrane and 500 ml. of oxygen insufflated through it. Tracheostomy is needed only on the rarest occasions.

TECHNIQUES OF ADMINISTRATION

1. Open Ether.—Atropine or scopolamine should be given as premedication. A Schimmelbusch mask (*Fig.* 63) is covered with fifteen thicknesses of gauze. After induction a gamgee pad with a hole for the nose and mouth can be allowed to separate the mask from the face, so cutting down air leaks. Because of the irritant properties of ether it is customary now to induce anæsthesia with halothane.

Halothane is the modern chloroform without the hazards of primary cardiac arrest and acute atrophy of the liver associated with the latter agent. The quantity of halothane that can be used safely in the fit adult is up to 4 ml. It is dropped on to the mask and the ether is commenced immediately the halothane is finished. Less than 4 ml. of halothane should be used for induction in the frail or shocked patient. One to two litres per minute of oxygen should be run under the mask by catheter to compensate for the reduction in oxygen tension due to displacement of atmospheric oxygen by carbon dioxide and by ether vapour. Concentrations of ether vapour up to 15 per cent are readily tolerated after halothane induction.

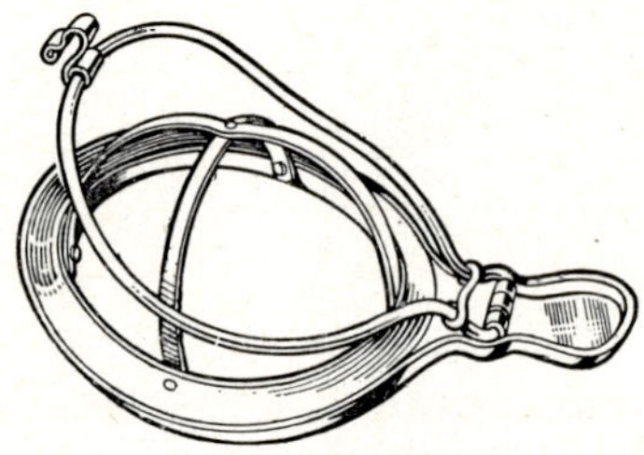

Fig. 63.—Schimmelbusch mask.

The optimal level of anæsthesia—to exist for the major part of most operations—is when the patient's pupils are centrally fixed and full ventilatory excursion of the chest occurs with each unobstructed breath (Stage 3, Plane 2). Ether is dropped steadily on to the mask to keep it damp (not saturated).

Anæsthesia by open mask results in considerable heat loss to the patient but the advantages of the method are its safety, cheapness, portability, and ease of administration.

The Risk of Explosion.—With ether this danger must always be borne in mind.

A self-fitting bag of the Ambu type (*Fig.* 64) should always be available in case ventilation should need to be augmented.

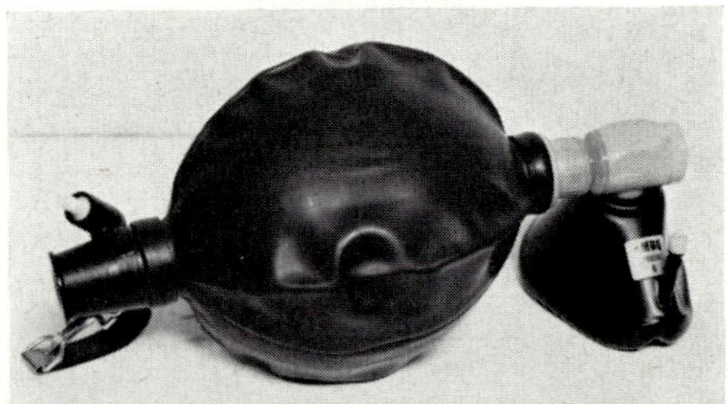

Fig. 64.—An Ambu bag for augmenting pulmonary ventilation or for artificial respiration.

2. Semi-closed Ether.—Continuous-flow machines such as the Boyle (*Fig.* 65) or intermittent-flow machines such as the Walton V or the Cyprane A.E. (*Fig.* 66) may be used. In the continuous-flow machines gases are delivered from cylinders and their rate is measured by flow meters. Gases can be directed over the surface or bubbled through the ether in the ether bottle. Wide-bore corrugated tubing, which prevents kinking, connects the machine with the face-piece, while near the machine is a reservoir bag, and near the mask an expiratory valve. After seeing that the cylinders of nitrous oxide, oxygen, and carbon dioxide are correctly coupled, unconsciousness is produced by a flow of 8 litres of nitrous oxide and 2 litres of oxygen and 0·5–1 per cent halothane from a flow and temperature-compensated vaporizer (*Fig.* 67).

The face-piece is held a couple of inches (5 cm.) away from the patient's face and hypnotic suggestion can with advantage be used. When consciousness is lost (as evidenced by absence of the eyelash reflex and failure to respond to a question), the mask is applied to the face and the ether tap is turned to its minimal

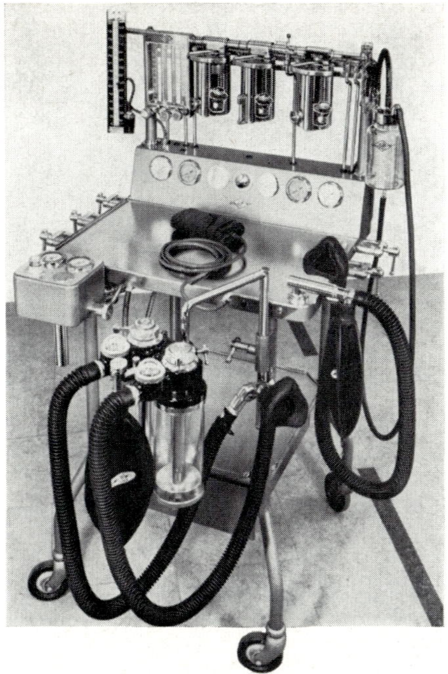

Fig. 65.—Boyle-Cavendish anæsthetic machine.

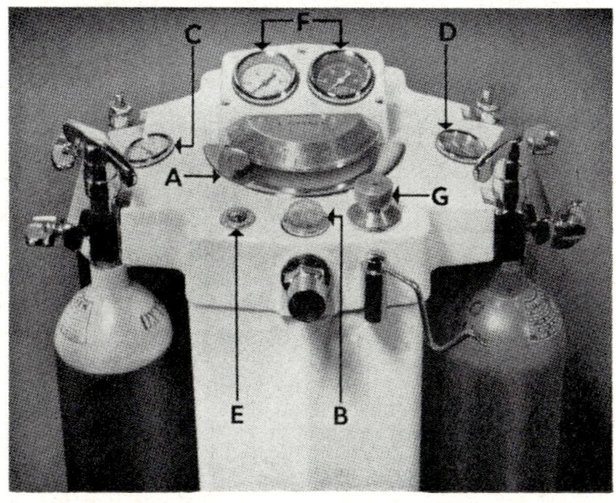

Fig. 66.—Cyprane, A.E. intermittent-flow anæsthetic machine. A, Mixture control. B, Breathing indicator. C, D, Cylinder pressure gauges. E, Emergency oxygen button. F, Delivery pressure gauges.

vaporizing position. The halothane may be increased to 2 per cent for a few breaths and then turned off while the ether tap is progressively turned every few breaths until it is full on, and then the plunger is depressed as fast as the patient will tolerate the increase in vapour strength. The addition of 0·5 litre

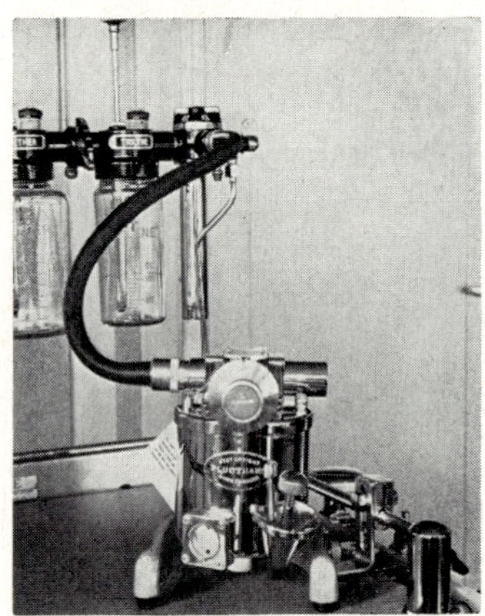

Fig. 67.—Flow and temperature-compensated vaporizer (Fluotec).

per minute of carbon dioxide will speed up the induction. Maintenance of anæsthesia can usually be smoothly carried along with the gases passing over the surface of the ether.

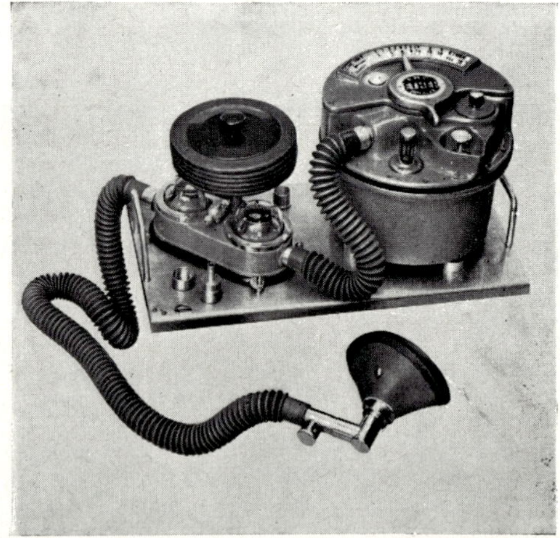

Fig. 68.—E.M.O. inhaler for the administration of ether vapour.

It is advisable that the total flow of gases should not be less than 8 litres and the oxygen percentage should be 25. This can be achieved by administering

6 litres of nitrous oxide and 2 litres of oxygen. The tension on the spring of the expiratory valve should be as light as possible.

If halothane is felt to be too expensive or is not available, anæsthesia may be induced with trichloroethylene before adding the ether.

Addition of Halothane or Trichloroethylene.—The nitrous oxide and oxygen from intermittent-flow machines are at predetermined pressures and of predetermined percentage, and are delivered to the patient only when he inspires when the pressure is zero. The gases can be diverted over halothane or trichloroethylene and then over ether in vaporizing bottles. For induction the pressure is set at 5 mm. Hg and 80 per cent nitrous oxide, 20 per cent oxygen, and a trace of halothane or trichloroethylene is delivered with the mask held 2 in. (5 cm.) from the patient's face as before, until consciousness is lost. Then the mask is applied

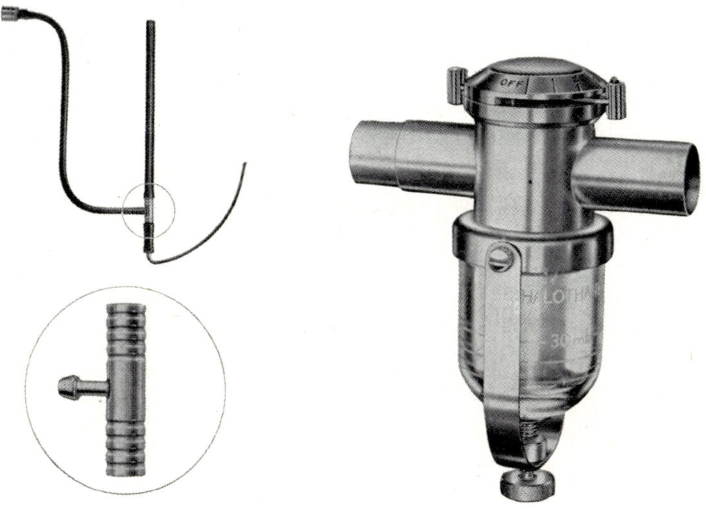

<table>
<tr><td>Fig. 69.—Ayre's T-piece.</td><td>Fig. 70.—Goldmann halothane vaporizer.</td></tr>
</table>

to the face and the ether pointer is turned to its minimal position. The recent introduction of premixed gases from a single cylinder and sensitive demand valves will probably replace the intermittent-flow machines.

The T-piece Technique.—This is used in infants and young children to prevent dilution of unexpired gases with air on the one hand, or rebreathing with carbon dioxide accumulation on the other hand. The total gas flow should be about twice the minute volume of the patient and the volume of the reservoir tube (*Fig.* 69) equal to about one-third of the tidal volume.

Draw-over Ether.—Here the E.M.O. (Epstein, Macintosh, Oxford) Inhaler is useful (*Fig.* 68). It will deliver a predetermined concentration of ether vapour in air, irrespective of changes in the temperature of the liquid anæsthetic, and is controlled by an automatic thermocompensator mechanism. A water compartment acts as a heat buffer. A Goldmann halothane vaporizer (*Fig.* 70) renders induction of anæsthesia speedy, safe, and smooth. If necessary, the air can be enriched with oxygen administered via a nipple attached to the machine.

The apparatus is useful in countries where nitrous oxide is not readily available or when portability is important.

For light anæsthesia with spontaneous respiration the patient should breathe ether in concentrations gradually increasing to 15 per cent, after which it may be reduced to 7 per cent for maintenance.

Controlled Respiration.—For controlled respiration induction with an intravenous barbiturate such as thiopentone is followed by intubation after using a non-depolarizing relaxant such as suxamethonium, and 5 per cent ether in air is then administered reducing to 3 per cent for maintenance which has proved to be very satisfactory.

Explosions have not been described during the administration of ether and air even when diathermy has been used.

3. Closed-circuit Ether.—With ether induction is quicker when a semi-closed circuit is used to begin with. The closed circuit is based on the principle that if sufficient oxygen is added to supply the body's basal needs and carbon dioxide is absorbed, the same mixture of gases can be used repeatedly as it is exhaled unchanged. Basal oxygen varies between 200 and 400 ml. per min. and the exhaled carbon dioxide is absorbed by soda lime as represented schematically in the following diagram:—

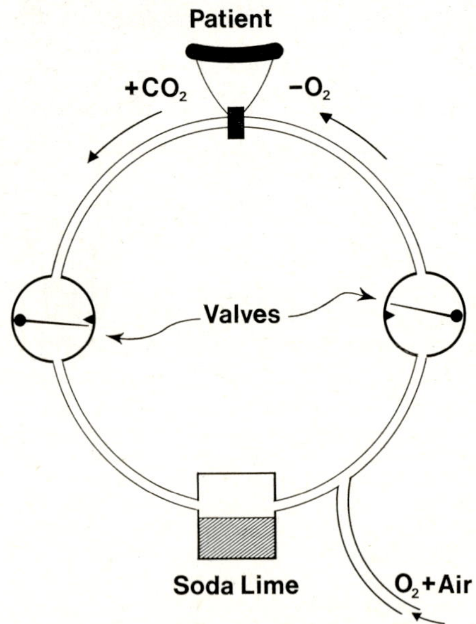

In the Marrett closed-circuit machine (*Fig.* 71) the ether vaporizer is *inside* the circuit so that the patient's respirations pass through it and a high concentration of vapour can be rapidly built up. In the Boyle's closed-circuit machine the ether vaporizer is *outside* the circuit and only the fresh gas flow passes over it. It is safer to use if controlled respiration is to be employed, as dangerously high concentrations of ether are less likely to be built up.

Warning.—Trichloroethylene must never be used in association with a closed circuit as it combines with soda lime to form toxic products, the most important being dichloracetylene which may produce paralysis of the cranial nerves or even death.

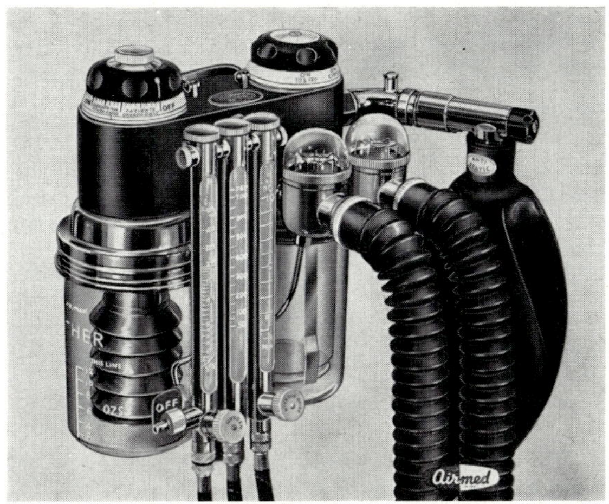

Fig. 71.—Marrett closed-circuit machine.

Generally speaking the occasional anæsthetist should eschew the closed circuit and restrict himself to the simpler methods discussed earlier, and become thoroughly familiar with just a few agents, such as nitrous oxide, oxygen, halothane, and ether.

SHOCK

Apart from the observation of the signs which indicate the depth of anæsthesia the patient must be carefully watched for the signs of developing 'shock'. These signs are similar in most cases to those in the conscious patient (p. 20) but may be masked by such agents as ether which dilate the skin vessels so that the development of pallor and coldness in shock is liable to be delayed. It is better to set up unnecessarily the apparatus for an intravenous drip infusion (p. 36) than to wait until it is obvious to all that such measures are required urgently. Blood-loss during major surgery should be continuously monitored as the operation proceeds and a near constant blood-volume maintained. A simple means of continuously monitoring the CVP, in addition to the pulse-rate, and systemic arterial pressure, is also desirable (*see* p. 24).

POSTURE

The anæsthetist should also pay attention to the patient's posture on the operating table. His heels should be raised by a support so that the calves are free, and a supporting pillow should be placed behind the knees. When an arm-board is used, the arm should be in the semi-prone position and at an angle less than a right-angle. No area of skin should be in contact with metal. A

Hewer's non-slip mattress with a bolster to support the lumbar region is useful; it also eliminates the need for shoulder supports.

ENDOTRACHEAL INTUBATION

This is a technique which every house officer should master, but expertise only comes with practice. It is indicated:—

1. In operations on the head and neck.

2. In many abdominal operations to ensure quiet breathing and absence of straining.

3. In thoracic operations.

4. In cases operated on in the prone position.

5. In cases of intestinal obstruction with regurgitant vomiting performed under general anæsthesia. In these cases, however, a large gastric tube should be passed prior to induction of anæsthesia, and pressure over the cricoid should be applied until a cuffed endotracheal tube is in situ and the cuff inflated.

6. In cardiac arrest (p. 2).

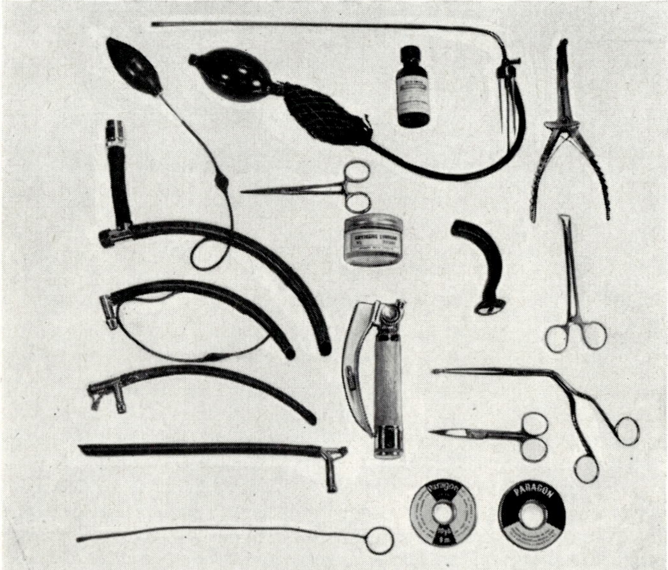

Fig. 72.—Endotracheal trolley layout showing: Lignocaine spray (*top*); endotracheal tubes, with metal angle piece, wire introducer (*left*); jaw gag, tongue forceps, and Magill's introducing forceps (*right*); forceps for clamping tube for inflating cuff, jar of lubricant, laryngoscope, oral airway (*centre*), and scissors; strapping 0·5 in. (1·25 cm.) wide.

Technique.—Before induction of anæsthesia all the necessary apparatus (*Fig.* 72) must be in readiness within easy reach. Intubation may be nasal or oral according to the nature of the operation. Nasal intubation may be performed blind or under vision.

Blind Nasal Intubation.—Gentleness should characterize the whole of this procedure, which is a knack only acquired by practice.

1. Examine the nares for patency by listening to the patient's breathing with each naris alternately occluded.

2. Select the largest tube that experience suggests will pass atraumatically through the larger naris. This usually ranges from size 6 to 9 in the adult.

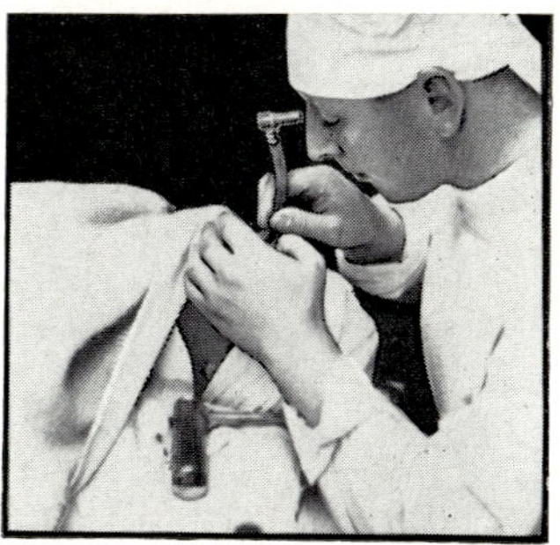

Fig. 73.—Blind nasal intubation.

3. The neck should be flexed and the head extended at the occipito-atlantal joint, a position referred to by Magill as that adopted when sniffing the morning air (*Fig.* 73).

4. Induce anæsthesia and produce hyperpnœa by allowing carbon dioxide to accumulate for a few breaths. A flow of 1 litre per minute is usually sufficient; a fairly deep plane of anæsthesia should be aimed at to allow plenty of time for intubation.

5. Insert a well-lubricated tube into the naris so that its concavity is directed to the patient's feet. Thrust the tube directly backwards. Movement of the bevel by rotation of the tube may be necessary to overcome resistance without trauma. The tube must be coaxed but never forced on its way.

6. Slightly elevate the lower jaw to lift the epiglottis away from the posterior pharyngeal wall. Occlude the opposite nostril so that all breathing is taking place through the tube. If the right naris is used, the head should be inclined slightly to the right and vice versa.

7. As the tube is inserted the patient must be breathing deeply. The ear is placed near the proximal end of the tube which is so advanced that the audible tubular breathing is maximal.

The anæsthetist's left hand may be able to move the larynx to meet the tube by manœuvring the thyroid cartilage. The fingers often feel a slight snap as the bevel passes between the cords, while there is usually some breath holding or cough, except in deep anæsthesia.

If the tube can be inserted to its full length and no breath-sounds can be heard, it is probably in the œsophagus.

An experienced worker can usually intubate blindly following an intravenous injection of propanidid or thiopentone and suxamethonium and this can save much time.

Errors.—Should the tube not be in the trachea it may be situated:—

1. In the œsophagus. This is because the tube is not sufficiently curved or the head is too flexed. It can be remedied by extending the head further and if necessary by resorting to a tube with a greater curvature.

6

2. On the anterior commissure of the larynx. This is because the tube is too curved and can often be corrected by withdrawing it a little, flexing the head, and then advancing the tube again.

3. In the vallecula. Rotation of the tube so that it slips down the lateral wall of the pharynx should overcome this obstruction.

4. In one or other pyriform fossa. This is overcome by rotating the tube, by moving the pharynx laterally to meet the tube, or by rotating the patient's head to the same side.

5. Curled up in the pharynx. This can only occur with soft, worn-out tubes. After several unsuccessful attempts to intubate blindly no more time should be wasted.

Direct-vision Nasal Intubation.—This is necessary if blind intubation fails and a nasotracheal tube is desirable. It is the preferred method of nasotracheal

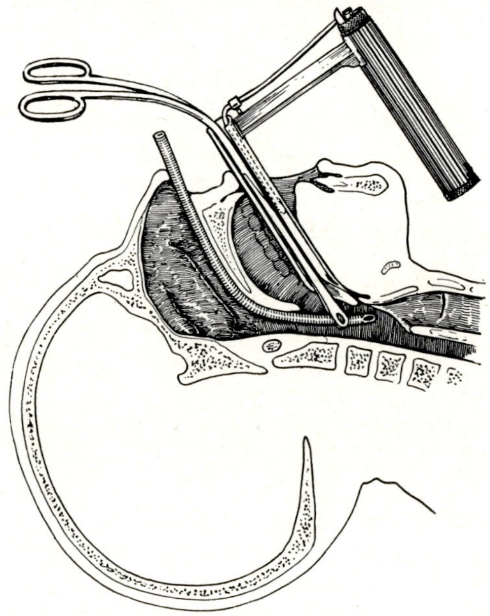

Fig. 74.—Direct-vision intubation.

intubation when using an intravenous barbiturate and relaxant. It is essential to have the head in the correct position and the jaw completely relaxed. The laryngoscope blade which should be lubricated is then inserted. The landmarks to look for are the base of the tongue, uvula, and the epiglottis (*Fig*. 74). If the laryngoscope has a straight blade, it passes behind the epiglottis; if a curved blade, in front of the epiglottis into the vallecula.

The base of the tongue is then lifted upwards and forwards, care being taken not to use the upper teeth or gum as a fulcrum by the laryngoscope blade. This manœuvre brings the rima glottidis into view and the tube is then guided past the vocal cords into the trachea with the aid of Magill's intubating forceps. If deemed necessary, the pharynx can be packed off at this stage with the aid of these forceps. The author finds tampax useful for this purpose as they rarely cause a sore throat. One is placed on either side of the endotracheal tube.

Cuffed Tube.—Working on the 'belt-and-braces' principle the author also prefers to use a cuffed endotracheal tube. A few millilitres of air are injected into the cuff to ensure a gas-tight fit with the trachea. The air is injected into the cuff via an inflating tube which is then clipped off.

The endotracheal tube is then attached to the tubing from the anæsthetic machine by means of an angle piece and catheter mount.

Direct-vision Orotracheal Intubation.—This technique is similar to that described for direct-vision nasal intubation. Magill's forceps are, however, not required and if it proves difficult to visualize the cords clearly a curved wire introducer inside the tube often facilitates the intubation. Such an introducer should always be available. Endotracheal intubation, like bronchoscopy, can be performed under topical analgesia.

EXTUBATION

Laryngeal spasm after extubation is sometimes seen, particularly in infants, so it is important to fill the lungs with oxygen before extubation, and to verify that breathing is free after the tube is removed. Extubation spasm can usually be prevented by the intravenous injection of 50 mg. of suxamethonium in the adult. Inflation of the apnœic patient with oxygen is then carried out for a few minutes until the return of normal breathing. This procedure, however, is not to be recommended if it involves the mixing of relaxants. It may, however, be justifiable after procedures where coughing and straining may ruin the surgical operation, e.g., after cataract extractions under general anæsthesia.

MUSCLE RELAXANTS

Suxamethonium.—This short-acting agent produces profound relaxation usually for about 4–5 minutes. The chief uses are in short procedures such as endotracheal intubation and electropexy. A single dose ranges from 30 to 100 mg. Following the injection, the patient's lungs must be inflated with air or oxygen. An Ambu bag or an Oxford oxygen inflator is useful for this purpose (*Fig.* 75). The relaxant is given following a sleep dose of an intravenous barbiturate such as 1 per cent methohexitone.

Warning.—There is no antidote to this relaxant and if respiratory paralysis is prolonged artificial respiration must be continued until the suxamethonium has been hydrolysed by the serum cholinesterase and respiration is again normal. In the occasional patient with an atypical serum pseudocholinesterase this may take several hours.

d-**Tubocurarine Chloride.**—This is the salt of the active principle of curare and is used in modern anæsthetic practice to produce muscular relaxation in conjunction with a light plane of general anæsthesia and controlled respiration.

The drug is soluble in water and the strength of the solution used is 10 mg. of *d*-tubocurarine chloride per ml. of sterile water. The initial dose is 3–4 mg. per stone (6·4 kg.) body-weight up to 40 mg. The duration of action is 30–40 minutes and increments of 5–10 mg. may be required after this time.

The antidote to curare is neostigmine, but as this drug has powerful muscarinic effects it is essential to combine it with atropine. It is customary to reverse the curarization at the end of an operative procedure by the intravenous injection

Tampax (Tampax Ltd., Havant, Hants).

of 2·5–5·0 mg. of neostigmine combined with 0·6–1·2 mg. of atropine, the dose depending on the degree of residual curarization.

Gallamine Triethiodide (Flaxedil).—This is a synthetic relaxant and 20 mg. of this relaxant are equipotent with 5 mg. of tubocurarine. Its duration of effect is shorter than that of tubocurarine and lasts about 20 minutes.

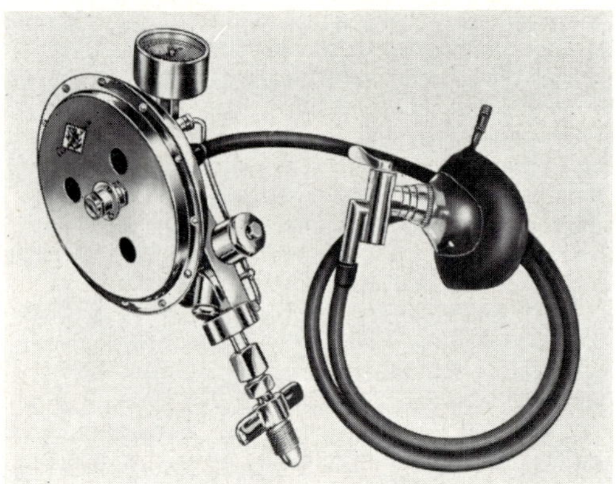

Fig. 75.—Oxford oxygen inflator.

The initial dose is 10–14 mg. per stone (6·4 kg.) body-weight. Further doses of 20–40 mg. will be required to maintain good muscular relaxation.

It has an atropine-like vagal blocking effect on the post-ganglionic nerve-endings in the heart which results in all patients developing some tachycardia.

The antidote is as for curare.

Excretion of both curare and flaxedil, unlike suxamethonium, is by the kidneys, so they should be used carefully in patients with renal impairment.

COMPLICATIONS OF INTUBATION

1. Epistaxis.—This looks messy but seldom causes post-operative discomfort. All blood must be swabbed out of the pharynx before attempting to proceed with the intubation.

2. Damage to Teeth.—This is liable to occur when intubation is attempted by direct vision with the jaw incompletely relaxed. If a tooth disappears, a radiograph must be taken, and if the tooth is found to be in a bronchus, it should be removed via a bronchoscope as soon as possible.

3. Kinking of the Tube.—The most probable site of kinking is just inside the nose where the metal angle-piece joins the rubber tube. Kinking causes an impaired airway and cyanosis results.

A flexometallic tube should be used when the surgical procedure or radiological investigation requires the head and neck to be postured in the manner which predisposes to kinking of the tube.

4. Obstruction by the Cuff.—Occasionally a cuff has been known to herniate over the end of the tube causing complete obstruction. When no obvious cause for an obstruction can be seen, the cuff should be deflated and a further attempt to ventilate the patient made.

Flaxedil (May & Baker Ltd., Dagenham, Essex).

5. Intubation of the Right Bronchus.—This may occur if the tube is too long, and is diagnosed by the hypoxic appearance of the patient and the absence of air entry into the left lung. A suitable length of tube is one which reaches from the upper border of the patient's ear to 1·5 in. (4 cm.) below the thyroid cartilage. When using a nasotracheal tube in the adult, doubling the distance from the tragus of the ear to the ala of the nose is a useful guide for tube length.

2. INTRAVENOUS ANÆSTHESIA AND ANALGESIA

Induction of anæsthesia by an intravenous agent has become the most popular method because of its simplicity, speed, efficiency, and pleasantness.

Two agents are now in common use, thiopentone (pentothal) and methohexitone (brietal), while a third, propanidid (epontol), has recently been introduced into clinical practice.

Thiopentone Sodium.—This is a thiobarbiturate containing a sulphur atom in its molecule. It is a yellow amorphous powder with an odour resembling hydrogen sulphide.

It is soluble in water and is made up into a 2·5 per cent solution (0·25 G. in 10 ml. of distilled water) with a pH of 10·81. A solution stronger than 2·5 per cent should never be used. If the solution becomes cloudy after standing at room temperature for some hours it should be discarded. The standard induction dose for a 70-kg. adult is 250 mg.

Methohexitone.—This is a methylated oxybarbiturate. It is two and a half to three times more potent than thiopentone, but complete recovery is in fact quicker with this agent. It is less irritating than thiopentone when injected into the tissues and causes less cardiovascular depression. It is soluble in water and is made up into a 1 per cent solution (0·1 G. in 10 ml. of distilled water) with a pH of 11·1. The aqueous solution, unlike thiopentone, is stable for several weeks. It may also be made up as a 2·5 per cent solution, but concentrations higher than this should not be used. The standard adult induction dose is 100 mg.

Because of its rapid elimination it is useful for induction of anæsthesia in the dental chair, and for operations on out-patients.

Propanidid.—This is a eugenol derivative, and is made up in a 5 per cent solution in a 20 per cent solution of polyoxethylated castor oil (cremphor E.L.), and is accordingly somewhat viscous necessitating the use of a larger needle. It is available in 10-ml. ampoules and has a pH of 7·8.

The period of narcotic action is shorter than with methohexitone and recovery is rapid and uneventful. A period of hyperpnœa occurs during induction. There is no laryngeal spasm, and unlike methohexitone no central stimulation; it may be used in porphyria. The standard adult induction is 500 mg.

Contra-indications to the Barbiturates.—

1. As with all intravenous agents:—

a. Absence of suitable veins.

b. Unavailability of apparatus to inflate the lungs or perform suction.

c. Out-patients who have to leave hospital alone.

d. Inadequate airway during induction, e.g., Ludwig's angina, status asthmaticus.

e. Factors liable to interfere with the airway during induction, e.g., recent food or drink or bleeding from the nose or throat.

2. Certain pathological conditions:—

a. Cardiac decompensation, e.g., constrictive pericarditis.

Thiopentone (May & Baker Ltd., Dagenham, Essex).
Pentothal (Abbott Laboratories Ltd., Queenborough, Kent).
Brietal (Eli Lilly & Co., Basingstoke, Hants).
Epontol (Bayer (Germany) F.B.A., Haywards Heath, Sussex).

b. Peripheral circulatory failure. The reduction of vasoconstrictor tone may precipitate acute cardiovascular collapse.

c. Impaired renal function, e.g., severe uræmia. Barbiturates are excreted by the kidney.

d. Impaired liver function, e.g., severe herbicidal poisoning. Barbiturates are detoxicated by the liver.

e. Low blood-pressure states, e.g., Addison's disease of the adrenal. Thiopentone in particular tends to lower the blood-pressure still further.

f. Porphyria. This inborn error of metabolism probably constitutes the only absolute contra-indication to the barbiturates. These are liable to precipitate a porphyric crisis which may result in an ascending paralysis and death.

Premedication.—This is not desirable or as a rule necessary when a patient is expected to return home shortly after regaining consciousness.

If the patient has to stay in hospital overnight then the rules for ordinary premedication referred to in the previous chapter should be observed.

TECHNIQUE OF INTRAVENOUS ADMINISTRATION

Vein.—The easiest and most accessible vein (*see* p. 37) should be chosen at one of the recognized sites:—

a. Antecubital fossa. The median cephalic rather than the median basilic vein should be chosen as the median nerve and brachial artery lie deep to the latter vein at this site.

b. Cephalic vein on the radial side of the forearm.

c. Internal saphenous vein, anterior to the medial malleolus. Varicose veins in the leg are unsuitable as the blood is stagnant.

d. Veins in the front of the wrist. Useful in the infant.

e. Veins on the dorsum of the hand.

f. External jugular vein.

g. Scalp veins. Useful in the neonate.

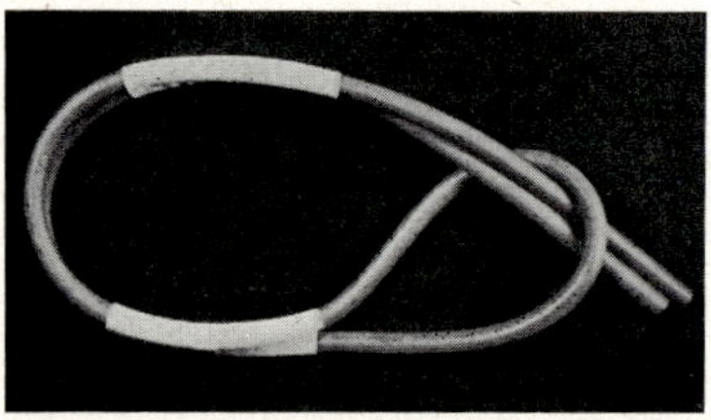

Fig. 76.—Quick-release tourniquet for occluding arm veins.

Application of Tourniquet.—A piece of soft rubber tubing (*Fig.* 76) or Velcro band is applied to the extended arm tightly enough to distend the veins without obliterating the arterial pulse of the wrist. A simple knot that can be released instantly by pulling one end of the tubing should be used.

Clasping and unclasping the fist and gentle slapping of the tissues in the region of the vein promote vasodilatation.

The syringe should be of the disposable or the all-glass type with an eccentric nozzle to allow the barrel to rest closely on the forearm, so that if the patient moves the forearm the relation of the needle to the vein will not be disturbed. The needle should be checked so that it is sharp with no barbs and is patent.

Insertion of the Needle.—The skin is cleansed. Air should be expelled from the syringe prior to venepuncture. Penetration is made with a needle of suitable size almost parallel to the vein, bevel downwards preferably; while doing so, the vein is steadied in position by stretching the skin that lies over it with the thumb of the left hand, which is grasping the patient's arm below the elbow (*Fig.* 77).

The skin is pierced a little to one side of the vein and the needle is advanced alongside it for about $\frac{1}{8}$ in. (3 mm.) before being inclined sufficiently to be introduced into the vein. This minimizes the risk of penetrating both walls of the vein. A sensation of 'give' is detected as the vein is entered.

Successful penetration of the vein is confirmed by raising the syringe and needle slightly with the right hand and gently withdrawing the plunger with the left hand, when blood will be aspirated into the syringe.

No injection should be made unless blood appears in the syringe.

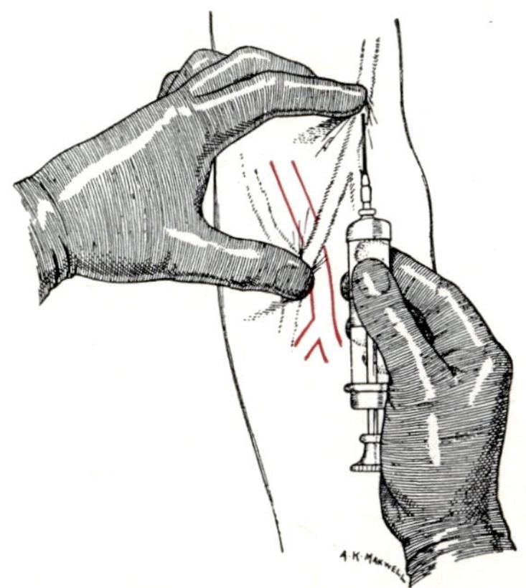

Fig. 77.—Method of stretching the skin and steadying the vein while performing intra-venous injection. The position of the brachial artery is shown in red.

The venous circulation is then restored by releasing the tourniquet, and pressure on the plunger by the thumb of the left hand is applied to give the injection. It should be noted that the grip of the syringe by the right hand remains unaltered throughout the procedure.

Rate of Injection.—A safe rate is 1 ml. every 5–10 seconds until the required depth of anæsthesia is attained. Each patient must be assessed on the dose necessary to produce sleep.

Anæsthesia can be continued with an inhalation anæsthetic. If intubation is necessary, anæsthesia may now be deepened to the required plane with halothane, followed by ether or a muscle relaxant given, and after adequate preliminary inflation with oxygen, intubation performed.

LOCAL COMPLICATIONS

1. Intra-arterial Injection.—Intravenous injection should be painless. Should injection be made into an artery the patient will immediately complain of severe burning pain in the hand. In this event the injection must be stopped, the needle left in situ and 10 ml. of 1 per cent procaine or preferably tolazoline hydrochloride (priscol) 50 mg. (5 ml. of 1 per cent solution) injected into the artery. To further eliminate spasm and thrombosis either a brachial plexus block or a stellate ganglion block should be performed. The operation should be abandoned if possible and the patient heparinized. The circulation in the limb must be kept under constant observation.

Priscol (Ciba Laboratories Ltd., Horsham, Sussex).

2. Perivenous Injection.—This may cause pain, redness, and swelling due to the alkalinity in the case of barbiturate solutions. Should the solution be deposited outside the vein 10 ml. of 1 per cent procaine should be injected into the area. This not only dilutes the anæsthetic solution but promotes vasodilatation and aids absorption. Hyaluronidase may also be added to facilitate absorption.

3. Thrombophlebitis.—This is due to chemical irritation of the vein wall. It is usually symptomless, but if painful should be treated by heat and rest.

4. Injury to Nerves.—The median nerve may be damaged if the injection is made into the medial side of the antecubital fossa.

5. Broken Needle.—As the fracture usually occurs at the junction of the hub with the shaft, at least 0·5 cm. of the latter should always be outside the tissues, otherwise the needle may be lost inside the vein.

GENERAL COMPLICATIONS

1. Respiratory Depression.—This is most likely to follow the injection of thiopentone in a premedicated patient and should be treated by ventilation with oxygen. Any associated respiratory obstruction must be corrected.

2. Circulatory Collapse.—This is usually due to a relative overdose causing vasodilatation and myocardial depression. Treat by elevating the legs, ventilation with oxygen, and the intravenous injection of a vasopressor, such as methoxamine (vasoxine) 10 mg.

3. Laryngeal Spasm.—This may result from: (*a*) direct local stimulation, e.g., by an airway or secretions; (*b*) stimulation of a reflexogeneous area, e.g., dilatation of the anal sphincter or cervix uteri; (*c*) part of a general anoxic spasm. Intravenous suxamethonium with oxygen under positive pressure may be necessary to relax the spasm.

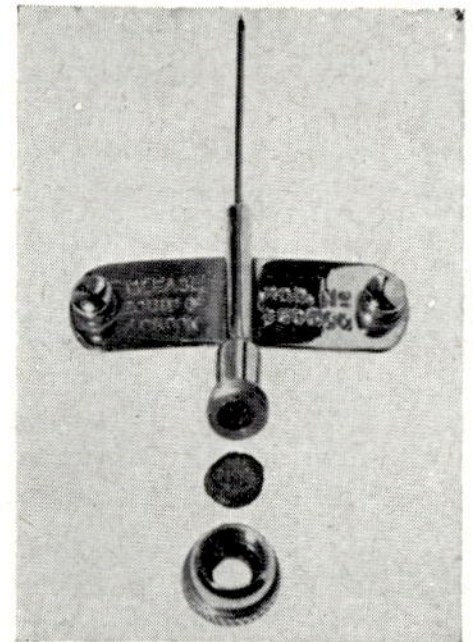

Fig. 78.—Gordh needle, dismantled.

The anæsthetist should always have access to the circulation and this can be maintained with: (*a*) an intravenous drip; (*b*) a Mitchell or Gordh needle (*Fig.* 78).

SPECIAL APPLICATIONS

Ultra-light Intermittent Techniques.—These are useful in out-patient surgery and are widely practised in chairside dental anæsthesia.

There is a state in the borderland between the first and second stages of anæsthesia referred to as *amnalgesia*, a hybrid term embracing amnesia and analgesia. In this state the respiration is automatic, the eyeballs tend to turn downwards and inwards, the eyelash and swallowing reflexes are present but the patient neither remembers nor feels pain.

Such a state can be produced by the intravenous injection of 1 per cent brietal or 5 per cent epontol. The apparatus used is illustrated in *Fig.* 79. It consists of a 250-ml. vial, a secondary venopak, an automatic two-way valve, a 10-ml. disposable syringe, and a disposable extension tube and needle. The latter is held in situ by a Velcro tourniquet. The arm is fixed to the adjustable arm-rest at the wrist by a strap.

Vasoxine (Burroughs, Wellcome Ltd., Euston Road, London, N.W.1).

The patient is asked to sniff and swallow to clear his nose and remove any saliva which may irritate the cords. An oral prop is inserted and then a sleep dose of 1 per cent brietal or 5 per cent epontol is injected slowly at the rate of 1 ml. every 10 seconds. Hypnotic suggestion is used until contact with the patient is lost when the dental procedure is started. If the patient moves a further increment is given, usually half the sleep dose, and at least 15 seconds should elapse before surgery is recommenced. Further increments are administered as required until the procedure is completed. In this way the dose is titrated to the individual patient's response rather than to his body-weight. The patient is usually, but not always, able to maintain a clear airway without jaw support. Efficient oral packing and the use of a high-volume low-pressure suction unit are essential.

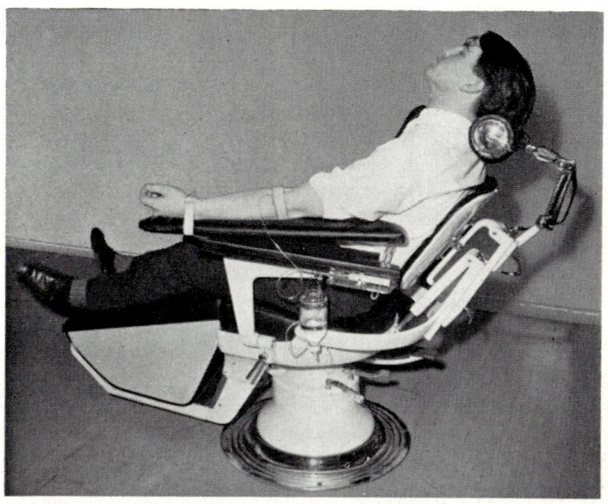

Fig. 79.—Chairside dental anæsthesia. The main vial and supplementary venopak are shown beside the chair with connexion leading to the needle in the medial cephalic vein.

If necessary, an assistant can use the sucker as a retractor to control tongue movements when the patient is very light. In this ultra-light plane patients will often obey commands during treatment and yet have no recollection of pain or discomfort on full recovery which speedily follows the termination of surgery. The absence of a nose piece greatly facilitates the surgeon's work and constitutes a very significant advantage.

About 7 per cent of patients receiving 1 per cent brietal become restless and move to a degree which interferes with the dental surgeon's work. Attempts to subdue such patients with further increments of brietal should be resisted as this results in prolonged recovery. In these cases recourse should be made to nitrous oxide and oxygen, and supplemented if necessary with halothane, either via a nose piece or a nasopharyngeal or an endotracheal tube.

While there appears to be no significant difference in the recovery time after using these drugs the "leaving time" is shorter in the case of epontol and the patients are more alert and ready for home more speedily than when brietal is used. It would seem that epontol is completely broken down in 2 hours by esterases in the blood and liver, whereas brietal is redistributed into the fat depots and not completely broken down for 12–24 hours. It would thus appear that patients who have received epontol could return to duty in a few hours, whereas those receiving brietal should not do so until the following day.

Intravenous Regional Analgesia.—This is also a useful technique for out-patient surgery particularly if the patient has had a recent meal. It involves the injection of a local analgesic solution into a vein of a limb which has been made ischæmic by a tourniquet. It is most useful for operations on the arms, but can be used also in the leg.

Technique.—A Mitchell or Gordh type needle is inserted into a vein on the dorsum of the hand or foot, and the limb is elevated to drain its blood content. If the limb is not painful this can be done more efficiently by applying an Esmarch bandage, but in doing so care must be taken not to dislodge the needle. A sphygmomanometer cuff on the upper arm or thigh is inflated to prevent arterial blood from entering the limb. The Esmarch bandage is now removed and 0·5 per cent lignocaine or preferably 0·5 per cent prilocaine solution is injected into the vein, up to 40 ml. for an arm and up to 100 ml. for a leg. The patient soon experiences tingling in the limb and muscular paralysis sets in. If the operation lasts more than 20–30 minutes, the patient complains of discomfort caused by the sphygmomanometer cuff, and a second cuff should be applied below the first one over the anæsthetized tissue and the first one removed. Alternatively a Hoyle's double cuff may be used. At the end of the operation the cuff is deflated and sensation and muscle tone return in a few minutes.

Toxic Effects.—Occasional toxic effects have been observed after lignocaine, but these are rare after prilocaine. However, their possibility should be borne in mind. The toxic manifestations include disorientation, twitching, and convulsions; there are occasionally cardiac arrhythmias. Treatment is by injecting 150 mg. thiopentone intravenously and instituting intermittent positive-pressure ventilation with oxygen through a tight-fitting mask or endotracheal tube; to facilitate the insertion of the latter suxamethonium should be used.

3. REGIONAL ANALGESIA

Local analgesic drugs may be used:—

1. Topically to anæsthetize mucous membranes, e.g., lignocaine gel (xylotox jelly) for the urethra; 4 per cent prilocaine (citanest topical) for the eye, nose, pharynx, and tracheobronchial tree. This is known as **surface analgesia.**

2. By infiltration to anæsthetize the nerve-endings at the site of operation. When a large area is involved, creating a zone of analgesia around the operating field, it is referred to as a **field block** (*Fig.* 80).

3. By **regional nerve-block**. This may be intraneural, as in the injection of the Gasserian ganglion in the treatment of tic douloureux, or paraneural, where local solution is deposited around the nerve or nerves as in stellate ganglion block, brachial plexus block (*Fig.* 81), and intercostal nerve block.

There are two special forms of regional nerve-block: (*a*) Epidural and caudal block where the local analgesic solution is deposited in the epidural space, and (*b*) spinal nerve-block where the local analgesic solution is deposited in the sub-arachnoid space. These techniques are not suitable for the occasional anæsthetist.

4. By intravenous injection as described in the previous chapter.

Adrenaline.—With the exception of cocaine (which has vasoconstrictor properties of its own) it is customary to add vasoconstrictor agents such as adrenaline to the local solution. Adrenaline keeps the solution in contact with the nerve

Xylotox Jelly (Willows Francis Ltd., Ashley Road, Epsom, Surrey).
Citanest Topical (Astra-Hewlett Ltd., Watford, Herts).

tissue for a prolonged time. This prevents toxic reaction from too rapid absorption and prolongs the duration of action of the analgesic.

Adrenaline or noradrenaline is not added to solutions applied topically, as in this situation it does not prolong the action of the analgesic solution. It is also usually avoided in epidural and spinal blocks, as spasm of a spinal artery may ensue, resulting in neurological sequelæ. It is also avoided where end-arteries are involved, e.g., digits and penis.

Combination of Local and General Anæsthesia.—At all times consideration should be given to the possibility of using local infiltration as a sole method or as a supplement to general anæsthesia. Even a partially failed block has an element which is helpful. For infiltration 0·5 per cent lignocaine or 0·5 per cent prilocaine is the agent of choice. Adrenaline 1–400,000 (0·25 ml. 1–1000 per 100 ml. in local solution) is added.

Maximum Dosage.—In all its injected concentrations the local anæsthetic should not exceed the maximum safe amount, e.g., in the case of prilocaine 50 mg. per stone (6·4 kg.) body-weight. In the very young and old one should try to stay well below this maximum amount by the use of more dilute solutions, e.g., 0·25 per cent.

Asepsis must be strictly observed with all blocks, and a good skin antiseptic should be used liberally. Patients should be supine during all local anæsthetic injections, however minor the procedure. A knowledge of the regional nerve-supply of the part to be blocked is essential.

Dangers.—Depending on the site the dangers are intravascular injection or, with special techniques, intrathecal injection and pneumothorax. Repeated aspiration during injections will avoid intravenous flooding with local solution. However, until the block has vanished a drug reaction may occur. This may be associated with hypotension and convulsions which may terminate in cardiac arrest. Treatment consists of: (1) artificial ventilation with oxygen; (2) intra-venous injection with a vasopressor drug, e.g., 10 mg. methoxamine; (3) intra-venous injection of suxamethonium or just sufficient thiopentone to control convulsions (100–150 mg.); (4) the routine treatment for cardiac arrest (p. 2).

REFRIGERATION ANALGESIA

This is the application of cold to a localized part of the body to block local nerve conduction and painful impulses. It is especially indicated in amputation of the leg for arteriosclerotic or diabetic gangrene, but melting ice makes it rather a messy technique. A tourniquet should be applied and the limb encased in ordinary ice for 2–3 hours. Analgesia persists for 1 hour if the tourniquet is kept efficiently (i.e., occluding the circulation) in place.

ABDOMINAL WALL BLOCK

1. For Herniorrhaphy.—

A strong 5 or 10 cm.-long needle with a diameter of 1 mm. is used for the main injection of 0·5 per cent lignocaine. First the skin is anæsthetized at points A and B (*Fig.* 80), by injecting 1 or 2 ml. of lignocaine subcutaneously with a hypodermic needle. Point A lies about 3 cm. up a line from the anterior superior iliac spine to the xiphisternum; point B is 2 cm. above the midpoint of the inguinal ligament.

The larger needle is now inserted through anæsthetized zone A and directed towards the inner lip of the iliac crest. Aspirating first before injecting to make sure no vessel has been entered, 10 ml. of lignocaine are now injected as the needle passes down to the bone; the needle is partially withdrawn and reinserted in radial fashion. This injection blocks the subcostal, the ilio-hypogastric, and the ilio-inguinal nerves as they lie between internal oblique and transversus abdominis muscles. Some local anæsthetic is also infiltrated subcutaneously towards the outer lip of the iliac crest.

A similar injection is then made at point **B** to anæsthetize the structures at the internal inguinal ring, including peritoneum and the genital branch of the

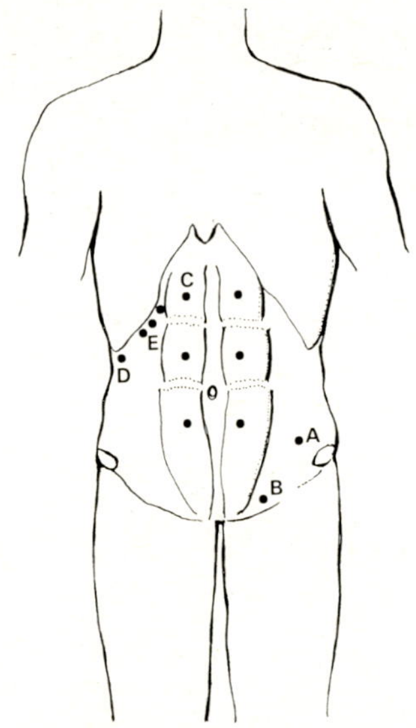

Fig. 80.—Abdominal field blocks. The sites of intermuscular injections are shown— **A** and **B** for herniorrhaphy; the points **C** in the rectus muscle compartments for midline and upper paramedian incisions; and **D** and the points **E** along the costal margin for more lateral incisions.

genitofemoral nerve. The injection is made at right-angles to the skin; the tendinous external oblique is easily recognized as it is pierced, and in an adult the needle may be inserted up to 3 cm. as 10 ml. of lignocaine is injected. In addition, the line of the skin incision is infiltrated subcutaneously, advancing the tip of the needle until it finally is about 2 cm. beyond the midline.

Warnings.—

1. Not more than a total of 40 ml. 0·5 per cent lignocaine should be used.

2. Wait at least 2 minutes before starting the skin incision.

3. Never put towel clips into unanæsthetized skin.

4. Be careful what you say during the operation—the patient can hear everything!

2. For Upper Midline or Paramedian Incision.—

Local anæsthesia is seldom employed for upper abdominal operations. Only when no anæsthetist is available or in a very ill patient might it be used, e.g., to insert a drain or to establish a feeding gastrostomy or transverse colostomy. Remember that the abdominal wall is supplied by both lateral and medial branches of the lower thoracic nerves, the medial branches emerging through the rectus abdominis muscle.

The equipment and precautions are as for a herniorrhaphy (*vide supra*). For a simple upper midline incision it is only necessary to infiltrate the line of the incision subcutaneously and then to inject the rectus muscle on both sides, and above and below the tendinous transverse intersections in these muscles. A 5-cm. 20 S.W.G. needle is inserted at right-angles through the points marked C (*Fig.* 80). A snap is felt as the anterior rectus sheath is pierced. The needle is advanced till the resistance of the posterior sheath is felt; 10 ml. of lignocaine are then injected into each muscle mass. Care must be taken not to penetrate the posterior sheath and peritoneum.

If a rectus muscle block is employed in an infant, e.g., for Ramstedt's pyloro-myotomy, not more than 12 ml. of 0·25 per cent lignocaine need be used.

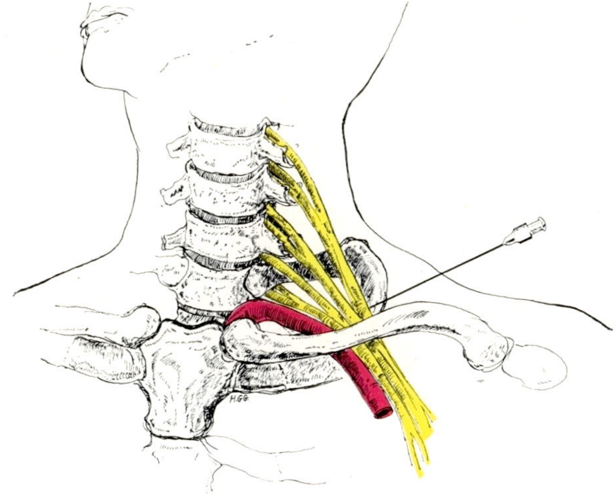

Fig. 81.—Brachial plexus block. The needle is inserted above the midpoint of the clavicle and directed towards the centre of the first rib.

For more laterally placed incisions an intercostal block is better than a local one, but is not suitable for the occasional operator. The 7th to 12th thoracic nerves can be blocked as they appear below the costal margin. To reach the 6th to 7th nerves the upper rectus sheath must be traversed; the 9th and 10th nerves are injected through points marked E, as they lie superficial to the transversus abdominis muscle; the 11th and subcostal nerves are reached by injecting just below the lower lateral corner of the costal margin, point D.

BRACHIAL PLEXUS BLOCK

The patient lies supine with his head slightly rotated towards the opposite side. First identify and if desired mark: (1) The subclavian artery; (2) the spinous process of T.3 behind. After scrubbing, putting on gloves, and cleansing the patient's skin, again locate the subclavian artery with a finger. Raise a weal in the skin with 0·5 per cent lignocaine just lateral to the finger-tip—this is usually about 1 cm. above the midpoint of the clavicle.

Keeping the subclavian artery depressed with the palpating finger, a 5-cm. needle is introduced through the weal and gently pushed backwards, slightly medially, and downwards towards the first rib—that is, in the direction of the tip of the T.3 spinous process. As the needle point reaches the plexus where it crosses the rib, paræsthesia may be felt down the arm. After aspirating to ensure that no vessel has been entered, 20–30 ml. of lignocaine are injected; the needle is withdrawn 1 cm. back from the rib, aspirated, and another injection made.

CHAPTER XII

PREPARATION FOR OPERATION

By ALLAN E. KARK and L. BURROWS

IN the past twenty years a gratifying decline in mortality and morbidity has occurred following major surgical operations, despite the fact that surgery has been extended to patients previously considered unacceptable risks. These advances have been made possible by progress in a number of areas: a greater understanding of surgical physiology, more detailed pre-operative evaluation, more precise diagnostic techniques, the development of monitoring equipment, refinements in anæsthesia, pharmacological advances, and improved operating-theatre techniques.

The importance of pre-operative care and assessment may be underestimated by a junior house officer, but the experienced surgeon recognizes it as a vital part of successful patient care. Indeed, in the aged, and in those undergoing complicated procedures, thoroughness of pre-operative preparation can spell the difference between life and death.

THE INITIAL EVALUATION

History.—While the chief complaints of surgical patients are often quite clear, for instance, blood from a body orifice, a palpable mass, or localized pain, complicated and chronic histories are equally common. Judgement in history taking is an art acquired through the practice of carefully worked-out routines; no detail should be overlooked, since any may offer the final diagnostic clue.

Table VII.—DRUGS COMMONLY USED IN MODERN MEDICAL PRACTICE FOR WHICH A HISTORY MUST BE ELICITED

> Adrenocortical steroids
> Amphetamines
> Androgens and œstrogens
> Antibiotics
> Anticoagulants
> Antidepressants and tranquillizers
> Antihypertensives
> Aspirin
> Barbiturates
> Chlorpromazine derivatives
> Digitalis, quinidine, etc.
> Diuretics, mercurials
> Insulin or oral hypoglycæmics
> MAO inhibitors (nardil, niamid, marplan)
> Narcotics
> Oral contraceptives
> Thyroid derivatives
> Vasodilators

In the majority of instances, a careful history will point to the diagnosis. On occasion, the history will obviate or clarify the need for surgical intervention, e.g., chlorpromazine ingestion in the presence of jaundice, or previous aspirin ingestion in a patient with upper gastro-intestinal bleeding.

With the widespread use of new drugs, careful questioning about previous drug usage or idiosyncrasy has become an essential part of a complete history. Has the patient ever taken rauwolfia compounds, phenothiazine derivatives, adrenocortical hormones, anticoagulants, diuretics, digitalis, etc.? Is there a history of penicillin, codeine, or iodine allergy or sensitivity reactions to iodine or adhesive tape? *Table VII* gives a list of drugs which are frequently used over periods of months and years, especially in the elderly, and which may play an important role when operation is undertaken.

The presence of serious secondary disease syndromes deserves careful consideration, e.g., diabetes, cardiovascular disease, hyperthyroidism, chronic bronchitis, renal disease, etc. Previous operative treatment should be confirmed whenever possible through direct communication with the original surgeon and hospital record.

Clues to a bleeding tendency must be sought, with particular attention to such symptoms as nose bleeds, menstrual bleeding, and easy bruising or undue oozing following dental extractions or brushing of teeth.

It may not be possible to obtain a complete history in the acutely ill, but the history from a relative or friend should elicit, at the least, specific causes for seeking emergency care, associated constitutional diseases, previous operations, and prior usage of drugs.

Any history of breathlessness, swollen ankles, precordial pain, or urinary difficulties should point to the necessity for the most careful examination of the cardiac, respiratory, and renal systems (pp. 138, 139).

Physical Examination.—A complete, thorough, and painstaking physical examination is essential. Too often emphasis is placed on the primary complaint while the remainder of the examination is of a perfunctory nature. A careful physical examination will frequently uncover small but significant positive findings such as the presence of an enlarged supraclavicular node in a patient with an abdominal mass. Thorough pelvic and rectal examination is necessary. The pulse-rate and blood-pressure always should be recorded and a thorough examination of the cardiovascular and respiratory systems performed.

Evaluation of the mental capacity and psychiatric state of the patient at this time is of practical importance. Any impairment of mental state serves as a warning of possible post-operative difficulties which might require extra supervision or sedation, and if diminished cerebral blood-flow appears to be a factor, special care must be taken to avoid even short periods of hypoxia during surgery.

The experienced clinician can make a shrewd initial assessment of an individual's general condition and the degree of surgical risk. This judgement must be substantiated by a properly performed, complete, and comprehensive examination. Close co-operation with the anæsthetist is desirable (p. 101).

LABORATORY TESTS

There are certain essential pre-operative laboratory examinations that must be performed as screening procedures. Excessive ordering of tests in the hope of finding a chance abnormality is poor clinical practice as well as being costly.

The following examinations should be done:—

1. A urine analysis including specific gravity, sugar, acetone, albumin, and an examination of the urinary sediment.

2. A complete blood-count, including hæmoglobin, hæmatocrit, white blood-count, and differential smear.

3. A blood typing and grouping.

4. A fasting blood-sugar, or 2-hour post-prandial blood-sugar.
5. A blood-urea nitrogen.
6. A chest X-ray.
7. An electrocardiogram in all patients over the age of 40.
8. A stool occult blood reaction.
9. Serum electrolytes concentrations (Na, K, Cl, CO_2).

A prothrombin time, bleeding time, and clotting time should be done in patients suspected of having bleeding or clotting abnormalities, e.g., cirrhotics. A further elaboration of tests will be included in subsequent sections.

Any abnormalities revealed by any of these tests should be fully investigated, evaluated, and treated before embarking on elective surgical procedures.

SKIN PREPARATION

A major source of wound infection comes from staphylococci harboured within the patient's own dermal crypts: repeated lathering of the operative area and surrounding skin with an antiseptic agent such as pHisohex is an essential preliminary. In the United States it is common on the days preceding the operation for the patient to shower, using this antibacterial cleanser with attention directed towards the operative site, scalp, face, axillæ, groin, anogenital area, and umbilicus. On the night before the operation, the operative site and surrounding skin should be wet shaved, using a disposable safety razor with care taken to avoid scratches and abrasions, from which infection may seed into the depths of the surgical wound. Apart from shaving, skin preparation the day *before* operation is no longer common practice in Britain.

This preparation should extend widely beyond the operative wound area. For an abdominal incision, the area should extend from the nipple line to the upper thighs and laterally to the prolongation of each mid-axillary line. The shaved areas should then be painted with an aqueous topical antiseptic, preferably of the povidone-iodine type (betadine), and the painted area covered with a sterile towel until the time of operating-room preparation. Skin preparation in an emergency case may, if necessary, await preparation in the operating room.

Note.—The presence of boils, eczema, or other skin inflammations should delay elective surgery for days or weeks until the skin condition has been treated and infection eradicated.

GASTRO-INTESTINAL PREPARATION

The extent of pre-operative preparation of the gastro-intestinal tract depends upon the type of procedure planned. In some patients, bowel cleansing is required to prevent post-operative soiling, impaction, and straining at stool: a soap or tap-water enema on the night before surgery is all that is needed. Purgation, with its dehydrating effect, is unnecessary and the pre-operative routine enema is less popular than formerly.

Where large-bowel surgery is planned, or if colon resection is likely, more intensive preparation is required. The aim is to cleanse the bowel by wash-outs and to decrease the bacterial population. A chronically constipated or partially obstructed patient requires more prolonged and intensive preparation.

The principles of large-bowel preparation include:—

1. *Diet*: A low-residue diet should be started about 4 days prior to operation. This should be replaced by a full fluid diet (*purée* food) approximately 2 days before surgery.

pHisohex (Bayer Products Co., Surbiton-on-Thames, Surrey).
Betadine (Berk Pharmaceuticals Ltd., Godalming, Surrey).

2. *Cathartics*: Mild catharsis is desirable. Daily mineral oil (liquid paraffin) or phosphate preparations should be started during the pre-operative week.

3. *Enemas*: Daily low tap-water enemas (p. 405) should be used beginning 3 days before operation. On the pre-operative day, high colonic irrigations should be administered in the morning and evening to cleanse the entire colon; the last of these should be continued until the return is quite clear.

4. *Antibiotics*: A diminution in large-bowel flora is desirable, and non-absorbable antibiotics in high dosage should be used beginning several days pre-operatively (*see* pp. 73, 77). A combination of a non-absorbable sulphonamide drug with neomycin is widely accepted. Sulphasuxidine (4 G. every 6 hours) or sulphathalidine (2 G. every 6 hours) is started 3 days before operation, and neomycin (6–7 G.) is administered in 1-G. doses on the pre-operative day. Recent work suggests that kanamycin alone is as effective as the above combination. There is a small incidence of serious staphylococcal enterocolitis secondary to overgrowth of this bacterium, especially following inadvisable prolonged pre-operative intestinal chemotherapy. Because bowel sterilization may eliminate the bacteria responsible for the production of vitamin K_1 and thereby lead to a bleeding problem, patients should receive daily parenteral vitamin K_1 (25 mg.) during the preparative period.

PRE-OPERATIVE INTUBATION

A nasogastric tube should be passed in patients undergoing major abdominal or thoracic procedures (*see* p. 348). Patients with œsophageal or gastric obstruction should have the tube passed twice daily pre-operatively for saline irrigation and cleansing, using a wide-bore Ewald tube if necessary. If small-bowel decompression is necessary, or if difficult intestinal surgery is expected, as in matted adhesions or ileitis, a long tube (Miller-Abbott, Kantor) can be of great help and should be put down a few days in advance. This form of intubation will decompress the bowel, facilitate exploration and closure, help define proximal and distal loops, and hasten re-establishment of small intestinal function (p. 342).

THE NIGHT AND MORNING BEFORE OPERATION

By this time, the surgeon and the resident house staff should have established rapport with the patient; he will have understood the need for surgery, its nature, and the expected post-operative pain and difficulties. The surgeon should reassure the patient and the family; any mutilating procedure, such as an amputation or ileostomy, should be discussed. It is comforting in such cases for similarly afflicted people who are fully rehabilitated to pay a visit to the patient. The 'Q.T.' Club* is an outstanding example of the value of such emotional preparation. Ex-patients are usually most anxious to help, especially if they faced their own ordeal inadequately prepared. Permission for operation should have been given by this time; if not, the form must be signed before any pre-operative sedation is administered (p. 102).

Intravenous Fluids.—If a procedure is scheduled for the afternoon, intravenous fluids (*see* p. 36) help prevent dehydration, and assist in bringing about a water and solute diuresis. The site of intravenous administration should be a forearm vein opposite the side on which the surgeon expects to operate. It is recommended that a sterile small polyethylene catheter be used which is introduced into the vein over a needle (angiocath).

---

* A lay organization of patients with ileostomies who meet and discuss their problems.

Pre-operative Orders.—On the night before surgery, the final pre-operative orders should be written. Though variation may exist in specific instances, certain basic orders are required for the majority of surgical procedures. These are:—

1. *Diet*: Nothing by mouth for at least 12 hours before operation; if afternoon operation is planned, a cup of sugared tea may be taken in the early morning.

2. *Skin preparation orders*: As outlined above and to include the limits of area to be shaved and treated.

3. *Enema orders*, now rarely necessary.

4. *Blood cross-matching*: The estimated number of units of blood that may be required during surgery should be indicated.

5. *Pre-operative medication*: The anæsthetist will have visited the patient pre-operatively to explain the details of anæsthesia and to write these orders (p. 103).

6. *Sedation orders*: A good night's rest the night before operation is important. One hundred mg. or more of a long-acting sedative (e.g., quinalbarbitone sodium) should be offered to allay anxiety and to aid sleep.

7. *Bladder*: The patient should be instructed to void just before the administration of pre-operative medication. An indwelling catheter should be inserted if major pelvic surgery is to be done.

8. *Nasogastric intubation orders.*

9. *Final weight* recording on the day preceding operation.

SPECIAL CONSIDERATION IN THE ELDERLY

Elderly patients respond surprisingly well to major surgery. However, the frequency of secondary degenerative disease leaves little leeway for post-operative complications. Episodes of tachycardia, fever, hypotension, or pneumonia are a setback in young vigorous individuals, but may prove fatal in the aged.

Careful evaluation of the cardiovascular system is required. An indication of *recent* coronary occlusion or myocardial damage demands a 2- or 3-month postponement of elective surgery.

Pulmonary emphysema with resultant hypercapnia and respiratory acidosis is common in the aged. Careful attention to tracheobronchial toilet and pre-operative breathing exercises can help prevent post-operative atelectasis and bronchopneumonia. The service of an enthusiastic physiotherapist is invaluable. The elderly are particularly sensitive to narcotics. As little as 10 mg. of morphine sulphate can cause severe functional hypoventilation and should be avoided.

A sluggish peripheral circulation is also characteristic of this age-group; these patients should be out of bed and if possible walking to prevent thrombo-embolic phenomena. This is particularly important if patients have been in bed for days or weeks before operation.

SPECIAL CONSIDERATION IN THE VERY YOUNG (*See also* Chapter XL)

At the other extreme of life, there are specific considerations in pre-operative management as well. The young child, removed from his protective environment, should be helped to adjust to his strange surroundings by all personnel involved in his care. The history obtained from parents is not always an accurate description of symptoms. The physical examination may also be inconclusive because of lack of co-operation.

In general, infants and young children have a vitality much beyond that expected of their size and age. Their organs have great powers of recovery, as the degenerative changes of ageing have barely started.

Children are especially liable to upper respiratory and exanthematous diseases and any possibility of these should be ruled out in the pre-operative preparation. Any unexplained fever or leucocytosis unrelated to the reason for surgical admission, or any recent exposure to an infectious exanthema is an indication for deferment of surgery.

The metabolic rate in infants and very young children is so high that frequent feedings are required to prevent glycogen depletion and metabolic acidosis. Feedings should not be withheld any longer than necessary before surgery. Within 2 hours after feeding, an infant's stomach is empty provided that no obstruction is present; consequently, these patients can be offered several ounces (60 ml.) of sweetened orange juice or its equivalent about 4 hours before operation. Older children can be given clear fluids (water, orange juice, ginger ale, etc.) up to 6 hours before surgery.

Infants do not tolerate wide variations in fluid and electrolyte imbalance. They have a relatively larger surface area per unit of weight than adults, so that fluid loss by perspiration occurs quickly and clinical manifestations of dehydration are more profound. The physiologically immature renal system cannot compensate for the variations in hydration as it can in later life. Therefore, extreme care should be taken in the calculation of fluid requirements in this age-group. Homeostatic fragility in the early days of life may also be due to an immature endocrine system and to the slow appearance of circulating steroids in response to stimulation.

Children with fevers do not withstand anæsthesia and surgery well. An operation upon a child with marked pyrexia is apt to be accompanied by an exceedingly high pulse-rate, collapse, or convulsion. The rectal temperature should be brought below 39° C. (102° F.) by the use of rectal aspirin, tepid water sponging, hydration, or the use of a cooling blanket.

By contrast, the relatively large surface area predisposes to excessive heat loss, and the infant should be kept warm *en route* to the operating theatre and during anæsthetic induction, with blankets, cotton-sheet wadding, or a heating pad.

The newborn requires daily vitamin K (2·5–5·0 mg.) to correct the mild bleeding tendency which is secondary to hypoprothrombinæmia. Vitamin C (25–100 mg.) should be administered to depleted infants to promote wound healing post-operatively.

CARDIAC DISEASE

The pre-operative preparation of the severe cardiac patient requires consultation with a cardiologist. Only life-saving procedures should be considered if congestive heart failure is present. Ample time should be allowed pre-operatively to attain optimal cardiac compensation before elective surgery. Pre-operative tests should include an electrocardiogram, central venous pressure determinations, and sometimes circulation time, cardiac fluoroscopy, and other special investigations that may be indicated.

Patients with rheumatic vascular disease or congenital heart disease should receive prophylactic antibiotics (e.g., penicillin) before, during, and after major surgery. If possible operation should be postponed in patients with active rheumatic fever.

The cardiac patient should be fed a strict low-salt (500 mg.) diet with a limited fluid intake. The judicious use of appropriate drugs such as digitalis glycosides, diuretics, quinidine, etc., may significantly lessen the operative hazard in patients with congestive heart failure or cardiac arrhythmias. The use of prophylactic digitalization in cardiac patients undergoing surgery is still debated, but recent evidence suggests that digitalis may aid the diseased myocardium whether congestive heart failure is present or not.

If the patient has been receiving anticoagulant drugs, the vitamin K and/or protamine sulphate should be administered pre-operatively in order to restore the prothrombin and clotting times to a normal range.

There are risks involved in operating on hypertensive cardiac patients who have been treated with antihypertensive agents such as the *Rauwolfia serpentina* drugs. These medications not only deplete cerebral and platelet serotonin but also lower catecholamine stores throughout the body. Reactive hypotension presents an operative hazard in patients receiving such drugs, so that *withdrawal of the drugs is preferable for at least 3 weeks before surgery*. Certain medications such as chlorthiazide diuretics induce hypokalæmia; they should be used judiciously in the pre-operative stage and be withdrawn at least 3 days prior to surgery, especially if hypokalæmia is noted.

RESPIRATORY DISEASE

A history or physical finding of pulmonary disease needs additional evaluation to avoid serious post-operative complications. The estimation of pulmonary function includes simple clinical tests such as the ability to climb at least two flights of stairs or blow out a lighted match held 6 in. away with a forced expiration. In addition, more sophisticated pulmonary function tests may be necessary, and the most valuable of these is the timed vital capacity which detects such obstructive ventilatory defects as are present in bronchitis or obstructive emphysema (*see* p. 164). Blood-gas analyses including arterial pH, P_ACO_2, and P_AO_2 may be required to establish the degree of hypoxæmia and respiratory acidosis present.

Sputum.—Tracheobronchial secretions should be cultured and antibiotic sensitivity tests performed. Where purulent sputum is present, pre-operative appropriate antibiotic therapy is indicated. Pulmonary efficiency should be improved by intermittent positive-pressure breathing devices containing aerosols and antibiotics, which the patient uses for 5–10 minutes hourly for several days. Breathing exercises should be carefully taught and supervised by a trained physiotherapist. Cigarette smoking must be stopped. Where active pulmonary disease persists, elective surgery should be postponed until infection and expectoration have been controlled.

URÆMIA

The presence of renal failure demands thorough preparation. Renal function can be improved by:—

1. Treatment of the associated congestive heart failure: Renal failure leads to diminished excretion of digitalis glycosides, and *decreased* maintenance digitalis dosage is required.

2. Treatment of the associated anæmia: Packed blood-cells should be administered until a hæmatocrit of 30–35 per cent is attained.

3. Correction of the fluid and electrolyte imbalance: Diuretic agents such as intravenous mannitol (250–500 ml. of 10 per cent mannitol) may promote a water-and-solute diuresis. Any accompanying metabolic acidosis can be

partially buffered with such agents as intravenous sodium bicarbonate; an 8·4 per cent solution contains 1 mEq. of sodium bicarbonate per 1 ml. (p. 26).

4. Control of hypertension: Rauwolfia compounds and ganglionic blocking agents are a hazard because of operative hypotension and must be used with caution and after due consultation with the cardiologist and anæsthetist.

5. Treatment of any urinary tract infection: Drainage of the lower urinary tract by catheterization and administration of antibiotics may both be necessary. In all such cases urine culture and sensitivity test should be used to determine the appropriate antibacterial agents. (*See* Chapter XXXIII.)

6. Correction of hyperkalæmia: Potassium exchange resins may be used (e.g., Kayexalate, 15 G. orally every 6 hours).

7. Renal dialysis: Peritoneal or hæmodialysis are effective means of controlling renal failure, and of preparing the ill patient for even major surgery (Chapter XXXI).

OBESITY

An obese person who undergoes elective major surgical procedure without adequate preparation poses problems of technical difficulty during the operation, and of increased incidence of post-operative pulmonary, cardiovascular, thrombo-embolic, and wound complications. The excessively fat individual should emphatically be advised to lose weight before any elective procedure; indeed the wise surgeon will often refuse to perform such procedures in patients over 200 lb. (90 kg.) unless and until they lose 20–30 lb. weight.

Any balanced weight reduction regimen is satisfactory. The basis is a low-calorie (1000–1500 cal./day), high-protein, low-fat diet with adequate amounts of vitamins and minerals. The hospital dietitian can offer valuable advice in the selection of a proper diet which may have to be adhered to for some months to achieve the required weight reduction.

ANÆMIA AND HYPOVOLÆMIA

Anæmia should be treated vigorously by specific corrective therapy. The most common type of anæmia encountered in surgical patients is the hypochromic, microcytic variety and is secondary to blood-loss and/or nutritional deficiency. Patients should not be operated upon with a hæmoglobin below 12 G. per 100 ml. It may be necessary to transfuse the patient pre-operatively to attain this level, but it should be emphasized that the unnecessary use of blood, with the dangers of serum hepatitis and allergic reactions, should be avoided. If time and circumstance permit, the patient should be placed on oral or parenteral iron therapy to raise the hæmoglobin level; the patient may be given ferrous sulphate 100–200 mg. thrice daily for 3 weeks. In the elderly patient, or in the cardiac where there is a distinct danger of overloading the circulation, packed cells offer a desirable alternative to whole blood.

With acute blood-loss, the hæmoglobin and hæmatocrit values are poor guides to therapy; hæmodilution may not yet have occurred, and the values may be misleadingly high. Central venous pressure measurement is essential by means of a catheter placed via an upper arm vein into the right atrium. As long as the central venous pressure remains below 10 cm. H_2O, overloading by intravenous fluids is not a danger (p. 24).

An estimation of the blood-volume deficit is required for accurate replacement therapy in chronic hypovolæmia. A semi-automatic instrument (Volumetron) based on radio-isotope dilution principles is of value in estimation of blood-volume deficit.

Volumetron (Atomium Corporation, Billerica, Massachusetts, U.S.A.).

THE DIABETIC

Prior to the introduction of insulin, operations on diabetics were followed by high morbidity and mortality. Though the risks of surgery have been considerably reduced by insulin therapy, there is still an increased incidence of complications in poorly controlled diabetics, e.g., fluid and electrolyte derangements, acidosis, infection, and cardiovascular accidents. Any source of infection tends to exacerbate the diabetic state, and diabetes in turn appears to worsen infections.

Local anæsthesia, spinal anæsthesia, and regional blocks may be very useful in diabetics.

The pre-operative management of a diabetic patient depends upon several factors: the severity of the diabetes in the past and in the present illness, the magnitude of the intended surgery, and whether this surgery is elective or urgent. A low carbohydrate diabetic diet should be given during the pre-operative phase.

1. Elective Surgery in Known Diabetics.—

a. Mild (those controlled by diet or oral agents).—Prepare these patients as if they were non-diabetics. The diet should contain 100 G. or less of carbohydrate. Neither oral hypoglycæmics nor insulin is required on the day of surgery. An intravenous solution of 5 per cent dextrose in water will adequately cover caloric needs in the immediate pre-operative period and prevent a tendency towards starvation ketosis.

b. Moderate (those requiring up to 40 units of insulin daily). Operations on these patients are best performed in the early morning when they normally take their food and insulin. Long-acting insulin preparations (e.g., Lente or N.P.H.) should be replaced on the day of surgery by regular insulin, which should be administered according to a sliding scale determined by 4-hourly urinalyses.

Thus:—

1 + sugar	5 units regular insulin subcutaneously
2 + sugar	10 units regular insulin subcutaneously
3 + sugar	15 units regular insulin subcutaneously
4 + sugar	20 units regular insulin subcutaneously

Immediately prior to and during surgery, intravenous 5 per cent glucose in water or 10 per cent fructose in water should be administered. Regular insulin should be added to the bottle in a ratio of 10 units to each 50 G. of sugar. No insulin need be added to the fructose solution because it does not have the same insulin requirements in its metabolic cycle. Fructose, because of its rapid peripheral uptake, has the further advantage of being antiketogenic and does not cause an osmotic diuresis as does glucose. Because of increased availability and reduced cost, fructose now is the sugar of choice in these surgical situations.

c. Severe (those patients requiring 40 units or more of insulin daily).—These patients have frequent episodes of ketosis and require high doses of insulin. On the day of operation, one-half the usual dose of long-acting insulin (Lente or N.P.H.) should be given. This type of insulin acts to prevent ketosis during and after surgery and also promotes a tendency towards anabolism and positive nitrogen balance. During and after surgery, intravenous solutions should be either 5 per cent glucose in water (with added insulin) or 10 per cent fructose in water. In addition, regular insulin is added every 4 hours depending upon the amount of sugar in the urine (as severe).

2. Emergency Surgery.—

a. Known Diabetics.—Acute surgical diseases requiring surgery exhaust carbohydrate stores so that ketosis frequently results. If the patient is not ketotic, the usual pre-operative rules for diabetics pertain. If ketosis is present, a vigorous effort should be made to reduce it before surgery. Only in the most desperate circumstances should emergency surgery under general anæsthesia be attempted *before* ketosis is controlled. With a severe infection, it may not be possible to abolish ketosis completely until the infection has been treated. The aim is to treat metabolic acidosis, correct electrolyte abnormalities, rehydrate the patient, and initiate antibiotic therapy if an infection is present. The severity of ketosis can be followed with serum acetone readings and when these fall to 2+ or below on a standard colorimetric scale, the operation can be scheduled. If the patient is known to be a severe diabetic, the initial dose of insulin should approximate twice his usual daily dose, and insulin administered at 2-hourly intervals depending upon blood-sugar determinations. An intravenous solution containing 5 per cent glucose should be used to protect against excess insulin dosage.

b. Newly Discovered Diabetic.—If the patient is a newly discovered diabetic, the initial dose of insulin should be 80–100 units if the urine shows 4+ sugar. Though severe ketosis is a relative contra-indication to surgery, the level of blood-sugar is in itself of little consequence. A 50 per cent glucose solution for rapid intravenous administration should be readily available in the event of insulin overdosage.

BLEEDING TENDENCIES

Surgery may be hazardous in patients with known or suspected bleeding tendencies. The general principles in the evaluation and treatment of these patients include identification of the missing blood-coagulation factor and, where possible, its replacement in sufficient quantity to afford protection against hæmorrhage during and after surgery. The assistance of a hæmatologist is advisable. Hæmophilia is considered on p. 485.

ORAL HYGIENE

An unclean mouth and the presence of dental sepsis favour the development of post-operative respiratory complications. Gum infections should be cleared, and infected teeth removed with sufficient time allowed for healing before elective surgery is planned. Dilute hydrogen-peroxide mouthwashes and frequent brushings of teeth should be used if mild dental hygienic problems are encountered. Dental consultations should be sought in any difficult situation.

ENDOCRINE ABNORMALITIES

The possibilities of adrenal insufficiency in the elderly patient or in persons who have been on cortisone therapy should be recognized. Serum or urine examinations for 17-hydroxysteroid levels after ACTH stimulation may offer conclusive proof of this disorder. If adrenal insufficiency is suspected, the patient should receive exogenous corticosteroids to cover the stress of operation. The exact dose and duration of corticosteroid therapy necessary to produce adrenal insufficiency and significant loss of pituitary reserve are not known, nor the time required for the functional recovery of these glands. It is recommended that for the patient who has been on corticosteroid therapy during the 2 years previous to admission, 300 mg. of intravenous hydrocortisone or its equivalent be given in the 24-hour period during which major surgery is performed. During the post-operative period, steroid administration is gradually diminished and eliminated when the clinical condition permits; the dose can usually be halved every second day. (*See also* Chapter XXXI.)

THYROID DISEASE

The hyperthyroid patient should be brought to a euthyroid state prior to a major operation by an acceptable method using antithyroid drugs and iodine. It is unjustifiable otherwise to operate on the thyrotoxic patient except in life-saving circumstances or for the surgical relief of medically uncontrollable hyperthyroidism. (*See* Chapter XXII.)

JAUNDICE

The risks of surgery in the jaundiced patient are related to the severity, duration, and cause of jaundice, as well as to the degree of liver failure. The patient with a severe degree of obstructive jaundice represents a serious surgical risk. Delay in relief of biliary tree obstruction is not well tolerated, and on balance early biliary decompression outweighs the benefits of time-consuming precise diagnosis.

The important considerations in the pre-operative management of these patients are:—

1. Restoration of adequate nutrition and liver glycogen stores: this enables the patient to withstand the stress of major surgery and is accomplished by a high-calorie diet, 70 per cent of the calories being derived from carbohydrate and the remainder from fat and protein. Concentrated carbohydrate can also be provided parenterally together with insulin to accelerate deposition.

2. Correction of any bleeding tendency: in obstructive jaundice, the absence of bile in the intestine leads to malabsorption of fat-soluble vitamin K, which in turn disrupts the clotting mechanism by preventing the formation of prothrombin by the liver. Excessive operative bleeding is unlikely to occur unless the patient's prothrombin time exceeds twice normal. Vitamin K_1 oxide should be given to all jaundiced patients. Large quantities of this vitamin are well tolerated; 25 mg. a day by intramuscular injection for 5 days will correct the deficiency unless extensive liver damage has resulted from prolonged common duct obstruction.

3. Correction of any anæmia, hypoproteinæmia, or blood-volume deficit with intravenous albumin and/or blood.

4. Avoidance of excess parenteral saline, since liver disease favours salt retention. During operation 500 ml. of 10 per cent mannitol may be given intravenously to prevent post-operative renal failure.

MALNUTRITION (*See* p. 46)

The surgical patient requires ample reserves of glycogen and protein as well as of normal fluid, electrolyte, hæmoglobin, and vitamin levels in meeting post-operative demands. A high-carbohydrate, high-protein, 4000-calorie/day diet will supply the malnourished individual with the energy requirements, and also the elements necessary for the synthesis of glycogen and its storage in the liver.

The period of pre-operative dietary preparation depends upon the degree of malnutrition. A patient with a weight-loss of 25 per cent or more should receive a minimum of 2 weeks of dietary preparation before major surgery. Progress can be measured in terms of daily weight-gain. If oral feeding is not possible and parenteral feeding does not provide adequate nutrition, a feeding gastrostomy or jejunostomy should be considered before subjecting the malnourished patient to major surgery.

Parenteral supplement in the form of intravenous glucose infusions may be required; these supply additional calories and nutrients and also provide a protein-sparing effect; intravenous albumin and blood transfusions are given for hypovolæmia or anæmia respectively. Anabolic steroids have not proven to be of value in pre-operative preparation. The use of intravenous fat with its hepatotoxic potentialities and of protein hydrolysate solutions is still experimental.

Vitamins.—Any prolonged period of parenteral therapy should include daily thiamine hydrochloride (vitamin B_1 50 mg. per day) to complement carbohydrate metabolism, ascorbic acid (vitamin C, 500 mg.) for subsequent tissue repair, and vitamin K_1 oxide (25 mg.), particularly if plasma proteins are deficient, to assure prothrombin activity.

CHAPTER XIII

ASSISTING AT OPERATIONS

By Albert Frankel and Allan E. Kark

Appreciation of the physiological mechanisms and pathogenesis of disease forms the essential basis of modern surgical treatment. Nevertheless, the culminating event in the management of the surgical patient is the operation itself, and the skills of the operating theatre—technical precision and attention to operative detail—remain the determining factors in limiting morbidity and mortality.

The operation should be carried out expeditiously without breaks in surgical technique. Adequate exposure is accomplished by anæsthetic relaxation, a carefully planned incision, and properly applied retraction. The illumination of the field should be bright, and instruments and ancillary monitoring equipment should be checked and in good working order. The operating team must be acquainted with the surgeon's methods and be able to anticipate his needs. Tissues must be handled gently, approximated accurately, and hæmostasis carefully secured, protecting from injury those structures outside the operative field.

The smooth co-ordination of these factors depends to a large part on the assistants' intelligence, forethought, and familiarity with the complexity of the modern operating theatre.

Zones in a Theatre Suite.—To minimize bacterial contamination, the operating theatre is divided into three zones. The *outer perimeter zone* encompasses those areas outside the operating theatre itself, used for sterilization of materials, scrubbing, and in some hospitals, induction of anæsthesia. The donning of sterile gown and gloves is often performed in this area, but is better carried out in the middle zone. In many modern suites this perimeter zone is separated from the rest of the hospital by an interchange area, where personnel must put on clean overshoes and gowns, and where ward bed linen is left.

The *middle zone* is the domain of the circulating nurse, the anæsthetist and his materials, and such non-sterile equipment as collection bottles, tubing, monitoring equipment, and the diathermy chassis. The circulating nurse delivers necessary supplies to the sterile field from storage areas, handles the non-sterile equipment needed in the operation, and keeps track of sponges, instruments, and specimens as they move to and from the operating table.

The *inner zone* is completely sterile and consists of the operative field, that portion of the patient draped by sterile sheets, the surgeon and his assistants, the instrument nurse, and the instrument table. Everything entering this area must be sterile as it comes into contact with the operative field.

Ideally all dirty and disposable materials leaving the theatre suite should do so by a separate passage having no connexion with the rest of the theatre.

Reducing Contamination.—In the modern operating theatre windows should be sealed, and temperature, humidity, and air-borne dust controlled and limited by air conditioners. Non-essential equipment should be stored outside the theatre and exposed surfaces and floors cleaned daily with bactericidal agents. Ultra-violet lamps can help to reduce the number of air-borne bacteria. The major threat of bacterial contamination comes from direct contact with and oral droplets from the operating team. Cutaneous or respiratory infections (including staphylococcal carrier states) should exclude an individual from the surgical team. An assistant who is ill, has a skin infection, or is exhausted should make his physical condition known to the surgeon and be excused from participation in the operation.

In order to minimize the bacterial inoculum inadvertently brought to the wound from the outside, certain standard practices should be adopted by the assistant. Ordinary clothing is exchanged for a freshly laundered, short-sleeved cotton suit. Many other fibres, including wool, silk, and most synthetic materials, tend to generate static electricity which can produce a spark leading to an explosion in the presence of combustible anæsthetic agents.

Electrically conductive shoes (or boots) reserved for the operating theatre alone should be worn, and covered with fresh cotton shoe covers before each new case. These shoe covers are made to maintain electrical conductivity to a conductive floor. A close-fitting cotton cap is worn to cover all exposed hair and prevent fall-out of dandruff into the field.

The most commonly used mask is made of multiple layers of cotton-gauze held over the nose and mouth by ties. Recently disposable masks made of synthetic fibres and plastics have been introduced and are more effective than the gauze. The mask should be changed before every case as it becomes more permeable to droplets when wet. A second type of mask which is non-porous and depends on posterolateral deflexion of exhaled air rather than filtration is also available. This type is less comfortable to wear and has not been enthusiastically received. Where the risk of droplet contamination is especially great, double masks should be worn.

Fogging of spectacle lenses can be prevented by shaping a lead insert along the top edge of the mask snugly around the nose, or taping the upper end of the mask across the bridge of the nose. Another very satisfactory method is to soap and polish the lenses, leaving a fog-resistant film. Proprietary anti-mist lotions and tissues are available.

DUTIES OF THE ASSISTANT

The functions of the assistant surgeon are:—

1. Checking the Patient, the Chart, and Pre-operative Investigations.—The patient must be identified before entering the operating room. A most satisfactory method is the plastic name bracelet which is kept on the patient's wrist throughout his hospital stay. The indication for operation and proposed procedure should be briefly reviewed by the surgeon and the rest of the team. In cases such as inguinal herniorrhaphy, the correct side to be operated on is confirmed. Great care in identification is needed for amputations and when operating upon digits. Special markings, such as those on varicosities of the lower extremities, should also be checked.

Appropriate radiographs should be on display. If radiological examination is likely to be required during the operation the radiologist must be contacted beforehand; likewise the pathologist for a frozen section.

The patient's chart must be checked to see that operative consent has been signed (p. 102) and the pre-operative orders (p. 136) have been carried out. It is becoming increasingly common practice to insist for medico-legal reasons on a brief note stating indications for, and the type of procedure intended, such as: 'Six-year history of duodenal ulcer with one previous hæmorrhage; vagotomy and gastrectomy recommended.'

2. Review with the Nurse.—The scope of and possible complications expected during the procedure must be briefly discussed with the Senior Nurse. This gives her an opportunity to prepare appropriate instruments and supplies. If a major vascular problem is likely to be encountered, a set of vascular instruments should be ready or, if opening of the chest is likely, a thoracotomy set should be available on a separate table.

A good nurse will tell a new assistant of locally used names for swabs, sponges, instruments, and local conventions.

3. Review with the Anæsthetist.—It is crucial to discuss the type of anæsthesia in relation to the need for electrocoagulation; where explosive agents are necessary, cautery must on no account be used.

Special problems such as a blood-coagulation deficiency should be described to the anæsthetist and appropriate medications, such as concentrated anti-hæmophiliac fraction, platelet concentrates, fibrinogen, etc., should be available. He should be informed of the number of units of blood cross-matched and where it is stored.

The anæsthetist should be warned of any likelihood of entering the pleural spaces so that positive-pressure ventilation can be assured.

Hypotensive anæsthesia, as is used in many neurosurgical procedures, can be arranged by prior consultation.

Where temporary, complete, or local occlusion of circulation is anticipated, hypothermia or extracorporeal circulation may be indicated (*see* p. 331).

4. Preparation of the Patient in the Operating Theatre.—Careful attention to the patient prior to incision contributes to a smooth operative course. The operative area should have been thoroughly shaved. Nasogastric tubes are checked for patency and position, and the stomach is aspirated.

Catheters.—Operations on the urinary tract or those involving pelvic structures usually require an indwelling urinary catheter. This may be placed after induction of anæsthesia, and strict aseptic technique must be observed (p. 448).

Where a large inflammatory or neoplastic lesion in the pelvis might carry dissection close to a poorly visualized ureter, or especially in reoperation in this area, insertion of a ureteral catheter via a cystoscope is of great help in identifying it during dissection. Care is taken to secure the catheter to the thigh with tape, and drainage is collected in a calibrated plastic bag to record intra-operative urine volume.

Patients undergoing surgery of the lower bowel benefit from an indwelling rectal tube which allows egress of retained gas and fluid. Its patency and position should be carefully checked by the assistant. An external irrigation set connected to this tube is helpful in providing final cleansing of stool, blood, and tumour cells prior to transection of the bowel.

Monitoring.—Extensive procedures, especially in the elderly and poor-risk patients, require continuous cardiocirculatory monitoring during the anæsthetic period. The most commonly used electrocardiographic monitors give a continuous audible and visual ECG representation. With many systems an alarm rings should a significant period of asystole develop. This is recorded from electrodes placed on the extremities. Other monitoring equipment such as the ear oximeter or electro-encephalogram may be used. Central venous-pressure-measuring equipment may be set up (*see* p. 24).

Positioning requires care in patients who have skeletal disease due to neo-plastic infiltration or demineralization, e.g., from advanced breast cancer or hyper-parathyroidism. Prevention of pathological fractures while turning the patient during the procedure requires padded splints or pre-operative padded plaster casts.

5. Proper Placement of Intravenous Infusions.—The correct placement of intravenous cannulæ constitutes a critical part of the operative preparation. These are not only used for blood and fluid replacement, but are the site of entry for anæsthetic agents or other medications. Ideally the infusion is placed in a vein of the upper extremity most distant from the operative field. When continuous or large volume replacement is required, multiple ports using large-bore plastic catheters should be used. One or more large-bore intravenous catheters can transport sufficient blood and fluid to maintain circulating volume in the face of massive hæmorrhage. These catheters can be introduced per-cutaneously through or around a large-bore steel needle. Where this cannot be accomplished, the catheter can be inserted via a phlebotomy incision. If possible, the catheter should not cross joint spaces where acute angulation may obstruct the infusion flow. These catheters must be secured to the skin with tape very carefully and a method allowing complete removal of the needle after placement

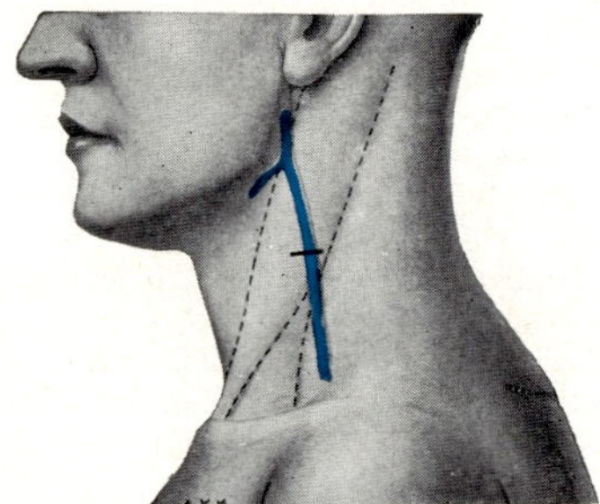

Fig. 82.—The external jugular vein, as it crosses the sternomastoid, can be exposed or cannulated easily for intravenous infusions or CVP measurement.

of the catheter is preferred. Instances of embolization of such catheters to the heart and pulmonary vascular tree have been reported where such a catheter has been accidentally severed or inadequately secured.

In general, use of the lower extremities should be avoided because of the high incidence of resultant thrombophlebitis. In an emergency, however, the greater saphenous vein is readily accessible subcutaneously, lying anterior to the medial malleolus at the ankle.

Since the site of potential intra-operative hæmorrhage can usually be antici-pated, infusion sites should be arranged so that transfused blood can reach the heart without traversing the damaged vessel. For example, in adrenalectomy where the inferior vena cava might be damaged, infusion sites should be in the upper extremity.

Venous and Arterial Pressure.—Where careful control of circulatory dynamics is important, the venous filling pressure of the heart (CVP) can be monitored by introducing a long catheter from the upper extremity or neck into the superior vena cava or right atrium, and leading it to a manometer (*see* p. 24). By use of three-way connexions this can also be used as an infusion site. These catheters can be introduced successfully via the brachial, cephalic, or external jugular veins (*Fig.* 82) in preference to percutaneous puncture of the subclavian vein, with its risk of intrathoracic bleeding and pneumothorax.

Where accurate measurement of arterial blood-pressure is necessary, as in cardiovascular surgery, cannulation of a peripheral artery, usually the radial, may be required. The catheter is led via extension tubing to a pressure-sensing transducer and recorder. These measurements are much more accurate than cuff techniques, but require careful calibration of recording equipment prior to surgery.

6. Intra-operative Radiography.—If intra-operative radiographs such as cholangiographs or arteriographs are anticipated, the nurse and anæsthetist must be informed, and the radiologist and his technician consulted beforehand. The appropriate part of the patient must be positioned over the film cassette holder.

7. Electrical Equipment.—A wide surface of the patient's skin should be in contact with the diathermy plate or patient electrode of the electrocoagulation device, but not with metallic parts of the table, since accidental burns may result from the skin contact with metal.

All power sources and lines should be checked and all electrically operated equipment demonstrated to work before proceeding. Auxiliary power sources and light should be available in case of a power failure.

8. Positioning of the Patient.—The assistant makes sure that the brake on a mobile theatre table has been applied.

The patient is positioned so as to facilitate exposure of the operative field. A trial of the effect of raising the elevating bridge or 'breaking' the table is worth while. Equally important is the protection of the unconscious patient from pressure and positional injury. The effects on ventilation, circulation, and nerve continuity must all be borne in mind. Undue sustained pressure on a peripheral vessel or nerve may result in thrombosis or palsy, and must be guarded against by attention to support and padding of the extremities. The use of muscle relaxants increases the possibilities of injury by removing the protective effect of muscle tone.

In the dorsal prone position the major strain is on the heels and low back. For prolonged procedures it is necessary to support these areas with padding. The restraining strap across the thighs should be padded and applied without

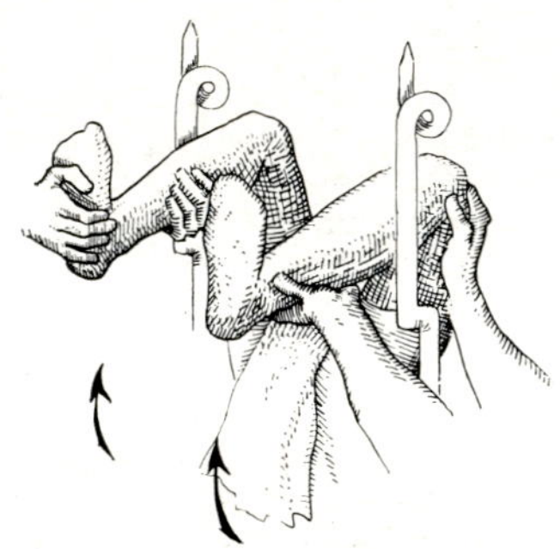

Fig. 83.—Lithotomy position. Both legs are raised or lowered simultaneously to avoid sacro-iliac strain.

constriction. The patient's hands may be placed alongside the thighs, but never under the buttocks.

The exposure of pelvic structures is facilitated by the Trendelenburg position, that is, the pelvis higher than the shoulders. Where this position is anticipated shoulder braces should be applied over the acromioclavicular joints. The braces should be wide and well padded to avoid pressure injury to the brachial plexus.

Procedures on the perineum and its orifices are often performed in the lithotomy position. Here the legs are flexed at the hips and knees with the patient supine. The feet and legs are supported in stirrups suspended from upright poles. The buttocks should be clear of the end of the table to facilitate exposure posteriorly. In using this position, the legs must be elevated and released simultaneously to avoid strain to the sacro-iliac area. (*Fig.* 83.) The vertical poles apply pressure to the lateral calves and this area must be amply padded. Both the lithotomy and Trendelenburg positions significantly reduce vital capacity by pushing the abdominal viscera against the diaphragm.

The lateral position is used for posterolateral thoracotomy, and flank incisions for exposure of lateral retroperitoneal structures. The arms are slightly flexed and the upper arm must be carefully padded and suspended from a suitable support such as the anæsthesia screen. Check the circulation in the lower arm. The lower leg is flexed and the upper one kept straight for stability. A large pillow should be placed between the knees. (*Fig.* 84.)

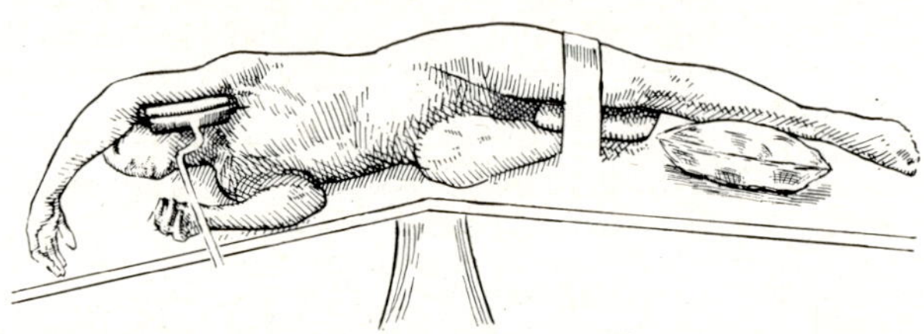

Fig. 84.—Lateral position. The lower leg is flexed for stability. The upper arm is extended and supported away from the chest to facilitate posterolateral thoracotomy incisions.

The arm carrying the intravenous infusion is often abducted to the side on a board which must not sag. The arm at the shoulder should not be extended to greater than 90° and the forearm is kept pronated. Because this extended position often interferes with the suitable positioning of the second assistant, the arms should be kept at the sides whenever possible and retained by the ends of the draw sheet. In this position, the arms are inaccessible during the operation, and therefore the infusion and blood-pressure cuff must be well secured and checked before positioning.

THE SURGICAL SCRUB

The forearms, hands, and nails are scrubbed at a deep-welled sink with faucets designed so that flow and temperature of water can be adjusted without using the hands. A sterile, firm bristle brush is used to scrub all areas from finger-tips to elbows. The nails are cleaned with a manicure stick or file. In many operating theatres brushes are delivered from a dispenser. Similarly, foot-pedal-operated dispensers are most suitable for delivering the skin cleanser.

Cleansing Agents.—The two enjoying the greatest popularity today are a 3 per cent hexachlorophene in detergent solution and a water-soluble iodine complex in a detergent base. Both these agents greatly reduce surface bacteria counts, but do not sterilize the hands. During the course of the operation, bacteria surviving in sweat-glands and hair follicles proliferate although inhibited by the antibacterial film left on the skin, and the bacterial concentration can be shown to increase again with time.

The initial scrub of the day is carried on for at least 5 minutes, while subsequent scrubs are of shorter duration depending on the cleanser used. Suds are rinsed from the hands and forearms, holding the hands above the elbows so that water will drain towards the elbows and not contaminate the hands. This position is maintained after the water is turned off until the hands are dried on a sterile towel received from the gowned nurse (*Fig.* 85). One end of the towel is used to dry one hand and forearm, and the other hand and arm are dried with the remaining sterile portion of the towel. The used area should never come in contact with dry areas.

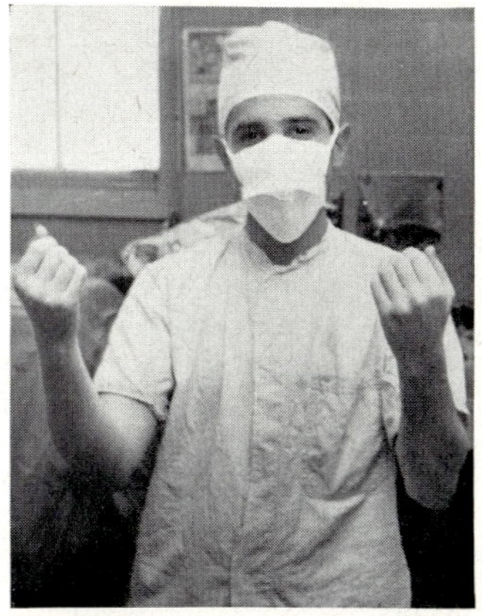

Fig. 85.—Position of hands until gowning.

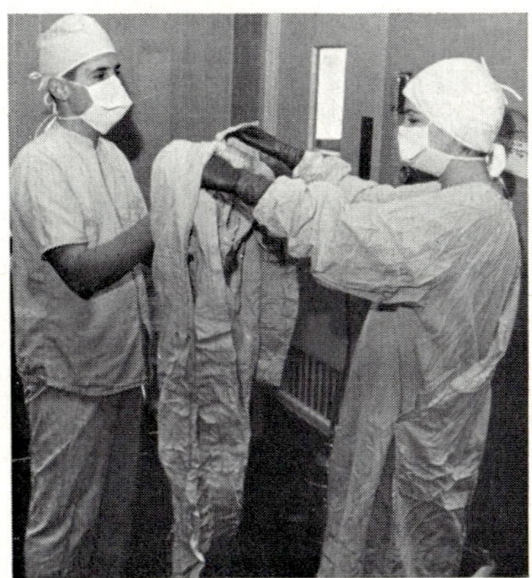

Fig. 86.—Gowning by the nurse.

Usually the scrub nurse will help the surgeon don the sterile gown by holding it near the shoulders with the inner side towards him (*Fig.* 86). The arms are inserted into the sleeves and the circulating nurse ties or clips the gown at the back. If the surgeon gowns himself, the inner surface is grasped near the neck, held away from the body, and allowed to drop open taking care not to let it touch the floor. The arms are then inserted upwards into the sleeves and are kept extended. The circulating nurse will grasp the inside of the gown near the shoulders from behind and pull the sleeves up over the wrists and the shoulders into the proper position. The gown will then be secured with snaps or ties.

Lastly the gloves are applied. These are supplied by half-sizes in sterile wrappings with the cuffs turned down. In America the scrub nurse holds the gloves open under the cuffs with palms towards the surgeon who slips his hands into them (*Fig.* 87). Her hands should not touch the surgeon's and she should glove the surgeon only when he is already gowned. In Britain the surgeon mostly gloves himself: the turned-down cuff representing the inner surface of the glove is grasped with the opposite hand (*Fig.* 88) in line with the palm and pulled onto the appropriate hand. The second glove is lifted from its container by placing the gloved fingers under the inverted cuff on the palm side and pulling it onto the remaining hand. The cuffs can be turned back (*Fig.* 89). In most instances where gloves are reused, a package of lubricating cream is enclosed and applied to the hands to lubricate and facilitate application of the gloves.

7

Disposable gloves do not require hand lubricants for ease of application since the gloves are not made sticky by autoclaving. The use of talc has been abandoned as a lubricant because of the risk of producing foreign-body granulomata. Other powders such as starch are widely used, but they tend to drift around the room and adhere to gloves, drapes, etc.

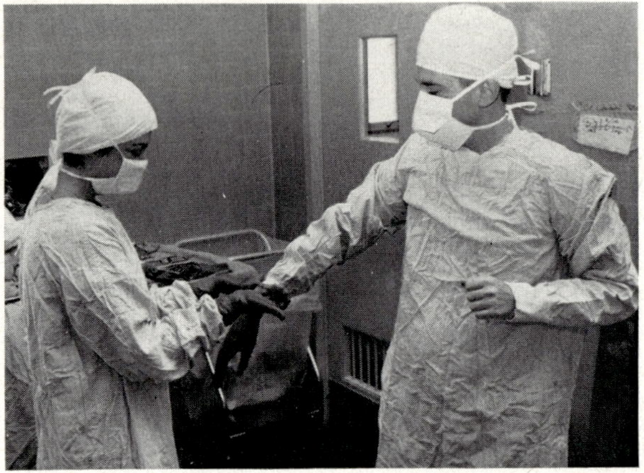

Fig. 87.—Gloving by the nurse.

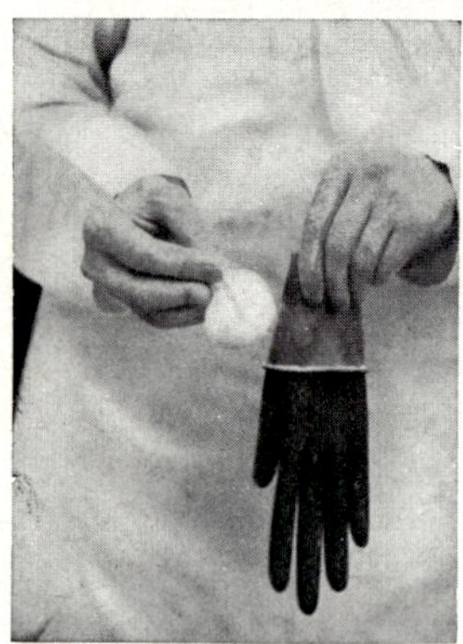

Fig. 88.—Gloving by the surgeon showing the method of holding the glove.

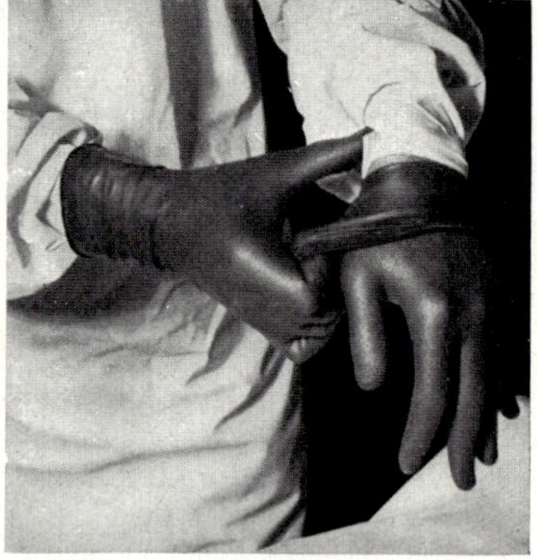

Fig. 89.—The final adjustment in putting on gloves—turning back the cuff so as to maintain sterility of the outer surface.

FINAL SKIN PREPARATION AND DRAPING

The final preparation of the patient's skin in the operating room is carried out on an area previously shaved and cleansed with antiseptic solutions. The area prepared should be extensive and well beyond the limits of the incision.

The assistant surgeon works from a separate 'prep' table using sterile sponges on long-handled sponge-holders dipped in appropriate cleansers and antiseptics (*Fig.* 90). A fat solvent such as ether may be used first to remove the surface film, but many operating theatres have now banned ether because of its explosive hazard. This is followed by detergent cleaner plus antiseptic or by a strong

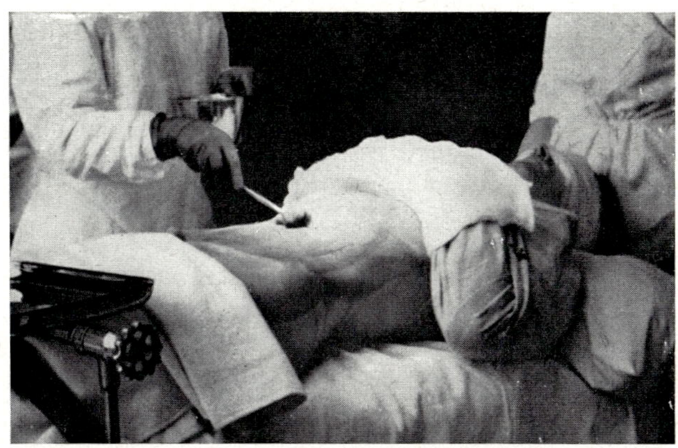

Fig. 90.—Preparation of the abdominal wall. With a gauze swab soaked in flavine in spirit and held with long forceps, a wide area has been prepared, the umbilicus being the last part to receive attention.

antiseptic alone. The antiseptic usually contains a dye so that the treated area can be easily identified. It is applied in concentric circles starting at the proposed site of incision and working outward to the periphery of the field. Intertriginous areas, the perineum, umbilicus, and other areas likely to be most heavily contaminated by bacteria are swabbed last. This also holds true for intestinal stomata or open wounds which may be present. In the case of a previously constructed colostomy or ileostomy, a gauze packing is placed into the stoma to eliminate soiling. For abdominal operations the skin preparation should extend from the nipple line to the pubis, and transversely between the mid-axillary lines. After completing the preparation—which must last 3–5 minutes—the assistant regowns and regloves.

Sterile Towels and Drapes.—The application of sterile drapes varies considerably from one institution to the other. Many have adopted the use of the self-adherent, thin, pliable, transparent polyethylene (plastic) sheet which when applied to the operative field adheres closely to the skin. This prevents skin contact with gloves and instruments, and prevents transmigration of skin bacteria through moist drapes. It is particularly useful for screening draining areas away from the new wound. The incision is then made directly through this sheet. The operative area, in any event, is framed with sterile towels and the entire patient, with the exception of the head (except for head and neck cases), is covered with sterile sheets which extend down below the operating team's knees on either side of the table and at the foot end. An overall final large drape with a 12-in. (30-cm.) hole in the centre is commonly used, but often two drapes, each with a half-circle cut-out at one end, are more useful as the overlapping half-circles provide an opening which can be tailored to any size of exposure needed (*Fig*. 91).

Position of Surgeon and Assistants.—The surgeon takes that position at the table from which he can most easily approach the operative field. This will mostly mean that he is on the same side as the lesion. But remember that some structures, such as the splenic flexure, are more easily approached from the

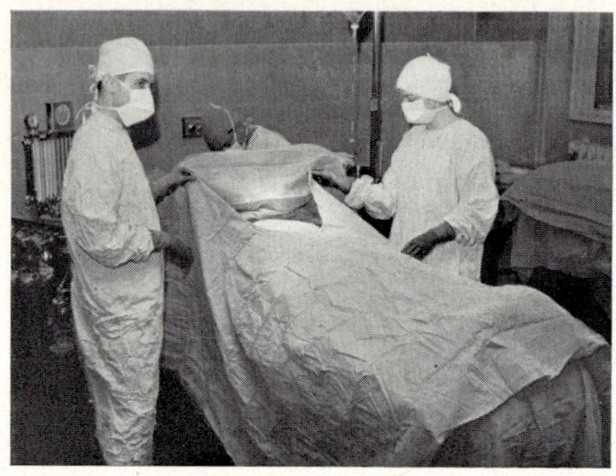

Fig. 91.—Draping the patient with half-circle sheets. The first such sheet is being placed and a second one will be put above to complete the circle   The size of the opening is determined by the overlap.

opposite side of the table. The first assistant stands directly opposite the surgeon, while the second assistant stands either above or below the surgeon depending on the direction of major retraction. The instrument nurse stands on the side opposite to the surgeon to facilitate passage of instruments.

The height of the operating table is adjusted for the comfort of the operating surgeon. This is generally to the level of the surgeon's xiphoid process. The table may be tilted in various directions during the course of the operation to facilitate exposure.

The operating light is designed to produce shadow-free illumination of the field. The light may be redirected by the circulating nurse or theatre orderly as the field of exposure changes during the operation. When the field to be illuminated is deep within a cavity, additional spot lights are available. Illumination should not be compromised and sufficient time should be allowed for the assistant staff to achieve optimal results. Special instrument lights may be sterilized and brought into the operative field to better illuminate or trans-illuminate deep structures.

ASSISTANTS' ROLE IN THE OPERATION

The function of the first assistant is to facilitate the progress of the operating surgeon by active aid in dissection, in securing of hæmostasis, and in other manœuvres. He should anticipate the moves and needs of the operator and respond accordingly. At all times he must ensure that the surgeon has a clear and unimpeded view of the structures being operated on. Above all, he must follow the instructions of the surgeon quickly and without debate. Suggestions may be made with discretion if they materially contribute to the smoothness of the operation without causing irritation to the surgeon.

The function of the second assistant is to carry out the instructions of the surgeon and his first assistant. This consists primarily in maintenance of proper retraction.

Conversation should be kept to a minimum as it is distracting and significantly contributes to droplet contamination of the field. Constant attention to the surgeon and the course of the procedure avoids lapses in exposure and resultant delay. A comfortable upright posture should be maintained to avoid fatigue and back strain. *Resting on the patient can be a cause of ventilatory embarrassment and nerve injury, and should be avoided.*

By and large, traffic through the inner two zones of the operating theatre should be restricted to essential personnel. Observers crowding around the operating team in an attempt to see the field significantly contribute to breaks in technique and bacterial contamination.

The assistants are responsible for keeping the operative field in an orderly fashion. Used and discarded instruments are passed back to the instrument nurse. In some hospitals instruments used in a carcinomatous field such as a radical neck dissection for carcinoma are discarded and reautoclaved prior to reuse. Soiled sponges and ends of suture material are promptly discarded into appropriate tableside containers. All needles, including disposables, are returned to the nurse for a final count. The assistant should never reach onto the instrument table to obtain or return an instrument. This table is set up so that the nurse can find requested instruments quickly and it might be disarranged and possibly contamined by the assistant.

The 'dirty-field' technique may be used in the course of an operation when contamination is likely to occur, such as in opening the colon. New sheets and towels, preferably in a different colour from the routine linen, are placed around the wound and the field carefully protected by pads. All instruments used thereafter are kept in a basin on the field. The nurse meticulously avoids contact with the surgeon's glove and handles all instruments with a forceps. At the completion of this portion of the procedure, all potentially contaminated drapes, towels, instruments, etc., are discarded and the surgeon and his assistants change their gloves. In this manner, the instrument nurse, her table, and remaining instruments remain uncontaminated. During glove changing, one member of the team remains at the side of the patient to guard against uncontrolled evisceration.

Regloving and regowning are often called for when breaks in technique are detected such as a hand accidentally brushing against the face of a hunched-over assistant. Anyone detecting such a break should immediately announce it.

Tears in the glove are common and require immediate replacement, whether obvious or appearing merely as a thin layer of blood seen under the translucent latex.

RETRACTION

Proper exposure of the deeply placed operative field depends upon proper use of retractors. Improperly used retractors can cause serious injury to structures in the field. The spleen and liver are especially prone to suffer such injuries. The tissues under a retractor should be carefully padded. The second assistant handling a retractor should regard it as he would the steering wheel of an automobile. He must maintain the placement as adjusted by the surgeon, but he should be constantly alert to the progress of the operation and prepared to readjust the retractors' position on command. The most effective exposure can be achieved if the surgeon permits the retractor holder to see what he is doing. Permission to see and touch the retracted tissues often transforms the day-dreaming retractor holder, frozen to the 'stick', to an active member of the team.

Sudden forceful pulls are never indicated. The force of pull required on the retractor varies with the surgeon's needs and can be judged by the alert assistant. A 'toeing-in' motion, by flexing the handle upward and thereby inclining the distal blade inward, is often more effective than increasing the force of pull. A constant hard pull is seldom necessary and usually indicates inadequate muscle relaxation which should be called to the attention of the anæsthetist.

Good retraction must be maintained right to the end of the operation. Often the closure of abdominal muscles and fasciæ is made difficult by the fingers of the tired surgeon becoming slippery through contact with subcutaneous fat. Skin and fat retraction expedites the closure and renders it more secure.

HÆMOSTASIS: SPONGING

An essential function of the assistant is to keep the field clear of blood. Sponging or blotting is carried out as a single motion with a firm but not forceful application of the sponge to the moist area, followed by rapid withdrawal of the sponge. Rubbing, wiping, or staccato motions should be avoided; sideways wiping movements often restart bleeding. When sponging a pumping vessel which quickly obscures the field, the sponge may slowly be rolled off until the site begins to appear and can be clamped. Hand sponges or swabs are not used in the major serous cavities and large gauze pads or abdominal packs are substituted. These have a large attached metallic marker which reduces the possibility of retention of a sponge. When sponging is inadequate and fluid wells up at a rapid rate, one or more suction tips are indispensable. The two basic types are those used for pin-point aspiration and those with a multi-perforated guard for use in areas where tissue such as omentum is likely to be drawn into a single point by strong negative pressure. Two or more suction tips may be required when blood or fluid fills the field rapidly, as in exposure of a lacerated vena cava or a tear in obstructed small intestine. Curved suction tips are ideal for exposing a massively bleeding duodenal ulcer through a gastro-duodenostomy incision.

Sponging in the depths of a wound is carried out by a folded sponge held in a long sponge-holder; these also make good dissectors for loose areolar tissue.

HÆMOSTASIS: LIGATION AND ELECTROCOAGULATION

Control of bleeding during an operative procedure is a team effort. At the initial incision, small bleeding points in the skin and subcutaneous tissues are temporarily controlled with firm pressure from a gauze swab or sponge. When the surgeon pauses to effect hæmostasis, these swabs are removed and remaining bleeding points are carefully secured with the point of a hæmostatic forceps. The vessel is taken with a minimum of surrounding soft tissue and is then either electrocoagulated or ligated.

Diathermy.—Electrocoagulation is accomplished by passing a dampened, intermittent oscillating current via a point electrode to the metal forceps holding the tissue. The patient is earthed by a large plate against the skin at a distant location. No other part of the patient should be touched by earthed metal. A sustained, undampened oscillating current has a greater disruptive force and less coagulating effect, and can be used for cutting soft tissues ('cutting' current). Effective coagulation requires a dry field and a small bite of tissue. Fat and long thin pieces of tissue form a poor return path for an electric current; vessels in them are often better ligated. Care must be taken that adjacent metal instruments (particularly if touching skin, bowel, etc.) are not in contact with the forceps to which the current is being applied.

Ligation.—When ligating a vessel held in a hæmostatic forceps, the assistant holding the handle aims the point at the nose of the person applying the ligature. The ligature is passed around the point of the clamp and a flat first throw applied and tightened down around the tissue as the assistant releases the instrument slowly and steadily. All important ties should consist of square knots (*Fig.* 92),

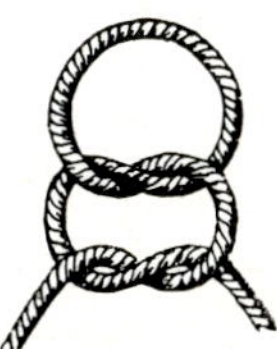

Fig. 92.—Reef (or square) knot.

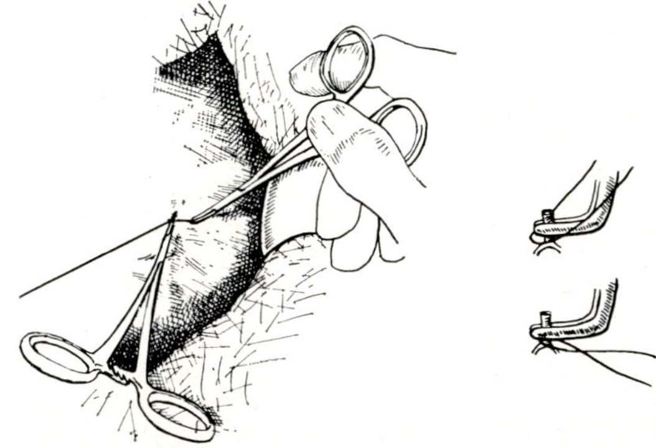

Fig. 93.—Ligating a vessel deep in the wound. The ligature is passed around the tip of the securing forceps with a long curved clamp; after encircling the pedicle a standard tie is made.

which do not slip. Awkward crossing of the hands over the field should be avoided by crossing the ends of the suture prior to throwing the loop of the tie. If fat or other constituent of the ligated mass is likely to fall between the first and second throws of the knot, the assistant should retake the apex of the mass with the hæmostats to prevent such interposition.

When ligating a vessel deep in a cavity, the ligature can be passed around the tip of the forceps with a long curved clamp (*Fig.* 93). When tightening down on the loop, one finger should be kept close to the knot, while the other hand pulls up so as to avoid avulsing the knot with the upward vector of force. When vessels in several different hæmostats have to be ligated, deal with the most superficial and accessible one first, so that there are no superfluous instruments when it comes to the deeper and more difficult ligatures.

Vascular pedicles, where the vessels are isolated, may be ligated in continuity before division. This is achieved by tying a ligature around the pedicle both above and below the desired point of division. The ligature may be either passed around the pedicle with a ligature carrier (an 'aneurysm' needle), or dissection around the pedicle may be carried out with a curved or right-angle forceps and the ligature then passed to the forceps which has found its way behind the pedicle.

Where the pedicle is thick and the vessels obscured by fat and lymphatic tissue, it is wise to secure the pedicle with a suture or transfixion ligature, as well as the tie in continuity. Simple ligature in continuity in this circumstance is inadequate, for when the thick pedicle is divided, the vessels can retract and slip through the tie.

Major bleeding from a large vessel which cannot be sacrificed is best secured by obtaining proximal and distal control with a non-crushing clamp or by pressure and closing the defect with a fine continuous suture on an atraumatic needle.

Sudden unexpected bleeding is best controlled by direct manual compression. Blind clamping in a pool of blood is ineffective and, more important, can lead to serious damage of adjacent structures. This is particularly true in areas such as the porta hepatis. With proper application of suction and rapid blood replacement, the pressure is released and the bleeding site accurately secured. Proximal compression of the offending vessel, e.g., the hepatic artery, with intermittent release, will enable the bleeding point to be accurately localized and dealt with.

In an operation, such as vagotomy, adrenalectomy, or sympathectomy, where many small vessels at some depth must be secured, stainless-steel clips may be used.

Hæmostatic Agents.—Bleeding from friable tissues or cellular organs which will not hold sutures or clamps can usually be controlled by pressure. Hæmostatic agents such as oxidized cellulose applied to such oozing surfaces promote clotting and may be left in place to be absorbed. In some difficult situations, a gauze packing may have to be left in place and brought out through the wound to be removed at a later time. Bleeding bone edges are controlled by hot wax applied to the oozing end. Crushed temporal muscle may be used on oozing brain surfaces.

Blood-loss Measurement.—When blood-loss is massive or continuous, careful measurement of loss should be instituted and prompt replacement started. All blood-soaked sponges and pads are weighed, and by subtracting their dry weight the amount of blood can be calculated. This is added to the amount accumulated in suction bottles as well as that estimated on the drapes. Dye-dilution techniques may also be used for estimating blood-loss.

Only if a large amount of blood must be infused *rapidly*, should it be warmed to body temperature prior to administration; this avoids unplanned hypothermias, and other circulatory derangements. A careful record is kept of blood and fluid balance during the operation.

Replacement of large volumes of blood is often complicated by coagulation defects. The addition of calcium to the infusion, however, is rarely indicated as only minute amounts are needed for the coagulation reaction and calcium is rapidly restored from bone sources. Deficiencies of platelets, fibrinogen, or other coagulation factors suspected during surgery may be evaluated by immediate hæmatological testing and replaced as necessary. Surgery on the lungs, prostate, and liver may be associated with circulating fibrinolysins and consequent failure of coagulation. This condition may be treated with epsilon amino caproic acid. Bleeding states are considered on p. 485.

LIGATURES AND SUTURES

Sutures are basically classified into two types: absorbable and non-absorbable. Absorbable suture of catgut is made from the connective tissue of the intestinal submucosa of sheep, which is processed into filaments and braided into strands of varied thickness and tensile strength. In the tissues it is gradually broken down and absorbed over the course of 4–7 days. Where slower reabsorption and greater staying power are desired, the catgut is impregnated with chromic acid. This chromic catgut lasts for approximately 3 weeks in the tissues, although survival time varies greatly depending on the response of the patient and the size of the suture.

Catgut is particularly useful in potentially infected areas because it is absorbed and does not remain as a foreign body which may perpetuate infection. It is generally useful on mucosal surfaces where permanent suture material might produce persistent granulomata and/or incrustations.

The most commonly used 'permanent' suture material is braided silk. Actually this material may be slowly absorbed over many years. Its advantage over catgut is greater tensile strength, less reaction in surrounding tissue, a more permanent hold, and greater pliability.

Other non-absorbable materials are: linen, cotton, and the newer, synthetic materials, including nylon, polyethylene, dacron, and teflon-coated materials. Stainless-steel and tantalum wire are also used and are even less reactive than the natural fibres, but may give rise to granulomata in the presence of infection. The metals have a tendency to break in the tissues and may produce cutaneous discomfort when placed subcutaneously in a thin individual.

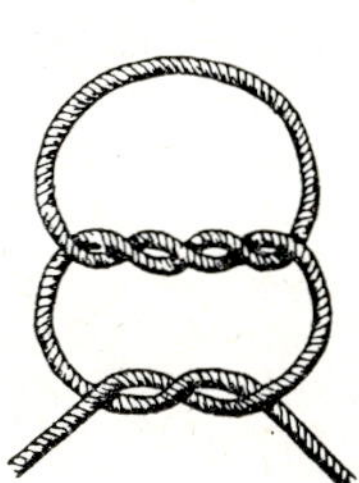

Fig. 94.—Surgeon's knot.

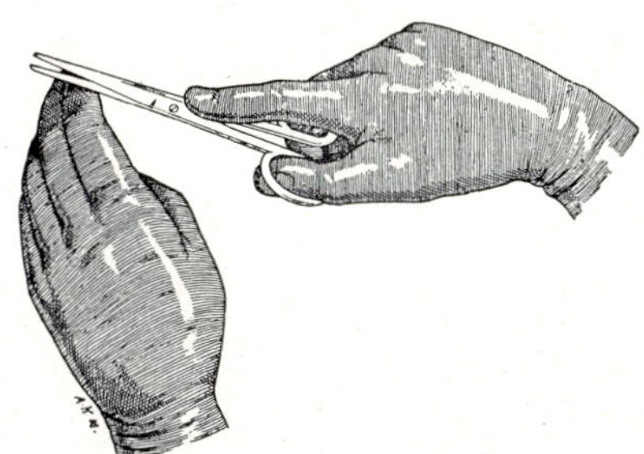

Fig. 95.—Cutting ligatures. Blades of scissors supported by fingers of the left hand.

Although a number of systems exist for describing the diameter of a suture, the most commonly used one proceeds from the digit zero. As sutures become finer they are designated as 00, 000, 0000, etc. Heavier sutures proceed upward from 0 to 1, 2, 3, etc. The most commonly used sutures range from 00000, used for the finest vascular and ophthalmic work, to 1, commonly used for ligating major blood-vessels.

The flat square knot is most reliable for securing a tie. Three throws are generally sufficient, although some of the synthetic plastic materials tend to unravel and are best secured by four or five throws (*Fig.* 94).

On completion of the tie, silk and other permanent materials are cut as close to the knot as possible in order to minimize the amount of suture material left in the patient (*Fig.* 95). Because catgut tends to imbibe fluid and swell, it is cut approximately $\frac{1}{8}$ to $\frac{1}{4}$ in. (3–6 mm.) from the knot to prevent unravelling. Extra length is advised for ligatures on major vessels, which may be ligated twice. Access to and visibility of a suture line may often be improved by temporarily leaving the ends of the first suture long and holding them taut with hæmostats.

The assistant should hold the distal end of a suture so that it is not completely pulled through the tissues after the needle; he should ensure that it does not become entangled with the handles of hæmostats, etc. Where several sutures are placed before tying they must be carefully kept in order.

Sutures are cut with a pair of blunt-nosed heavy-duty scissors. Delicate tissue scissors should not be used, as their edges are rapidly dulled on sutures. One blade of the scissors is placed against the suture ends and slid down the taut upheld suture until the knot is reached; the scissors is then tilted and the cut carried out near the scissor tip, care being taken to avoid inclusion of adjacent tissues. If the second assistant cannot clearly see and reach the suture to be cut, he should relinquish the task to the first assistant.

Needles.—These are available with both round and cutting shanks. The cutting shank has one sharp edge which facilitates passage through dense tissues such as skin, fascia, cartilage, and scar. Round needles are used in softer tissue such as bowel, vessels, muscle, etc., since they produce the smallest hole. Most suture material is now available on an atraumatic needle, to which it is permanently swaged, thus avoiding the increased diameter of the threading eye. As each suture is used the needle must be discarded. Atraumatic sutures are particularly useful in bowel, exocrine ducts, blood-vessels, and parenchymatous organs.

Needles are available in a variety of sizes, thicknesses, and curvatures ranging from straight to full circle. Curved needles are used with a needle-holder and are most manœuvrable within a cavity or at a depth. On the surface, straight needles which can be handled with the fingers will speed the placement of sutures.

INSTRUMENTS

Familiarity with the types and proper names of instruments available at a particular hospital greatly facilitates the operation. The popular name applied to an instrument generally varies from hospital to hospital, even in the same community.

The basic surgical instruments include:—

1. Surgical Knife (Scalpel).—This is the razor-like cutting instrument used for incision and dissection. It is available as a separate handle to which is coupled a disposable blade. Both the handles and blades come in a variety of sizes and shapes. To ensure optimal control and safety, only a very keen-edged, fresh blade should be used. Contact with dense tissue and metallic materials will quickly dull the razor edge and calls for replacement with a fresh blade.

2. Scissors.—Different types of scissors are available for dissection, division of tissues, and cutting of sutures. The character of the tissue being dissected dictates the size and sturdiness of the scissors selected. Those with curved blades lend themselves to dissection while those used for cutting sutures are generally straight with blunt tips.

3. Tissue Forceps (Thumb Forceps).—These tweezer-like instruments are available with a variety of grasping tips, ranging from gently serrated ones to those with interlocking (mousetooth) teeth. These are used for grasping tissues, sponges, sutures, needles, etc. Newer types are available with fine teeth for atraumatic but secure handling of delicate tissues.

4. Hæmostatic Forceps (Spencer-Wells).—These are hinged clamps with a ratchet lock device in the handle. They are available in various sizes, both straight and curved. The interlocking serrated blades are used to hold and compress blood-vessels for control of bleeding. They are often used for blunt dissection or grasping of tissues. Most varieties crush the tissue within their jaws; however, atraumatic vascular clamps are also available which occlude a vessel's lumen without injuring its wall.

5. Retractors.—These are instruments used to provide exposure by distracting wound edges and adjacent structures from the operative field. The two basic rigid types include the hand retractor and the self-retaining retractor. Each type consists of a handle and retracting blade. The form and size of the blades vary considerably, allowing for application in a wide range of anatomical situations. They vary from small rake-like retractors for drawing back sub-cutaneous tissue to those with long, broad, flat, convex blades for retracting viscera deep within the abdominal cavity.

Self-retaining retractors depend on the bidirectional or multidirectional pull of opposing blades to effect retraction and to maintain their position. They are fixed in position and therefore are less flexible than the hand variety which can be relocated with ease. Nevertheless, they are invaluable in such locations as the thoracic wall or lower abdominal wall, and in situations where there is a shortage of surgical assistants.

6. Needle-holder.—This instrument is similar to the hæmostatic forceps, with the jaws modified to securely hold and guide the curved surgical needles.

7. Other Specialized Surgical Instruments.—This group includes blunt dis-sectors, sponge-holders, tenaculæ, suction tips, stapling devices, hæmostatic clips and clip-holders, intestinal clamps, ligature carriers, etc., and should be familiar to the surgical assistant.

DISSECTION

Dissection by the surgeon is facilitated by the manœuvres of the assistant. Dissection is performed sharply with a knife or scissors, or bluntly with finger, gauze pledget, or a variety of forceps and blunt dissecting instruments.

Application of the various techniques to varying situations can only be learned by practical experience and time spent in the operating theatre. Familiarity with various tissues and their responses together with a tactile sensibility achieved by practice produces expertise in surgical dissection.

The major principle of dissection is the distraction of tissues by the application of traction and counter-traction so that a plane of separation can be identified and entered by the dissection instrument. Ease of dissection is further enhanced by bringing the tissues to be dissected as close to the operator as possible. Applying counter-traction to tissues held by the surgeon is a key role of the assistant. Accurate dissection is not possible unless the assistant assiduously keeps the field clear of blood at all times.

DRAINS
(*See* pp. 64 and 395)

EMERGENCIES

During the course of an operation the assistant should be alert to emergency situations. A peculiar absence of bleeding or a darkening of the blood may signal circulatory collapse or cardiac arrest, and should be immediately reported to the anæsthetist. The course of action for cardiac arrest is discussed on p. 2. Cardiac massage and inflation of the lungs with oxygen are commenced at once and the assistant must be familar with the approved drill and location of equip-ment.

Should the assistant be cut or pricked by an instrument during the course of the operation or become nauseated or otherwise ill, he should immediately notify the surgeon and withdraw from the operation.

COMPLETION OF OPERATION

Swab Count.—At the completion of the operation prior to closure of the wound, all sponges, pads, and instruments are accounted for by the nurse and should be confirmed verbally by the assistant.

Check of Hæmostasis and Drains.—All operative areas are re-examined for completeness of hæmostasis and proper placement of any drains employed. Drains should be secured to the skin with suture as they may be extruded or lost within a cavity as a result of muscular movement.

The Method of Closure.—This is determined by the particular preference of the surgeon. Full-thickness retention sutures should be strongly considered in patients having poor nutritional states, malignant disease, or abdominal distension or with contaminated and potentially infected wounds. These sutures are placed loosely, as post-operative swelling and distension will increase their tension.

Prior to approximating the skin, in dirty cases, the subcutaneous layer should be thoroughly irrigated with saline or an antibiotic solution. This serves to remove loose fat, devascularized debris, and clots. Intraperitoneal antibiotics are rarely used. Neomycin, kanamycin, and streptomycin have been reported to cause respiratory paralysis when used with curariform drugs intra-operatively.

The skin is carefully coapted with an everting, fine, non-absorbable suture or Michel clips. In contaminated or infected wounds, it is advisable to pack the wound open, placing sutures for a secondary closure.

Wound Dressing.—Sterile absorbent gauze, if desired, is applied to the wound, and the gloves are removed before the application of the adhesive strapping. Prior application of tincture of benzoin adjacent to the dressing protects the skin and helps secure the tape. Where a known allergy to standard adhesive strapping is known, a number of hypo-allergenic and non-reactive substitutes are available.

Where pressure to the wound is required, elasticized tape is applied, but should be checked within 24 hours as it may produce desquamation with painful burns. Internal suction drainage has replaced compression dressings in many such instances, e.g., radical mastectomy wounds.

Where adherence of the dressing to exudate is to be avoided, as over skin-grafts, both fine- and coarse-mesh gauze impregnated with petroleum jelly or oil are available as a surface cover.

In the Recovery Room.—The assistant should remain in the operating theatre to help move the patient to the stretcher. Careful supervision is essential to ensure that important tubes and infusions are not dislodged.

The assistant should examine the patient in the recovery room. The patient is usually conscious at this stage, and encouragement and assurance that the operation has been successful are appreciated and may greatly reduce restlessness. It is also important at this early stage to insist on repeated deep breathing and arm movements. Minor atelectasis can be appreciably lessened by so doing.

Labelling Specimens.—The second assistant should be responsible for labelling the surgical specimen. Unusual specimens should be photographed. Bacteriological cultures taken during surgery must be accurately labelled and incubated. Small specimens such as lymph-nodes should be sectioned and fixed in formalin. Where bacteriological studies are indicated, part of the specimen should be placed in sterile saline, making it available for guinea-pig inoculation or culture study.

Notes and Instructions.—The first assistant records a written note in the patient's chart describing the major features of the operation. An anatomical sketch is of great help in portraying clearly the operative procedure; it is of inestimable value in the follow-up clinic in later years.

After prior consultation with the surgeon, the post-operative orders are written by the first assistant or the anæsthetist. Specific instruction regarding the recording of vital signs, handling of drainage tubes and infusion, diet, position of the patient, therapeutic drugs, and analgesics should be made. Routine orders regarding catheterization of the urinary tract should be avoided. Catheterization should be ordered only after examination and if the patient is uncomfortable and unable to void. This will reduce the incidence of iatrogenic urinary tract infections.

In many ways, the assistant is the key intermediary in the total operative process. It is his prime responsibility to ensure that all pre-operative orders including placement of tubes and intravenous infusion have been completely carried out; his tactful review with nurse, anæsthetist, and junior assistant or student makes for an interested and integrated team. His skill at the operating table can make of any operation, especially the difficult procedures, a relaxed technical challenge rather than an uncoordinated and perhaps unrewarding exercise.

CHAPTER XIV

POST-OPERATIVE PULMONARY COMPLICATIONS

By F. Dudley Hart

Post-operative pulmonary complications are an ever-present source of anxiety to the surgeon. In Britain they may develop in up to 25 per cent of patients undergoing abdominal surgery and account for 30 per cent of post-operative deaths. Laparotomy temporarily reduces both total lung capacity and mechanical efficiency, the breathing being more rapid and shallow than normal. Much can be accomplished both in the prevention and cure of these complications provided a timely and thorough examination of the thorax is undertaken and the patient is questioned carefully concerning previous respiratory disorders. In arranging a date for an operation often too little attention is paid to the following:—

Physical Examination of the Respiratory and Cardiovascular Systems.—This must be thorough and the patient questioned as to previous respiratory and cardiovascular illnesses. The worst subject for operation is an elderly male with chronic bronchitis and/or sluggish circulation, possibly with a degree of cardiac decompensation. He must be questioned as to his exercise tolerance, for it should be remembered that a man with an apparently normal heart who cannot walk up ten stairs without pausing for breath is a worse subject for operation than a man with cardiac murmurs but an excellent exercise tolerance.

On examination the shape of the chest is important. The barrel-chested bronchitic with hyper-resonant percussion note, chest held in inspiration, and diffuse râles on auscultation, has a much reduced vital capacity, and an abdominal operation, particularly an upper abdominal operation, will further diminish this capacity.

It is of paramount importance to know that in a comparatively young person persistent post-tussive crepitations in the upper zones nearly always mean pulmonary tuberculosis, and an X-ray should be taken to verify this and to ascertain the extent of the disease. Coarse basal crepitations, more marked in, or confined to, one base, usually signify bronchiectasis. Finer moist sounds at both bases are found often in elderly subjects with a degree of pulmonary congestion. The fingers should be examined for clubbing, and the position of heart and trachea noted, for established bronchiectasis is commonly complicated by a collapsed lower lobe, with displacement of heart and mediastinum to the affected side.

Cyanosis and dyspnœa should be looked for. A mild degree of cyanosis is best seen in lips and nail-beds, and a lilac colour of the latter should suggest cardio-respiratory disease. Mild dyspnœa may be brought out by the exertions of examination. Pallor of the ears, nail-beds, and palms of the hands indicates a degree of anæmia.

Although routine radiography of the thorax is often carried out before any major operation, this does not absolve the clinician from making a thorough clinical examination; these two examinations are complementary, not supplementary. If, as a result of the patient's history or this examination, any of the conditions just alluded to is even suspected, the house-surgeon should inform the surgeon and the anæsthetist. A physician may then be consulted. An accurate assessment of the patient's ventilatory capacity can be made by measurement of the peak expiratory flow rate (PEFR) using Wright's flow-meter (*Fig.* 96). Improvement or deterioration can then be followed. Blood gases

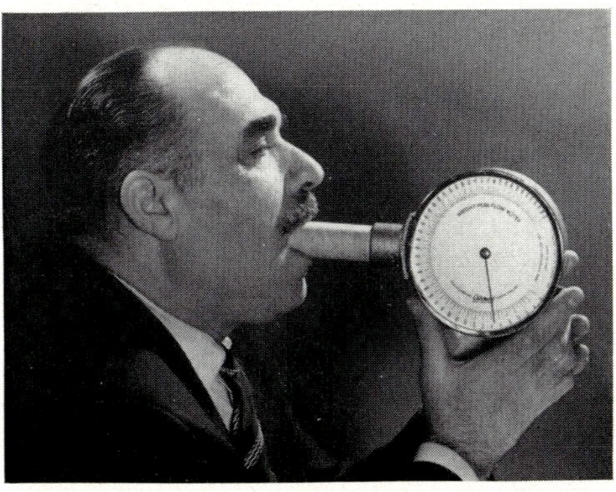

Fig. 96.—A Wright peak flow-meter.

may be determined and, if there is already evidence of hypoxæmia or hypercapnia, a prophylactic tracheostomy may be deemed advisable.

Unless the operation is particularly urgent it is more than likely that it will be postponed for a sufficient time to allow pre-operative prophylactic measures which reduce the incidence of post-operative pulmonary complications to be carried out.

PRE-OPERATIVE PROPHYLACTIC MEASURES

1. An Emergency Operation is required.—Obviously there is no time to carry out planned prophylactic treatment, but if the physical examination of the thorax reveals that the patient belongs to one or other of the groups described above, the incidence of post-operative pulmonary complications will be reduced by close attention to the following facts:—

a. Atropine dries up the bronchial secretion and tends to make the sputum of a bronchitic subject more tenacious and less likely to be coughed up. Atropine *should not be given after operation.*

b. Postural drainage (*see Fig.* 99, p. 172), if it can be carried out, will empty the bronchi of a bronchiectatic subject and make him a better subject for anæsthesia of any sort.

c. Morphine should be given as little as possible pre-operatively as it tends to depress the cough reflex.

d. The cough test: The type of cough evoked by the request to clear the throat is most informative; responses vary from an innocent dry bark to a prolonged paroxysm of coughing followed by wheezing and dyspnœa.

e. Any sputum is cultured for organisms and their sensitivities determined.

2. An Elective Operation is to be performed.—In non-emergency cases in hospital for some days before operation, much can be done to improve the patient's condition.

Group 1 (Pulmonary).—Patients with *chronic bronchitis* and *emphysema* are given intensive breathing exercises to improve the vital capacity and to aerate all parts of the lung. It is in the elderly male who smokes and suffers from bronchitis that the risk of complications is greatest.

Smoking should be stopped or rigidly curtailed except for an early morning 'chest emptier' which acts as the morning dose of expectorant; these instructions regarding curtailing smoking should be given to the patient when he is first seen in the out-patient department, for it is usually several weeks before much beneficial effect is noted. If the cough is wearing out the patient and is not productive of sputum, linctus of codeine or methadone (amidone) may be used.

Subjects with *bronchial spasm* may be given ephedrine tablets 30 mg. t.d.s., or sublingual isoprenaline tablets, but both these drugs should be used with caution in elderly patients; in an elderly male, occasionally ephedrine causes or precipitates retention of urine. Methyl ephedrine, which is less likely to give rise to this complication, is therefore advised in these subjects. Alternatively, choline theophyllinate (choledyl), which is a bronchodilator as well as a mild coronary dilator and a diuretic, can be recommended.

Inhalation of 1 per cent isoprenaline using a hand inhaler thrice daily causes dilatation of the bronchi and reduction of mucosal swelling; postural and postural-percussion drainage for fifteen minutes subsequently is thus rendered more effective. Five to seven days of such pre-operative treatment given thrice daily will greatly improve most 'chronic chests'. With a recent exacerbation of symptoms in such patients, it is wise to delay operation until the condition improves. In some cases antibiotics are useful adjuncts in improving the condition of the chest before operation; usually penicillin plus streptomycin (Chapter VI) is effective, but any known sensitivities are followed.

Group 2 (Cardiovascular).—In many elderly patients an element of *cardiac decompensation* is present. In these, pulmonary congestion causes the shortness of breath and the cough. Such patients may show no signs of venous congestion elsewhere (œdema of the legs, distended veins in the neck, hepatic enlargement, etc.), and the cardiac insufficiency may be confined to the left ventricle. Usually these patients have *high blood-pressure*. Rest, propping up on several pillows day and night, digitalis, and an oral diuretic such as chlorothiazide usually effect a remarkable improvement; mersalyl may occasionally be necessary.

Post-operative Thrombosis.—The 'vascular' members of this group who require watching with especial care are elderly patients with low blood-pressure and atheroma of the arteries, for post-operative venous thrombosis is relatively common and may lead to pulmonary embolism. Clotting in the ilio-femoral and leg veins with its attendant dangers also occurs readily in recumbent patients with cardiac disorders. Elderly subjects also are more prone to spontaneous arterial thrombosis during periods of operative and post-operative hypotension. In this instance the three lines of preventive treatment are therefore:—

1. To relieve the pulmonary congestion by graded rest.

2. To improve the peripheral circulation by active and passive movements of the legs, raising and depressing them for several minutes many times a day, taking the level of the 4th rib anteriorly as the horizontal plane for rest.

3. By elastic bandaging of the legs to divert the superficial venous circulation through the deep veins, and so avoid deep venous stasis.

Choledyl (Allen & Hanburys Ltd., Bethnal Green, London, E.2).

Obese patients should be encouraged to reduce weight substantially and remain active before elective operations. They are particularly liable to thrombo-embolism.

PROPHYLACTIC MEASURES *AFTER* OPERATION

The house-surgeon should carefully examine each patient's chest daily for several days, especially after an upper abdominal operation.

In reducing the incidence of pulmonary complications, prophylactic measures after operation are of even greater importance than those taken before operation.

'Don'ts' for the House-surgeon after Operation

1. Don't apply an abdominal binder so tightly that it interferes with respiration.
2. Don't immobilize the patient, but encourage simple movements of limbs and trunk.
3. Don't allow knee pillows or other obstructions to impede venous return in the legs.
4. Don't depress the cough reflexes unnecessarily.
5. Don't allow the patient to become constipated.

For the patient there are three main 'do's':—

1. Do cough if you feel there is something to bring up; hold the wound with both hands and cough up the sputum. A few early voluntary coughs may save thousands of involuntary ones later, and it is the latter which break wounds down, not the former. Practise deep breathing from the time you come round from the anæsthetic.

2. Do keep your legs moving. The nursing staff should be instructed either to provide a cradle under which leg movements can be carried out, or to strip back the bedclothes several times a day for ankle, calf, and knee exercises.

3. Do take deep breaths every 10 minutes to aerate the basal parts of the lungs.

High-risk Patients.—There are two classes of patient to watch with special care: (1) The bronchitic or 'bubbly' subject, particularly if aged and stout, recovering from an upper abdominal operation; (2) The patient with sluggish circulation.

The former group should be encouraged to expectorate his sputum and to use all parts of his lungs as much as possible. Breathing exercises should be instituted to encourage basal expansion and abdominal (diaphragmatic) breathing. The patient should be encouraged to move about in bed. Intermittent inhalation of oxygen may be helpful. Postural-percussion drainage (*see Fig*. 99, p. 172) thrice daily, perhaps preceded by isoprenaline inhalations, may be given in selected cases. The first inhalation should always be given slowly as pallor, tachycardia, and restlessness sometimes occur, and isoprenaline, because of its adrenaline-like action, should never be used in patients who have cardiac asthma, coronary disease, or hyperthyroidism. Morphine should only be given if pain is severe and exhausting. Atropine should never be given. A linctus is useful if the cough is very troublesome.

In some cases the patient may remain 'bubbly' and somewhat cyanosed for several hours after operation. Such patients may die of asphyxia if their condition is not relieved. Much can be done in such cases by intubation and tracheo-bronchial aspiration. If conscious, surface analgesia is necessary, the throat and nose being sprayed with 2 per cent lignocaine (xylocaine). The house-surgeon

Xylocaine (Astra-Hewlett Ltd., Watford, Herts).

on his night round after the afternoon's operation list should be on the look-out for such cases and deal with them there and then.

The second group should continue with those measures started before operation—exercises and movements. A careful watch is kept for signs of thrombosis in the legs; note *any* rise in pulse or temperature as these may be slight and easily overlooked.

Expose the legs daily and note the skin temperature of each leg; look for tenderness in the groin or calf. These two signs may be the only ones, or there may develop pain, œdema, and cyanosis with fullness of the small superficial veins in the affected leg.

POST-OPERATIVE PULMONARY COMPLICATIONS

Pulmonary Complications which may follow operation range from slight tracheitis to pulmonary embolism. Such complications are due to a variety of causes, as set out in *Fig*. 97.

Post-operative Bronchitis.—
This is usually an exacerbation of a pre-existing bronchitis. Precipitating factors are a badly administered anæsthetic, chilling and exposure on the trolley or operating table, and limitation of respiratory excursions by pain of an operation incision and/or tight bandage. Cough, sputum production, and substernal discomfort usually commence within 36 hours following an operation.

Often there is general distress, and there may be a rise of temperature. As coughing causes pain in the abdominal wound, the tendency is for the patient to cough less than he should, and so remain unduly bubbly. The physical signs are those of an ordinary bronchitis—diffuse rhonchi and crepitations. If the larynx is affected hoarseness or aphonia is present. A dry, very hacking cough indicates tracheitis.

Further Complications.—Bronchopneumonia; collapse of the lung.

Treatment.—Relieve pain as much as possible. Usually the more common analgesics, such as aspirin, suffice. Fluids are given generously, and the patient is encouraged to move about in bed to some extent. Sleep should be sound but not stuporous; therefore sedatives such as the milder barbiturates are given accordingly. If the cough is very irritable and non-productive, a soothing linctus, such as linctus of codeine or methadone, is given occasionally. If there is respiratory distress a steam kettle may give relief. Usually appropriate anti-biotic therapy is advisable, but is less important than securing adequate aeration of all parts of the lungs. Care is taken to avoid constriction of the chest. If the breath-sounds become weaker at one base in a chest full of moist sounds it is wise to stimulate respiration (and thereby expectoration) by giving vigorous breathing exercises or postural-percussion drainage, with preceding isoprenaline inhalation. Oxygen and 5 per cent CO_2 inhalations may be given to stimulate deep and full respiratory excursions. In this way the supervention of pulmonary collapse (*see* p. 171) can often be avoided.

Unless expectoration is satisfactory there should be no delay in resorting to bronchoscopy and aspiration of the bronchial tree. A temporary tracheostomy for the same purpose is advisable in more severe and refractory cases (*see* p. 16).

Acute Tuberculous Pulmonary Lesions.—Following an operation, particularly gastrectomy, a quiescent tuberculous focus in the lung can be transformed into an active one. Even if a most inactive-looking lesion can be demonstrated in the

FACTORS INVOLVED IN THE PRODUCTION OF POST-OPERATIVE ATELECTASIS

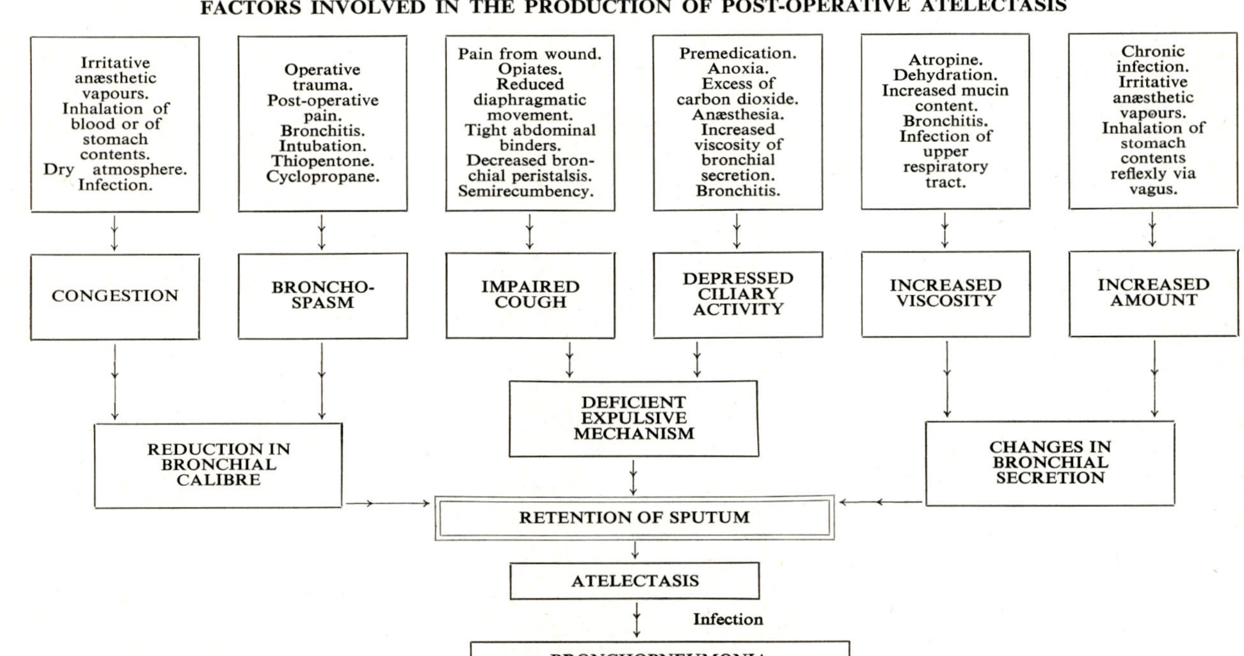

Fig. 97.—Post-operative pulmonary complications: factors in their ætiology.

pre-operative radiograph of the chest a close watch should be kept on the patient's chest afterwards and post-operative radiographs taken routinely.

Acute Pulmonary Œdema.—

1. Pulmonary Œdema due to Excessive Intravenous Fluid Therapy.—Fluid replacement is a two-edged weapon, for misuse or excessive use of it may cause water intoxication, pulmonary œdema, or sudden congestive heart failure in patients with a pre-existing slight degree of decompensation (*see below*). Before fluid of any kind is given intravenously signs of cardiac decompensation should be looked for.

The immediate treatment of pulmonary œdema due to overloading the circulation may involve emergency venesection and oxygen administration (*see* p. 301) and the use of potent diuretics.

2. Pulmonary Œdema due to Cardiac Failure.—

a. Failure confined to the Left Heart manifests itself as dyspnœa, abundant and often extensive moist sounds in the lungs, and in most cases (but not in all) bronchial spasm. This is the so-called 'cardiac asthma'. Morphine, 15 mg. by subcutaneous injection, breaks the vicious cycle: pulmonary congestion → dyspnœa → reduction of mean intrathoracic pressure → greater inflow into the right ventricle → increased congestion, by depressing respiration.

*b. Failure Secondary to Mitral Stenosis.—*Acute pulmonary œdema also occurs characteristically in sufferers from mitral stenosis, sometimes soon after operation or childbirth, or in the presence of acute respiratory infection. Treatment is with digitalis, diuretics, and oxygen administration.

*c. Failure following Coronary Thrombosis.—*Although, usually, coronary thrombosis announces itself by sudden precordial oppressive pain, this is not invariable. In the elderly such pain often is light, or even absent, while at any age the typical radiation of the pain into the neck and arms may be absent. When in doubt electrocardiographs should always be taken.

Prophylaxis.—To prevent the development of acute pulmonary œdema the patient with even a moderate degree of cardiac decompensation should be treated by digitalis and diuretics. Morphine given early in an attack of cardiac asthma will often curtail that attack satisfactorily. On no account should morphine be given in bronchial asthma or in acute severe infections of the lungs, because it depresses respiration. Finally, beware of overloading the circulation, particularly of cardiac sufferers and the elderly, with fluid of any kind, or in an effort to correct anæmia.

Post-operative Pneumonia.—

Bronchopneumonia.—The sooner bronchopneumonia sets in after an operation the more severe it tends to be; in a weak subject it may develop within a few hours of leaving the operating table. More commonly it becomes manifest several days later, often superimposed upon chronic bronchitis.

Treatment is largely symptomatic, the most useful measures being:—

1. Oxygen therapy for the cyanosed, distressed patient (*see* p. 301);

2. Strict rest and skilful nursing—the patient is kept as still as possible propped up on several pillows;

3. Penicillin, 50,000 units every 6–8 hours by intramuscular injection, or an appropriate wide-spectrum antibiotic, e.g., ampicillin, 250 mg. 6-hourly;

4. Plentiful dextrose drinks and other fluids;

5. Brandy or whisky as a sedative;

6. Tepid sponging, to reduce high temperatures;

7. Oral hygiene;

8. Reduction or elimination of abdominal distension.

Careful watch must be kept for cardiac or peripheral circulatory failure. If congestive cardiac failure supervenes, venesection often is helpful. Tracheostomy may be advisable and should not be delayed (*see* p. 16).

Pneumococcal Lobar Pneumonia is a rarity after operation, and a consolidation of one area alone should suggest pulmonary collapse rather than pneumonic consolidation; indeed, pulmonary collapse following operation is much more common than post-operative lobar pneumonia.

Pulmonary Collapse.—

Pulmonary collapse (atelectasis; collapse-pneumonitis) occurs post-operatively from inhalation of mucus in an incompletely aerated or ventilated lung with impaired basal (diaphragmatic) movement. It can also follow fracture of ribs and other thoracic injuries.

Often the symptoms are slight or absent, but if the collapse is extensive, there may be severe discomfort in the side with dyspnœa. An unproductive cough and cyanosis are not uncommon. Physical signs include restricted movement with, in some cases, impaired resonance, absent or impaired breath-sounds, and not infrequently a shift of the heart and/or of the trachea towards the affected side, and raising of the diaphragm on that side. Sometimes pulmonary collapse may be difficult to distinguish from pneumonia, but the onset of the former is more acute and it tends to occur within the first 48 hours after operation. As inflammatory changes coexist in most areas of collapse, collapse-pneumonitis is a better title. Commonly the temperature rises abruptly at the onset. A radiograph will verify the diagnosis, and should always be taken if the condition is suspected.

Pneumonia or Pulmonary Collapse?—So frequently are these two conditions confused that it is well to contrast and compare them. Correct and immediate diagnosis is essential because the treatment of the two conditions is entirely different.

Pneumonia	*Collapse of the Lung*
Gradual onset.	Sudden onset.
Occurs usually after fifth day.	Occurs almost always within 72 hours of operation.
Physical signs of consolidation (air entry somewhat reduced, breath-sounds bronchial, vocal resonance and fremitus increased).	Physical signs of SILENT consolidation (markedly diminished or absent air entry, vocal resonance and fremitus decreased).
No mediastinal displacement. Sterno-mastoid sign negative.	Mediastinal and diaphragmatic displacement often apparent.
Patient toxic.	Patient rarely toxic.
Treatment: Immobility.	Treatment: Mobility.

The last point of contrast is of cardinal importance. The patient with pneumonia is treated by rest, whereas the patient with pulmonary collapse is encouraged to turn from one side to the other, and to move the arms and legs.

Prophylactic Treatment of Pulmonary Collapse.—The measures outlined on pp. 166 and 167 are all-important—movement, breathing exercises, postural drainage, fluids, and perhaps isoprenaline or 5 per cent CO_2 inhalations. In bad-risk patients a prophylactic tracheostomy may be performed at the end of the operation.

Treatment after Collapse has occurred.—Similar measures are employed at once, with the patient so postured that the segment of the lung particularly affected receives the maximum vibratory percussion:—

1. Roll the patient onto the sound side so that the affected lung is the highest part being raised on pillows, and the head is low (*Fig.* 98). Encourage the patient to cough, and with the left hand flat over the collapsed lung strike

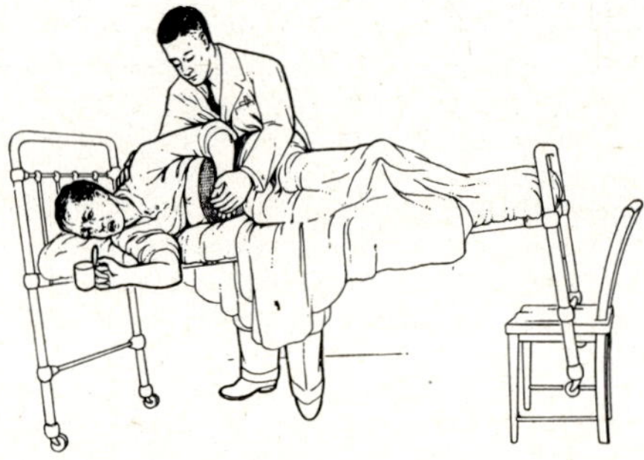

Fig. 98.—The knees are drawn up and the foot of the bed is raised on a chair. An abdominal binder, the patient's hand, and the clinician's hand all guard the abdominal incision. The clinician's other hand keeps the patient on his sound side. This hand also detects the clearing of rhonchi as mucus is coughed up.

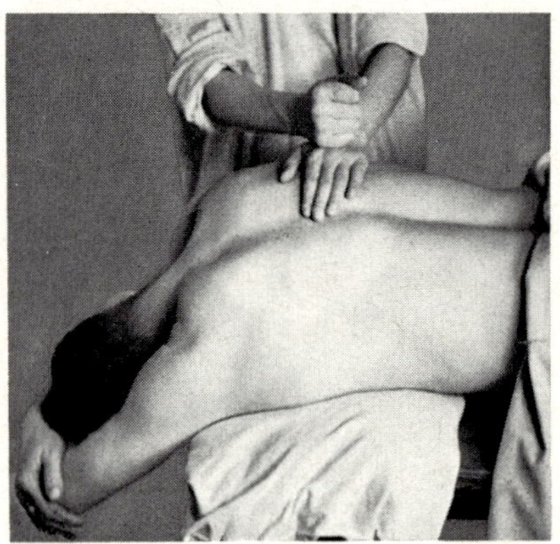

Fig. 99.—Postural-percussion drainage in collapse of the lung.

smartly with the right fist on the back of the left hand (*Fig.* 99). This postural-percussion drainage, if practised soon after collapse has occurred, loosens the plug of mucus, which is dislodged towards the trachea sand coughed up, allowing re-expansion to occur. Laying the patient flat and rolling him first to one side of the bed and then to the other, a dozen times, often proves useful and may be repeated at intervals of four hours. Isoprenaline inhalations may be given beforehand.

2. With postural percussion, combine overbreathing, to expand the lungs.

3. Antibiotics are given in most cases. Send a sputum specimen for bacterial sensitivities.

4. If the collapse be caused by a foreign body, bronchoscopy and removal is the obvious treatment, but if mucus or soft tissue has been the cause, it is so rapidly sucked into the smaller bronchi that anything but immediate bronchoscopy is generally useless.

Pulmonary Suppuration.—

Five forms occur:—

1. Diffuse Suppurative Pneumonitis is uncommon, and to all intents and purposes is indistinguishable from severe bronchopneumonia. The patient is very ill and the prognosis is bad. A course of the appropriate antibiotic in full doses should be commenced as soon as possible. Occasionally the condition progresses to a chronic form—necrozing pneumonitis.

2. Necrozing Pneumonitis occurs at variable times, often several weeks, after operation, and is characterized by progressive cavitation of the lungs. In some cases necrozing pneumonitis is due to clostridia, in others to *Staph. aureus* or to an anaerobic streptococcus. Areas of lung break down to form scattered pulmonary abscesses. The profuse expectoration is extremely foul-smelling, and sometimes blood-stained. The pleura overlying a cavity is liable to become involved with the formation of a pocket of thin, offensive pus. The patient is extremely ill, the pulse- and the respiratory-rate rise slowly but relentlessly, while the temperature remains between 38° and 40° C. (101° and 104° F.). The prognosis is grave. The best that can be expected is a prolonged convalescence and residual symptoms of bronchiectasis.

Treatment.—An appropriate antibiotic is given 6-hourly, the total daily dose being 1–2 mega units or more, and continued for so long as there is a favourable response. Any pleural pockets of pus must be aspirated completely and filled with a solution containing 50,000–100,000 units of sodium penicillin. Transfusion of fresh blood is helpful.

3. Lung Abscess occurs either as a blood-borne infection or (more often) from the inhalation of a foreign body or a piece of the patient's infected tissue detached during the course of an operation, most often an operation on the nose, the throat (tonsillectomy), or the mouth (particularly scaling of teeth or dental extractions). Usually abscesses due to inspiration of infected material are solitary or two in number; embolic pulmonary abscesses are multiple.

As a rule the onset of symptoms and signs occurs 7–17 days after operation. The patient sweats profusely, looks ill, and exhibits tachycardia and high temperature. A cough, at first unproductive, develops; in many instances a sudden expectoration of foul pus in large amounts leads to spontaneous resolution. In these circumstances a particularly foul odour of the breath emanates. Slight hæmoptysis may occur. The physical signs are dependent on the position of the abscess and the condition of the rest of the lung. Radiographs—anteroposterior, lateral and tomograms—should be taken to verify the diagnosis and to locate accurately the collection of pus.

Treatment.—A waiting period of 2–3 weeks is commonly advocated, with postural-percussion drainage (*see* p. 172) and antibiotic therapy. If complete resolution occurs no further action is required, but if the lesion ceases to improve the advice of a thoracic surgeon is sought. Bronchoscopy is advisable to exclude a primary bronchial neoplasm. If copious expectoration occurs and the abscess becomes an open one, draining into the bronchus, postural drainage is performed, the position of the patient depending on the site of the abscess.

4. Empyema is uncommon. When it occurs after abdominal operations it may be secondary to a subphrenic abscess or to a small lung abscess previously overlooked. The treatment of empyema is given on p. 313.

5. Subdiaphragmatic Abscess.—*See* p. 392.

PHLEBOTHROMBOSIS AND PULMONARY EMBOLUS

Pulmonary Embolism is the most dangerous of all post-operative pulmonary complications. It is most common in rather inactive patients over 45 years of age, particularly if they are obese. As a rule the embolus originates from femoral or iliac thrombosis, though there may be no obvious signs of such thrombosis in the affected limb. Usually pulmonary embolism is preceded by a slight rise in temperature and pulse-rate. Large emboli usually arise from a thrombus in the iliofemoral venous segment—its exact site may be determined by venography.

There are three main types of pulmonary embolism:—

Type 1—Massive Embolus.—A large embolus lodges in the bifurcation of the pulmonary artery, and temporarily occludes one (commonly the right) or both branches thereof. The onset is dramatic in its suddenness. The patient in a moment becomes very shocked, pale, and sweating, with a sense of impending death and a strong desire to defaecate. The blood-pressure falls, the pulse becomes rapid and often irregular, and may become imperceptible. If the right heart fails, cyanosis replaces pallor. Central venous pressure rises and is visible in the neck veins. A sense of constriction or actual pain is felt in the centre of the chest, and the patient feels himself rapidly 'slipping away'. Death often occurs within a few minutes, but may be delayed for hours or days. Permanent recovery is possible, but too often the patient seemingly recovers only to die from a second embolus at some time during the succeeding fortnight.

Treatment.—If the heart has stopped external cardiac massage is started and oxygen is administered (*see* p. 2). Treat the shock, but at the same time keep the patient as still as is humanly possible. Unless the risk of bleeding from the site of operation is very great, the administration of anticoagulants (*see* p. 79) must commence as rapidly as possible. In centres with the necessary equipment, rapid connexion of the patient to a cardiopulmonary by-pass machine (p. 332) (right atrium to ascending aorta) and pulmonary embolectomy may be possible.

Type 2—Small Embolus.—A smaller embolus, which passes through the pulmonary artery usually without causing symptoms, lodges in a lung and produces symptoms and sometimes signs of pulmonary infarction with overlying pleurisy. The right base is the site of election. On taking a deep breath, or on coughing, the patient experiences pain in the affected area, and often a small fragment, or fragments, of blood-clot is coughed up within 48 hours of the onset. At other times the onset is more gradual. The physical signs vary from none to those of consolidation with overlying pleurisy. Characteristic radiological findings are clouding of the affected lung field, with obliteration of the costophrenic angle and elevation of the diaphragm on the affected side, but unfortunately sometimes there are no radiological signs of pulmonary embolism whatever.

Treatment.—Bed-rest and analgesics are essential. Local heat to the thoracic wall may be employed. Anticoagulant therapy is instituted if there is no contra-indication. Removal of thrombi should be considered. (*See* Chapter XXXVII.)

Type 3—Recurrent Emboli.—Showers of small emboli pass from the site of thrombosis into the circulation, and become arrested in the lungs. They may so fill the lung as to cause failure of the right side of the heart. Cases belonging to this group are the most difficult to diagnose correctly.

Treatment.—A surgeon may advise ligation of the affected vein proximal to the thrombosis. It is a grave decision to take, but consultations should be started if a second pulmonary embolus is diagnosed. Alternatively, thrombectomy with suction through a Foggarty balloon catheter may also be tried; it is possible to clear thrombus from the iliac veins and lower inferior vena cava. Anticoagulants are indicated in most cases.

FAT EMBOLISM

Every year several examples of fat embolism occur in every general hospital, yet unless the staff of that hospital is diagnostically aware of the condition, none will be diagnosed correctly. Should the patient die of fat embolism, unless the pathologist also is aware of the possibility of the condition and, in relevant cases, has sections of (at least) the lungs and the brain prepared and suitably stained for fat, death will be attributed to some other cause.

Classically (and frequently) the condition follows a fracture of the femur or of the tibia. It can also arise as a result of various orthopædic procedures and severe injury to soft parts, particularly that due to burns.

Fat embolism following trauma has a special predilection for chronic alcoholics.

Clinical Picture.—Fat embolism arises much earlier than venous pulmonary embolism, viz., during the second day rather than the second week after the operation or the accident. The initial symptoms are those of shock accompanied by pulmonary, and a little later by cerebral, symptoms.

The pulmonary symptoms include stertorous breathing, dyspnœa, and cyanosis, sometimes slaty rather than blue, but always accompanied by venous congestion as seen in the veins of the neck. White froth at the mouth and the nostrils is characteristic.

The cerebral symptoms are typified by clouding of the sensorium, to which soon is added the noisy restlessness of cerebral irritation. Rarely are there localizing signs.

In patients who survive until the third or fourth day petechial hæmorrhages sometimes appear over the upper part of the trunk, particularly in the axillæ and over the lateral aspect of the chest, and occasionally in the conjunctivæ and the retinæ. Such petechiæ are of grave diagnostic significance. At this time signs of patchy bronchopneumonia are usually present, and a radiograph of the thorax often shows a bilateral pulmonary 'snowstorm'.

Confirmation of the Diagnosis.—

1. A rapid and profound fall in the hæmoglobin value of the blood is a constant and a reliable test.

2. Fat droplets in the urine are diagnostic, but they are seldom detected, mainly because they are not sought. Using a non-oily lubricant, a catheter specimen of urine is obtained and stained with Sudan III for fat droplets.

3. Fat droplets in the circulating blood *provided they are at least between* 10 *and* 15 μ in diameter are also diagnostic, but special skill is required for these measurements.

4. Fat in the form of tiny droplets is nearly always present in the pneumonic sputum of those who have suffered fat embolism.

Prophylaxis.—The need for particularly gentle handling and early splinting of fractures, especially those of the lower extremity, will be brought home to the reader previously comparatively unfamiliar with this condition.

Treatment.—

1. Remove the patient to a side ward, if possible.

2. Treat shock (p. 20).

3. Give 5 per cent dextrose solution with 5 per cent alcohol intravenously (*see* p. 50). Intravenous alcohol is an excellent sedative; it is also a fat solvent.

4. Early heparinization (*see* Chapter VII) is an extremely good and often a life-saving treatment.

5. If the patient will tolerate the mask, give oxygen therapy.

6. In cases of right heart failure and threatened pulmonary œdema rapid digitalization is strongly indicated.

If diagnosed and treated early, the prognosis of even severe cases of fat embolism is rendered hopeful by the above régime.

CHAPTER XV

APPLICATION OF BANDAGES

By Miriam A. Gough

A BANDAGE is defined as a piece of material used to cover, support, immobilize, or exert pressure to a part of the body. Good and effective bandaging can be learned only by frequent practice. It is worth mastering, for a well-applied bandage is greatly appreciated by the patient.

Bandages are used for many purposes: as a first-aid measure in the treatment of the injured, particularly to control bleeding; to immobilize a part or restrict its movement; to afford support, to hold splints securely, and to prevent or reduce swelling. They are also used to protect a surgical wound against infection, to hold surgical dressings or other local applications in place, and to assist in the correction of a deformity.

Before applying a bandage the following considerations must be kept in mind:—

1. The purpose of the bandage.
2. The comfort of the patient.
3. The most natural position of the part to be bandaged.
4. The neatness and the economy of the bandage.

Table VII.—Guide to Approximate Dimensions of Bandages used for Various Parts

| | Length | | Width | |
Part	Yards	Centimetres (approx.)	Inches	Centimetres (approx.)
Toe or finger	1–3	90–270	$\frac{3}{4}$–1	1·8–2·5
Head	6	540	2 –4	5–10
Arm	6	540	2 –2$\frac{1}{2}$	5–6·25
Leg	6–9	540–810	2$\frac{1}{2}$–3	6·25–7·5
Trunk	6–9	540–810	4 –6	10–15

ROLLER BANDAGES

There are many new proprietary bandages available which are proving effective and easy to apply. However, some roller bandages still have a place in hospital and general medical practice, and for this reason are included in this chapter. A roller bandage is defined as a length of material wound into a compact firm roll.

1. Size.—Various lengths and widths are used according to the part to which the bandage is to be applied and the need (*Table VII*).

2. Material.—A roller bandage may be improvised from any material torn into strips, but the most commonly used material is cotton. Other materials include calico, flannel, and domette, each of which has a particular use. Special bandages will be described later in the chapter.

An open-wove cotton bandage is light, soft and—because it is porous—cool. It is pliable and can be adjusted to fit any part of the body, though it offers little support. It is available with a frayed or woven edge. The 'Kling' bandage —a relatively recent product—is an open-mesh cotton conforming bandage which is effective and in Britain is replacing the open cotton woven bandage. The crêpe bandage, which is also made of cotton, is light and woven in such a way as to allow considerable elasticity. It can be applied easily so that uniform pressure is maintained over the area covered and it provides good support.

3. Application.—Before starting to apply a roller bandage the patient should be placed in a comfortable position and the part to be bandaged should be in the natural position if permitted. The person applying the bandage should stand in front of the patient and the part to be bandaged. A tightly rolled bandage should be used and only a short length, not more than 2–3 in. (5– 7·5 cm.) unrolled at a time so that full control of the bandage is maintained.

The outer surface of the bandage is placed next to the skin and a firm start is made, usually below the part to be covered. The bandage should be applied in an upward direction whenever possible and from within outwards for a limb. Absorbent cotton-wool should be placed between two skin surfaces to absorb perspiration and to avoid friction. All prominences should be well padded. Particular care should be taken that the bandage is applied with even tension over the whole area. It should be borne in mind that the degree of pressure required will vary according to the purpose for which the bandage is used. One-third of each turn of the bandage should be left uncovered.

The bandage should be finished with a complete turn and fixed securely—with a strip of adhesive strapping or Sellotape; with the end of the bandage, which is split and tied; with a safety-pin, taking care that it will not cause harm; or by sewing the end with needle and cotton.

Mistakes.—When applying a bandage every effort should be made to avoid the following:—

a. A wet bandage, as it will shrink when dry.

b. Uneven tension of the bandage as it is being applied—a very tight bandage will interfere with the circulation of blood and cause death of tissue—a loose bandage will become displaced.

c. Reverse turns over a prominence or wound as they will not give at all and can cause the patient discomfort and pain.

d. Use of too much bandage which will cause discomfort and is expensive.

e. Incorrect securing of the end of the bandage, which may do harm.

4. Basic Turns.—There are five turns commonly used in roller bandaging.—

a. Circular.—When the bandage is carried horizontally around the part. It is used mainly for securing a bandage at the beginning and end. It should not be used around a limb as it could interfere with the circulation of blood.

b. Spiral.—When the bandage is carried spirally up the limb. It is applied over parts that are of uniform thickness as for the finger and the upper arm. (*Fig.* 100.)

c. Reverse Spiral.—When a spiral bandage has a reverse turn. It is used for parts of varying dimensions, as for the forearm. (*Fig.* 101 A, B.)

d. Figure-of-eight.—When each complete turn of the bandage forms a figure-of-eight. It consists of overlapping turns, each of which crosses at a mid-point and ascends or descends alternately. It is used over joints and as an alternative to the reverse spiral. A spica is a modification of the figure-of-eight turn when

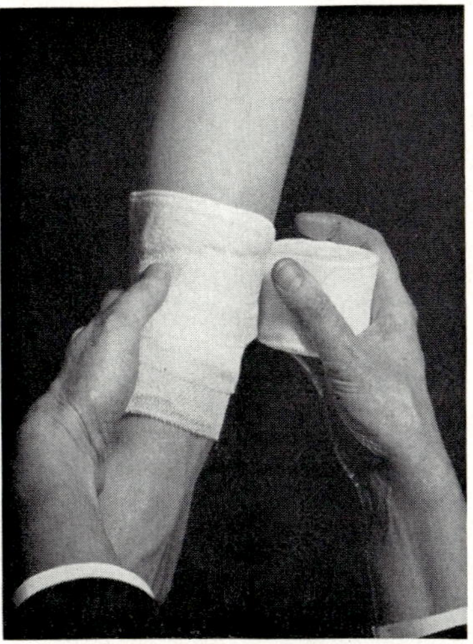

Fig. 100.—A spiral turn.

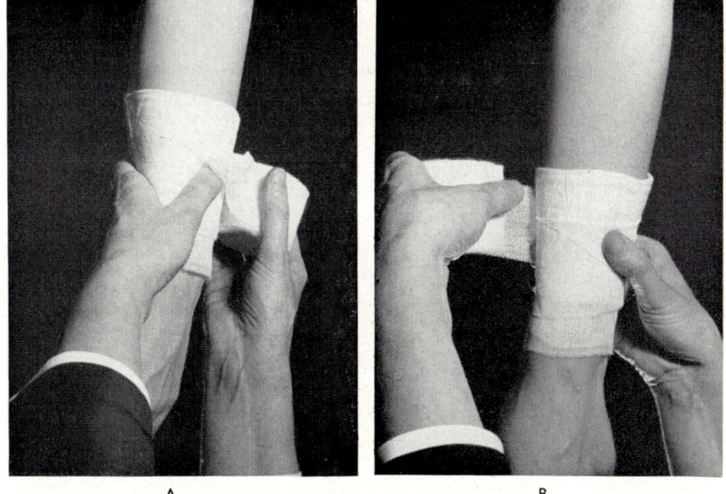

A   B

Fig. 101.—A, B, A reverse spiral turn.

one loop is much larger than the other. It is so named because the appearance of the pattern of the completed bandage suggests an ear of barley. (*Fig.* 102.)

e. Recurrent.—When a series of alternating turns are made. After one or two spiral turns the initial turn is made across the middle of the area to be covered and the succeeding turns pass to and fro over the end on first one side, then the other, of the initial turn until the entire area is covered. Finally, the

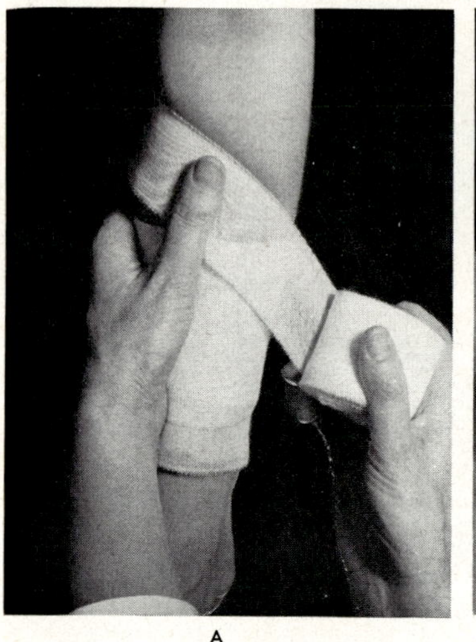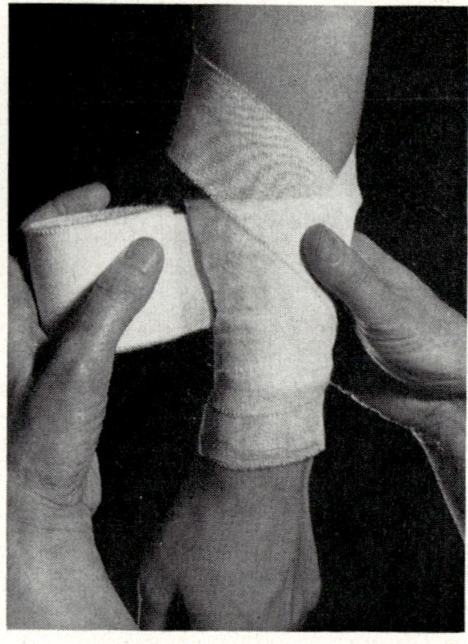

A   B

Fig. 102.—A, B, A figure-of-eight turn.

bandage is completed with one or two spiral turns. This pattern is useful when applying a bandage to the stump of an amputated limb, or to the head (*Fig.* 103).

5. Removal.—If a roller bandage is to be used again it is unfastened and taken off by gathering it loosely together and passing it from one hand to the other whilst unwinding. It is then washed, rewound, sterilized, and stored under cover until required. Alternatively, a bandage which cannot be used again is removed by cutting along its entire length on the side away from the injury or wound. The ends of the bandage are then carefully gathered and the bandage destroyed.

INDIVIDUAL BANDAGES

Although tending to be supplanted by adhesive bandages, roller bandages are still used for:—

HEAD BANDAGE

A 2–4-in. (5–10-cm.) cotton or crêpe bandage is required. An assistant will be needed to support the head and hold in place the recurrent turns unless the patient is fit to co-operate fully. Ensure that the dressings are in position and insert cotton-wool behind the ears.

Commence with a horizontal turn around the head, beginning at the right ear, carry it backwards low on the occiput and forward over the left ear, across the forehead to the starting point. Repeat. Over the starting point make a reverse turn and guide the bandage over the centre of the head to the left ear. (Sometimes the central bandage is continued down the left side of the head under the chin and up the right side of the head over the right ear, up over the head to one side of the first turn to the left ear and then continued as already described.) Here reverse the bandage again and guide it back over the head to one side of the central bandage to the right ear. Pass the succeeding turns to and fro over the head on first one side then the other of the central bandage until the head is covered. Finish with two horizontal turns round the head and fix in front with a safety-pin or adhesive strapping. (*Fig.* 103.)

This bandage is frequently used in neurosurgical units.

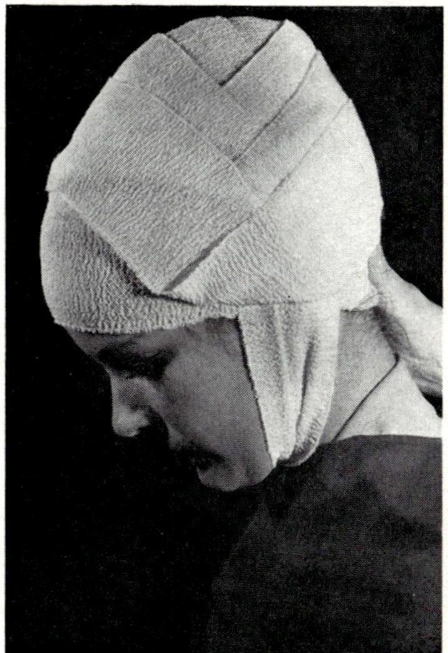

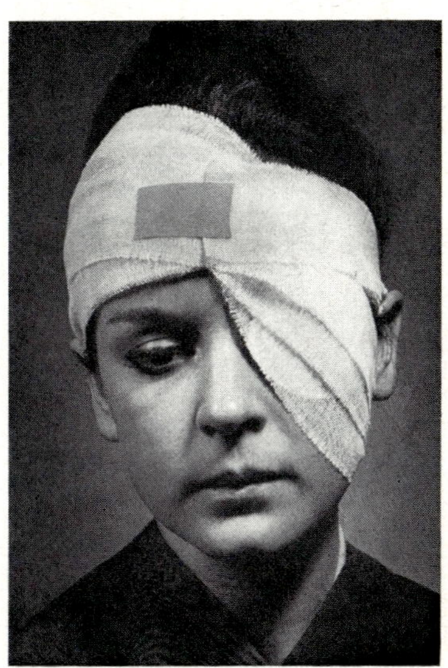

Fig. 103.—Recurrent turns when applying bandage to the head.

Fig. 104.—Bandage to left eye.

EYE BANDAGE

A 2-in. (5-cm.) woven edged bandage is used. The 'Kling' bandage is suitable for children. Place the bandage against the forehead above the affected eye, pass it horizontally around the head towards the sound eye and above the ears, bringing it low on the occiput and forward to the starting point. Here, take it over the back of the head under the ear on the affected side and up over the inner edge of the dressing to the centre of the forehead. Care is needed to keep the edge of the bandage clear of the sound eye. Take the bandage obliquely across the side and down the back of the head and again up over the eye. Finally, after two or three such turns make one horizontal turn around the head and secure the end of the bandage on the forehead. Crêpe bandages are used when pressure is needed. (*Fig.* 104.)

EAR BANDAGE

Take a 2–2½-in. (5–6·25-cm.) bandage; cut off a length of approximately 9 in. (22·5 cm.) and lay it vertically across the patient's forehead. Fix, by placing the free end of the bandage over the dressing and taking one and a half turns around the head; then carry the bandage from a point above the ear on the sound side obliquely downwards low on the occiput and forwards to cover the lower edge of the dressing on the affected side. Continue to carry the bandage forwards and upwards across the horizontal turn and over the front and side of the head. Repeat the complete turn, bringing the first part a little higher each time over the dressing, and the second part a little nearer the forehead over the head. Finish with a complete horizontal turn around the head. The strip is then tied tightly to fix the end of the bandage and to prevent any slipping. (*Fig.* 105.)

The application of the single ear bandage to each side in turn is most practical when both ears require dressings.

If used for a mastoidectomy a crêpe bandage may be applied for the first 24 hours when it can be replaced by a cotton open-wove bandage for a few days.

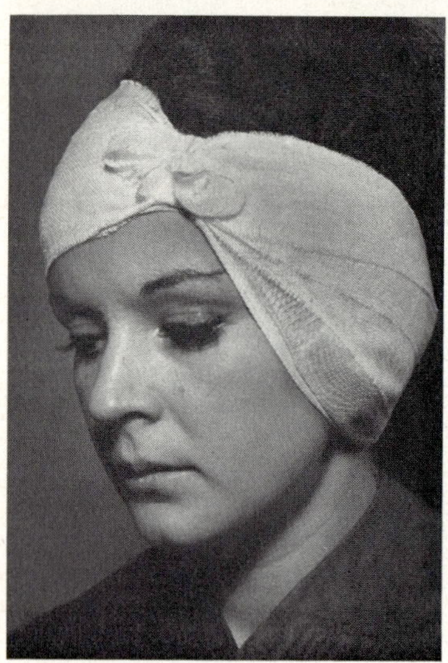

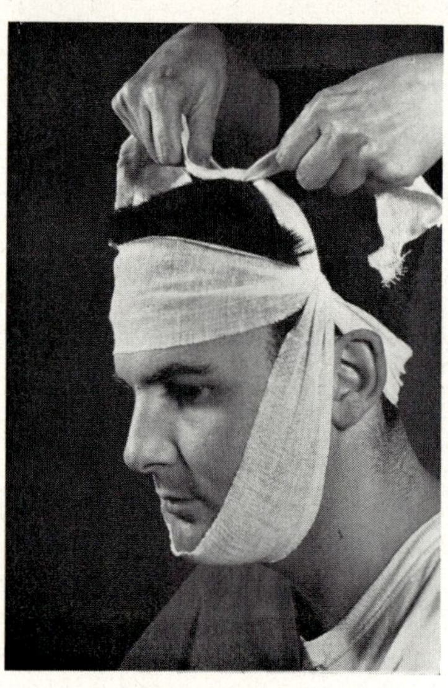

Fig. 105.—Bandage to left ear.   *Fig.* 106.—A barrel bandage.

BARREL BANDAGE FOR FRACTURED JAW

A barrel bandage is used for a fractured jaw. Take approximately 60 in. (150 cm.) of a 2½–3-in. (6·25–7·5-cm.) bandage and place the centre under the chin, carry the ends to the top of the head and tie with the first loop of a reef knot; loosen and separate the loop bringing one half over the forehead and the other low on the occiput. The ends are now taken to the top of the head and tied securely with a reef knot. (*Fig.* 106.)

NECK BANDAGE

1. Front.—Place a pad of absorbent cotton-wool in each axilla. Take a 2½-in. (6·25-cm.) bandage and make a turn around the neck to cover the upper edge of the dressing; carry the bandage across the chest, under the axilla, across the back, under the other axilla, and over the chest, crossing the previous turn in the centre of the chest. Continue these figure-of-eight turns until the dressing is covered. Finish the bandage on the front of the chest and secure. This bandage is still used occasionally to cover a thyroidectomy dressing. (*Fig.* 107.

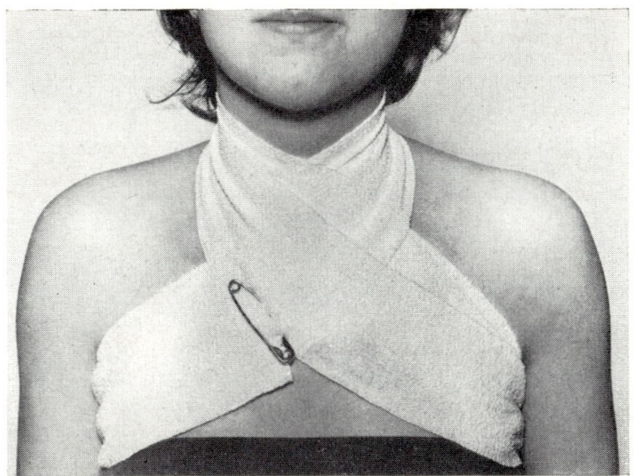

Fig. 107.—Bandage to front of neck.

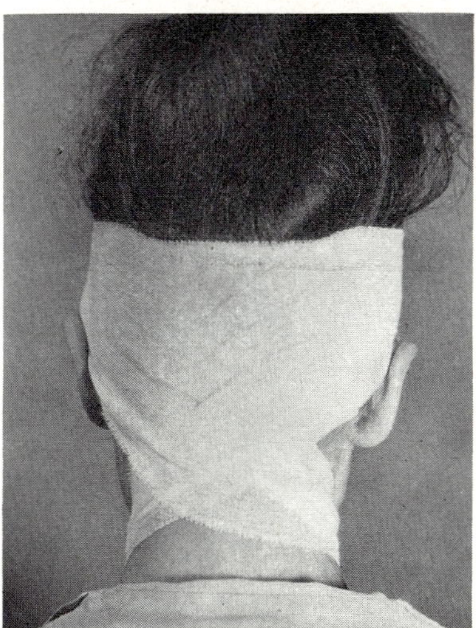

Fig. 108.—Bandage to back of neck.

   2. Back.—Place the end of a $2\frac{1}{2}$–3-in. (6·25–7·5-cm.) bandage on the forehead and take a horizontal turn around the head. Then bring the bandage backwards above the ear and take it obliquely across the back of the neck below the other

8

ear, around the front of the neck up at the back and around the forehead. Repeat these turns until the dressing is covered, taking the bandage lower down each time it crosses at the back. Fix the bandage on the forehead. This bandage is usually used for a carbuncle of neck. (*Fig.* 108.)

SHOULDER BANDAGES

There are two ways of applying a spica to the shoulder. If the dressing is low over the joint the ascending spica is used; conversely, if the dressing is high on the shoulder a descending spica should be used.

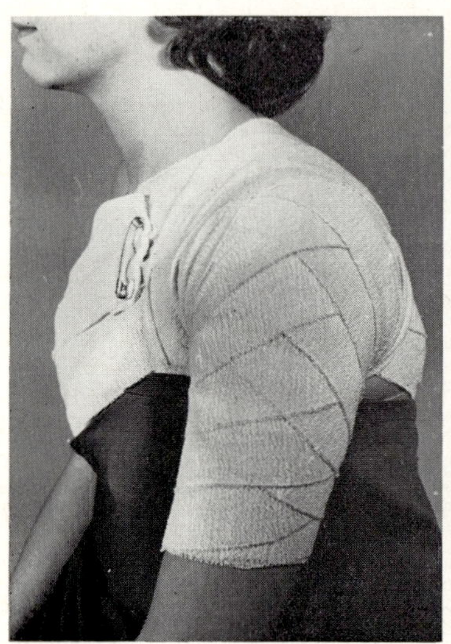

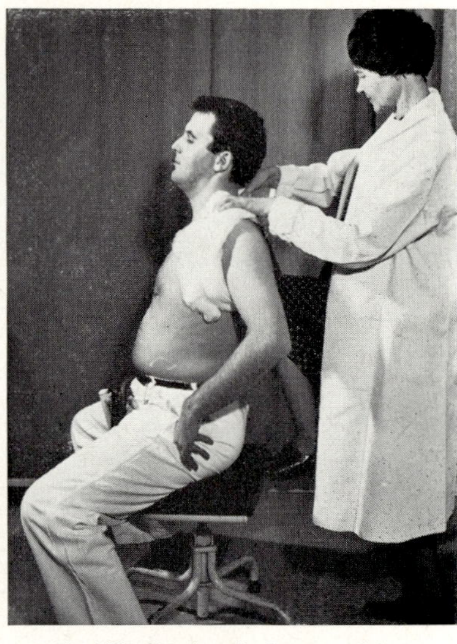

Fig. 109.—Bandage to left shoulder—ascending spica.

Fig. 110.—Bandage for fracture of the clavicle.

1. Ascending Spica.—Insert a pad of absorbent cotton-wool in each axilla. A 3-in. (7·5-cm.) bandage is used. Commence by taking a spiral turn around the upper part of the arm on the affected side, follow with two reverse spirals and carry the bandage across the back and under the opposite arm well below the axilla, across the front of the chest and over the shoulder. Then take the bandage under the arm from behind forwards, up over the shoulder and across the back again. Repeat these turns until the dressing is covered and secure in front. If the dressing is not extensive the reverse spiral turns on the arm can be omitted. (*Fig.* 109.)

2. Descending Spica.—The bandage is similar to that already described for an ascending spica but the figure-of-eight turns work downwards to cover the entire dressing and it is secured on the arm.

BANDAGE FOR FRACTURE OF THE CLAVICLE

Use a 4–5-in. (10–12·5-cm.) domette (i.e., cotton and wool weft) bandage. The patient sits with shoulders braced back, arms flexed and hands resting on hips. The person who is applying the bandage stands behind the patient. Place

large pads of wool over the shoulders and under the axillæ. Start in front of
the sound shoulder. Take the bandage across the back, under the axilla, and
up in front of the affected shoulder. Continue across the back under the axilla
and up in front of the sound shoulder to complete a figure-of-eight. Repeat
these turns until a firm bandage, which draws the shoulders well up and back,
has been applied. Secure in front. Support on the affected side in a sling.
Reapply bandage every few days over a 3–4-week period. (*Fig.* 110.)

BANDAGE FOR THE BREAST

For the left breast the patient's left arm is flexed and supported. Use a
4–6-in. (10–15-cm.) bandage. A 'Kling' conforming bandage is suitable for this
purpose. Begin by placing the bandage over the lower edge of the dressing
and carrying it towards the left side. Make a complete turn around the body
and then carry the bandage from the right side obliquely across the chest, over

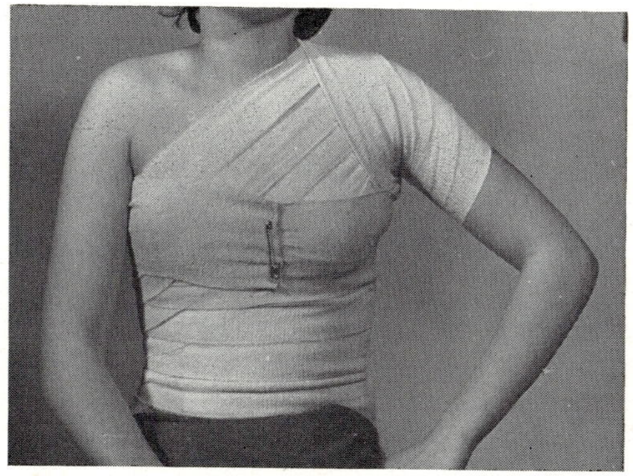

Fig. 111.—Bandage to left breast.

the left shoulder and around the left arm, covering the extreme margin of the
dressing. Next carry the bandage obliquely across the back and forward under
the right axilla at a higher level than the first turn around the body. Repeat these
turns in an upward direction until the dressing has been completely covered,
and secure in front. This bandage is occasionally used following a radical
mastectomy. (*Fig.* 111.)

HIP AND GROIN BANDAGE

Use a 3–4-in. (7·5–10-cm.) bandage to form a spica for hip or groin.

1. Ascending Spica.—The patient needs to be supported by a pelvic rest with
the knee on the affected side slightly flexed. Take a spiral turn around the thigh
from within outwards, then make two reverse turns. Carry the bandage across
the front of the groin outwards, behind the hip and across the back. Then
bring it around the front of the body, crossing the last turn, and leaving a third
of it uncovered. Continue these turns, working upwards until the dressing is
covered and secure in front. If necessary the reverse spiral turns on the leg
can be omitted. (*Fig.* 112.)

2. Descending Spica.—The bandage is similar to that already described for an ascending spica but the figure-of-eight turns work downwards to cover the entire dressing and it is secured on the thigh.

These bandages are being used less frequently because of the risk of contamination and disturbance of the bandage when a urinal or bed-pan is used.

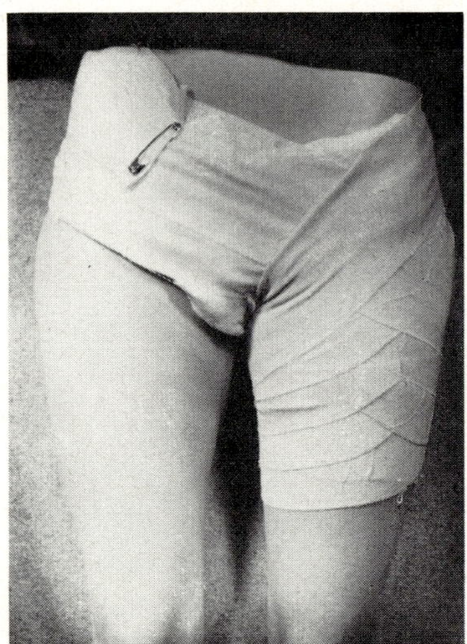

Fig. 112.—Bandage to left hip—ascending spica.

BANDAGES FOR THE UPPER LIMB

1. Whole Arm.—A $2\frac{1}{2}$-in. (6·25-cm.) bandage is used. Turn the hand palm downwards and bend the elbow. Start with a spiral turn around the wrist, from within outwards. Then fix the bandage by taking one turn around the hand followed by a figure-of-eight turn, one loop being around the knuckles and the

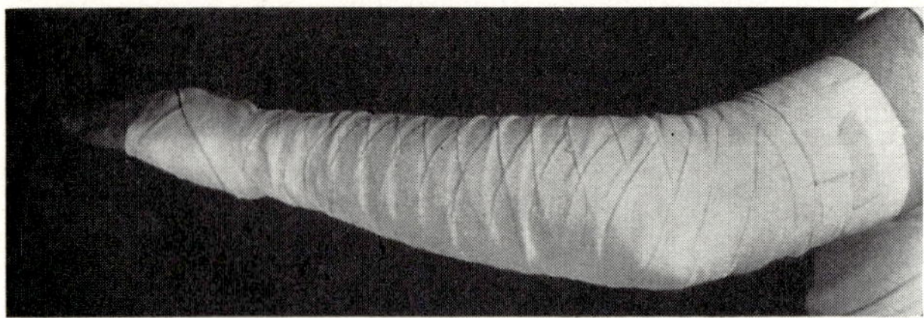

Fig. 113.—Bandage to left arm.

other around the wrist. Now make one spiral turn around the wrist and begin to reverse. Continue up as far as the elbow, keeping the turns near the centre of the arm to avoid pressure on the bone (alternatively, figure-of-eight turns can be used). Change to figure-of-eight turns over the elbow. Either continue these turns to the top of the arm or reverse again after the elbow is passed. Finish with a spiral turn and secure. (*Fig.* 113.)

2. Spica of Elbow.—Use a 2½-in. (6·25-cm.) bandage. Start with two spiral turns around the elbow so that the point of the elbow rests in the middle of it. Continue the bandage with figure-of-eight turns, working above and below the point of the elbow until the dressing is covered. Finish above the elbow with a spiral turn and secure. (*Fig.* 114.)

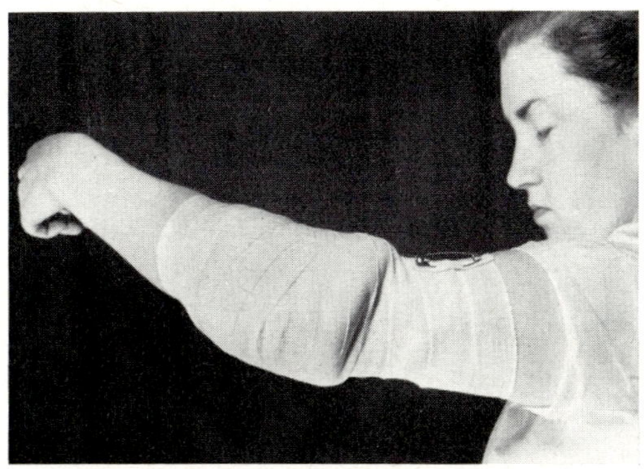

Fig. 114.—Bandage to elbow—spica.

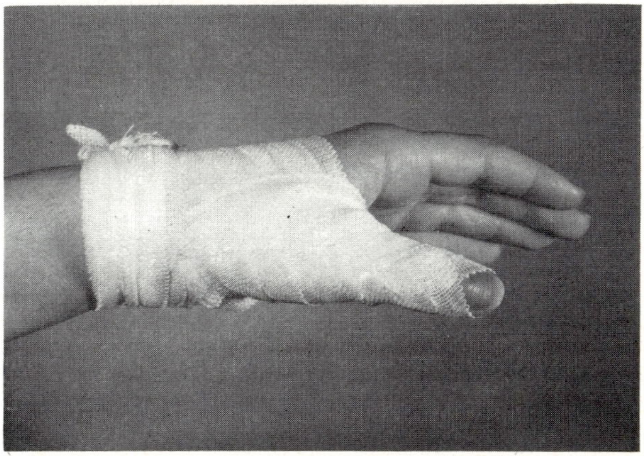

Fig. 115.—Bandage to thumb of left hand—spica.

3. Spica of Thumb.—Use a 1-in. (2·5-cm.) bandage. Turn the palm of the hand downwards. Commence with a turn around the wrist, then carry the bandage across the back of the thumb between the thumb and the first finger. Encircle the thumb. Then bring it across the back of the hand and under the wrist and again around the thumb, covering two-thirds of the previous turn.

Continue these figure-of-eight turns until the thumb is covered; finish with a turn around the wrist and secure. (*Fig.* 115.)

BANDAGES FOR THE LOWER LIMB

1. Whole Leg and Spica of Knee and Heel.—A 2½–3-in. (6·25–7·5-cm.) bandage is used. A similar technique is employed as described for the upper limb.

2. Knee Pressure Bandage.—A 3-in. (7·5-cm.) domette bandage is used. The patient lies in the dorsal recumbent position with knee extended and his heel resting on a wedge. Wrap a thick layer of wool around the knee. Apply two or three firm circular turns of the bandage around the knee, add another layer of wool, then two or three more firm circular turns of bandage. Repeat until a firm unyielding bandage has been applied. This bandage is used to control and reduce swelling for immobilization of the knee following injury, and as a post-operative measure.

3. Sprained Ankle.—A 2½-in. (6·25-cm.) bandage is used. The patient is seated and an assistant supports the foot in an elevated position and at right-angles to the leg. For maximum effect the bandage is applied from without

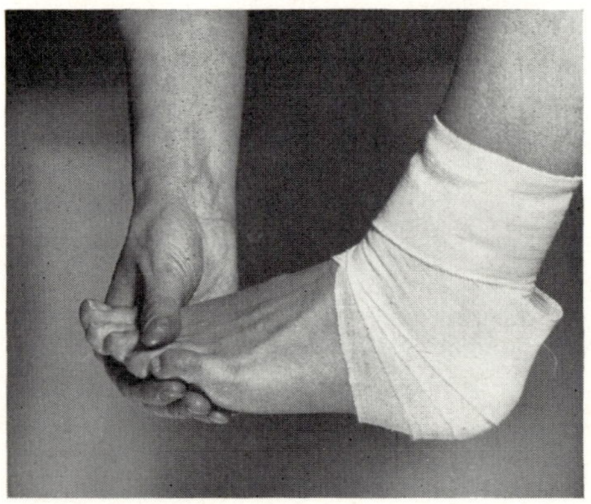

Fig. 116.—Bandage to sprained ankle.

inwards. Begin above the external malleolus. Make a complete turn, carry the bandage down the inner side of the heel, under the heel, up on the outer side of the heel and then around the leg covering the first turn above the malleoli. Repeat this figure-of-eight turn around the heel and ankle three or four times. Finish with a turn around the ankle and secure. The bandage (*Fig.* 116) is used as a temporary measure only, and has been replaced by the more effective application of adhesive strapping bandage (p. 202).

BANDAGING AN AMPUTATION STUMP

Use a 3–4-in. (7·5–10-cm.) bandage according to the size of the stump. A crêpe bandage is particularly suitable for this purpose. For an amputation of the leg above the knee, the aim is to apply a bandage which will produce a conical stump upon which an artificial limb can be worn. This is effected by applying the bandage firmly from below upwards, the pressure around the stump being gradually eased as the bandage is continued upwards. Begin by placing the free end of the bandage in the centre of the anterior aspect of the limb about 5 in. (12·5 cm.) above the end of the stump. Then carry the bandage over the centre to a similar position on the posterior aspect and hold it there with the thumb. Repeat these recurrent turns over the end of the stump until it is completely covered. Continue up the sides of the stump with figure-of-eight turns until the dressing is covered. Finish with a spiral turn and secure (*Fig.* 117).

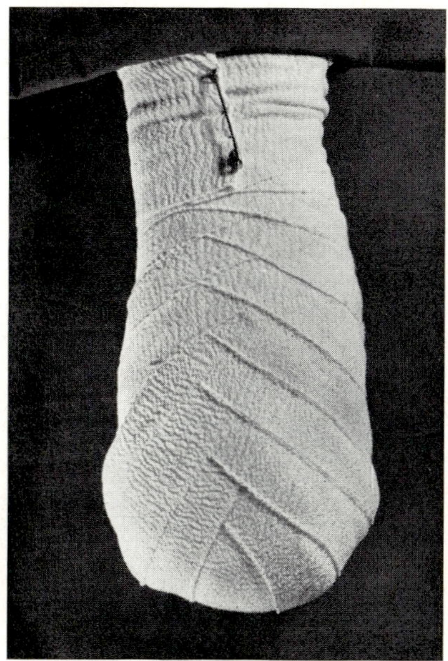

Fig. 117.—Bandage to the stump of an amputated limb.

To be really effective the bandage will need to be reapplied frequently. A hip spica incorporated in the bandage renders the dressing more secure following a high amputation of the lower limb. Flexion of the stump must be prevented.

SPECIAL BANDAGES

The Many-tailed Abdominal Binder.—This is still occasionally used:—
1. To keep a dressing in place and for support after major abdominal surgery.
2. To exert pressure following paracentesis abdominis.
It is very comfortable and adapts itself easily to the shape of the body.
It consists of long strips of material, usually flannelette, overlapping each other for two-thirds of their width, the size and number of strips varying according to the area which requires to be covered. The centres of the strips are sewn to a piece of the same material of appropriate size.
The binder is placed so that the centre of it lies under the middle of the patient's back; the other strips are folded over from below upwards in a slightly

oblique direction, and the uppermost one is fixed with a safety-pin. **Perineal** stirrups may be used to prevent the bandage from riding up. (*Fig.* 118.)

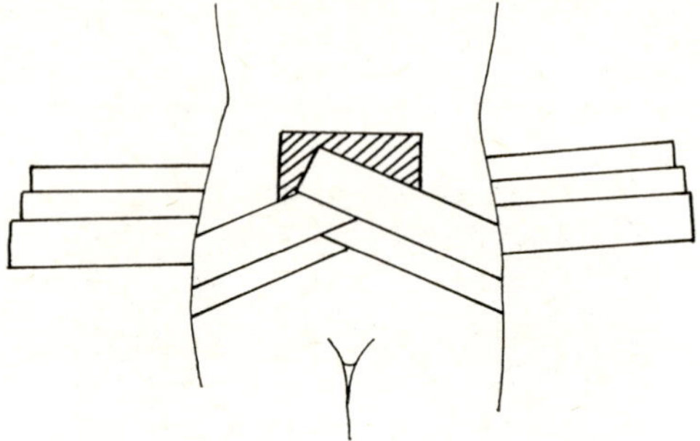

Fig. 118.—Diagram of a many-tailed abdominal binder.

The T-bandage.—This bandage may have one tail (single) or two tails (double) attached to a belt. The belt is passed around the waist and secured. The single or double tails are passed between the legs, which are extended, and tied or

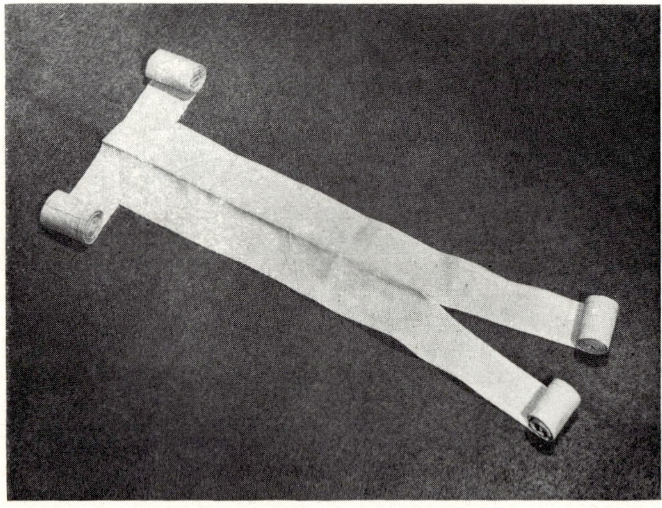

Fig. 119.—A T-bandage.

pinned to the belt. T-binders are used for fixing dressings on the perineum and in the groin, e.g., after hæmorrhoidectomy or abdominoperineal excision of the rectum. (*Fig.* 119.)

The Moorfields' Bandage.—This bandage is the most effective one for fixing dressings over both eyes as it can be applied and removed with the minimum of movement of the patient's head. It is made of a rectangular piece of firm material of double thickness, and a small notch is cut in the lower border to fit over the nose. The tapes are carried around the head and carefully tied on the front of the forehead. (*Fig.* 120.)

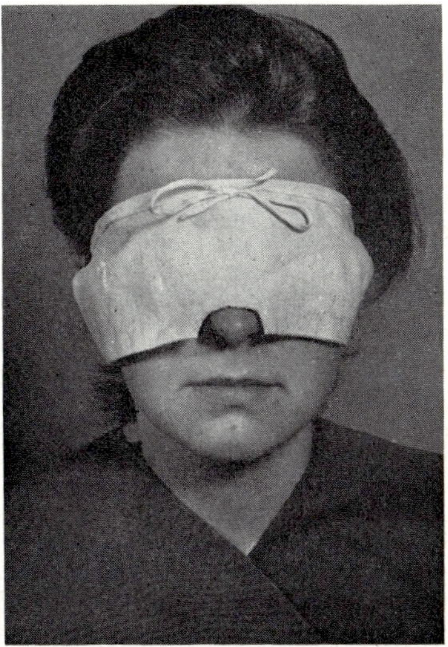

Fig. 120.—The Moorfields' bandage.

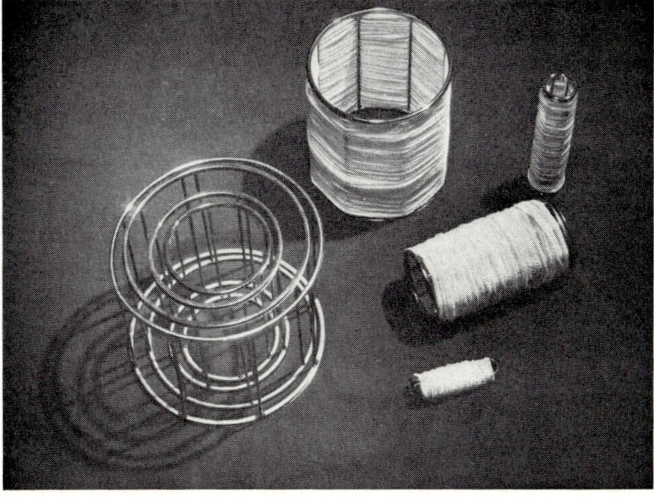

Fig. 121.—Loaded and unloaded tubegauz applicators.

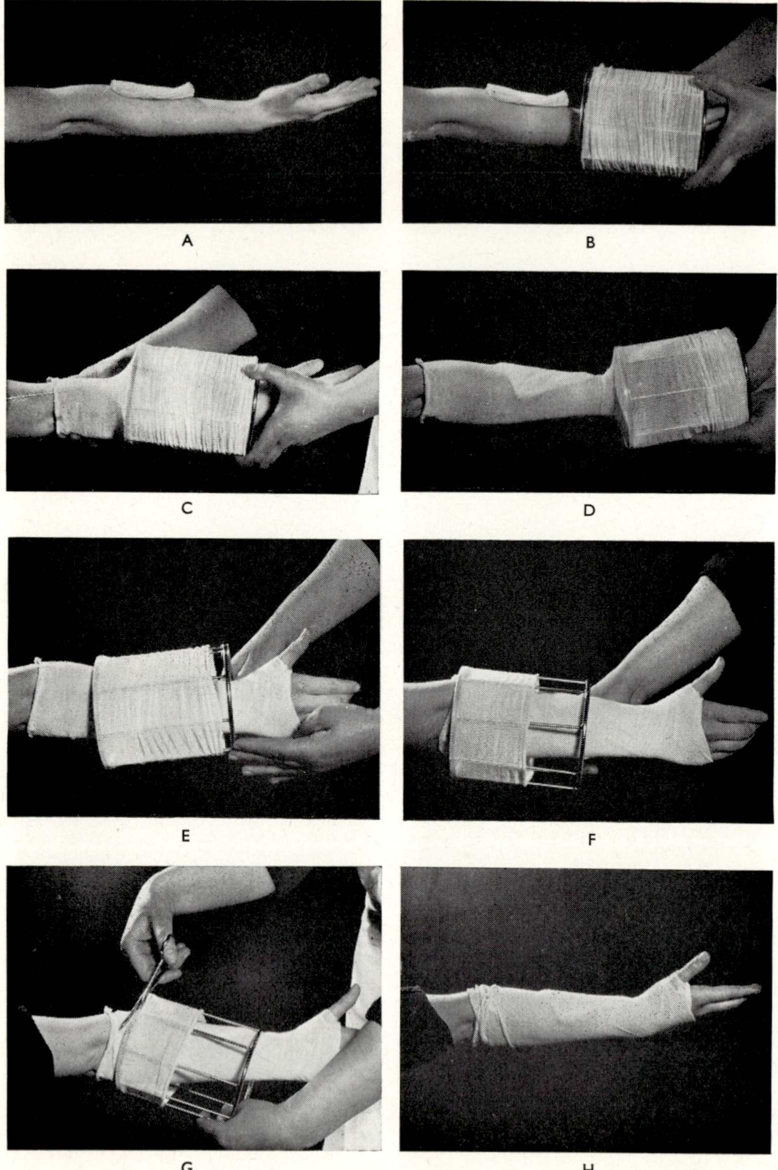

Fig. 122.—A–H, The application of tubegauz bandage to forearm.

Tubular Gauze.—Tubegauz is a seamless tubular gauze available in rolls of standard size: the bandages are supplied with specially designed applicators (*Fig.* 121). The following table sets out the sizes of the applicators with indications for their use. Each applicator is clearly marked both with its size and the size of the bandage with which to load it.

Bandage	Applicator	Uses
01	0, 00, and 1	Fingers and toes, children and adults
12	1 and 2	Large fingers, over large dressings
34	3 and 4	Children's arms and hands. Small adults' hands and arms
56	5 and 6	Arms and legs of adults and children
78	7 and 8	Head, thigh, legs
T.1	—	Hips and thighs of adults. Trunks of children
T.2	—	Trunk of adults

Since tubegauz can be used quickly and effectively with or without applicators and the bandage can be adapted to fit any part of the body, it is commonly used in hospital practice, particular in casualty departments, fracture clinics, and dermatological units.

Technique.—The required amount of tubegauz is cut from the roll and eased on to the applicator of suitable size. Half-way along the part to be covered, the bandage is drawn over the rim of the applicator and held lightly on the dressing. The applicator is then rolled and at the same time carried down the limb. The simple rolling movement is continued whilst the applicator is carried upwards and downwards over the area to be covered according to the number of layers required. The method of finishing is to cut the tubegauz around the channelled rim of the applicator, split the edge of the bandage, and tie. If a surgical dressing is being covered the loaded applicator will need to be sterilized. (*Fig.* 122.)

If pressure is required it can be applied effectively by adopting a method similar to that which has been described, the only difference being in the degree of control over the discharge of tubegauz from the applicator and the amount of rotation used. A constant tension on the bandage and on every continuous rotary movement will produce pressure that is uniform throughout. As for roller bandages, the application of tubular gauze can be learned only by frequent practice. It is extremely important that the person applying tubular gauze bandages must master the technique of rolling the applicator correctly so that an overtight bandage which will interfere with the circulation of blood is avoided.

Further details of the uses and methods of applying tubegauz are found in the booklet *Practical Bandaging with Tubegauz* issued by The Scholl Manufacturing Co. Ltd., 182–204 St. John Street, London, E.C.1.

BANDAGES IMPREGNATED WITH MEDICAMENTS

Various impregnated bandages are available (*Fig.* 123). They are made of cotton which may be impregnated with one of the following:—

1. Hydrocortisone acetate B.P., 1 per cent (cortacream); silicone fluid, 10 per cent; in an emulsified base.

2. Ten per cent w/w zinc oxide B.P. (viscopaste) in an emulsified non-gelatinous base.

Tubegauz (The Scholl Manufacturing Co. Ltd., 182–204 St. John Street, London, E.C.1). Cortacream, Viscopaste (Smith & Nephew Pharmaceuticals, Welwyn Garden City, Herts).

3. Two per cent ichthammol B.P. in a zinc oxide and gelatin paste (ichtho-paste).

4. Prepared coal tar B.P.C. 3 per cent, in a water-miscible paste (coltapaste).

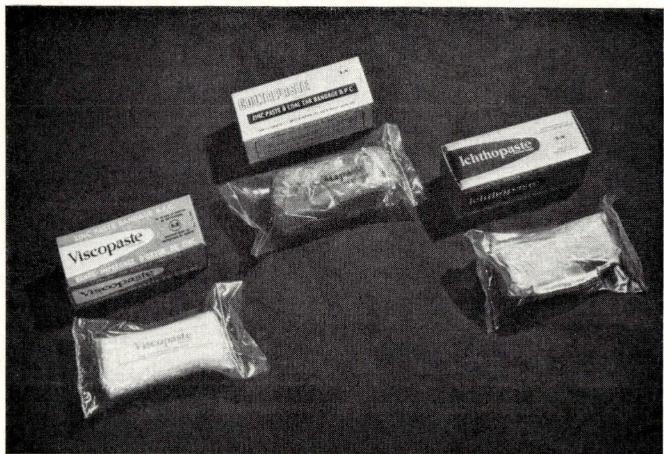

Fig. 123.—Bandages impregnated with medicaments.

These bandages are used to protect and soothe the skin and to promote healing of wounds, particularly for chronic conditions of the leg, e.g., varicose ulcers, when they are applied in conjunction with a roller or adhesive bandage.

A similar technique is used as for strapping. Detailed instructions are supplied with the bandages.

COTTON CRÊPE (ELASTOCREPE)

This is a smooth-surface cotton crêpe bandage which provides greater com-pression and support than the ordinary crêpe bandage. It stretches to nearly twice its length but regains its original length readily. This elasticity gives firm but controlled compression, and is particularly useful for this purpose when applied in conjunction with the impregnated bandages already described.

Cotton incorporated with Rubber Threads (Elastoweb).—This is a bandage incorporating strong rubber threads which provides even greater compression and support than the cotton crêpe (elastocrepe) bandage. It is fitted with a special foot loop.

Method of application of this bandage for varicose veins of the leg: The patient is seated and an assistant supports the foot at right-angles to the leg. Place the loop over the foot with the edge level with the base of the big toe. Pull the bandage well out during application, especially when covering the lower third of the leg. As the bandage ascends pressure on the limb is lessened gradually. Carry the bandage over the tendo Achillis and then over the dorsum of the foot so that the loop is overlapped by at least two-thirds. Repeat the turns around the foot and the heel, ensuring that the overlapping is constant, and continue up the leg. Finally, finish below the knee and secure. The bandage should be taken off at night and reapplied each morning. (*Fig.* 124.)

Ichthopaste, Coltapaste (Smith & Nephew Pharmaceuticals, Welwyn Garden City, Herts).

ADHESIVE BANDAGES

An adhesive bandage is usually made of cotton and it may or may not be extensible. The bandage is usually rolled, wrapped, and supplied in a sealed tin or other suitable container; it should be stored in a cool place.

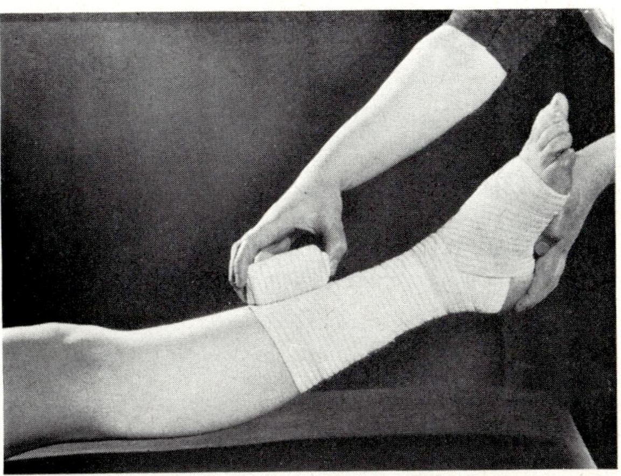

Fig. 124.—The application of elastoweb bandage to right leg.

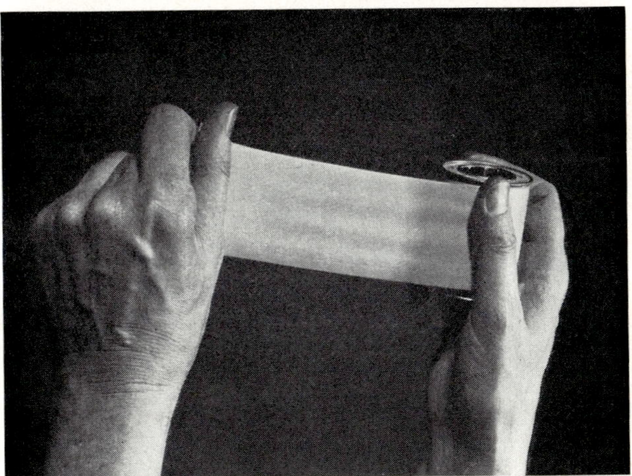

Fig. 125.—Waterproof adhesive strapping.

1. Purpose.—Adhesive strapping is used for almost all the conditions given in the previous paragraphs for a roller bandage and is tending to replace the latter. It is, however, particularly effective in providing:—

a. Pressure and support for chronic conditions of the legs, e.g., varicose veins and ulcers.

b. Support for sprains and strains.
c. Immobilization of fractures.
d. Skin traction in the treatment of fractures and diseased joints.
e. Protection of wounds.

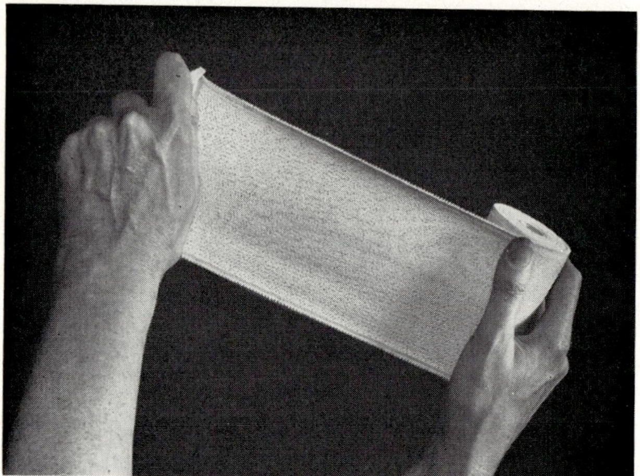

Fig. 126.—Porous adhesive strapping.

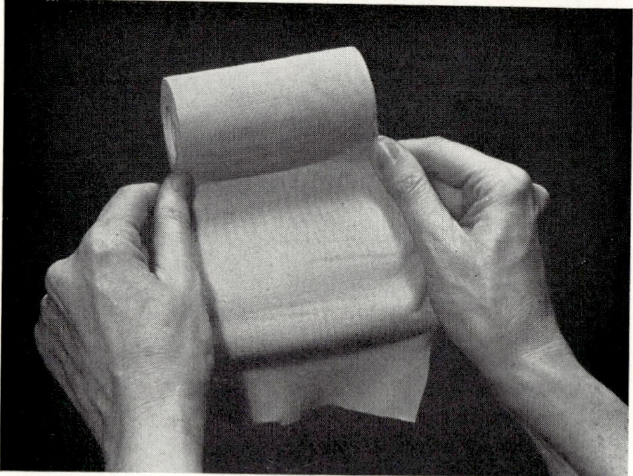

Fig. 127.—Extension adhesive strapping.

2. Types.—The three types in common use are:—

a. Waterproof.—This is made from a thin, pliable plastic film spread with adhesive plaster. It is ideal as a temporary protection of wounds or of normal skin, for example, when the bandage is placed over the surfaces and edges of plaster-of-Paris casts. (*Fig.* 125.)

b. Porous.—This type of bandage is spread with an adhesive in such a way that it permits free circulation of air, evaporation of sweat from the skin, and avoidance of skin irritation without loss of efficiency. (*Fig.* 126.)

c. Extension.—This is similar to the porous bandage, but the material is made so that it is rigid lengthways and extensible crossways. It is used for the application of skin traction. (*Fig.* 127.)

3. Application.—Adhesive bandages have many advantages if they are applied correctly. They are prepared for immediate use, are quickly and easily applied, effective, neat, and patients find them comfortable. Adhesive strapping should adhere to the skin, be free of creases, and not be so tight as to cause discomfort, pain, or impairment of function. The bandage is applied more effectively if it is split at each end.

Precautions.—Irritation of the skin is one potential hazard which can be minimized if the person who applies the bandages takes heed of the following directions:—

a. The area to be covered should be clean, dry, and hairless.

b. Sensitive skin should be protected by being painted with compound tincture of benzoin before application of the bandage.

c. The bandage should remain untouched unless the patient complains of discomfort or pain.

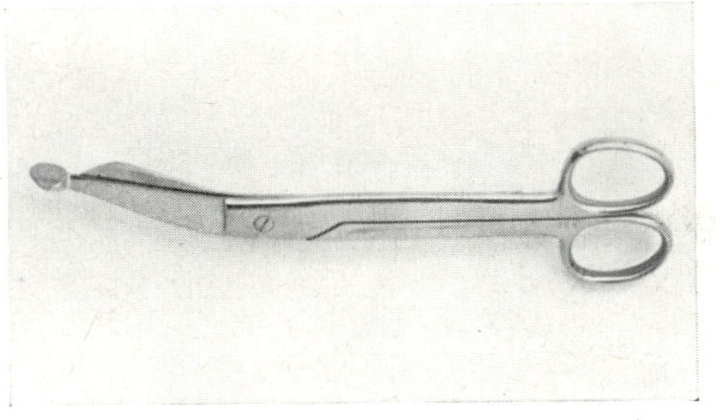

Fig. 128.—Lister's scissors for cutting adhesive strapping.

4. Technique.—When strapping is applied to protect a wound: Unroll 4–5 in. (10–12·5 cm.) of strapping. Split the free end as required and apply to the skin some distance from the dressing. Hold in place with the palm of the hand until it has adhered firmly. Ask the patient, if able, or an assistant, to keep the stuck end of the strapping in place and then draw the roll of adhesive firmly over the dressing to the other side. Similarly, keep the adhesive in position on both sides of the dressing while cutting, splitting, and applying the other end of the strapping firmly to the skin. Maintain pressure until the ends are stuck securely. Further lengths of strapping are applied as required.

5. Removal.—The strapping should be removed with care by: (*a*) Peeling it off gently and slowly with ether or a special commercial non-inflammable plaster solvent (Zoff); (*b*) using special scissors, one blade of which is probe-pointed, and cutting along the entire length of the bandage in the same way as described for a roller bandage. (*Fig.* 128.)

INDIVIDUAL ADHESIVE STRAPPING BANDAGES

Extensible adhesive strapping is used for the following bandages unless otherwise indicated.

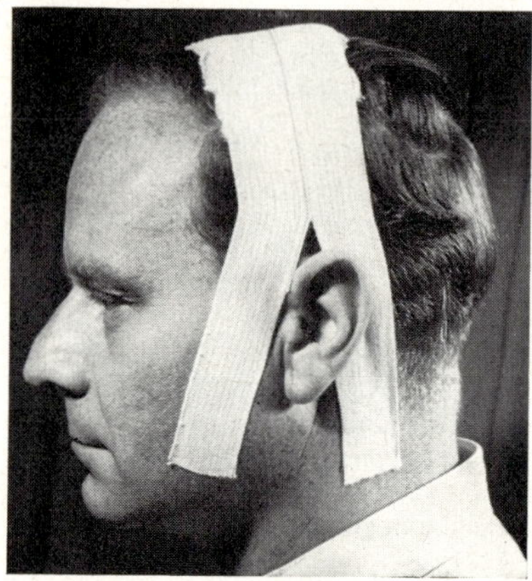

Fig. 129.—Adhesive strapping to head.

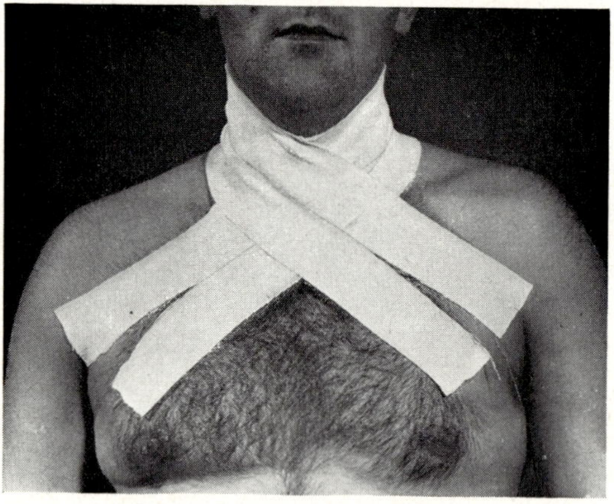

Fig. 130.—Adhesive strapping to neck.

HEAD

A strip 3 in. (7·5 cm.) wide is required. Cover the adhesive surface which will come in contact with the hair with gauze. Split each end for 3 in. (7·5 cm.). Place the centre of the strip over the dressing on top of the head and stretch outwards so that the split ends adhere to the skin on either side of the ears. It can be easily adapted to cover dressings on any part of the head. (*Fig*. 129.)

NECK

A strip 3–4 in. (7·5–10 cm.) wide is required. Cover with gauze the adhesive surface of the part of the strip that will be placed around the back of the neck. Place the centre of the strip at the back of the neck and bring the ends (which may be split) forwards so that they cross over the dressing in front of the neck. This is a simple and effective method for fixing a dressing over a thyroidectomy wound. (*Fig.* 130.)

AXILLA

A strip 3–4 in. (7·5–10 cm.) wide is required. Raise the arm on the affected side and support it. Split the ends of the bandage. Fix the ends posteriorly

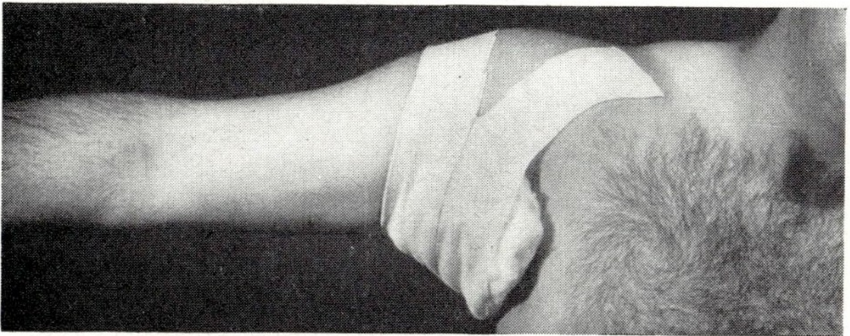

Fig. 131.—Adhesive strapping to axilla.

approximately 4 in. (10 cm.) apart on the shoulder and the upper arm, bring the strip (kept taut) forwards under the axilla to cover and secure the dressing and fix the ends anteriorly in a like manner. (*Fig.* 131.)

BREAST

Several lengths 4 in. (10 cm.) wide are required. Flex the arm on the affected side and support. Place the end of the strapping well back under the axilla. Apply overlapping strips exposing one-third of the width either horizontally or obliquely over the chest on the affected side so that the dressings are covered. The strips can be adjusted for a radical mastectomy, when they should pass around and beyond the opposite breast. If used to support the breast or to fix a dressing over a wound after removal of a fibro-adenoma, the nipple should be left uncovered. The bandage should not interfere with normal breathing. (*Fig.* 132.)

RIBS

Use either extension crosswise strapping or adhesive non-extensible plaster 2–4 in. (5–10 cm.) wide. Sit the patient in an upright position with the arm raised and the hand resting upon his head, giving assistance if necessary. Apply the end of the first strip approximately 2 in. (5 cm.) below the nipple on the unaffected side. Instruct the patient to breathe out to the fullest degree and carry the strip towards the affected side around the trunk, and fix at a point beyond the vertebral column so as to encircle three-quarters of the trunk. Apply further strips during expiration in a similar way so that each one overlaps the preceding one by a third of its width, to a level 2 in. (5 cm.) approximately above the injured area. This bandage is used only occasionally for fractured ribs when the patient complains of severe pain and discomfort. (*Fig.* 133.)

ABDOMEN

Lengths varying according to purpose for which they are to be used, each 4 in. (10 cm.) wide, are needed. Split the ends. Apply overlapping strips horizontally, obliquely, or vertically over the abdomen as required. These

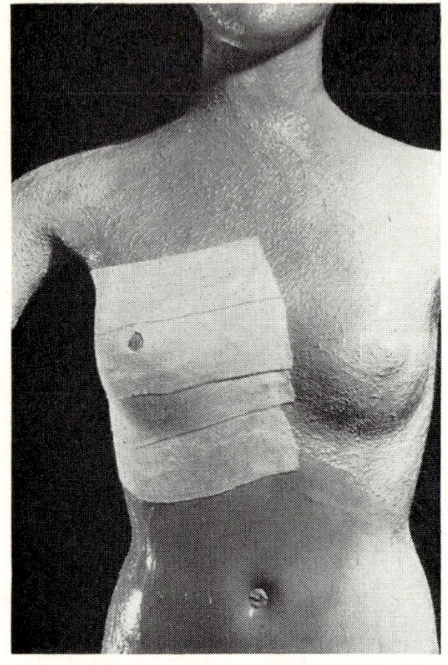

Fig. 132.—Adhesive strapping to breast.

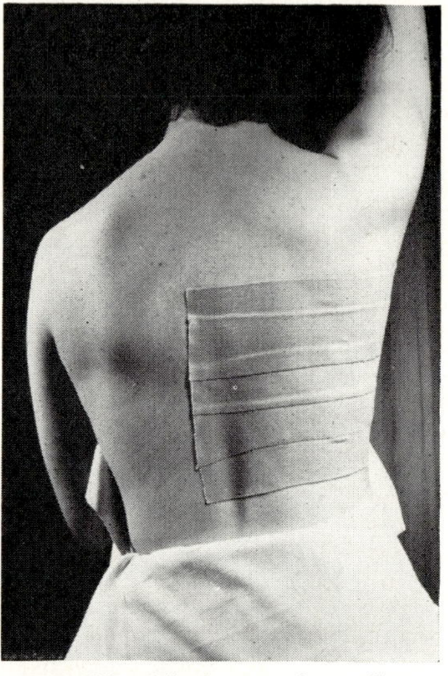

Fig. 133.—Adhesive strapping to ribs.

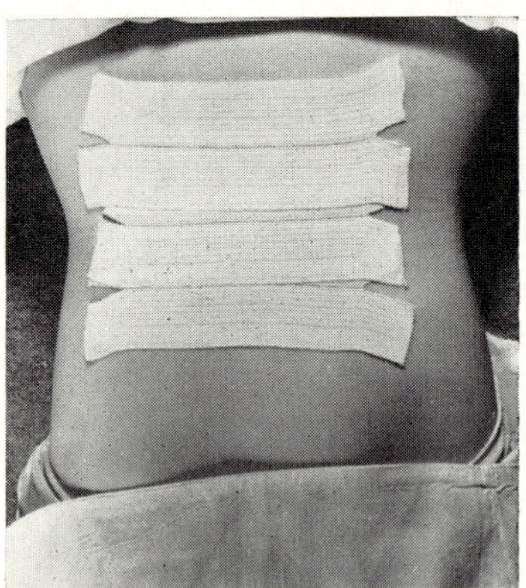

Fig. 134.—Adhesive strapping to abdomen.

bandages are commonly used after abdominal surgery. The bandage should be applied with only moderate stretch if discomfort is to be avoided. (*Fig.* 134.)

The following varieties of bandages are recommended as an abdominal support for patients submitted to abdominal surgery who have a persistent cough or weak abdominal muscles, and also for approximating the edges of abdominal wounds:—

1. Tongue and Slot.—Two strips, each long enough when stretched to encircle two-thirds of the body, and 4 in. (10 cm.) wide, are required. Apply the strips against the patient's back and bring forwards on either side. Make a transverse slit so that when in position the slit lies near the edge of the wound. Turn in the lateral edges of the free end of the other strip and manœuvre it through the slit. Then pull the ends across in opposite directions, having instructed the patient to take a deep breath, and securing the adhesive surfaces of the free ends while still taut to the strapping beneath. (*Fig.* 135.) This type of strapping may be used for small umbilical hernias in infants.

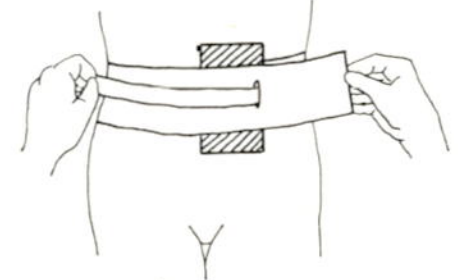
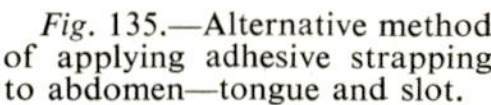

Fig. 135.—Alternative method of applying adhesive strapping to abdomen—tongue and slot.

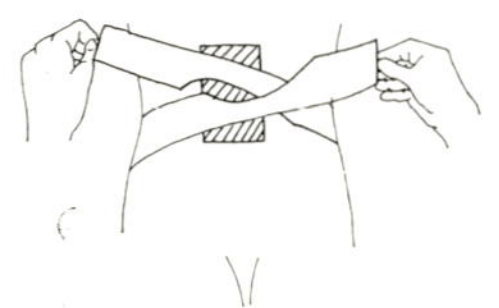

Fig. 136.—Alternative method of applying adhesive strapping to abdomen—interlocking cut-outs.

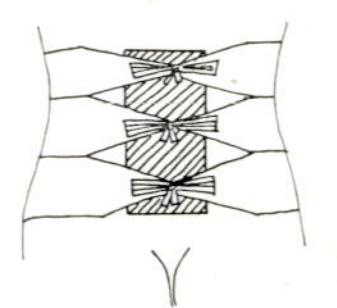

Fig. 137.—Alternative method of applying adhesive strapping to abdomen—abdominal corset.

2. Interlocking Cut-outs.—Use two strips 18 in. (45 cm.) long and 3 in. (7·5 cm.) wide. Cut out a semicircle half the width of the bandage 6 in. (15 cm.) from the end of each strip. Place a prepared strip against either side of the patient's trunk and draw together so that the semicircles face and fit into each other. Secure both ends while the bandage is still taut. (*Fig.* 136.)

3. Abdominal Corset.—Two or more strips 4 in. (10 cm.) wide are required. Fold back one end of each strip and cut holes 0·5 in. (1·5 cm.) from the folded edge. Secure the strips to the skin on each side of the wound, and lace up with tape. This forms a corset which can be adjusted to any part of the body. (*Fig.* 137.)

A very effective abdominal support which does not ride up is

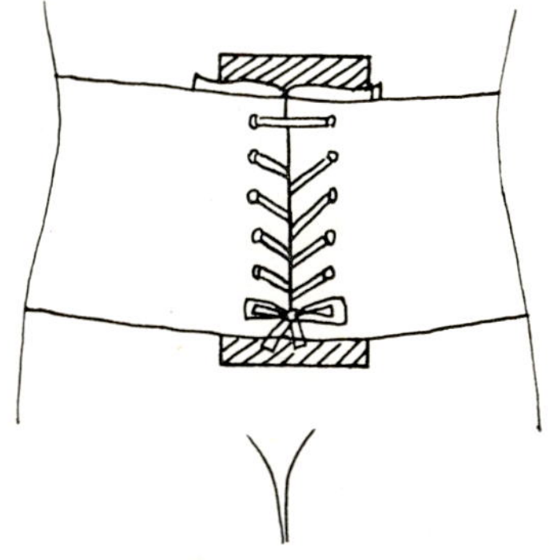

Fig. 138.—Alternative method of applying adhesive strapping to abdomen—many-tailed corset.

a many-tailed binder. It is made by taking six 12-in. (30-cm.) lengths of 3-in. (7·5-cm.) wide bandage and attaching tapes at the end of each length. The three lengths are applied to the body from each side and the tapes are tied over the abdominal dressing. (*Fig.* 138.)

LEG

Elevate the leg and support the foot at right-angles. Apply four vertical strips of bandage 3 in. (7·5 cm.) wide smoothly over the area from the foot as far as the tibial tuberosity. Start the bandage at the base of the big toe and apply four circular turns from within outwards to cover the foot, enclose the heel with the fifth turn, being particularly careful that there are no creases. Continue with the circular turns up as far as the lower third of the leg, exposing one-third of the width of the bandage to effect the required support. Continue up the leg lessening the pressure slightly by exposing gradually up to half the width of the bandage. (The coloured centre thread running through the length of bandage should not be visible anywhere.) Finish the bandage below the bend of the knee to avoid any rucking on movement. This compression bandage is used for varicose veins and ulcers. Its success depends on the application of the correct tension over the whole area and avoidance of any creases. (*Fig.* 139.) Outlets in the form of holes may be necessary when there is a copious discharge.

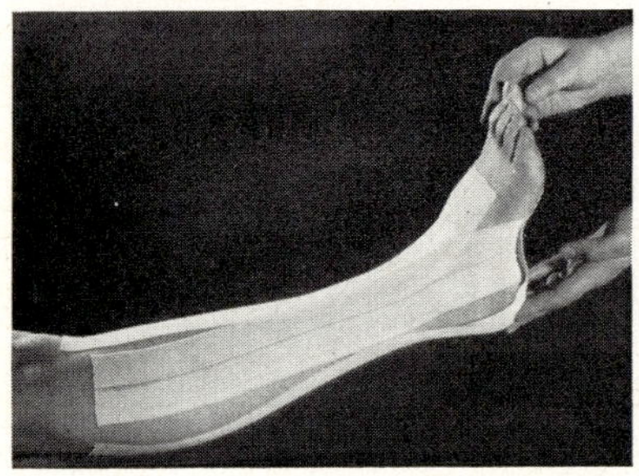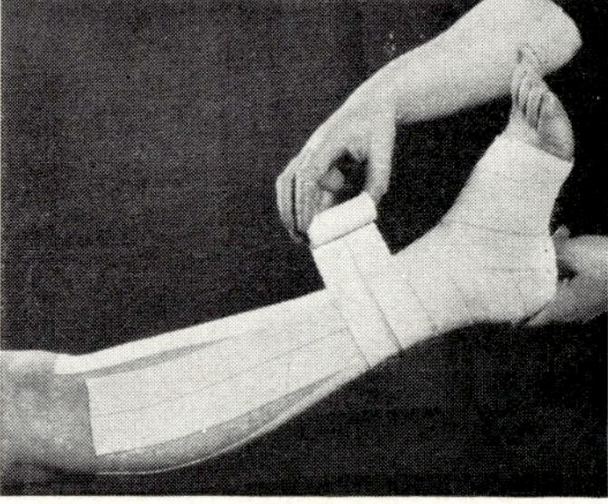

A   B

Fig. 139.—A, B, Application of adhesive strapping to leg for varicose ulcers.

This bandage may be applied from below the knee downwards, especially for women who can then pull on their stockings without fear of rucking the edges of the bandage.

A bandage to the leg can be applied with the adhesive surface outward. It is not easy to apply and is only used for a patient with a particularly sensitive skin.

ANKLE STRAPPING

Use a 3-in. (7·5-cm.) bandage. The patient is seated and an assistant supports the foot in an elevated position and at right-angles to the leg. Apply a stirrup, using moderate tension, from above the malleolus, around the sole of the foot, to a point at the same level on the other side of the leg. Take two or three turns around the foot, and working from without inwards and below upwards, make three or four figure-of-eight turns each with one loop around the ankle and the other around the foot, finishing with two turns round the leg. This provides a firm support for a sprained ankle. It is greatly appreciated by patients as it is comfortable and they can walk with no danger of stretching the injured ligament.

Further information on the application of strapping for a variety of conditions is found in a booklet *Elastoplast Technique* published by Smith & Nephew Ltd., Welwyn Garden City, Herts.

CHAPTER XVI

GENERAL PRINCIPLES IN THE TREATMENT OF FRACTURES

By Sir Reginald Watson-Jones

In the emergency treatment of fractures at the site of the accident the advice contained in the maxim 'Splint them where they lie' should be followed where possible. Before the patient is moved from the site, suspected fractures should be immobilized by splints constructed of strips of wood, walking-sticks, or folded newspapers. The splints should extend beyond the joints above and below the level of injury. The whole limb should be immobilized. In the case of thigh injuries, first-aid splints of this type must obviously extend over the trunk as well as over the whole lower limb, and added fixation may be secured by tying the two lower limbs together. Inflatable splints are described on p. 52.

If a Thomas's splint is available it is the best emergency splint for lower-limb injuries. It may be applied before the boot or trousers are removed and before the wound is dressed. Traction is applied to the limb so that it can be raised without angulating the fragments, and, while traction is maintained, the ring of the splint is guided over the foot, leg, and thigh, and pressed firmly against the pelvis. The foot may be fixed to the notch at the lower end of the splint by means of a bandage round the ankle.

GENERAL MANAGEMENT

In the general management of fractures—whether closed or open—there are three principles, all of equal importance, which must be in the mind of the surgeon from the first day of injury until the last day of recovery:—

1. *Reduction.*—To correct displacement perfectly and maintain replacement of the fragments, always using X-ray control.

2. *Immobilization.*—To fix the fragments completely and without interruption until the fracture is firmly united.

3. *Functional Activity.*—To preserve movement in joints which need not be immobilized, by the patient's own active exercise, but never by passive stretching. To maintain the tone of muscles even in the parts immobilized, and to encourage use of the limb, as far as possible, throughout the period of immobility.

REDUCTION

Manipulative Reduction.—The technique of reducing the displacement of fractures consists simply in inspecting radiographs to see where the fragments lie, replacing them by direct pressure or by traction, and X-raying to see that the object has been achieved. In other words, it is merely a question of putting the bone back into the position it was in before injury. Occasionally manipulative reduction may fail by reason of anatomical difficulties or undue delay. Operative reduction may then be needed.

Reduction should be effected by guarded measured strength rather than by sudden jerking force. This is important in fractures of the shafts of the long bones where considerable leverage is possible: it is particularly important in greenstick injuries, which must be reduced by gentle moulding, taking care not to convert the injury into a more difficult complete fracture. In fractures near the ends of the long bones, especially when impacted, much more force may be necessary. Frequently in fractures of the ankle, and sometimes in other fractures, the radiograph will show that the fragments lock when fully reduced, so that over-reduction is impossible.

Manipulation under Anæsthesia.—No displaced fracture should be manipulated without an anæsthetic; to do so is unfair to the patient and unfair to the surgeon. Even the most fragile patients can, with proper preparation, be given a general anæsthetic with safety.

Standard of Reduction.—How perfectly must the fragments be replaced? Is an anatomical 'hair-line' reduction necessary? The standard of end-result must be a limb clinically indistinguishable from normal—one which has normal function and which looks normal. The alinement must always be perfect, and there must be no rotational displacement. Slight lateral displacement may be of no significance in fractures of the shafts of the humerus and of the femur, but if lateral displacement exceeds a certain minimum, bony thickening impairs the cosmetic result, particularly in subcutaneous bones such as the tibia. Furthermore, when there is marked lateral displacement reduction may be unstable. X-ray examination is therefore essential after every manipulation, and the surgeon must be satisfied that the position, though not necessarily anatomically perfect, is compatible with perfect function and appearance.

Ideal Time for Reduction.—The fracture which is seen within about half an hour of the injury should be reduced under anæsthesia and immobilized at once. If it is feared that subsequent swelling may be of such severity that a complete encircling cast would be dangerous, a plaster slab may be applied over half to two-thirds of the circumference of the limb and held in place by a bandage which can be cut at once if required. The encircling cast is completed the following day.

If the fracture is reduced and plaster applied when the limb is already severely swollen, redisplacement very often occurs a few days later as the swelling subsides and the plaster becomes loose. In this event it may be better not to anæsthetize the patient unnecessarily, but without preliminary manipulation to immobilize the fracture by a plaster slab and put the patient to bed with the limb elevated. Two or three days later the swelling will have subsided and the fracture is then manipulated under anæsthesia and completely immobilized.

Subsequent Check Radiographs.—If a fracture has been reduced and plaster applied over a swollen limb, a check radiograph is essential seven to ten days later before the new plaster is applied, in order to be sure that the fragments have not been redisplaced. Every time that plaster is reapplied, a further radiograph should be taken through the new plaster, however unlikely it may appear that the position has altered; slight but important changes in the position of the fragments often occur during the reapplication of plaster.

IMMOBILIZATION

The repair of fractures takes place by the development of a delicate osteoid tissue between the fragments which calcifies to form callus. Tearing of this granulation tissue delays repair. The slightest shearing or rotational strain interrupts the continuity and causes continued de-ossification of the bare ends. If movement continues a fibrous bridge develops, and the final process of re-ossification occurs, not in a continuous callus between the fragments, but across the bone-ends which become densely sclerosed so that non-union is established. Operative treatment by bone-grafting is then needed.

The more complete the immobilization, the more rapid is the union. Plaster casts must be carefully moulded to the contour of the limb. Complete immobilization should be continued until the fracture is united, and even if the average period has been exceeded there should still be no interruption of the immobilization. Many factors account for slow repair and delayed union: they do not cause non-union if the immobilization is suitably prolonged: but if immobilization ceases, non-union becomes established.

The accepted periods of immobilization should be recognized only as minimum periods, to be exceeded in any case where clinical and radiographic tests show a slower rate of repair. Most fractures are united in children in two months and in adults in three months. Fractures of the lower limb weight-bearing bones must be immobilized for the whole of this time; in the upper limb a shorter period of protection is necessary, particularly if the fracture lies near the joints so that leverage strains are reduced.

In general it may be said that fractures near the ends of long bones need to be immobilized for about four weeks (although in the weight-bearing joints, for example the ankle, at least twice that length of time is needed) whereas fractures of the shafts of long bones which are subjected to much greater stresses, especially in the femur and tibia, need to be immobilized for much longer periods. It can be said only that *a fracture must be immobilized until it is united*—whether the period is of four or five weeks, four or five months, or even longer.

FUNCTIONAL ACTIVITY

No joint should be immobilized unnecessarily. Complete fixation of the fracture is essential, so that immobilization of the joints immediately above and below the injury cannot be avoided—but no other joint must be covered by splints, plaster, strapping, or bandage. *It is not enough that these joints are free; it is the surgeon's duty to see that they are actively mobilized by the patient's own exercise.*

Stiffness of the Fingers.—Recovery should be complete after a Colles's fracture of the radius within about two months of injury. If the finger-joints have been allowed to stiffen it will be at least twelve months before the patient can use the hand, and the limb may even be permanently crippled. This stiffness may develop within a few days, especially if the fingers are swollen and œdematous. The patient believes that swelling indicates a very severe injury, and that aggravation is to be avoided by guarding against the slightest movement of any part of the limb. Exactly the opposite treatment is urgently indicated: *the more swollen the fingers the more imperative is active exercise.* The patient must flex the interphalangeal joints by bending the fingers tightly into the palm, flex the metacarpophalangeal joints by reaching towards the front of the wrist with the finger-tips, extend all the joints until the fingers are fully spread, and repeat the exercises for at least five minutes every hour of the day (*Fig.* 140).

In every upper limb injury the first step when the patient recovers from the anæsthetic is to teach the patient finger exercises. The patient must be seen daily until movements are perfect, and any patient who through anxiety or lethargy fails to regain movement rapidly must be referred to a physiotherapy department—not for massage, but for daily supervision of the exercises. If the swelling of the fingers is so severe that movement is difficult the patient must be admitted to hospital, the limb elevated, and exercises supervised every hour.

Finger exercises are equally important in fractures of the hand, wrist, or fore-arm in plaster, for fractures of the elbow or shoulder in a collar-and-cuff sling, or for fractures of the clavicle in bandage or strapping.

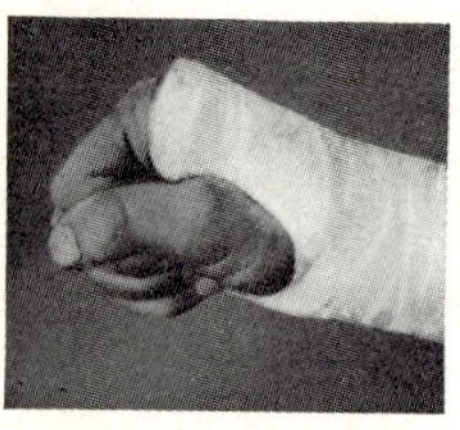

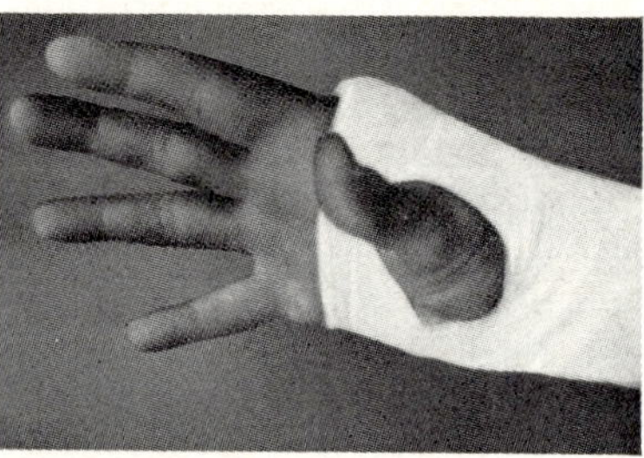

Fig. 140.—Full finger exercises must be practised although the fractured wrist is immobilized in plaster.

The Danger of Passive Movement.—It is of vital importance that the exercise should be done by the patient himself, and that there should be no stretching or passive movement of any type.

Passive stretching not only causes unnecessary pain, but it has exactly the opposite effect of that for which it was intended. The stretching injures the joints, tears the capsule, increases the exudation, and aggravates adhesion forma-tion. If stiffness of the fingers is threatening, the one way to make certain that the stiffness will be serious or even permanent is to force the joints.

Stiffness of the Shoulder.—In fractures of the hand, wrist, and forearm, shoulder exercises are also important. Several times a day the shoulder must be fully externally rotated, fully abducted, and internally rotated, by lifting the arm with its plaster until the hand is behind the neck, over the opposite ear, and in the small of the back (*Fig.* 141).

Fig. 141.—Exercises for the shoulder whilst the limb is encased in plaster.

Functional Use of the Upper Limb.—As a rule no sling should be worn after the first day or so. In many cases the patient may use the limb for dressing, eating, and for household duties. This activity prevents stiffness of the fingers, and it maintains the tone of the muscles within the plaster; promotes a normal circulation, and minimizes adhesion formation around the immobilized joints so that subsequent recovery is more rapid (*Fig.* 142).

Wasting of the Quadriceps.—In lower-limb injuries the thigh muscles waste very rapidly, especially when the knee is injured. This wasting occurs so quickly that many months of treatment may be required to regain the losses of only two or three weeks. No injured knee should be immobilized without at the same time teaching the patient 'quadriceps drill'. Smooth rhythmic contraction and relaxation of the muscle is continued for five or ten minutes every hour of the day. The muscle must be braced as tightly as possible and in doing so the knee must be *fully* extended. It is only during the last two or three degrees of extension movement that the vastus medialis comes into play and this muscle will continue to waste rapidly and seriously despite leg-raising exercises unless the knee is braced quite straight.

Functional Use of the Lower Limb.—In many fractures and dislocations of the foot and ankle, patients may safely walk with the limb immobilized in closely fitting plaster casts. With certain fractures weight-bearing may begin

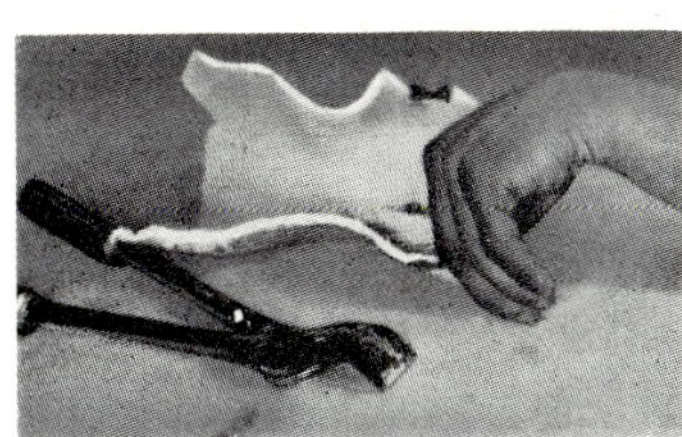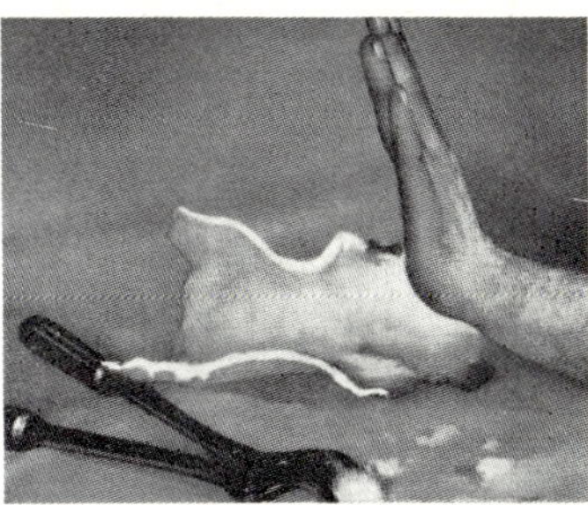

Fig. 142.—The range of wrist movement possible immediately the plaster is removed after six months' immobilization for a fracture of the scaphoid. Functional activity and finger exercises have prevented adhesion formation round the joint despite immobility.

within two or three days, but as a rule, especially when there was marked swelling of the foot at the time that the original plaster was applied, weight-bearing is deferred for two or three weeks until the new plaster has been applied. The exercise maintains the tone of the leg muscles, it minimizes disuse decalcification of the bones, and it prevents circulatory stasis with resulting œdema and adhesion formation. When walking the patient should not allow the foot to rotate outwards at each step, a tendency which causes harmful rotational stresses at the site of the healing fracture. Instruction in how to walk properly with a plaster may be necessary.

OPEN WOUNDS AND COMPOUND FRACTURES

An open wound or fracture is a surgical emergency. The open wound may be contaminated, but it must not become infected (*see* p. 211). Operative treatment is urgent. The patient should be taken at once to the operating theatre. The operation to be performed is not a simple stitching which can be done on a casualty couch; it is a complete excision of all devitalized tissues followed by primary skin closure, either by suture or by skin grafting when suture is not possible.

PRINCIPLES OF WOUND EXCISION

The purpose of the operation is to excise dead and dying tissue, to remove grossly contaminated matter, and to divide both skin and fascia in the longitudinal axis of the limb so that tension will be relieved and free circulation maintained, thus securing a wound lined only with living tissues, freely supplied with blood, and capable of destroying bacteria.

Technique of Wound Excision.—The wound is left covered with sterile dressing until surrounding skin has been cleaned with a detergent or an antiseptic. It is then screened off with sterile towels. No tourniquet is used.

The wound edges are lightly trimmed with a scalpel and the wound is enlarged in the long axis of the limb 2–3 in. (5–7·5 cm.) above and 2–3 in. below. The deep fascia is similarly trimmed and freely divided throughout the extent of the wound. Each layer of tissue is then trimmed with curved scissors—first the superficial muscles, then the deep muscles, and finally the periosteum. All dead, crushed, and non-contractile muscle should be excised; none must be left behind. No bone fragments are to be removed unless they are widely displaced and completely loose; the less bone removed the better. Hæmostasis is secured by pressure forceps twisted off, larger vessels being tied with fine catgut. The wound is then flat and saucerized and no recesses remain, so that it is obviously impossible to insert drainage-tubes; they would fall out. Penicillin is given in doses of two million units a day, continued for several days.

MULTIPLE INJURIES

After multiple injuries have been sustained it is of the greatest importance that the management of the patient should be in order of priorities, and in general this should be on the following lines:—

1. Immediate establishment of a clear airway, either by an endotracheal tube or when this is impossible or impracticable then by tracheostomy, and oxygen should be administered when cyanosis is present.

2. The treatment of shock and replacement of blood-loss by transfusion (*see* p. 43). This comes second in the order of priority because it is pointless to transfuse blood into a person who cannot oxygenate it.

3. A short period of observation (including X-ray examination when indicated) in order to discover a head, intrathoracic, or intra-abdominal injury which may not be apparent at the first examination, and provisional immobilization of fractures to lessen pain and shock on movement.

4. Intramuscular or intravenous antibiotic cover in the case of open wounds.

5. Craniotomy, thoracotomy, or laparotomy, after resuscitation, in order to deal with hæmorrhage or ruptured viscera in these cavities.

6. Reduction and immobilization of fractures and the closure of skin wounds.

Early liaison and close co-operation with the other specialists concerned, especially anæsthetists, is essential for successful management.

In the case of babies and very small children, where an obvious fracture is present, the presence of other injuries may well be overlooked, particularly when an inadequate or reluctant history of injury is given by the parents (the battered baby syndrome). For these reasons it is of the greatest importance that examination of the infant should be a full one and not merely confined to the presenting fracture, and that in any case of doubt the child should be admitted for careful observation in order to discover at the earliest possible moment any progressive intracranial, intrathoracic, or intra-abdominal injury.

COMPLICATIONS OF FRACTURES

Every patient with a fracture or dislocation must be examined at regular intervals for several days after the injury in order to confirm that: (1) reduction is complete; (2) there is no undue friction at the margins of the plaster; (3) bandages or strappings are not too tight; (4) the circulation is normal; (5) there is no undue œdema of the fingers or toes; (6) the patient is practising exercises adequately.

If the patient has not been admitted to hospital explicit instructions (printed if possible) must be given that he is to report the next day, and *if there is pallor, cyanosis, numbness, tingling, or immobility of the fingers or toes, he must then return at once whatever hour of the day or night.* When the danger of complications is over, the patient is examined weekly until recovery is complete.

LOCAL COMPLICATIONS

Œdema.—During the first two or three days after injuries of the wrist and ankle there is usually swelling of the fingers and toes, especially when local swelling is prevented by a plaster cast. If the circulation is brisk, and there is no cyanosis or anæmia, the swelling is of little significance. The limb must be elevated until it has subsided. Active exercises to prevent joint stiffness are even more important than usual, and patients must be disillusioned of the belief that "the fingers are too swollen to move".

Gangrene.—When there is not only swelling but also impairment of the circulation, the position is much more serious. If any limb is encased in plaster or splints the circulation must be tested frequently by compressing the tip of each digit, and seeing that the area made anæmic rapidly flushes with blood when pressure is released. If pressure is not released and the vascular obstruction is not relieved, gangrene may develop and necessitate amputation.

Volkmann's Ischæmic Contracture.—Occasionally in fractures of the elbow and forearm, even when all external pressure has been relieved, the limb remains pallid or blue and the radial pulse is weak or absent. Compression of the brachial artery in the antecubital fossa, or injury to the walls of the brachial, radial, or ulnar arteries, must be suspected. The resident medical officer must inform the surgeon at once. The surgeon must not await the development of contracture of the fingers before establishing the diagnosis; if he does he will be too late and there will be permanent crippling. He must diagnose Volkmann's ischæmia by the pallor or cyanosis of the fingers.

The five symptoms are pain, pallor, paræsthesia, pulselessness, and paralysis—but the most important are pain in the fingers and pallor of the fingers. If the surgeon waits for pulselessness or paralysis he will be far too late.

If the circulation is not restored within about six hours the flexor muscles of the forearm die and are replaced by fibrous tissue which shortens so that the fingers contract at the interphalangeal joints. The contracture may occur in a localized form, affecting only one or two fingers. It must be looked for in all

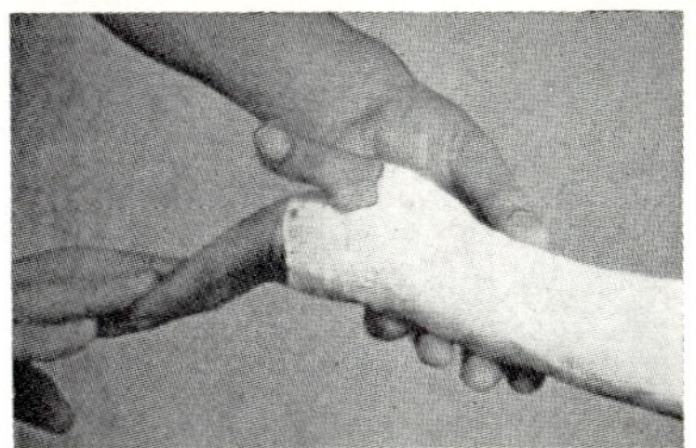

Fig. 143.—Testing for Volkmann's ischæmic contracture in a fracture of both forearm bones immobilized in plaster.

forearm and elbow injuries during the first few days, especially when there has been circulatory impairment, by testing the ability of the patient to extend the fingers fully (*Fig.* 143). The fully developed contracture causes serious and permanent crippling, and it may be associated with paralysis of the ulnar and median nerves.

These serious consequences can be avoided only by prompt treatment during the first few hours. The surgeon must first satisfy himself that there is no pressure on the artery.

Pressure may arise from: (1) tight bandages, strapping, or plaster; encircling bandages must be cut, and if there is an encircling plaster the front half must be removed; (2) flexion of a swollen elbow-joint; in elbow fractures the only safe position may be 20° or 30° below the right angle; (3) displacement of a supra-condylar fracture, the vessels being stretched over the lower end of the shaft; the displacement must be reduced, and the position maintained by a posterior plaster slab.

If all these factors can be excluded and there is still pallor or cyanosis and absence of the radial pulse, the artery has been damaged and immediate opera-tion is urgently needed. It may be found that the artery is not actually severed but is in spasm, which is often relieved by simple exposure of the vessel and cleaning of its walls with a warm moist saline swab or the local application of 2·5 per cent papaverine sulphate or 1 per cent procaine. If the artery is partly severed a segment of it should be excised in order to remove all vasoconstrictor nerves.

Nerve Lesions.—Injuries to the nerves are usually sustained at the time of the original injury. Primary nerve lesions are particularly common in injuries of the elbow, humerus, and shoulder; in most cases the paralysis is incomplete and due to simple bruising of the nerve-trunk.

Pressure Sores.—These may develop from undue pressure over bony promi-nences by splints, bandages, or plaster.

Plaster sores may be due to: (1) pulling one turn of the plaster bandage too tightly; (2) careless moulding of the plaster; (3) application of a plaster slab which instead of being wet and sloppy has begun to harden, so that it does not adapt itself smoothly to the contour of the limb; (4) movement of a joint during the setting of the plaster so that a ridge is formed; (5) before the plaster has firmly set, allowing it to rest on a hard surface so that it is flattened over a bony prominence (especially the back of the heel in leg plasters, and over the sacrum in trunk and hip plasters); (6) pushing coins, heads of knitting needles, small wads of wool, or other foreign bodies down between the plaster and the limb; (7) delay in repairing a crack in the plaster near the joint, so that there is friction from the broken margins.

The patient may complain of persistent localized discomfort and pain. In other cases the skin and subcutaneous tissues become anæmic and anæsthetic, and there is no complaint of pain. The first sign may then be the typical smell of accumulated secretions and discharge.

As soon as a pressure sore is suspected, a window must be cut in the plaster. The gap should afterwards be filled with a pad of wool firmly bandaged into position.

Skin Blistering.—This is very common during the first twenty-four hours in the region of severe elbow, leg, and ankle fractures. The blisters arise from traumatic œdema and exudation into the cuticle, the exudate sometimes being hæmorrhagic. They can develop only where the skin is unsupported. The blisters should be emptied by pinching the overlying cuticle. Plaster may then be applied in the usual way.

Joint Stiffness.—Stiffness of the joints from adhesion formation is to be avoided by active exercises and early functional activity. If any stiffness does develop, it must be overcome by the patient's own exercise and not by massage or stretching.

Stiffness of the elbow-joint is very commonly due to passive stretching. When a child is seen with an elbow injury, the parents must be warned at once that the recovery of movement may be slow, but that it will be most rapid and most complete if it is allowed to develop at its own rate. *No elbow injury should be treated by massage; there must be no single stretching movement; the patient must not be allowed to carry buckets of water or heavy weights with the object of straightening the joint.* The range of movement should be estimated and recorded week by week by means of an angle measurer (*Fig.* 144).

Myositis Ossificans.—This is due to the ossification of subperiosteal hæmatomata, and occurs most commonly in children, where the periosteum is easily stripped, and after dislocations, where ligaments and muscles are avulsed with their periosteal attachments. It is most common at the elbow (*see* p. 221) but it may also occur at the shoulder, hip, knee, or ankle. The complication may be avoided by prompt reduction of dislocations, and by avoiding all passive stretching which interferes with the re-attachment of the periosteum to the bone.

Delayed Union of Fractures.—At the conclusion of the usual minimum period of immobilization, union is tested (*a*) clinically by very gently 'springing' the bone, and (*b*) it is estimated radiographically. If the fracture is not firmly united, plaster is reapplied for a further four to six weeks, when

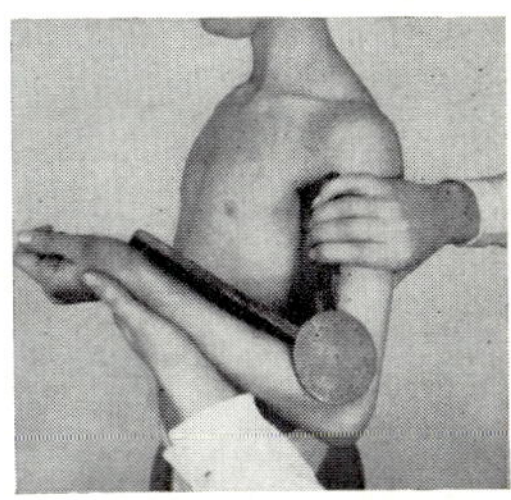

Fig. 144.—The range of joint movement must be measured accurately and recorded.

union is again tested. In cases of delayed union this routine is repeated as long as may be necessary up to twelve months or longer, or until it is decided that operative treatment, namely bone-grafting, is essential.

INFECTED FRACTURES

If by reason of failure of primary treatment there is infection of an open fracture the wound must be drained and laid widely open. No layer of the wound is sutured. The cavity is then lightly filled with sterile gauze and the fracture is immobilized either by means of a complete plaster cast or by a splint with traction. Appropriate antibiotic treatment is given.

In late cases, when infection has been present for many weeks or months, care must be taken to remove all fragments of sequestrated dead bone. The deep layers of the wound and the fascia are still not sutured, but the skin margins are. If all sequestra have been removed, healing is often secured almost by first intention. Immobilization of the fracture by splints or plaster must continue until union is sound. It is sometimes necessary to continue immobilization for many weeks in order that bone destroyed by infection may be bridged, and sound union secured. Occasionally a secondary bone-grafting operation is advisable some weeks after complete healing of infection. In such cases, lest there might be a flare of infection, the grafts should consist solely of cancellous bone chips. No compact bone which would sequestrate, and no screws or other metallic foreign body which would act in the same way as a sequestrum, should be included.

Gas Gangrene.—(*See* p. 70).

GENERAL COMPLICATIONS

Rise of Temperature.—An increased temperature is not uncommon for a day or two after severe fractures, even though there is no compound injury and no infection. The febrile reaction disappears as the blood-clot undergoes absorption.

Hypostatic Pneumonia.—This may occur in old people, especially those who are somewhat emphysematous. It is due to congestion, and its onset is favoured by keeping these patients on their backs. The rule, therefore, in treating fractures in elderly people should be never to allow them to remain flat on the back unless there is some very special reason to the contrary. They should be well propped up with pillows.

Delirium Tremens.—This is a cerebral disorder, precipitated in patients who have taken alcohol in excess, by an injury such as a fracture or dislocation. There may be hallucinations with delusions, especially the hearing of sounds. It arises from vitamin deficiency and should be treated by intravenous injections of vitamins B and C.

Fat Embolism.—This is an occasional cause of death after fracture. The emboli consist of fat globules which may be liberated from the medulla of the fractured bone, or be derived from the fat of blood-plasma broken down from the normal state of emulsification. Localized fat emboli in the lungs give rise to the symptoms of bronchopneumonia, but more often they are scattered throughout the body, and embolism of the brain gives rise to cerebral irritation, coma, and death on the third or fourth day. Symptomatic treatment only is indicated.

*　　*　　*　　*　　*

In the three chapters which follow, Chapters XVII, XVIII, and XIX, the common fractures of the upper limb, spine, and lower limb are described and the appropriate treatment outlined. Many patients, and particularly those with the commoner fractures of the upper limb, may be treated in Accident Centres or Casualty Departments as out-patients; they should receive printed instructions on the care of their plasters and on the warning signs of complications before they are sent home.

After a period of instruction many of the treatments may be carried out by a senior house officer or registrar. However, the more difficult fractures and dislocations, e.g., Monteggia and Bennett's fractures, should be handed over to an experienced orthopædic surgeon as soon as possible. Likewise, when there is evidence of complications, e.g., Volkmann's contracture or nerve palsy, a senior colleague should be informed. Most fractures of the long bones of the lower limb will require in-patient treatment under a consultant orthopædic surgeon.

CHAPTER XVII

FRACTURES AND DISLOCATIONS OF THE UPPER LIMB

By Sir Reginald Watson-Jones

FRACTURES AND DISLOCATIONS OF THE CLAVICLE

Fractures of the Clavicle occur most commonly in the middle third of the bone. There is usually overriding of the fragments, the inner being displaced upwards by the pull of the sternomastoid muscle, and the outer displaced downwards and forwards by the weight of the arm. The fragments can only be re-alined and replaced by pulling the whole shoulder-girdle upwards and backwards.

The figure-of-eight bandage is simple and effective. The patient sits on the front of a stool, the operator standing behind with one foot on the stool and his knee between the patient's shoulder-blades. A large pad of wool is placed in front of each shoulder, extending into the axilla. Several long bandages 5 or 6 in. (12·5 or 15 cm.) wide are then applied in the form of a figure-of eight, passing in front of the shoulders under the axillæ, and crossing between the shoulder-blades. With each turn of the bandage the shoulder-girdles are pulled backwards and upwards as strongly as possible without compressing the axillary vessels (*Fig.* 145). The bandages may be stitched together to prevent slipping, or alternatively they should be reapplied every second or third day for the first fortnight. For the first ten days the shoulder is elevated by a triangular sling tied over the opposite side, but after that time it is left free for

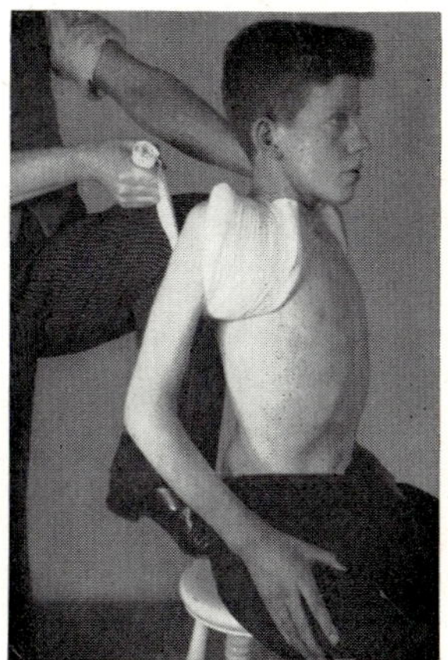

Fig. 145.—Fracture of the clavicle immobilized by figure-of-eight bandage over large axillary pads. The limb is supported in a triangular sling for ten days.

exercises. The fingers, wrist, and elbow must be exercised frequently from the first day. The figure-of-eight bandage may be discarded after three weeks when there is clinical evidence of union; there is no necessity to wait for radiographic evidence of union, which is much more delayed.

The only indication for operation in recent fractures is the exceedingly rare complication of compression of the brachial plexus or subclavian vessels by displaced fragments.

Dislocation of the Acromio-clavicular Joint.—If the ligaments of the acromio-clavicular joint are torn, the weight of the arm displaces the shoulder-girdle and acromion downwards below the level of the outer end of the clavicle. Incomplete dislocations (subluxations) are common; more rarely the acromion lies entirely below and in front of the clavicle. The dislocation is easily reduced by elevating the whole arm and shoulder-girdle, but the weight of the limb tends to reproduce the displacement. It is for this reason that strapping the arm in the elevated position is seldom successful. Left untreated a full, painless range of shoulder movement is obtained within a few weeks after injury.

DISLOCATION OF THE SHOULDER

Dislocation of the shoulder seldom occurs before the age of twenty. The capsule is torn from the glenoid on its anterior surface and the head of the humerus slides below the glenoid fossa, or in front of the glenoid beneath the coracoid process.

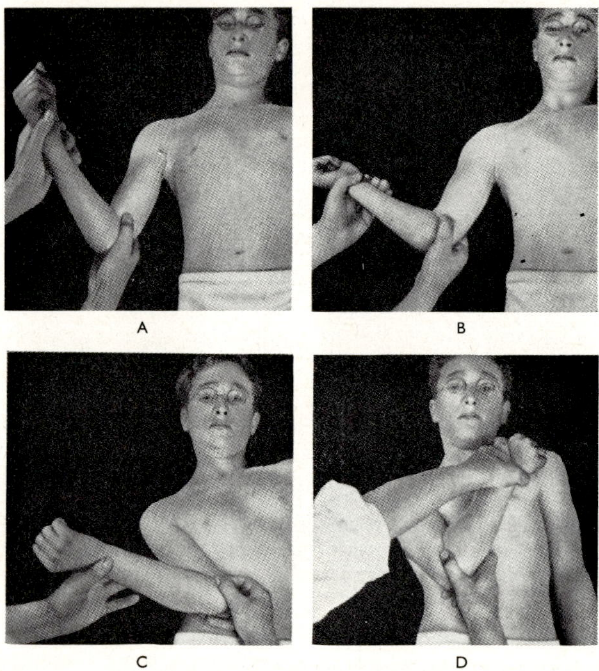

Fig. 146.—Kocher's method of reducing a dislocation of the shoulder. A, Traction is applied; B, The humerus is slowly externally rotated; C, It is adducted across the chest; D, It is internally rotated.

The limb must be examined carefully for nerve injuries. The deltoid muscle is often paralysed by injuries to the circumflex nerve, the posterior cord, or the outer trunk of the plexus. The examiner palpates the muscle belly with one hand, and instructs the patient to attempt abduction movement against the resistance of his other hand over the patient's elbow. If the nerve-supply is uninjured the muscle is felt contracting although the shoulder is not actually moved.

Method of Reduction.—The head of the humerus is held in its inwardly displaced and inwardly rotated position by the tension of the subscapularis. To reduce the dislocation this muscle must be stretched slowly and gradually by Kocher's manipulation. For a dislocation of the right shoulder, the surgeon takes the elbow in his right hand and the wrist in his left (*Fig.* 146). Strong, smooth traction is applied to the humerus by pulling with the right hand. The arm is then very slowly and gently externally rotated, by moving the wrist outwards, until the normal limit of 90° external rotation is reached. Keeping the limb in full external rotation, the limb is adducted across the chest. Finally the limb is internally rotated and the hand brought over to the opposite shoulder. The manipulation is performed so smoothly that the head of the humerus glides into position, and the surgeon does not know at which stage the dislocation reduced. There should be no click or sudden jerk. It is essential that the accuracy of reduction should be confirmed, not only clinically, but also by radiographs taken in two planes.

If the dislocation is not reduced by Kocher's manipulation at the first attempt the method first described by Hippocrates should be used. The surgeon grasps the wrist with both hands and places his stockinged foot between the upper arm and chest just short of the axilla. With knees and elbows straight he leans backwards and thus applies traction. He slowly externally rotates the limb and then adducts it over the leverage of his foot. The manipulation is essentially the same in the two manœuvres but more power is available by the Hippocratic method and there is no greater danger of injury to the axillary artery or nerves; indeed, the danger may be less and there is certainly less danger of fracturing the neck of the humerus by direct traction than by forcible external rotation of the arm. The limb is immobilized across the chest for three weeks by a collar-and-cuff sling and body bandage. Immobilization for a shorter period than three weeks predisposes to recurrent dislocation as the tear in the anterior capsule does not heal soundly until three weeks after injury. The fingers, hand, and wrist must not be covered, and they are exercised constantly. After three weeks the patient regains movement at the elbow and shoulder by his own exercise.

Dislocation with Fracture of the Tuberosity.—Radiographs may show that a large fragment of the great tuberosity has been torn off at the time of the dislocation. As a rule the fragment is in perfect position when the dislocation is reduced and treatment is continued as for an uncomplicated dislocation.

Danger of Recurrent Dislocation.—After every simple dislocation of the shoulder the limb must be strapped and bandaged over the chest and held rigidly in this position, with no single external rotation movement, for three weeks. This does not cause permanent stiffness, but, on the other hand, failure to use such early immobilization is the cause of recurrent dislocation of the shoulder.

FRACTURE OF THE NECK OF THE HUMERUS

Three types of fracture must be distinguished: (1) Contusion crack fractures; (2) Adduction fractures; and (3) Abduction fractures (*Fig.* 147).

Contusion Crack Fractures.—The injury follows a fall on the outer aspect of the shoulder, and the crack across the neck of the humerus is often associated with a comminuted fracture of the tuberosity. Complete immobilization is not necessary. The limb should be supported in a sling for a few days, after which active exercises are practised.

Adduction Fractures.—These occur equally commonly in adults and in children, and the fragments are impacted in such a way that the shaft is adducted on the head. If the displacement is not corrected, abduction movement is permanently limited by a degree corresponding with the degree of angulation. In elderly patients this is unimportant and the impaction should not be broken down by manipulation. Treatment is carried out exactly as for contusion crack fractures.

In younger patients the displacement is reduced by traction on the limb in the abducted position, so that the adduction angulation is corrected. After this

9

has been done, the normal anatomical relationship remains when the arm is brought down to the side. After three weeks' rest in a sling, active exercises are begun.

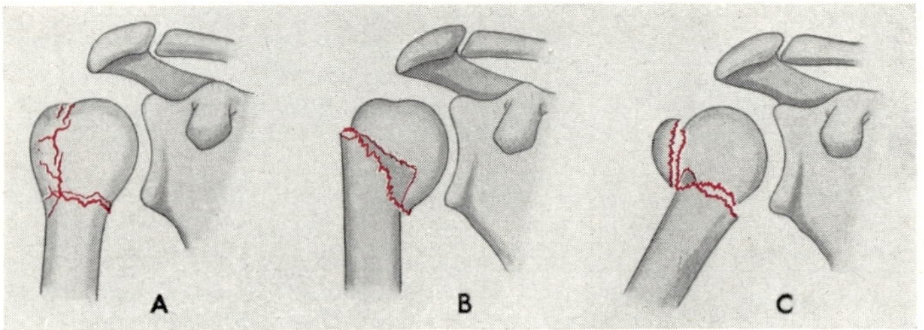

Fig. 147.—Fractures of the neck of the humerus: A, Contusion crack fracture; B, Adduction fracture; C, Abduction fracture.

Abduction Fractures.—These fractures occur less commonly in children than in adults. The shaft is slightly abducted on the head and the great tuberosity is pinched off by compression between the head and the outer margin of the shaft. The injury is treated in the same way as simple crack fractures by protection in a sling for a few days followed by active exercises.

STIFFNESS OF THE SHOULDER DUE TO ADHESIVE CAPSULITIS

Fractures and dislocations, or simple contusions and sprains of the shoulder, are often followed by painful limitation of shoulder movement.

It is the limitation of external rotation which is of significance. The normal shoulder cannot be abducted beyond a right angle if the humerus is held internally rotated; outward rotation is an essential component of abduction. Every upper limb which is supported in a sling is immobilized with the shoulder in full internal rotation. The resulting limitation of outward rotation may be demonstrated with the elbow to the side and the forearm and hand directed forwards. Normally it is possible to rotate the limb outwards through almost 90°, so that the forearm and hand point sideways. If this movement is completely limited, it is a waste of time to practise abduction exercises: external rotation exercises must first be practised, by keeping the elbow to the side and turning the forearm more and more outwards. The patient must also try to reach the back of his neck. As this movement recovers, he endeavours to reach over the top of the head to the opposite ear. The exercises must be performed by the patient himself five minutes hourly throughout the day. Many patients require encouragement and stimulation, *but there must be no passive stretching by a physiotherapist or relative. The exercises must be done smoothly, without sudden jerking or forcible movements. The patient must not hang by the affected arm from overhead beams or parallel bars so that body-weight exerts passive stretching.*

FRACTURE OF THE SHAFT OF THE HUMERUS

Fractures of the shaft of the humerus which are adequately reduced show little tendency to redisplacement. For this reason it is usually sufficient to use a simple collar-and-cuff sling, with a plaster-of-Paris gutter splint.

Radial Nerve Palsy.—If the radial nerve has been damaged, stretching of the extensor muscles of the forearm should be prevented by supporting the wrist in moderate dorsiflexion. A long cock-up splint which immobilizes the finger-joints in the fully extended position must not be used, because it so often causes serious stiffness of the fingers, and this may prove even more disabling than the paralysis itself. If there is no sign of recovery of the nerve lesion within six weeks, exploration is advisable, because the nerve-trunk may have been severed by the sharp bone fragments and nerve suture is essential.

SUPRACONDYLAR FRACTURES OF THE HUMERUS

Types of Fracture.—There are two types of supracondylar fracture—the usual type where the lower fragment is displaced backwards, and the less common type in which it is displaced forwards. In the common form the line of fracture

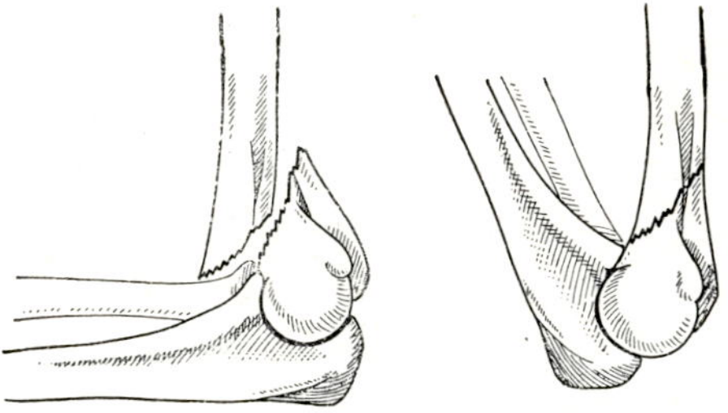

Fig. 148.— Supracondylar fracture of the usual type, with backward displacement of the small fragment. Reduction is stable only if the elbow is flexed.

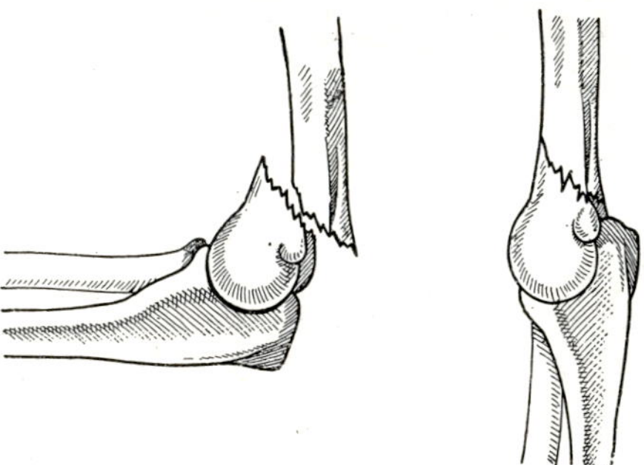

Fig. 149.—The less common type of supracondylar fracture, in which there is forward displacement of the lower fragment. Reduction is stable only if the elbow is fully extended.

runs obliquely upwards and backwards; the displacement is reduced by applying traction to the limb, and while traction is maintained flexing the elbow. In this position the fragments lock securely (*Fig.* 148). In the other type the fracture line is oblique downwards and backwards. If the elbow is flexed the displacement is increased, and the fragments lock only in the extended position

9*

(*Fig.* 149). It is obviously wrong to treat all supracondylar fractures with the elbow flexed. The common type must be treated in this position, but the opposite type must be treated in the opposite position.

Importance of Perfect Reduction.—Accurate reduction with complete correction of tilting of the lower fragment is of the utmost importance. If the fragment unites with forward tilting, extension of the elbow will be permanently limited by a corresponding degree. If the fragment unites with backward tilting, there will be a greater range of extension than normal, and flexion will be permanently limited. If lateral tilting remains uncorrected, the carrying angle of the forearm is altered and there is obvious deformity. These angulations do not undergo correction with subsequent growth of the bone.

Supracondylar Fracture with Backward Displacement.—In no circumstances should the deformity be first increased, thus imperilling the vascular supply, with the mistaken idea that only thus can the fractured surfaces be brought into apposition. The most gentle traction on the limb, in the position in which it lies, will always succeed. In the common type with backward displacement, while traction is maintained, the elbow is gradually flexed to almost 45° above the right angle. Lateral displacement is then corrected. An assistant holds the limb by the wrist, keeping the elbow flexed, and the surgeon applies direct lateral pressure with one hand over the shaft of the humerus and the other hand on the opposite side of the limb over the displaced fragment itself. The circulation is at once tested, and if the swelling of the joint is so severe that 45° of flexion has compressed the radial artery or the veins, the elbow must be extended until the pulse and venous return are normal. A plaster back slab is applied over the back of the limb and lightly bandaged into position, avoiding any pressure over the front of the joint. The limb is slung from the neck by a collar and cuff.

An immediate check X-ray with a portable machine is essential, and if the displacement is not completely corrected, the fracture is at once remanipulated. Full general anæsthesia should be used, so that anatomical perfection is obtained.

Supracondylar Fracture with Forward Displacement.—If the fracture is of the opposite type, traction is applied and the limb is extended until the elbow is quite straight. Lateral displacement is corrected as before, and a plaster back slab applied from below the shoulder to just above the wrist.

FRACTURE OF THE LATERAL CONDYLE OF THE HUMERUS

This injury occurs usually in children of 5–15 years of age. A perfect recovery can be achieved, but failure to apply the correct treatment leads inevitably to non-union, to an appalling deformity, and sometimes to ulnar paralysis supervening ten to twenty years later due to increasing valgus at the elbow. The separated fragment includes the capitulum and outer part of the trochlea; the external lateral ligament and the extensor muscle origin remain attached to it. The tension of the muscle tilts the fragment out of the elbow-joint, and rotates it so that the fractured surface is directed outwards (*Fig.* 150).

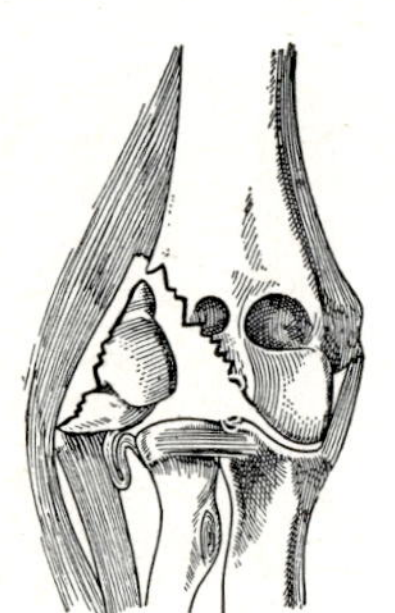

Fig. 150.—Fracture of the lateral condyle of the humerus. The condylar fragment is tilted out of the joint by the pull of the extensor muscles.

Sometimes it turns completely upside down, and the articular surface of the fragment lies opposite the fractured surface of the shaft of the humerus. In these circumstances bony union is obviously impossible, and a weak fibrous union results, with a completely unstable elbow.

As years go on, the forearm bones become displaced more and more to the outer side of the humerus, until the carrying angle may be as much as 60° or 70°. Gradual stretching of the ulnar nerve round the inner side of the elbow accounts for the delayed ulnar palsy.

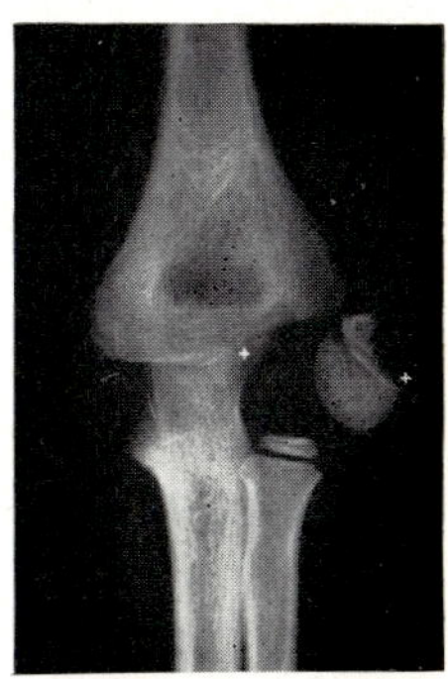

Fig. 151.—Displacement of lateral condylar epiphysis which is tilted and rotated so that its flat surface is no longer in contact with the humerus.

The displacement is easily seen in the antero-posterior radiograph (*Fig.* 151). In children, where the epiphyses are not yet fully ossified, it must be recognized that the fragment shown in the radiograph is merely the ossific nucleus of a very much larger cartilaginous fragment.

Manipulative Reduction.—This may be possible within a few days of the injury. An assistant holds the limb by the wrist with his other hand on the inner aspect of the elbow, and gently opens the joint on the outer side so that the limb is in slight cubitus varus. The surgeon places one or both thumbs beneath the fragment and pushes it upwards and inwards, tilting it into the joint. The elbow is then flexed, and the two condyles of the humerus are strongly compressed laterally so that the fragment is firmly pressed into its bed. Reduction is usually stable, but a plaster cast may be used in addition to a collar-and-cuff sling. The after-treatment is the same as for supracondylar fractures.

Operative Reduction.—If the fragment is not perfectly replaced, the joint must be opened on the outer side, the fragment replaced, and held in position by catgut suture. There is no necessity to peg or screw the fragment to the humerus.

FRACTURES OF BOTH CONDYLES OF THE HUMERUS (T AND Y FRACTURES)

This injury consists of a high supracondylar fracture, with a second vertical fracture line extending into the joint, separating both condyles. It is sometimes comminuted, and usually occurs in elderly patients from a fall on the point of the elbow.

The displacement is reduced by traction and direct lateral compression of the fragments. A plaster cast is applied, well moulded to the inner and outer aspects of the joint, in order to prevent recurrent tilting of the fragments with distortion of the joint surface.

As a rule the elbow is held in right-angled flexion and the limb is suspended by a collar-and-cuff sling. In some cases the flexed or right-angled position tilts the condylar fragments forwards so that extension movement of the joint would remain limited. In this event the cast must be applied with the elbow fully extended.

Since the injury occurs in elderly patients, it is particularly important to preserve full finger and shoulder movements. Only if a plaster cast has been used, in addition to a collar-and-cuff sling, can early shoulder exercises be practised with safety.

FRACTURE OF THE MEDIAL EPICONDYLE OF THE HUMERUS

The medial epicondyle of the humerus may be fractured by direct violence, but more often the epicondyle or its epiphysis is avulsed by the common flexor group of muscles (*Fig.* 152). Slight displacement of the fragment is of no significance, and operative treatment is not necessary; union of the fragment may be fibrous and not bony, but this does not usually impair the functional result. If the fragment is widely displaced, or rotated away from the humerus, it should be

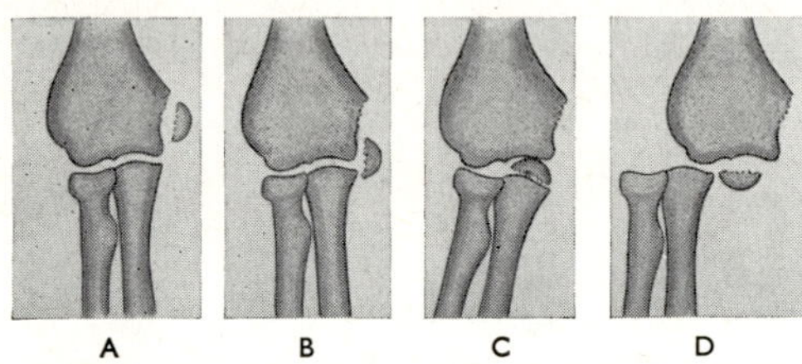

Fig. 152.—Separation of the epiphysis of the medial epicondyle. A, Minimal displacement; B, Marked displacement—operative fixation is usually advisable; C, Inclusion within the elbow-joint—operative replacement is imperative; D, Displacement associated with dislocation of the elbow-joint—care must be taken in reducing the dislocation not to include the epiphysis within the joint.

replaced through a short incision and fixed with catgut sutures. The associated traumatic synovitis of the joint necessitates immobilization by a collar-and-cuff sling for three weeks and movement is then regained by the patient's own exercise. The recovery of full extension is sometimes a slow process, and even twelve months may elapse before movement is normal. Passive methods, or manipulation under anæsthesia, must be avoided because they delay the recovery still more.

Inclusion within the Elbow-joint.—If the fragment is displaced into the elbow-joint its immediate replacement is imperative. In early cases it may be dislodged from the joint by manipulation, but in other cases operation is necessary. The fragment should not be pinned or nailed into position; any foreign body other than absorbable catgut causes irritation of the elbow-joint, with recurrent exudation and dense adhesion formation.

Ulnar Nerve Palsy.—Since the epicondyle is displaced by the stretching open of the inner side of the joint there is frequently a coincident traction injury of the ulnar nerve, with paralysis which is usually incomplete. Transposition of the nerve from the irregularly thickened post-condylar groove to the front of the joint is sometimes necessary.

DISLOCATION OF THE ELBOW

As a rule both radius and ulna are dislocated backwards, either directly backwards, backwards and outwards, or backwards and inwards. The injury is often associated with avulsion of the medial epicondyle or its epiphysis. It is important to recognize this complication before reducing the dislocation, in order to avoid imprisoning the small fragment within the inner side of the joint. In other cases there may be a comminuted fracture of the head of the radius. Forward dislocation of both radius and ulna together with a fracture of the olecranon is rare.

Reduction and After-treatment.—Backward dislocations are easily reduced by applying traction to the forearm and gradually flexing the elbow. The wrist is suspended from the neck by a collar-and-cuff sling, and the joint is immobilized for three weeks; throughout this time movements of the fingers and shoulder must be practised. Radiographs *must* be taken after manipulation to confirm the accuracy of reduction, to be sure that the medial epicondyle is not displaced within the joint, and to exclude fracture of the head of the radius necessitating operative treatment (*see below*). Movement of the elbow is regained by the patient's own gentle exercise, with no massage, no passive stretching, and no weight-carrying. The range of movement should be measured and recorded week by week.

Myositis Ossificans.—This complication is due to ossification of a hæmatoma beneath periosteum which has been avulsed by muscles or capsule. It is still occasionally seen after dislocation of the elbow when passive stretching has been employed. But it should never occur to such degree as to cause stiffness. If forceful passive stretching is avoided, subperiosteal hæmatoma ossification is never important. 'Myositis ossificans' is not a spreading invasion of osteoblasts into muscles. It is no more than subperiosteal ossification which does not arise if active movement as opposed to passive stretching is relied upon.

The first sign of the complication is the radiographic evidence of a cloudy shadow in the front of the joint. The shadow gradually becomes more dense and consolidated, but since the hæmatoma is continually absorbing, the final bony mass is much smaller than the original shadow.

In the treatment of myositis ossificans, the absolute immobility sometimes recommended is neither necessary nor advisable. The tearing away of periosteum and the hæmatoma formation are the result of passive stretching, not of active exercise. The only treatment necessary is to prohibit passive stretching. Recovery is no more rapid if active exercise is prohibited and the joint completely immobilized in plaster. On the other hand, complete immobility allows consolidation of the adhesions which have also occurred from the passive stretching, and stiffness and limitation of extension are then inevitable.

FRACTURES OF THE HEAD OF THE RADIUS

Fractures of the head of the radius may appear insignificant but they are of considerable gravity. If treated inexpertly even simple marginal chips may cause serious incapacity. The injury follows a fall on the outstretched hand and is often overlooked. The diagnosis is based on the tenderness over the head of the radius, limitation of extension of the elbow, and pain on radio-ulnar movement.

Crack Fractures without Displacement.—These require rest by means of a triangular sling, or collar and cuff, for two or three weeks, followed by active exercises. The fracture involves the joint surfaces of the elbow, and passive stretching is disastrous. Stretching for only three or four weeks often causes permanent limitation of extension movement.

Displaced Marginal Fractures.—If a marginal sector of the head of the radius is displaced so that the radio-humeral joint surface is broken up and irregular, early operative removal of the head of the radius is advisable. It will often be found that the articular surface of the capitulum opposite the head of the radius is also damaged and loose fragments may be separated. The ideal time for operation is within the first ten days, but when the fracture occurs as a complication of dislocation of the elbow-joint it is wise to defer the operation for three weeks, by which time the avulsed ligaments, tendons, and periosteum will be sufficiently healed to prevent myositis ossificans.

Comminuted Fractures.—If the whole head of the radius is comminuted, there is breaking up of the radio-ulnar as well as of the radio-humeral joint surfaces. Unless the head of the radius is removed within the first two or three weeks, there will be permanent limitation of pronation and supination as well as of extension.

Post-operative Treatment.—After operation treatment is continued as for fractures of the head of the radius without displacement. The recovery of movement may be very slow, but the temptation to accelerate recovery by massage, stretching, or manipulation under anæsthesia must be rigidly avoided. However slow recovery may be, it will be still more slow if these measures are permitted, and permanent limitation of extension movement will result.

FRACTURE OF THE OLECRANON

Fractures of the olecranon process extend into the sigmoid notch and involve the elbow-joint surface. If the gap between the fragments is not closed and a smooth joint surface restored, stiffness of the elbow and painful movement remain. If the fragments are not immobilized in perfect apposition for at least four to six weeks, fibrous union will result, with impairment of active extension of the elbow against resistance.

Operative Treatment.—Fractures of the olecranon must be treated by operation. Sometimes the fragment may be replaced and fixed with a screw or nail; but it is often wise to excise the detached fragment and suture the triceps tendon to the ulna. Active movements may be started within about three weeks.

FRACTURES OF THE SHAFTS OF THE RADIUS AND ULNA

One or both forearm bones may be fractured in any part of the shaft. If a fracture of the radius lies above the insertion of the pronator teres, the proximal fragment is fully supinated by the unopposed action of the supinator and the biceps. The distal fragment must therefore be held in a similar position, and the limb is immobilized in full supination. If the fracture of the radius lies below the insertion of the pronator teres, the proximal fragment has both supinator and pronator muscles attached to it. The limb must then be immobilized in the position midway between full supination and full pronation. As a rule the elbow is held at the right angle. Accurate reduction and proper immobilization of the forearm bones are difficult to achieve.

Method of Reduction.—Overriding and angulation of the fragments is reduced by traction. Counter-traction should be arranged by passing a sling of calico bandage over the front of the arm just above the flexed elbow. An assistant takes the patient's fingers in one hand and the thumb in the other, and pulls steadily. The surgeon applies direct pressure to the fragments and moulds them into position. An unpadded plaster cast is then applied from the upper arm just below the shoulder to the knuckles, not extending into the palm beyond the oblique skin creases (*Fig.* 153).

After-treatment.—During the first few days the hand is elevated with the fingers pointing to the ceiling in order to minimize reactionary swelling. The circulation and movements of the fingers must be carefully watched, because of the danger of Volkmann's contracture (*see* p. 209). If there is cyanosis or pallor of the fingers, or difficulty in fully extending them, the plaster is at once cut longitudinally from the front of the wrist to above the elbow. When the circulation is again normal the plaster may be repaired. The average minimum period of immobilization is six weeks in children and ten weeks in adults. Full movements of the fingers and shoulder are practised throughout.

Non-union of the Shaft of the Ulna.—Non-union is sometimes seen in fractures of the shaft of the ulna at the junction of the middle and lower thirds, but it is always due to inadequate immobilization or immobilization for too short a period. In some cases a below-elbow plaster cast which does not prevent rotatory movement of the fragments has been relied upon. In other cases a complete cast above the elbow has been replaced after six or eight weeks by a below-elbow plaster. The union which had developed during the first few weeks was broken down by the rotatory movements subsequently permitted. The complete cast from the upper arm to the knuckles must be retained until there is radiographic evidence of union of the fracture. It is sometimes necessary to operate and promote more vigorous bone growth by implanting cancellous bone-chip grafts cut from the crest of the ilium.

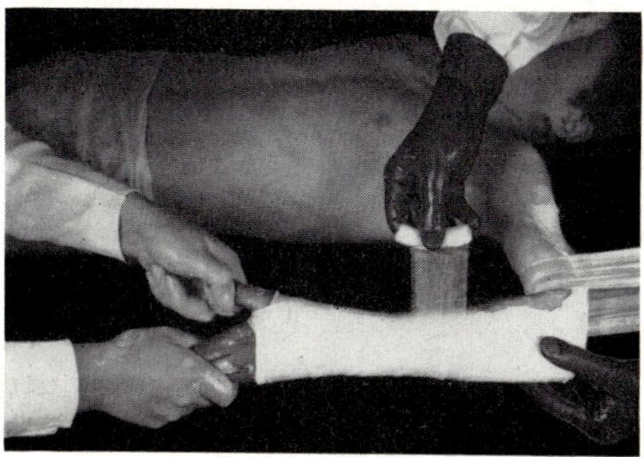

Fig. 153.—Reduction of fracture of shafts of both forearm bones.

Fractures of the Upper Third of Both Bones.—When the fracture lies high in the forearm the flexed position of the elbow may tend to produce a similarly flexed position of the fragments—a backward angulation. In these circumstances the elbow should be fully extended and plaster applied with the limb in this position.

Fractures of the Upper Shaft of the Ulna with Dislocation of the Head of the Radius.—*In every fracture of the upper shaft of the ulna the surgeon should suspect that there may also be a dislocation of the head of the radius.* The dislocation is often overlooked, and a very serious permanent disability then remains. The combined injury—the Monteggia fracture-dislocation—is one of the most difficult of all bone injuries and none except the most experienced should embark upon the treatment of it. The case should be transferred at once to an expert. He will probably perform an intramedullary nailing of the fractured ulna, possibly with excision of the head of the radius if it has been seriously fractured.

Fracture of the Lower Shaft of the Radius with Inferior Radio-ulnar Dislocation.—This is a relatively common injury, and there is a marked tendency to redisplacement, the radius angulating towards the ulna, and the inferior radio-ulnar joint again dislocating. It must be reduced by traction on the radius applied through the thumb. The limb is immobilized with the wrist deviated as far as possible to the ulnar side. The plaster must be closely moulded round the radius and wrist-joint, and carried well down the radial side of the hand over the thumb and index metacarpals.

COLLES'S FRACTURE OF THE RADIUS

This very common fracture is usually the result of a fall on the outstretched hand; the lower fragment of the radius is displaced upwards, backwards, and to the radial side.

Method of Reduction.—It is possible to correct both backward and outward displacement by one simple movement which pronates the lower fragment; but it is more satisfactory to correct each displacement separately by two distinct manœuvres. To reduce a right Colles's fracture, the surgeon grasps the lower fragment in his left hand, securing a grip between his thenar eminence on the

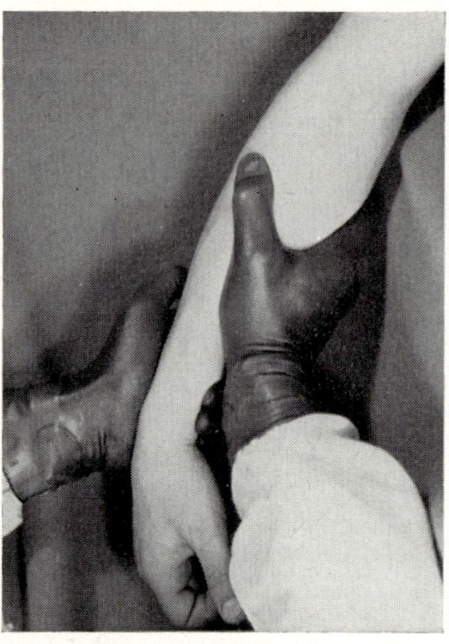

Fig. 154.—Reduction of Colles's fracture. Correction of backward displacement.

back of the fragment and his finger-tips on the front (*Fig.* 154) and pulls. An assistant steadies and provides counter-traction on the upper arm. By pressure with the surgeon's other hand on the front of the forearm, the fragment is tilted and pushed forwards as strongly as possible. A new grip is then taken to correct the radial displacement. The surgeon places his right thenar eminence over the patient's radial styloid process, and his finger-tips over the ulnar side of the joint, and with his other hand on the opposite side of the limb the radial fragment is tilted and pushed inwards towards the ulna (*Fig.* 155). It is impossible to over-correct the displacement however strongly the surgeon manipulates.

An assistant holds the limb, taking the patient's thumb in one hand and fingers in the other, and maintains strong traction. The surgeon applies a dorsal plaster slab directly to the skin, from the back of the knuckles to just below the fold of the elbow. An encircling plaster bandage may also be applied. The plaster must extend over the radial side of the thumb metacarpal to the base of the thenar eminence, and over the front of the wrist-joint to below the scaphoid tubercle, but not actually into the palm. While the plaster is setting, the surgeon must again grasp the wrist and mould the plaster very closely round the radius, reproducing the normal concavity of the lower end, and pushing the carpus and lower radial fragment forwards and inwards (*Fig.* 156). The wrist should be in the neutral or rest position—neither strongly dorsiflexed nor palmar-flexed. Unless the plaster is closely moulded to the bone, redisplacement will occur and the fracture will unite with radial deviation.

After-treatment.—The hand is lightly bandaged or strapped to the dorsal plaster. There must be nothing in the palm except strapping or bandage, and full finger and shoulder exercises are practised at once. If the fingers are swollen the limb is elevated until the œdema has subsided. A sling may be worn for 24–48 hours; the arm is then put through the sleeve of the clothes and used in the

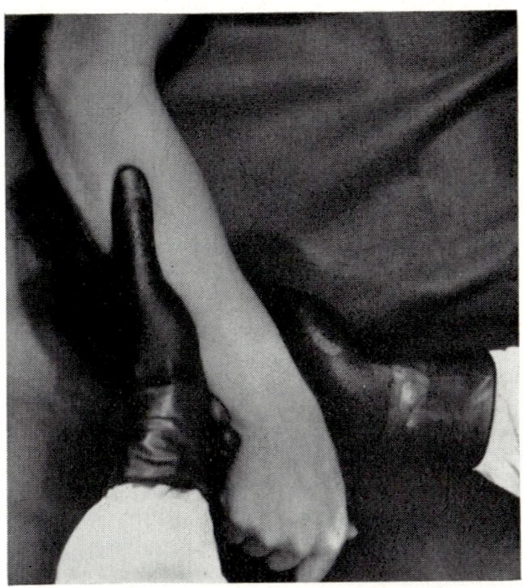

Fig. 155.—Reduction of Colles's fracture. Correction of radial displacement.

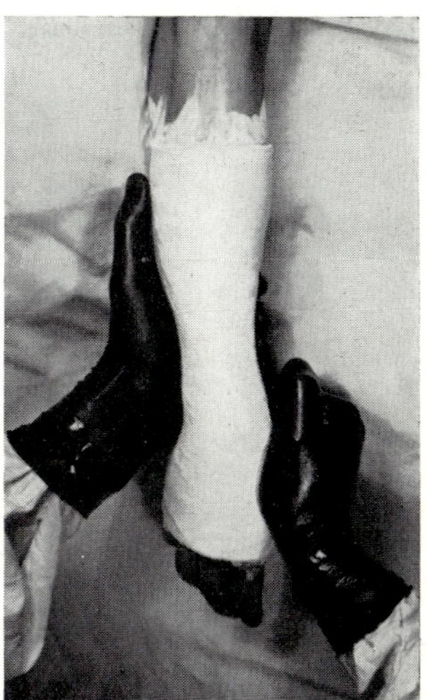

Fig. 156. — Reduction of Colles's fracture. While the plaster is setting the radial concavity is reproduced by the fingers of the left hand and the lower fragment is pushed forwards and towards the ulna with the right hand.

ordinary way for light activities. The plaster must be retained for five weeks. If the limb was very swollen when the fracture was reduced, a new plaster is necessary seven to ten days later (*see* p. 203). Wrist and forearm movements recover by the patient's own activity within a few weeks of removing the plaster.

Reversed Colles's Fracture.—In more uncommon cases the lower fragment of the radius is displaced forwards and not backwards. The displacement is reduced by pushing the fragment backwards and dorsiflexing the wrist. A plaster cast is applied in the usual way and the wrist immobilized for five weeks.

Displaced Lower Radial Epiphysis.—The same injury sustained in children causes a backward and outward displacement of the lower radial epiphysis. The clinical signs, method of reduction, and after-treatment are the same as for Colles's fracture. The injury is to be regarded as a fracture adjacent to the epiphysial line. It seldom causes arrested growth of the radius such as occurs after compression of the epiphysial disk.

Spontaneous Rupture of Thumb Tendons.—The extensor pollicis longus tendon lies in a groove on the back of the lower end of the radius. A sharp spicule of bone in this groove may cause fraying and spontaneous rupture of the tendon. If this happens, the extensor indicis, or one of the radial carpal extensor tendons of the wrist, should be transferred to the distal part of the tendon of extensor pollicis.

FRACTURE OF THE CARPAL SCAPHOID BONE

Fracture of the scaphoid bone is a frequent injury in boys and in young men. If it is properly treated perfect recovery is possible within three or four months. If treatment is delayed the incapacity period is prolonged to six or twelve months. If the wrist is not immobilized at all non-union is inevitable, the wrist is permanently weakened, and arthritis with a very serious disability may supervene years later. Early diagnosis is therefore of great importance. Unfortunately the injury is often regarded as a sprain and the fracture is overlooked.

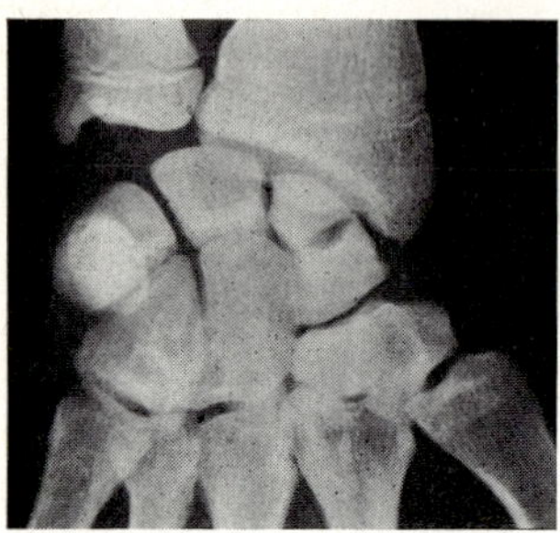

Fig. 157.—Two-months-old fracture of the carpal scaphoid bone; there is cavitation at the site of fracture.

Diagnosis.—Sprain of the wrist is almost an unknown injury. Nearly every so-called sprain is actually a fracture. *Every patient who injures the wrist and complains of pain and tenderness over the radial side of the joint must be assumed to have sustained a fracture of the scaphoid until radiographs prove otherwise.* The radiograph may show only the very finest hair-line crack. The crack may be obvious only when seen through a magnifying lens. Nevertheless, this is a complete fracture and must not be ignored. If the wrist and thumb are not immobilized, even the finest crack will gradually widen until a gap appears (*Fig.* 157) and non-union develops. If a fracture of the scaphoid is suspected three radiographs must be taken, including an oblique view at right angles to the floor of the 'anatomical snuff-box' as well as the classic anteroposterior (*Fig.* 158) and lateral views. If the crack does not appear even in the oblique view,

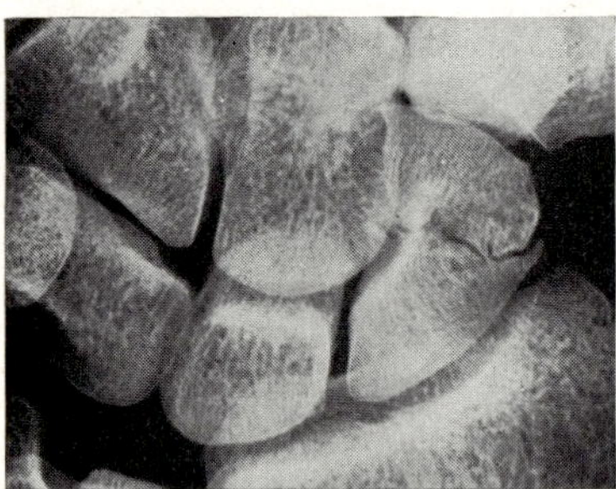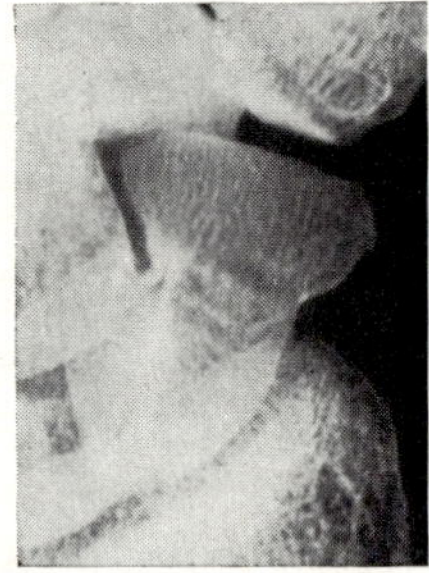

Fig. 158.—Recent fracture of the carpal scaphoid bone. Although it is a hair-line crack, complete immobilization is essential.

the surgeon should still not be satisfied. A further series of three radiographs must be taken two weeks later. If there is any fracture, it will show clearly after this interval.

Treatment.—The wrist must be immobilized until there is radiographic evidence of union. Every single shearing movement of the fragments retards the process of repair, and if the movement is repeated often enough the fracture will never unite. A cock-up splint does not afford sufficient immobilization. A plaster slab must be moulded to the limb from the metacarpal heads to the upper forearm, extending far enough round the radial and ulnar margins to prevent side-to-side movements of the hand. The wrist is in slight dorsiflexion and the thumb in opposition. The plaster extends round the radial side of the index and thumb metacarpals, and must not fall short of these metacarpal heads. The slab is then secured by encircling turns of plaster bandage which are very closely moulded in the palm of the hand so that wrist movement is completely limited. The plaster must not extend beyond the skin creases of the palm. The patient must report at once if the plaster shows signs of cracking at the wrist, and he must not allow it to become wet. With these reservations he may undertake any activity, and may return to work.

Duration of Immobilization.—Most fractures of the tubercle of the scaphoid are united in four weeks, and most recent fractures of the waist in eight to ten weeks. *If the fracture is not united at that time, strict immobilization must be continued until it is united.* If occasional movements have been permitted, it may be necessary to continue for three or four months. If there was any delay in the institution of immobilization, six to twelve months may be required.

DISLOCATION OF THE LUNATE BONE

Clinical Signs.—The lunate bone is dislocated forwards into the very confined space beneath the anterior annular ligament. This space is already almost fully occupied by the flexor tendons of the fingers and the median nerve. The typical clinical signs are, therefore, immobility of the semiflexed fingers, median paralysis in 50 per cent of cases, and swelling and painful limitation of wrist movement, with no obvious deformity.

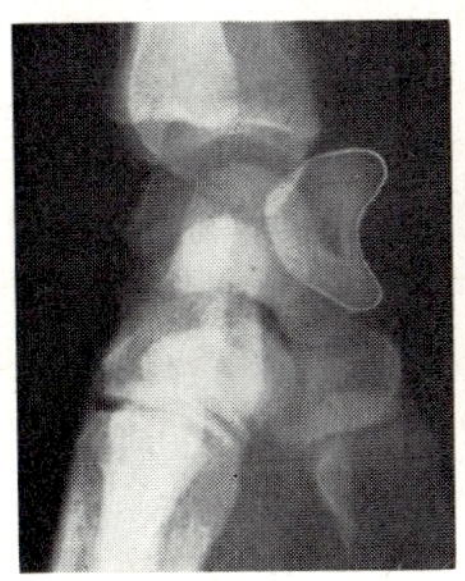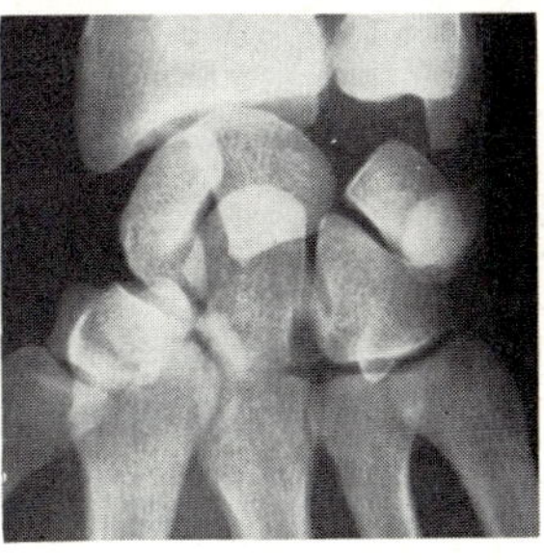

A   B

Fig. 159.—Dislocation of the carpal lunate bone. A, In a lateral view the cup of the lunate is tilted forwards and the capitate lies behind it. B, The anteroposterior view. The normal quadrilateral-shaped shadow of the lunate is now triangular.

X-ray Diagnosis.—The radiographic appearances are quite typical, but are often misinterpreted. In the lateral view it is evident that the head of the capitate no longer lies in the cup of the lunate (*Fig.* 159 A), but is displaced behind it. As a rule the lunate is tilted so that its cup is directed forwards instead of downwards. This 90° tilt accounts for the different shape of the X-ray shadow in the anteroposterior view (*Fig.* 159 B). Whereas normally the bone outline is quadrilateral, when it is dislocated it appears triangular.

Method of Reduction.—Manipulative reduction is seldom difficult. The surgeon presses over the front of the semilunar with one thumb. With the other hand grasping the patient's fingers he applies strong traction to the remainder of the carpus, pulling the capitate away from the radius and gradually flexing the wrist so that the head of the capitate is pulled into the cup of the lunate (*Fig.* 160).

After-treatment.—The wrist is immobilized by a dorsal plaster cast, in 45° of palmar flexion, for seven days. The plaster is then changed, no anæsthetic being used, and immobilization is continued with the wrist in the mid-position for a further two weeks.

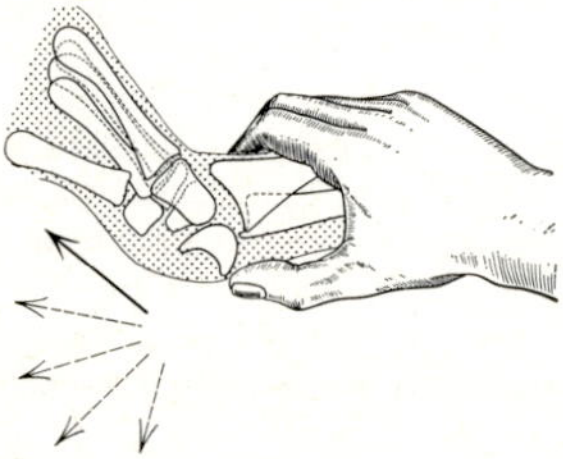

Dislocation of the Lunate with Half of the Scaphoid.—Fracture of the waist of the scaphoid may be combined with dislocation of the lunate which carries the proximal half of the scaphoid with it. The distal half of the scaphoid remains attached to the capitate and other carpal bones, and is displaced backwards and to the radial side. The dislocation is easily reduced in the usual way. The wrist is then immobilized for as many weeks or months as may be necessary to secure bony union of the fractured scaphoid.

Fig. 160.—Manipulative reduction of dislocation of the lunate.

Operative Treatment.—Old unreduced dislocations of the lunate and half-scaphoid should be treated by operative excision of the displaced bone. Operative reduction is not advisable, because if the dislocation is of long standing the blood-supply of the displaced bones is so impaired that avascular necrosis supervenes, with stiffness of the wrist.

FRACTURES OF THE METACARPAL BONES

The metacarpals may be fractured at the base, in the middle of the shaft, or at the neck. There is usually no displacement and the hand is simply immobilized for four weeks by a dorsal plaster cast similar to that used for fractures of the carpus. The finger-joints must be left free for movement. The old method of strapping the fingers over a roll of wool or bandage in the palm must not be used.

If there is angulation of a fracture of the shaft or neck of the metacarpal, with displacement of the metacarpal head forwards into the palm, the displacement must be reduced. This must not be attempted by hyperextension of the metacarpo-phalangeal joint because the manœuvre will fail and immobilization of the fingers in this position causes permanent stiffness. The metacarpo-phalangeal and proximal interphalangeal joints are flexed to a right angle; if the phalanx is then thrust backwards, the metacarpal head is pushed backwards and the angulation thereby corrected. The finger is immobilized with both joints flexed 90°.

BENNETT'S FRACTURE-DISLOCATION OF THE THUMB

In this injury a marginal fragment is broken off the base of the thumb metacarpal. This fragment, however, remains in its normal position, and it is the metacarpal itself which is displaced. The base of the metacarpal is partly or completely dislocated from the trapezium, and lies to the radial side of the carpus (*Fig.* 161). If it is unreduced, abduction movement of the thumb is lost, the span is reduced, the thumb is greatly weakened, there is an ugly deformity, and arthritis of the carpo-metacarpal joint may supervene.

The oblique articular surface of the trapezium coincides with the line of fracture and forms a sliding plane. The dislocation is reduced by traction and strong, firm pressure over the prominent base of the metacarpal while the thumb is held in abduction. A plaster cast is applied closely moulded over the base of the metacarpal and the reduced position held while the plaster sets. This difficult fracture-dislocation is immobilized for three weeks.

INJURIES OF THE FINGERS

The finger-joints are the most important joints of the upper limb; a workman with completely stiff fingers is very little better off than a workman with an amputated arm. These joints are particularly susceptible to injury; they stiffen very readily, and even minor sprains may cause months of incapacity. Every finger injury must therefore be treated with great respect, and if serious and possibly permanent incapacity is to be avoided certain principles of treatment must be observed:—

1. *The injured finger must be immobilized for at least two or three weeks.* This applies even to joint sprains.

2. *The finger must be immobilized in the flexed position.* This is the position in which reduction is usually most stable; it is the position in which the injured finger will stiffen least; and it is the only position which will allow bending movement of the other fingers. If one finger is held fully extended it is quite impossible to flex the others.

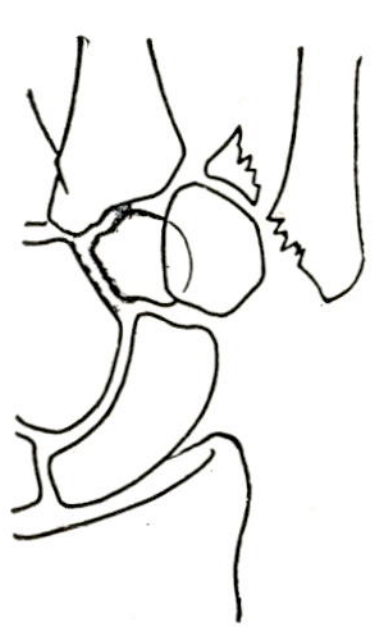

Fig. 161. — Bennett's fracture - dislocation of the thumb metacarpal.

3. *Every finger except the injured one must be left free of splints, strapping, or bandage.* There must be no restriction of any sort to full movements of the normal fingers.

4. *The patient must move every uninjured finger throughout its normal range many times a day.* It is not enough to 'waggle' the finger in the middle range of movement. The limits of flexion and extension must be reached.

5. *Passive stretching and manipulation must never be permitted.* Massage is a waste of time; if the fingers are stiff active exercise is the essential measure; if the fingers are swollen elevation of the limb will relieve the swelling.

Sprain of a Finger-joint.—The joint is acutely painful and swollen. Radiographs may show small bony chips detached from the joint margin by avulsion of the capsule. In other cases the capsule itself is torn. Many finger sprains have been actual dislocations, spontaneously reduced at the moment of injury. The joint should be immobilized in moderate flexion for two or three weeks.

Dislocation of the Fingers.—Dislocations are usually due to hyperextension injuries. A triangular fragment may be chipped from the base of the distal phalanx. Reduction is easily accomplished by traction and flexion of the joint. The finger is immobilized for three weeks by a small plaster cast with all joints flexed at least 30° to 40°. Reduction is sometimes unstable, and check radiographs must be taken seven days after reduction. If the detached fragment is a fairly large one and carries one-third or more of the articular surface of the joint, there is a strong tendency to recurrence of the dislocation. This injury is comparable with Bennett's fracture-dislocation of the thumb, and may require internal fixation; expert advice should be sought.

Dislocation of the Thumb.—Dislocations of the metacarpo-phalangeal joint of the thumb are also produced by hyperextension, and are sometimes difficult to reduce because the tendons of the short thenar muscles slip round the sides of the metacarpal head. The sesamoids may be interposed between the two articular surfaces. If manipulative reduction fails, operative reposition is necessary.

Fractures of Phalanges.—These usually occur in the shaft of the bone. The proximal fragment is flexed and the distal fragment tilted backwards (forward angulation). The displacement is reduced by traction and flexion of the joints.

The digit is immobilized by a small plaster cast. If the fracture is oblique and there is considerable overriding, traction may be necessary.

Mallet Finger.—The extensor tendon is avulsed from the base of the terminal phalanx with or without a small flake of bone.

The terminal joint is flexed and, although passive extension is possible, active extension is lost. Failing suitable treatment a severe mallet-finger deformity develops. The whole of the power of the extensor tendon is then concentrated

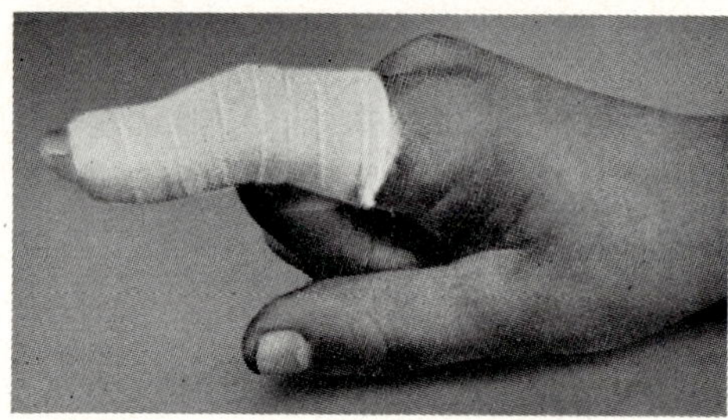

Fig. 162.—Application of plaster cast for mallet finger. A small slab is moulded to the flexor surface by means of ribbon-gauze bandage. While it is setting the surgeon holds the terminal joint in full hyperextension. This is a very difficult plaster to apply and much practice is needed. Try it first on a normal finger.

on the proximal interphalangeal joint. A hyperextension deformity at this joint is therefore added to the flexion deformity at the terminal joint. The finger must be immobilized by a plaster cast, with the proximal interphalangeal joint flexed and the terminal joint hyperextended for at least six weeks (*Fig.* 162). It is sometimes wise to do an early operative repair within the first 48 hours, retracting fibres of the extensor tendon interposed in the back of the terminal interphalangeal joint and suturing them accurately in position.

CHAPTER XVIII

FRACTURES AND DISLOCATIONS OF THE BONES OF THE FACE, SPINE, AND PELVIS

By Sir Reginald Watson-Jones

FRACTURES OF THE BONES OF THE FACE

Nasal Bones.—The nasal bones or cartilages and the nasal septum may be fractured by direct violence, and even minor degrees of displacement cause serious disfigurement. Asymmetry due to lateral displacement should be corrected by direct pressure over the fragments. An instrument such as a pair of straight artery forceps covered with thin rubber tubing may be inserted into the nostril to correct lateral deviation of the septum and to elevate depressed fragments. Reduction is usually stable; it is seldom necessary to use any splint, and the nose should not be plugged.

Malar Bone.—Fractures of the zygomatic arch and malar bone are usually depressed; if the fragments are not elevated facial disfigurement persists. There is sometimes anæsthesia of the cheek and lip from compression of the infra-orbital nerve. Replacement can be effected by an elevating instrument inserted through a half-inch incision placed within the hair margin above and behind the zygomatic arch.

FRACTURES AND DISLOCATIONS OF THE LOWER JAW

Fractures of the Lower Jaw.—Almost every fracture of the body of the jaw is compound into the mouth, and frequent antiseptic mouthwashes are necessary. A fluid diet is prescribed, and soft foods may be taken after a week or ten days. If there is no displacement of the fragments the jaw is supported by means of a four-tailed bandage for about ten days. If the fragments are displaced and occlusion of the teeth is inaccurate, the co-operation of a dental surgeon should be sought. After reduction of displacement the jaw may be immobilized by: (1) an interdental splint cemented on to the teeth; (2) wires secured round the teeth which fix upper and lower jaws together. Co-operation with the facio-maxillary and/or dental surgeon is desirable (*see* p. 610).

Dislocation of the Lower Jaw.—This may be bilateral, when both condyles slip forward on to the articular eminences, or may be unilateral, when one condyle slips forwards and pushes the jaw and chin towards the opposite side. To reduce the dislocation the operator stands in front of the patient, and, with his protected thumbs passed into the mouth, presses the angle of the jaw downwards, at the same time raising the chin with his fingers outside the mouth. The jaw is supported by a four-tailed bandage kept in position for two weeks, the patient meanwhile being fed on fluids and soft foods.

FRACTURES OF THE SPINE

Transport in Suspected Spinal Fractures.—Patients with suspected fractures of the spine should be moved with particular caution because damage to the spinal cord may cause permanent paralysis. If a patient with a fractured spine is lifted face upwards by the shoulders and hips, sagging of the trunk between the two points of support forces the injured area into flexion. The spine above and below the fracture forms such a powerful pair of levers that this apparently simple movement may crush the spinal cord or the cauda equina. If no other means of transport is available it is better to roll the patient carefully on to his face and lift him in the prone position. This is less dangerous because the spine then sags into extension. It must be recognized, however, that even this position is not entirely safe because sometimes a fracture of the spine is complicated by interlocking of articular processes and the spinal cord is then in no less danger of traction by hyperextension movement than of compression by flexion movement. The only safe procedure is to avoid both flexion and hyperextension strains and to keep the spine in the *neutral position*. As the patient lies on his back, slings of roller towels, bandages, or strong handkerchiefs are passed under the neck, shoulder-blades, loin, buttocks, and thighs. The slings are grasped on each side and the patient is carried to a firm stretcher. If no stretcher is available broad planks from a building site or a carriage door from a wrecked train may be used. When the patient is safely on a stretcher he should not be moved from it until radiographic examination in hospital is completed.

Special precautions are necessary when it is suspected that there may be an injury in the cervical spine. Having passed many slings under the patient, tied them to wooden rods on each side of the trunk, and arranged for two bearers to lift and carry the patient, the doctor himself should hold the patient's head firmly in traction and permit no single flexion, extension, or rotation movement. His supervision must continue until the patient is safely in hospital.

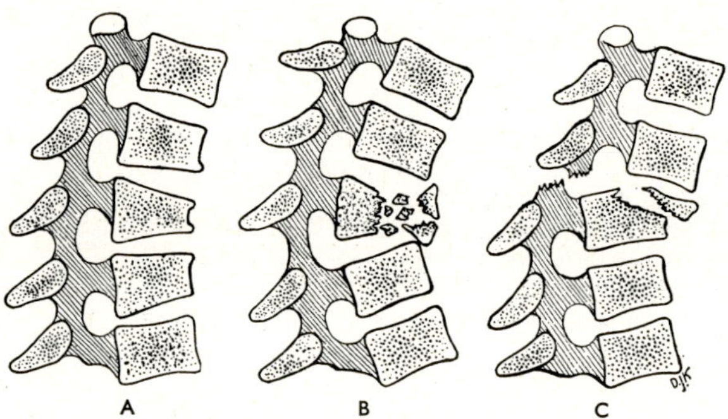

Fig. 163.—Three types of crush fracture of the spine: A, Wedging of one or more vertebral bodies; B, Comminuted fracture of a vertebral body; C, Fracture-dislocation.

Types of Fractures (*Fig.* 163).—There are three types of flexion fracture: (1) simple wedge compression of one or more vertebræ; (2) comminuted fracture of one vertebral body due to more localized and acute angulation; (3) fracture-dislocation.

Diagnosis.—The deformity may not be obvious on inspection, but is easily felt when the examining finger passes down the line of spinous processes. The patient usually, but not always, complains of pain in the back. Every patient who falls, even from a moderate height, in the sitting or standing position, and has pain in the back, should be X-rayed.

X-ray Examination.—The lateral radiograph discloses the injury more clearly than the anteroposterior film. Even the slightest wedging of a vertebral body must be accepted as a complete fracture. In severe angulation in young people, the deformity should be reduced by hyperextension of the spine and maintained in a plaster-of-Paris jacket for three months. However, this is not commonly necessary, the majority of compression fractures only requiring a brief period of rest followed by extension exercises.

The patient may be more comfortable when lying in bed if fracture boards are used—that is to say ordinary 1-in. (2·5-cm.) thick planks of wood slightly longer than the width of the bed placed across and under the mattress to keep it firm. But the patient must not think that he is to be kept inactive. He should start extension exercises from the beginning. In all spinal fractures, injury to the spinal cord must be excluded by noting the power, sensation, and reflexes of the lower limbs, and the functions of the bladder and rectum.

Method of Reduction and Immobilization.—The patient is rolled on to his face, so that when he is lifted the spine will be extended and the dangerous movement of flexion avoided. A double layer of stockinet 8 in. (20 cm.) wide is pulled over the trunk and fixed over the shoulders and in the perineum. Each anterior superior iliac spine is protected by adhesive felt, and a larger piece of felt, 4 × 6 in. (10 × 15 cm.) applied over the spinous processes at the level of fracture. Two tables, one 10–12 in. (30 cm.) higher than the other, are placed end to end with a space between them slightly greater than the length of the patient's trunk. The patient is then lifted into position so that his head and arms are resting on the edge of the higher table (*Fig.* 164). The lower table supports the lower limbs to the level of the upper thigh, but must fall short of the symphysis pubis by several inches.

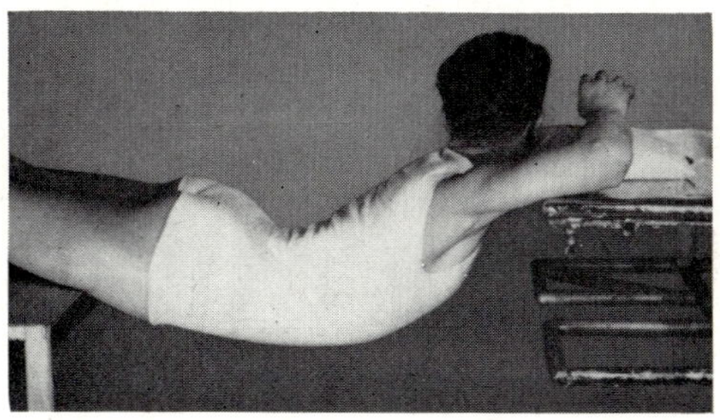

Fig. 164.—Reduction and plaster fixation of a crush fracture of the lumbar spine. The pelvis is entirely clear of the lower table and there is no ventral sling, so that the lumbar spine is fully extended.

Plaster is at once applied, and successive layers are rubbed into each other firmly. This degree of pressure is sufficient to complete the reduction; there must be no manipulation and no forcible thrusting over the kyphos. The plaster must extend from the groin to the clavicles.

After-treatment.—Until the plaster is thoroughly dry the patient lies with pillows beneath the concavity in the arch of the spine. The position is then changed every few hours during the day, to avoid hypostasis and congestion of the lungs. The patient may sit up at once, and if there is no nerve complication, walking may be resumed within a day or two. Exercises are taught to maintain the tone of the spinal and abdominal musculature; they are, furthermore, an essential part of the much commoner 'functional treatment' of compression fractures (*vide infra*).

After removal of the plaster movement of the spine is regained by the patient's own exercise. It is seldom necessary to manipulate the spine, and full movements should be regained within about two months of discarding the jacket.

'Functional Treatment' of Minor Wedge Compression Fractures of the Spine.—
When there is minor wedge compression of a vertebral body, and radiographic
examination proves that there is no subluxation of the posterior interarticular
joints, no rupture of the posterior interspinous ligament, and no rupture of the
intervertebral disks, so that the spine is stable and displacement will not increase,
no plaster jacket need be used. Hyperextension exercises are instituted within
a few days or at the latest within 2–3 weeks. This régime is nearly always indicated
in old patients who sustain minor compression in consequence of senile osteoporosis.

FRACTURES AND DISLOCATIONS OF THE CERVICAL SPINE

Subluxation of the Cervical Spine.—Crush fractures of vertebral bodies seldom
occur in the cervical region, but subluxation of one interarticular joint is a
frequent injury. There is often pressure on the adjacent nerve-root causing
pain, tingling, or numbness in one or both arms. Reduction may not be possible
except by skull-traction from calliper-splints which are inserted into the temporal
region of the skull with a light weight suspended from the calliper over the head-
end of the bed. After four to six weeks of traction the callipers should be
removed and the cervical spine immobilized in plaster-of-Paris for three months.

SPINAL FRACTURES WITH PARAPLEGIA

Recoverable and Irrecoverable Paralysis.—Fractures and fracture-dislocations
of the cervical, dorsal, or lumbar regions may be associated with injury to the
spinal cord or cauda equina and paralysis of the lower limbs, bladder, and rectum.
The cord injury may be a simple contusion, a compression by the bony walls of
the spinal canal, or an actual severance of the nerve-fibres. If the cord is severed,
no recovery is possible whatever treatment is undertaken. On the other hand,
paraplegia due to simple compression will recover if the compression is relieved.

During the first few hours the types cannot always be distinguished by neurological tests. In all cases, therefore, immediate steps should be taken to relieve
pressure. It is better to maintain the neutral or slightly extended position by
means of pillows on a firm mattress.

Special care must be taken to recognize fracture-dislocations with interlocked
articular processes. These must never be hyperextended. Open operative reduction of the interlocked processes is necessary, often with internal fixations by
plates and screws applied to the spinous processes after reduction.

FRACTURES AND DISLOCATIONS OF THE PELVIS

The bone injury is often unimportant, but the associated injury to soft tissues
may be serious or even fatal. Injuries to the urethra, the bladder, the vagina, the
rectum, the nerve plexuses, and even to the diaphragm must be excluded. Concealed blood-loss from hæmorrhage into the soft tissues can be very great and
in severe injuries is often fatal.

Injuries to the Urethra or Bladder.—If injury to the urethra or bladder is even
suspected, arrangements should be made immediately with the surgeon in charge
of the case to carry out the necessary investigation in the operating theatre.
Sounding of the urethra and similar procedures should not be carried out except
in an operating theatre where asepsis can be assured and, if necessary, operation
undertaken immediately. If urgent relief of retention of urine is needed before
these facilities are at hand, catheterization is still contra-indicated; the bladder,
if full, should be emptied by suprapubic aspiration. In cases of rupture of the
urethra, the patient must not under any circumstances even attempt to pass urine.

Treatment of the Bone Injury.—The common injuries to the pelvis are fractures of one or both pubic rami, slight separations of the symphysis pubis, and fractures of the body of the ilium. No special treatment is necessary other than bed-rest for about three weeks.

Disruption of the Pelvis (*Fig.* 165).—The one injury that requires special treatment is disruption of the pelvis from compression in the anteroposterior axis. One half of the pelvis is rotated outwards, carrying with it the corresponding

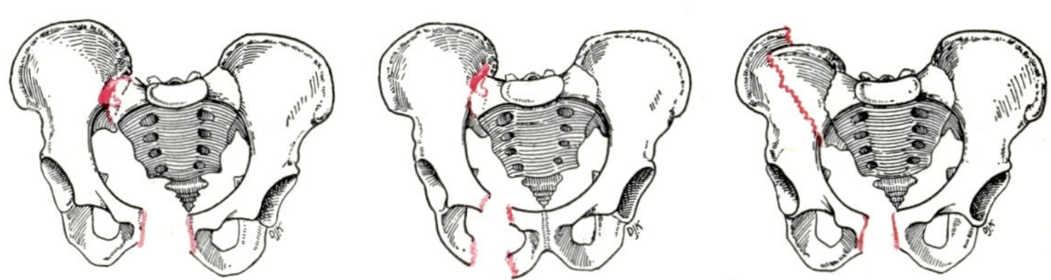

Fig. 165.—Three types of fracture-dislocation and disruption of the pelvis.

lower limb. Radiographs show wide displacement of the fragments of the pubis, but much less obvious displacement of the sacro-iliac joint. Nevertheless, there may be a traction injury to the lumbo-sacral nerve plexus.

While the patient lies on his back, gravity and the weight of the lower limb maintain the outward rotation of the dislocated half of the pelvis. A dislocated pelvis is like a partly opened oyster: when laid on the hinge at the back, gravity keeps the two halves apart, but when laid on one side the two halves tend to close. Similarly with the dislocated pelvis, if the patient lies on one side the two halves of the pelvis sometimes fall together. When separation is severe, some degree of reduction may be obtained by passing a canvas sling behind the pelvis at the level of the sacrum, and connecting each end of the sling to a weight-and-pulley traction system (attached to an overhead beam) which is pulling upwards and across towards the opposite sides of the body.

CHAPTER XIX

FRACTURES AND DISLOCATIONS OF THE LOWER LIMB

By Sir Reginald Watson-Jones

DISLOCATION OF THE HIP

Traumatic dislocation of the hip was at one time very rare but with the increasing hazards of collision of motor vehicles it has become increasingly common. Reduction is a matter of urgency.

Method of Reduction.—The object of the manipulative procedure is to flex the hip and rotate it so that the femoral head lies just below the acetabulum and then to lift the head into the acetabulum. Reduction is easily accomplished by gentle

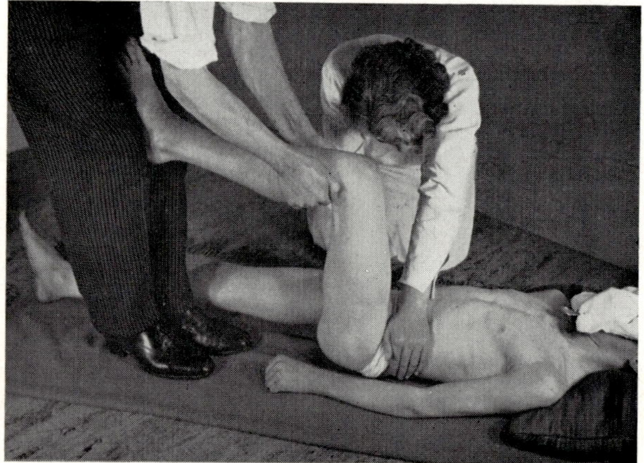

Fig. 166.—Reduction of a traumatic dislocation of the hip. The femoral head is rotated to the neutral position and lifted into the acetabulum.

manœuvring; forcible manipulation and vigorous traction are unnecessary and dangerous. The anæsthetized patient is laid on blankets on the floor so that the surgeon can more easily hold the limb. An assistant kneels by the patient and steadies the pelvis with both hands. The surgeon stands over the hip, and with both the hip and knee flexed to a right angle, he slowly rotates the limb from the position of deformity into neutral rotation, and then lifts it with firm steady traction (*Fig.* 166). This simple procedure will usually reduce all types of dislocation.

If it fails, the surgeon again applies traction to the flexed hip, and circumducts the limb through the position opposite to that of the deformity, into neutral extension, so that it lies by the side of its fellow. In the commoner dorsal dislocation where the hip is adducted and internally rotated, it is flexed, traction is applied, the hip is moved into abduction and external rotation, and then into the neutral position. In the rarer anterior dislocation where the hip is abducted and externally rotated, it is flexed, traction is applied, the hip is moved into adduction and internal rotation, and then brought down to the side of its fellow limb.

Marginal Fracture of the Acetabulum.—Marginal fragments of the acetabulum which are displaced with the head of the femur are often replaced fairly accurately when the dislocation is reduced, but it is sometimes necessary to perform an operative reduction. If there is tilting of a marginal fragment associated with sciatic nerve paralysis, operative replacement is urgently needed. The urgency is just as great as that of any abdominal emergency.

FRACTURE OF THE NECK OF THE FEMUR

Every elderly patient who after slight injury to the hip complains of pain, or is found to lie with the limb in external rotation, must be assumed to have sustained a fracture of the femoral neck until anteroposterior and lateral radiographs prove otherwise.

Three types of fracture must be distinguished: (1) abduction cervical fractures; (2) adduction cervical fractures; and (3) basal fractures (intertrochanteric and pertrochanteric).

Abduction Cervical Fracture.—This is a high cervical or subcapital fracture with true impaction (*Fig.* 167). The femoral shaft and neck are abducted in relation to the proximal fragment in the coxa valga position. Moreover, the fracture lies in a relatively horizontal plane (*Fig.* 168). It follows, therefore, that weight-bearing and muscle pull impact the fragments more closely and do not give rise to shearing stresses. These fractures usually unite perfectly well without operative treatment. But it must be recognized that this is the first stage of a rotational stress on the femoral neck which with excess strain could go on to a completely displaced 'adduction' fracture. Usually the only treatment needed is rest in bed for 3–4 weeks. But some surgeons prefer to take the safety course of nailing even these fractures.

Adduction Cervical Fracture.—In this common injury the distal fragment is adducted, the plane of fracture is relatively vertical, and the line of force of muscle pull and weight-bearing is more or less parallel with the

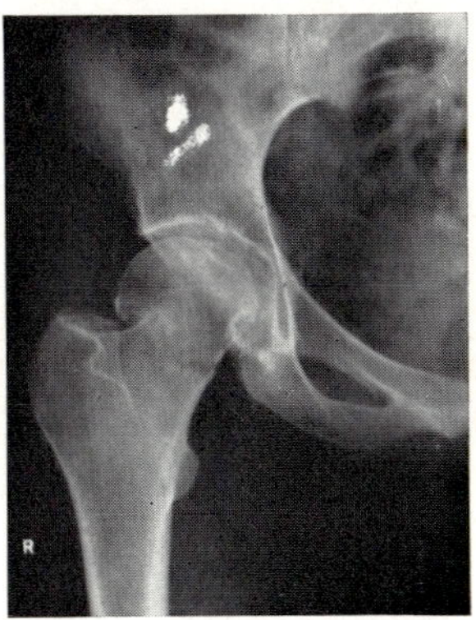

Fig. 167.—Abduction fracture of the neck of the right femur.

fractured surfaces, so that there is shearing strain (*Fig.* 169). Even if the fragments appear to be impacted, continued shearing strain prevents bony union, and there is progressive absorption of the bone of the femoral neck. The displacement must be corrected, the fragments impacted in slight abduction, and a three-flanged stainless-steel nail driven through the neck of the femur into the head. In elderly patients it is now advised that the head of the femur should be removed and be replaced by a stainless-steel prosthesis.

After operation the patient sits up at once and is encouraged to move freely in bed. Weight-bearing should not be resumed until about three months after operation.

Basal Fractures.—If the fracture lies at the intertrochanteric line, the bone on the distal side of the fracture is too thin to afford a secure grip for the nail.

In these cases a nail with an attached plate must be used; the plate is screwed to the shaft of the femur. Alternatively the limb may be supported in a Thomas's splint which is slung in the position of abduction, the patient being encouraged to sit up and move about in bed from the beginning with the aid of an overhead sling.

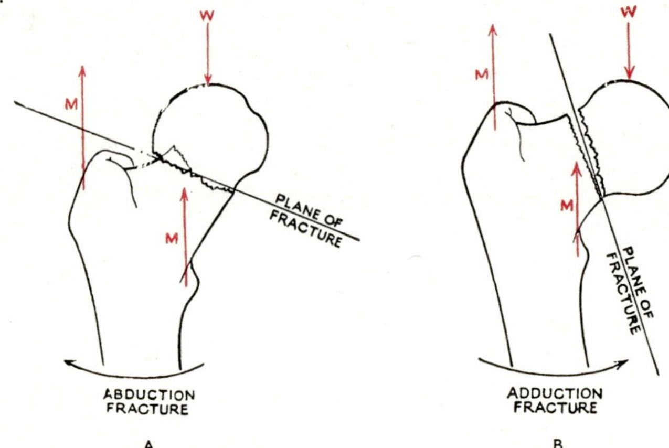

Fig. 168.—A, In abduction injuries the fracture is in the relatively horizontal plane. Muscle retraction (M) and weight-bearing (W) impact the fragments and bony union occurs spontaneously. B, In adduction fractures there is shearing stress from muscle retraction and weight-bearing. Non-union occurs unless perfect immobility is secured by a nailing operation.

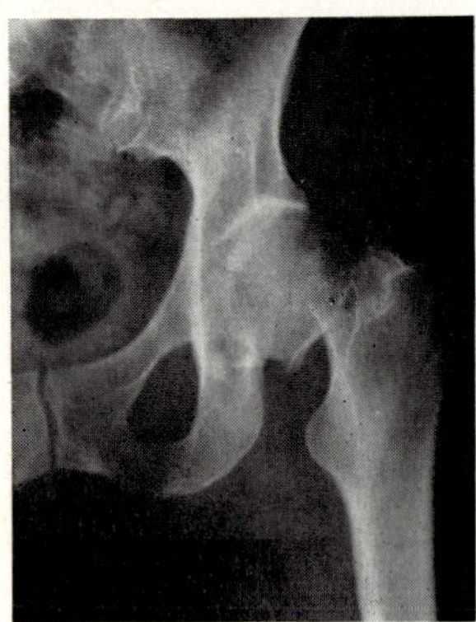

Fig. 169.—Adduction fracture of the neck of the left femur.

DISPLACED UPPER FEMORAL EPIPHYSIS

This injury, like high fractures of the femoral neck, is liable to interfere with the blood-supply of the femoral head. Forcible manipulations and open operations are therefore to be avoided. In acute displacements of a few days' duration, reduction by gentle abduction and internal rotation of the limb and immobilization in a plaster spica may be safe, but in long-standing displacements even this degree of trauma precipitates avascular necrosis and stiffness of the hip. In such cases internal fixation should be carried out.

FRACTURES OF THE SHAFT OF THE FEMUR

The essentials of treatment are to preserve full length and to prevent rotation or angulation of the fragments; accurate apposition of the fragments is less important. Since the muscles of the thigh are so long-bellied and powerful that there is a strong tendency to overriding and shortening, traction on the limb throughout the period of immobilization is essential.

Treatment by Fixed Traction.—The best routine treatment of shaft fractures is immobilization in a Thomas's knee splint with skin traction.

General anæsthesia is used. The foot and ankle are held by an assistant, who pulls strongly and steadily on the limb so that he can elevate it without damaging the soft tissues by the sharp bone fragments. Three-inch (7·5-cm.) wide brown holland strapping, warmed to make its surface adhesive, or 'one-way stretch elastic strapping', is applied on each side of the limb from just above the malleoli to the level of the fracture. The outer strip is centred a fraction

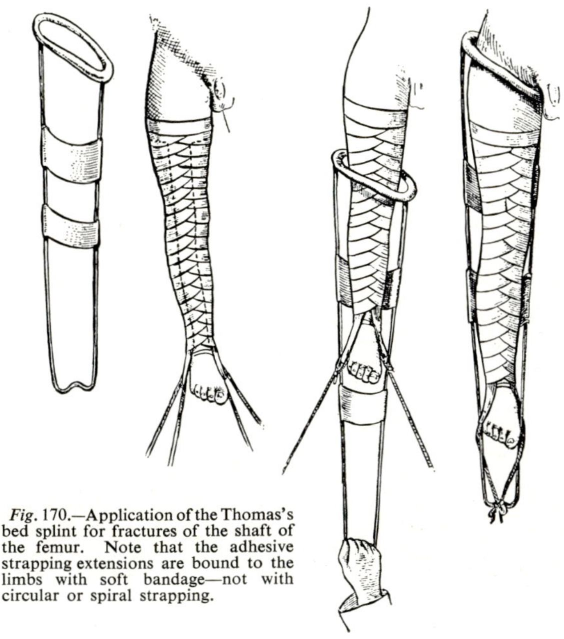

Fig. 170.—Application of the Thomas's bed splint for fractures of the shaft of the femur. Note that the adhesive strapping extensions are bound to the limbs with soft bandage—not with circular or spiral strapping.

behind the midline and the inner strip in front, so the limb will lie slightly more in internal than in external rotation. *The extension strapping must not be bound to the limb by circular or spiral turns of adhesive strapping, but by soft bandage.* If strapping is applied in a spiral or circular manner, pressure sores will result in later weeks when it slides down the limb. For the same reason the malleoli, ankle, and back of the heel must be protected by thick pads of wool under the extension tapes, and the encircling bandage must stop short 2–3 in. (5–7·5 cm.) above the malleoli.

The ring of the splint is then threaded over the limb (*Fig.* 170). If the ring of the splint is too big a pad of wool or felt is fixed between the outer part of the ring and the outer aspect of the thigh so that the inner part of the ring lies snugly against the adductor region and does not encroach on the perineum. The limb is supported in the splint by means of a wide metal gutter splint held in position by strong bandage slings placed at the top and bottom. The normal forward curve of the lower shaft of the femur must be preserved by keeping at least two-thirds of the limb in front of the side bars and only one-third behind.

To the lower free end of the extension strapping, strong linen tapes are secured by firm knots. The outer tape is passed over the outer bar of the splint, the inner tape under the inner bar, the padded ring of the splint is pushed well up against the ischial tuberosity, and the extension tapes are tightened and fastened securely over the cross-bar at the end of the splint. While the patient is still under the anæsthetic, and while strong, steady traction is applied, the fragments are manipulated into good apposition by direct pressure. Radiographic control is used.

AFTER-TREATMENT.—The position of the fragments is confirmed radiographically, with a portable X-ray apparatus, every second or third week. Throughout the period of immobilization the patient must practise toe and foot exercises; for five minutes every hour of the day the foot is dorsiflexed, inverted, and circumducted. There is no need for a foot support on the splint. After a few weeks the thigh muscles should be exercised by smooth rhythmic contraction and relaxation.

After about twelve weeks the degree of union is estimated clinically. When the fracture is clinically firm, and is no longer tender, and the callus shown in the radiographs is ossifying soundly, the patient may be allowed to get up with the

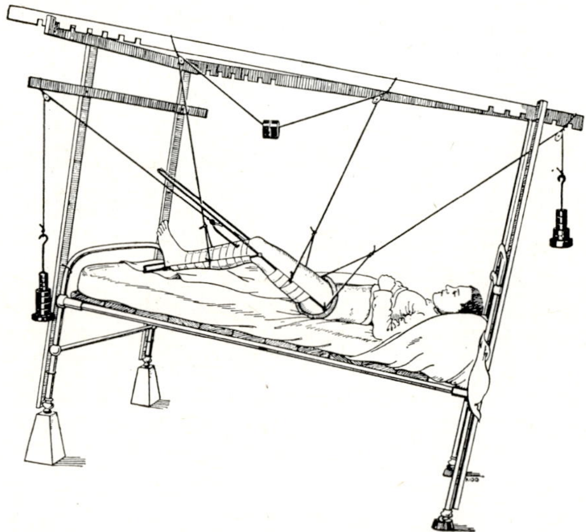

Fig. 171.—Balanced traction and suspension for fracture of the shaft of the femur. The traction pin is in the tibial tuberosity—*not the femoral condyles.* Great care is necessary to avoid overpull and distraction of the fragments.

use of crutches to protect weight-bearing, at the same time practising exercises of the knee-joint repeatedly throughout the day by bending the limb over the side of the bed and exercising the quadriceps muscle.

Treatment by Balanced Traction.—A Steinmann's pin is driven through the tibial tubercle, and a stirrup is fixed to the pin (*see* p. 241). Infection of the pin track must be avoided by taking all aseptic precautions in the insertion of the pin, and by fixing the pin securely so that it cannot rotate or move in its track through the bone. A Thomas's splint with a Pearson's flexed-knee attachment is guided over the limb and suspended from an overhead beam with weights. A cord from the tibial pin stirrup passes over a pulley at the foot of the bed to a 10-lb. (4530-G.) weight. The foot of the bed is raised on blocks. (*Fig.* 171.)

It is most important to avoid excessive weight and distraction of the fragments. The slightest overpull, even if it causes no more than a third of an inch (0·8 cm.) of distraction of the fractured surfaces, and even if corrected within a few days, adds many months to the necessary period of immobilization. A fracture of the femur which would otherwise unite in two or three months may then unite only after ten or twelve months. Excessive traction is now the commonest cause of slow union of fractures. Half an inch (1·25 cm.) of shortening due to underpull is far less serious than half an inch of lengthening with slow union due to overpull.

Treatment by Intramedullary Nailing.—One of the great problems in treating fractures of the shaft of the femur is the prevention of outward bowing, because of course the abductor muscles are all attached to the upper fragment in the region of the trochanter, whereas the equally strong adductor muscles are all attached to the distal fragment in the region of the adductor tubercle on the medial side of the lower shaft. Then no matter how carefully the early treatment in a Thomas's splint is controlled, and no matter how skilfully any other conservative method of treatment is pursued, there is always danger of late recurrence of outward angulation when early exercise and weight-bearing are permitted. Thus many fractures of the shaft of the femur are treated by the intramedullary insertion of a nail, usually driven down from the trochanter across the site of fracture into the distal fragment. The nail can be left in position for one or more years, thus protecting the bone from late angulation. It must be said, however, that even with such an intramedullary nail, there should usually be protection from the strains of weight-bearing for the first two or three months. It is still wise, even with the nail, to use a Thomas's splint or a plaster spica in the early stages.

Stiffness of the Knee-joint after Fracture of the Femur.—Attempts have been made to avoid stiffness of the knee by permitting early movements of the joint after internal fixation of the fracture, or by encouraging movement while using supracondylar skeletal traction. Very often the only effect of these measures has been to convert temporary stiffness into permanent stiffness. The adhesions between the capsular plications of the joint and between the muscles of the thigh which result from immobility alone are easily overcome within a few months by the patient's own exercise. Recovery is facilitated and accelerated by instituting regular quadriceps drill within a few weeks of fracture while the limb is still immobilized.

Suitable sites for insertion of a pin for skeletal traction have been narrowed down to the upper or the lower end of the tibia.

Technique.—The operation, which can be carried out in the patient's bed, is conducted under general anæsthesia, methohexitone (brietal) being sufficient for the purpose. All apparatus necessary for splinting and traction must be to hand before the operation is commenced. The skin is sterilized with great care. Steinmann's pin (*Fig.* 172) is used widely. The bony landmarks having been determined, the skin is drawn proximally with the forefinger and thumb. A skin incision is made with a tenotome just large enough to admit the pin. The pin is driven through the bone strictly at right angles to the long axis of the

Brietal (Eli Lilly and Co. Ltd., Basingstoke, Hants).

limb, boring the pin through with the attached handle; at the start the Steinmann's pin requires a blow with a mallet to drive the point through the cortical bone. When the point of the pin appears on the contralateral side, the skin is nicked and the pin advanced appropriately. The details of technique in the varying sites are as follows:—

1. *Through the Upper End of the Tibia.*—The point chosen should be ¾ in. (1·8 cm.) behind the crest, just below the level of the tubercle of the tibia

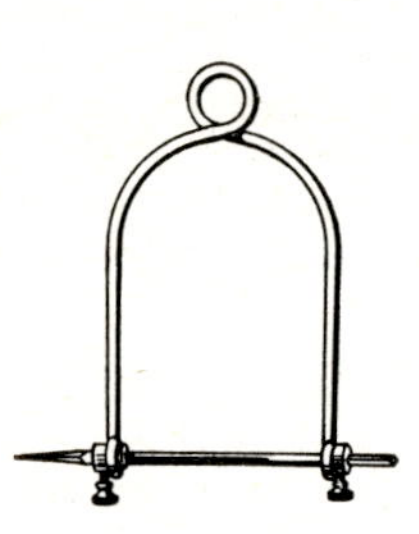

Fig. 172.—Böhler's swivel stirrup affixed to a Steinmann pin.

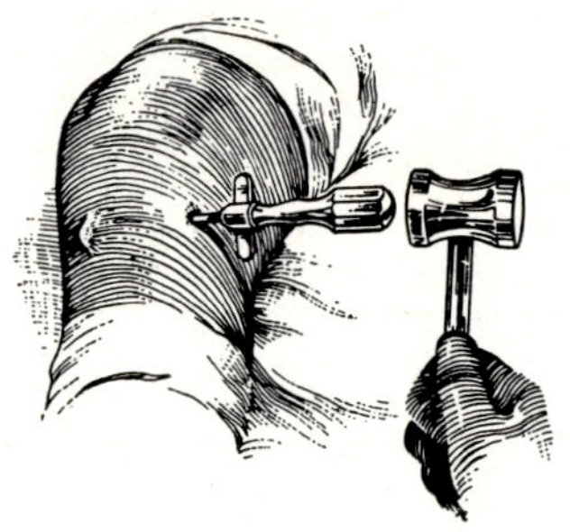

Fig. 173.—Inserting a pin through the upper end of the tibia.

(*Fig.* 173). A criticism of this site is that the knee-joint is liable to become overstretched. Provided the knee is kept flexed and the distracting force is not excessive, the knee-joint will suffer no harm.

2. *Through the Lower End of the Tibia.*—Here the bone is penetrated about 2 in. (5 cm.) above the ankle.

The pin having been inserted, pledgets of sterile cotton-wool are used to cover the sites of entry and exit. Some advise no covering at all; others advocate smearing the puncture wounds with tinct. benzoin co.

The Removal of a Pin.—The stirrup is detached and the entrance and exit wounds, together with the pin itself, cleansed meticulously with spirit. The pin can be pulled out with pliers, and, as it is loose, an anæsthetic is unnecessary. The entrance and exit wounds are swabbed, this time with iodine or some other skin antiseptic, covered with a small piece of sterile gauze, and sealed with flexible adhesive plaster. Healing should take place within a fortnight.

RUPTURE OF THE EXTENSOR APPARATUS OF THE KNEE

Avulsion of the Quadriceps.—The radiograph shows no bone change, and for this reason the injury is sometimes overlooked. Loss of active extension against gravity with tenderness at the upper margin of the patella in elderly patients is sufficient to establish the diagnosis. It is usually possible to feel the gap between the muscle and the bone. If the quadriceps is not stitched back, ossification occurs in the hæmatoma between the retracted muscle and the patella, giving rise to the condition described as 'myositis ossificans of the quadriceps'. The muscle should be firmly reattached with catgut mattress sutures. Plaster-of-Paris splintage is necessary for a few weeks. A full range of movements should be regained within four to six months.

Fracture of the Patella with Displacement.—When the patella is fractured by muscular action it must be recognized that the fracture is only a part of the rupture of the extensor tendon; there is also a rupture of the quadriceps expansion on each side of the bone. The upper fragment is retracted by the quadriceps muscle, and the aponeurosis from the front of the patella falls inwards over the fractured surfaces. Unless operative treatment is carried out fibrous union results, and because there is a gap between the patellar fragments with lengthening of the quadriceps tendon, full active extension is permanently lost.

At operation the fragments of the patella are sutured with catgut or stainless-steel wire and the quadriceps expansion is repaired. A plaster cast is applied with the knee almost fully extended. Weight-bearing may be resumed within a few days. The plaster cast is removed after six or eight weeks. Flexion movement of the knee is regained by active exercises practised for a few minutes hourly throughout the day.

Excision of the Fractured Patella.—In comminuted fractures with serious damage to the articular surface the bone fragments should be excised before the quadriceps tendon is repaired. Active knee movements are begun within three or four weeks, and weight-bearing may be resumed within five or six weeks.

Avulsion of the Ligamentum Patellæ.—The ligament must be stitched back to the bone. Since the injury occurs in younger patients, there is no danger of permanent stiffness of the knee. It is therefore quite safe to immobilize the joint in extension by a plaster cast for eight weeks.

Fracture of the Patella without Displacement.—Crack fractures may occur from a direct blow over the bone. The fracture may lie transversely, or one of the angles of the patella may be separated by an oblique crack. This injury is quite different from the other type of patellar fracture; in this case there is no rupture of the quadriceps expansion. Operative treatment is unnecessary. It may be advisable to immobilize the knee by a posterior plaster slab for a few weeks. After a more severe contusion the whole bone may be comminuted and crushed, and excision of the patella is often advisable.

DISLOCATION AND ALLIED INJURIES OF THE KNEE

Traumatic Dislocation of the Knee.—The ligaments are torn or severely stretched, and the head of the tibia is displaced backwards, forwards, or laterally. The popliteal vessels and nerves may be damaged. Manipulative reduction usually offers no difficulty. The joint must be immobilized in a plaster cast from the toes to the groin for not less than ten weeks. Recovery depends on the tone of the thigh muscles. Even if the ligaments remain lax, if muscle control is perfect there will be little disability. No trace of wasting of the muscles must be permitted, and from the first day after reduction quadriceps drill should be practised for five minutes hourly. Weight-bearing may be resumed within a few days. After the plaster is removed it is inadvisable to use a knee cage because it encourages wasting of the quadriceps. Muscle redevelopment is still the most important treatment.

Rupture of the Medial Ligament of the Knee.—Minor sprains of the medial collateral ligament are treated by regular quadriceps drill, bandaging the joint until the effusion has subsided, and raising the inner border of the heel and sole of the shoe $\frac{1}{4}$ in. (0·6 cm.) to prevent valgus strains of the knee.

There has in recent years been increasing recognition of the importance of recognizing avulsion of the medial ligament with retraction of the fibres and in-curling which can be corrected only by immediate operative treatment. More and more of these injuries will be treated by operation; but nevertheless the redevelopment of the quadriceps muscle is still paramount.

FRACTURE OF THE TIBIAL TUBEROSITY

A severe abduction strain of the knee may not only rupture the medial collateral ligament, but also crush the outer tuberosity of the tibia. As a rule the tuberosity is split vertically by the impact of the outer margin of the lateral femoral condyle (*Fig.* 174). A lateral marginal fragment is displaced outwards, and the tuberosity itself is comminuted and depressed. The displacement must be reduced to correct the knock-knee deformity and to restore the smoothest possible articular surface. While strong traction is applied in the long axis of the limb, the tibial tuberosities are laterally compressed manually. The knee is held in as much varus as possible, and a closely fitting plaster cast is applied from the toes to the groin. The ligamentous rupture is no less important than the bone injury. Regular quadriceps exercise must be instituted at once, and the immobilization continued for not less than ten weeks. Usually a new cast is necessary in four to six weeks, after the swelling has subsided, before weight-bearing is resumed. Development of the quadriceps muscle must continue throughout every stage of the treatment.

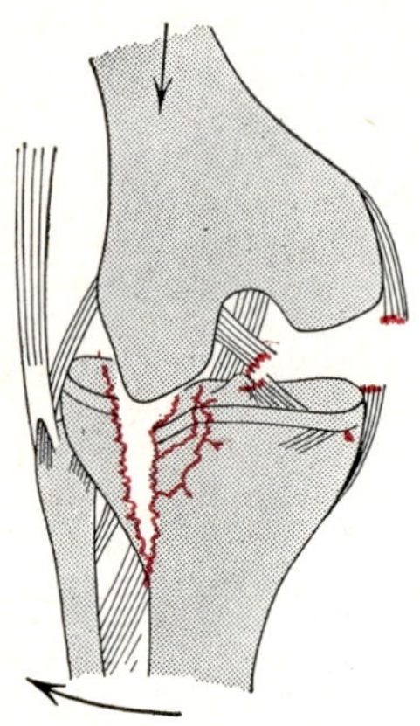

Fig. 174.—Comminuted fracture of the lateral tuberosity of the tibia due to severe valgus strain. The cruciate and medial collateral ligaments are ruptured.

FRACTURES OF THE SHAFTS OF THE LEG BONES

Fractures without Overriding.—Greenstick and subperiosteal crack fractures of the shafts of the tibia and fibula occur fairly commonly in children. Similar fractures may occur in adults where there is no serious loss of apposition but merely slight angulation of the fragments. A plaster cast is applied with the limb hanging over the end of a table in the line of gravity. Angulation and rotatory displacement are corrected. When the plaster from the toes to the tubercle of the tibia is hard, the knee is almost fully extended and the cast is continued to the groin.

Fractures with Overriding.—When the fractures are complete and the fragments are disengaged, simple manual reduction is more difficult. The position is checked by radiographs taken with a portable apparatus, and a cast is applied from the toes to the knee. When it is hard, the plaster is extended to the groin with the knee slightly flexed. Care must be taken that rotation displacement is completely corrected, so that the toes and patella point in the same direction.

Wedging the Plaster.—Radiographs must be taken through the plaster, and if there is the slightest angulation of the fragments this is corrected by wedging. A linear cut is made around two-thirds of the plaster at the level of the fracture on the concave side of the angle. A very short anæsthetic may be given; the linear division is opened to a wedge and a small block of wood placed between the two cut edges (*Fig.* 175). The block of wood must be exactly opposite the angle—in front of the leg for backward angulation, on the inner side for outward angulation, half-way between the two for combined backward and outward angulation, and so on. Another radiograph is taken, and the degree of correction may be increased or decreased by inserting larger or smaller blocks of wood.

When the alinement is quite perfect the gap in the plaster is filled and reinforced. The wedging method allows absolute control and accurate correction of minor degrees of angulation. Caution is necessary when more severe angulation is corrected. Gross wedging may so increase the pressure of the plaster on the limb,

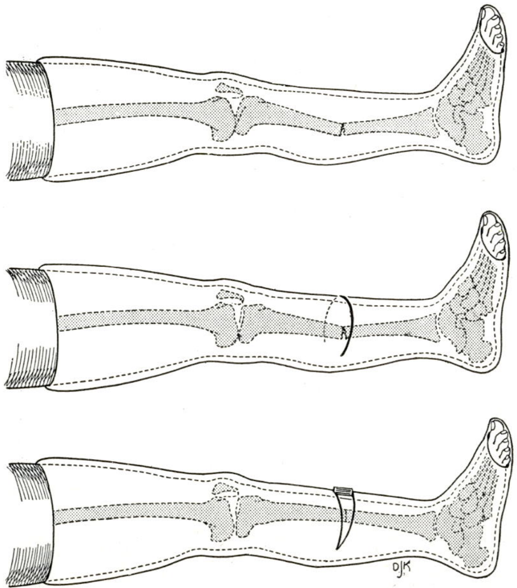

Fig. 175.—Angulation of fragments corrected by wedging the plaster.

even a considerable distance above and below the level of the wedge, that pressure sores may develop unless this possibility is borne in mind and discomfort relieved by cutting windows.

AFTER-TREATMENT.—If the toes are swollen the limb is kept elevated. Regular toe exercises, especially flexion at the metatarso-phalangeal joints, must be practised to prevent rigid hyperextension contracture and rigid transverse flat-foot. If the limb was already swollen when the plaster was applied, a new cast is necessary three weeks later. In all cases check radiographs should be taken three weeks and six weeks after reduction, because there is frequently a tendency to redisplacement within the plaster.

After ten weeks the union may be tested clinically. If there is tenderness over the fracture, and elasticity or pain when the fracture is strained, a new cast is applied, again from the toes to the groin. As a rule, at this stage weight-bearing is safe. A pad of sorbo rubber is fixed to the heel and the foot of the plaster is covered with a cloth boot or golosh. Union is tested at four-weekly intervals and immobilization is continued by walking plasters until union is firm. Occasionally it is necessary to continue immobilization for several months.

When the plaster is removed active exercises are practised for the knee and ankle.

SPRAINS OF THE ANKLE AND DISLOCATION OF THE ANKLE

Many believe that it is worse to sprain an ankle than to fracture it. If all ankle sprains are treated by simple strapping and early weight-bearing this is true, for a certain proportion of ankle sprains which show no bone injury in ordinary radiographs are actually dislocations of the joint. Two types of injury to the lateral ligament of the ankle must be distinguished.

A simple sprain is a tearing of a few fibres of the ligament by inversion strain. There is swelling, œdema, and ecchymosis below the lateral malleolus, pain on inversion movement, but no instability of the joint. This is a relatively minor injury, and if adhesion formation is prevented recovery should be complete within a few weeks. On the other hand, the anterior and middle bands of the lateral ligament may be completely ruptured. The swelling, œdema, and ecchymosis below the lateral malleolus are still more severe, and the ligamentous injury is then so complete that on inversion movement of the foot the talus tilts within the joint, and there is obviously excessive mobility. Ordinary anteroposterior and lateral radiographs show no abnormality, but radiographs taken with the foot in maximum inversion show that the talus is subluxated, or even dislocated from within the tibio-fibular mortice. Unless the joint is completely immobilized in plaster, for at least ten weeks, recurrent dislocation is inevitable. When the patient walks over rough, irregular surfaces and the foot is suddenly inverted, there is no ligamentous protection, the talus again dislocates, the ankle gives way, and the patient may even fall to the ground.

Sprain of the Lateral Ligament of the Ankle.—If the ankle is already swollen, the limb is firmly bandaged over wool and elevated until the swelling has subsided. The foot and lower leg are then strapped with elastoplast or brown holland strapping, applied from the inner side of the sole of the foot, across the outer side of the joint on to the leg, so that the ankle tends to be everted. Non-weight-bearing exercises are practised at once, but only within the limit of pain. After a few days weight-bearing should be resumed. The strapping is retained for at least two to three weeks. If there is still swelling or œdema, an elastic anklet must be worn. Recurrent œdema aggravates the tendency to adhesion formation, and must be prevented by elastic support and active exercise.

If after two or three months there is still pain below the lateral malleolus on plantar flexion and inversion movement, and the radiograph shows no evidence of subluxation or dislocation of the talus on inversion, it is evident that adhesions have formed. The joint should be manipulated under anæsthesia, and the patient must practise regular active exercise until recovery is complete.

Complete Rupture of the Lateral Ligament of the Ankle (Dislocation of the Ankle-joint).—A plaster cast must be applied from the toes to just below the knee, with the heel slightly everted. No anæsthetic is necessary. If there is already severe swelling, a new plaster is necessary in two to three weeks. Weight-bearing in the plaster may be resumed at once. The plaster is retained for ten weeks, and if clinical examination shows normal stability of the joint, weight-bearing is then permitted with a viscopaste dressing which is worn until the tendency to œdema has subsided. If there is still instability of the ankle, shown by rocking of the talus on inversion movement, or by subluxation of the bone shown in radiographs taken in maximum inversion, an outside crooked elongated heel should be worn for several months, or even if necessary an inside iron and outside T-strap.

Elastoplast, Viscopaste (Smith & Nephew Pharmaceuticals, Ltd., Hull and Welwyn Garden City, Herts).

If, through failure to recognize this condition, or through inadequate treatment, recurrent dislocation is allowed to occur, new ligaments must be constructed
from free fascial grafts or from the peroneus brevis tendon.

FRACTURES AND FRACTURE-DISLOCATIONS OF THE ANKLE

Varieties.—Four types of malleolar fracture should be distinguished: (1)
External rotation fractures; (2) Abduction fractures; (3) Adduction fractures;
and (4) Fractures from vertical compression.

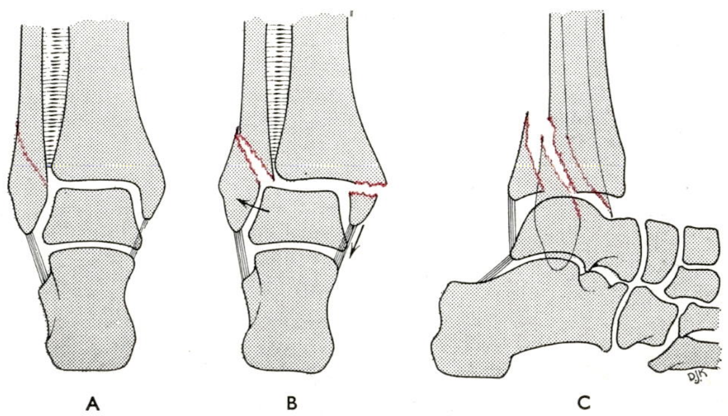

Fig. 176.—External rotation fractures of the ankle. A, 1st degree—Fracture of the
lateral malleolus without displacement. B, 2nd degree—Bimalleolar fracture with outward dislocation. C, 3rd degree—Trimalleolar fracture, with outward and backward
dislocation.

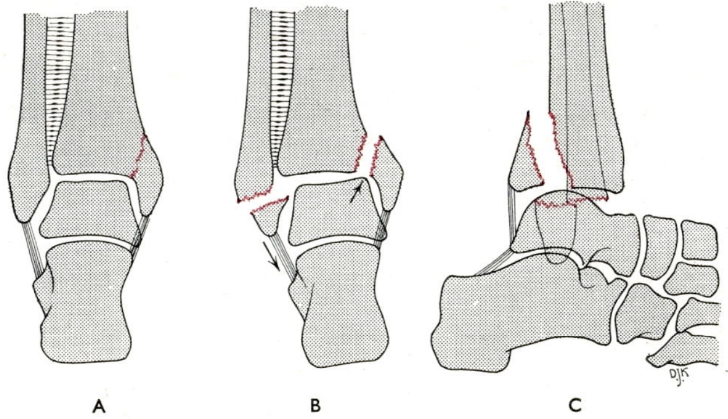

Fig. 177.—Adduction fractures of the ankle. A, 1st degree—Fracture of the medial
malleolus without displacement. B, 2nd degree—Bimalleolar fracture with inward dislocation. C, 3rd degree—Trimalleolar fracture with inward and backward dislocation.

1. External rotation fractures: In this type of injury the foot is externally
rotated in relation to the leg. External rotation injuries produce spiral fractures
of the lateral malleolus at the level of the tibio-fibular joint. There are three
degrees of displacement (*Fig.* 176). Relatively minor force results in a subperiosteal fracture of the lateral malleolus without displacement. If the injury

is more severe, the medial ligament or a fragment of the medial malleolus is avulsed from the tibia, and there is outward displacement of the talus and foot. In the third degree there is not only fracture of both malleoli with outward dislocation, but also fracture of the posterior margin of the tibia with backward dislocation.

2. Abduction injuries cause transverse fractures at any level in the lower two-thirds of the fibula. There are again three degrees of displacement: (1) Fractures of the lateral malleolus with no displacement; (2) Bimalleolar fractures with outward dislocation; (3) Trimalleolar fractures with outward and backward dislocation. The only difference between these injuries and external rotation fracture-dislocations is that the inferior tibio-fibular ligament is often torn so that special care must be taken that there is no redisplacement within the plaster. A new plaster cast must be applied after two or three weeks and immobilization should be continued even longer than the usual period of ten weeks.

3. Adduction fractures are due to forcible inversion of the foot, which drives the talus against the medial malleolus. There are again three degrees of displacement (*Fig.* 177). The least serious injury is the subperiosteal fracture of the medial malleolus without displacement. This fracture is easily distinguished radiographically from avulsion injury of the medial malleolus due to abduction. The abduction injury avulses a relatively small flake. The adduction injury compresses the malleolus at its base, and the line of fracture runs almost vertically upwards from the inner angle of the ankle-joint. If the injury is more severe, the lateral ligament, or a fragment from the lateral malleolus, is avulsed and the foot is dislocated inwards. Still more gross violence causes fracture of both malleoli, and of the posterior margin of the lower end of the tibia, with inward and backward dislocation of the foot.

4. The vertical compression type of injury is usually due to a fall from a height, so that the foot is driven forwards and upwards. There is an anterior marginal fracture of the tibia and forward dislocation of the ankle-joint (*Fig.* 178).

Unless grossly swollen many first-degree ankle fractures can be treated on an out-patient basis.

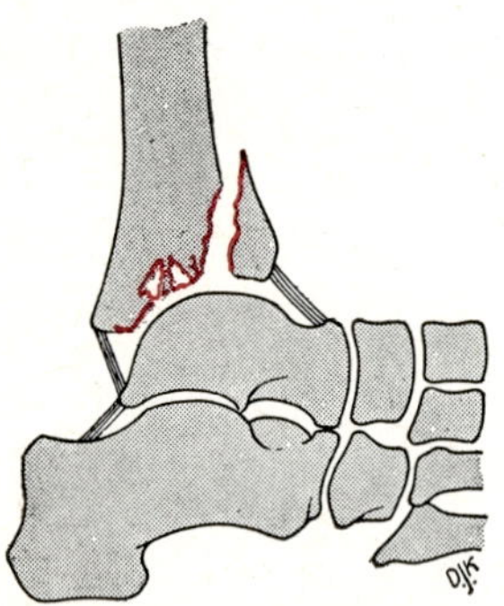

Fig. 178.—Anterior marginal fracture of the ankle with forward dislocation.

Fracture of the Lateral Malleolus without Displacement.—There is tenderness, œdema, and slight ecchymosis over the lateral malleolus, and the radiographs show a subperiosteal crack fracture without displacement. Some surgeons treat these cases by the simple protection of strapping, but it is better to apply a walking plaster for a few weeks.

Fracture of the Medial Malleolus without Displacement.—A walking plaster is applied for a few weeks.

Bimalleolar Fracture with Outward Dislocation.—In this injury there is an actual or potential outward dislocation of the foot. Even if there is no evidence of outward dislocation in the initial radiograph, if further radiographs taken in maximum eversion show that the talus displaces outwards, plaster immobilization for not less than ten weeks is essential. With the limb hanging over the end of a table, an unpadded plaster cast is applied from the toes to just below the knee, with the foot at right angles to the leg, and neutral to inversion and eversion (*Fig.* 179 **A**). Whilst the plaster is hardening, the surgeon supports the forefoot with his knee to keep it at right angles to the leg, and he uses both hands to push the talus inwards as far as possible towards the medial malleolus. In the case of a fracture of the left ankle, his left hand is placed over the lower shin, and his right hand over the outer side of the ankle and heel

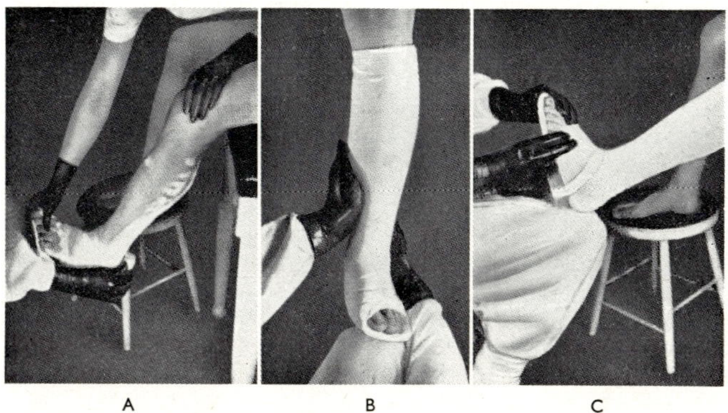

Fig. 179.—Reduction and plaster fixation of abduction fracture-dislocation of the ankle. **A**, Application of the plaster. **B**, While the plaster is hardening, the forefoot is supported by the surgeon's knee and the talus is pushed strongly inwards. **C**, The transverse arch must be moulded up and the metatarso-phalangeal joints flexed. Note the sorbo heel in position before the final turns of plaster are applied.

(*Fig.* 179 **B**). Firm steady inward pressure is applied over the malleolus itself; it is usually quite impossible to over-reduce. No attempt should be made to maintain the position by twisting the foot inwards, adducting the forefoot, and inverting the heel; all the force will be expended on the tarsal joints.

Trimalleolar Fracture with Outward and Backward Dislocation.—This is again reduced by direct pressure over the malleoli and heel, and not indirectly by twisting the forefoot. The limb hangs over the end of the table so that the knee is flexed and the calf muscles relaxed. For a fracture-dislocation of the right ankle the surgeon places his right hand over the front inner aspect of the lower shin, and his left hand over the outer aspect of the ankle, with his fingers curved round the back of the heel. The foot is pulled strongly forwards and pressed strongly inwards. An assistant steadies the foot by holding the toes while the plaster cast is applied. This must be done as quickly as possible, and before the plaster has begun to harden the surgeon again takes the same grip and holds it strongly and firmly until the plaster has set. When there is a posterior marginal fracture of the tibia, reduction is often unstable, and backward dislocation may recur while the plaster is hardening. It is usually impossible to over-reduce, however strong the pressure which is applied.

Accuracy of reduction must be confirmed radiographically. If the talus is even slightly tilted or displaced outwards, or there is the least trace of backward displacement, the plaster must be removed and a new cast applied. Reduction and immobilization should be carried out as soon as possible after injury. If the limb is already swollen, a new unpadded plaster is necessary in two to three weeks.

AFTER-TREATMENT.—Immobilization for at least ten weeks is essential. If the plaster is removed earlier, displacement will recur. Check radiographs are taken during the third and sixth weeks. With a sorbo rubber heel and a plaster boot the patient is encouraged to walk. If the limb was already swollen at the time of reduction, weight-bearing must be deferred until the new cast is applied after two to three weeks. During the last six weeks the patient should walk about five miles a day. After ten weeks the plaster is removed and radiographs are taken in the oblique axis to determine the degree of union of the lateral malleolus. If the patient is heavy and the firmness of union is doubtful, plaster immobilization should be continued for a few weeks longer.

Adduction Fractures and Fracture-dislocations.—The principles of treatment are exactly the same as in abduction fractures and fracture-dislocations. Fractures with actual or potential inward dislocation, or with inward and backward dislocation, must be immobilized in plaster for ten weeks. The talus is replaced by strong outward pressure applied over the medial malleolus and inner side of the heel. Imperfect reduction is often seen; surgeons are so often impressed by the fallacy that because the everted position of the foot is a position of weakness, the inverted position must be one of strength, that they hesitate to push the heel outwards strongly enough. If the talus is allowed to remain tilted either outwards or inwards, there will be persistent pain and ultimately arthritis of the joint. The only position of strength is the normal position, and this is attained in adduction fractures only by very strong outward pressure on the heel (*Fig.* 180). It is practically impossible to over-reduce.

Anterior Marginal Fractures with Forward Dislocation.—A large fragment is broken off the front of the lower end of the tibia, and displaced with the talus and other tarsal bones forwards and upwards. The more the foot is dorsiflexed the more it dislocates forwards. It must be reduced by pushing the tarsus backwards and downwards, and immobilized in plaster with the foot in moderate plantar flexion. Reduction is often unstable and it is necessary to use operative reduction and internal fixation.

DISPLACED LOWER EPIPHYSIS OF THE TIBIA

Abduction strains of the ankle-joint in children may cause outward displacement of the lower tibial epiphysis. Reduction, immobilization in plaster, and after-treatment are carried out as for abduction fractures in adults. Adduction fractures may also occur, and these are more serious because the inner half of the lower tibial epiphysis is crushed and its growth is therefore arrested. The outer half of the epiphysis and the lower fibular epiphysis continue to grow and gradually force the foot into the inverted position. The deformity must be corrected by osteotomy, or prevented by operative fusion of the undamaged part of the epiphysial lines.

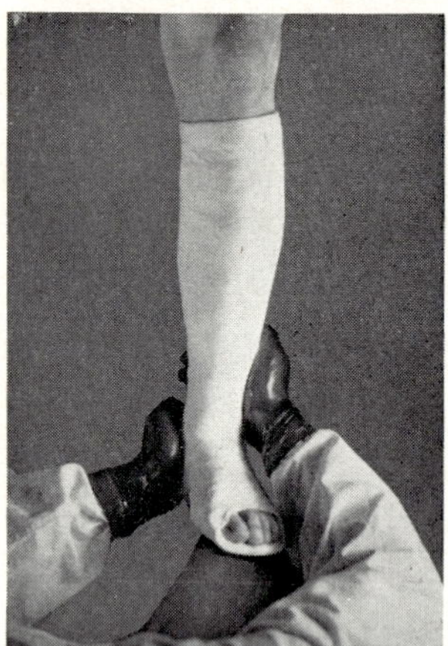

Fig. 180.—Reduction of an adduction fracture-dislocation of the ankle. While the plaster hardens, the talus is pushed strongly outwards.

FRACTURES OF THE TALUS

Fracture of the Neck of the Talus is important because the true nature of the injury is so often overlooked. Unless radiographs are examined with great care the injury appears to be a simple fracture without displacement, whereas in fact there is almost invariably a dislocation of the posterior half of the subtaloid joint, and unless this is corrected, painful stiffness of the foot persists as a serious permanent disability. The clue to the displacement lies in the fact that when the body of the talus is separated by fracture from the other tarsal bones, it always tilts into the plantar-flexed (equinus) position. If the foot is not held in a similar degree of equinus, but is immobilized in the usual right-angled position, there is no normal apposition between the body of the talus and the head of the bone in front, or the calcaneus beneath. The foot must be fully plantar-flexed and, as a rule, everted; it must be immobilized in plaster in this position for six or eight weeks. After that time, when the fracture is uniting, a new walking plaster is applied in as much dorsiflexion as can be secured without straining the site of fracture. Two or three weeks later a third plaster is applied with the foot in the right-angled position. This is discarded after several weeks.

Fracture of the Talus with Dislocation of the Body is a surgical emergency. The body is dislocated backwards and lies under tightly stretched skin behind the medial malleolus. If it is not reduced promptly the skin sloughs. Every effort should be made to reduce the dislocation by manipulation, but operative reduction is sometimes necessary. Excision of the body of the talus and total removal are to be avoided.

FRACTURES OF THE CALCANEUS

The weight of a patient falling from a height on to his heels frequently crushes one calcaneus or both. The bone is spread laterally, so that the heel feels unduly broadened. The subtaloid joint is usually involved, causing pain and limitation of inversion or eversion movement of the heel. The back of the calcaneus is displaced upwards. If this remains uncorrected, the power of the calf muscles is reduced by the relaxation of the tendo Achillis.

Some surgeons believe that the best treatment is simple bed-rest with early exercise and elevation for the first two or three weeks and then walking with the support of a crêpe bandage. At most, gross valgus deformity and spreading of the heel should be corrected by moulding and immobilization in plaster. If the articular surfaces are seriously fragmented and comminuted, early arthrodesis of the subtaloid and mid-tarsal joints is advisable.

FRACTURES OF THE METATARSALS

The shafts of the metatarsals may be fractured by a direct crushing injury, or indirectly by twisting strains sometimes sustained almost spontaneously after strenuous marching. The base of the 5th metatarsal may be fractured by the pull of the peroneus brevis tendon during a sudden inversion strain of the foot. If these fractures are not immobilized in plaster, union is delayed, callus may be excessive, and the disability period is prolonged. An unpadded plaster cast in which the patient may walk at once should be retained for six weeks.

Marked displacement of the fragments should be corrected by manipulation. This is particularly important in fractures of the necks of the metatarsals, where imperfect reduction always causes permanent disability.

10

FRACTURES OF THE TOES

The most common injury to the toes is a comminuted fracture of the terminal phalanx of the great toe due to crushing by a weight. Serious displacement of the fragments is rare, but there is extreme swelling and ecchymosis. The toe should be protected for a week or two by means of a collodion gauze dressing. A heavily soled boot is the best splint. If necessary, the toe-cap may be cut out, and it is sometimes advisable to fit a metatarsal bar in order to avoid weight-bearing through the great toe.

CHAPTER XX

PLASTER-OF-PARIS TECHNIQUE

By F. P. FITZGERALD

PLASTER-OF-PARIS bandages are made in varying widths, and usually are 3 yd.*
long. Immediately before use the bandage selected is placed in a bowl of water
with half a turn of the bandage unwound (*Fig.* 181) so as to prevent the free
end of the bandage from adhering to the roll, and thus making it difficult to
find and unfurl quickly. The bandage remains submerged until bubbles cease
to rise, then the *ends* of the soaked bandage are gripped firmly, and it is lifted
out of the water: traction (*Fig.* 182) with moderate torsion is exerted on the

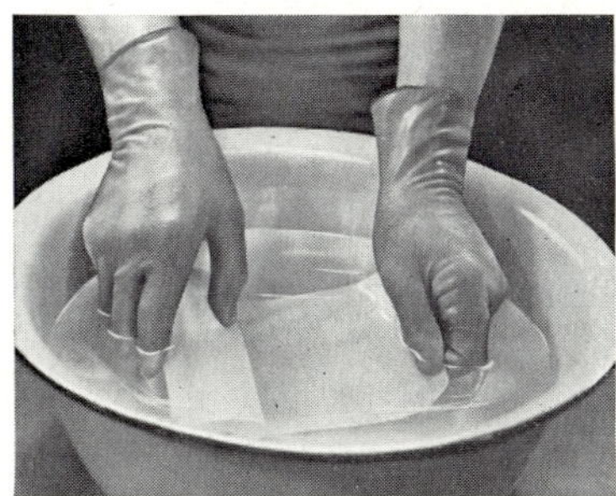

Fig. 181.—The bandage is placed in the
water. The end is free.

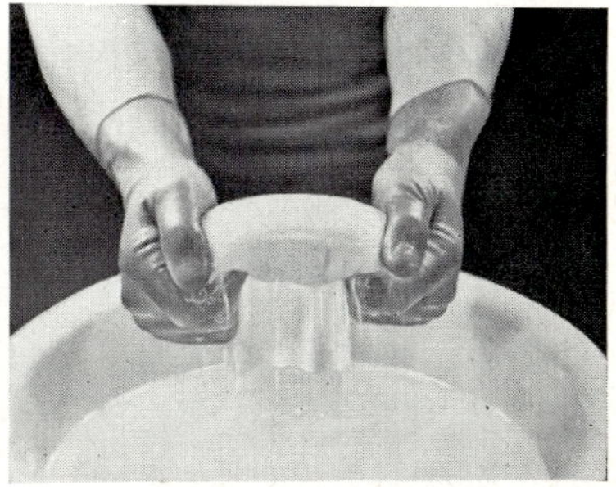

Fig. 182.—The bandage is grasped by its
ends and excess water is expelled.

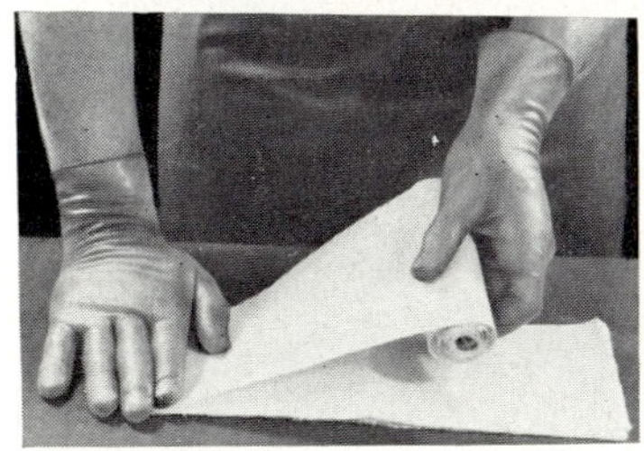

Fig. 183.—Method of making a plaster slab.
Preferably the bandage should be dry.

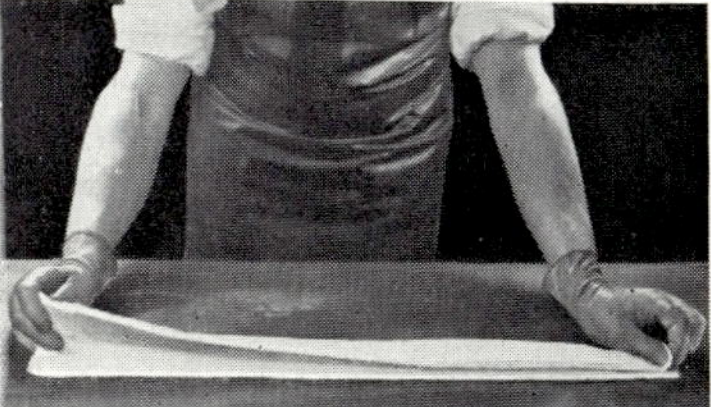

Fig. 184.—Method of folding a slab on itself.

ends so as to squeeze out excess of water, and yet retain the plaster. The
temperature of the water varies as to whether slow or quick setting is required.
The plaster sets more quickly when hot water is used; as a rule a temperature
of 35° C. (95° F.) will provide the optimum setting time.

---

* For conversion of the lengths and breadths of bandages given in this chapter, from
imperial measurements to those of the metric system, *see* inside front cover.

Plaster bandages can be applied either in the manner of a roller bandage or placed upon the part in the form of a slab made by unrolling a specific length of bandage and superimposing layer upon layer (*Fig.* 183) to the required thickness *before* it is moistened. A 'dispenser' of ready-made slabs is now available, and is useful in large departments.

A narrow slab is made quickly by making a thin slab from bandage twice the required breadth, and then folding it longitudinally (*Fig.* 184). A slab is fixed to the limb by a circularly-applied, dry, open-wove gauze bandage. When necessary moist plaster bandages are put on over this.

Rules for the Application of a Plaster Bandage.—

1. Apply the bandage evenly as a spiral without reverses.

2. Leave 1 in. (2·5 cm.) between the tops of the turns so that the plaster cast will be the same thickness throughout.

3. Do not allow any creases next to the skin.

4. Do not twist the bandage or attempt to do 'figures of eight'.

5. Remember that a plaster cast does not contract while setting.

Padded or Unpadded ?—Both padded and unpadded casts have their uses.

A *padded cast* is separated from the skin by stockinet or wool, or both.

An *unpadded cast* is applied directly to the skin without the intervention of any buffering.

It is important that the latter definition should be qualified, for while it is true that plaster and skin *are* in contact, the *entire* limb surface should *not* be so encased. A plaster slab is applied, encasing approximately two-thirds of

THE UNPADDED PLASTER CAST

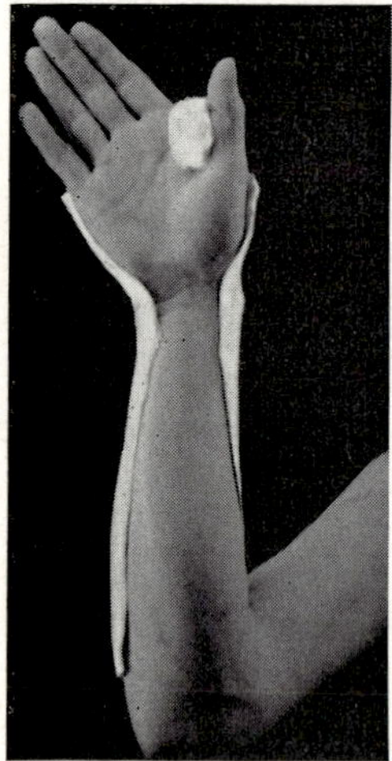

Fig. 185.—The plaster slab is applied directly on to the skin, but does not encircle the limb completely. Note ulnar deviation for Colles's fracture.

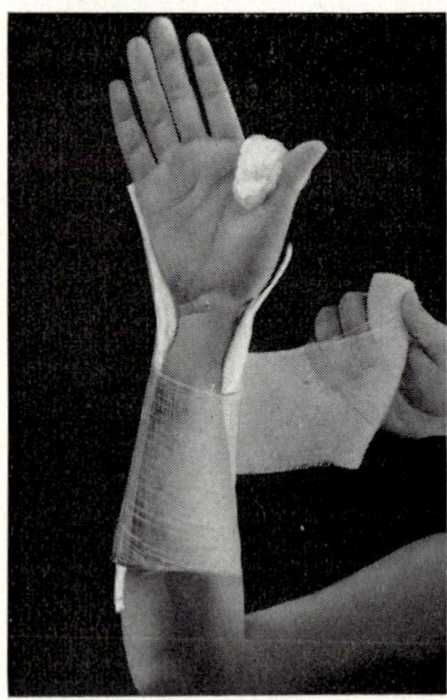

Fig. 186.—Application of a dorsal slab. Note: (1) pad of wool separating index finger and thumb; this helps to keep the thumb abducted and therefore permits full flexion of fingers; (2) the slab does not include anterior one-third of wrist; (3) dry gauze bandage being used to fix slab.

the limb at its narrowest part (*Fig.* 185). This is kept in position by a dry gauze bandage *six yards long and six inches wide*, in adults (*Fig.* 186). The latter is put on loosely and provides a layer of padding about ¼ in. (6 mm.) thick over at least one-third of the limb's surface. *In no circumstance should a circumferential skin-tight plaster be applied.*

Instructions to the Patient.—*A patient should not be allowed to leave hospital without written instructions as to how to recognize circulatory obstruction, and what to do if it should occur.*

INSTRUCTION CARD

1. If the fingers or toes become painful, swollen, or blue, elevate the limb.
2. If there is no improvement after half an hour, come back to hospital or call in a doctor.
3. If it is impossible to obtain medical advice, remove the plaster with a knife or saw. Soaking in water softens plaster.

APPLICATION OF PLASTER IN SPECIAL REGIONS
THE WRIST OR HAND

Materials:—
1. Two plaster bandages 3 yd. by 6 or 4 in. ⎫ depending on the size of
2. A gauze bandage 6 yd. by 6 or 4 in.   ⎬   the limb.
3. A 4-in. band, for counter-traction.   ⎭

Position of Patient.—When traction is necessary the patient lies on a table with the humerus abducted to 90° and the elbow at a right angle. The band is passed round the arm above the elbow over a pad of wool, and fixed to some immovable object such as a staple fixed to the wall. If the fracture is above the wrist a piece of elastic adhesive strapping is wrapped around the thumb, and

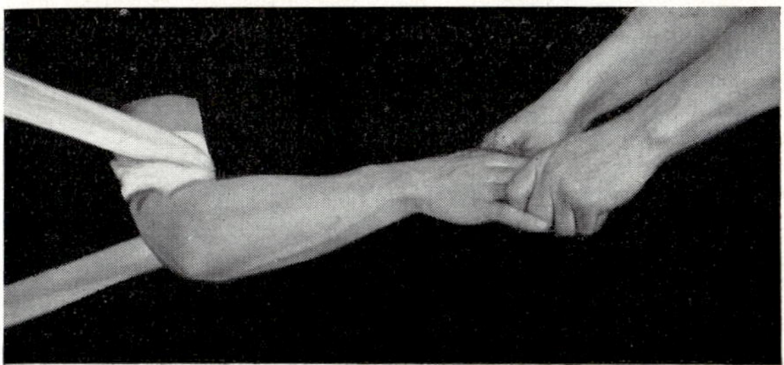

Fig. 187.—A counter-traction band is applied to the upper arm over a pad of wool.
Manual traction is maintained on the fingers and thumb.

another piece fixes the radial three fingers together. An assistant then grasps the thumb in one hand and the three radial fingers in the other, and pulls in the opposite direction to the counter-traction band (*Fig.* 187).

Techniques.—

The Wrist.—The distance from olecranon to knuckles is measured. A plaster slab of this length is laid along the dorsum of the forearm, wrist, and hand, as far as the knuckles. It is moulded to the limb, covering it dorsally and at the sides, but at no point does it encircle the limb completely. A small pad of wool is placed between the thumb and the index finger, and the cast is bandaged on evenly, but not tightly, with the gauze bandage, two turns of which hold the

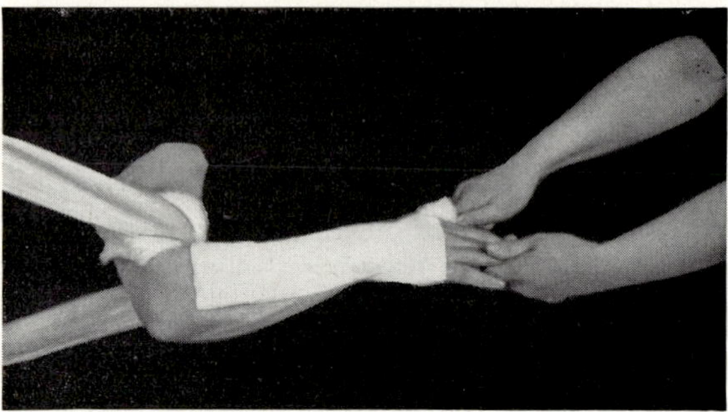

Fig. 188.—The slab extends from elbow to knuckles, and is moulded to the contour of the wrist.

wool in place. A moist plaster bandage, applied circularly, is now superimposed and the cast (*Fig.* 188) is allowed to set. Any excess can then be trimmed.

The Hand or a Digit.—A small slab is made to cover the dorsum of the hand and the finger. The slab is retained in position by a narrow gauze bandage. Over this sufficient roller plaster bandage (of similar width) is applied to make a light

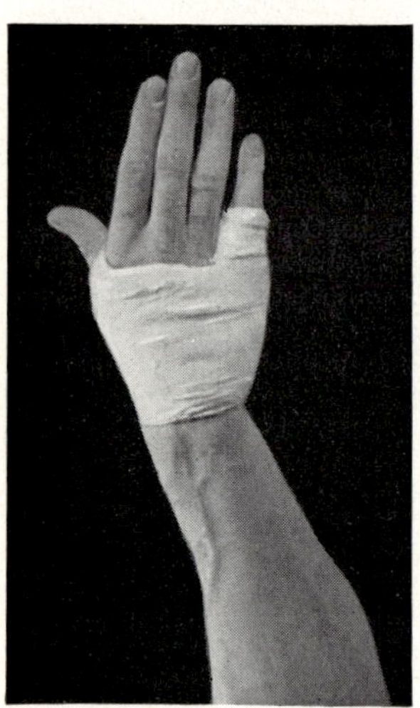

Fig. 189.—Only the metacarpophalangea joint of the affected digit is immobilized.

cast. It is important to leave the end of the digit visible so that the integrity of the blood-supply can at all times be ascertained. Should the lesion be situated in the region of a metacarpophalangeal joint, the plaster cast extends no farther than is shown in *Fig.* 189. When the lesion is more proximal, the wrist-joint must be included.

THE ELBOW AND FOREARM

Materials:—
1. Four plaster bandages 3 yd. by 6 or 4 in.   }   depending upon the size of
2. One gauze bandage 6 yd. by 6 or 4 in.   }   the limb.
3. Band for counter-traction, with wooden spreader.
4. Small pad of wool.

Technique.—The position of the patient is the same as that described for the wrist cast (*see* p. 255). The limb is measured from the insertion of the deltoid to the knuckles. A slab of this length is applied from the knuckles along the dorsum of the forearm, behind the elbow, and along the extensor surface of the upper arm. At the elbow, cuts are made into the slab at each side (*Fig.* 190) and the edges folded accurately over each other. Wool is placed between the

finger and thumb and in front of the elbow-joint, and the slab is retained in position by a dry gauze bandage. The wooden spreader widens the loop of the counter-extension band to allow the slab to pass through (*Fig.* 191). Two moist plaster bandages are now applied in a circular fashion and the cast is allowed to set. The extension band is then removed from the arm, and that region is reinforced by turns of one more plaster bandage.

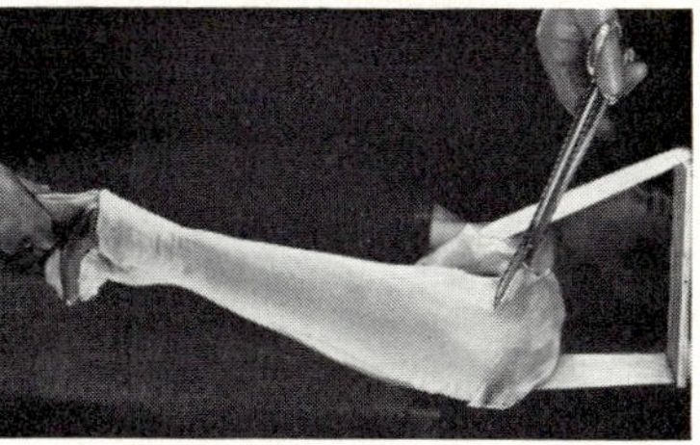

Fig. 190.—The slab is incised at the elbow, and the edges are folded over neatly to prevent a sore.

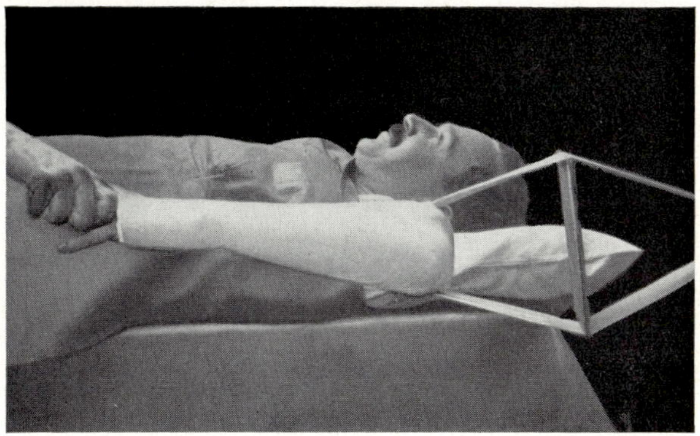

Fig. 191.—Application of cast for elbow or forearm injuries. Note: (1 manual traction; (2) fixed counter-traction; (3) spreader separating loop of traction band.

THE UPPER ARM

Materials:—
1. A strip of felt 2 in. wide.
2. One gauze bandage 6 yd. by 6 or 4 in. } depending upon the size of
3. Three plaster bandages 3 yd. by 6 or 4 in. } the limb.
4. A cuff-and-collar sling.

Technique.—The strip of felt is placed around the upper arm close to the axilla. A slab long enough to extend from the acromion round the elbow and up to the axilla is made from a plaster bandage 6 in. wide. It is folded on itself to make a 3-in. slab (*see Fig.* 184). The slab is then applied to the medial and lateral surfaces of the arm in the form of a U (*Fig.* 192). It is moulded to the contour of the limb and fixed in place by the gauze bandage and the remaining two plaster bandages.

The forearm is supported by a collar-and-cuff sling with the elbow-joint at a right angle. In fractures with even moderate displacement it is advisable to increase the weight of the plaster by the addition of a forearm cast. Other good reasons for this addition are: (*a*) when the patient's arms are fat, so as to obviate

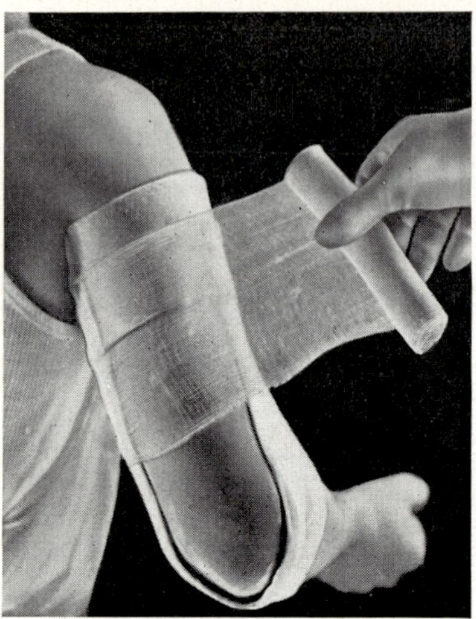

Fig. 192.—The U-shaped slab is placed along the medial and lateral aspects of the arm and held in place by a gauze bandage.

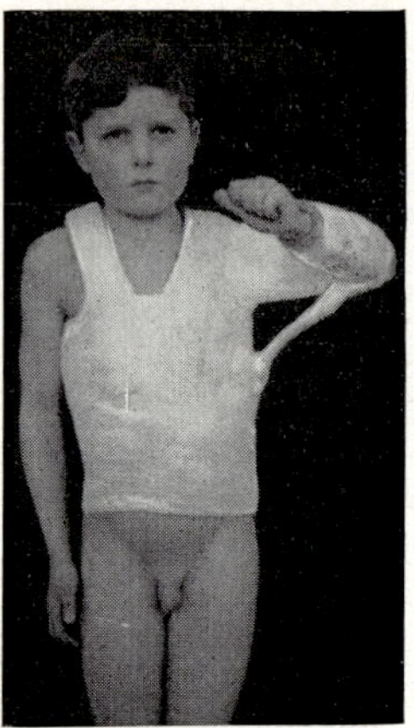

Fig. 193.—Shoulder spica. The cast should extend lower over the iliac crests.

the plaster edge cutting into the skin; and (*b*) to prevent swelling below the elbow-joint.

Lesions of the shoulder-joint or transverse fractures of the middle third of the humerus may require an abduction splint or a plaster shoulder spica.

THE SHOULDER SPICA

This spica is rarely used in Britain nowadays. However, if a ready-made lightweight abduction frame is not available a shoulder spica may be made as follows:—

Materials:—
1. Stockinet, wide and narrow.
2. Wool.
3. Two gauze bandages 6 yd. by 6 in.
4. Twelve plaster bandages, four 3 yd. by 8 in., eight 3 yd. by 6 in. Or, for a child, four 3 yd. by 6 in., eight 3 yd. by 4 in. plaster bandages.

Position of Patient.—Sitting on a stool or standing, the arm is abducted to a right angle and is 30° in front of the coronal plane. The elbow is flexed to a right angle, and the forearm is placed midway between pronation and supination.

Technique.—A length of wide stockinet, long enough to extend from the neck to the pubis, is cut from the roll. At the shoulder level, on either side, a hole is cut to allow the arms to be passed through, as in a sleeveless vest. A suitable length of the narrower stockinet is drawn over the arm, from the knuckles to the shoulder, like a sleeve. Pads of wool, ½ in. thick when compressed, are placed along both iliac crests, over each shoulder, and along the spine, and are held in place by gauze bandages.

Two wide moist plaster bandages are made to encompass the iliac crests, the abdomen, and the thorax, from whence they are brought across both shoulders. Plaster slabs (made from the narrow bandages) flank the cast from the axillæ to below the iliac crests, over which they are moulded accurately. These slabs are held in place by one wide encircling bandage. This completed, another wide bandage is employed as a shoulder spica. A long slab is placed along the extensor aspect of the arm and forearm as far as the wrist, and retained in position by a gauze bandage, followed by three narrow plaster bandages. Next a narrow bandage is made into a slab and folded longitudinally, so as to act as a prop or flying buttress. This is placed (*a*) over the lower two-thirds of the cast covering the trunk in the mid-axillary line, and (*b*) along the under surface of the forearm from the elbow to the wrist, the intervening portion forming the bracket shown in *Fig.* 193. This slab is bound to the trunk and to the forearm respectively by the remaining two bandages. The edges are trimmed and the stockinet is folded over the margins of the cast. A Z is cut out of the cast over the manubrium sterni. *Note*: It is important for the cast to extend below both iliac crests, otherwise it will sag, and give rise to a pressure sore or sores.

THE LEG

Materials:—
1. A high chair, table, or a traction apparatus.
2. A strip of felt 1 ft. by 4 in.
3. Five plaster bandages 3 yd. by 6 or 4 in. } depending on the size of
4. One gauze bandage 6 yd. by 6 or 4 in. } the limb.
5. A walking iron or sorbo rubber.

Position of Patient.—The patient sits on a high chair or table, the operator sitting on a low stool with the patient's foot resting on his knee. The sound leg is supported on a stool or chair.

The piece of felt is placed around the leg immediately below the flexed knee-joint (*Fig.* 194, inset A).

Method I (Complete Plaster Cast).—A long slab is made and folded on itself longitudinally (*see Fig.* 184, p. 253). This is applied from the medial condyle of the tibia, along the medial aspect of the leg, beneath the heel, and along the lateral aspect of the leg to the lateral condyle of the tibia (*Fig.* 194, inset A). Another slab is made long enough to extend from the back of the knee-joint, passing behind the heel, to beyond the toes. After this has been superimposed (*Fig.* 194, inset B) a transverse cut is made on either side of the heel and the

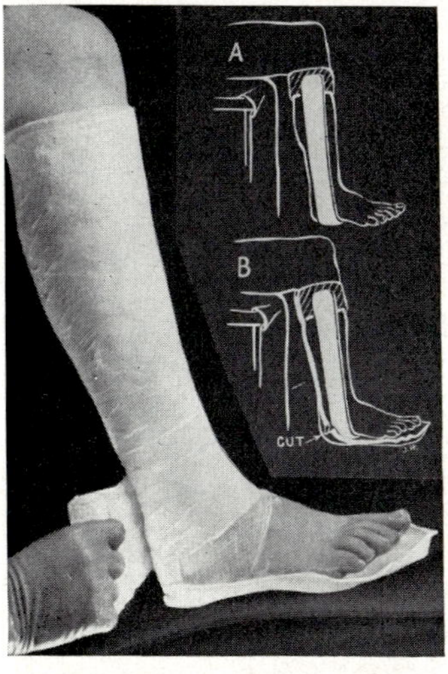

Fig. 194.—Leg plaster nearing completion. Showing also, *inset* A, position of the rim of felt and the first slab; *inset* B, the same with second slab superimposed.

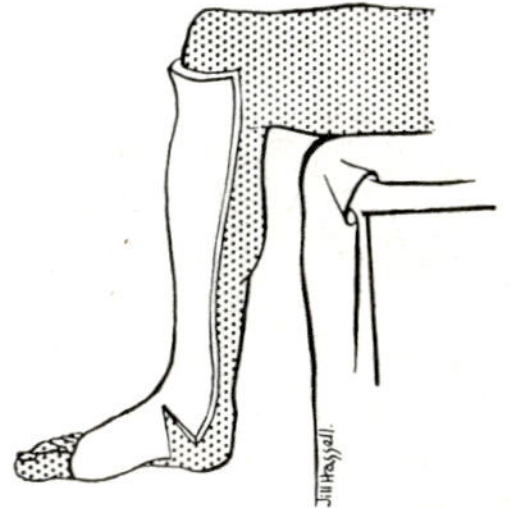

Fig. 195.—The anterior shell leg plaster completed.

cut edges are imbricated upon one another evenly. These slabs are fixed in position by a dry gauze bandage. Moist plaster bandages are then rolled on from above downwards. The plaster is trimmed so that the dorsal surfaces of the toes are free. A vertical cut 1 in. (2·5 cm.) long over the upper end of the fibula prevents pressure on the peroneal nerve.

Method II (Anterior Shell).—An anterior slab is applied from below the insertion of the patellar ligament to the base of the toes. It is moulded accurately to the contour of the leg and a V-shaped piece is removed as shown in *Fig*. 195, the better to allow the plaster to lie without wrinkles on the dorsum of the foot. The slab is fixed with a gauze bandage, over which is superimposed a cast made from covering the area with three plaster bandages. After this plaster

FITTING A SORBO SOLE TO THE CAST

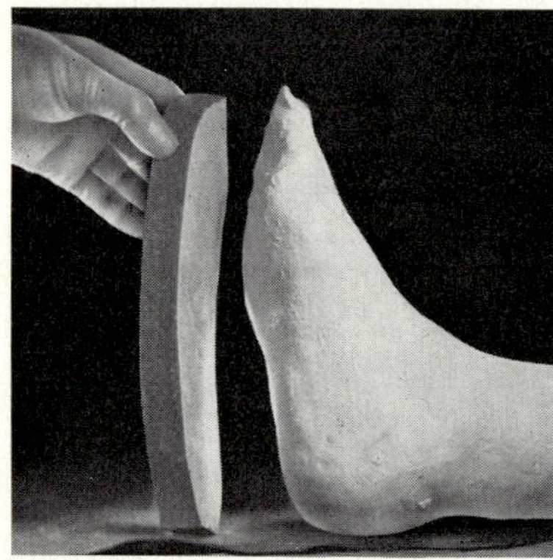

Fig. 196.—Sorbo rubber is cut to fit the sole of the cast.

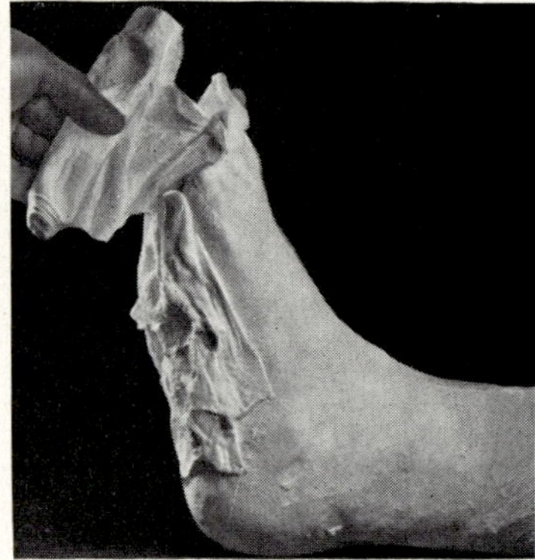

Fig. 197.—The sole of the cast is reinforced with a deliberately rough foundation.

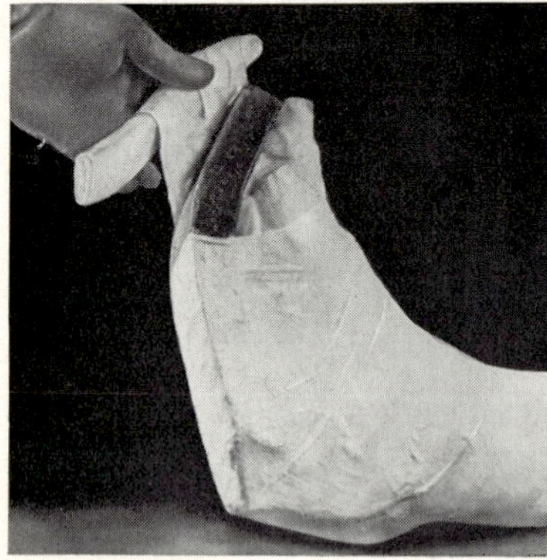

Fig. 198.—The rubber sole is incorporated in the cast by the superimposition of a further plaster bandage.

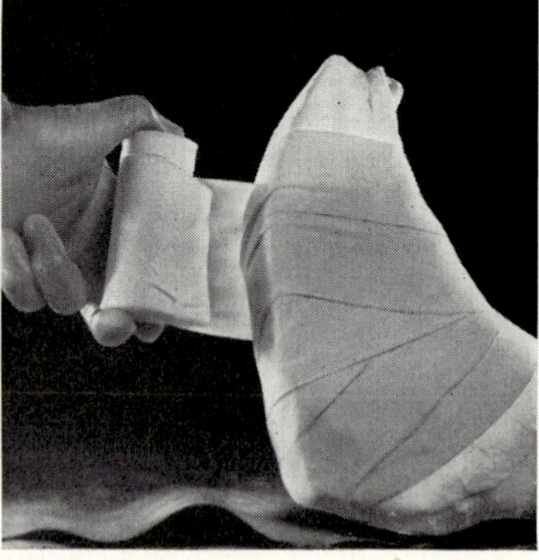

Fig. 199.—When the cast is dry the application of elastic adhesive strapping helps to prevent wear and is 'non-skid'.

cast has been completed the fact that it is an anterior slab cast should be recorded in indelible pencil on the plaster, so that when the time comes for it to be removed the cut can be made on the posterior aspect. *The anterior shell leg plaster is unsuitable for fractures about the ankle-joint because it does not regularly prevent the displacement recurring.*

Devices for enabling a Patient with a Leg in a Plaster Cast to use that Limb for Walking.—

Application of a Rubber Sole.—A piece of sorbo rubber is cut to a paper pattern of the outline of the sole of the cast (*Fig.* 196). As a foundation for the rubber sole a wet plaster bandage is unwound back and forth over the plaster sole, so as to make a bed for the rubber sole—*the bed is rendered rugged (Fig.* 197) *deliberately*, in order that its craggy exterior will bind better with the sorbo sole laid upon it. This accomplished, the sorbo sole is lashed to the foundation with a moist plaster bandage (*Fig.* 198). When the case is moderately dry, that portion of the cast covering the foot is enwrapped with elastic adhesive strapping (*Fig.* 199) which protects the thin shell binding the sponge to the sole; it also renders the surface upon which the patient will walk less slippery.

An Iron Heel must be attached to a cast *exactly in the line of the leg,* and not tilted backwards or forwards. The stirrup upon which the patient walks extends 1½ in. (3·8 cm.) below the plaster cast. To fix the iron heel in place, a turn of moist plaster bandage is taken around the leg. The iron is then placed in position, and the next turn of bandage passes once round the leg over the side bars, and then the bandage is hitched over the free end of one of the cross-bars, as shown in *Fig.* 200, the direction of the encircling bandage being then

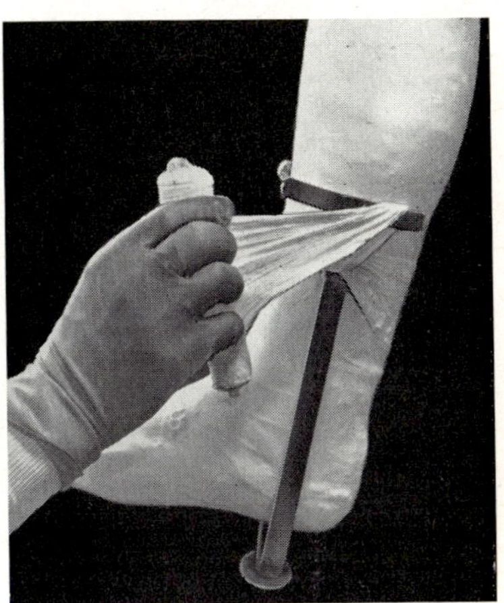

Fig. 200.—Application of an iron heel. The long axis of the heel must be in the line of the leg.

reversed. One-and-a-half more turns will bring the bandage in the vicinity of the cross-bar on the opposite side, over which the bandage is hitched and reversed. This process is repeated until the iron frame is fairly stabilized. At this stage the soft cross-bars are moulded firmly against the cast, after ensuring that the side-bars are exactly in the line of the leg before doing so. Two turns of bandage are taken over the cross-bars and the bandage is continued over the side-bars down the leg to the ankle. The attenuated bandage is passed through the loop of the iron and anterior and posterior slings again are constructed, care being taken to ensure that the iron is still in the line of the leg.

When in use outside the house the plaster can be kept clean by wearing a canvas or plastic 'drizzle' boot over it, an aperture being cut in the right place to permit the stirrup to project outside the cover.

The 'Wide Loop' Heel.—For fractures of the calcaneus an iron heel with a very wide loop (*Fig.* 201) is employed. The wide loop permits inversion and eversion of the foot and regular exercises of this character are advantageous. Weight-bearing is prevented entirely—one form of treatment of a fracture of the calcaneus.

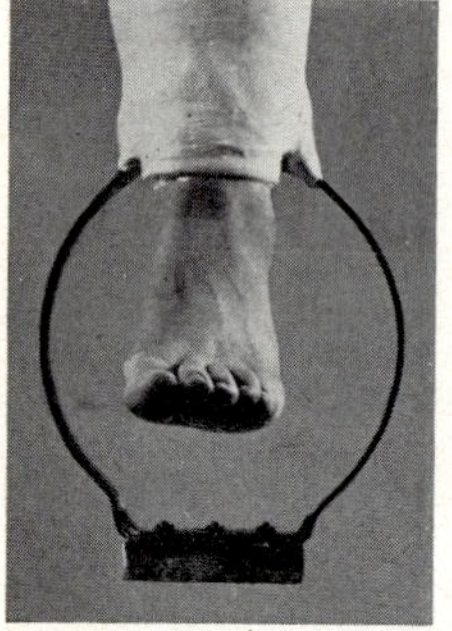

Fig. 201.—The 'wide loop' heel.

Method.—Felt pads are applied immediately *below* the condyles of the tibia and just *above* the lateral and medial malleoli. Short slabs are applied on either side from pad to pad, and are fixed with a gauze bandage, followed by three plaster bandages. The wide-loop heel is incorporated in exactly the same way as detailed for an ordinary iron heel.

THE THIGH AND LEG

Materials:—
1. Eight plaster bandages 3 yd. by 6 or 4 in. ⎫
2. Two gauze bandages 6 yd. by 6 or 4 in. ⎬ depending upon the size of the limb.
3. Iron or sorbo heel. ⎭
4. Strip of ¼-in. adhesive felt 1 in wide.

Technique.—The strip of felt is placed round the limb at the upper limit of the thigh. A gauze bandage is wrapped round the knee. The limb is measured from the fold of the nates round the heel to the toes. A slab is made from two 6-in. bandages and is applied along the thigh, calf, and sole to the toes. It is cut at right angles at the heel on either side and the edges are overlapped and moulded carefully. The slab is bound on by a gauze bandage and four circular plaster bandages. A heel may be fixed as described above.

LEG CYLINDER

A plaster cylinder is used when it is not necessary to include the foot, e.g., for patella and knee injuries. It is made like the thigh-and-leg plaster except that, distally, circular felt pads are fixed just above the malleoli. A long back slab is fixed from proximal to distal felt pads and completed as in the long-leg plaster above.

THE SHORT HIP SPICA

Materials:—
1. Ten plaster bandages 3 yd. by 8 in., and four 3 yd. by 6 in. In a child, six 3 yd. by 6 in., and four 3 yd. by 4 in.
2. Stockinet, wide and narrow.
3. Gauze bandage 6 yd. by 6 in.
4. Wool.
5. Pelvic rest or an orthopædic table.

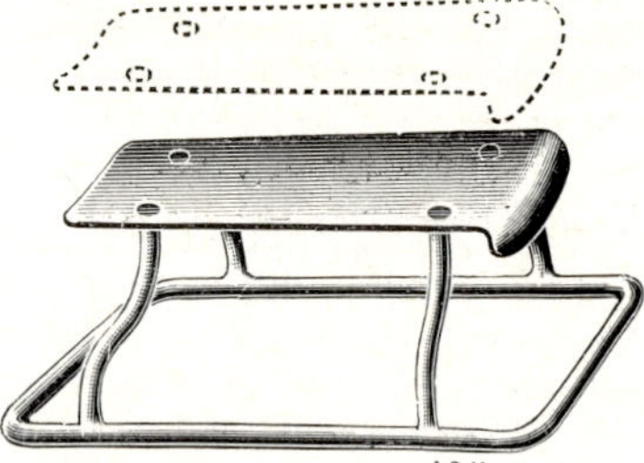

Fig. 202—Muirhead Little's pelvic rest.

Preliminary Measures.—A piece of wide stockinet is drawn over the head and shoulders and reaches from the groin to pye nipples. The narrower piece is drawn over the affected limb and reaches from groin to knee. Pads of wool, ¾ in. (1·8 cm.) thick when compressed, are placed over the anterior superior spines, the iliac crests, the sacrum, and around the adductor region. All the pads are fastened into position by the gauze bandage.

Position of Patient.—The patient is placed on the pelvic rest (*Fig.* 202) or an orthopædic table. If an orthopædic table is used, the feet are bandaged to the sole-plates. The knee is suspended by a bandage from the cross-bar to avoid extension of the hip and hyperextension of the knee. The table is then 'let down', so that the patient is suspended by the shoulders, pelvis, and feet (*Fig.* 203).

Technique.—Two wide plaster bandages are applied to the lower chest and abdomen and then as a spica over the pelvis and upper thigh. Two slabs made from narrow bandages are applied, one along the lateral aspect and the other in front of the hip. A wide bandage holds these in place, and then a slab is placed along the back of the thigh, from the back of the hip to the knee. The remaining wide and narrow bandages are applied circularly above and below. During the application of the cast it should be moulded deeply above and below the iliac crests and around the greater trochanter so that visible grooves are formed. The cast is then cut out in the form

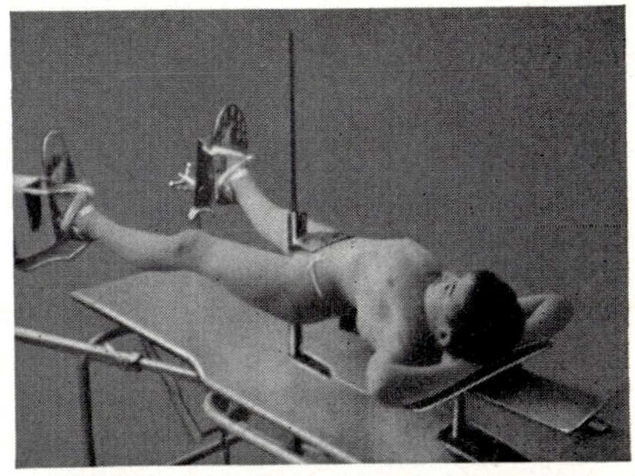

Fig. 203.—Position for application of hip spica. The knees have not yet been suspended.

of a V or half-moon over the upper abdomen, leaving it high at both sides. The plaster is cut away at the upper border of the pubis, and on the sound side along the thigh to allow the thigh to flex to a right angle (*Fig.* 230). Then the patient is taken off the table, turned on to the face, and an area cut out behind to expose the upper limit of the natal cleft.

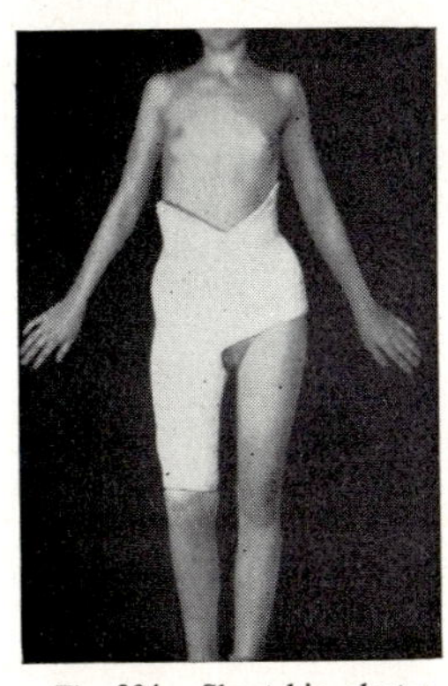

Fig. 204.—Short hip plaster. Note the moulding over the ilium and greater trochanter. On the left side it is cut away to allow the hip to flex to a right angle.

THE LONG HIP SPICA

Materials:—
1. Sixteen plaster bandages, six 3 yd. by 8 in., ten 3 yd. by 6 in. Or in a child, six 3 yd. by 6 in., ten 6 yd. by 4 in.
2. Three gauze bandages 6 yd. by 6 in.
3. Stockinet, wide and narrow.
4. Wool.
5. Pelvic rest or an orthopædic table.

Technique.—The position of the patient is the same as in a short spica (*see Fig.* 203), and the same routine is followed as far as the knee. Then a slab is made to extend from the mid-thigh to the lower third of the leg and covered with one gauze and two plaster bandages. Another slab reaches from the middle of the calf to the tips of the toes, and is fastened with one gauze and one plaster bandage. In an active child or heavy adult, the cast may need extra strength. This can be achieved by making a slab from a 6-in. bandage, folded on itself to make a 2-in. plaster rope, and incorporating it along the lateral aspect of the thigh from above the hip to below the knee. The cutting out and moulding are as before. On the plantar aspect the plaster is cut flush with the tips of the toes; on the dorsum it is trimmed along the line of the webs.

THE PLASTER JACKET

Materials:—

1. Ten plaster bandages, six 3 yd. by 8 in., four 3 yd. by 6 in. Or for a child, six 3 yd. by 6 in., six 3 yd. by 4 in.
2. Stockinet.
3. Gauze bandage.
4. Wool.

A stockinet vest as in a shoulder spica is worn; if the neck is to be included, the vest should be allowed to extend above the head during the application of the cast, and have spaces cut out for the eyes and mouth. Felt or sorbo rubber adhesive strips ½ in. thick, or else doubled plastic foam sheeting, are placed over the iliac crests and the shoulders, and along the spine and sacrum. In a cervical case a padding layer is wound around the neck. These pads are retained in position by the gauze bandage.

Position of Patient.—This varies according to the lesion. If a fracture of the dorsal or lumbar vertebræ is being treated, the cast is applied in a position of extension, the weight being taken by a band round the chest and attached to a block and tackle, or between two tables (*see* p. 233). For cervical caries the child is placed in a special frame. Shoes are strapped to the feet, and these are in turn screwed to the floor-boards of the frame. A sling is attached under the chin and occiput, and most of the body-weight is taken by a cord over a pulley on the overhead cross-bar.

Technique.—

Thoracic or lumbar case: Two wide plaster bandages are wrapped around the chest and abdomen, extending to the sternal notch above and the pubis below. Four slabs made from narrow bandages are now applied. One on each side extends from the axilla to 3 inches below the iliac crest, another from the sternal notch to the front of pubis, and the fourth along the spine posteriorly to the upper limit of the natal cleft. These are fixed by two more wide bandages and then circular slabs made from narrow bandages are applied around the upper and lower margins of the cast. Two wide plaster bandages complete the cast. An area the size of a dinner plate may be removed over the upper abdomen. At the groin the plaster is cut on either side to allow flexion of the thighs to a right angle. It is essential that these casts be moulded accurately over the iliac crests, the lumbar lordosis, the pubis, and the sternum.

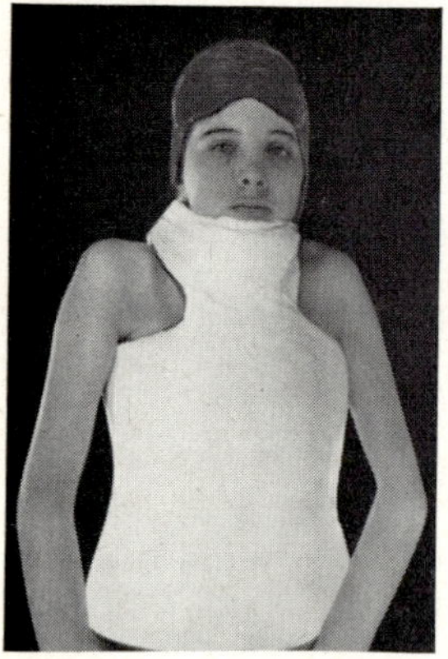

Fig. 205.—A plaster jacket for a lesion of a cervical vertebra.

Cervical case: The routine is the same, except that alternate turns of the circular bandages are taken over the shoulders. Two circular bandages are then wound round the neck and shoulders, including the chin, skirting the lower borders of the ears, and extending up on to the occiput posteriorly.

A slab is applied from the occiput to the upper part of the thorax, and fixed by two wide circular bandages. The plaster is cut along a line running parallel to and half an inch *above* the lower border of the mandible (*Fig.* 205), just below the ears, and along the line of the occipital bone. The stockinet is then folded back and fixed with a narrow plaster bandage (*Fig.* 205).

Plaster Bed.—The construction of a plaster bed is too specialized to be included in this book. The reader is referred to works on orthopædic surgery, and especially to English's *Plaster of Paris Technique*.

FINISHING PLASTERS

A good finish to a plaster can be obtained by rubbing the plaster while it is setting with clean, moist hands, followed by polishing the surface with a wet roll of plaster bandage.

The edge or the edges of the cast must be rendered free from projecting irregularities. Major projections are amputated with strong scissors or plaster shears, according to their thickness; minor irregularities can be hammered down before the plaster has hardened.

If a stockinet vestment was put on before constructing the plaster cast, the cut edge of the stockinet is seized and pulled upon sufficiently to allow it to be folded over the entire circumference of the trimmed plaster edge. Here it is retained by a narrow plaster bandage.

REMOVING PLASTERS

The task of removing modern light plaster casts (such as those described in this chapter) is not nearly so laborious as it was when thicker casts were employed. Even so, it must be recalled that when the more senior members of

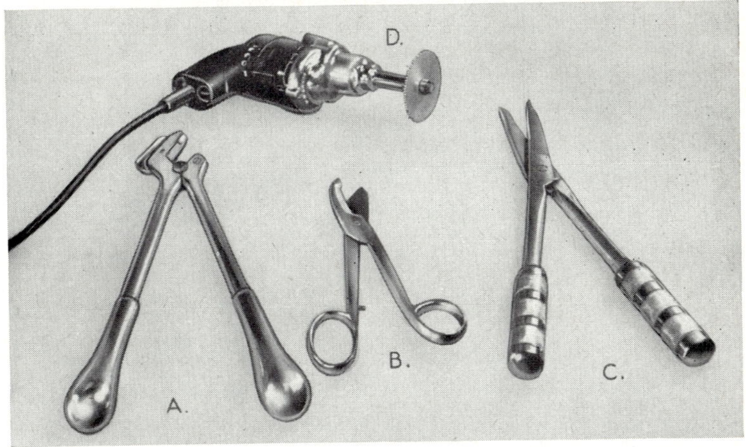

Fig. 206.—Instruments for removal of a plaster. A, Stille's shears; B, Böhler's scissors; C, Lloyd's plaster opener; D, Desoutter's plaster cutter.

the profession received their training the only instruments with which they could be provided to split or to remove a plaster cast were a butcher's saw, Hey's saw, a pair of bone-cutting forceps, and a motor-tyre lever. Needless to say,

English, Marian, *Plaster of Paris Technique*, 1957, Edinburgh.

the saws required frequent setting and the blades of the forceps frequent sharpening. It is no exaggeration to say that to be provided with latter-day plaster-removing instruments halves the toil.

Instruments (*Fig.* 206).—Stille's shears, Böhler's scissors, and Lloyd's plaster opener constitute the standard plaster removing equipment. The last is a particularly useful instrument when a plaster has been cut through and the

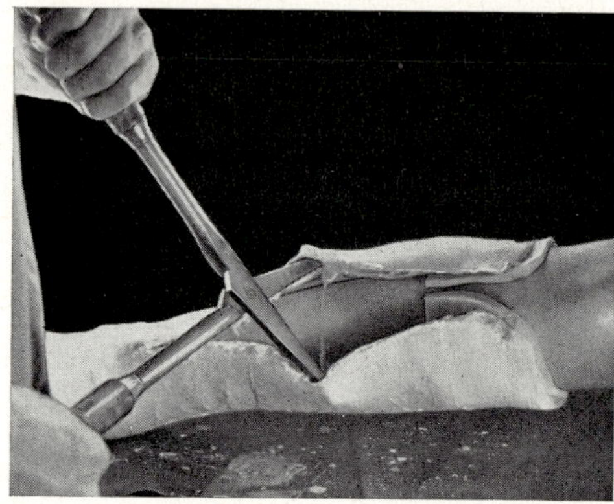

Fig. 207.—When a plaster has been cut through, Lloyd's plaster opener, by spreading apart the cut edges, facilitates removal of the cast.

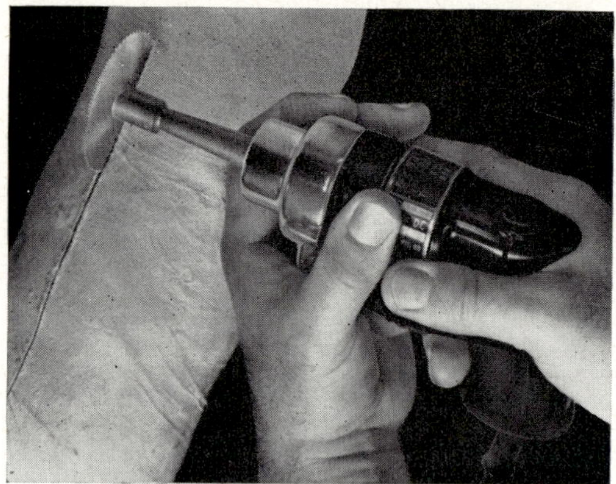

Fig. 208.—The Desoutter electric plaster cast cutter in use.

two edges have to be prised apart (*Fig.* 207). In some large orthopædic departments an electric plaster cast cutter is provided. This expedites splitting the cast. The Desoutter electric plaster cutter (*Fig.* 208) is a very effective instrument; the saw does not rotate, but vibrates, thus limiting the risk of cutting the skin.

Useful Information concerning Removal of Plasters.—Never cut over a bone. It is amazing how often the plaster is cut along a line where a slab has been applied instead of choosing a portion of the circumference where the cast is perhaps half that thickness. In order to prevent this frequently enacted paradox it is recommended that on completing the application of a plaster cast the position (or positions) that a reinforcing slab (or slabs) occupies in relation to the periphery are marked in indelible pencil with an X. In passing, the reader is reminded always to write the date on which the plaster was applied on the cast. Obviously it is best to cut the plaster where it is thinnest. In the case of a leg plaster, cut vertically in a downward direction between the tibia and the fibula along the antero-lateral aspect of the cast.

When special instruments for removing plasters are unobtainable, when the shape of the plaster is awkward, or when the patient is a frightened child, the cast can be softened by soaking it in warm water before removal is attempted. If the plaster has to be split immediately after its application the best method is to place next to the skin, or, if stockinet has been used, next to the stockinet, a copper strip (and, if the cast is to be converted into one that takes on and off, a second copper strip diametrically opposite this) and to apply the plaster bandages over this strip until the cast is completed. While the plaster is still soft, using a sharp scalpel, a cut is made along the entire length of the cast over the line of the strip. The line of the copper strip can be followed by allowing the extremities to protrude above and below the edges of the cast. When the bandage has been split the copper strip is removed by pulling on one extremity, and thus withdrawing it.

ELASTICIZED PLASTERS AND THE POST-OPERATIVE MANAGEMENT OF MID-THIGH AMPUTATION STUMPS

When the flaps are being closed the surgeon normally leaves in some type of suction drain (p. 65); this is removed after 48 hours. A sterile dressing is applied over the suture line and if possible is left undisturbed till the stitches are removed.

If a pylon is to be fitted at once, the stump is moulded into conical shape by applying elasticized plaster bandages. These are applied firmly from below upwards. In the distal end of the plaster a lightweight metal socket is incorporated. When the patient gets up a tubular metal pylon is inserted into this. The patient can bear weight on the second or third day.

The natural tendency for a thigh amputation stump is to assume a flexed and slightly abducted position. It is therefore important to start stump exercises early—on the second or third day—the physiotherapist paying particular attention to strengthening the adductor and extensor muscles of the hip. When in bed, the patient should lie prone for part of the day to prevent flexion deformity.

When the immediate fitting of a pylon is not contemplated, the stump is moulded by the firm application of 6-in. crêpe bandages. These must be reapplied each day. Active exercises for the stump are practised assiduously. The skin stitches are removed on the twelfth to fourteenth day: a suitable elastic stump sock may be applied but these are less popular than formerly. If the patient's general condition is satisfactory he is now fitted with a temporary lightweight pylon and commences walking exercises between parallel bars. A permanent prosthesis is fitted once the stump has shrunk to its final size. Nearly all long-leg prostheses require shoulder straps.

In countries where specially made artificial limbs are not available, the simplest prosthesis is a leather gaiter for the stump, fashioned by a local handyman, to the distal end of which a wooden or metal peg leg is attached.

Complications.—Hæmatoma and infection in the wound and necrosis of the skin flaps with protrusion of the bone end are the commonest complications that the house-surgeon must look for. Careful operative technique and adequate drainage do much to prevent them. Early physiotherapy lessens the incidence of troublesome phantom limbs.

If a hæmatoma does develop it should be evacuated under aseptic conditions after cutting one of the skin stitches. Established infection is dealt with in similar fashion, taking a swab for culture from any infected material present and then commencing the patient on the appropriate antibiotic (*see* p. 72).

CHAPTER XXI

HEAD INJURIES

By J. F. MULLAN

'No head injury is so slight that it should be neglected or so severe that life should be despaired of.' (Hippocrates.)

HIPPOCRATES' aphorism is one of the very few ancient medical sayings that is still true in the second half of the twentieth century. The management of any head injury is always a serious responsibility, calling for sound judgement, detailed and frequently repeated examination, and a correct sense of priorities. The commonest single cause of head injuries today is road-traffic accidents. These frequently result in multiple injuries. More than half the deaths are caused by injuries to the head, although in point of time respiratory obstruction or massive intra-abdominal hæmorrhage may kill the patient more quickly.

CLASSIFICATION

A head injury may be localized or generalized (*Fig.* 209). The localized injury is usually caused by a small object moving at moderate velocity. It expends most of its force upon a small area of the scalp and skull, and may even penetrate the skull, dura, and cortex without causing loss of consciousness. These injuries require early débridement and suture of all scalp wounds and intradural débridement with dural repair when the bone is depressed and the dura torn. Depressed bone in infants without skin or dural tear also requires elevation. The generalized injury damages the whole brain by compressing the total skull until it cracks, thereby compressing the underlying brain, or by creating accelerating and decelerating forces which set up shearing strains within the brain, contuse the surface against bony promontories of the skull, and avulse bridging veins. Generalized injury usually results in loss of consciousness. Many injuries exhibit both localized and generalized features.

There are three large groups of unconscious head-injured patients (*see Fig.* 213, p. 277):—

1. Those with mild injury who quickly regain consciousness with little medical help.

2. Those with extensive laceration who quickly deteriorate and die, and are beyond medical help.

3. Those with brain swelling who must be nursed through many days or weeks of coma.

In addition, there are three small groups with very special problems:—

4. A few patients will develop acute extradural (epidural) or subacute subdural hæmatomata, and their lives will be saved by early diagnosis and removal of these blood-clots.

5. A few will develop intracranial infections from basal fractures (which allow cerebrospinal fluid to leak into the nasopharynx or middle ear) unless ascending infection is prevented by the use of antibiotics.

6. Lastly, there is a group of patients who, often with minimal trauma, develop chronic subdural hæmatomata weeks or months later.

CLINICAL MANAGEMENT

Clinically the patient who does not respond to the spoken word is unconscious. The head-injured patient when first seen may be:—

1. Conscious without having been unconscious.

2. Conscious, either alert or drowsy, but having been unconscious for a short period.

3. Unconscious.

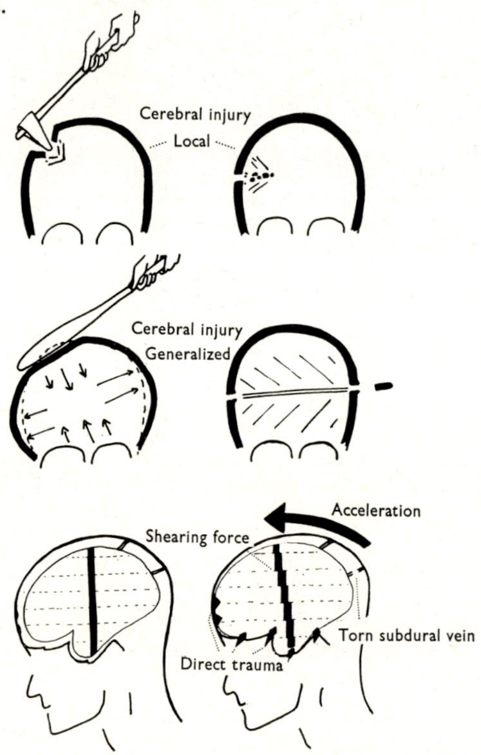

Fig. 209.—Types of injury: *Top*: Local injury. Damage limited to a small area of cortex. *Middle*: Generalized crushing and explosive injuries. Damage widespread. *Bottom*: Generalized accelerating or decelerating injury. Damage widespread.

The first group (*see* p. 281) presents no immediate problem, the second (*see* p. 280) must be observed for at least 24 hours in case an extradural hæmatoma develops, and the third group needs immediate attention. This group will be described first.

A. THE UNCONSCIOUS PATIENT

1. Initial Management.—

Immediately and sequentially he needs:—

a. MAINTENANCE OF THE AIRWAY.—This is of the utmost importance. Many with head injuries die before reaching hospital because of an obstructed airway.

Anoxia and excess carbon dioxide produce brain swelling. The tongue of the comatose patient in a supine position must be regarded as a foreign body in the oropharynx. Oropharyngeal secretions, vomitus, or copious blood and cerebral spinal fluid leak from a nasopharyngeal fracture may add to the obstruction. Extension of the head and elevation of the jaw (by its angles) will raise the tongue out of the posterior oropharynx. Stove-in fractures of the middle third of the face and double fractures of the mandible constitute special hazards and the assistance of a facio-maxillary specialist should be sought *after* clearing the airway. Secretions are removed by nasopharyngeal and oral suction. If the patient is deeply comatose an oro- or nasopharyngeal air tube should be inserted, and this will help maintain a good airway. If this is insufficient an endotracheal airway is needed. If the coma is light the use of a suction tube or indwelling airway in the oral pharynx may stimulate vomiting and add to the obstruction. An endotracheal tube may produce distressing coughing. In such cases tubes are not used and the patient is turned on to the three-quarter prone position to enable the secretions to fall out by gravity while the angles of the jaw are held forward to maintain the airway (*Fig.* 210). Patients with laryngeal stridor or

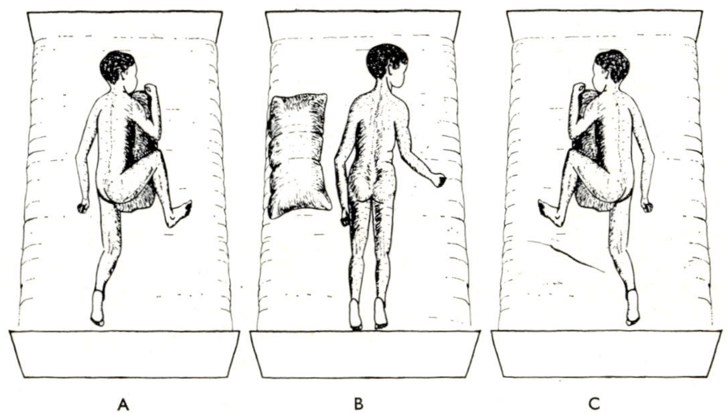

Fig. 210.—The three-quarter prone position. A, The right arm and leg are supported by a large pillow or pillows. The head automatically assumes the three-quarter position. B, To turn the patient, pull out the pillow. This allows the body to fall completely prone. C, Next turn the head to the left side, raise the left arm and leg upon the pillow, and the head will again assume the three-quarter position. One person can turn a heavy patient in this manner without help.

obstruction subsequent to aspiration of secretions or vomitus, and those with an extensive fracture of the jaw may require an early tracheostomy (p. 16). Many patients thought to be moribund improve dramatically when good aeration is secured.

  b. EMERGENCY CONTROL OF SCALP HÆMORRHAGE.—As a general rule, scalp hæmorrhage has ceased by the time the patient is admitted to the hospital. If not, a gauze sponge of suitable size is placed over the wound and secured to the skull by means of a moderately firm bandage. (Rarely, a spurting artery is seen in scalp or muscle and is controlled by application of a sterile hæmostat.)

  c. EXAMINATION FOR MAJOR BODY INJURY.—The blood-pressure is next taken and it will quickly determine if shock is present (p. 20). If shock is present, then there is extensive body injury to some part other than the head. Brain injury does not cause oligæmic shock. The volume of blood-loss sufficient to produce shock greatly exceeds the volume of intracranial blood necessary to cause death. Blood-loss into the abdominal cavity from a ruptured liver or spleen may be suspected by abdominal palpation and confirmed by diagnostic four-quadrant abdominal puncture with a No. 18 lumbar puncture needle. Intrathoracic hæmorrhage may be determined by inspection, percussion, and auscultation of the chest, and confirmed by a chest radiograph. Shock from intrapericardial hæmorrhage is rare because these patients do not usually reach hospital alive. It is suspected by the diminution or absence of audible heart-sounds. Retro-peritoneal hæmorrhage from a ruptured kidney may be difficult to determine but is suspected by the presence of blood in the urine. Severe external hæmor-rhage from a laceration of the scalp may have occurred before the patient was admitted to hospital and is a cause of shock, especially in the aged.

The fracture of a major bone such as a femur may be associated with sufficient extravasation of blood into the tissues to cause shock, again especially in the aged. Pain from the untreated fracture may cause restlessness.

A low blood-pressure is sometimes present without loss of blood. A neck fracture, with cord compression and interruption of sympathetic fibres carrying vasomotor tone, may allow blood to pool in the dependent part of the body. Pain due to a fracture sometimes causes reflex lowering of the blood-pressure, but in this situation the pulse is not accelerated as it is in oligæmic shock. One should also beware of the presence of a compensated oligæmic shock manifested by a normal blood-pressure and a fast pulse since decompensation sometimes sets in rather abruptly.

Oligæmic shock, when severe, will cause coma because of insufficient blood-supply to the brain. It is distinguished from blood-pressure failure in the late stage of brain injury by the relatively light coma level in the presence of a very low blood-pressure, by the fast pulse, sweaty skin, and rapid deep, but regular, 'air hunger' respirations.

Priority in Controlling Hæmorrhage.—If oligæmic shock is present then its treatment usually takes precedence over specific management of the head injury. Immediate replacement of blood-volume by plasma and quick replacement of whole blood by transfusion are required together with control of the source of hæmorrhage, for example, a ruptured spleen. Although a general anæsthetic may raise the intracranial pressure unless very expertly administered and will mask the development of neurological signs, it is best to get on with the control of severe hæmorrhage and accept the risks to the central nervous system that exist. A spinal anæsthetic in expert hands will allow continuous observation of the brain injury but tends to increase the degree of shock by relaxing vaso-motor tone.

If the head-injured patient is not in shock there is no point in inserting intra-venous needles and catheters at this stage for the purpose of administering fluids. These only immobilize the limbs and interfere with an accurate examina-tion of the neurological state. In all patients, whether shock is present or not, a systematic examination is made of the limbs, thoracic cage, and spine by inspection and gentle palpation to determine the presence or absence of a fracture. These will determine the ease with which the patient can be moved about in bed and turned from side to side.

d. EXAMINATION OF THE HEAD.—A systematic examination of the external surface of the head may reveal lacerations and hæmatomata of the scalp.

Hæmatomata are circular or oval and have an elevated, thickened edge. Their centre is soft and fluctuant, and may be depressed by touch. This must not be confused with a depressed fracture. Depressed fractures are not diagnosed by palpation, which is unreliable and dangerous. They may be visibly depressed in an open wound but, as a rule, they are diagnosed by radiography. The most important scalp swelling is that which may be found in the temporal region in relation to an extradural hæmatoma. This is due to hæmorrhage through the fracture site beneath the temporal muscle. It gives a soft boggy swelling which does not pit on pressure. A soft swelling of the scalp which pits on pressure is due to local injury in the skin. Both may be present in the same area.

Subconjunctival hæmorrhages extending back behind the eye suggest a fracture of the anterior fossa. Continued bleeding or loss of cerebrospinal fluid from the nose or ears represents fractures of the base. Skin discoloration behind the ears, which may not be obvious at an early stage, represents fracture of the temporal bone.

The external auditory meatuses should be inspected for bleeding and any blood present may be gently removed by cotton-wool pledgets soaked in hydrogen peroxide. Relatives may be able to supply information about any pre-existing chronic middle-ear or sinus disease. Undisplaced fractures of the mandible or cervical spine are not uncommon but are frequently overlooked.

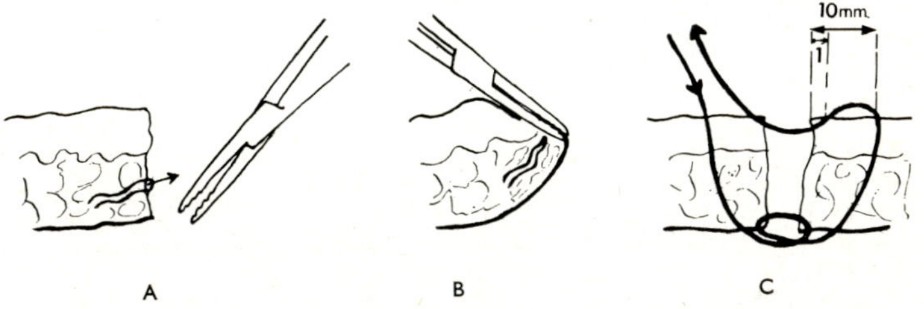

Fig. 211.—Control of scalp hæmorrhage. **A,** The hæmostat is applied to the galea deep in the spurting artery. **B,** It is then turned back over the skin. The artery is compressed between the hæmostat and the galea. **C,** Single-layer closure with tight galea approximation. The needle follows the direction of the arrow. This is particularly useful if scalp hæmorrhage persists. Otherwise a simple mattress stitch is sufficient.

In almost all cases hæmorrhage from the scalp wound will have ceased by the time the general examination is completed. If an arterial spurter continues then this can be controlled by compressing the section of scalp involved against the underlying bone by the pulps of the fingers. If a depressed fracture is suspected, pressure must be exerted at a distance from the wound. Pressure is continued for a minimum of 5 minutes. If a sterile hæmostat is available, hæmostasis may be achieved by everting the scalp edge by means of this hæmostat applied to the galea (*Fig.* 211 A, B). One must not probe blindly into the centre of a wound with an artery forceps because this may only start more hæmorrhage than it stops. It may also damage the brain when a depressed fracture is present.

e. NEUROLOGICAL EXAMINATION.—The nuances of a good neurological examination are lost in the presence of coma. Examination consists in observing spontaneous movement and movement elicited by pin-prick stimulation to each limb, eliciting reflexes, in recording pulse-rate, respiratory rate, respiratory depth and rhythm, and in examination of the reaction of the pupils to light. These observations must be charted clearly so that continuity of care is maintained from one observer to the next.

Levels of Consciousness.—Coma is distinguished from the lighter states of impaired consciousness in that in the former the patient makes no response to the spoken word. In the latter there is some response. When consciousness is deeply clouded commands may need to be repeated and reinforced by gestures; when it approaches normality there may only be slight disorientation for time and place.

There are four degrees of coma: light coma, deep coma, the premoribund state, and the moribund state (*Fig.* 212).

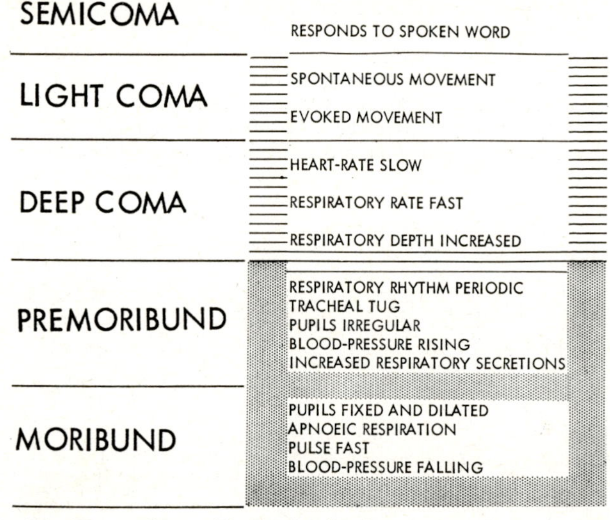

Fig. 212.—Degrees of coma. The boundary lines between the various stages are somewhat arbitrary. Deterioration is a dynamic process, not a series of changes from one static level to the next.

i. *Light coma*: The patient moves spontaneously and moves his limbs on stimulation by pin-prick. It is best to stimulate the same area with the same intensity at each examination in order to estimate improvement or deterioration. The ulnar border of the hands and the sole of the feet are convenient. These movements indicate paresis or paralysis of one side if the other side moves better. Absent movements indicate that the patient has suffered spinal cord trauma in addition or is already in the premoribund state. Increased movement on serial examination usually means that the patient is awakening. Sometimes an increase in spontaneous movement may only mean that he has pain or discomfort from a full bladder, from a fracture, or because manual restraints have been mistakenly used to control restlessness. Rarely increased spontaneous movements, especially rubbing the head, indicate that the patient is actually deteriorating, that in fact he is experiencing a headache due to an accumulating intracranial hæmatoma. While the patient remains in a light coma, there is no alteration in the pulse or respiration.

ii. *Deep coma*: Spontaneous and evoked movements decrease, the pulse slows, and a subtle change occurs in respiration. Its rate quickens and its depth increases. These are very serious signs.

iii. *The premoribund state*: Spontaneous movements have practically ceased. Evoked movements are sluggish. The rate and depth of respiration continue to increase. The patient's trachea seems to be drawn down into his chest with each respiration (the ominous tracheal tug). The respiratory rhythm becomes irregular with alternating fast and deep with slow and shallow periods (Cheyne-Stokes respiration). The pupils constrict and become unequal in size. The blood-pressure commences to rise. Secretions in the pharynx become a problem (the well-known death-rattle).

iv. *The moribund state*: There is no response to pin-prick. The pupils are fixed and dilated. There are periods of apnœa at the end of each slow cycle. The pulse-rate accelerates to about 160. The blood-pressure, which may have reached a level of about 200 mm. Hg systolic, begins to fall and may remain, for a time, at a level well below the normal systolic. Respirations deteriorate into inspiratory gasps, the blood-pressure falls further, and respirations cease before the heart stops. Blood-pressure collapse from head injury differs significantly from that due to shock. It is characterized by the absence of response to pain, by fixed dilated pupils, and by a very slow or very irregular respiration.

DIFFERENTIAL DIAGNOSIS.—One might pause at this point to remember that, while a combination of coma and external signs of injury almost always indicate head injury, this is not invariably so.

a. Coma causing Body Injury (*with or without Head Injury*).—The comas of epilepsy and drunkenness are often associated with external signs of injury. Patients such as automobile drivers and steel erectors who are exposed to physical danger may sustain signs of external injury if they suffer sudden collapse due to a coronary thrombosis, intracranial hæmorrhage, or diabetic coma. The epileptic patient wakens within a few minutes and can be aroused, even if he appears drowsy for 30 minutes or more. The drunk may give more difficulty because he wakens more slowly, but in his case improvement is also continuous. Other types of coma independent of head injury must be considered on the basis of the history available.

b. Coma resulting from Body Injury.—Shock as a cause of coma has already been discussed. It produces a relatively light somewhat restless coma with ashen pallor, cold clammy skin, and a deep sighing respiration, as well as a fast pulse and low blood-pressure. Fat embolism associated with a recent injury to bone or fatty tissue also produces a rather characteristic coma—light and very restless, as though the patient was just about to wake up.

2. Management during the First Few Hours after Injury (*Fig.* 213).—
This stage is separated from the first day to emphasize the fact that all patients who are very rapidly deteriorating from head injury need not be rushed off to the operating theatre for unavailing bur holes. Unless there is a history of a lucid interval or unless the nature of the trauma was disproportionately light considering the depth of present coma, an extradural hæmatoma is unlikely. Rapid deterioration in the very early hours of a head injury is more likely to be due to extensive cerebral laceration than to extradural hæmatoma. For these rapidly deteriorating patients there is little to be done. A good airway must be continued. Urea, 200 ml. of 30 per cent, and mannitol, 250–500 ml. of 20 per cent

solution, intravenously, are of questionable help. If in doubt it is reasonable to try them.

For the less seriously injured this is a period of detailed observation during which the surgeon gets to know the patient well, gets a feeling of the dynamic situation of improvement or of worsening, and during which he prepares for an extended period of very intensive care. The steps to be taken during this period are:—

a. MAINTAIN THE AIRWAY.—Usually this is accomplished by turning the patient into the three-quarter prone position (*see Fig*. 210). The 'upper arm' and leg are supported by means of a pillow or pillows. The head is turned to the side and secretions run out through the mouth. Some extension of the head is advisable. The patient is turned to the other side at least every 2 hours by simply pulling out the pillows and allowing him to fall prone, turning his head to the opposite side, and raising the opposite arm and leg upon pillows (*see Fig*. 210). A few who do not maintain a good airway in the three-quarter prone position may require a tracheostomy. These are often patients who have had a vomitus with partial aspiration and in whom the larynx is in partial spasm.

b. RESTLESSNESS is managed by padding the sides of the bed and by covering the hands with a soft bandage in a manner which will prevent the patient grasping objects such as his catheter, intravenous apparatus, or the sides of the bed. No sedative drugs are used, and in particular morphine is avoided.

c. CATHETER.—During the first few hours it is usually wise to insert an indwelling Gibbon catheter into the bladder. A quick estimation of kidney function should be made against the anticipated use of the cerebral dehydrating agents, urea and mannitol. A fluid-balance chart is started. A blood-urea or non-protein nitrogen estimation is performed.

d. MEDICATION.—

i. *Antibiotics*.—Patients with evidence of a fracture at the base of the skull leaking cerebrospinal fluid and blood into the nasopharynx or into the middle ear should have antibiotics to prevent an intracranial infection. Elderly patients and those who have aspirated vomitus should have antibiotics to prevent pneumonia. When a catheter is inserted it is common practice to administer a low-dosage sulphonamide to help prevent urinary infection (*see* Chapter VI).

ii. *Anticonvulsants*.—During the stage of coma a single convulsion may jeopardize a patient's life by the short period of anoxia and of excessive carbon-dioxide build-up. Both of these factors cause acute swelling of the brain. For this reason it is often advisable to administer a non-hypnotic anticonvulsant such as diphenyl hydantoin, 100 mg. three times daily.

e. HYPERPYREXIA.—Hyperpyrexia is a serious complication as it increases the metabolic requirements of a brain unable to cope with normal metabolism. Patients should be kept at a normal temperature by means of a cooling mattress or by means of a cold tent. Hypothermia used extensively over the past 15 years does not seem to have provided much specific help and is now being used with decreasing frequency.

f. SERIAL NEUROLOGICAL EXAMINATION.—The frequency depends upon the skill of the doctors and nurses present, and ideally one skilled medical observer should be in continuous attendance. Observations at least every 15 minutes must be regarded as a minimum. Pulse-rate, blood-pressure, and respiratory rate are best recorded graphically on a chart.

The attending nurse should call the house doctor if:—

i. The degree of restlessness changes or the level of consciousness deepens.

ii. The pulse-rate either quickens or slows.

iii. The respiration alters in rate or in rhythm.

iv. The size of the pupils changes.

v. The temperature exceeds 39° C. (101° F.).

vi. Convulsions or abnormal movements (mainly the extension of decerebrate rigidity) occur.

vii. The blood-pressure changes.

g. X-RAY OF THE SKULL.—This should be taken for two purposes: (i) to detect the presence of a depressed fracture and (ii) to detect the presence of a linear fracture over the territory of the middle meningeal artery or over a major dural sinus. A fracture in these critical sites indicates the likelihood of an extradural hæmatoma. The size of the fracture on a radiograph is not a good measure of the severity of the head injury *per se*.

h. DEFINITIVE SUTURE OF SCALP WOUNDS.—This may be attended to at any convenient time and the technique is described below.

3. Management during the First Day (*Fig.* 213).—

This is a period of maximum suspicion of *extradural hæmorrhage*, though it may present at any time during the first few hours or days. Often the patient has

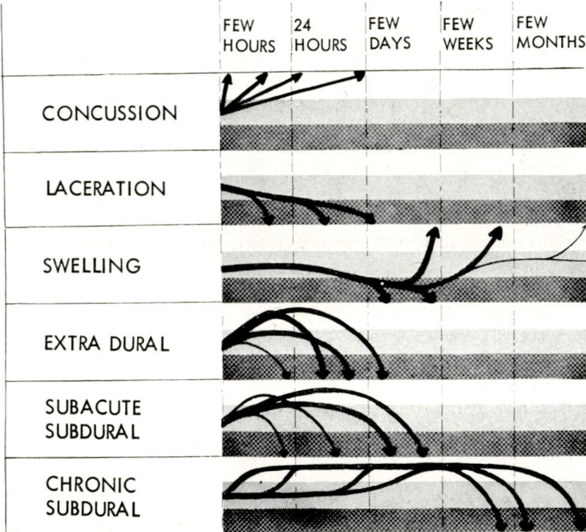

Fig. 213.—Opposite each of the six pathological states some probable courses are indicated by arrows. The time factors relate to the time of injury (not time of admission to hospital). The non-shaded areas represent states of confusion and of full consciousness. The lightly shaded areas represent the stages of light and deep coma in which the patient no longer responds to the spoken word. The darkly shaded areas represent the premoribund and moribund states with severe disturbance in the vital regulatory function of the brain-stem.

not been admitted until several hours have elapsed and the valuable observations of the early hours are missing. If the history, physical examination, and radiographic appearance are those of a severe crushing injury or through-and-through gun-shot injury, it is probable that deterioration is mostly due to laceration of the brain. If the history, external evidence of trauma, and radiographic appearance are those of a lesser injury, then any deterioration must be regarded as possibly due to an extradural hæmatoma. Laceration of the brain and extradural hæmatoma may, of course, occur together. Diminished response to pin-prick and a slow pulse-rate with or without altered respiration are the signs which must be watched. Paresis or paralysis may also appear and may be on the side contralateral to the hæmatoma or on the same side (false localization). If a fracture of the skull overlies the middle meningeal artery, the suspicion is heightened. If the patient has had a period of temporary improvement in conscious level or if there is a soft boggy swelling in either temporal fossa, diagnosis is virtually definite. The soft boggy swelling is characteristic. It is due to accumulation of blood beneath the temporal muscles and therefore does not pit on pressure as a cutaneous abrasion or subcutaneous hæmatoma would do. A classic lucid interval simplifies but is not essential to the diagnosis.

If a lucid interval is present diagnosis of extradural hæmatoma should be made during the ensuing period of drowsiness. If the suspicion of extradural hæmatoma should be entertained before or during the period of deepening coma, it can be confirmed or ruled out by an arteriogram. If entertained during the premoribund stage, then the diagnosis should be made by an immediate bur hole. If entertained during the moribund stage, then evacuation of the hæmatoma is almost invariably too late. A very few cases in whom fixed dilated pupils developed while preparation for operation was already under way have recovered following evacuation of the clot. If the patient is in the premoribund or moribund state, then the rapid intravenous administration of 300 ml. of 30 per cent urea in 10 per cent travert (invert sugar) or of 500 ml. of 20 per cent mannitol in water will temporarily shrink the brain and lessen the severity of cerebral displacement while preparations for operation are being made. Ordinarily these drugs are not given in the presence of impaired renal function, but in these desperate situations they may be given unless there is a history of definite renal incompetence. One must not confuse the results of these drugs with true improvement and delay definitive treatment on that account.

Children may show sudden and profound deterioration of conscious level at an early stage and may reach a state of fixed dilated pupils with one or more attacks of decerebrate rigidity and may yet recover spontaneously. Sometimes they do this quite promptly and sometimes more slowly. Such an acute deterioration in them may be due to swelling or may be due to an intracranial hæmatoma, and in all instances when the dilemma exists it must be settled by arteriography or bur holes according to the stage reached rather than by speculation. Sometimes before the preparations for these procedures are completed there is a perceptible improvement. In such cases delay is justified.

4. Management during the First Week (*Fig.* 213).—

If the patient is not conscious within 24 hours, he may remain unconscious for several days or even weeks. The main problem with these patients is the management of cerebral swelling. Deterioration from late extradural and from subacute subdural hæmatomata occurs and must be watched for. Anterior and posterior fossa extradurals usually present late. The posterior fossa variety is characterized by lower cranial nerve palsies and by cerebellar signs.

a. Maintain the Airway.—It is difficult to maintain a good airway over a prolonged period. Continued nasopharyngeal and oral suction traumatizes the oral pharynx with swelling and hæmorrhage, and this increases obstruction. In most instances it is advisable to perform a tracheostomy if there are no signs of an early awakening.

b. POSITION.—The patient should be nursed, if possible, on an intermittent pressure mattress. He is slightly turned to one side and should be turned at least every 2 hours in order to empty secretions from the lungs.

c. FLUIDS.—It should be noted that during the first 24 hours no attention has been given to the administration of fluid. The average hydrated patient will withstand dehydration for 24 hours without difficulty. If there is evidence of dehydration or if the climate is warm, then fluids must be given during this period. Fifteen hundred ml. of fluid are required each day and are administered intravenously, preferably through a long intravenous catheter so strapped that it cannot easily be pulled out (p. 36). All intake and output are charted.

d. MEDICATION.—Antibiotics and anticonvulsants are continued if it is felt they are indicated.

e. ENEMA.—It is as well to begin the use of olive-oil retention enemata early so that a massive fæcal impaction does not develop by the end of a week or 10 days.

f. TREATMENT OF CEREBRAL ŒDEMA.—Cerebral œdema following brain injury is often maximum by the third or fourth day. If it is apparent that the patient is going to remain unconscious for several days then it is possible that cortisone, 300 mg. daily, or dexamethasone 12 mg. daily, will minimize œdema. This is anti-swelling therapy, not replacement therapy, and the dose therefore greatly exceeds that used in replacement therapy. Hypothermia has been tried in the past but probably is of little avail. Apparently it delays the evolution of œdema rather than prevents it. Hypertonic urea and mannitol will reduce swelling for a few hours but are of little value in treating prolonged œdema. The main treatment consists in maintaining a good airway and in preventing the aspiration of vomitus by adherence to the three-quarters prone position if a tracheostomy has not been performed.

g. SERIAL NEUROLOGICAL EXAMINATIONS.—These are continued in order to detect late extradural hæmatomata and subacute subdural hæmatomata. Again observations should ideally be continuous. Serially detailed examinations should be made at least every hour. The differentiation of these hæmatomata from swelling is especially difficult. The presence of a period of improvement or the development of lateralizing paralysis is usually in favour of the presence of a clot rather than of swelling, but both can be present in cases of swelling which, in some instances, is maximum in a single lobe, especially the temporal lobe (pulped lobe syndrome). Again differentiation is made during the stage of deep coma by means of arteriography and during the premoribund phase by bur holes. While temporal bur holes usually locate an extradural hæmatoma, one requires bifrontal, biparietal, and bitemporal bur holes to exclude all subdural hæmatomata. The subdural hæmatoma at this stage may be quite solid and require a craniotomy or craniectomy for removal according to the urgency of the condition. Occasionally continued deterioration due to a 'pulped lobe' demands excision of that lobe.

5. Management during Subsequent Weeks.—

Airway problems have now stabilized. Nutrition must be provided; this is best done by intragastric feeding (p. 46). A continuous unattended drip method which is suitable for the conscious patient is unsuitable for the unconscious patient. The tube should be passed and withdrawn three times a day. The nurse must ensure that the tube has entered the stomach (and not the bronchi) either by aspirating bile-stained gastric juice or by injecting air down the tube and listening with a stethoscope over the stomach for the resultant gurgling. The patient should be closely watched for 15 minutes after each feeding has been delivered. Each feeding consists of 500 ml. containing 500 calories and appropriate vitamins. If a patient is not observed immediately following feeding or if the gastric tube is kept permanently in place, vomiting may occur causing obstruction of the airway and death.

B. PATIENT WITH CLOUDED CONSCIOUSNESS

These patients respond to the spoken word and may be graded as mild, moderate, or severe according to the ease of that response. Basically they are managed in a manner similar to that of the patient in coma. They are observed for the appearance of extradural hæmatoma, subacute subdural hæmatoma, pulped lobe, and generalized swelling. Both management and observation are easier. There is usually little difficulty with the airway; there may or may not be need for catheterization. Restlessness is more of a problem, but again is managed by means of the padded bed sides and not by restraints or drugs. Simple reassurance and a gentle manner help greatly. Pain relief can be given by aspirin or by one of the simple analgesics. It should be remembered that increasing headache may be a symptom of awakening or of an expanding hæmatoma. Observation is mainly a matter of response to questions and commands. Is it getting better or worse? Voluntary limb movement is added to the frequent serial neurological examination and so also may cranial nerve functions such as the fields of vision. Sensory examination may be possible. The greatest difficulty, especially in children, lies in distinguishing ordinary sleepiness from pathological drowsiness. The patient must simply be roused sufficiently, despite protest, to make this distinction clear. In pathological states a slow pulse-rate may be present while the patient still responds (although this has previously been listed as a feature of coma). Diagnostic action by echo-encephalogram or arteriography should be taken in the presence of deterioration before the patient passes into semicoma. Restlessness during arteriography should be overcome by an appropriately designed head-holder rather than by a general anæsthetic—this would mask continuing neurological change and might increase the intracranial tension if not expertly administered.

C. THE ALERT PATIENT WHO HAS PREVIOUSLY BEEN UNCONSCIOUS

Even a short period of unconsciousness indicates that a severe brain injury was sustained and the possibility of developing an acute extradural or subdural hæmatoma exists. The patient should have an X-ray examination of his skull. If there is a fracture line along the middle meningeal artery or across a major sinus, it is absolutely essential that he remain in hospital for 24 hours. Observation consists of determining if the patient is becoming drowsy. Observation must be made at least every 30 minutes. This means that the patient gets little sleep for 24 hours in most instances. If no fracture is present an exceptionally alert family may elect to assume responsibility for this 24-hour period of observation with the understanding that the patient does not sleep for more than 30 minutes at a time and that he will be returned to hospital if headache develops or increases, or if drowsiness develops. If in any doubt, admit to hospital without question. In all instances, once it has become apparent that the patient is really drowsy and not just sleepy, arteriography should be performed. Not all patients who deteriorate after this interval of consciousness have hæmatoma. Many, as already noted, have swelling or have a pulped lobe. Arteriography is required to differentiate these.

D. THE PATIENT WHO HAS NEVER BEEN UNCONSCIOUS

The vast majority require simple reassurance. There is no need of radiographs unless there is a scalp laceration and a depressed fracture is suspected. A depressed fracture can be present in an infant (and very rarely in an adult) without a scalp laceration. The history of the trauma is important. Small sharp objects such as a pencil or nail can penetrate deeply into the skull of a child, especially in the temporal region, leaving only a minimal stab in the skin. A penetrating fracture of this type may not always be evident upon radiographs. Patients without fracture are allowed to go home. They are told that a small amount of headache and some lack of energy are not unusual after a mild bump upon the head and that these symptoms may last for a few days or a few weeks. If headache is severe, and not relieved by simple analgesics, they should return for examination. Patients with unusually severe post-concussion headaches must be suspected of developing signs and symptoms of a chronic subdural hæmatoma at a later date. Most do not and they lose their headache in a few weeks. A few, motivated by factors of industrial compensation and fears of loss of mental function, develop functional headaches. The cause of many post-concussional headaches, dizziness, and loss of memory is not understood. Recent work suggests they may be related to changes in cerebral circulation.

E. LATE COMA IN A PATIENT WHO HAS HAD ANTECEDENT HEAD INJURY

The previous head injury may have produced a long or short period of unconsciousness or no unconsciousness at all, or, indeed, it may have been totally unremembered. There may be a history of deteriorating mental function, drowsiness, or headache, or any combination of these. Papillœdema is rare, especially in the aged. There may or may not be lateralizing neurological signs.

This coma must be differentiated from others which present without immediate signs of external injury. They are acute poisoning, commonly barbiturate or carbon monoxide, acute encephalitis, meningitis, abscess, acute intracerebral hæmorrhage, acute subarachnoid hæmorrhage, and acute decompensation of a brain tumour. The relatives of patients in diabetic, hepatic, and uræmic coma can usually provide an adequate antecedent history. A coma of barbiturate poisoning is a very quiet one, like an exaggeration of normal sleep, with a slow depressed respiration quite unlike the irregular distressed respiration of brain-stem decompensation. A diagnosis of carbon-monoxide poisoning depends largely upon the history (and upon the bright-red complexion). Neck stiffness occurs with subarachnoid bleeding and meningeal infections, as well as with broken necks, and may occur with the late stage of brain-stem impaction due to either a tumour or subdural hæmatoma. A lumbar puncture will diagnose subarachnoid hæmorrhage and the infections. Intracerebral hæmorrhage is characterized by very sudden coma in a patient previously quite well and by marked lateralizing neurological signs.

In all of those patients in whom a definite diagnosis of the cause of coma cannot be made, a subdural hæmatoma must be suspected. An angiogram up to a stage of deep coma and bur holes in the premoribund stage will establish the diagnosis.

In infants and young children there may or may not be a history of head injury and there may or may not be a skull fracture. Listlessness, anorexia, vomiting, anæmia, and seizure are common. A seizure may precipitate coma. In sudden coma of this type one considers lead poisoning and poisoning by aspirins or by various household poisons. Acute meningitis, encephalitis, and abscess are also possibilities, so are acute subarachnoid hæmorrhage from arteriovenous malformation and acute decompensation from a posterior fossa tumour.

Before the age of 2 the presence of retinal hæmorrhages without elevation of the optic disks is pathognomonic of subdural hæmorrhage (or of leukæmia). Before the anterior fontanelle closes, diagnosis and emergency treatment are easily made (if neurosurgical help is not immediately available) by a subdural tap. A short No. 22 needle is inserted obliquely beneath the dura at the external angle of each fontanelle. If subdural fluid is present it will flow out freely. Not more than a total of 30 ml. should be removed on the first occasion.

TECHNICAL PROCEDURES

1. Scalp Laceration.—The hair should be widely shaved (at least 3 in., 7·5 cm.) from the margins of the incision. The adjoining hair should be matted with soap or petroleum jelly so that it will not float loosely into the clean area. Using full aseptic techniques, the wound is loosely packed with gauze and the surrounding area cleansed by gentle washing with soap and water for a period of about 10 minutes. Using a new set of gloves, gowns, and instruments an

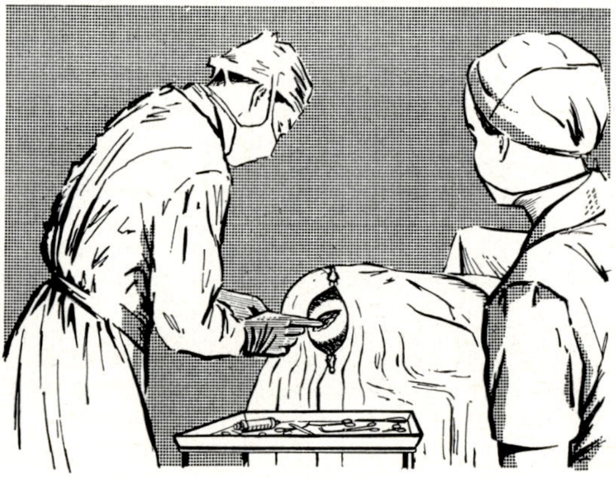

Fig. 214.—Exploration of a head wound. Showing the isolation of the area with sterile towels. Surgeon and instrument nurse masked and wearing sterile gloves.

ellipse of skin surrounding the wound is anæsthetized by intracutaneous injection of 1 per cent procaine or 1 per cent lignocaine which is injected into the skin and not subcutaneously. An intradermal injection blanches the skin, whereas a subcutaneous injection merely elevates it. The patient need feel only one pinprick during this process. Each subsequent needle puncture is made into the periphery of the blanched analgesic area and the fluid spreads from that point into the adjoining skin without pain. The wound is draped with self-adhesive plastic or with skin towels sewn into the anæsthetized margins. The operator dons new sterile gloves and gown (*Fig.* 214). The wound is now painless and is cleansed by sterile saline and sponge. Devitalized tags of skin are trimmed away (*Fig.* 215). If the wound is more than 12 hours old or if it is grossly contaminated with dirt that cannot be washed away, then the skin edges should be excised. This will start fresh bleeding for the control of which artery forceps on the galea or cautery to the bleeding points are required. Underlying periosteum should not be disturbed unless there is some ingrained dirt. If periosteum is removed, bleeding from the bone is best stopped by packing and waiting for at least 5 minutes. If it still persists, bone wax and cautery may be used, but

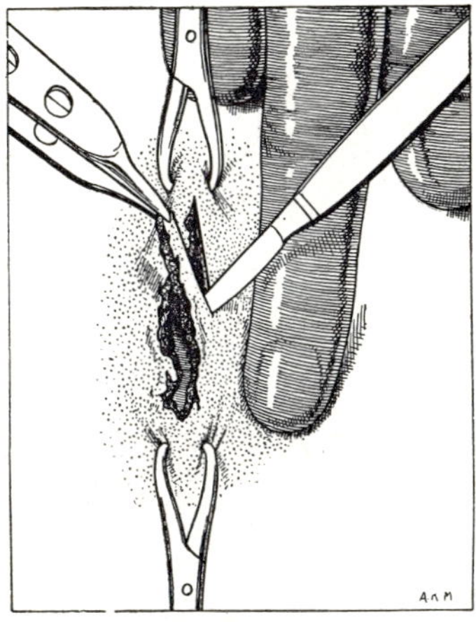

Fig. 215.—A method of excising a
wound of the scalp.

neither of these is desirable. One remains as a foreign body, the other produces necrotic tissue in a potentially infected wound. Underlying temporal muscle may have to be trimmed of devitalized fragments. Penetrating injuries should be traced through the muscle to the bone.

Surgical scalp incisions are closed in two layers, one permanent row is placed in the galea and one removable row in the skin proper. Scalp injuries are usually closed in one row of inverted mattress sutures so that no foreign body will be left in a potentially infected wound. Hæmorrhage from the scalp is sometimes better controlled by a stitch which grips the galea (*see Fig.* 211 C, p. 273). A monofilament material such as steel or nylon is preferable. Drains are not used. Hæmostasis must be adequate. Patients with severe contusion of underlying muscle or with neglected wounds involving muscle should have tetanus booster if previously inoculated or tetanus antiserum if not previously inoculated (p. 67). If some skin is missing the wound cannot be closed easily. It is possible to approximate the edges by various plastic procedures, but it should be remembered that the scalp is extremely vascular and it is better for the inexperienced operator to pack the wound and await expert help rather than get involved in extensive vascular mobilizations of skin.

2. Subcutaneous Hæmatomata.—If soft and fluctuant and painful their contents may be aspirated but usually it is best to leave them alone.

3. Depressed Fracture.—Wounds in which dural tear is presumed require débridement and repair of the dura by a competent neurological surgeon. A

11

minimal depression may not tear the dura but the position on the radiograph, after the bone has sprung back, may be deceptive in that it does not reveal the depth of penetration of bone at the moment of injury. Unskilled attempts to elevate the depressed fractures may further lacerate the brain and may cause profuse hæmorrhage by lifting a fragment of bone out of a dural sinus. Anti-biotics will control the infection problem until adequate help is available. The wound may be packed or temporarily sutured.

Skilled elevation (local anæsthesia) begins with surgical toilet of the scalp wound, and a bur hole in the edge of adjoining bone allows the operator to get an instrument under the depressed bone. A small amount of normal bone may be rongeured away to allow the depressed bone to float free. The depressed bone is not elevated by physical force. If the depression involves a dural sinus, the sinus is exposed above and below the depression so that hæmorrhage from it (as the bone is removed) may be controlled. The dural tear is inspected and contaminated or devitalized cortex, together with local blood-clot and any foreign material, are removed. The dura is sewn with silk sutures. If deficient, it may be patched by splitting it into two layers, thereby swinging the superficial layer over the defect. Loose bone is discarded. The skin is closed.

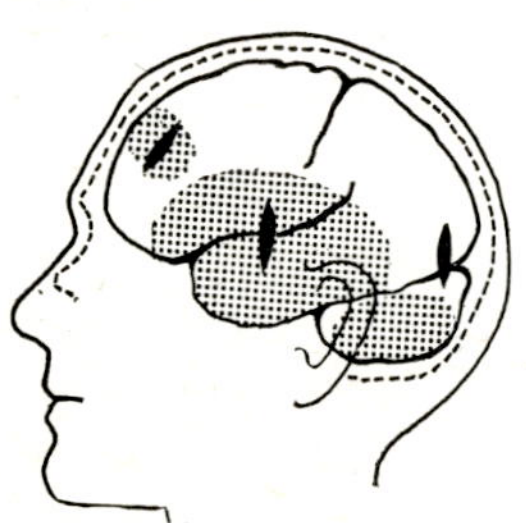

Fig. 216.—Sites of predilection of extradural hæmorrhage.

Closed depressed fracture in infants and small children should be elevated at any convenient time by making a bur hole along the rim of the depression and elevating with a blunt instrument.

4. Extradural Hæmorrhage.—This is also a lesion for the skilled neurosurgeon and carries an appreciable mortality. Occasionally a situation arises where a patient's life may be saved by prompt evacuation of the clot by a doctor with less experience. The sites of predilection are shown in *Fig.* 216. Once the diagnosis has been made, the side is usually evident from the site of fracture and the temporal swelling. The early development of ipsilateral pupillary abnormality is also fairly reliable, but the early development of contralateral hemiparesis is not so reliable because of the possibility of false localization. Anæsthesia is usually unnecessary in these desperate situations but skin infiltration by local solution may be needed if the coma is still sufficiently light. A straight 4-in. (10-cm.) incision is made, 1 in. (2·5 cm.) in front of the external auditory meatus, its lower margin coming down to the bottom of the zygoma. Skin bleeding is controlled by artery forceps on the galea or may be ignored temporarily if the situation is very grave. Muscle incision is in the same line, and skin and muscle are retracted by automatic retractors of the mastoid type. An area of bone of about 2½ in. (6 cm.) in diameter is exposed. This is penetrated by a perforator and then by a bur. The end point of penetration of each of these instruments is determined by a tactile feel of increased resistance which comes to the operator by experience. The inexperienced should remember that these instruments may plunge excessively and should concentrate upon the rotatory rather than upon the perforating aspect of the instrument. Further bone is removed by a rongeur or other available instrument. The clot is sucked out. The bleeding point should be located and controlled by a cautery if in dura or by wax if in bone. If the bleeding point is not located, the wound may be packed until competent help arrives. The volume of external blood-loss rarely requires transfusion.

5. Subacute Subdural Hæmorrhage.—Patients deteriorating during the first week from subacute subdural hæmorrhage usually have a solid blood-clot, not a liquefied one. This cannot, as a rule, be evacuated through a bur hole and requires an expert craniotomy. In a desperate situation a wide lateral craniectomy is acceptable.

6. Repair of Cerebrospinal Fluid Leak.—Most cerebrospinal fluid leaks from the base of the skull will cease within three weeks. Infection is prevented during this time by antibiotics. Patients are advised not to blow their nose. Those few which fail to seal may require repair by an intracranial operation.

7. Chronic Subdural Hæmatoma.—Again this is an operation for the skilled neurosurgeon except in an absolute emergency. The head is completely shaven. Local anæsthesia is used. Through a small linear incision over each parietal eminence, a bur hole is made using the perforator and bur. In the presence of a subdural hæmatoma the dura is seen to be blue and tense. The dura and underlying external subdural membrane are cauterized in a cruciate fashion and then opened. Dark liquid blood will pour out. The skin is closed in two layers. If the hæmatoma is not found in the parietal areas, further bur holes are required in both frontal and in both temporal regions.

CHAPTER XXII

THE MANAGEMENT OF NECK AND FACE CASES

By JOHN A. PALMER

SOFT-TISSUE INJURIES OF THE NECK

BECAUSE of the complex anatomical arrangement of structures in the neck, perforating or penetrating wounds in this region may produce extensive damage to major blood-vessels, the air-passages, and the pharyngo-œsophagus. Massive bleeding, hæmatoma formation, and suffocation, mediastinitis, or fatal emphysema may result. However, with adequate care, even the severest of wounds may be treated successfully.

Emergency Care.—Control of hæmorrhage and the provision of an airway are the two important considerations.

Bleeding is best controlled by direct finger or hand pressure over the site of injury to compress the vessels against the vertebral column. Visible clots should not be disturbed or foreign bodies removed. The blood-volume should be restored as quickly as possible (*see* pp. 23 and 43).

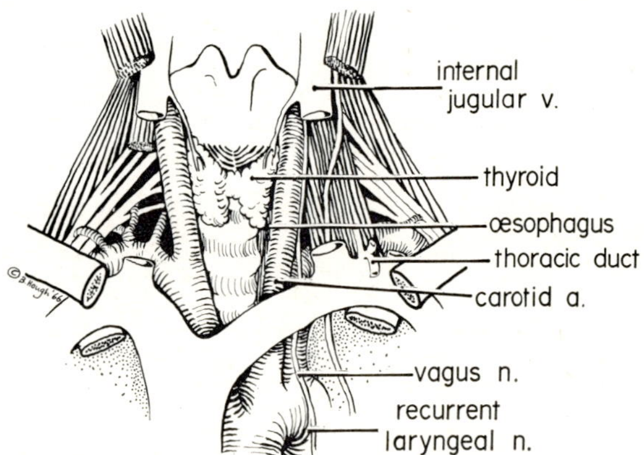

Fig. 217.—Structures in the front of the neck liable to be damaged in cut-throat injuries.

Emergency tracheostomy (*see* p. 16) or endotracheal intubation will relieve airway obstruction, produced by aspiration of blood through an opened larynx or trachea, external tamponade by air or blood, or gradual obstruction by œdema secondary to trauma.

Repair.—Except for lacerations superficial to the platysma, deep or penetrating wounds should be explored under general endotracheal anæsthesia. If tracheostomy is considered necessary but not urgent, it can be done at leisure at the end of the operation with the endotracheal tube in place.

Adequate exposure and a knowledge of the local anatomy are necessary (*Fig.* 217). In general, incisions around wounds should be extended in the long axis of the vessels likely to be involved.

All veins in the neck may be ligated. Air embolism can be prevented by applying pressure on the vein, which is then ligated while positive venous pressure is maintained by the anæsthetist. The common and internal carotid arteries should be repaired (p. 529); if this is not possible, proximal and distal ligation can be carried out, but incurs a significant risk of anoxic hemiplegia. All other vessels may be ligated with impunity.

Injuries of the trachea, larynx, pharynx, and œsophagus should be repaired with end-to-end sutures of either silk or wire. The area should be drained and a tracheostomy done. A broad-spectrum antibiotic is given post-operatively for 4–5 days.

INFECTIONS OF THE NECK

Serious infections in the neck usually take the form of a cellulitis. The tissue spaces in close relation to the mouth and pharynx may be directly infected and the spread of the infection in the loose areolar pathways, extending from the base of the skull into the mediastinum, may be particularly rapid.

General Principles.—

1. Bed-rest is necessary and, except for superficial infections, so is close observation in hospital.

2. Antibiotics are valuable in the treatment of spreading infections and those with systemic effects, but are unnecessary in small localized abscesses. They should seldom be used beyond a few days if there is no clear-cut clinical improvement because of the danger of masking a smouldering deep infection.

3. Localized abscesses should be incised and drained. In certain areas it may be necessary to decompress a space when the development of inflammatory œdema has endangered the airway.

Anæsthesia.—General anæsthesia with endotracheal intubation is employed.

SUBMANDIBULAR SPACE INFECTIONS (LUDWIG'S ANGINA)

Infection in this area is usually related to dental or periodontal inflammation, and involves the environs of the submandibular gland. The tongue becomes greatly swollen, and is pushed superiorly and posteriorly against the palate. There is bulging of the submandibular area, with pain, trismus, inability to swallow, and respiratory distress.

Treatment.—Antibiotic therapy is begun immediately and, if the swelling gets larger, surgical decompression of the area may be required even if an abscess has not yet formed. A tracheostomy is frequently necessary because of the difficulties of intubation due to distortion and œdema of the glottis and surrounding structures.

The area is approached through a transverse incision, just above the level of the hyoid bone; this is extended through platysma to the mylohyoid diaphragm (*Fig.* 218). By blunt dissection laterally and deep to the anterior bellies of the digastric muscles, channels for adequate drainage are opened.

The area is loosely packed open. Antibiotics are continued for a further 24 hours or longer, depending on local and systemic factors. The packing is removed in 24–48 hours. A wick of gauze, soaked in 1 per cent hypochlorite solution diluted 1–10, is inserted into the cavity daily to ensure progressive healing from its depths to the surface.

PARAPHARYNGEAL SPACE INFECTION

Infection in this area is usually related to inflammation of the tonsils or pharynx. The space lies between the pharynx medially, and the submandibular gland, mandible, and the parotid gland laterally. The three diagnostic signs of such infection are: (1) trismus, (2) bulging of the tonsil and lateral wall of the pharynx, and (3) swelling between the mastoid process and the angle of the mandible.

Treatment.—The same general principles of treatment are followed, with surgical drainage for persisting infection.

The approach is through the submaxillary triangle. A transverse incision is made 1 in. (2·5 cm.) below the horizontal ramus of the mandible and extended

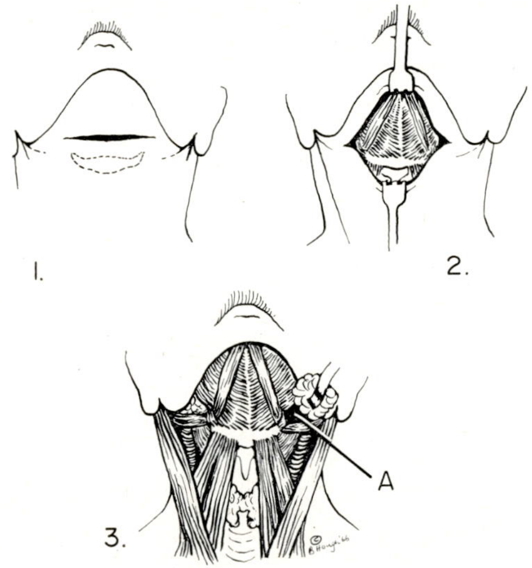

Fig. 218.—The steps 1, 2, and 3 illustrate the drainage of a submandibular infection. A shows the approach to the parapharyngeal space. The submandibular gland is elevated and the deeper tissues are separated by a finger or a blunt instrument.

to the submaxillary gland. The gland is elevated by blunt dissection, and the space deep to the gland entered (*Fig.* 218, 3A). After-care is the same as for submandibular infections.

ACUTE PAROTITIS

Factors predisposing to this complication are:—
1. The aged patient.
2. Dehydration from any cause, including fever.
3. Excessive pre-operative medication with atropine.
4. Infections in the mouth; in particular, dental caries.

The initial complaints are pain and tenderness in the region of the parotid gland. There is progressive swelling, tenderness, and trismus associated with increasing pain and fever.

Treatment.—The prompt administration of a broad-spectrum antibiotic is the most effective measure (*see* p. 74). Proper hydration and improved oral hygiene are important. Radiation therapy is no longer necessary.

Persistent and progressive pain, swelling, and fever longer than 48 hours denote the development of an abscess which requires incision and drainage.

A vertical incision, through skin and subcutaneous tissue only, is made in front of the ear and over the most prominent aspect of the abscess (*Fig.* 219).

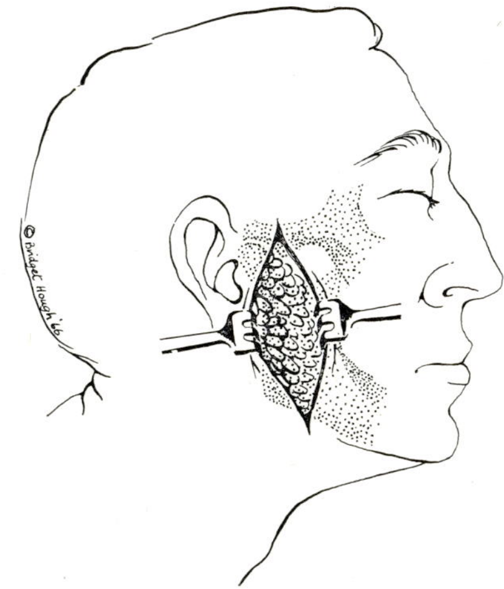

Fig. 219.—The incision for drainage of acute suppurative parotitis; it is usually 4–5 cm long, centred over the most prominent part of the gland.

The deeper tissues are then carefully separated transversely with a blunt instrument until the abscess cavity is opened. A loose gauze pack is left in the cavity for 24–48 hours.

TUMOURS OF THE HEAD AND NECK

The cancers of the oral cavity involve the following areas in decreasing frequency: lip, tongue, floor of mouth, buccal mucosa, alveolus, palate, tonsil, and pharynx. These tumours are usually squamous-cell carcinomata, although less common lesions may occur, e.g., minor salivary gland tumours and lympho-epithelioma. The tumour usually presents as an ulcerating lesion or may only be suspected when metastatic disease develops in the cervical lymph-nodes.

Diagnosis.—Any ulcerating or papillary growth in the mouth should be regarded as carcinoma until *biopsy* is done to establish the diagnosis. If the lesion is small, atypical, and appears to be benign, a biopsy should be taken if it has not healed after 3 weeks of conservative treatment. A generous biopsy (0.5×0.5 mm.) should be obtained from the margin of the lesion. Because the base of the ulcer is frequently covered by a non-specific inflammatory exudate, a superficial biopsy taken from this area may not reveal the underlying carcinoma.

If carcinoma is suspected because of the development of a lump in the neck, a careful search must be made for the primary tumour. This search will include the oral cavity, naso- and hypopharynx, and skin of the face and scalp (particularly for a melanocarcinoma); indeed, the primary tumour may be found anywhere in the body. If at all possible, do not excise the suspected lymph-node because this may compromise subsequent surgical treatment.

The full blood-picture and Wassermann reaction should be determined.

Rationale of Treatment.—

1. The disease tends to remain localized to the head and neck. Distant metastases are unusual and occur only late in the course of the disease.

2. Hæmatogenous spread is unusual. Because lymphatic spread is mainly by tumour emboli, rather than by lymphatic permeation, primary and secondary tumours can be treated separately.

3. Squamous-cell carcinomata, as a group, tend to be radiosensitive. Because these tumours are accessible for radium implants and accurate beam direction, the primary lesion can be treated effectively by radiation.

4. Metastatic tumour in lymph-nodes is best treated by radical excision.

Treatment.—

1. Radiation therapy for the primary lesion.

2. If the primary lesion persists or recurs after radiation, surgical excision should be performed.

3. Radical *en bloc* neck dissection if one or more lymph-nodes are clinically involved by tumour.

4. Combined excision of the primary tumour in continuity with a radical neck dissection, if the primary tumour is uncontrolled and cervical lymph-nodes are involved.

5. Arterial infusion with methotrexate as a palliative measure.

Care before and during Treatment.—

1. *Radiation Therapy.*—The local and systemic effects of radiation are usually underestimated. Radical radiotherapy may profoundly affect an already debilitated person. Anæmia and concurrent infections should be improved before treatment. Carious teeth should be removed and, if external radiation is necessary, even healthy teeth near the tumour should be removed to reduce the risk of radionecrosis of the underlying mandible. During therapy, mouthwashes should be used after eating, and, when necessary, oral penicillin to reduce local infection and xylocaine (lignocaine) viscous to relieve the discomfort of local radiation reaction.

2. *Surgical Therapy.*—The majority of patients with oral cancer are elderly and frequently have cardiorespiratory and liver disease. Careful pre-operative assessment and treatment of these associated conditions are advisable.

Blood transfusions may be required pre-operatively and certainly during the operation, except for the minor surgical procedures.

Post-operative Treatment.—With adequate blood replacement and a good airway, maintained if necessary by tracheostomy, even elderly and frail patients withstand these major procedures well.

Heavy sedation should be avoided because pain is not severe; codeine, 60 mg., or morphine, 10 mg., is adequate. Deep breathing and coughing to clear tracheobronchial secretions, and early ambulation are encouraged. If the primary tumour has been resected, mouthwashes and gentle warm saline irrigations should be ordered. After post-anæsthetic nausea has passed off, oral fluids should be encouraged and a soft diet offered in 3–4 days. If fluid and food intake are inadequate, a temporary gastrostomy (*see* p. 350) is preferable to

Xylocaine (Astra-Hewlett Ltd., Watford, Herts).

prolonged intravenous therapy. A course of broad-spectrum antibiotics (usually tetracycline 1 G. daily) is given after the radical combined operation.

Avoid bulky dressings. The exposed incisions are kept free of crusts by daily suture-line care, using cetavlon or hydrogen peroxide.

Post-operative Bleeding.—The most common post-operative complication is bleeding under the skin-flaps with its associated problems of blood-loss, airway obstruction, and delayed healing. Suction drains, routine for major operations, will handle minor bleeding. However, if bleeding is excessive and there is tense bulging of the skin-flaps, the patient should be returned to the operating room and anæsthetized again, the skin-flaps opened, collected blood removed, and the bleeding point identified and ligated. If a tracheostomy has not already been done, it is usually necessary during the secondary operation. Occasionally, massive, secondary carotid artery bleeding may occur a few days or weeks after operation. The most common cause is wound breakdown from tissue necrosis after excision of a previously irradiated cancer. Bleeding is controlled by finger or hand pressure over the site of hæmorrhage, the blood-loss is rapidly replaced, and personnel and facilities are prepared for carotid artery ligation. In the operating room, the local pressure is not released until everything is ready and the surgeon takes control of the bleeding area. Ligatures are placed around the normal artery well away from the site of bleeding.

ARTERIAL INFUSION WITH CHEMOTHERAPEUTIC AGENTS

Chemotherapeutic agents can be introduced into a tumour-bearing area via its arterial blood-supply (*see* p. 737). Thus a tumour can be bathed in a high concentration of an anti-metabolite such as methotrexate while the systemic

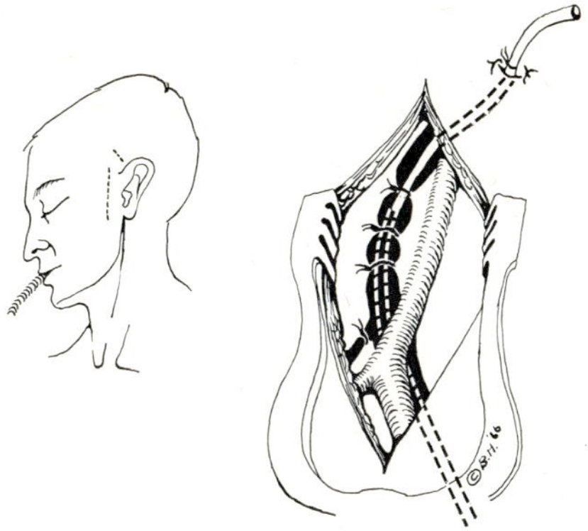

Fig. 220.—Intra-arterial infusion: the catheter is inserted into the superficial temporal artery in front of the ear and after proper positioning is secured as illustrated.

effect of the agent is minimized by the intermittent intramuscular administration of an antidote such as citrovorum factor. Satisfactory palliation is obtained in at least one-third of patients with head and neck cancer, and occasionally the results are striking.

Method.—General anæsthesia is employed. A polyethylene or teflon catheter is inserted into the superficial temporal artery, through a small incision in front

Cetavlon (I.C.I. Ltd., Pharmaceuticals Division, Macclesfield, Cheshire).

of the tragus of the ear (*Fig.* 220). The catheter is inserted far enough so that its tip will reach the bifurcation of the common carotid artery or immediately above this. Then 5 ml. of fluorescein dye are injected into the catheter and the resultant area of fluorescence is assessed in the darkened room under ultraviolet light. If the area of distribution is satisfactory, the catheter is secured in the artery and continuous infusion begun (*Fig.* 221).

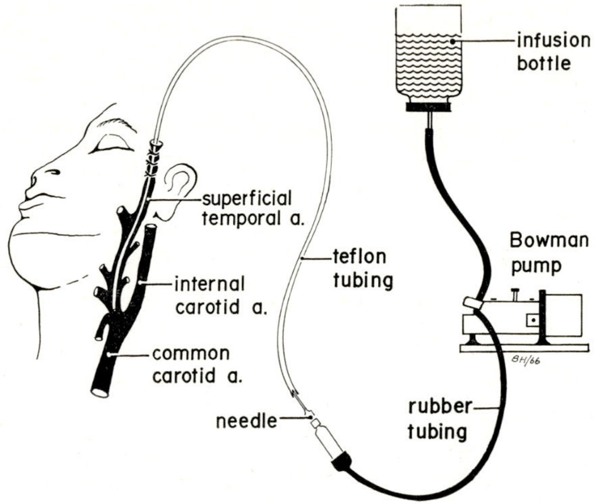

Fig. 221.—Diagram of the catheter assembly. A gravity flow method may be used as an alternative to the pump.

Management during Infusion.—Careful supervision is required to maintain continuous infusion and prevent complications when this technique is used in the treatment of head and neck neoplasms, or those situated elsewhere in the body.

1. *Catheter.*—A blocked catheter can be cleared by forcing 1–1000 heparin solution through it with a tuberculin syringe. If the infusate leaks around the catheter, the infusion should be stopped and the catheter removed, otherwise local infection and secondary hæmorrhage may occur.

2. *Hemiplegia.*—Hemiplegia may develop from the embolism of air introduced while changing the infusate bottles, or it may gradually develop due to drug-induced cerebral irritation. Such hemiplegia is usually temporary and clears when the infusion is stopped. Occasionally if the catheter has been inserted directly into the carotid artery or via the superior thyroid artery, there may be a major slough of the carotid arteries. Emergency carotid ligation is then necessary.

3. *Systemic effects* are mainly related to the effect of the drug on the hæmopoietic system. The dosage of the drug is limited by this factor. A daily monitoring of the white cells and platelets is essential. A progressive decrease in these levels can be expected and the daily dosage of the drug modified accordingly. If the leucocyte count drops to 1500 per c.mm. or below, or the platelets to

75,000 per c.mm., the drug should be stopped. The infusion is started again when the blood-counts return to normal levels.

4. *Dosage.*—The average daily dosage is 50 mg. of methotrexate in 1000 ml. of 5 per cent glucose in water and 6–8 mg. of citrovorum factor, intramuscularly every 6 hours. When treatment is over the catheter can be flushed with heparin and its distal end heat sealed to allow further treatment, or it can be removed. Bleeding is controlled by simple pressure over the exit wound.

THE MANAGEMENT OF THYROID CASES
INVESTIGATION OF THYROID DISORDERS

Thyroid disease may present as: (1) simple goitre, diffuse or nodular; (2) as hyperthyroidism, exemplified by the young agitated female, sweating, with finger tremor and probably exophthalmos; (3) hypothyroidism, either post-surgical, post-irradiation, or possibly the result of auto-immune phenomena—it causes a slowing down of the metabolic processes; and (4) a steadily enlarging lump, arousing suspicion of carcinoma of the thyroid. The clinical differentiation of these different conditions is mostly straightforward and elaborate tests are not necessary. But sometimes there is an admixture of the features of several groups in one patient; in this type of situation, in particular, the clinical diagnostic index (*Table IX*) and the following investigations will be of value:—

Special Tests: A. Hyperthyroidism.—

1. *Radio-iodine,* [131]I, *4-hour Uptake.*—This test, normally carried out by the Isotope Department, is the most valuable single test, the gland uptake being greatly increased in hyperthyroid states. The results may be altered by iodine pools outside the thyroid, and no iodine-containing drugs or radio-opaque dyes should have been given for some days before the test.

2. *Tri-iodothyronine Suppression Test.*—The administration of 100 μg. daily for a week should lower the ^{131}I uptake by 50 per cent. However, this may not occur with a secreting adenoma of thyroid ('hot nodule').

3. *Protein-bound Iodine at* 48 *Hours.*—The increased binding in hyperthyroidism constitutes a most helpful test, particularly when it is considered along with the ^{131}I uptake. The normal range is 3·5–8 μg. per 100 ml. of plasma. The use of radio-opaque contrast media and of oral contraceptive pills during the preceding months may give falsely elevated readings, while mercurial diuretics and long-term salicylate therapy may lower the values obtained.

4. *Therapeutic Trial.*—When isotope laboratory facilities are not available and there is clinical doubt, a trial with an antithyroid drug for at least six weeks is often helpful.

The Thyroid Lump—Benign or Malignant.—

A rapidly growing, firm, fixed thyroid mass is 'manifest carcinoma', is easily diagnosed clinically, and requires prompt biopsy and treatment. However, the clinically solitary thyroid lump is difficult to assess in regards to incidence of malignancy or potential for malignant change.

Factors to Consider.—

i. History of rate of growth, if known.

ii. Age of patient—there is an increased chance of a solitary nodule being malignant in the young patient.

iii. The clinical assessment of the size and consistency of the lump is difficult to relate to the presence or absence of malignancy. However, if there are multiple nodules the likelihood of one being carcinoma is small (less than 1 per cent).

Special Investigations.—

i. Thyroid Scan.—Radio-iodine, ^{131}I, is the most commonly used isotope, although technitium 99 may prove to have some advantages. The scan is the most useful single test for the assessment of a thyroid nodule. If the lump shows a normal or increased intake (hot nodule), it is rarely malignant (less than 1 per cent). However, a cold nodule may be malignant in 10–15 per cent of cases.

A scan is also useful in the identification of thyroid tissue whether in the tongue, neck, or mediastinum, and particularly in the differentiation of a mediastinal goitre from other tumours in this area.

Table IX.—CLINICAL DIAGNOSTIC INDEX FOR HYPERTHYROIDISM

The points shown are awarded according to whether the symptoms and signs listed are present or absent. The total score is then calculated; if it is over 19 hyperthyroidism is diagnosed, while if it is less than 11 the patient is euthyroid.

SYMPTOMS OF RECENT ONSET AND/OR INCREASED SEVERITY	PRESENT	ABSENT	SIGNS	PRESENT	ABSENT
Dyspnœa on effort	+1		Palpable thyroid	+3	−3
Palpitations	+2		Bruit over thyroid	+2	−2
Tiredness	+2		Exophthalmos	+2	
Preference for heat (irrespective of duration)		−5	Lid retraction Lid lag	+2 +1	
Preference for cold	+5		Hyperkinesis	+4	−2
Excessive sweating	+3		Finger tremor	+1	
Nervousness	+2		Hands: Hot Moist	 +2 +1	 −2 −1
Appetite: Increased Decreased	+3	−3	Casual pulse-rate: Less than 80/min. More than 90/min. Auricular fibrilla- tion	 +3 +4	−3
Weight: Increased Decreased	+3	−3			
Totals			Totals		
Total symptoms score			Total signs score		

Total score

ii. Vocal Cords.—Paralysis of a vocal cord is relatively common in carcinoma of the thyroid. Their function should be noted on the patient's chart prior to thyroidectomy.

iii. Radiographs of neck and upper thorax may show tracheal compression or displacement, and radiographs of the chest may reveal metastases.

iv. Needle Biopsy.—Because of the danger of needle implants of carcinoma, this procedure is not advised for the routine assessment of thyroid nodules. It may be helpful in the histological diagnosis of inoperable carcinoma and thyroiditis.

B. Auto-immune Thyroiditis.—

1. *Precipitin Test.*—Precipitation takes 3–7 days.
2. *Tanned Red-cell Hæmagglutination Test* (TCH).
3. *Complement Fixation Test* (CFT).

For each of these tests 5 ml. of blood are required. Interpretation of results needs an expert knowledge of the incidence of positive results in various types of thyroid disease; the immunologist should be consulted. The TCH test measures antibody to thyroglobulin and is positive in 80 per cent of Hashimoto's thyroiditis and 40 per cent of hyperthyroid cases. The CFT against thyroid cytoplasm gives a similar percentage of positive results in thyroiditis and 40 per cent positive in patients with pernicious anæmia. The precipitin test is almost always negative in simple goitre, carcinoma, and hyperthyroidism.

C. Hypothyroidism.—

1. *Radio-iodine Uptake.*—In hypothyroid states it is necessary to measure results after 24 or 48 hours or after TSH stimulation.

2. *Protein-bound Iodine.*—5 ml. of clotted blood required.

3. *Serum Cholesterol.*—Send 5 ml. of blood to the laboratory.

4. *ECG.*—An electrocardiogram is also required in any patient with fibrillation or in whom there is reason to suspect cardiac damage.

Thyroidectomy is an effective method of treatment for selected cases of hyperthyroidism, nodular goitre, and thyroid carcinoma.

HYPERTHYROIDISM

Preparation for Thyroidectomy.—Successful surgical management requires that the patient be restored to a normal (euthyroid) state before operation. An excess of circulating thyroid hormone produces changes in many organs. The heart muscle is most seriously affected, producing tachycardia and dyspnœa; auricular fibrillation is seen in about 10 per cent of patients and, not infrequently, heart failure. Nervousness, excitability, and emotional instability are common and there may be muscle weakness, particularly in the lower limbs. The nutrition of the patient is impaired. These changes, which reflect the increased metabolic rate, call for an adequate pre-operative course of therapy with an antithyroid drug. The agents in common use and their daily doses are:—

Propylthiouracil	300– 400 mg.
Methylthiouracil	100– 300 mg.
Methimazole (tapazole)	20– 60 mg.
Potassium perchlorate	600–1000 mg.

The daily dose should be divided and given in 6–8-hourly equal portions. The patient is seen weekly to assess the response to treatment and to watch for complications. This examination should include a leucocyte count. The thiouracil drugs produce a leucopenia in 4–5 per cent of patients, which may progress to agranulocytosis, particularly if treatment is prolonged or the dosage excessive. Potassium perchlorate is a useful alternative for those sensitive to thiouracil. *Iodide* in the form of Lugol's iodine (10 drops three times daily in milk) is usually given during the week before operation. It is believed to reverse the vascularity and friability of the gland produced by thiouracil.

Pre-operative Sedation.—Pentobarbital sodium (nembutal), 100–200 mg., or a similar preparation should be given in the evening preceding operation, to allay apprehension. Morphine, 10 mg., and hyoscine, 0·4 mg., are given 1 hour before operation.

Post-operative Management.—Complications are uncommon when the patient is euthyroid and the operation is meticulously performed, with identification and preservation of the parathyroid glands and the recurrent laryngeal nerves. Among the possible complications are:—

Nembuta (Abbott Laboratories Ltd., Queenborough, Kent).

HÆMORRHAGE.—If bleeding is persistent and significant, the patient should be reanæsthetized, the incision opened, the bleeding controlled, and a tracheostomy done if necessary. The main danger is a tamponade of the airway; the house-surgeon must be prepared hastily to remove a few skin stitches in the ward and evacuate blood and clot.

AIRWAY OBSTRUCTION.—The patient should not leave the operating room until an unobstructed airway is assured. The function of the vocal cords should be assessed when the endotracheal tube is removed. If one or both nerves are damaged or if œdema is marked, tracheostomy is usually necessary.

PARATHYROID INSUFFICIENCY.—Hypoparathyroidism is rare after thyroid lobectomy, uncommon after subtotal thyroidectomy for hyperthyroidism, but is a significant problem after total thyroidectomy for carcinoma, with or without radical neck dissection. It can be avoided by identifying and preserving one or more of the glands. (For treatment *see* p. 297.)

THYROID CRISIS.—Since the introduction of the antithyroid drugs, acute thyrotoxicosis is rarely seen. However, it occurs occasionally after an acute illness or an emergency operation in a patient with unrecognized or uncontrolled hyperthyroidism. The patient is acutely toxic, extremely restless, and confused. Tachycardia and pyrexia are marked.

Treatment.—Treatment is supportive and includes:—

1. *Hydration*: Intravenous glucose in water and saline is administered in sufficient quantity to replace the fluid loss, but care must be taken to avoid overloading the circulation.

2. *Sedation*: Heavy sedation with barbiturates and chlorpromazine is required.

3. *Hypothermia*: The body is cooled with ice packs or a hypothermia blanket.

4. *Cortisone* should be administered intravenously in large doses (1·0 G. in the first 24 hr.).

5. *Iodine* is given intravenously, a solution containing 1 G. sodium iodide every 4 hours.

In the absence of these complications, the post-operative management of a patient after routine thyroidectomy is relatively simple. Intravenous fluids are given for 12–24 hours. Pain is not marked and can be controlled by codeine or morphine. The drain can be removed in 24–48 hours. Sutures or Michel clips are removed early, after 3 to 5 days, to reduce the incisional scar.

THE MANAGEMENT OF THE PATIENT RECEIVING RADIOACTIVE IODINE

In *investigative studies* previous iodine consumption, for example in cough mixtures, in cholecystograms and pyelograms, interferes with radioactive uptake results and those of neck scanning. For this reason, all iodine should be excluded for 6–8 weeks before these studies. The amount of radioactivity involved in these examinations is not a health hazard.

If radioactive iodine is used in the *treatment of hyperthyroidism*, the only necessary precaution is the disposal of the urine down a flush toilet for the first 24 hours. In the *treatment of thyroid cancer* the dose is increased by ten times or more and the patient's excreta are a potential health hazard. For the first 24 hours the patient is confined to a single room and young or pregnant visitors and attendants are excluded. Urine and vomitus are stored in a shielded area for at least 24 hours and disposed of when the radioactivity count falls to a sufficiently low level.

There is a high incidence of hypothyroidism after the treatment of hyperthyroidism with [131]I. Such patients must be followed carefully and given thyroid hormone replacement (*l*-thyroxine 0·3 mg. daily) as necessary.

THE MANAGEMENT OF PARATHYROID CASES

1. HYPERPARATHYROIDISM

Hyperparathyroidism is much more common than generally believed. The diagnosis would be less frequently missed if accurate serum-calcium determinations were done as part of the investigation of all patients with renal calculi, skeletal abnormalities, peptic ulceration, pancreatic disease, and emotional disorders.

Serial serum-calcium estimations are by far the most important step in making a diagnosis of hyperparathyroidism. First ascertain what value your laboratory accepts as being the upper limit of normal (usually about 5 mEq./l.). Then take blood samples on three or more mornings when the patient is fasting. Only occlude the vein momentarily before the needle enters it, to prevent stagnation; and check that the plasma proteins are normal quantitatively and qualitatively (electrophoretic strip). Serum-phosphate levels are also determined.

Numerous complicated tests such as calcium-balance studies and calcium-infusion tests have been devised for the diagnosis of parathyroid hypersecretion. Their popularity has generally been short-lived and their usefulness less than that of repeated fasting serum-calcium estimations.

When bone disease is suspected, radiographs of the hands and skull give the earliest evidence of bone resorption. The serum-alkaline phosphatase level should be determined.

If renal calculi are present a full urological work-up is necessary (*see* Chapter XXXI). When there is azotæmia, the serum calcium may not be as high, nor the phosphorus as low, as might otherwise have been the case.

Parathyroid exploration is advisable in patients with hypercalcæmia in whom other causes have been excluded, e.g., sarcoidosis, multiple myeloma, metastatic carcinoma, and certain renal disorders.

Pre-operative Management.—The most common complication of this disease is renal calculi and varying degrees of kidney damage, secondary to obstruction or renal calcinosis. Except for the relief of ureteric obstruction by bilateral stones, parathyroid exploration should be done first. The renal complications are dealt with later. If the urine is infected, the antibacterial agent most lethal to the principal organisms should be administered. Matched blood should be available because it is occasionally necessary to explore the anterior mediastinum, as well as the neck, for ectopic parathyroid glands.

Post-operative Management.—With the exception of thyroid crisis, the same complications may follow parathyroidectomy as follow thyroidectomy. Their treatment is given on p. 296. A serum-calcium estimation should be done daily to assess the effect of operation and to guide treatment of parathyroid insufficiency. Serum magnesium should be checked on the third day if there has been skeletal demineralization.

2. HYPOPARATHYROIDISM

This complication, unusual after thyroidectomy, is not uncommon after parathyroid exploration, particularly in patients with marked skeletal disease. The symptoms—nervousness, tingling and numbness of the lips, nose, and extremities

—usually appear 2–3 days after operation. The diagnosis is confirmed by eliciting Trousseau's sign (*Fig.* 222) and by the finding of a low serum calcium.

Immediate Treatment of Tetany.—Calcium gluconate, 10 ml. of a 10 per cent solution, is given intravenously. This is followed by an intravenous infusion of 100 ml. of 10 per cent calcium gluconate in 1 litre of 5 per cent glucose and water given over a 4-hour period.

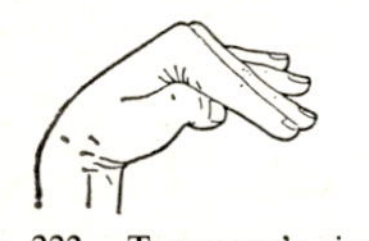
Fig. 222.—Trousseau's sign.

Then give calcium chloride solution by mouth (100 mg. calcium per ml.) at a dosage of 4–8 ml. four times daily. To avoid gastric irritation, this should be diluted with milk or water and not given on an empty stomach. An alternative but more expensive preparation is calcium effervescent tablets (calcium sandoz), each equivalent to 4 G. calcium gluconate and given three times daily.

The serum-calcium levels usually return to normal within 7–14 days.

Vitamin D.—This is unnecessary if hypoparathyroidism is temporary, but may be required, in addition to calcium supplements, for chronic hypoparathyroidism. The usual dose is 50,000 units daily. Vitamin D has a cumulative action, so that the maximum effect of a given daily dose may not be manifest for several weeks. It is advisable to observe the effects of any given dose for a month or two before the dose is increased.

The patient and his serum-calcium levels must be followed until normal, and indefinitely when a diagnosis of chronic hypoparathyroidism has been established. Hypoparathyroidism, frequently with borderline serum calciums, may give rise to persistent paræsthesias, cramps, mental depression, eczema, falling hair, and cataracts. Suitable maintenance doses of calcium and vitamin D are needed. There is a danger of hypervitaminosis D if the dose is excessive, resulting in renal dysfunction, nephrocalcinosis, and metastatic calcification. Thus the need to follow hypoparathyroid patients carefully, with particular attention to serum-calcium determinations, is stressed.

THE MANAGEMENT OF HARE-LIP AND CLEFT-PALATE CASES

Hare-lip and cleft palate are relatively common congenital abnormalities. One or both defects may occur in the same patient. When present they are associated with an increased incidence of other congenital abnormalities.

HARE-LIP

Time of Operation.—10–10–10 (10 lb., 10 weeks, and hæmoglobin 10 G.).

Pre-operative Management.—Breast feeding is encouraged; if unsuccessful use either a teat with a large hole, a Brecht feeder, or a pipette.

The Operation.—This requires a general endotracheal anæsthetic. It is designed to correct the associated nasal deformity and to lengthen the cleft segment of the lip to normal by the use of the Z-plasty principle (*Fig.* 223).

Post-operative Management.—Complications to be aware of are: wound sepsis and breakdown, pneumonia due to atelectasis and aspiration, and upper respiratory infections including otitis media.

The care of the sutured lip includes:—

1. A Logan's bow is attached to the cheeks to prevent rubbing and tension on the suture line.

2. A restraining jacket provides further protection.

3. Nasal and oral secretions are suctioned frequently.

Calcium Sandoz (Sandoz Products Ltd., 23 Great Castle Street, London, W.1).

4. The suture line is kept clean with mild antiseptic.

5. A sugar solution (10 per cent glucose and water) is given by a sterile rubber-tipped medicine dropper for 48 hours; then the pre-operative formula is used.

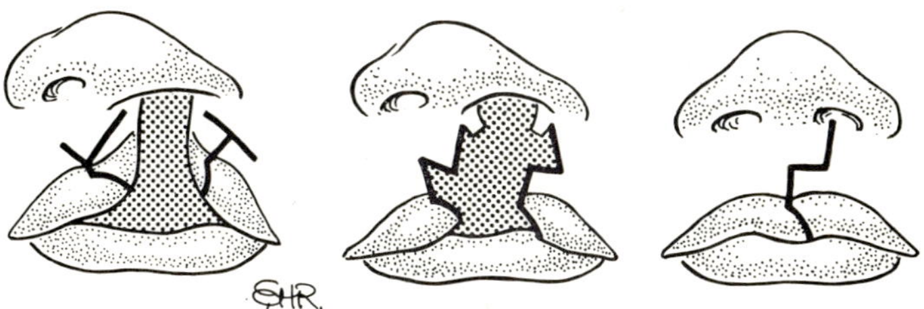

Fig. 223.—Cleft lip: the LeMesurier method of lip repair. The incision is marked out (*left*), the edges of the defect pared (*centre*) and sutured (*right*).

6. To prevent aspiration, solid foods and oily preparations should not be given until the fifth or sixth day. The chest should be examined regularly.

7. Sutures are removed in 5 or 6 days.

8. Oral antibiotics are given if infection occurs.

CLEFT PALATE

Time of Repair.—16–18 months.

Pre-operative Management.—The child should be free of carious teeth and upper respiratory infection. Blood should be available for transfusion. An intravenous infusion of Ringer's lactate solution or normal saline should be running before the operation is begun.

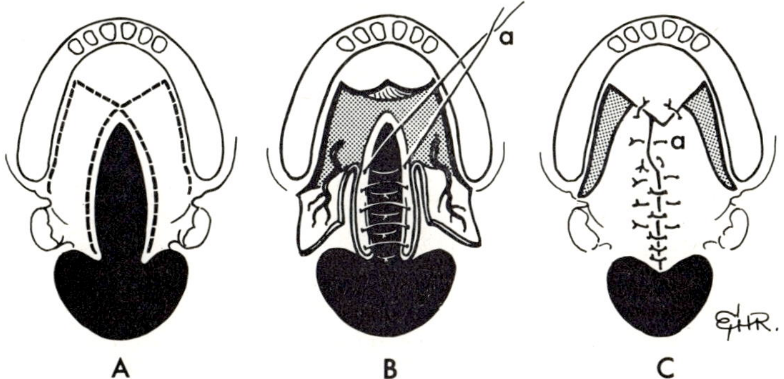

Fig. 224.—Cleft palate: a method of closing the midline defect and lengthening the palate. The muco-periosteal flaps (A) are mobilized posteriorly (B) and sutured (C).

Operation.—An endotracheal tube is inserted through the mouth. Care must be taken to maintain the airway following the extension of the neck and the insertion of the mouth retractor. Blood-loss should be measured and replaced if the loss is greater than 10 per cent of the blood-volume (calculated as 80 ml. per kg. of body-weight). The average loss is 45–50 ml. or 5 per cent of the blood-volume.

The purpose of the operation is to create a functioning partition between the nasopharynx and oropharynx, by a shift of the lateral segments of the cleft palate to the midline, and posteriorly (*Fig.* 224).

Post-operative Management.—Complications to be aware of are: upper respiratory infections, otitis media, and pneumonia due to aspiration or atelectasis. Persistent bleeding or secondary hæmorrhage may require reoperation and suture control of the bleeding point. If wound dehiscence occurs it is usually related to a poor nutritional state or an oral or respiratory infection. Until these are corrected and the child is thriving, reoperation should be delayed.

1. Following operation a restraining jacket is applied.

2. The mouth and nose are sucked out gently and frequently.

3. Sugar solution (10 per cent glucose in water) is given by medicine glass for 48 hours; thereafter milk is given by glass, and puréed foods by spoon.

4. The ears and chest should be examined frequently.

5. The non-absorbable sutures are removed under a general anæsthetic on the tenth post-operative day.

SUBSEQUENT MANAGEMENT OF THE HARE-LIP AND CLEFT PALATE

The initial operation on the lip and palate is the beginning of a programme which is prolonged and involves the plastic surgeon, orthodontist, prosthodontist, and speech therapist. Occasionally consideration must be given to revisions of the lip and nose, the closure of residual palatal defects by surgical or prosthetic methods, pharyngoplasty, and the assessment and treatment of speech problems. The parents should be advised that further treatment will be necessary and arrangements made for this to be done in a centre adequately equipped and staffed by personnel interested in these problems.

CHAPTER XXIII

THE MANAGEMENT OF SURGICAL THORACIC CASES

By T. Holmes Sellors

OXYGEN THERAPY

The indications for the use of oxygen are many and varied, and the method of administration will depend on the circumstances. For example, a high concentration for a short period will be required in an anoxic emergency, while a lower flow-rate over a prolonged period is more suitable in cases of chronic respiratory or circulatory insufficiency.

There are certain basic considerations that apply to the use of oxygen in surgery as opposed to medicine. It is frequently required in the post-operative phase when the semiconscious patient is intolerant of any apparatus that encloses or restricts him, and it is also desirable that there should be free access to the patient for nursing purposes.

METHODS OF ADMINISTRATION

The two methods by which oxygen can be given is to enclose the patient completely in an atmosphere of oxygen—the oxygen tent—or to administer the gas by a face-mask or nasal catheters. The rate of oxygen flow will vary according to the circumstances—a high flow-rate of 6–8 litres a minute is necessary for the oxygen tent, but lower rates of 2–4 litres are adequate for masks or catheters. The oxygen may be humidified by rebreathing at low flow-rates, but it is normally kept moist by passing over or by bubbling through water. A blast of cold, dry oxygen on to the patient's mucous membranes is undesirable as well as uncomfortable.

A continuous supply of oxygen has to be ensured either from piped oxygen to the wards or by relays of cylinders. A standard 120 cu. ft. cylinder delivering 6 litres a minute will last approximately 9 hours; at 2 litres it will last up to 28 hours. All cylinders should have an attached flow-meter to register the amount being delivered.

Oxygen Tents.—These are satisfactory for continuous administration at a comparatively high concentration and are suitable for cyanotic heart conditions, severe post-operative lung complications, and respiratory insufficiency.

In spite of transparent panels patients complain of stuffiness and heat, and show signs of claustrophobia. From the nursing point of view, the tent imposes a psychological and physical barrier to the finer points of nursing care.

A minimum flow of 8 litres per minute is required and the humidification and temperature levels are achieved by passing the oxygen over ice (of which large quantities are required). The oxygen content of the gases in the tent should be regularly measured.

The capital outlay and maintenance of the equipment are overcome in some centres by hiring.* Regular practice in setting up the tent should be carried out so as to be ready in emergency.

---

* Oxygen tents can be hired from Oxygenaire Ltd., Basingstoke, Hants. (Branches in most cities in Britain.)

Incubators.—These small 'oxygen' boxes are specially designed for the nursing of premature babies and small infants. They are completely transparent, heated, and give easy access to the patients, as well as maintaining the appropriate oxygen concentration.

Nasal Catheters.—A simple flexible tube passed into one nostril will give a concentration of 20–25 per cent oxygen in the inspired air with a flow of 2–3 litres per minute. The tube has to be fixed with fine adhesive strips to the face or forehead to avoid it falling out and, even if smeared with local anæsthetic ointment, it may be irritating to the patient.

Bilateral nasal catheters which just enter the nares have become increasingly popular (*Fig*. 225). These tubes are light, easily adjusted, and well tolerated with oxygen flows of 2–3 litres per minute. Above this figure the jets of oxygen become irritating and possibly traumatic to the nasal mucosa. The openings of

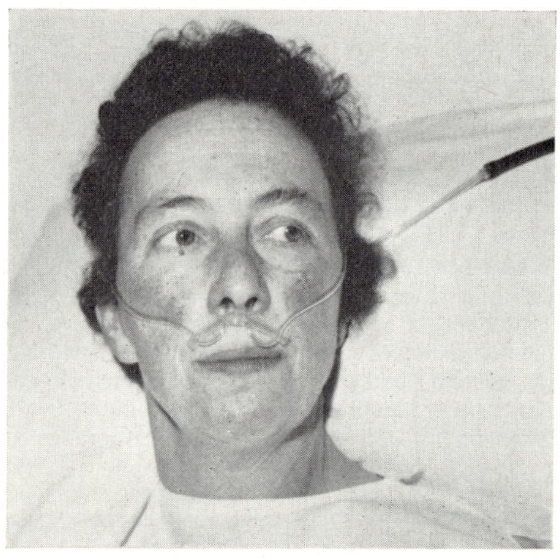

Fig. 225.—Nasal tubes for oxygen administration. These are disposable and light with minimal inconvenience to the patient.

the tubes should be directed almost horizontally well into the nares to ensure that the oxygen is actually inspired and not simply blowing over the face. Humidification over warm water is necessary.

These catheters are admirable for long-term low flow-rates and enable the patient to eat and sleep without disturbance.

Oxygen Masks.—Oxygen masks have stood the test of time both in medicine and at high altitudes, but the original forms such as the B.L.B. or Barach-Eckmann have been replaced by disposable, lightweight, transparent types, of which many varieties have been produced.

The essential features for any mask is that it should be light, that the face piece should fit well (even in an edentulous elderly patient), and that it should be tolerated well with reasonably high flows of oxygen. Humidification is necessary for any long-term use.

The description of three types does not exclude the use of other models that meet the necessary specifications.

The M-C (Catterall) Mask is a highly efficient apparatus with a small, firm transparent face piece padded with plastic foam (*Fig. 226*).

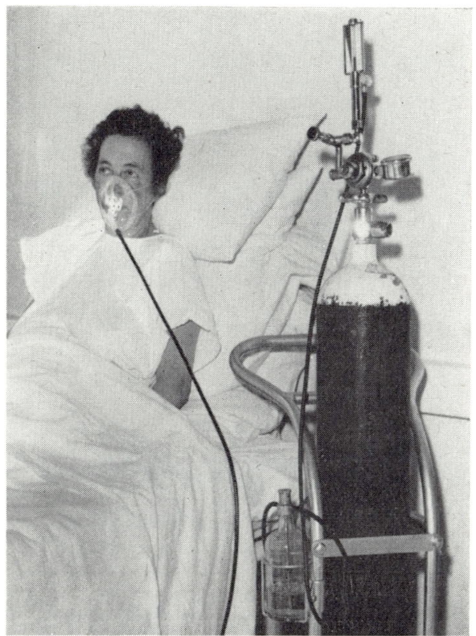

Fig. 226.—Oxygen mask. M-C pattern—showing oxygen cylinder, flow-meter, and humidifier.

At low flow-rates, 2 litres per minute, humidification is not necessary as the moisture comes from rebreathing and a 40 per cent oxygen concentration is achieved in the inspired air. A 6-litre flow produces 60 per cent and 8 litres gives 70 per cent concentration.

In an emergency it is recommended that high flow and full humidification is used for 1 hour and the oxygen flow is then gradually reduced to 2 litres.

This is probably the most satisfactory mask in current use, but, in unconscious patients who are sweating, care must be taken to avoid pressure ulceration on the bridge of the nose.

The Ventimask acts on the Venturi or injector principle and delivers a fixed oxygen concentration which is stamped on the apparatus. There are two patterns: one delivering 27 per cent at 4 litres per minute, the other 35 per cent at 8 litres. In spite of its appearance it is light and well tolerated. Its great advantage is that, by not raising the oxygen concentration too high, it prevents hypoventilation with a subsequent build-up of carbon dioxide.

The Polymask (*Fig.* 227) has many advantages in being light and fitting well with a self-inflating cuff, but it has one grave disadvantage. Being made of soft

M-C mask (Bakelite Xylonite Ltd., Darton, nr. Barnsley, Yorks).
Ventimask (Oxygenaire Ltd., Basingstoke, Hants).
Polymask (British Oxygen Co., Hammersmith House, London, W.6).

plastic it can collapse or be sucked in on the patient's face if the oxygen inlet tube is obstructed or kinked. No unconscious patient should be left unattended with one of these masks. They are, however, valuable for transport from operating theatre to ward or where there is constant attention.

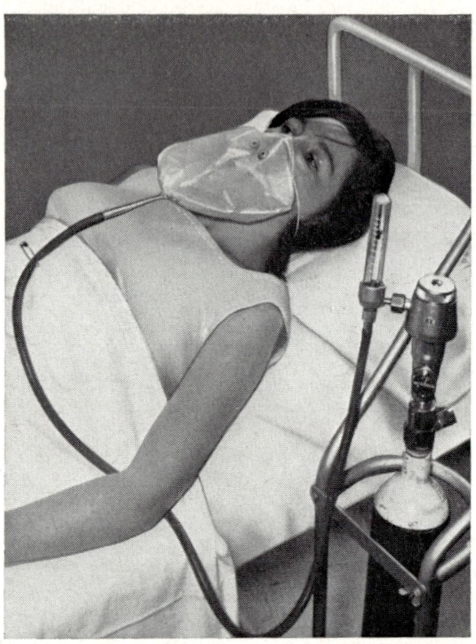

Fig. 227.—The polymask. This is only to be used if there is constant supervision to avoid the danger of sucking the mask over the air-passages.

Dangers.—Methods of administration of oxygen have made great progress since the days in which a funnel attached to a small oxygen cylinder blew the gas over the patient's face. At the present time the extensive use of oxygen should not be so haphazard and the risks of (*a*) oxygen poisoning, or (*b*) its inflammability, must not be overlooked.

Warning.—Oxygen itself does not burn, but in its presence any inflammable object burns more vigorously than in air. Consequently all oxygen administration is open to the grave risk of fire and explosion; many of these explosions have proved fatal. All forms of spark, fire, or combustibles must be kept away.

The following are examples of what must be avoided: smoking, matches, electric light and power switches, night lights, sparking toys, static sparks from combing the hair vigorously, gas rings, and gas lighting. The most dangerous practice of all is to grease the screw-fitting of any oxygen cylinder. Oxygen and grease under pressure do not merely burn—they explode.

PRINCIPLES OF TREATMENT IN THORACIC SURGERY

Nearly every thoracic operation involves opening into the pleural cavity. This temporarily destroys the physical conditions under which the lungs are kept fully expanded. When the operation is completed, it is essential to restore the normal conditions of the pleural cavity and not to allow the lung to remain collapsed.

Inflation of the lung by the anæsthetist ensures expansion of the lung, but there must be an escape route for air and/or fluid that may collect after closure of the chest wall.

This is achieved by aspiration (p. 307) or closed drainage (p. 310) of the pleural cavity. Either method ensures removal of air and fluid, and brings the surface of the lung into apposition with the parietal pleura and obliterates the dead space.

Any thoracotomy is followed by a collection of blood-stained effusion which may amount to 300–600 ml.; in addition, any air leak that may be occasioned in lung resection operations may persist for some days before it seals off. For this reason closed suction drainage is commonly used for 24 or 48 hours at least, until no bubbles of air appear and the lung is radiologically fully expanded. The only exception to this is pneumonectomy, where effusion and air are used to fill up the dead space occasioned by removal of the lung. After a lobectomy the residual lobe or lobes will stretch or overexpand to fill in this dead space.

Under no circumstances should open drainage be used where the pleural cavity is free.

TENSION OR PRESSURE PNEUMOTHORAX

Apart from injury to the lung surface at operation, spontaneous rupture of a bulla or cyst from a lung fringe may occur. Commonly, as the lung collapses with the ensuing pneumothorax, the leak is self-sealing, but, should it persist, it will not only collapse the lung, but will ultimately press on the mediastinum.

The onset is usually marked by some pain in the chest and breathlessness which may subside, but if tension develops there will be intense respiratory distress and cyanosis. The signs of pneumothorax (absent breath sounds and hyperresonance) will be present, but they give no indication as to the extent of the condition. Pushing over of the mediastinum and trachea in the suprasternal notch is indicative of 'tension' which can be confirmed by X-ray examination.

Treatment.—Tension constitutes a major urgency which is simply treated in the first instance by aspiration of air. In an emergency a needle can be thrust into the pleural cavity through the 2nd interspace anteriorly and connected to a length of fine rubber tubing whose open end lies in a bowl of water where the escaping bubbles can be observed.

The more formal method is to use an artificial pneumothorax apparatus (*see* p. 668) and to measure the amount of air removed, as well as to record the pleural pressure. The Maxwell pattern has the advantage of being compact and portable. After introduction of the needle, air is sucked out until no more can be removed and there is a 'negative' pressure in the pleural cavity. The pressures should be confirmed after an interval of some minutes, and should they have altered the presence of a persistent leak may be inferred—and this may require continuous tube drainage rather than aspiration.

HÆMOTHORAX

Blood within the pleural cavity remains fluid and can be removed by aspiration. It occurs most commonly as the result of closed or penetrating chest injuries, but may also occur as a result of neoplastic or tuberculous invasion.

The reason for the blood remaining fluid is not the result of any clotting failure, but follows defibrination of the blood as a result of cardiac and pulmonary movements which whip out the fibrin. A large hæmothorax may amount to 2·5–3 litres and produce 'tension' signs, but by the time treatment is instituted the hæmoglobin content may have fallen as much as 25–30 per cent below that of the circulating blood in a few hours. This is due to irritation of the pleura and the formation of a secondary effusion which dilutes the blood. What appears to be pure blood may actually contain as little as 10–20 per cent hæmoglobin. The effusion carries an additional factor in the form of fibrinogen, which increases to such an extent that it is higher than the blood level at the end of a week or ten days. In this event the whole mass may form a secondary clot. This is strictly not a clotted hæmothorax but a clotted effusion stained by blood.

Treatment.—Early removal of fluid blood by aspiration avoids a much more detailed and complex procedure that has to be used when clot has formed.

All hæmothoraces should be completely evacuated within 24–48 hours of an injury no matter what their size, and the aspiration repeated daily if there is any evidence of further fluid. The presence of clot or organization of fibrin on the lung and chest wall leads to delayed expansion and loss of function.

PLEURAL INFECTION

Two stages can be recognized in the process of pleural infection:—
1. Diffuse suppurative pleurisy.
2. Localized pleural abscess or empyema.

Though empyema is much less common than formerly due to the reduction of lung infection, it does occur and, if early treatment has not been initiated or is unsuccessful, the chronic state can be prolonged and cause great disability. The early recognition and treatment of pleural infection may save months of ill health.

The earliest evidence of pleural infection is a clear effusion teaming with bacteria, but whose signs are masked by the underlying lung infection. Within a day or so the fluid is turbid due to leucocytes and dead bacteria, and at this stage it can be aspirated. By the end of a week or ten days thin pus is present and, though this can be aspirated, the presence of fibrin flakes may obstruct the needle. When this occurs it can be assumed that fibrin deposit is beginning to line the infected area and to localize it, and, when the pus is thick or 'frank', the diffuse stage has been converted into a localized abscess.

Treatment.—There are two principles in treatment:—
1. Removal of breakdown and toxic products.
2. Closure of the abscess cavity.

It is the closure of an empyema that causes so much trouble. The lung tends to retract from the parietes and the chest wall is too rigid to fall into the dead space. 'Negative' pressure or suction, either intermittent (aspiration) or continuous (closed drainage), is required to remove the contents and to encourage the lung to expand and obliterate the cavity.

When aspiration fails, closed drainage is indicated and must be continued until there is a thick-walled abscess cavity. At this stage open drainage can be used (for the only time in thoracic surgery). The use of antibiotics has confused the issue to the extent that the abscess can be sterilized, but, if a space still remains, it must be closed by drainage or pleurectomy and not left alone to become more and more fibrous and rigid.

ASPIRATION OF THE CHEST

Clinical and radiological examination indicates the most likely site for exploration. This is commonly the 8th or 9th space, one hand-breadth away from the midline.

Position of the Patient.—The patient should lean forwards with arms resting comfortably on a hospital type of bed-table (*Fig.* 228). When the arms are

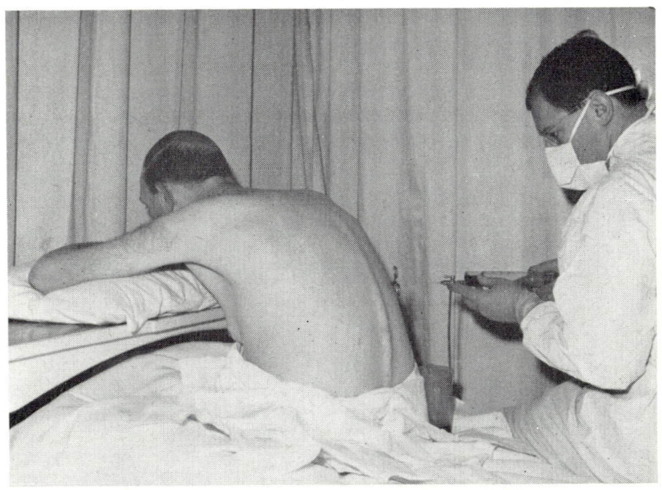

Fig. 228.—Aspiration of the pleural cavity. The patient is leaning forward and is well supported. A 50-ml. syringe with a two-way tap is being used.

carried forward, the scapulæ are carried away from the region of the paravertebral gutter. Because the procedure may take time, the operator as well as the patient must be comfortable.

Anæsthesia.—A small quantity of local anæsthetic solution is injected under the skin with a very fine needle. With a somewhat larger needle the deeper tissues are infiltrated with particular attention to the area outside the actual pleural membrane. About 7–10 ml. of dilute local anæsthetic will be needed.

Apparatus (*Fig.* 229).—A variety of needles and a 20- or 50-ml. syringe are the basic requirements, but, to ensure that there is no leak of air into the system, lock-on or bayonet catch joints are desirable. There should also be a two-way tap between the needle and syringe so that the syringe can be emptied without having to disconnect it and run the risk of admitting air.

Technique.—After waiting a few minutes to give the anæsthetic time to work, the skin is nicked with a tenotomy knife and a large-bore needle is inserted through this incision. (If the skin is not incised there is a risk of carrying a core of infected dermis into the pleural cavity.) The syringe attached to the needle can contain a few ml. of the local anæsthetic solution and, as suction is exerted by the piston of the syringe, the needle is advanced through the intercostal space into the pleural cavity. It is possible to gauge the thickness of the membrane which, in normal circumstances, is no thicker than a piece of thin paper but, when inflamed, becomes appreciably more tough and with advanced pleural infection gives a rubber-like or woody sensation.

Findings.—

1. *Gas is withdrawn.*—If, instead of fluid, gas appears in the syringe, it may be due to one of three causes:—

a. A leak in the needle-syringe outfit.

b. Puncture of the lung.

c. Air in the pleural cavity. There may be an air leak—spontaneous pneumothorax—but this should have been recognized previously. Offensive gas may be produced by anaerobic organisms.

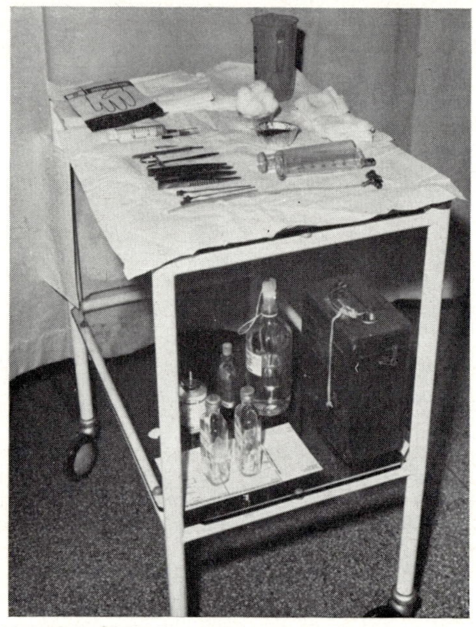

Fig. 229.—Apparatus for aspiration of the chest, including a large tight-fitting glass syringe and a two-way tap, with a selection of aspirating needles.

2. *Fluid is withdrawn.*—Clear fluid, usually straw-coloured, indicates a pleural effusion whose origin will have to be determined by bacteriological or cytological examination. Fluid that quickly forms a clot when removed from the body indicates a high fibrin content.

3. *Blood is withdrawn.*—It is essential to note the colour and character of the first few drops of fluid that appear in the syringe. If they are initially clear, the later appearance of blood suggests trauma arising from puncture of the lung or of a chest-wall vessel. Blood-stained fluid should be estimated for its hæmoglobin content and not interpreted as being pure blood. Fluid the colour of port wine may show as little as 10 or 15 per cent hæmoglobin content. The presence of a heavily blood-stained effusion is suggestive of a new growth or tuberculosis. Withdrawal of pure blood suggests puncture of the heart or, in

some cases, puncture of the liver. If aspiration is performed as a post-operative procedure, the fluid will certainly be blood-stained.

4. *Pus is withdrawn.*—The character of the pus withdrawn into the syringe should be noted in respect of its viscosity and colour. At least two specimens should be provided, one to leave in a test-tube to observe the amount of deposit in 12 hours, and the other for bacteriological examination. Direct film staining may give a clue to the organism without having to wait for cultures or sensitivities to antibiotics.

The site and depth at which pus was obtained must be carefully noted and, wherever possible, the pleural cavity should be emptied of its contents as completely as possible. Should the aspirating needle become blocked, it indicates that fibrin flecks are present and that the pleural inflammation is certainly 7–10 days old. Use of a wider-bore needle or flushing out the needle may allow the operation to continue, but once a needle has become blocked from this cause blocking is likely to be repeated.

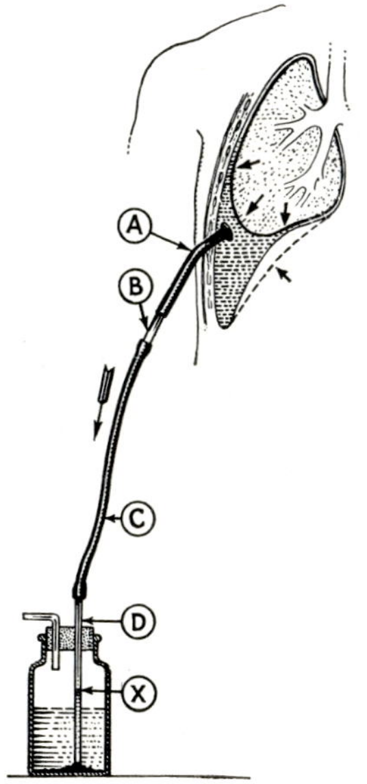

Fig. 230.—The principles of 'closed' drainage (*see text*).

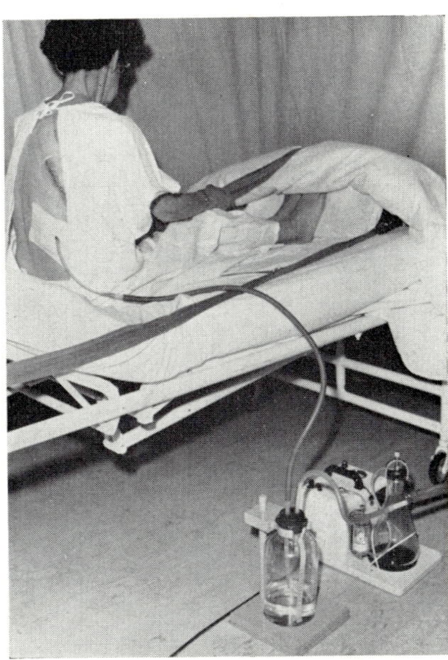

Fig. 231.—Post-operative closed drainage. Note drainage tube leading (without loops) to drainage bottle, in the front of which is a small suction motor.

Failure to find pus on one aspiration should be followed by further attempts, angling the needle slightly from one side to another and up and down. It may be that aspiration has been performed too low, in which case a further attempt in a higher place can be tried. More often the failure to aspirate and find fluid in the pleural cavity is due to inadequate localization, which should have been confirmed by postero-anterior and lateral radiographs. Failure to find fluid where it is suspected should lead to reappraisal of the situation, with possible further attempts the following day.

CLOSED WATER-SEAL DRAINAGE

When the end of a pleural drainage tube is placed under water, air cannot be sucked back into the pleural cavity. Respiration and coughing continue to eject air and fluid along the tube and help the lungs to expand.

Apparatus.—The apparatus required is simple and is illustrated in *Fig.* 230. The drainage tube (A) which leaves the chest wall through a stab wound is connected (B) by further tubing (C), which is attached to glass or plastic tubing (X) dipping *below* the surface of water in a large-capacity bottle. Alterations in the pleural pressure lead to the fluid swinging up and down the glass tube (X) and, if the patient coughs and any air is still present, it will blow bubbles into the bottle. Suction may be applied to the small outlet tube from the bottle (*Fig.* 231).

A free and unkinked closed drainage system will continue to conduct fluid into the bottle until the lung has fully expanded and the pleural space is obliterated. The efficiency of the system is governed by its narrowest part, usually

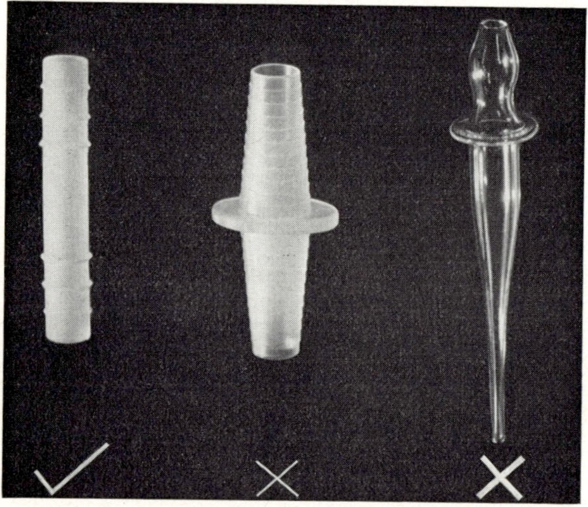

Fig. 232.—Connexions. The straight tube is acceptable, the other two are not. Connexions should be made of plastic in preference to glass and must have the widest possible lumen.

the connexions (*Fig.* 232). These must not be unduly tapered and should have an internal lumen as wide as the chest tube, otherwise blood-clot or fibrin may occlude the system. Further weak spots in a system can be kinking or angulation of the chest tube by the patient lying on it or from pressure of bedclothes, and looping of the intermediate length of tubing or its kinking.

If the system has become blocked (absence of oscillation of the fluid level in the bottle) the tubing should be inspected for elementary mechanical errors and the intermediate tubing (C) can be 'milked' downwards. This may dislodge clot or fibrin, but if the block persists it may be for the desirable reason that the lung has fully expanded and has occluded the tube openings within the chest.

At this point, if full expansion is noted radiologically also, the tube can be removed.

Cautions.—The water-seal system can at no time be disconnected without having doubly clamped the chest tube with hæmostats. This will only be necessary for changing the bottle and measuring the amount of drainage.

Free bubbling into the bottle suggests a leak in one of three places—the apparatus and connexions, the pleural cavity and the outer air, or the pleura and the air-passages.

Leakage.—Normally there is an air-tight joint between skin and drainage tube, but if the tube has to be left in situ for more than 10 days there is a risk of leaking alongside the tube and consequent failure of the closed system, with sucking of air into the pleural cavity. If the cavity has become adherent the damage is minimal, but with a free space (and a total pneumothorax) the tube must be removed and another air-tight one inserted nearby.

INTERCOSTAL DRAINAGE

After any intrathoracic operation the pleural cavity is drained for at least 24 hours by a tube that is passed through an intercostal space via a stab wound. The tube is held in place by a skin-stitch tied firmly round it, and a long loose stitch is passed through the skin edges to be tied when the tube is withdrawn.

The tube is connected to a closed water-seal before the chest wound is finally closed and the lung is fully expanded by the anæsthetist to remove air.

Removal of the Tube.—This is carried out by cutting the holding stitch and having the loose stitch ready to tie after clamping the tube. The tube is then taken in one hand by the operator, who holds in his other hand a sterile pad of petroleum jelly gauze or tulle gras which is firmly placed over the stab incision as the tube is smartly withdrawn. The loose stitch is then tied under the pad which is covered by a short length of adhesive. At the moment of withdrawal the patient is instructed to cough to prevent any chance of air entering the chest. The procedure is much less alarming and more painless than might be imagined.

Continuous Drainage.—There are occasions when intercostal drainage is required to drain off a rapidly accumulating effusion—usually of streptococcal origin. Aspiration will have failed to keep pace with the collecting fluid and a more continuous form of aspiration is required. In such a case an intercostal tube, inserted via a trocar and cannula and connected to a closed water-seal system, may prove invaluable.

The technique for this procedure is similar to that of aspiration, except that considerably more generous injection of local anæsthetic is required and an incision 1 cm. long is made over the selected space. The trocars and cannulæ, which are made in three sizes, are designed to take a Malecot or de Pezzar catheter. The trocar-cannula is inserted through the anæsthetized skin incision and is guarded carefully with the index finger to avoid too deep penetration into the pleural cavity. The trocar is then withdrawn and the catheter stretched on its introducer is passed into the cavity so as to lie 2–3 cm. within the chest. Holding the catheter steady, the cannula is withdrawn and the catheter is connected *with the minimum of delay* to the closed water-seal system and held in place with a skin-stitch.

This form of drainage may be life-saving when there is a rapid accumulation of an effusion, but it should not be persisted with if the drainage becomes obstructed by fibrin flakes. The internal diameter of the tube is the limiting factor.

RIB RESECTION

Removal of a short length of rib over an empyema cavity has two main advantages—the cavity can be explored and a *wide* drainage tube can be inserted.

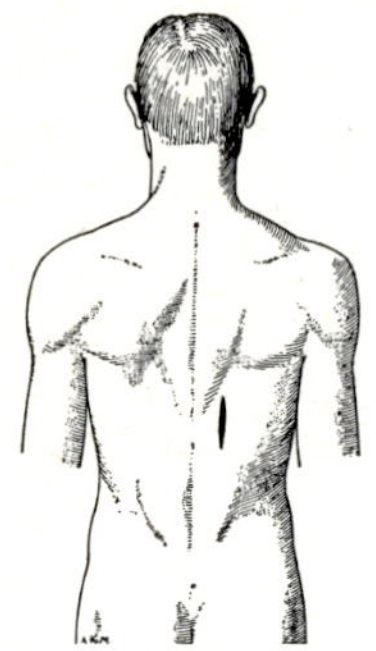

Fig. 233.—A vertical incision allows access to more than one rib, and is recommended in case the original localization by the needle is inaccurate.

Technique.—There is no constant site for this operation, which should be carried out with the patient in a sitting posture in case the existence of an unsuspected bronchopleural fistula should lead to flooding of the lungs with pus. Local or light general anæsthesia can be used. Careful localization with the aspirating needle must determine the lowest and most posterior point of the empyema cavity, so that drainage will occur by the action of gravity and, because the site of drainage is in the lowest part of the cavity, undrained pools will be avoided. The most usual place for drainage is through the bed of the 8th or 9th rib at the posterior angle of the rib just outside the sacrospinalis muscular mass. A vertical incision (*Fig.* 233) allows access to more than one rib in case the original localization by needle has not been accurate. After sub-periosteal resection of 2–2½ in. (5–6·3 cm.) of the appropriate rib, the empyema is opened through the rib bed, and pus flows out. The use of a mechanical sucker is advantageous.

The cavity is then explored through this small incision, first with the finger, in order to remove any fibrin or 'lymph' mass. If a special illuminator is available the interior of the cavity is inspected and all pockets of pus sucked dry.

A wide-bore tube is used for drainage, so placed that the inner opening lies within the cavity, but does not project so far that it impinges on the lung (*Figs.* 234, 235). Skin and muscle are loosely closed around the tube which is cut short externally and transfixed with a safety-pin (*Fig.* 236). The safety-pin is fastened to the drainage-tube in order to prevent it from slipping into the chest. It is prevented from coming out of the wound by anchoring the safety-pin to the chest wall with a narrow adhesive tape (*Fig.* 236),

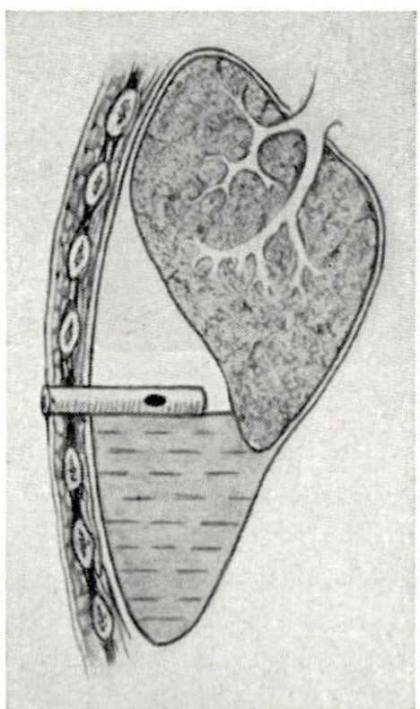

Fig. 234.—Faulty 'open' drainage. Tube too small and inserted too high.

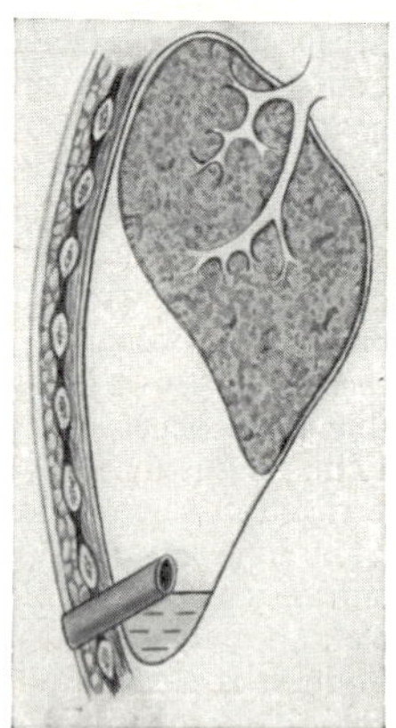

Fig. 235.—'Open' drainage. Large tube placed correctly.

and the whole is covered by light dressings. Circumferential binders do not always prevent the dressing from slipping, and tend to restrict respiratory excursions. Corsettage (*Fig.* 237) is the method which should be employed.

THE MANAGEMENT OF AN EMPYEMA DRAINAGE-TUBE

Chronic empyema is a most disabling condition which entails months of continuous treatment. In nearly all cases it can be prevented by a proper understanding and careful management of the drainage-tube.

Contrast Radiographs or Pleurograms.—As it is impossible to determine the progress of healing from outward appearances and straight radiographs, and as it is essential to know the size and shape of the cavity, especially during the later stages of treatment, contrast radiographs at regular intervals (every two

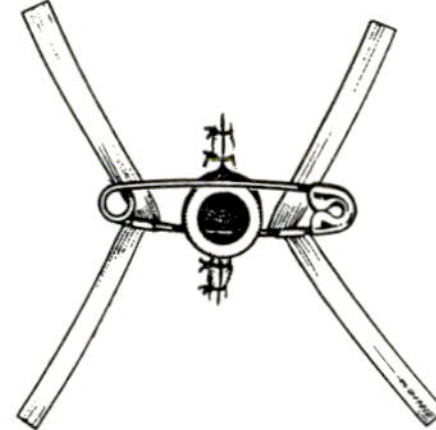

Fig. 236.—Method of anchoring an open empyema drainage tube.

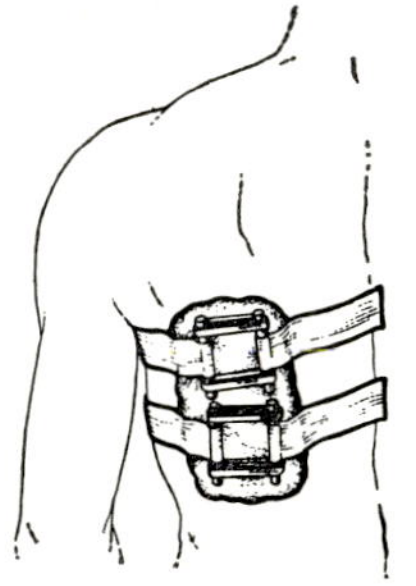

Fig. 237. — Learmonth's method of corsettage is particularly suitable for maintaining an empyema dressing in position.

to three weeks) are indispensable. Having first excluded the presence of a gross communication of the empyema cavity with the bronchial tree, opaque oil (neohydriol or lipiodol) is allowed to gravitate into the cavity, the patient lying with the drainage opening uppermost. Radiographs in the anteroposterior and lateral planes are taken, it being particularly important not to ignore the lateral view. In this way a good estimation of the cavity can be gained and compared as successive films are taken at, say, bi-weekly intervals.

Irrigation of an Empyema Cavity is not recommended. If the cavity has been drained properly, it is unnecessary. Should a bronchopleural fistula be present, it is dangerous. To pour fluid into a cavity which opens into the air-passages is to invite an uncontrollable fit of coughing, and possibly death from drowning.

Test for a Bronchopleural Fistula.—A few ml. of a harmless dye such as dilute methylene blue are injected into the cavity. If the patient coughs up sputum stained blue, it is obvious that a pleurobronchial communication is present.

When should the Drainage-tube be removed?—Clearly it is a mistake to remove the tube if there is a suppurating cavity still requiring drainage. Temptation to remove the tube must be resisted when the discharge has almost ceased and the patient's condition obviously is good. Healing cannot be guaranteed until the whole empyema cavity has become obliterated; consequently the tube must remain in place until the capacity of the cavity is less than 5 ml. As the cavity closes, the tube must be shortened appropriately until the empyema is virtually nothing more than a chest-wall sinus. This point cannot be stressed too strongly; many chronic empyemata are seen as the result of too early removal of the drainage tube. *An 'open' drainage-tube should never be removed from an empyema cavity, only from a track in the chest wall!* It is safe to leave the original tube *in situ* only until such a track remains, but it may add to the patient's comfort to substitute a somewhat smaller one when the process of healing is well advanced. *The practice of removing a tube to have it washed and boiled each day is to be deplored.* If the tube is removed frequently, invariably a point is reached when the contraction of the opening prevents the original tube being re-inserted without pain and a smaller tube is usually placed in the sinus; at later dates the process is repeated until the external opening is totally inadequate. This error in management is still too frequent, and is often caused by the surgeon relegating the entire after-treatment to inexperienced junior staff.

Factors requiring Special Attention.—As a result of the pleurograms and other data, it will become evident that certain cases require special measures if chronicity is to be avoided.

Mechanically Imperfect Drainage.—When confronted with a case where the external opening has been allowed to contract prematurely, steps must be taken to stretch it sufficiently to allow the re-insertion of a tube of adequate calibre by: (*a*) the passage of graduated bougies; or, preferably, (*b*) the insertion of a laminaria or sea-tangle tent for twenty-four hours, but care must be taken to have a string attached to the tent for purposes of withdrawal. When these measures fail the cause of the external narrowing is usually due to osseous regeneration, and operative measures to ensure a sufficiently large opening are required.

It is only by contrast radiographs that unsuspected pockets and tracks can be visualized. If the gravity drainage of these is inadequate further operative treatment is essential, otherwise the infection may be perpetuated and ultimate healing postponed indefinitely. From time to time the bacteriology of the discharge should be ascertained. If an otherwise straightforward case is becoming unduly tardy, special examinations for tubercle bacilli and *Actinomyces* should be made. The possibility of a hitherto unsuspected neoplasm also should be considered.

An offensive discharge or continuing profuse pus indicates imperfect drainage and points to the necessity of a full review of the case. If the contrast radiographs show that the cavity is not draining at its most dependent point, the patient must either be placed in such a position that the opening is able to drain with the aid of gravity, or, if this is improbable or inefficient, operative measures must be invoked.

Persistent Pain.—If other factors have been excluded intercostal neuritis may be the cause. This often responds temporarily to an injection of lignocaine, but if the neuritis soon returns, alcohol injection or resection of the affected intercostal nerve is required.

Breathing Exercises.—The importance of aiding re-expansion of the lungs by means of breathing exercises cannot be over-estimated. Blowing water from one bottle to another is the traditional procedure. Unfortunately, the indispensable effort in expansion is not expiratory, but inspiratory. Supervised exercises, preferably conducted by a physiotherapist, must therefore be directed towards improving the tone of the inspiratory mechanism, i.e., not only the tone of the musculature of the lower chest, but also that of the diaphragm. The exercises should be started within a day or two of the drainage of the empyema and must be persisted with until, and even after, the wound has healed.

General Treatment must not be overlooked.—

1. The Correction of Anæmia.—In many cases of empyema a severe degree of anæmia is present and this, if untreated, will result in delayed healing. Repeated blood examinations are advisable and, in addition to iron preparations, blood or packed red-cell transfusions may be required.

2. A High Protein Intake is required.—There is a steady drain of body protein in the purulent discharge, and to counter this a high-protein diet is necessary; in severe cases of malnutrition the advisability of giving intravenous infusions of plasma or protein hydrolysate should be considered (*see* p. 46).

3. Early Ambulation is most necessary.—Once the empyema has been properly drained there is no need to keep the patient bedridden. A 'closed' drainage system necessitates some restriction of activity, but at the earliest opportunity the patient can be allowed to sit out of bed and, to start the process of physical rehabilitation, movements of the limbs are encouraged.

CHAPTER XXIV

THE MANAGEMENT OF ŒSOPHAGEAL CASES

By R. H. Franklin

PRE-OPERATIVE MANAGEMENT

BEFORE a major operation upon the œsophagus is undertaken the patient must be prepared with great care to counter the extreme wasting that so often accompanies œsophageal obstruction. This consideration applies particularly to sufferers from carcinoma of the œsophagus, but often considerable loss of weight also is evident when the cause of the dysphagia is benign.

Improving Nutrition.—At the preliminary examination the patient should be weighed, and the result recorded; a specimen of blood should be obtained with the special objects of ascertaining the red cell and hæmoglobin values. When necessary, blood transfusion is carried out. Should dysphagia be so complete that even fluids cannot be swallowed, it may be necessary to carry out temporary gastrostomy or jejunostomy, but this course should never be followed unless it is absolutely essential. A patient in whom dysphagia is to all intents and purposes complete when he is first admitted to hospital, after a period of rest afforded by rectal and/or parenteral administration of fluid, not infrequently improves sufficiently to permit the swallowing of thickened fluids. If the full benefit is to accrue from a liquid diet it is essential that solid food be prohibited.

Fortified milk or Complan must be placed at the patient's disposal throughout the day and night so that a few sips can be taken whenever he feels able to do so. The importance of taking all the nourishment he can must be explained to the patient who usually will co-operate readily when he understands that it is vital to his recovery.

The basis of the fortified liquid is milk, and to 1000 ml. (2 pints) of milk are added the following:—

> 2 eggs
>
> 60 G. (2 oz.) of sugar
>
> 1 teaspoonful of salt
>
> 60 G. (2 oz.) of National dried milk (full cream)
>
> 30 G. (1 oz.) of butter.

This mixture can be flavoured with brandy or fruit juice, or either of these may be taken as a separate drink. The aim should be for the patient to drink at least 2500 ml. of the mixture during the day.

Vitamins and ferrous sulphate are administered independently.

Pulmonary System.—Careful examination of the thorax often reveals evidence of bronchiectasis or fibrosis. Treatment in the form of postural drainage and breathing exercises may improve the condition. As soon as the patient feels strong enough he should be encouraged to take exercise daily, preferably in the open air. Smoking should be restricted and stopped completely two or three days before the operation.

Complan (Glaxo Laboratories Ltd., Greenford, Middlesex).

Dental Sepsis.—It is a mistake to embark on the extraction of unsound teeth because infection stirred up thereby takes many weeks to eradicate, and the treatment of the œsophageal condition does not permit this delay. Extractions should be restricted to loose teeth; those that remain should be scaled by a dental surgeon and cleaned, particular attention being paid to the treatment of gingivitis, if present. A good method is for the patient to rub moist salt on his gums with the forefinger.

Mitigating Local Debris.—Sipping dilute hydrogen peroxide solution (liquor hydrogen peroxide 1 part, water 8 parts) clears debris from the growth and exercises a mild antiseptic action.

Other Measures.—Constipation is usual in patients who have been undernourished for a considerable time. It is therefore essential to carry out a rectal examination. If hard scybala are present and all are not expelled after enemata on two consecutive days, the remainder must be removed manually.

In elderly patients it is not unusual for some degree of chronic urinary obstruction to be present and, although no action is advisable at this stage, the information may be of value during the post-operative period.

As a result of this pre-operative régime most patients improve considerably and some gain in weight. Often the patient feels stronger and more hopeful about the outcome of the operation. Two or three weeks are well spent in preliminary preparation and the delay in removing the growth is more than compensated by the patient's greatly increased chance of survival.

Antibiotic therapy for the patient's chest, usually with a combination of penicillin and streptomycin, is commenced three days before the operation.

POST-OPERATIVE MANAGEMENT

From the moment the operation is completed until two or three weeks have elapsed, a patient who has undergone a major œsophageal operation requires unremitting attention, and for this reason operations of this nature should never be attempted unless proper nursing facilities are available. At the end of the operation the anæsthetist should aspirate the bronchial tree carefully. If the anæsthesia has been kept light, an injection of morphine 10 mg. is administered. The use of repeated small doses of morphine, or the corresponding amount of pethidine, is the keynote of the post-operative sedation. Sufficient sedative should be given to enable the patient to breathe without undue pain, but a large dose which would suppress respiration must be avoided rigorously. Whenever possible the patient's bed should be brought to the operating theatre to avoid unnecessary movement and lifting from the bed must be carried out with particular gentleness. The intercostal drainage-tube is connected to a water-sealed bottle (*see Fig.* 230, p. 309) while the patient is still in the operating theatre.

Intravenous fluid therapy is continued for some days (*see* p. 34). The patient is sat up in bed as soon as his condition permits.

Care of the Lungs.—Preferably on the second, but not later than the third postoperative day regular, supervised breathing exercises are commenced. It is very important that emphasis on proper breathing is not confined to the daily visits of physiotherapists. Throughout the day the nurse and the house-surgeon should make sure that the patient is doing his best to breathe properly and he should be encouraged to cough up any accumulated secretions. It is a help to hold the chest firmly in order to lessen the pain produced by coughing and to change the patient's position at frequent intervals. Breathing a mixture of carbon dioxide and oxygen for a few minutes also stimulates coughing. As a rule the above measures are sufficient to keep the air-passages clear. Bronchoscopic aspiration is rarely necessary. If the bronchial secretion is very viscid and the patient unable to cough, a temporary tracheostomy may be of very great value (p. 16).

To lessen the risk of thrombosis and pulmonary embolism movement and massage of the legs should be undertaken regularly. It is important to endeavour to arrange that the lung and leg exercises are carried out concurrently at given sessions so as to avoid repeated disturbances and to allow periods of rest that are so essential for the patient's recovery.

Radiographic Control of the Thorax.—It must be appreciated that *both* pleural cavities may have been opened during the course of the operation. In order to ensure that an accumulation of air or fluid in either pleural cavity has not been overlooked a daily X-ray examination of the thorax is most advisable. The glass terminal of the intercostal drainage-tube passing into the water-sealed bottle (p. 310) is watched to see that the whole system is airtight and that the column of fluid moves with respiration and maintains a negative pressure of 3–5 in. (7·5–12·5 cm.) of water. If the column of fluid oscillates excessively, the rubber tube should be partially occluded by a clamp; on the other hand, if the column becomes stationary 'milking' the tube is carried out to ensure that the lumen is not blocked by blood-clot. In the event of sudden breathlessness the patient's chest should be explored with an aspirating needle connected to a syringe, even though the radiograph appears comparatively normal. Daily radiography of the thorax must be continued after the withdrawal of the drainage-tube and any accumulation of air or fluid aspirated.

Removal of the Intercostal Drainage-tube is not undertaken until the risk of intrapleural bleeding is believed to have passed—as a rule this is on the third post-operative day, but in patients whose pre-operative blood-pressure was high and/or when the water in the water-sealed bottle becomes coloured after changing it, the removal is postponed for a further 24 or 48 hours.

An excellent method of preventing air from entering the thorax at the time of the removal of the tube is to spread a piece of lint thickly with zinc and castor oil ointment, and to wrap it around the base of the tube and hold it there during the removal of the tube.

Resumption of Feeding.—In the immediate post-operative period the fluid requirements of the patient are supplied intravenously. During the operation a neoplex gastric tube was passed through the patient's nose and its tip was guided beyond the anastomosis. In order to minimize the development of ileus hourly aspiration through this tube is carried out for at least 24 hours. After the patient has passed flatus per rectum, provided there is no undue abdominal distension, the tube is used for feeding purposes and following a satisfactory trial with water, fortified milk is introduced at two-hourly intervals. After continuing in this way for 5 days, sips of half-strength saline solution are allowed, and satisfactory ingestion is the signal that the gastric tube can be removed. On the seventh post-operative day Benger's food is substituted for the half-strength saline solution and thereafter the diet is increased gradually, but solids are not allowed until the tenth post-operative day.

POST-OPERATIVE COMPLICATIONS

Leakage from the Anastomosis.—Should a leak from the anastomosis develop, the pleural drainage-tube must be kept in position and all feeding by mouth stopped. An intravenous drip is set up once more. Through the gastric tube

Neoplex gastric tube (Porges, Paris; Sole Agents for Great Britain, Endoscopic Instrument Co., Ltd., London, W.9).
Benger's food (Benger Laboratories Ltd., Holmes Chapel, Cheshire).

(re-introduced, if it has been removed) aspiration is carried out at hourly intervals. If after 24 hours the pleural drainage is diminishing it is permissible to give some soft solid food by mouth while continuing with the administration of fluid by the intravenous route. Should the œsophageal fistula show no signs of closing, jejunostomy must be performed (*see* p. 351).

There is a danger of overlooking certain complications, the signs of which are less evident in a patient in a low general condition, particularly:—

Intraperitoneal Hæmorrhage which sometimes occurs from a bleeding point on the diaphragm, or

Strangulation of the Small Intestine may follow herniation through the diaphragmatic incision or through the opening in the transverse mesocolon. Unrecognized, either intraperitoneal hæmorrhage or intestinal strangulation is likely to prove fatal: both require immediate operation, but surgical intervention at this stage is clearly a matter of extreme seriousness. It is apparent that very great care should be taken to prevent these complications and this can be done only by meticulous attention at the time of operation. Every bleeding point must be secured in the diaphragm. When closing the incision in the diaphragm, in addition to interrupted sutures of thread, it is a wise precaution to add a running suture of catgut. With regard to herniation through the diaphragm or mesocolon, the complication is best avoided by attaching the diaphragm or the mesocolon at several points to that part of the stomach or intestine which is brought through either of these openings.

Later Complications.—If the stomach has been used to restore continuity, there is a risk of reflux œsophagitis occurring. This risk is minimized by carrying out a pyloroplasty at the time of the operation, and the higher the anastomosis has been made the less is the risk of œsophagitis developing. The patient should be advised to sleep with the head and shoulders raised, and also always to chew food thoroughly. The wearing of corsets or tight belts should be avoided.

CHAPTER XXV

THE MANAGEMENT OF CARDIAC CASES

By A. K. Basu

The scope of cardiac surgery has made phenomenal progress in the past 20 years. Intracardiac lesions which in the recent past were accepted as well beyond the realm of operative management are now routinely and successfully corrected. From the management point of view, there are two types:—

1. Lesions which are best corrected by closed cardiac surgery.

2. Lesions for which an open cardiac operation, necessitating use of extra-corporeal circulation, is required.

In the following vignettes of correctable cardiac lesions the house-surgeon is first reminded of some of the essential points in the clinical diagnosis of each. Many investigations are routine and common to all; they are listed below. In addition, special investigations are sometimes necessary and are described under the appropriate lesions. While techniques are steadily improving and new operations being devised, currently accepted operative procedures for each type of defect are indicated.

Many of the points in the post-operative management of cardiac surgical patients are dealt with in the section on mitral stenosis and are not repeated in later sections. In addition the house-surgeon must be vigilant and active in the prevention of pulmonary complications (*see* p. 164) and know the details of thoracic surgical management (*see* p. 301). Cardiopulmonary by-pass and hypothermia are highly specialized techniques, whose use is confined to a few centres; more information on them is given on pp. 331–334.

ROUTINE INVESTIGATION AND ASSESSMENT

The pre-operative assessment of patients about to undergo closed cardiac surgery should include the following:—

1. Complete case history with systemic inquiry, with particular reference to recent rheumatic symptoms, and full physical examination.

2. Blood group. Forewarn the blood bank of likely requirements.

3. Erythrocyte sedimentation rate.

4. Hæmoglobin and full blood-count.

5. Urinalysis.

6. Chest radiograph.

7. Electrocardiogram.

8. Serum urea and electrolytes.

9. Cardiac catheterization with determination of pressure gradients, etc., as indicated (*see* p. 335).

Further investigations may be suggested by facts revealed in the history and physical examination, or by abnormalities in the routine investigations, e.g., proteinuria and a raised serum-urea level, due to impaired renal function, may contra-indicate operation; a significant degree of anæmia would require investigation and correction prior to operation.

LESIONS CORRECTABLE BY CLOSED SURGERY
MITRAL STENOSIS

Correction of this lesion is the commonest cardiac operation. The cusps of the mitral valve are affected by rheumatic endocarditis, resulting in commissural fusion. Diagnosis of this condition is fairly straightforward and depends on the following:—

1. *Symptoms.*—These are due to (*a*) low cardiac output (effort dyspnœa, small pulse), (*b*) pulmonary congestion (recurrent bronchitis and hæmoptysis), and (*c*) right-sided cardiac overload (prominent neck veins, enlarged liver).

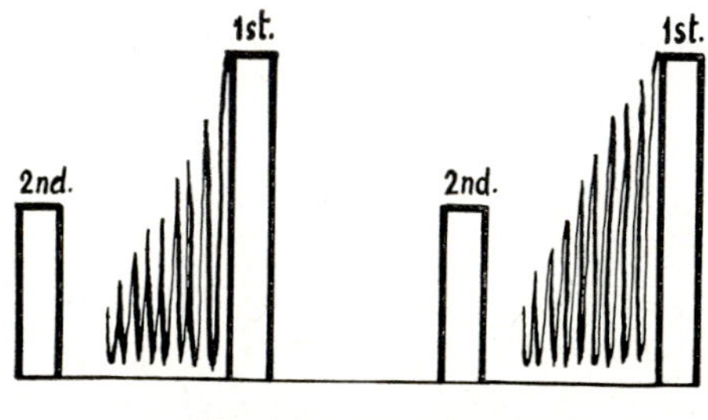

Fig. 238.—Mitral stenosis 'crescendo' murmur.

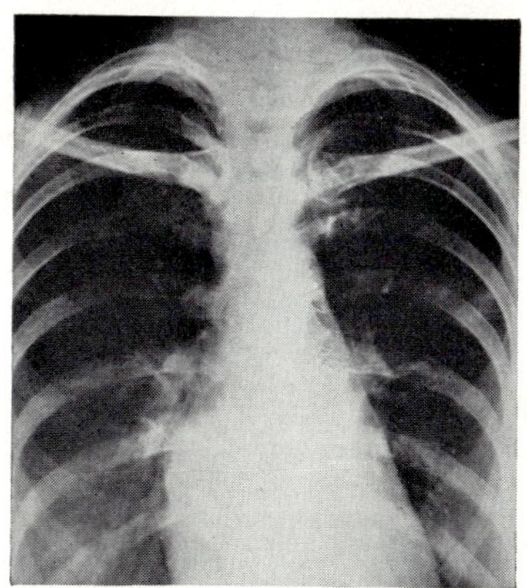

Fig. 239.—Postero-anterior view radiograph of the heart in a case of mitral stenosis showing 'straightening' of the left border and double contour.

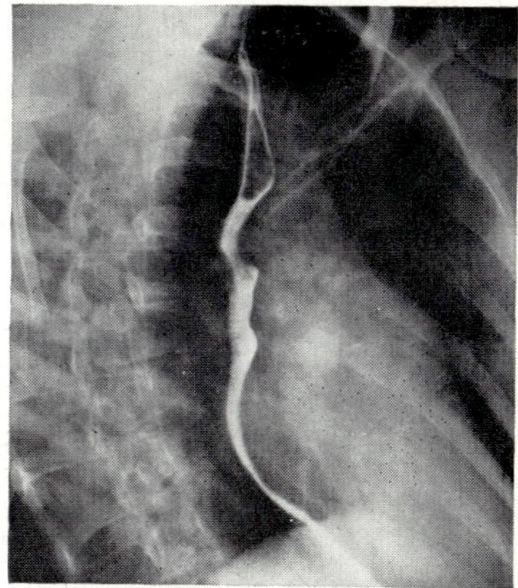

Fig. 240.—Lateral view radiograph of a case of mitral stenosis showing œsophageal impression due to enlarged left atrium.

2. *Auscultation of the Heart.*—A well-established mitral stenosis murmur is very characteristic. The murmur starts in mid-diastole, increases in intensity in presystole, and ends sharply in a loud first sound. It is called 'crescendo' murmur (*Fig.* 238).

3. *Radiology.*—Postero-anterior and lateral views of the heart with barium swallow (*Figs.* 239, 240) will probably reveal:—

    a. Small aorta.

    b. Straightening of the left border of the heart.

    c. Double contour—hypertrophied left atrium.

    d. Uplifted apex—right ventricular hypertrophy.

    e. Pulmonary congestion.

4. *Electrocardiography.*—

    a. Right axis deviation.

    b. Right ventricular hypertrophy.

    c. P mitrale.

Preparation for Operation.—

1. *Age.*—The optimal age is between 20 and 40 years. Before 20 years, recurrence of rheumatic activity is common after operation. However, in many countries in the tropics mitral stenosis is well established even at 15 years and consequently patients have to be accepted for operation at earlier ages.

2. *Absence of rheumatic activity* should be ensured by finding a normal ESR, and by the absence of fever, joint pains, and tachycardia.

3. *Absence of other cardiac abnormalities* such as mitral insufficiency or aortic valve lesions should be determined. Mobility of the cusps of the mitral valve as judged by the presence of an opening snap is an added advantage.

4. *Pre-operative Rest and Preparation.*—The patient should be prepared by a period of rest—in the tropics for 7 days before operation; salt intake should be low during this period; he should be digitalized by giving 0·25 mg. of digoxin tablet twice a day. A course of oral penicillin tablets is also indicated. Breathing exercises should be practised. If signs or symptoms of congestive failure are present, the patient will need longer intensive pre-operative medical preparation.

5. *Atrial Fibrillation.*—Patients who are fibrillating before operation present difficult problems. They usually have thrombi in the auricular appendix and the incidence of post-operative embolic complications is high in such cases. These patients should be even more carefully digitalized.

Post-operative Care.—

1. *Blood-loss Replacement.*—Most cases of mitral commissurotomy require 250–500 ml. of blood replacement depending on the amount lost during the operation. Subsequent transfusion will depend on the amount lost during the first 24 or 48 hours of the post-operative period.

2. *Drainage-tube.*—A radiograph is routinely taken on the morning after the operation to check that the lung is fully expanded. If the post-operative drainage is not too much (over 400 ml.), the water-seal drainage-tube is removed 24 hours after operation. If much fluid subsequently accumulates in the chest it is removed with a broad-bore needle, using a local anæsthetic and preventing air from entering the chest (p. 307).

3. *Digitalization.*—Digitalis should be administered in the same dosage as before the operation. However, the ECG should be checked periodically and if necessary the dose of digitalis may have to be adjusted. Some patients may start fibrillating during or after commissurotomy. A cardiologist should be consulted in such cases.

If the post-operative fibrillation continues, quinidine should be administered after the tenth day and under the supervision of the cardiologist. Quinidine is sometimes given over a period of 7 days in divided doses, the individual dosage gradually increasing each day from 200 mg. 4-hourly to 600 mg. 4-hourly on the last day.

An ECG should be taken after the last dose of quinidine each day and, if there is evidence of quinidine toxicity such as bundle-branch block or ventricular conduction disturbances, quinidine should be withheld the following day.

Post-operative atrial fibrillation can also be converted by administering counter-shock to the heart by a DC defibrillator. In many centres this method is preferred to quinidine defibrillation.

After restoration of normal sinus rhythm, the patients will require to be put on a maintenance dose of quinidine (200 mg., three or four times daily).

4. *Embolic complication* may develop during and following mitral commissurotomy. All the peripheral pulses should be carefully palpated at the end of the operation. Embolectomy may be indicated in rare cases. If any neurological deficit is detected after operation, embolic complication should also be suspected. Consultation with a neurologist would be necessary in such cases.

5. *Post-commissurotomy Syndrome.*—Some patients develop precordial distress, tachycardia, and unexplained fever in the post-operative period. This syndrome may last for as long as 3–4 weeks. The most probable cause is presence and organization of effusion in the pericardial sac. To prevent this condition developing, it is good practice to make a large dependent incision on the left side in the pericardial sac which will allow free drainage after the main pericardial incision is closed. The condition, when it develops, needs no specific treatment and usually settles down in time. Administration of corticosteroids has been recommended when the syndrome persists.

PATENT DUCTUS ARTERIOSUS

Diagnosis.—The presence of a continuous machinery 'Gibson' murmur at the base of the heart (second left intercostal space), associated with a continuous thrill and wide pulse-pressure, is very characteristic of this congenital anomaly. However, in some cases the systolic element may only be audible. On radiography the pulmonary artery is prominent and the lung fields are plethoric. There may be 'hilar dance' on fluoroscopy.

Pre-operative Care.—

1. Most cases do not require any specific preparation. Bacterial endocarditis is a possible complication in PDA. When suspected it should be confirmed by repeated blood-cultures and the antibiotic sensitivity of the organism determined. Most commonly it is treated by heavy doses of penicillin, 2 to 4 mega units of crystalline penicillin daily for 3 weeks.

2. The presence of pulmonary hypertension should be suspected in elderly cases or in patients with a large ductus. This can be confirmed by cardiac catheterization. When the hypertension is very severe (pulmonary artery pressure 60–80 mm. Hg) and particularly if cyanosis develops on exertion, operation is fraught with severe risk.

Post-operative Care.—Most cases do well and the operative mortality is no more than 1 to 2 per cent. Little blood is lost during the operation and so there is little need for replacement. Management of the chest drain is as detailed under mitral stenosis. If the ductus is simply ligated, the incidence of post-operative recanalization is said to be about 5 per cent.

COARCTATION OF THE AORTA

Diagnosis is made by the presence of superior extremity hypertension and absent or feeble pulses in the lower extremity. The patients may complain of headache and throbbing pulses in the neck. There may also be symptoms of intermittent claudication in the legs. The patient's left ventricle hypertrophies in an attempt to overcome the aortic obstruction and collateral channels open up.

Pre-operative Care.—

1. *Radiography.*—To know the exact site and the extent of the coarctation, aortography is necessary (*see* pp. 526, 720). A plain radiograph will show (*a*) prominent ascending aorta, (*b*) 'double' aortic knuckle with an intervening area of constriction, and (*c*) rib notching indicating enlarged and tortuous intercostal arteries. There may be left ventricular enlargement.

Angiography: Seldinger's catheter should be introduced percutaneously into the ascending aorta through the right brachial artery. Injection of 20–40 ml. of 70 per cent diodone solution under pressure will show the coarcted segment and its relation to the left subclavian artery. The post-stenotic dilated segment will also be visible.

2. *ECG* study will indicate the degree of left ventricular hypertrophy.

3. *Age of Operation.*—The optimum age is between 5 and 15 years. Beyond the age of 25 years the wall of the aorta becomes inelastic and friable, and does not take sutures kindly.

The operation requires good exposure and considerable mobilization of the aorta. There are numerous enlarged tortuous collateral vessels in the chest wall which may be cut across during the operation. The assistant must watch for and help control these bleeding vessels. There may be more than average blood-loss and arrangements must be made for adequate blood replacement during the operation. On an average about 1000 ml. of blood should be got ready for the operation.

Post-operative Care.—Average operative mortality is 5 to 10 per cent, depending on the severity of the case. Usually patients do well. Blood-pressure in the upper extremity comes down and equalization takes place with that of the lower extremity.

Complications.—The possible complications are:—

1. Leaking from the suture line or from the graft surface when used. If the leakage is sizeable, there will be excessive drainage from the chest and a fall in blood-pressure; re-exploration may be necessary.

2. Injury to the spinal cord. If more than three pairs of intercostal vessels have been sacrificed during the anastomosis, ischæmia of the spinal cord may supervene; the house-surgeon should check the neurological state of the lower limbs.

3. Rupture of cœliac or mesenteric vessels has been reported. This is a remote possibility; there are acute abdominal symptoms and the blood-pressure falls. Laparotomy is necessary.

PERICARDITIS

1. ACUTE PYOGENIC PERICARDITIS

Diagnosis.—Retrosternal pain, high swinging fever, tachycardia, together with the shadow of a large pear-shaped cardiac outline on a radiograph should suggest the diagnosis. Treatment is by pericardial aspiration.

Aspiration.—

a. Position of Patient.—The patient is supported by a backrest and partially sits up in bed at an angle of 45° (*Fig.* 241).

b. Needle.—A special trocar with cannula is available. It is short and bevelled. But any cannula about 15 cm. long and 3-mm. bore can be used.

c. Site of Puncture.—Under local anæsthesia, the needle is introduced beside or close to the xiphoid process and pushed upwards and backwards at an angle of 45°. About 4 cm. from the skin, the thickened pericardium is encountered.

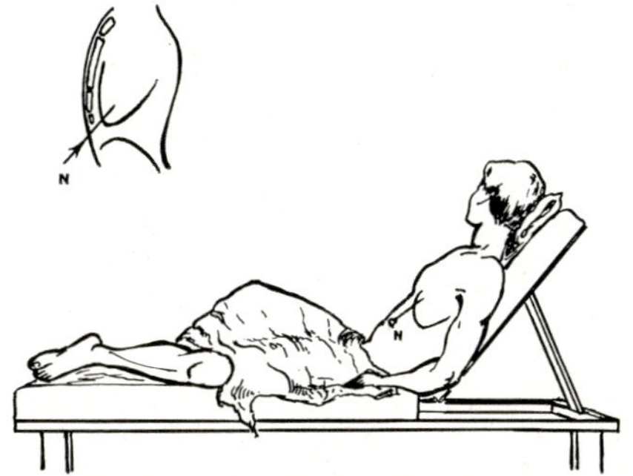

Fig. 241.—Position of the patient for aspiration of the pericardium.

The pericardium is punctured and a sudden loss of resistance indicates penetration. The trocar is withdrawn; emergence of pus indicates successful penetration. The cannula is connected to a suitable syringe and all the pus is withdrawn. In cases requiring prolonged drainage, a blunt-ended polythene tube with multiple side-holes is threaded through the cannula and is led into the pericardial cavity while the cannula is being withdrawn. The polythene tube is then fixed to the skin and is connected to a water-seal receptacle. Strict aseptic measures are maintained. After withdrawal, the pus should be cultured and the sensitivity pattern of the offending organism determined. The patient should then be given the appropriate antibiotics.

2. CARDIAC TAMPONADE

When fluid or blood rapidly accumulates in the pericardial cavity, the patient will develop acute dyspnœa, hypotension, distension of the neck veins, and even circulatory collapse. There may be 'pulsus paradoxus'—with diminution of the pulse volume during inspiration and increase during expiration. Paracentesis of the pericardium is urgent. If blood is aspirated in massive quantity (for example, after a penetrating missile injury), rapid blood transfusion is necessary and, if the bleeding continues, exploratory operation will be urgent to save the life of the patient.

3. CONSTRICTIVE PERICARDITIS

Diagnosis.—Dyspnœa on exertion, prominence of the neck veins, fullness of the face, ascites, and enlargement of the liver are characteristic signs and symptoms. The blood-pressure is usually low and the peripheral pulses are small. On auscultation the heart-sounds are feeble. Fluoroscopy shows diminished pulsation of the heart; radiographs show alteration of its contours. Calcification may be seen. In the ECG study, all the complexes are of low voltage; T waves may be inverted. The venous pressure is elevated.

Pre-operative Care.—

1. The patient should have adequate antituberculous treatment prior to operation as the majority of the cases are due to infection by *Mycobacterium tuberculosis*.

2. For about 2 weeks prior to operation, the patient should be on a low salt diet; diuretics (*see* p. 664) should be given on alternate days and, if necessary, fluid in the pleural and the peritoneal cavities should be aspirated.

Post-operative Care.—Depending on the state of the myocardium, the degree and the duration of the constriction, the patients have either easy or stormy post-operative courses. Some cases develop hypotension, and right- or left-sided congestive failure, which will have to be treated by adequate resuscitative measures, viz., vasopressors, blood, or diuretics and venesection (*see* p. 663). Patients developing atrial fibrillation should be treated by digitalis.

The long-term results are excellent. Ascites subsides in 2–3 weeks' time. Paracentesis is seldom necessary after decortication.

ANEURYSM OF THORACIC AORTA

Pre-operative Investigation.—Most aneurysms result from atherosclerotic or degenerative causes, but in all cases active syphilis must be excluded by blood tests. If the aneurysm involves the ascending aorta or the arch, it poses extremely difficult problems and will require extracorporeal circulation for adequate management. If the aneurysm involves the descending thoracic aorta, it can be repaired more easily. To obtain exact diagnosis about the site, extent, and the type of aneurysm, good aortography is essential (*see* pp. 526, 720). The aneurysm may also be of the dissecting type; dissection can start either in the ascending aorta or the arch.

Saccular aneurysms can be repaired by lateral excision and repair. For cylindrical aneurysms and for dissecting aneurysm, resection of the aneurysm and bridging of the defect by a dacron vascular graft will be necessary.

Post-operative Hazards.—These are similar to those following correction of a coarctation of the aorta; possible coagulation defects may follow the use of an extracorporeal circulation.

LESIONS CORRECTABLE BY OPEN HEART SURGERY

When involved in the treatment of patients requiring this type of surgery, one of the main duties of the house-surgeon is to act as a co-ordinator. Once the probable date of the operation has been fixed he must ensure that all members of the large team involved—surgeon, anæsthetist, cardiologist, technicians, bio-chemist, blood-transfusion officer, and others—know and have all necessary preparations made. Large quantities of blood will likely be required, both to prime machines and also to replace operative loss and correct any coagulation defects that may subsequently appear.

Outlines of cardiopulmonary by-pass and hypothermia techniques, and details of necessary tests and possible complications are given on p. 331.

When talking to relatives of patients about to undergo open heart surgery, the house-surgeon should warn them that there are still considerable risks involved. However, many of the patients will certainly die without operation.

AORTIC STENOSIS

Stenosis may occur at the valve level or at the supravalvular or subvalvular level. The valve stenosis may be corrected by closed transventricular valvotomy, but here again open heart operation is preferable. The fused, diseased commissures may be repaired by plastic procedures or the valve totally replaced by a prosthetic valve such as the Starr-Edward ball-and-socket valve (*Fig.* 242).

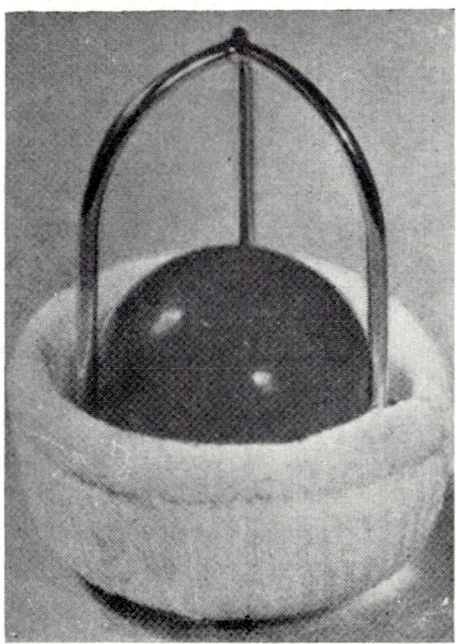

Fig. 242.—Starr-Edward prosthetic valve.

Pre-operative Investigations.—

1. *Determination of the Pressure Gradient across the Aortic Valve.*—This can be performed by direct left ventricular and brachial artery punctures. For left ventricular puncture, a long 18-gauge needle is introduced under local anæsthesia directly over the apex and the needle advanced slightly backwards at an angle of 35° towards the right second costochondral junction. The left ventricle is soon felt and punctured by a sharp tap. The pressure is recorded by electromanometer. The brachial artery is simultaneously punctured by the arterial needle and the pressure recorded. To obtain a withdrawal pressure tracing across the aortic valve, a fine polythene tube can be passed through the ventricular needle and manipulated through the aortic valve into the ascending aorta. This is indicated by the appearance of the diastolic pressure level in the tracing. The tube can then be slowly withdrawn into the left ventricular cavity and the actual level of obstruction thereby determined.

The same information can be obtained by introducing the Seldinger catheter percutaneously in the femoral artery, and advancing it through the abdominal and thoracic aorta to the aortic valve and then through the valve into the left ventricle (p. 338). A withdrawal tracing is obtained by slow and gradual withdrawal of the catheter.

Aortic commissurotomy would be indicated when the pressure gradient across the aortic valve exceeds 60 mm. of Hg.

2. *Angiography* of the left ventricular outflow tract will delineate the site of obstruction. This may be very helpful in selected cases.

AORTIC INCOMPETENCE

Diagnosis.—An early diastolic murmur down the left sternal edge, high bounding 'water-hammer' or 'Corrigan' pulse, and wide pulse-pressure (high systolic and very low diastolic) characterize the condition. Radiographs show a large left ventricle and ECG reveals left ventricular hypertrophy. To confirm the diagnosis and to note the degree of incompetence, retrograde aortography by the Seldinger catheter can be performed.

Pre-operative Care.—These cases are most satisfactorily treated by replacement of the aortic valve. Currently the Starr-Edward prosthetic valve is most commonly used. Homografts of the aortic valve have also been inserted with success. Before the operation, the patients should have adequate treatment for congestive failure and close co-operation with the cardiologist is essential.

MITRAL INSUFFICIENCY

Diagnosis.—The majority of cases coexist with mitral stenosis. A systolic murmur at the apex conducted to the axilla, left ventricular hypertrophy in the electrocardiography, and the presence of a giant left atrium on a radiograph confirm the diagnosis.

In some patients the diseased, shrunken cusps may be repaired, but in most cases replacement with a prosthetic mitral valve (Starr-Edward) is the operation of choice.

Pre-operative Care of Patients needing Valve Replacement.—All patients in whom the normal valve has been replaced by a prosthetic valve will need to take anticoagulants on a long-term basis. The prothrombin time will have to be adjusted at twice the normal value and frequent (fortnightly) check estimations of the prothrombin time will have to be made. Dindevan is a suitable drug to use (*see* p. 79). One tablet (50 mg.) twice a day is the usual dose. When homograft valves are used, anticoagulants are not necessary.

ATRIAL SEPTAL DEFECT

Diagnosis.—This is one of the commonest congenital defects in the heart. It is a well-tolerated anomaly of the heart and symptoms may not become manifest before 10 to 15 years. The apex beat is right ventricular in type. There is a soft systolic murmur over the pulmonary area. An ECG shows right ventricular hypertrophy and partial or complete bundle-branch block. On a radiograph, the pulmonary artery is large, the apex of the heart is uplifted, the lung fields are plethoric, and the aorta is small. The diagnosis is confirmed by catheterization, which shows oxygen lift (increase in oxygen content) in the right atrial blood sample. The size and location of the defect can be accurately delineated by a balloon-tipped catheter (*Fig.* 243) or by passing a loop of catheter through the defect (*Fig.* 244). This common foramen secundum type has to be distinguished from the rare foramen primum type in which the symptoms appear early; the axis of the heart is left sided and there may be left ventricular hypertrophy.

Pre-operative Care.—Patients can be operated on under moderate hypothermia with inflow occlusion or with extracorporeal circulation. Most cases do not need any special pre-operative care; exceptions are those with high pulmonary hypertension.

VENTRICULAR SEPTAL DEFECT

Diagnosis.—An isolated defect of the ventricular septum is a very common congenital cardiac anomaly. It can, in addition, be part of a complex type of

Dindevan (Duncan, Flockhart, & Evans Ltd., Birkbeck Street, London, E.2).

defect such as Fallot's tetralogy, transposition of vessels, etc. Diagnosis is made by the presence of a lowly situated systolic murmur (third intercostal space). The apex beat is of the left ventricular type. On a radiograph, left ventricular enlargement, prominent pulmonary artery and pulmonary plethora, and left

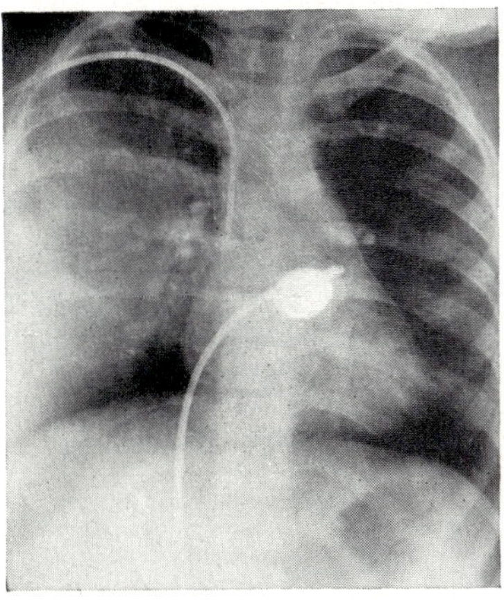

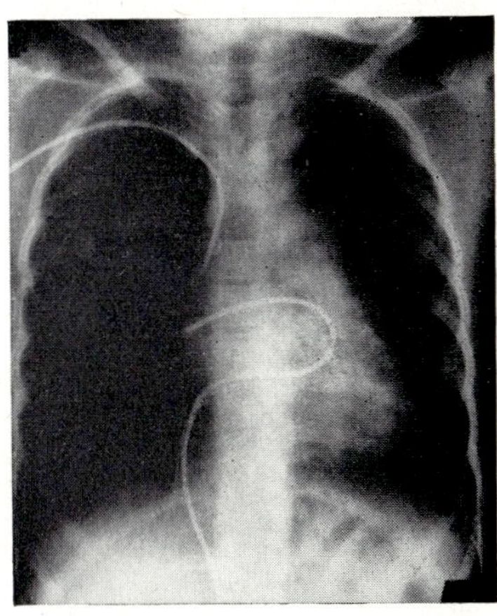

Fig. 243.—Balloon-tipped catheter passed through the atrial septal defect to show its position and approximate size.

Fig. 244.—Looping of the cardiac catheter through the atrial septal defect to show its position and approximate size.

atrial enlargement may be seen. There is left ventricular hypertrophy on ECG study. Diagnosis is confirmed by oxygen lift in the right ventricular blood sample in the catheterization study.

Pre-operative Care.—The defect is repaired with the help of an extracorporeal circulation. No special care is necessary apart from that already outlined for routine open heart surgery. The optimum age for operation is between 5 and 15 years. Small defects have been known to close spontaneously within the first 5 years.

Post-operative Care.—The most important complication that may arise is partial or complete heart block due to inclusion of the right bundle branch in the sutures to close the defect. The management of this condition will be referred to later.

PULMONARY STENOSIS

Diagnosis.—Congenital stenosis of the pulmonary valve may exist alone or in association with other congenital defects such as ventricular septal defect. There is a harsh, high-pitched ejection type of systolic murmur over the pulmonary area and the pulmonary second sound is single. Radiographs show post-stenotic dilatation of the trunk of the pulmonary artery. The lung fields are oligæmic (*Fig.* 245). An ECG shows right ventricular hypertrophy. Diagnosis is confirmed by cardiac catheterization which shows high right ventricular pressure (50–80 mm. Hg) and low pulmonary artery pressure. The exact outline of the pulmonary outflow tract and the pulmonary valve may be delineated by angiocardiography (*Fig.* 246).

Results of closed transventricular pulmonary valvotomy are not always reliable. More effective valvotomy can be achieved by open operation with the help of moderate hypothermia and inflow occlusion, or with extracorporeal circulation.

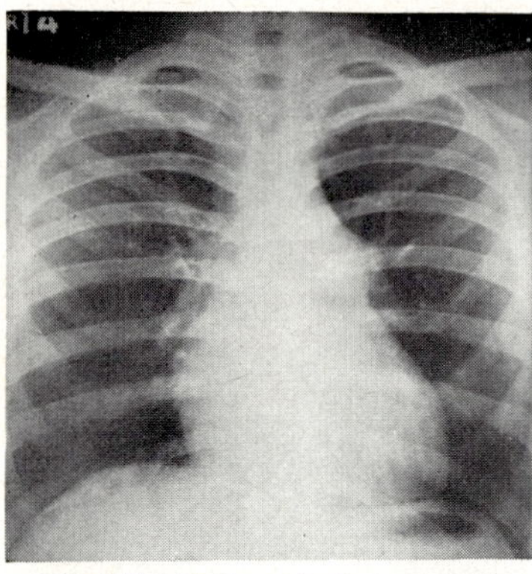

Fig. 245.—Radiograph of a case of pulmonary stenosis showing post-stenotic dilatation of the pulmonary artery and oligæmic lung fields.

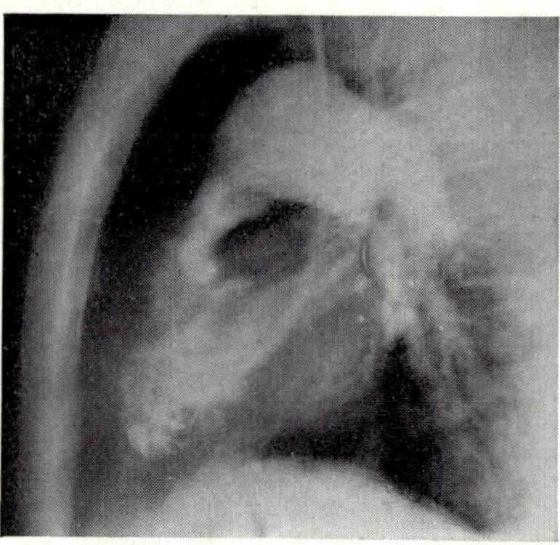

Fig. 246.—Selective angiography of the pulmonary outflow tract in a case of pulmonary stenosis: lateral view showing the narrowing anteriorly.

FALLOT'S TETRALOGY

Diagnosis.—The patients are young children, deeply cyanosed, with clubbing of their fingers and toes. They frequently squat and become dyspnœic on slight

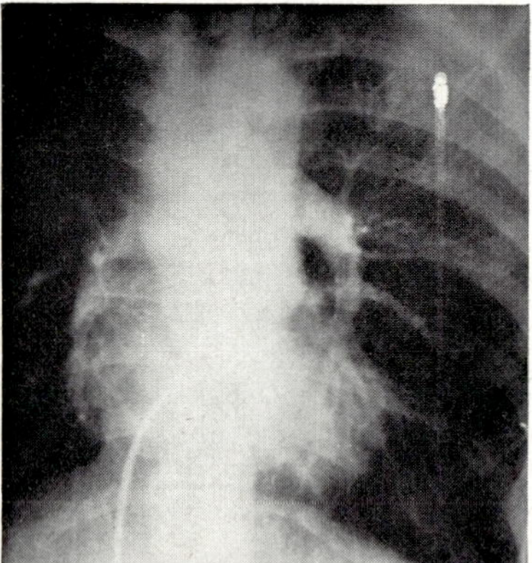

Fig. 247.—Angiocardiography in a case of Fallot's tetralogy showing simultaneous opacification of aorta (centre) and pulmonary artery.

exertion. There is a systolic murmur over the pulmonary area accompanied by a thrill. An ECG shows a boot-shaped heart (*cœur-en-sabot*) with uplifted apex and constricted pulmonary conus. The aortic arch is sometimes right sided. The lung fields are oligæmic. Diagnosis is confirmed by cardiac catheterization and angiocardiography. The latter is very characteristic and shows a dextroposed aortic root, narrowing of the pulmonary outflow tract, and simultaneous opacification of the pulmonary artery and aorta (*Fig.* 247).

Treatment.—If the patients are below 4 years of age and are intensely cyanosed, the best procedure to adopt is a palliative Blalock-Taussig operation (anastomosis of the subclavian to the pulmonary artery). Before this operation is undertaken, the position of the aortic arch and the size of the left subclavian artery should be determined by angiocardiography.

The Brock operation of direct right ventricular infundibulectomy by closed punching procedure is practised by some surgeons.

The best operation is total correction of the anomaly (closure of the ventricular septal defect and enlargement of the right ventricular outflow tract) by open heart operation. However, the mortality and morbidity associated with this operation are still very high.

TECHNICAL PROCEDURES
HYPOTHERMIA

In this procedure, the temperature of the body is reduced by artificial cooling. Hypothermia reduces body metabolism, oxygen consumption, and all enzymatic activities. The greater the fall of body temperature, the greater is the reduction of oxygen consumption (*Fig.* 248).

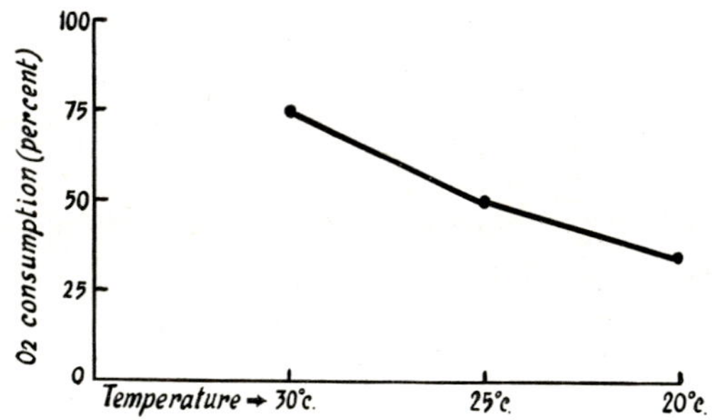

Fig. 248.—Reduction in normal oxygen consumption as the body temperature is reduced from 30° to 20° C.

In surgical practice, two ranges of fall of temperature are used:—
1. Moderate hypothermia—32°–28° C.
2. Profound hypothermia—20°–15° C.

Below 28° C. there is an increasing risk of ventricular fibrillation, so that surface cooling is limited to 28° C. Below this temperature a heart–lung machine must be used. Moderate hypothermia is commonly employed during by-pass procedures as it permits lower flow rates to be used.

With the help of moderate hypothermia, the circulation can be arrested for 6–8 minutes. With profound hypothermia, circulation can be arrested for 30–45 minutes. This latter method, however, is hazardous and is restricted to a few centres only.

Two types of *congenital defects* are suitable for correction with moderate hypothermia—closure of an atrial septal defect and pulmonary valvotomy. Aortic stenosis may also be dealt with under hypothermia. Pre-operative diagnosis must be accurate and precise.

Method of Cooling.—Cooling is usually performed by immersion in cold water with ice packs surrounding the body. Cooling is stopped at 32° C.: there is an after-drop of about 2°–3° C.

Alternatively the patient may be placed between blankets containing tubes through which cold water circulates.

Post-operative Care.—There may be a hæmorrhagic tendency after hypothermia procedures which can be prevented by:—

1. Early rewarming of the patient. This can be started at the commencement of the thoracotomy by circulating warm water through the hypothermia blanket. The temperature of the circulating water must not exceed 44° C. After the intracardiac procedure is completed and while the chest is open, warming may be accomplished by application of infra-red lamps to the chest cavity or to other parts of the body and the heart may be warmed by application of warm saline. After the chest is closed and the wound covered by waterproof dressings, the patient may be immersed again in warm water in the bath tub.

2. Adequately ventilating the lungs before and after inflow occlusion so that metabolic acidosis is minimized as far as possible.

The acid-base status (pH), P_{CO_2}, and CO_2-combining power of the blood should be checked. Acidosis should be corrected by an intravenous injection of 8·4 per cent sodium bicarbonate solution. If the loss of blood is significant, the patient should be returned to the theatre. The source of the bleeding—either from the chest wall or from the atrial incision line—should be controlled.

EXTRACORPOREAL CIRCULATIONS

No attempt will be made to describe the working of the heart–lung machine in detail. However, the essential principle consists of withdrawing the venous return of the heart by cannulating the two venæ cavæ, oxygenating the blood by bringing it in contact with an atmosphere of oxygen, and pumping the oxygenated blood back into arterial circulation after filtering it (*Fig.* 249). During this process the blood must be prevented from clotting by the use of anticoagulants (heparin), and from foaming and bubbling by the use of antifoam agents. After the by-pass, the effect of heparin is neutralized by protamine (*see* p. 81).

Pre-operative Care.—

1. The patient's weight and surface area should be measured or calculated.

2. The patient's blood group should be determined and the blood bank should be given adequate notice to arrange for a suitable number of donors of the same group. Heparinized blood is collected on the day of the operation from the donors and each sample of blood is carefully cross-matched with the patient's blood, as also with each other to ensure complete compatibility.

3. The clotting mechanism of the patient's blood should be determined in detail.

4. Arrangements should be made for the determination of the following during and after operation:—

    a. pH of blood.

    b. P_{CO_2} of blood.

    c. CO_2-combining power of blood.

    d. Arterial pressure.

e. Central venous pressure (*see* p. 24).
f. ECG.
g. In some centres EEG.
There is an increasing tendency for many of these parameters to be continuously monitored by automatic equipment.

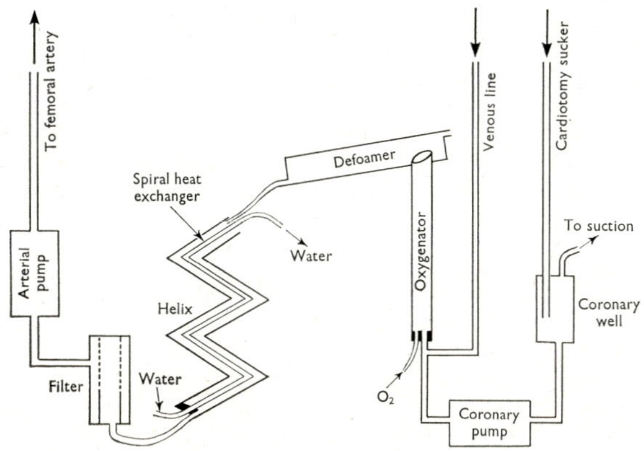

Fig. 249.—Extracorporeal circulation. The input (including blood sucked out of the cardiotomy) is on the right. After passing through the oxygenator, defoamer, and heat exchanger, the blood is pumped into the arterial line (left).

Post-operative Care.—
Recovery Ward.—The patient is received in the intensive care unit or the recovery room, which should be well lighted, spacious, and equipped with the following:—
a. Humidified oxygen supply.
b. Positive-pressure ventilator.
c. ECG machine with oscilloscope.
d. Suction equipment.
e. Cardiac resuscitation set—including syringes charged with the necessary drugs (*see Table I*, p. 5).
f. Tracheostomy and bronchoscopy set.
g. Emergency thoracotomy set.
h. Portable X-ray set.
Monitoring.—For the first 24–36 hours after operation, the patient should remain connected to the ECG machine, and the arterial and venous pressure monitors. pH, P_{CO_2}, and CO_2-combining power should be checked every 3 to 4 hours.
The urine excreted should be drained by an indwelling catheter and the amount measured hourly. The stomach is aspirated periodically by a nasogastric tube.
Blood and Fluid Replacement.—Blood-loss should be carefully estimated and adequate replacement made, taking the arterial and venous pressures into consideration. Additional fluid lost should be estimated, including insensible

and metabolic losses, but is less important than blood replacement. Saline, $N/3$ in 5 per cent glucose, is recommended for the replacement of this fluid loss. If the urine output falls much below 100 ml. per hour, 500 ml. of 10 per cent mannitol should be given.

Clotting Abnormalities.—Excessive blood-loss may be due to clotting disturbances or to an unobserved source of bleeding. If the former, it is best managed by giving a transfusion of fresh blood and intravenous injections of 1 ampoule of 10 per cent calcium gluconate for every 2 bottles of citrated blood. In some cases injection of fibrinogen or epsilon amino caproic acid (EACA) will be life-saving. If loss of blood is due to a missed bleeding source, thoracotomy and control of the bleeding source will be necessary.

Respiration.—In most cases the respiratory effort of the patient is inadequate in the immediate post-operative period and needs to be supported by intermittent positive-pressure ventilation for 18–24 hours. Many varieties of ventilators are available for this purpose.

Hypotension.—This is often a problem. The cause should be carefully ascertained. It may be due to undertransfusion or to overtransfusion, or there may be myocardial insufficiency or vasomotor failure. Cardiac tamponade is also a possible cause. If the cause can be accurately determined and treatment directed accordingly, results will be gratifying.

Ambulation.—If everything goes well, patients can be made to sit up in bed after 48 hours and are usually out of bed after a week. Many patients develop anæmia after the operation. This will need to be corrected by iron and vitamin C.

HEART-BLOCK

Partial or complete heart-block is sometimes a complication after intracardiac operations or may occur by itself in ischæmic heart disease. It is due to interference with the bundle of His. If incomplete, some of the atrial impulses get

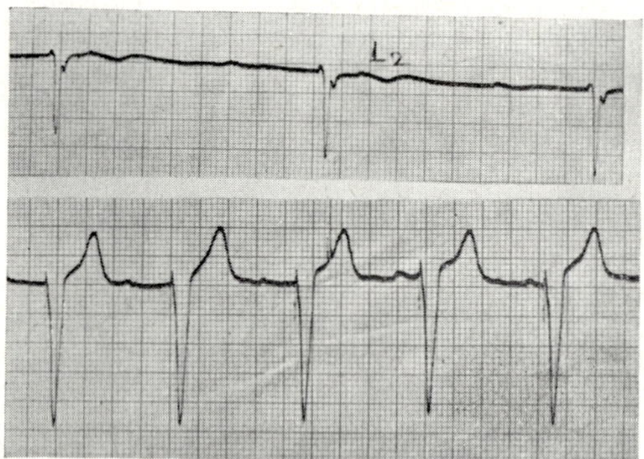

Fig. 250.—Heart-block. Electrocardiogram showing infrequent ventricular complexes (above) and effect of implanting a pacemaker (below).

through into the ventricle. If complete, there is total dissociation of the atrial and ventricular rhythm (*Fig.* 250). When there is marked slowing of the ventricular contraction and long periods of asystole, Stoke-Adams syndrome develops and may end in death. In early cases the patients should be treated by sympathomimetic drugs (ephedrine or isoprenaline). These have beneficial effects in many cases.

In severe cases, use of an artificial pacemaker will be necessary. In an emergency and for temporary use, external pacemakers, in which all the electrodes are put on the body surface, may suffice. For long-term use, internal pacemakers will be required. Here, the internal electrode is fixed to the surface

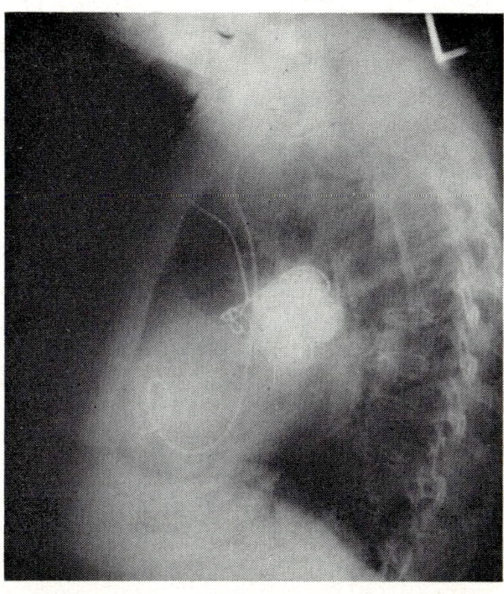

Fig. 251.—Radiograph of a pacemaker implanted on the lateral thoracic wall. The electrode passes to the ventricle via the internal jugular vein.

of the heart after thoracotomy or attached to the endocardium of the right ventricle after introducing it through the jugular vein (*Fig.* 251). Stimulation is effected by a transistorized battery complex which is placed in a subcutaneous pocket in the chest wall. The life of these pacemakers is said to vary between $1\frac{1}{2}$ and 5 years.

CARDIAC ARREST

Cardiac arrest may occur during (1) any operative procedure under general or local anæsthesia, (2) any non-operative manipulation such as reduction of fractures or cardiac catherization, (3) following trauma, and (4) electrical shock.

It is considered in detail in Chapter I. If arrest or ventricular fibrillation occurs during cardiac surgery, recognition and treatment are much easier as the heart is exposed.

CARDIAC CATHETERIZATION

Cardiac catheterization is performed as part of the investigation of congenital or acquired disease of the heart and great vessels. It allows pressure measurement in, and blood sampling from, the cardiac chambers and the vessels, also the injection of foreign substances such as radio-opaque solutions, dyes, ascorbic acid, radioactive material, ice-cold saline, etc., for diagnostic purposes.

Apparatus Required.—This includes:—

1. An ECG amplifier with oscilloscope display for continuous monitoring of the patient's cardiac rhythm throughout the procedure.

2. A low-volume-displacement strain gauge for pressure measurement, with its associated amplifier, oscilloscope display, and a recording device with at least two channels for permanent recording of pressure and ECG simultaneously —this may be photographic, ultra-violet, or direct writing. In certain circumstances simultaneous measurement and recording of two or more pressures may be necessary.

3. Suitable catheters, e.g., Cournand, NIH, or Goodale-Lubin, are shown in *Fig.* 252. Commonly used sizes are 6–9 F for adults and 5–7 F for infants and children; NIH catheters with closed ends and side-holes, in a variety of sizes, are used for injection of radio-opaque material for angiography.

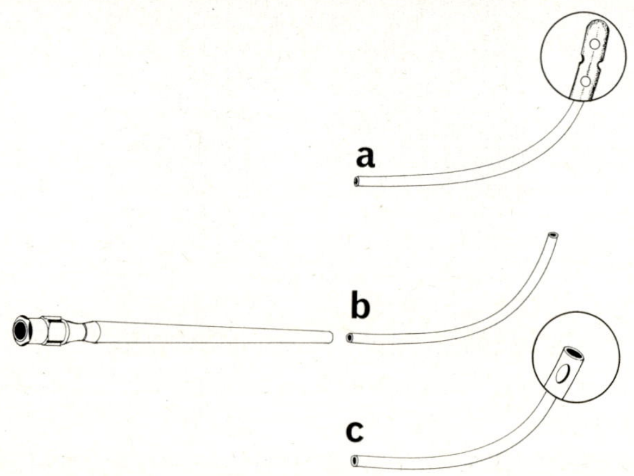

Fig. 252.—Cardiac catheters. In the centre is the Cournand catheter (*b*) with simple open end. The enlargements show the tips of (*a*) the NIH and (*c*) the Goodale-Lubin catheters. Cardiac catheters can be obtained in lengths ranging from 50 cm. to 125 cm. and sizes 5 F to 10 F.

4. Radiographic screening equipment, preferably with image intensifier and facilities for taking angiograms.

5. Riley or Cournand needles for arterial puncture.

6. Equipment for performing cut down on a vein for insertion of catheter.

7. Apparatus for analysis of oxygen and carbon dioxide in expired air, and also for estimation of oxygen content of the blood.

8. DC defibrillator.

9. Intravenous infusion set.

10. Heparinized syringes for collection of blood samples.

11. Mouthpiece, non-return valves, and plastic bag or spirometer for collection of expired air.

RIGHT-HEART CATHETERIZATION

Right-heart catheterization is performed by introducing a radio-opaque catheter into the median cubital or basilic vein in the right arm, or the saphenous vein in the groin, and advancing it via the superior vena cava or inferior vena cava into the right atrium, right ventricle, and pulmonary artery. If an atrial septal defect or a patent foramen ovale is present, the catheter, particularly if passed via the saphenous vein, may be made to traverse the atrial septum so that the left-heart chambers may be entered also; similarly, if a ventricular septal defect or persistent ductus arteriosus is present, the catheter may, more rarely, be passed through this into the left ventricle or aorta respectively

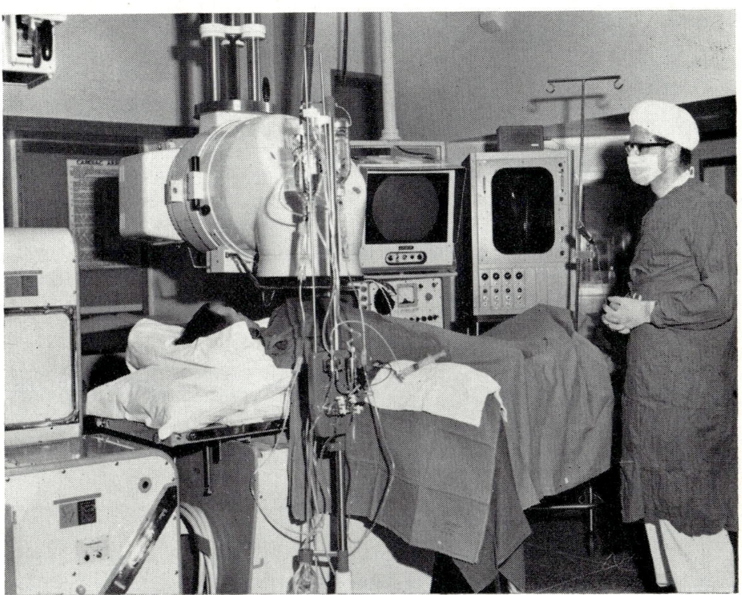

Fig. 253.—Cardiac catheterization in progress. Sterile precautions are observed. The patient lies under the X-ray image intensifier. Pressure transducers (centre) are attached to the catheter, while on the right are monitoring screens for pressure and the electrocardiogram. A multi-channel recorder (not shown) is also attached.

Method.—The patient should be given prophylactic penicillin to reduce the risk of subacute bacterial endocarditis. This may be given in the form of 1 mega unit intramuscularly 1 hour before the catheterization, followed by oral penicillin 6-hourly for the next 72 hours. If the patient is sensitive to the drug, another antibiotic may be used. A sedative should also be given beforehand.

The procedure is performed under strict aseptic conditions, the operator having scrubbed up and wearing lead apron, cap, mask, and gown (*Fig.* 253). The skin of the patient's arm or groin is cleansed with antiseptic solution, sterile towels are applied, the chosen site is infiltrated with local anæsthetic, the skin is incised, and the vein is exposed by blunt dissection. Ligatures are placed around the vein to control bleeding and with a small pair of scissors the vein wall is opened. Using a fine pair of forceps to keep the aperture thus made open, the appropriate size of catheter is inserted in the lumen of the vein and advanced up it towards the heart. The catheter tip has a preformed bend and, by appropriate rotation of the shaft of the catheter, it may usually be made to advance in the desired direction, thus entering the chambers of the right heart and the pulmonary artery and its branches. The lumen of the catheter is kept patent by a slow infusion of heparinized saline (strength, say, 10,000 units per litre). Pressures in the heart chambers are measured by connecting the catheter lumen temporarily to the strain gauge and blood samples may be taken by aspiration through the catheter, first discarding the saline in the lumen. If a needle is inserted in a systemic artery, e.g., brachial or femoral, then by measuring the patient's oxygen consumption and taking simultaneous blood samples from pulmonary artery and systemic artery, and measuring their oxygen content, the cardiac output may be estimated by the Fick principle. If a left to right shunt is present, the magnitude of this may be estimated by the same method and the site of shunt detected by taking serial blood samples all the way from the pulmonary artery to the superior vena cava and inferior vena cava, and analysing their oxygen content.

Cardiac output and shunts may also be estimated by injecting a foreign indicator, e.g., dye, through the catheter and, by means of a suitable detecting device, inscribing a dilution curve from some downstream site, usually a systemic artery or the capillary bed of the ear lobe.

Angiograms may be performed by replacing the Cournand or other open-ended catheter by a closed-ended NIH catheter with side-holes through which radio-opaque dye is injected under high pressure. It is usual for the patient to have a short general anæsthetic for the angiogram, especially if a child.

LEFT-HEART CATHETERIZATION

This is usually a more difficult technique, and several approaches are possible:—

1. During right-heart catheterization, when the left heart is entered via an atrial septal defect, foramen ovale, ventricular septal defect, or persistent ductus arteriosus.

2. By piercing the atrial septum, using a long needle introduced through a catheter inserted into the saphenous vein.

3. By puncture of the left atrium via the right main bronchus, using a long needle introduced through a bronchoscope.

4. From the back, by inserting a needle to the right of the vertebral column and directing it forwards and to the left into the left atrium. A fine catheter can be introduced through this towards the left ventricle.

5. By direct puncture of the left ventricle through the chest wall, inserting the needle either just lateral to the cardiac apex or below the xiphoid process, in which case the needle traverses the right ventricle to enter the left ventricle.

6. Using the suprasternal approach in which a long needle is passed through the aorta and pulmonary artery to enter the left atrium (the Shish-kebab technique).

7. By retrograde arterial catheterization: This is the safest technique for the occasional operator. Methods (2)–(6) should only be attempted by those with extensive experience of cardiac catheterization.

RETROGRADE ARTERIAL CATHETERIZATION

Retrograde arterial catheterization will usually be performed in conjunction with right-heart catheterization and the general points of technique are as described for that procedure. The artery (usually brachial, axillary, or femoral) may be entered in one of two ways:—

1. By the Seldinger method in which the vessel is punctured by a needle through which a guide wire is inserted, the needle withdrawn, and the catheter then advanced over the guide wire. A small incision in the skin facilitates insertion of the catheter.

2. By cut-down on the artery, bleeding being controlled by tapes and bulldog clamps, and the incision in the arterial wall closed afterwards by fine sutures. This method has the advantage that closed-ended NIH catheters can be inserted for rapid injection of radio-opaque contrast material without a tendency for the catheter tip to recoil or for a jet to penetrate the myocardial wall. However, it is now possible to obtain an occluder, mounted on the end of a thin wire, to close off the end-hole of an open-ended catheter with side-holes, as used in Method 1. Entry into the left ventricle through the aortic valve may be difficult and is sometimes facilitated by having a pre-formed pigtail loop at the catheter tip.

COMPLICATIONS

Cardiac arrhythmias are very common, particularly when the tip of the catheter lies in the right or left ventricle. These, however, are usually transient and may be terminated by adjustment of the catheter position. Rarely, more serious arrhythmias such as ventricular tachycardia or fibrillation may occur, so that facilities for prompt DC counter-shock should be available.

Arterial thrombosis may sometimes occur after catheterization of the vessel and may necessitate further arteriotomy and removal of the clot.

Other complications include venospasm, local sepsis, phlebitis in the vein used, and blockage of the catheter by clot. Air embolism could in theory occur, but should not happen if the catheter end is kept closed off by connexion to an intravenous infusion, to a syringe, or to the strain gauge.

CHAPTER XXVI

THE MANAGEMENT OF GASTRODUODENAL CASES

By James Kyle

IN a general surgical ward the majority of patients will be suffering from abdominal complaints. The management of biliary and pancreatic cases is described in Chapters XXVII and XXVIII, and renal cases in Chapter XXXII, while problems peculiar to infants and young children are considered in Chapter XL. In the present chapter the pre-operative investigation and preparation and the post-operative care of patients with acute and chronic lesions of the stomach and duodenum are described. The surgeon will expect his house-surgeon to have a knowledge of the general management of abdominal cases and of the post-operative complications which may arise.

GENERAL PREPARATION

Many patients undergoing elective abdominal surgery, e.g., herniorrhaphy, and who are otherwise fit will require very little preparation. Other patients such as those about to have gastric or intestinal resections require much more detailed evaluation, particularly of their nutritional status.

1. Cardiorespiratory System.—Every patient who is going to have an abdominal operation under general anæsthesia must have: (i) his blood-pressure measured; (ii) the rate and regularity of his pulse checked; and (iii) his chest examined by auscultation. If any abnormality is revealed then further investigations, e.g., ECG or radiography of the chest, are needed. When there is a history of chronic chest infection it is advisable to have a specimen of sputum submitted for culture before operation.

2. Blood-picture.—(*a*) A hæmoglobin estimation is essential when it is known or suspected that a patient has been bleeding and when pallor is noticeable. With some chronic gastro-intestinal diseases there may be a slow fall in hæmoglobin over months or years; it is desirable to correct this loss before operation. (*b*) WBC counts are mainly of value in the diagnosis of acute inflammatory conditions, e.g., appendicitis. (*c*) ESR is determined to assess the activity of and response to treatment in conditions such as ulcerative colitis and regional enteritis. These three investigations can all be performed in the side-room of the ward (*see* p. 695). (*d*) Plasma proteins—electrophoretic strip determinations may be valuable in colitis, enteritis, severe liver disease, and malnutrition.

3. Blood Transfusion.—When a gastric or intestinal resection is contemplated, a blood sample should be sent for cross-matching. More severe degrees of anæmia (Hb below 10 G. per cent) should be corrected before elective operation (*see* p. 43).

4. Urinalysis.—All patients must have their urine checked for the presence of sugar and/or protein. Traces of either substance are frequently found in the urine of patients with acute abdominal conditions and should not delay operative treatment. The presence of larger amounts calls for more detailed investigation.

When urinary tract infection is suspected, organisms and pus cells may be looked for in a spun-down sample of urine in the side-room. If present, a mid-stream specimen is then sent to the laboratory for determination of organism type and sensitivity. Pelvic operations may flare up a latent cystitis.

5. Serum Electrolytes.—Many otherwise healthy patients *do not* require pre- or post-operative determination of serum electrolytes and urea. To submit daily requests for every abdominal case is to subject the laboratory service to an insupportable load. Patients who (*a*) have lost fluid and electrolytes, e.g., by vomiting and diarrhœa, or (*b*) are known to have renal disease, and (*c*) patients over 60 years of age should have their serum sodium, potassium, chloride, and urea estimated. Likewise when there is clinical evidence of dehydration, when the veins are collapsed (hyponatræmia) or the patient is drowsy, drooping, and distended (hypokalæmia) biochemical analysis should be performed (*see* p. 132). Daily electrolyte checks are necessary when fluids are given intravenously. Remember that both hypotension and hypertension may seriously interfere with renal function and that otherwise satisfactory kidneys may not be able to compensate for incorrect types and amounts of fluid administered intravenously.

6. Bowels.—Pre-operative bowel preparation is seldom necessary except for patients undergoing colonic surgery (*see* p. 136). If a barium-meal or enema examination has been carried out within 3 days preceding operation an enema saponis may be given to clear the bowel of barium which may tend to solidify.

7. Weight.—A record of the patient's pre-operative weight is a useful base-line against which to measure progress in many gastro-intestinal diseases.

8. Skin Preparation.—*See* p. 135. For abdominal cases the skin should be shaved from the nipple line above to the lower border of the pubis below, and from one mid-axillary line to the other. For an inguinal herniorrhaphy the upper half of the thigh should also be shaved.

9. Nasogastric Intubation.—*See* p. 348.

10. Rest, Sleep, and Relief of Pain.—Amid the rapidly developing science of surgery, the young doctor should never forget the enormous benefits conferred on a patient by adequate rest, sound sleep, and relief of pain (*see* pp. 103–107).

POST-OPERATIVE CARE

The care of patients after abdominal operations inevitably varies with the magnitude of the surgery that has been performed. Some procedures, e.g., herniorrhaphy, are simple and straightforward and the patient may return to his home the same evening. Other operations, e.g., pancreatico-duodenectomy, involve extensive resection and reconstruction; the patient needs intensive medical and nursing care for many days and is unlikely to leave hospital in less than 18 days. Furthermore, individual surgeons may have preferences based on personal experiences which differ from those contained in the advice given below; the house-surgeon should ascertain such individual variations early in his appointment.

The house-surgeon must see each patient every day, check that his temperature and pulse are normal, his abdomen soft, and his fluid intake–output are in balance. If any abnormality is found he must take steps to find the reason and to correct it.

1. Food and Drink.—Eating and drinking are the natural and pleasurable ways of getting nourishment and fluid into the body. After operation, the patient should be allowed to return to these necessary pleasures as soon as he is able and it is safe for him to do so. Intestinal peristalsis is scarcely interfered with at all by simple laparotomy. Even when the stomach and intestine are handled and sutured, propulsive activity in the intestine is resumed within 6–8 hours, although gastric emptying may take a little longer.

A. Oral Fluid.—After an inguinal herniorrhaphy, a healthy patient can have a cup of tea (200 ml.) in about 6 hours, and next day can take normal diet if he feels like it. When some intra-abdominal procedure has been carried out, before commencing oral fluid it is customary to check that:—

i. The abdomen is soft—no peritonitis, and
ii. The patient has felt borborygmi or passed flatus, or
iii. Bowel-sounds are heard on auscultation.

Before saying that bowel-sounds are absent it is necessary to listen for 2 minutes over each quadrant of the abdomen in a quiet room. A verdict based on a stethoscope bell sitting on top of a dressing for 15 seconds is valueless. In applying the above criteria common sense must also be exercised—it is absurd to deny a drink to a patient who looks and feels well, has a soft abdomen, and is sitting up in bed reading his paper.

After most gastric and intestinal operations it is usual, once there is confirmation of peristaltic activity, to commence with small amounts of fluid hourly. Fifteen ml. of water are drunk hourly; if no ill-effects, such as vomiting, are obvious in 3–4 hours, the amount is increased to 30 ml. hourly and soon to 60 ml. hourly. The latter rate is generally achieved on the day following operation and, allowing for some hours of sleep during the night, represents a fluid intake of about 1000 ml. per 24 hours. Progression to 120 ml. per hour and then free fluids is rapid thereafter.

Type of Fluid.—Tap water is advisable at first but taken hour after hour it tastes singularly insipid. Water can be flavoured with lime or lemon juice, which also stimulates salivation. Orange juice and milk tend to leave the mouth sticky. Aerated drinks should be completely avoided as they may cause abdominal distension and colic. A small cup of tea or coffee is welcomed by the patient not only for its thirst-quenching properties, but also as a first sign of a return to normality.

Contra-indications to Early Oral Fluids.—

a. Operations for gastric or intestinal obstruction. It is advisable to proceed more slowly.

b. Peritonitis, which may prevent the resumption of propulsive activity (paralytic ileus) or render it ineffective (mechanical obstruction).

c. Doubt about the integrity of gastro-intestinal suture lines. Keeping the stomach empty reduces peristaltic frequency and slightly diminishes the volume of secreted juices reaching the doubtful area.

d. Large gastric aspirates—over 60 ml. per hour. By themselves such aspirates are not a contra-indication—the nasogastric tube may be too far down and should be drawn back. But if combined with nausea and a rapid pulse, large aspirates indicate that gastroduodenal contents are not progressing caudally in a satisfactory manner. Very large aspirates should arouse suspicion that the patient is swallowing his mouthwash or other fluid.

B. Food.—Once a patient who has had a standard gastric or intestinal operation is taking 120 ml. of fluid hourly by mouth, it is safe to give him soft solids such as jelly, ice-cream, scrambled eggs, and creamed potatoes. Few patients feel like eating much until their bowels have acted; then the diet can rapidly be increased, but the patient should be warned to chew solids such as meat and oranges thoroughly before swallowing them.

2. Intravenous Fluids.—Patients undergoing simple laparotomy do not need intravenous fluids although, being deprived of oral fluids for 24 hours, their urinary output may be halved during that period. After straightforward operations such as vagotomy plus pyloroplasty or right hemicolectomy, intravenous fluids may be stopped after 24 hours; indeed if the operation has been performed in the morning, the drip may be stopped that night.

In uncomplicated cases, an intravenous infusion should always be stopped within 36 hours unless there is a clearly defined reason for its continuance.

When intravenous fluids have to be given for more than 24 hours, the serum electrolyte concentrations should be checked. Large volumes of fluid may have to be given in intestinal obstruction and prolonged intravenous therapy, often with supplementary potassium and sodium, given for chronic losses, e.g., from fistulæ or a malfunctioning ileostomy.

3. Nasogastric Aspiration.—Many abdominal patients do not require such aspiration. Often when a tube is left in position after operation it is there simply as a safety valve, to ease the surgeon's mind rather than for any actual good that it confers on the patient. Furthermore, a transnasal tube is unpleasant for the patient and predisposes to respiratory infection. Consequently there are good reasons for the early removal of nasogastric tubes.

In the immediate post-operative period the tube is aspirated hourly, the amount obtained and its colour—brown or clear, bile- or blood-stained—recorded on the fluid balance sheet. Once oral fluids are started, the tube is aspirated once in 4 hours; if the volume obtained is less than twice that swallowed, the tube can be removed.

4. Bowels.—These often act spontaneously on the third or fourth post-operative day. Eating a normal diet will generally expedite the process. When there is a previous history of constipation or intestinal anastomoses have been fashioned, it is advisable to give a gentle laxative on the second and third nights, e.g., liquid paraffin emulsion, 15 ml., or senna pod extract (senokot), 14 mg.—2 tablets or 1 teaspoonful of granules. If no bowel action has been obtained by the evening of the fourth day a bisacodyl (dulcolax) suppository is inserted into the rectum. A good house-surgeon regularly checks and if need be ensures that a patient's bowels act at the appropriate time.

Ambulation.—The patient can sit out in a chair for a short time on the first post-operative day. Once the intravenous drip is removed he can go to the toilet and thereafter become increasingly active. However, patients who have had large direct or bilateral herniæ may benefit from 2–3 days in bed; common sense and compassion are displayed in dealing with the frail and elderly.

Smoking.—The period covering an operation is an excellent time for a patient to stop smoking permanently. If he will not do so, he should at least refrain from restarting till the third or fourth post-operative day.

Prevention and management of pulmonary complications, common after upper abdominal operations, are dealt with on p. 164.

CARE OF THE INCISION

Some surgeons leave abdominal incisions completely uncovered, without detriment to wound healing and with increased comfort to the patient. More often the incision is covered by sterile gauze and perforated adhesive. These should be left undisturbed unless there is: (*a*) an unexplained fever; (*b*) unexpected pain in, or (*c*) discharge from the incision. In these circumstances the dressing should be removed, using a no-touch, aseptic technique, and the incision

Senokot (Westminster Laboratories, Hull, Yorks).
Dulcolax (Boehringer Ingelheim Ltd., Isleworth, Middlesex).

is inspected. If there is localized redness and tenderness a stitch may be removed, and a swab for bacteriological investigation is taken from any discharge.

Normally the skin stitches in an inguinal hernia or gridiron appendicectomy incision are removed on the seventh post-operative day. Skin stitches from most other types of abdominal incision are removed on the tenth day although they may be left to the twelfth day in obese subjects.

Deep nylon *tension stitches* should generally not be taken out before the fourteenth day. The surgeon will only have inserted them when:—

a. The abdominal wall is unusually thin, or subjected to excessive strains, e.g., by distension or coughing.

b. Healing is likely to be poor on account of advanced age, malnutrition, or carcinomatosis.

c. Catgut sutures may be attacked by bacterial, pancreatic, or intestinal enzymes.

Management of Abdominal Drains.—These are now used much less frequently than was at one time the case. The various types are described on p. 395. Even though several hundred millilitres may be discharged in the first 24 hours, in most cases the drainage thereafter rapidly diminishes. The drain can then be shortened 2 in. (5 cm.) on the second and third days, and be removed by the fourth or fifth day. Only when copious amounts continue to be discharged should the drain be left in place longer; it is rotated daily and the amount of fluid collected in the bedside bag or bottle recorded on the fluid balance chart.

COMPLICATIONS AFTER ABDOMINAL OPERATIONS

The complications which the house-surgeon must be on the look out for after abdominal surgery fall into three groups:—

1. Those that may follow any operation, e.g., phlebothrombosis (p. 174) and pulmonary atelectasis and infection (p. 164). The latter is commoner after upper abdominal operations while pelvic inflammation, dehydration, and obesity predispose to phlebothrombosis.

2. Complications that may result from laparotomy and a variety of intra-abdominal procedures.

3. Those peculiar to specific operations, e.g., on the stomach. The commoner ones are outlined on p. 356.

POST-OPERATIVE NAUSEA AND VOMITING

People vary greatly in the ease with which feelings of sickness or actual vomiting are induced. Children vomit more readily than adults, and a nervous patient will do so much more readily than a more stoical individual.

Allowing for such variations, nausea and vomiting after operation should always arouse suspicion, particularly of commencing intestinal obstruction.

A careful search for a possible cause should be made.

Causes.—

a. Anæsthetic Agents.—Modern anæsthetic agents do not often cause nausea afterwards. But open ether used to be a common cause and one well known to the public. The resulting fear of an anæsthetic may induce sickness.

b. Drugs.—Morphine and opiates make many people feel sick and are best avoided, being replaced after operation by pethidine or physeptone. Nitrofurantoin produces nausea in about one-third of the patients to whom it is given; large doses of digitalis preparations and stilbœstrol may have a similar effect.

c. Excessive Drinking.—A patient feeling dry and thirsty after operation may on his own initiative drink fluid that he is not meant to take. Guilt frequently prevents him admitting his error.

d. Commencing Intestinal Obstruction.—This is the cause for which the house-surgeon must constantly be on the lookout. The obstruction may be mechanical or paralytic in type (p. 389).

e. Pregnancy, a sometimes forgotten cause of nausea and vomiting in a young woman in a surgical ward.

Treatment.—The treatment of the above causes is obvious or is given on the pages indicated. When no cause can be found treatment has to be non-specific. Sedation with barbiturates or chlorpromazine will calm the nervous patient. Stemetil (prochlorperazine) 5 mg., sparine (promazine) 25 mg., or maxolon (metoclopramide) 10 mg., may be given three times per day; sparine may be injected intramuscularly.

Acute Dilatation of the Stomach.—Thirty years ago a chapter on the management of abdominal operations would have included a lengthy section on this topic. But in the past twenty years the writer has not seen a single undoubted example. It now seems probable that many of the cases in reality were simply the result of injudicious administration of fluid orally, or had unrecognized pyloric stenosis, or the symptoms heralded the onset of paralytic ileus. The stomach was distended with over a litre of 'storm-water' fluid; treatment consisted of removing this fluid by nasogastric suction and by giving intravenous fluids.

HICCUP

Persistent hiccup is a harrowing complication sometimes encountered after abdominal operation, but by no means rare in uræmic subjects. Apart from the distress to the victim, it is upsetting to the other patients and distracting to the nursing staff.

Morphine sometimes controls it for a time, but persistent hiccup is almost untouched by this or any other drug. Carminatives have a place in treatment; unfortunately it is a very small one, and after a transitory feeling of relief, and perhaps bringing up some wind, the spasms return, but a drop of anæsthetic ether on a lump of sugar for the patient to suck should be tried.

Management.—It will be assumed that carminatives and holding the breath have been tried without avail. Commence by doing three things:—

a. Pass a gastric aspiration tube to ensure that the stomach is empty.

b. Ascertain the urinary output and in relevant cases collect a specimen of blood for a blood-urea estimation.

c. Examine the thorax, with special reference to pleurisy, and if there is any supporting evidence, have the diaphragm screened for the presence of a subphrenic abscess. The inhalation of 5 per cent CO_2 from a pre-mixed gas cylinder may stop the hiccup at least temporarily when no cause can be found. For longer-term control, chlorpromazine 25 mg. over 6 hours is recommended.

Injection of the phrenic nerve as it lies on the scalenus anterior in the root of the neck is rarely required.

COMPLICATIONS OF A LAPAROTOMY

Admittedly some complications are unforeseeable or are an almost inevitable complication of the lesion for which operation was performed, e.g., perforated appendicitis. Nevertheless, many complications are the direct result of errors in surgical judgement or technique. Their appearance should be regarded as a

Stemetil (May & Baker Ltd., Dagenham, Essex).
Sparine (John Wyeth & Brother Ltd., Taplow, Maidenhead, Berks).
Maxolon (Beecham Laboratories Ltd., Brentford, Middlesex).

reproach to the whole surgical team and active steps taken to determine their cause and to ensure that there is no repetition.

DEHISCENCE (BURST ABDOMEN)

This is the most dramatic disaster to follow a laparotomy but it is fortunately uncommon, occurring in only 1–2 per cent of patients.

Causes.—In a small proportion of cases dehiscence occurs quite unexpectedly in an apparently fit young patient. In most instances, however, there have been predisposing factors. These are the same as those (p. 344) which lead the surgeon to insert deep tension stitches—advanced age, malnutrition, poor tissues, obesity, distension, and coughing. Unfortunately, breakdown is sometimes the result of bad technique in closing the incision—failing to suture the peritoneum properly, wrong choice of or frayed suture material, wide gaps between stitches or reliance on continuous sutures when interrupted ones would be more appropriate.

Extent.—Part of the peritoneal closure has always given way and the edges have been pushed apart by herniating small intestine or omentum. The musculo-aponeurotic layers also separate; then only the skin stitches prevent complete breakdown which occurs once they are removed.

Time.—Usually between the fourth and the twelfth post-operative day. It is often precipitated by straining, e.g., on coughing or at defæcation.

Symptoms.—Often the patient has felt something giving way. Pain and shock are frequently slight or completely absent. Blood-stained peritoneal fluid escaping from the skin incision is an almost pathognomonic warning sign. Intestine may then prolapse onto the abdominal wall.

In less complete forms, an omental mass around which pinkish fluid is exuding may be seen between the slightly parted skin edges. The house-surgeon should not mistake this for subcutaneous fat and must appreciate that it represents almost complete breakdown of all the deeper layers of the incision.

Treatment.—Reassure and sedate the patient. Place a sterile abdominal pack or dressing over any prolapsed intestine, holding it in place with adhesive strapping. Then alert the surgical team and operating theatre, as repair is necessary.

When breakdown is incomplete, the partially separated muscles can be drawn together by firmly applied strapping (p. 201), but once the stomach is empty, surgical repair is still necessary.

About one-quarter of patients with dehiscence eventually die (usually from the predisposing cause rather than the dehiscence itself). Another quarter are likely to develop an incisional hernia, but in the remainder healing is mostly surprisingly sound and rapid.

PERITONITIS

Peritonitis may already be present at the time of operation, e.g., perforated appendicitis, and continue during the post-operative period or it may develop some days after operation as a result of leakage from faulty intestinal suture lines or necrosed bowel. The latter group is preventable. The diagnosis and management of all forms of post-operative peritonitis can be difficult—few conditions so clearly reveal the difference between the experienced clinical surgeon and the pure surgical scientist. Every aspect of the patient's clinical condition must be assessed day after day and in particular his abdomen must be repeatedly examined with great care and gentleness.

Clinical Features.—

Pain.—This is an almost constant symptom, but may be confused with early post-operative discomfort and the pain caused by the incision. It is constant, renders the patient rather immobile, and may be generalized or more local depending on the extent of the peritoneal involvement. Colic suggests mechanical intestinal obstruction and is often accompanied by restlessness.

Appearance.—The patient looks ill and worried. Drawn features are usual after several days. The skin may be flushed if there is a high fever; toxæmia or interference with diaphragmatic movements cause cyanosis, with laboured breathing.

Temperature and Pulse. There is almost always some elevation of the temperature, with a rapid and frequently thready pulse. When intra-abdominal abscesses begin to form or septicæmia supervenes the temperature may spike to 40° C. (104° F.).

Vomiting.—Anorexia is almost invariable and vomiting not uncommon. If a nasogastric tube is still in position, aspirates will remain large—over 60 ml. per hour.

Abdominal Examination.—Initially the abdomen may be retracted and board-like but after a few hours there is usually some distension. Tenderness and guarding are marked over the affected areas, and the patient is apprehensive of being examined—often his free hand hovers near the surgeon's examining hand. With generalized peritonitis, bowel-sounds are absent (paralytic ileus).

The discharge of fæcal material into the peritoneal cavity and gross purulent peritonitis cause profound *shock* in addition to the above manifestations.

Management.—Sound judgement based on experience is invaluable. When a surgeon is worried about a patient it is much more difficult for him to refrain from reopening the abdomen than to do so. But many patients with post-operative peritonitis do not require a second laparotomy. Another operation should only be done if:—

a. There is mechanical obstruction;

b. An abscess requiring drainage has formed;

c. Intestinal contents are freely entering the peritoneal cavity.

Active treatment is as follows:—

1. Fluid and electrolytes—maintain proper balance. Intravenous fluids are needed, and the volumes of urine passed, gastric contents aspirated, and discharges from drains must be accurately recorded. An adequate supply of calories must be ensured (p. 46). For management of shock *see* p. 20.

2. Gastric aspiration—necessary with general peritonitis, certainly for the first day or two. With localized peritonitis it is probably not needed unless there is vomiting or abdominal distension.

3. Laboratory tests: (*a*) Serum electrolytes and urea daily; (*b*) WBC count at intervals to check on the resolution of the inflammatory process; (*c*) Blood gases (p. 13) if there is evidence of cardiorespiratory failure and toxæmia.

4. Antibiotics—most cases are due to *Escherichia coli* and *Streptococcus fæcalis*. Tetracycline can be given into the intravenous infusion—500 mg. into the first bottle, thereafter 250 mg. Sensitivity tests on a swab taken at the initial operation may indicate another antibiotic as being appropriate.

5. Temperature, pulse, and respiration—record 4-hourly.

6. Relief of pain—pethidine 50 mg. may be given i.m. Although morphine sulphate 10 mg. may interfere with peristalsis it promotes sleep and mental tranquillity in addition to relieving pain.

13

7. Oxygen therapy (p. 301) if there is cyanosis; tracheostomy (p. 16) may be advisable in gravely ill and feeble patients.

8. Frequent abdominal examination for evidence of intestinal obstruction or abscess formation.

Finally, remember that a patient who has had peritonitis will afterwards require a longer convalescence and more intensive efforts to restore his nutrition than are needed after uncomplicated operations.

Residual Abscesses.—*See* p. 392.

Intestinal Obstruction.—*See* p. 389.

GASTRIC SURGERY

The management of uncomplicated operations on the stomach, e.g., for carcinoma or duodenal ulcer, is as outlined on p. 340. In the present section the techniques of using nasogastric tubes are explained. The three tests of gastric secretory function—pentagastrin, augmented histamine, and insulin tests—are described in detail. Brief accounts are given of the management of bleeding and of perforated peptic ulcer and of pyloric (duodenal) stenosis. There are a few complications which are peculiar to or are commoner after operations on the stomach; their diagnosis and treatment are described at the end of the section.

NASOGASTRIC TUBES

In surgical practice the passage of a nasogastric tube may be required for:—

a. Diagnostic tests of gastric function;

b. Therapeutically to empty the stomach and keep it empty;

c. For intragastric feeding.

The presence of a nasogastric tube is technically of assistance in performing abdominal vagotomy, and after operation may give early warning of bleeding should it occur.

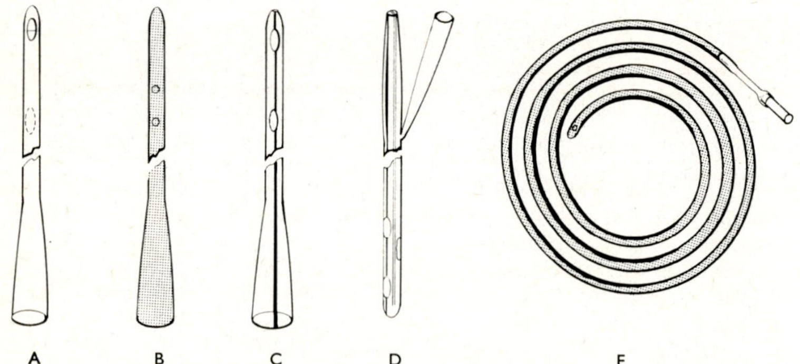

Fig. 254.—Nasogastric tubes (*see* text). A, plastic; B, Ryle; C, Levin; D, Salem; E, Plexitron.

Types of Tubes.—In Britain nearly all the tubes now in use are made of plastic and are pre-sterilized. The old style of Ryle's tube made of red rubber was often too small in calibre to provide effective gastric aspiration, while larger sizes were irritant to the mucosa and sometimes caused late strictures of the œsophagus.

The plastic tube illustrated in *Fig.* 254 **A** is that most commonly used. It is 75 cm. long and available in various sizes—a 14 or 16 F is the size most often used. Large sizes, e.g., No. 32 F, passed through the mouth, may, however, be needed for aspirating food, and for lavage, e.g., in pyloric stenosis or poisoning.

The Ryle-type tube illustrated in *Fig.* 254 **B** is radio-opaque; the exact position of its tip in the stomach can easily be checked radiologically. An opaque marker is incorporated in the

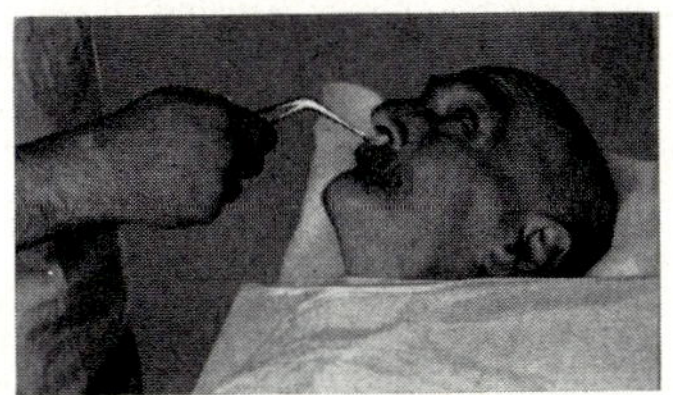

Fig. 255.—The patient sits up in bed with his head supported at the angle shown. The wider nostril is cleaned and packed with wool soaked in 2 per cent anethaine.

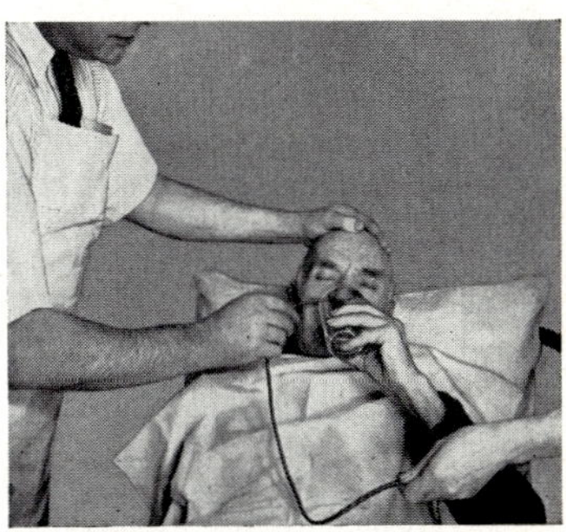

Fig. 256.—A tumbler of water is handed to the patient. After the cotton-wool has been removed the tube is passed down the nostril. Steadying the patient's head while he drinks, the tube is pushed onwards.

Levin-type tube (*Fig.* 254 **C**) which is 120 cm. long and rather more rigid than the previous type of tube. While it may be slightly less comfortable for the patient, it is easier for the radiologist to position it exactly under fluoroscopic control.

The Salem sump suction type of tube (*Fig.* 254 **D**) has an additional air inlet and is useful for continuous aspiration of the stomach. The fine No. 8 F Plexitron tube (*Fig.* 254 **E**) is used for nasogastric drip feeding and may be left in position for some days.

Passing the Tube.—First explain to the patient what you are going to do and what he can do himself to ensure that the tube goes down easily. A very nervous or uncooperative patient may have his nasopharynx sprayed with 2 ml. of 4 per cent lignocaine (or citanest) or be given an intramuscular injection of 100 mg. phenobarbitone half an hour before the tube is passed. The terminal portion of the tube is lubricated with sterile liquid paraffin. The patient sits up comfortably in bed with the head supported at the angle shown in *Fig.* 255. The nostrils are inspected, and if there is obvious deviation of the septum, the wider nasal passage is selected. This nostril is cleaned with a pledget of cotton-wool moistened with a bland antiseptic, e.g., weak flavine solution, the pledgets being applied on forceps. This complete, the tip of the nose is held between the finger and thumb of one hand while the tube is pushed gently horizontally along the floor of the nose. The passage past the inferior concha is facilitated by tilting the tip of the nose upwards. When the pharynx is entered, retching occurs; repeatedly urge the patient to swallow. If, instead of swallowing, retching continues, call upon the patient to sip and swallow some water (*Fig.* 256); a glass half-filled with water should be at hand. Once the end of the tube has passed the region of the cricoid cartilage, as a rule the passage of the tube along the œsophagus is straightforward.

Plastic stomach and Ryle-type tube (Messrs. W. Warne & Co., Ltd., Barking, Essex).
Levin-type tube and Salem sump suction tubes (Brunswick Corporation, St. Louis, Mo., U.S.A.).
Plexitron tube (Messrs. Baxters, Illinois, U.S.A.).
Citanest (Astra-Hewlett Ltd., Watford, Herts).

Apart from œsophageal obstruction, the only condition that may arrest the tip of the tube is chronic contraction of the diaphragm with tight embracement of the terminal portion of the œsophagus by the diaphragmatic crura which occurs when the upper abdomen is intensely rigid. With the less flexible pattern of tube usually resistance due to muscular spasm can be overcome.

That the end of the tube has reached its destination can be ascertained by withdrawal of some of the gastric contents by means of a syringe. Alternatively, some air can be injected down; with a stethoscope its arrival in the stomach is denoted by bubbling sounds in the left upper abdomen. When the tube is correctly positioned, secure it in position by looping the centre of a strip of zinc-oxide strapping round the tube at the external nares and sticking the ends to each side of the nose.

Unconscious Patients (without a swallowing reflex).—The easiest way to introduce a gastric aspiration tube in an unconscious patient is to pass a Magill's endotracheal tube. The Magill's tube, well lubricated both inside and out, is passed through the nose past the pharyngeal sphincter. Through the Magill's tube is passed the gastric aspiration tube. When the latter has reached the stomach the Magill's tube is withdrawn. That the tube has reached the stomach and has not entered the trachea is proved by aspirating gastric contents. On the other hand, if no fluid is withdrawn one should listen at the end of the tube for a blowing sound; impingement of air upon the ear is proof-positive that the tube has entered the air-passages.

Care of the Tube.—The house-surgeon should check that gastric aspiration is functioning efficiently. It is best performed by hand, at stated intervals. If no aspirate has been obtained on several occasions try injecting 10 ml. of air or water down the tube to see if it is patent. Once patency is demonstrated, if gastric contents are still not aspirated it means that the tip of the tube is not in the most dependent part of the stomach—often it is curled up in the fundus. Try withdrawing it 5 cm. and aspirate; if this fails, reinsert it rather further and aspirate again, or pass a new tube.

Nasogastric tubes should be removed as soon as their presence is no longer essential (p. 342). Once they have been in place for 2–3 days they may cause rhinitis with some encrustation around the tube—the part traversing the nares should be smeared with naseptin or other antibiotic cream.

GASTROSTOMY FOR ASPIRATION AND FEEDING

When a patient objects to or is unable to swallow a nasogastric tube, the stomach can be kept empty after operation by inserting a small Foley bag catheter. Before closing the abdominal incision a small stab is made in the left upper abdominal wall and the tip of the Foley catheter brought through it into the peritoneal cavity. A 1-cm. incision is then made on the anterior wall of the stomach, the catheter introduced and secured in position by two purse-string catgut stitches. The bag on the catheter is then inflated with 5–10 ml. of water and omentum wrapped loosely around the shaft of the catheter—the stomach does *not* need to be stitched to the parietal peritoneum.

The catheter is aspirated like a nasogastric tube during the post-operative period. After 5–7 days, the bag is deflated and the catheter removed. In other circumstances the Foley catheter gastrostomy may be used for supplementary alimentation; feeds of 2500 ml. are dripped in each day (p. 49).

An alternative type of catheter is the combined aspiration and feeding Kay catheter (*Fig.* 257). It contains a second channel, prolonged for 20 cm. beyond

Naseptin (Imperial Chemical Industries Ltd., Alderley Park, Cheshire).

the normal tip as a fine tube which is passed into the upper jejunum; through it dextrose-saline may be infused, while the larger channel is used to aspirate the stomach. This catheter is particularly useful in centres where there are not enough trained nurses to properly supervise intravenous infusions.

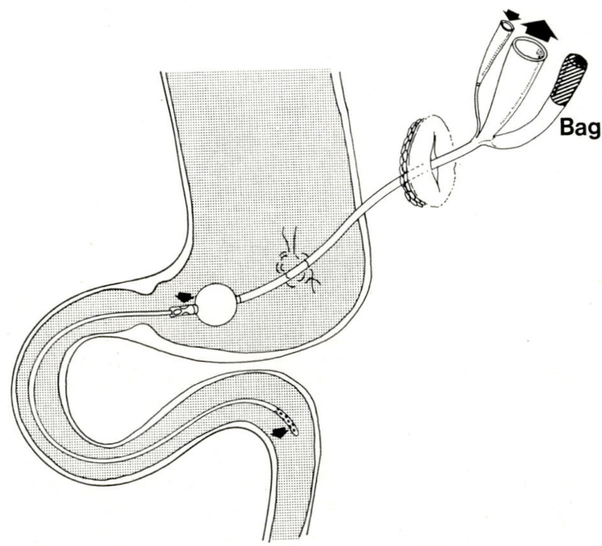

Fig. 257.—Kay's combined gastric aspiration and feeding catheter.

Jejunostomy Feeding.—A Foley catheter inserted by a technique similar to that described above is suitable for a feeding jejunostomy. Hepovite and complan can be added to the feeds shown on p. 49 which contain fat emulsion (prosparol).

DUODENAL ASPIRATION

This is seldom performed except for special tests of pancreatic secretion (*see* p. 387). The duodenal tube is 125 cm. long—it is approximately 75 cm. from the external nares to the papilla of Vater. The tube is passed in a similar fashion to a nasogastric tube until 55 cm. have been inserted. The patient then lies on his right side and the tube is advanced very slowly, at the rate of 1 cm. per minute, for 20 minutes. The tip should now be in the duodenum; its position is checked radiologically.

INTESTINAL ASPIRATION

The use of long Miller-Abbott or 18 F Cantor tubes for intestinal decompression is rare in Britain. It is relatively simple to pass the well-lubricated, mercury-loaded bag of a Cantor tube (*Fig.* 258) through the nose and pylorus of a healthy person, but much more difficult in a patient with paralytic ileus who might benefit from it. Once the stomach is reached, the procedure for negotiating the pyloric canal is the same as for a duodenal tube; it may take up to 2 hours and exhaust

Hepovite, Prosparol (Duncan, Flockhart, & Evans, Ltd., Birkbeck St., London, E.2).

an ill patient. Continuous suction is applied once the upper jejunum is reached. A large free loop of tube must be left beside the patient's head so that the loaded tip can advance with the return of peristaltic activity in the decompressed intestine.

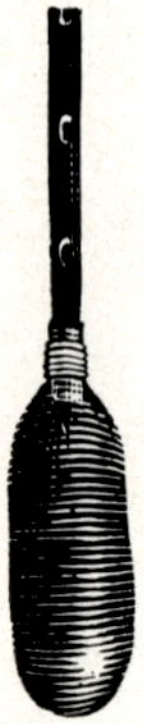

PENTAGASTRIN TEST OF GASTRIC SECRETION

Synthetic pentagastrin is used as the stimulant of gastric secretion. The test is the most helpful one to use before operations for peptic ulcers.

Technique.—

1. Overnight fast of 12 hours.

2. Nasogastric tube size 14 F or 16 F is passed 55–57 cm., and its position checked radiologically.

3. Patient lies supine or slightly on his left side and the stomach emptied by aspiration.

4. Pentagastrin 6 μg. per kg. body-weight is injected i.m. into the quadriceps muscle.

5. Aspirate gastric contents every 10 minutes for half an hour, either by hand or else by continuous suction (−2·5 cm. Hg), injecting a little air periodically to ensure patency. The position of the tube may have to be adjusted occasionally to ensure that it taps the pool of gastric secretion.

6. Titrate juice collected between 10–30 minutes after pentagastrin injection against 0·01 N sodium hydroxide to phenolphthalein end-point (total acid). This acid output (10–30 minutes) in mEq. $\times$ 3 is the peak acid output per hour.

Fig. 258.—To the distal end of the Cantor tube is attached a small, thin rubber bag. This is partially filled with mercury.

The pentagastrin causes no side-effects and consequently is more pleasant for the patient than the augmented histamine test. The maximum acid output (between 10–30 minutes) occurs 15–20 minutes sooner than after histamine injection, but the peak acid output per hour is approximately the same for pentagastrin and histamine tests—from 20 to 30 mEq. per hour in normal subjects, 30–60 mEq. per hour for many males with duodenal ulcers.

THE AUGMENTED HISTAMINE TEST

The method is as follows:—

1. The patient is fasted for 12 hours.

2. A 16 F stomach tube is introduced into the stomach and using a 50-ml. syringe the entire fasting contents are aspirated. This procedure is facilitated by altering the position of the tube and the patient until the gastric pool is located. The position of the tube is verified by an X-ray. The tube is then fastened in position around the nostril and the patient kept in the same position (usually on the left side, semi-upright) throughout the test.

3. The spontaneously secreted juice, which is the *basal secretion*, is now aspirated continuously, or by intermittent hand suction, for 60 minutes. The total volume is measured, the free and total HCl titrated (with Topfer's reagent and phenolphthalein, respectively) and expressed as the number of milliequivalents secreted in this period. During the test saliva is sucked out or expectorated.

4. Four ml. (100 mg.) of mepyramine hydrogen maleate (anthisan) are injected intramuscularly, 30 minutes after the start of the basal juice collection.

5. Four body-weight doses of histamine acid phosphate (a body-weight dose is 0·1 mg. per 10 kg.) are injected subcutaneously.

Anthisan (May & Baker, Ltd., Dagenham, Essex).

6. The gastric secretion is continuously aspirated for one hour after giving histamine or, alternatively, is collected as four 15-minute specimens and the free and total HCl titrated. The weight of HCl produced in this 60-minute period is an expression of the maximum parietal cell response to stimulation.

INSULIN TEST

This is used as a test for the completeness of vagotomy. The hypoglycæmia induced should actuate the vagus brain-stem centres to stimulate the secretion of acid gastric juice if any nerve pathways remain undivided.

Technique.—

1. Overnight fast of 12 hours.

2. Nasogastric tube passed and its position checked radiologically. Saliva is expectorated.

3. Patient lies supine or slightly on his left side.

4. Stomach aspirated until empty—*fasting juice*; then basal juice collected for 2 hours.

5. Take a blood sample for blood-sugar estimation.

6. Inject slowly intravenously 15–20 units soluble insulin (0·2 unit per kg. body-weight).

7. Aspirate gastric contents every 15 minutes for 2 hours; measure and label each of the eight samples. Before each aspiration 10 ml. of air may be injected to ensure patency.

8. Take blood-sugar samples every 30 minutes.

It is advisable to have available a 50 per cent solution of glucose suitable for intravenous administration. The test is only likely to be valid if at least one blood-sugar reading falls below 40 mg. per cent, a level which sometimes produces unpleasant hypoglycæmic symptoms. If present, these develop about 20 minutes after the insulin injection and about 20 minutes before maximal stimulation of acid secretion.

Interpretation of results is difficult as mostly there is a new opening in the bottom of the stomach through which alkaline bile regurgitates. If there is more than 0·75 mEq. of HCl in the 2 hours after insulin compared to the 2-hour basal secretion, vagotomy is probably incomplete.

HÆMATEMESIS AND MELÆNA

Eight out of ten instances of hæmatemesis and melæna in Britain are the result of duodenal or gastric ulcers or erosions. The only other cause that is at all frequent is hiatus hernia; portal hypertension is uncommon.

Nine out of ten patients will *not* require an urgent operation. In fact many patients have already stopped bleeding by the time they are admitted to a medical ward. A few will continue to bleed moderate amounts or have recurrent stutter hæmorrhages in hospital. Massive hæmorrhage with blood pouring from mouth and rectum is dramatic and unforgettable but it is very rare.

Management.—

1. Obtain a history (from patient or relative) of peptic ulceration, hepatitis, alcoholism, or of the ingestion of aspirin or other gastric mucosal irritants. Was there any pre-existing hypertension or blood dyscrasia?

2. Measure blood-pressure and pulse-rate. If bleeding is continuing chart the values every 30 minutes. In other cases 2-hourly will suffice.

3. Palpate abdomen gently—mainly to exclude a gastric tumour, enlarged spleen, and liver.

4. Gastric aspiration—pass a nasogastric tube, size No. 16 or 18, and aspirate half-hourly to get early warning of recurrent bleeding. Many patients have stopped bleeding and show no evidence of hypovolæmic shock.

5. Take blood samples for: (*a*) Hæmoglobin determination; (*b*) Blood grouping; (*c*) Blood-urea.

Indications for Blood Transfusion.—

1. Blood-pressure under 100 mm. Hg systolic;
2. Hb below 66 per cent;
3. Pulse-rate persistently over 100 per min.;
4. Blood-urea over 100 mg. per cent.

When it is decided that transfusion is necessary then: (*a*) Give at least two bottles of blood—1000 ml.; (*b*) Inform the surgeon whose services may eventually be required. He may request an emergency barium meal and/or gastroscopy.

Medical Treatment.—

1. Careful supervision for evidence of further bleeding. Because of its later appearance, melæna is more treacherous than hæmatemesis; it often causes turbulent bowel-sounds.

2. Bed-rest.

3. Sedation, e.g., phenobarbitone injection 60 mg. i.m. every 8 hours or amylobarbitone 60 mg. orally. The patient should be kept continuously slightly drowsy.

4. Hourly milk feeds, 60 ml., which are rapidly increased when there is no active bleeding.

5. Watch the urinary output and check haemoglobin daily at first.

Indications for Urgent Operation.—Apart from those with massive hæmorrhage in most patients with moderate or recurrent bleeding a number of factors must be considered before deciding on an urgent operation. Factors in favour of operation are a patient over 45 years old, a known gastric ulcer, other complications, and recurrence of bleeding in hospital.

PERFORATED PEPTIC ULCER

In Britain there are more perforated duodenal ulcers than gastric ones—some of the latter may be perforations in carcinomatous ulcers. The onset is sudden. Upper abdominal pain is the outstanding symptom and once the diagnosis is made, its relief is the house-surgeon's most urgent task.

Diagnosis.—

1. Abdominal examination: board-like rigidity of the upper abdomen is characteristic. The patient lies still, and diaphragmatic movement may be interfered with.

Percussion sometimes reveals loss of liver dullness.

2. Exclude: (*a*) Tabes dorsalis; (*b*) Basal pneumonia; (*c*) A posterior myocardial infarct.

3. X-ray of upper abdomen with the patient erect shows free gas under the diaphragm (p. 705).

4. Serum amylase—is often raised above 200 units, but rarely reaches the acute pancreatitis range, above 600 units.

Treatment.—Nearly all patients require operation, usually simple suture of the perforation. When the patient is fit and there are sound pre-existing reasons for surgery, a definitive operation may be performed.

Preparation.—

1. Nasogastric tube, hourly aspiration.
2. Intravenous glucose-saline infusion.

3. Fluid balance chart.

4. Blood for: (i) Serum electrolytes; (ii) Cross-matching if definitive surgery likely.

Antibiotics are not usually necessary to begin with—for some hours the peritonitis is chemical rather than bacterial. But patients with perforations are particularly prone to post-operative chest infections (p. 164).

NON-OPERATIVE TREATMENT OF PERFORATED PEPTIC ULCER

Indications.—Nearly all perforations are treated by operation—either simple suture or definitive surgery for the ulcer. In the following rare circumstances a non-operative régime may have to be adopted:—

1. No operating facilities available, e.g., on board ship.

2. Patient refuses operation.

3. Grave medical contra-indications to operation.

Non-operative Régime.—

1. *Position.*—The patient lies flat, with head supported on one pillow.

2. *Intravenous Fluids.*—These are necessary for 3 or 4 days. They must be adjusted frequently, charted, and the amounts given kept in balance with the urine output and other fluid losses.

3. *Gastric Aspiration.*—This should be performed hourly, by hand, by a special nurse. Continuous suction systems are liable to block.

4. *Pulse, Temperature, and Respiration.*—These are charted every 4 hours, as in the non-operative treatment of appendicitis (*see* p. 390). A progressive rise in these parameters indicates that the method is failing.

5. *Abdominal Examination.*—Twice daily at first, by an experienced clinician, to detect increased tenderness, distension, and ileus. After a few days a rectal examination is performed to ascertain if there is any pelvic infection.

6. *Drugs.*—Having decided on the line of treatment the patient may be given not more than 10 mg. morphine or 100 mg. pethidine slowly, intravenously. Failure to gain relief within 2 hours should lead to a reassessment of the diagnosis. Narcotics are not required on subsequent days.

7. *Antibiotics.*—Tetracycline 250 mg. i.v. or i.m. every 6 hours.

8. *Repeated radiographs* must be looked upon as an essential part of the non-operative treatment. In addition to the first diagnostic radiographs others should be taken 12, 36, and 48 hours after admission. If the perforation becomes sealed by fibrinous lymph, the subdiaphragmatic shadow of air diminishes slowly in size; conversely, if the shadow increases in size (usually the patient is an air swallower) after the passage of a stomach-tube to allow air in the stomach and the peritoneal cavity to escape, then, if practicable, operation should be performed without further delay.

9. *Diet.*—Oral fluids may be started (*see* p. 342) about the third day if there are bowel-sounds audible and the abdomen is soft.

A point that merits particular attention is that aspiration treatment is nearly always fatal in patients severely ill with diffuse peritonitis. Consequently, it must not be used in the very type of case that on a *prima facie* acquaintance with the subject one would think is more suitable for non-operative treatment than almost any other. Persistent air swallowers are also unsuitable for non-operative treatment.

PYLORIC STENOSIS

Advanced stages of pyloric stenosis are now seldom seen in Britain, but may still be encountered elsewhere, causing very serious losses of body fluids and electrolytes.

Management.—

1. Empty the stomach with an indwelling No. 18 nasogastric tube. Aspirate hourly. Saline injections down the tube will help to flush out thick mucus and undigested food.

2. Serum electrolyte and urea estimations daily.

3. Urinary output carefully checked. Aim at a 24-hour output of over 1000 ml., with a SG below 1015.

4. Intravenous fluid: A patient with obvious dehydration—dry tongue, sunken eyes, and collapsed veins—may already have a fluid deficit of 4 litres, to which must be added the body's normal daily fluid requirement of 2–2·5 litres, and any measured losses. About half this total should be given in the first 12 hours and replacement is usually complete in 36–48 hours.

5. Electrolytes: Vomiting for 2–3 days depletes the body of sodium, and so at first alternate bottles of normal saline and of 5 per cent dextrose are infused. More prolonged vomiting reduces the potassium reserves and may cause alkalosis and tetany. Potassium chloride, 1 G. per 500 ml. of 5 per cent dextrose, may be given, but not more than 6 G. of KCl should be administered in 24 hours.

By the second day it is often possible to give some gastrografin orally, and, by radiographing the patient, determine whether or not pyloric obstruction is complete. (The organic narrowing is usually in the first part of the duodenum.) Frequently there is an element of spasm or œdema which will subside on the above management. If so, the patient is placed on an anti-ulcer régime and prepared for definite surgical treatment, which is always necessary with genuine cases of pyloric stenosis.

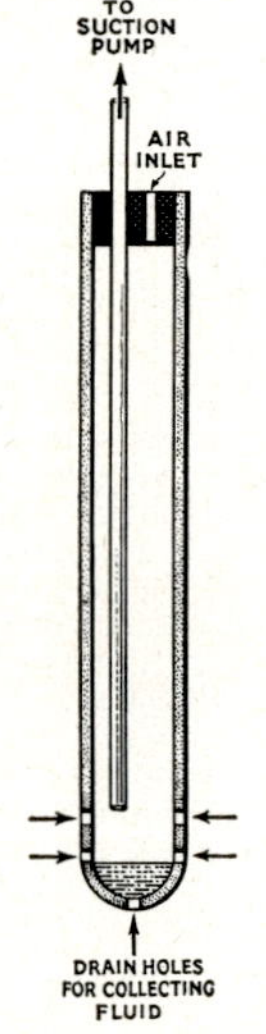

Fig. 259.—Cleland's plastic sump drain.*

COMPLICATIONS OF GASTRIC SURGERY

Modern gastric surgery is remarkably safe. There are only three complications peculiar to it which occur with any frequency.

1. Pancreatitis.—This usually appears on the second to fifth day. The pain follows and merges with the immediate post-operative discomfort, making evaluation difficult. The patient is restless, has a low fever and fast pulse. There is upper abdominal pain, tenderness, and guarding, and sometimes back pain. The serum amylase is over 600 units.

Treatment.—Trasylol intravenously, 200,000 units in the first bottle of 5 per cent dextrose, followed by 200,000 units per 24 hours. This treatment and gastric aspiration are given until all symptoms subside.

2. Bleeding.—After elective surgery on the stomach some bleeding from the suture line occurs in perhaps 2 per cent of patients and is revealed by gastric aspiration or even a hæmatemesis.

Treatment.—With sedation and a slow blood transfusion bleeding mostly ceases. If it continues after 4 hours, or if there is evidence of hypovolæmic shock (systolic BP under 100 mm. Hg; pulse over 100 per minute) or if clots are being brought up, then re-exploration of the suture line is necessary.

3. Blown Duodenal Stump.—After a Polya-type gastrectomy the closure of the duodenal stump may suddenly give way, classically about the fourth day. Often the operation was difficult and the post-operative course stormy. There is sudden severe right upper abdominal pain, collapse, and bile-stained duodenal contents may issue from any drain that was left in place.

---

* Made by Portland Plastics Ltd., Hythe, Kent.

Trasylol (F.B.A. Pharmaceuticals Ltd., Haywards Heath, Sussex).

Treatment.—It is essential to secure good drainage. This usually means making a small incision through which to insert a sump suction drain (*Fig.* 259) down to the duodenum. Continuous suction is applied to this drain, and the skin around it is protected with a liberal application of aluminium paste. At the same time a feeding jejunostomy (p. 351) may be established; otherwise fluid and electrolytes are given intravenously. The stomach is kept empty by aspiration and the patient nursed when possible on his left side. Check the serum amylase and treat pancreatitis if present (*vide supra*). In any case propantheline bromide, 15 mg. every 8 hr., may be given to reduce pancreatic secretion, but it may precipitate parotitis or retention of urine.

ABDOMINAL TRAUMA

Trauma is unselective and different parts and systems of the body may be injured in the same accident. When confronted by a patient who has sustained an abdominal injury, the house-surgeon must make certain that no other injuries are present. Fractures of long bones and skull are usually obvious, but fractures of jaw, cervical spine, and ribs are easily overlooked initially. Appropriate radiographs must be taken; when life is immediately threatened by severe head injuries or respiratory obstruction it may be necessary to bring the X-ray apparatus to the patient, not vice versa. Other specialists who may be involved in the care of the multiply-injured patient should be notified at once.

The liver and spleen are the intraperitoneal viscera most frequently injured; renal trauma is dealt with in Chapter XXXII. The possibility of delayed rupture of abdominal organs must always be borne in mind; it can have fatal consequences for the patient and serious legal consequences for the young doctor. Closed abdominal injuries involving the intestines are particularly treacherous; the senior surgeon must always be notified and the patient re-examined at frequent intervals. Needle paracentesis may be helpful (p. 384) in doubtful abdominal injuries.

Open penetrating wounds which appear to involve peritoneum always require laparotomy. Operation is also essential for rupture of solid viscera and for perforation of hollow viscera. Blood transfusion is arranged for and an intravenous infusion set up. A central venous pressure monitor (p. 24) is valuable in assessing the need for and rate of fluid replacement; pulse, blood-pressure, and respiratory rate are charted every 15 minutes and the urinary output watched —a catheter may have to be inserted. As bowel may have been ruptured, tetracycline, 250 mg. every 6 hours, is given parenterally.

CHAPTER XXVII

THE MANAGEMENT OF BILIARY AND HEPATIC CASES

By William Burnett

BILIARY tract disease is common throughout the world and every house-surgeon must have a thorough understanding of its management. Jaundice is a frequent diagnostic challenge and constitutes a serious hazard to life. Although hepatic disease is less common, skilful management is necessary if life is to be saved and health restored.

THE MANAGEMENT OF ACUTE CONDITIONS OF THE BILIARY TREE

GALL-STONE COLIC

Gall-stone colic arises when a stone impacts in the neck of the gall-bladder, in the cystic duct, or in the bile-duct. The pain can begin gradually or very suddenly and is felt as repeated spasms, usually in the right hypochondium, or less often in the epigastrium, with radiation to the interscapular region. It may, on occasion, be referred to the right shoulder. It may last only a few minutes or may go on for many hours. Traditionally, morphine has been used to relieve gall-stone colic, but it is often found that the pain is not relieved as much as might have been expected. The reason is that morphine causes spasm of the sphincter of Oddi, thus increasing intrabiliary pressure and consequent pain. Morphine is therefore contra-indicated in biliary disease, since it increases any biliary-tract obstruction, raises the possibility of super-added pancreatitis, and may result in further liver damage. The most suitable drug for relieving pain and biliary colic is pethidine hydrochloride (B.P.),* which should be given in doses of 50 or 100 mg. An initial dose of 50 mg. should be given intravenously for rapid action; if found insufficient, a further 50 mg. may be given. This can be repeated 4-hourly, but if the pain returns 1–2 hours after the first injection, the dose may be repeated at that time. It will often be found that the skin of the right hypochondrium has been burnt superficially by local application of hot-water bottles by the patient prior to admission to hospital. Further local heat may be comforting, but should not be required in hospital if adequate analgesics are given.

ACUTE CHOLECYSTITIS

Diagnosis.—

1. *Clinical.*—The onset may be quite sudden or may be preceded by a history of chronic gall-bladder disease. The upper abdominal pain is often sharp but continuous, and there may be a superimposed element of biliary colic. Gradual fading of the pain may signify either resolution of the condition or the development of a quiet perforation of the gall-bladder. Tenderness is usual in the right hypochondrium and there is often enough rigidity to prevent palpation of an enlarged gall-bladder. Tachycardia is moderate and the temperature is commonly about 38° C. (100° F.). If the temperature rises to 39·5° C. (103° F.) and

---

* Known as demerol in the U.S.A.

particularly if associated with rigors, cholangitis should be suspected. Leuco-cytosis is usually present but can be absent in the elderly. If jaundice develops, a stone may be present in the bile-duct, but jaundice may also be due to a localized inflammatory mass involving the bile-duct, with cholecystadenitis, cholangitis, or pancreatitis around the bile-duct termination.

The most important conditions to be differentiated are perforated peptic ulcer, acute pancreatitis, appendicitis, and intestinal obstruction. The condition may also resemble myocardial infarction, pneumonia, and diaphragmatic pleurisy.

2. *Radiological.*—A plain abdominal radiograph may show the outline of a distended gall-bladder or gall-stones may be seen. Ten per cent of all gall-stones are radio-opaque. The plain abdominal radiograph also excludes gas under the diaphragm from a perforated hollow viscus, pancreatic calcification, and the 'sentinel loop' of intestine seen in acute pancreatitis. Oral cholecystography is not of much value in acute cholecystitis, but a normally functioning gall-bladder in fact eliminates cholecystitis. Intravenous cholangiography is preferred to cholecystography, since it can be carried out much more quickly and gives valuable information with regard to the bile-duct. (*See* Chapter XLVII, p. 712.) In some cases where clinical diagnosis is difficult, intravenous cholangiography may prove useful in separating acute cholecystitis from acute pancreatitis and other acute abdominal conditions.

Conservative or Surgical Treatment?—Acute cholecystitis nearly always sub-sides spontaneously, but occasionally a patient's condition so deteriorates that operation becomes essential. Unfortunately, it is very difficult to predict the need for surgery when the patient is first seen. Definitive treatment of acute cholecystitis by early elective operation was first recommended 30 years ago, and since then there has been continuing controversy. The advocates of early surgery believe that it is the logical treatment for an acute process because it eliminates the possibility of later complications such as gangrene of the gall-bladder and perforation, while it also reduces the duration of the illness and hospitalization. Those who prefer conservative management believe that definitive surgery can be carried out more safely at a later stage after the acute process has subsided. They point out that the risks of perforation (1 per cent) are considerably smaller than have been stated. There are also difficulties associ-ated with the necessity for making a correct early diagnosis if early surgery is being advocated. However, the divergence between the two schools of thought is not as great as might at first be presumed. Early operation is no longer advised by the more radical group until diagnosis is certain, and the patient has been adequately evaluated and prepared. On the other hand, the conservative group emphasize the importance of extreme vigilance in the non-operative treatment, and advise immediate surgery should the patient's condition deteriorate.

Indications for Immediate Laparotomy.—Laparotomy should be carried out at once if (1) the patient has a WBC count greater than 15,000 per c.mm., (2) develops a palpable mass, and (3) has rigidity in the right hypochondrium. This indicates an unrelieved outlet obstruction of the gall-bladder, carrying a relatively high perforation and mortality-rate.

Indications for Delayed Laparotomy.—If the pulse-rate and temperature do not fall with conservative management, if the pain persists, or gets worse, and if tenderness and rigidity increase, or a larger mass develops in the hypochondrium, empyema or perforation of the gall-bladder should be suspected and prepara-tions for operation should be made forthwith. Mucocele of the gall-bladder is recognized by the presence of a large, relatively non-tender gall-bladder swelling in the absence of pyrexia or leucocytosis. It is impracticable to persist with conservative management in these circumstances and cholecystectomy should be carried out. If the local signs indicate that the gall-bladder has ruptured into the general peritoneal cavity, immediate operation is required. If acute typhoid cholecystitis is diagnosed, operation is recommended because in this condition the gall-bladder is rather liable to perforate.

Management of Acute Cholecystitis (*see also* p. 390).—

1. Rest in bed.
2. Sedation.
3. Fluid and electrolyte balance.
4. Nasogastric suction.
5. Antibiotic therapy.
6. Careful record of vital signs.

Whether or not early surgery is preferred, a patient with acute cholecystitis is treated by rest in bed, sedation adequate to control his pain, and the fluid and electrolyte balances are maintained. If nausea and vomiting prevent oral administration, fluids should be given intravenously and nasogastric suction instituted. Pethidine is preferable to morphine as the latter drug has the more marked effect in causing spasm of the sphincter of Oddi. An antibiotic should be given from the start. Unfortunately, it is rarely, if ever, possible to know

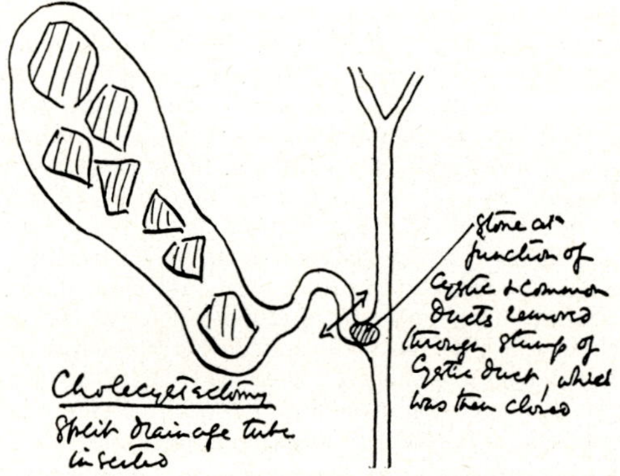

Fig. 260.—Fascimile of a record of the operation of cholecystectomy to supplement the full case record description which is preferably typed.

the sensitivity of the organisms concerned at the start of the illness when an antibiotic is being selected. However, since most of the infecting organisms are of bowel origin, it is wise to use a broad-spectrum antibiotic such as tetracycline. The basic dosage is 1 G. per day orally in divided doses of 250 mg., but if vomiting makes the oral route impracticable it should be given in the intravenous drip. The patient's temperature and blood-pressure are recorded every 2 hours. The outline of any hypochondrial mass is marked on the skin, and a record kept of the patient's pain, the amount suf sedation required, and any increase or resolution of the physical signs. When the pulse, temperature, and local physical signs show that the inflammation is subsiding, oral intake of fluids can be stepped up. In the great majority, complete resolution will occur within a week.

If conservative management has got the patient over the acute phase of his illness—as happens in most cases—the patient should then go home and return for cholecystectomy after some months. Local conditions will not have subsided fully in much under 3 months, and some inflammation may be present even then. However, a decision has to be taken to operate reasonably soon, otherwise recurrence of acute cholecystitis may take place. The patient should be put on a reducing diet for the intervening 3 months if there is marked obesity, so that both surgery and post-operative care will become relatively much easier.

Operation Records.—It is important that a full description of the details of the emergency or elective operation be entered in the patient's records and that this is checked by the surgeon who carried out the procedure. All details of the pathology found and the operation carried out are necessary in the record. When a patient has a recurrence of biliary symptoms it is frustrating not to have all the relevant details of previous procedures. A diagram included in the records can add to their value (*Fig.* 260). It is of great value if a note can also be added about the condition of the œsophageal hiatus, stomach, duodenum, pancreas, and liver, as other pathology may declare itself later.

PRE-OPERATIVE PREPARATION FOR BILIARY SURGERY

Nutrition.—Many patients requiring surgery for gall-stones are grossly overweight. Unless severe pain, infection, or jaundice make early surgery mandatory, it is in the patient's interests that he should reduce his weight to normal limits for his height and build. A suitable reducing diet should be laid down for the patient and he should be instructed to keep a weekly record of his weight taken under standard conditions. Such a patient should be seen monthly to ensure that the diet is being followed. If he can succeed in reducing to near-normal limits, surgery is technically much easier and the patient's post-operative progress becomes much smoother.

On the other hand, some patients have lost a considerable amount of weight because of their disease. Patients who have been jaundiced for some time are liable to be suffering from malnutrition and there may be evidence of considerable loss of weight. If it is possible to delay surgery for a short time, the patient will benefit from an intensive effort to improve his nutrition, as the liver parenchymal cell is working at a disadvantage from the effects of obstructive jaundice, and every effort should be made to improve its function by the use of a high-calorie diet. This diet should contain large amounts of carbohydrate in the form of glucose, together with adequate protein. Full vitamin supplements should be given, especially vitamin C in a dosage of 500 mg. per day. Unfortunately, the patient may well suffer from nausea and find it difficult to maintain an adequate intake by mouth. Transnasal gastric tube feeds may often help, but, if necessary, the intravenous route should be used (p. 46).

Increased Tendency to Bleeding.—In post-hepatic jaundice, the absence of bile-salts from the alimentary canal decreases the absorption of the fat-soluble vitamins including vitamin K. The shortage of vitamin K impairs the synthesis of prothrombin by the liver. This results in a tendency to bleed; formerly this made biliary surgery in obstructive jaundice very hazardous. Any increased bleeding tendency can be estimated pre-operatively by the prothrombin time. If this is elevated, vitamin K should be given in the form of K_1 intravenously. A dose of 20 mg. is followed by a rapid return to a normal prothrombin time within 12–24 hours if the liver is normal. If the first observation of prothrombin time shows an elevation, a further test should always be carried out after giving vitamin K to ensure that conditions have indeed returned to normal before operation. Vitamin K in a dose of 10–20 mg. should be given daily intravenously or intramuscularly until operation takes place. It is usually unnecessary to continue the administration of vitamin K post-operatively. When there is severe hepato-cellular damage the parenteral administration of vitamin K_1 will not bring the prothrombin time back to normal, as prothrombin cannot be made by a badly damaged liver cell. The only other source of prothrombin in these circumstances (to permit of safe operation) is dried plasma, or plasma frozen after separation from the red cells. Prothrombin activity is retained in these plasma fractions for several months. Stored whole blood contains little or no prothrombin.

The Elderly Patient.—With the improvement in anæsthetic and surgical techniques and a rise in the age of the populace, a steadily rising percentage of elderly patients are being subjected to operations on the biliary tract. Many of these patients suffer from ischæmic heart disease, and while this may, from time to time, give rise to certain difficulties in diagnosis (because biliary pain and the pain of myocardial ischæmia can be confused), it is also of the greatest importance that the elderly patient be so investigated (*see below*) and prepared for operation on the biliary tract that he has the best possible chance of avoiding cardiopulmonary complications in the post-operative period. One very important factor is the maintenance of full oxygenation to the heart. Thus the correction of any pre-operative anæmia becomes of great importance; the hæmoglobin should always be estimated and, if significantly lowered, an attempt made to get this to a pre-operative level of 80–90 per cent, if necessary, by blood transfusion. Many of the patients have chronic bronchitis and emphysema, and are especially liable to post-operative atelectasis because of the viscid nature of their sputum and the atrophic condition of the mucosa of their bronchial tree. Pre-operative physiotherapy and, if necessary, postural drainage should be carried out to prepare the patients for the further use of these measures post-operatively when their movements will not be so free (*see* p. 164).

Pre-operative Investigations.—The following investigations should always be carried out prior to any surgery on the biliary tree:—
1. Chest radiograph.
2. ECG.
3. Hæmoglobin.
4. Serum bilirubin and liver-function tests (*see* p. 369).
5. Serum electrolytes.
6. Blood-urea.
7. Blood grouping and cross-matching of 2 pints (1000 ml.) of blood.

This routine group of tests should highlight any cardiopulmonary, hepatic, or renal dysfunction, so that it may be corrected pre-operatively. It also acts as a satisfactory base-line in case any post-operative complications occur in these particular systems. If jaundice has been present during the previous few weeks, the tests enumerated on p. 369 should also be performed.

POST-OPERATIVE MANAGEMENT

If post-operative complications are to be avoided, it is most important that certain detailed observations be made by the house-surgeon during the first 24 hours after operation:—
1. When the patient has been returned to bed, he should check that the airway is clear and that the patient is being well oxygenated.

2. The temperature, pulse-rate, and blood-pressure should be noted, and these should be recorded hourly for the first 4 hours, and then, if progress is uninterrupted, 4-hourly records should suffice.

3. Any drains which have been inserted at the time of operation should be examined to ensure that they are not kinked and that drainage is free, and drainage tubes should be connected to their appropriate receptacles. Care should be taken that the drains are not displaced from these containers in periods of restlessness during the recovery phase (*see* pp. 365, 395).

4. If nausea and vomiting occur, nasogastric suction should be instituted; this is *not* normally necessary after biliary-tract operations, unless there have been incidentally any direct procedures on the upper gastro-intestinal tract.

5. Patients should be instructed to breathe deeply and to cough up any retained secretions. Physiotherapy should be available to assist in this. Suction should be used if a patient finds difficulty in clearing retained secretions from his trachea or throat. This is particularly necessary in the elderly.

6. Pain should be controlled by adequate amounts of pethidine (50–100 mg.). Morphine should not be used.

7. All patients should be encouraged in early movement. They should sit up during the first 24 hours on the edge of the bed and swing their legs freely. Early mobilization out of bed should be carried out consistent with comfort. A patient should not be forced into early ambulation before he feels up to it.

8. If there is any evidence of pulmonary infection, the appropriate antibiotic should be started without delay. Again, this is particularly important in the elderly patient so that bronchopneumonia does not become established.

9. After operations on jaundiced patients urinary function may be impaired. Maintenance of a normal blood-pressure during operation is important in prevention. During the course of the operation 500 ml. of mannitol 10 per cent should be given intravenously to increase urine output.

Post-operative Complications.—With pre-operative care and preparation, these are fortunately now much less common. Nevertheless, with an increasing percentage of elderly patients undergoing operation, there will continue to be post-operative difficulties for some. These complications may be related to the general anæsthetic, to upper abdominal surgery in general, or specifically to technical difficulties encountered at the operation on the biliary tract. The older and frailer the patient the more liable he becomes to myocardial damage, impaired liver function, and renal infection or failure. It is presumed that any cardiac arrhythmias, heart failure, diabetes, etc., which may have been discovered will have been treated adequately before operation. Post-operatively, it is particularly important that detailed observation be kept on the elderly, the obese, and those with chronic bronchitis and emphysema for early signs of pulmonary atelectasis, bronchopneumonia, and phlebothrombosis with pulmonary infarction (*see* p. 168).

Complications Related to Surgery.—

1. *Hæmorrhage.*—After biliary operations, hæmorrhage may arise from the gall-bladder bed, the liver, the cystic artery, from vessels around the bile-duct, or from the abdominal wall. The symptoms will be those of internal hæmorrhage. It is very rare for much obvious blood-loss to issue along the drainage track. The patient should be adequately transfused and then the abdomen opened without delay. The blood and blood-clot should be removed and an inspection carried out to find the bleeding point. In many cases no bleeding point will be seen, but it is important to remove all the blood from the peritoneal cavity as this, especially when contaminated by bile, easily becomes infected, resulting

14

in the formation of a subhepatic abscess. Prophylaxis of bleeding consists of the proper pre-operative preparation of jaundiced patients with vitamin K and careful hæmostatic technique during the operation.

2. *Leakage of Bile.*—This can arise from the gall-bladder, cystic duct, or bile-duct, or from the liver. It may result in a localized subhepatic abscess, a general peritonitis, or in fistula formation to the outside. A sudden escape of bile may lead to general peritonitis and shock. The affected patient should be given intravenous plasma sufficient to raise the blood-pressure and prepare him for urgent laparotomy to remove the bile from the peritoneum and deal with the leaking point to prevent further extravasation. More common, however, is the subhepatic accumulation of bile resulting from a slow leak and which is walled off by omentum and colon (*Fig.* 261). The fluid under the liver is generally a mixture of blood, bile, and lymph from divided channels in the gall-bladder bed or the neighbourhood of the bile-duct. The patient complains of subhepatic pain, the temperature and pulse-rate rise, and there may be some leakage of bile along the drainage track. As a prophylactic measure, it is generally regarded as essential to put a soft drain down to the bed of the liver after cholecystectomy. Most biliary-tract operations should be drained to the outside, using a drain which comes directly through the abdominal wall. In some cases formed subhepatic collections do not settle spontaneously and it may be necessary to re-open the abdomen and drain the subhepatic collection.

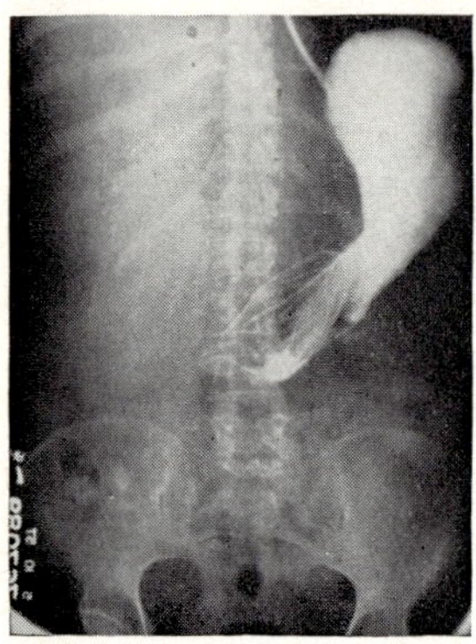

Fig. 261.—Radiograph showing displacement of the stomach in a case of subhepatic accumulation of bile.

3. *Jaundice.*—Jaundice which appears rapidly after operation may well be due to operative injury to the bile-duct. On the other hand, it may be due to a cholangitis which had been present pre-operatively but had flared up as a result of the operative manœuvres. Jaundice may also be due to the use of old blood for transfusion or, rarely, to a mismatched transfusion. If this is so, then renal shutdown is very likely, followed by tubular necrosis—a very serious complication for a jaundiced patient after biliary-tract surgery, in some necessitating the use of renal dialysis. Finally, jaundice which either occurs or becomes worse post-operatively may be due to pathology in the bile-duct such as a residual stone or a missed carcinoma.

4. *Pancreatitis.*—This complication may occur after biliary-tract operations, particularly when there has been manipulation near the lower end of the duct, which facilitates regurgitation of infected bile up the pancreatic ducts. Though often minor, post-operative pancreatitis can be fatal if it extends to become hæmorrhagic pancreatic necrosis. Diagnosis is made by the serum amylase estimation, when values over 1000 Somogyi units may be found (*see* p. 382).

EVALUATION OF POST-CHOLECYSTECTOMY SYMPTOMS

Residual Stone in the Bile-duct.—About 3 per cent of patients undergoing operation for simple cholelithiasis may leave the theatre with a stone in the bile-duct, whereas residual stone after choledocholithotomy may occur in 10 per cent or more. Residual duct stone should be suspected if (1) pain, (2) jaundice, or (3) leakage of bile occurs after a T-tube has been clamped, or (4) an external biliary fistula develops after its removal. In some, symptoms may not appear for a year or more. Intravenous cholangiography is usually diagnostic.

Carcinoma of the head of the pancreas, the ampulla of Vater or the bile-duct, can coexist with cholelithiasis and may not be noticed at the primary cholecystectomy. If pain or jaundice recurs, or if a fistula develops, the possibility of malignant stricture should be kept in mind.

Stricture of the bile-duct may arise following clamping of the duct or placing of the cystic duct ligature too close to the bile-duct. Poor positioning of a T-tube may also be responsible, or overzealous attempts to bougie the ampulla of Vater. Fibrosis of the sphincter of Oddi may follow pancreatitis, previous inflammation from a nearby stone, or injury by instrumentation at choledochotomy. It may also be a primary disease of the sphincter. The patient presents with biliary pain, nausea, and vomiting, and there may be mild jaundice, and elevated serum bilirubin and alkaline phosphatase levels.

Investigations.—If symptoms develop after cholecystectomy, the patient's history should be carefully reviewed together with the pre-operative findings, the details of the operation carried out, and the sequence of the events leading to the present disability. If there is no jaundice, intravenous cholangiography should be carried out. This examination can be very helpful, although it often fails to demonstrate the lower end of the duct where so many lesions are suspected. Many other lesions can mimic biliary conditions and, indeed, the lesion responsible for the symptoms may have been present pre-operatively or could have developed as a new and unrelated condition after operation. Amongst these, the most common are peptic ulcer, hiatus hernia, appendicitis, diverticulitis, urinary-tract infections, and ischæmic disease of the heart. Barium-meal and other appropriate investigations may help with the clinical history in unravelling the precise diagnosis.

The Problem of Biliary Dyskinesia.—Much has been written on biliary dyskinesia, which is defined as an imbalance of autonomic control in the biliary tree, leading to so-called 'hyperkinetic' or 'atonic' forms. There is no doubt that pathological lesions, such as stone, infection, and cancer, can give rise to symptoms from secondary biliary dyskinesia, but these symptoms subside with treatment of the primary condition. However, the consensus is that *primary* dyskinesia is very rare, and there is nearly always a valid organic cause for symptoms arising after cholecystectomy.

DRAINAGE AFTER BILIARY-TRACT PROCEDURES

Drainage Tubes.—A tube or other form of drain (Penrose, corrugated rubber, etc.) draining the gall-bladder bed is shortened on the third day, and removed on the fourth or fifth day, unless there is an undue discharge of bile or blood, in which event the tube is shortened a little day by day, but left in place until the drainage ceases or becomes minimal.

MANAGEMENT OF THE T-TUBE

Selection of Appropriate T-tube.—A soft flexible tube of suitable size is usually chosen. It should lie freely in the bile-duct, which is closed round it by a bile-tight catgut suture. There is no need for the short limbs of the T-tube to be longer than 1·0 to 1·5 cm. A V is generally cut out of the T-tube on the wall of the tube opposite the long limb (of the T-tube), and a gutter removed from the length of the short limbs, involving one-third to a half of the circumference of the tube (*Fig.* 262). This improves drainage down the bile-duct, past the

T-tube, and also facilitates removal of the tube. A stitch of 000 catgut anchors the T-tube to the wall of the duct. This will become absorbed by the time appropriate for removal of the tube. The T-tube is brought out directly through the abdominal wall, and a certain amount of slack should be left within the abdomen so that there is no danger of the tube being pulled out of the bile-duct by a sudden movement of the patient. The T-tube is also secured by a stitch to the skin, tying the stitch firmly around the tube in criss-cross fashion, but not kinking or otherwise obstructing it (*Fig.* 263).

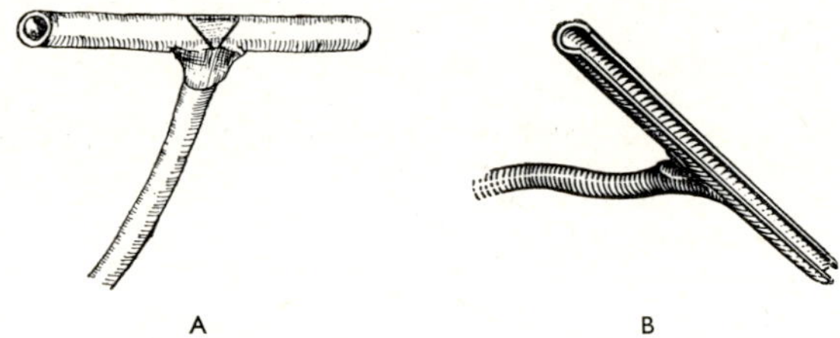

A   B

Fig. 262.—**A,** If a V is cut out of the tube, as shown, the tube is more easily withdrawn, or **B,** Half the circumference can be cut away with the same objective, viz., facile withdrawal.

Management of a T-tube in the Bile-duct.—Bile usually drains freely in the early post-operative days because of œdema in the distal end of the bile-duct and spasm of the sphincter, consequent upon passage of instruments during operation. This temporary obstruction normally subsides during the first week and, provided there is no jaundice and the 24-hour total of the recorded quantity of the bile fistula drainage has lessened in amount, the tube may be clamped with a screw clamp for 4 hours on the seventh day. The clamp should be opened if the patient has any abdominal pain. If no pain occurs, the T-tube is again clamped for 12 hours on the following day, and for 24 hours on the ninth day. At this stage a post-operative cholangiogram can be performed. If the cholangiogram is normal, the T-tube may be removed about the twelfth or fourteenth day.

Removal of the Tube.—After cutting the skin suture attached to the tube, the T-tube may be removed by a steady pull. If it cannot be extracted with moderate tension, a hæmostat may be applied to the tube, close to the abdominal wall, and the patient permitted to walk about. This often allows the tube to come away; if it fails to do so, the manœuvre should be repeated on the following day. After removal of the T-tube there may be a small amount of biliary discharge for the first 24 or 36 hours, but often there is little or no discharge and the drainage tract heals rapidly.

Contra-indications to the removal of the T-*tube.*—
1. Jaundice.
2. Fever.
3. Recurrence of pain after clamping the tube.
4. Leakage of bile around the tube after clamping.

COMPLICATIONS ASSOCIATED WITH CHOLEDOCHOTOMY

As there is a tendency for the sphincter of Oddi to be held closed post-operatively, increased biliary pressure arises if free drainage is not possible through the T-tube. Leakage will occur through divided small ducts in the gall-bladder bed, around the choledochotomy opening when there is a T-tube in position, and even through the small stitch-holes in the bile-duct used for closing the incision in the bile-duct. A Penrose or similar drain should always be used to drain the subhepatic region.

Occluded T-tube.—In the early post-operative period the tube may become blocked by blood-clot or by biliary mud. Gentle syringe irrigation with isotonic sterile saline will usually restore patency. When a T-tube has been retained in the common duct for a long period, it sometimes happens that the lumen becomes occluded by encrustation. Again, saline irrigation should be employed rather than chemical solvents which are not recommended.

Dislodgement of T-tube from the Duct.—This can occur if a stuporose or restless patient pulls the tube completely out, or if the tube is caught by the patient's clothes or bedding while he is turning in bed or attempting to sit up. Much more often, and with greater resulting peril, the T-end of the tube can be dragged

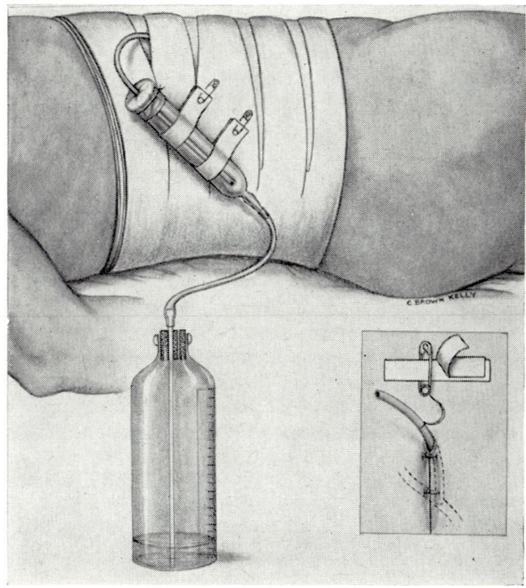

Fig. 263.—Precautions to minimize accidental dislocation of a T-tube from the common bile-duct.

out of the bile-duct into the peritoneal cavity by some apparently innocent movement of the patient in bed. The particular danger of this form of dislodgement is that it is not marked by any symptom or sign other than the cessation of bile drainage from the tube. This may pass unnoticed until bile peritonitis supervenes, or the dressing becomes yellow and saturated by a copious escape of bile along the side of the tube. The shorter the lapse of time between operation and the extrusion of the tube, the more serious are the consequences; the abdomen must be reopened, bile sucked out of the peritoneal cavity, and a new T-tube inserted.

Precautions that minimize the Accidental Dislodgement of T-tube.—The following procedure is in use at the Lahey Clinic and is very effective:—

1. At the conclusion of the operation a length of black silk is tied around the emerging limb of the T-tube sufficiently tightly to stop just short of narrowing the tube lumen. The silk is then anchored to the abdominal wall (*Fig.* 263, *inset*).

2. The point of a hæmostat is forced from within outwards through the dome of an amputated thumb of a rubber glove and its jaws are opened to grasp the distal end of the tube which is drawn through the puncture. The base of the cap is insinuated over the rim of the barrel of an old glass syringe. A rubber band or a ligature is used to hold the cap in place. The tube is adjusted so that its orifice lies about 2 cm. above the nozzle end of the barrel. A many-tailed bandage is applied to the abdomen and the newly constructed interceptor is suspended from this (*Fig.* 263).

It will be appreciated that if subsequently the patient rolls from one side to another any drag on the tube will shift the tube within the glass barrel and spare displacement of the tube from the duct. It is true that soiling of the bedclothes by bile is liable to result, but assuredly, in spite of the work this entails, the knowledge that it has spared soiling of the peritoneum is rewarding. A satisfactory compromise is to dispense with the drag-taker on the fifth post-operative day.

MANAGEMENT OF A CHOLECYSTOSTOMY TUBE

The tube is led into a sterile bottle (*Fig.* 264) or, better still, into a sterilized bag of the type used for collecting urine. In profoundly jaundiced patients liver function is at a low ebb and the flow of bile during the first 48 hours is often discouraging. The bile is very thick and the house-surgeon can very gently irrigate the interior of the gall-bladder through the tube using not more than 30-60 ml. of sterile saline. A flow of bile usually recommences when rehydration of the patient is complete, provided that the obstructing stone has been removed from the neck of the gall-bladder at operation, allowing free flow of bile from the biliary ducts through the gall-bladder and cholecystostomy tube.

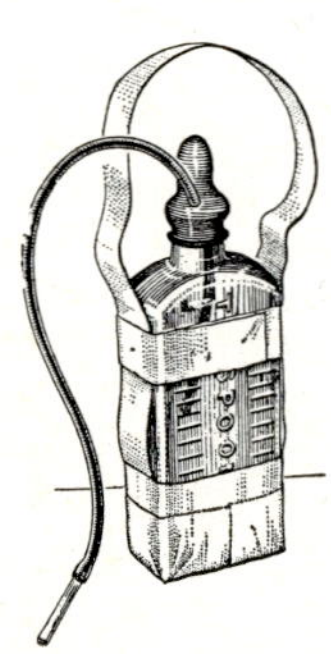

Fig. 264.—A medicine bottle, a rubber teat, and adhesive plaster make a convenient sterile receptacle for bile.

After any acute inflammatory process in the gall-bladder has settled postoperatively, cholangiographic examination of the biliary tree can be carried out by instilling a radio-opaque medium through the cholecystostomy tube. The tube should never be removed early; in most cases it is preferable to cut the retaining stitch on about the tenth day and allow the tube to be extruded spontaneously.

MANAGEMENT OF PATIENTS WITH OBSTRUCTIVE JAUNDICE

The critical decision in every case of jaundice is whether or not to advise operation. The temptation to operate may be great when a patient presents with deep jaundice, acholia, and bilirubinuria. However, unnecessary laparotomy under general anæsthesia can produce as big a surgical tragedy in severe hepatitis as can failure to diagnose and operate on a patient with an impacted stone in the bile-duct. Judgement based on clinical experience is all-important, and a correct diagnosis can be made by this means alone in 80–90 per cent of jaundiced patients.

However, even experienced clinicians can be misled by symptoms and signs in a jaundiced patient and it is therefore advisable to use to the full all ancillary aids to diagnosis, particularly radiology, hæmatology, and liver-function tests. Always question the patient carefully about recent drug ingestion.

Classification of Jaundice.—
1. Pre-hepatic:—
    a. Hæmolytic.
    b. Non-hæmolytic.
2. Hepatic:—
    a. Hepatocellular.
    b. Hepatocanalicular.
3. Post-hepatic:—
    a. Obstruction complete.
    b. Obstruction incomplete.

The term 'obstructive jaundice' is not specific enough, as both 'hepatic' and 'post-hepatic' obstruction can give the same clinical and biochemical picture of obstructive jaundice. Mixed features are common.

DIAGNOSTIC AIDS IN JAUNDICE

1. Radiology (*see* p. 711).—A good soft-tissue radiograph will show an enlarged liver or spleen and also will demonstrate any radio-opaque gall-stones. Barium-meal examination may disclose œsophageal varices, an alimentary tract cancer if the jaundice is metastatic in origin, or a widening of the duodenal loop if there is a cancer of the head of the pancreas. Suitable films of the second part of the duodenum may show an ampullary carcinoma. Oral cholecystography and intravenous cholangiography are valueless in clinical jaundice as the medium cannot be excreted by the liver in adequate amount to visualize the biliary tree.

2. Hæmatology.—The house-surgeon should have (*a*) the hæmoglobin, (*b*) red blood cell-count and film, (*c*) fragility where indicated, (*d*) white blood cell-count, and (*e*) clotting time determined. In pre-hepatic hæmolytic jaundice, spherocytosis and reticulocytosis are common. Leucopenia with relative or absolute lymphocytosis is usual in viral hepatitis, whereas polymorphonuclear leucocytosis is a feature of cholangitis. Anæmia is common in cirrhosis and is usually microcytic, although it may be macrocytic, and megaloblastic marrow change is sometimes seen. Hypersplenism is reflected as neutropenia and a low platelet count. In jaundice associated with cirrhosis coagulation defects are also found. The deficiencies are usually multiple and can involve prothrombin, fibrinogen, Factor V, and Factor VII. Fibrinogen deficiency is rather uncommon, but fibrinolysins have been demonstrated. The prothrombin time estimation is of value in differential diagnosis; if elevated, a good response to intravenous vitamin K is evidence of post-hepatic jaundice, whereas the absence of a response favours hepatic jaundice.

3. Liver-function Tests.—As the parenchymal cell has many different functions, and each liver-function test measures only one aspect of liver function, it follows that a number of tests are required. It should be remembered that the liver has a high functional reserve and patchy lesions of the liver may show no abnormality in the function tests until 80 per cent of the liver has been destroyed. All tests are of value only if the clinician appreciates both the normal and pathological range for each individual test and the various possibilities for error in the laboratory methods used.

In a jaundiced patient the tests shown in *Table X* will normally be carried out (the quantitative urobilinogen tests may be omitted).

Table X.—BASIC GROUP OF LIVER-FUNCTION TESTS USEFUL IN THE DIAGNOSIS OF JAUNDICE

Serum bilirubin	Mean = 0·65→1·5 mg. per cent	Objective record of the jaundice
Fæcal urobilinogen	50→200 mg./24 hours	Very useful
Urinary urobilinogen	0→2·5 mg./24 hours	Very useful
Serum albumin	3 G. per cent	Useful diagnostically if depressed below normal
A/G ratio	>1	
Serum electrophoresis		Essential
Cephalin cholesterol flocculation	0→1+	Valuable aids to diagnosis
Thymol turbidity	0→4 units	
Thymol flocculation	0	
Serum alkaline phosphatase	3–13 KA units	Useful
Serum transaminase (GPT)	<40 Karmen units/ml.	Valuable index of recent cell damage
Response of prothrombin time to parenteral vitamin K		Valuable diagnostic aid if prothrombin time elevated

SERUM BILIRUBIN.—The total serum bilirubin is an objective index of the depth and progress of jaundice, and so it is valuable to repeat this observation every 3 or 4 days. The normal mean total bilirubin is approximately 0·6 mg. per cent with an upper limit of 1·5 mg. per cent. In jaundice a fall in the level is a favourable sign, whereas a sudden rise should be viewed with some concern. Partition of serum bilirubin into the direct and indirect fractions is often done, but the direct van den Bergh reaction is given by both the mono- and diglucuronides of bilirubin which regurgitate into the blood in both hepatic and post-hepatic jaundice. Thus, estimation of these fractions is of no value in the differentiation of hepatic from post-hepatic jaundice. However, the indirect fraction is high in pre-hepatic jaundice.

URINARY AND FÆCAL PIGMENTS.—Persistent acholia is typical of jaundice due to cancer of the head of the pancreas or the bile-duct. However, it should be remembered that acholia of shorter duration can occur in hepatitis or in calculous jaundice. A normally coloured stool in a deeply jaundiced patient suggests liver disease, while a very dark stool is a feature of pre-hepatic hæmolytic jaundice. Quantitatively, the fæcal urobilinogen is under 5 mg. per 24 hours in cancer, and can rise to 2000 mg. in hæmolytic crises. Normal values are less than 200 mg. per 24 hours.

Bilirubinuria is found in both hepatic and post-hepatic jaundice, and so cannot be used in differentiating these two groups. Normally, the urinary urobilinogen is under 2 mg. per 24 hours. Complete absence over a week or more suggests carcinoma. In viral hepatitis excess urobilinogen is present early, even in the pre-icteric stage, vanishes during the period of intrahepatic cholestasis when the jaundice is at its height, and reappears as the jaundice fades. As much as 300 mg. urobilinogen may be excreted daily in haemolytic anæmia, but similar large amounts may be found after release of an impacted stone in the bile-duct. The house-surgeon should note that estimations of fæcal and urinary urobilinogen are invalid if the patient has been receiving a broad-spectrum antibiotic, as intestinal organisms are required for the degradation of bilirubin to urobilinogen.

SERUM PROTEINS IN JAUNDICE.—The classic findings in hepatic jaundice are a low albumin, increased globulin, and a reversed A/G ratio. A value of under 3 G. per cent for albumin is significantly low. It should be remembered that values of this level will occur only in the minority of patients with hepatic jaundice, even when estimated electrophoretically (which is the preferable method as it is more accurate than the older chemical methods).

FLOCCULATION AND TURBIDITY TESTS are used to distinguish hepatic from post-hepatic jaundice. In general, results are positive in hepatic jaundice and negative in post-hepatic jaundice. The tests reflect certain alterations in circulating plasma albumin and globulins. Of the many flocculation tests which have been introduced, the following remain the most consistently popular and useful tests in the differential diagnosis of jaundice:—

a. Cephalin Cholesterol Flocculation.— Here, flocculation depends on a low or altered albumin, and an increased gamma-globulin. Positive results are found in hepatitis in 90 per cent and in cirrhosis in 60 per cent of cases.

b. Thymol Turbidity and Flocculation.— This is one of the most widely used tests in the diagnosis of jaundice. The turbidity is due to a protein–thymol–phospholipid complex. Positive results are found in hepatitis in 80–90 per cent and in cirrhosis in nearly 70 per cent. *Thymol flocculation* is merely a variant of the test in which flocculation is estimated in the turbidity test-tube after it has stood for 18 hours. It is more sensitive than thymol turbidity, and has the further merit of not requiring

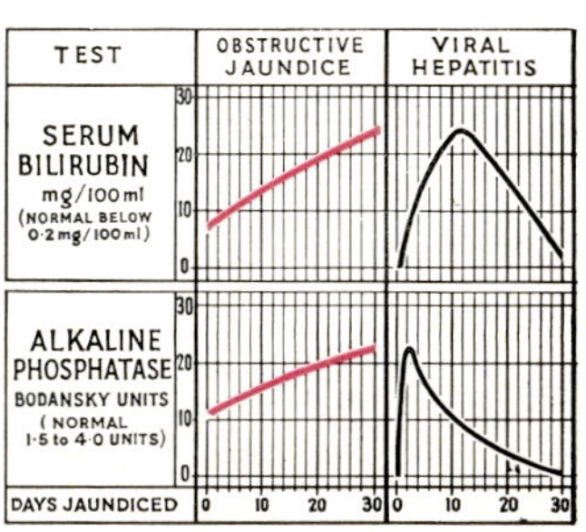

Fig. 265.—Charts showing the typical curves of the serum-bilirubin and alkaline phosphatase estimations in obstructive jaundice and viral hepatitis.

the use of units as it is recorded merely as positive or negative. In considering the results of the thymol turbidity test, the normal range for the particular hospital laboratory concerned should be ascertained.

c. Zinc Turbidity.—This test depends on the amount of gamma-globulin present. A negative test in long-standing jaundice is very nearly specific for post-hepatic jaundice.

A major problem in the interpretation of flocculation tests is the negative or typical post-hepatic or 'surgical' type of result given in hepatocanalicular jaundice due to viral hepatitis or to the exhibition of certain drugs such as chlorpromazine. Positive results of the 'hepatic' jaundice type are also found in severe cholangitis and care must be taken not to be misled by this.

LIVER ENZYMES.—

a. Serum Alkaline Phosphatase.—This is a mixture of several phosphatases originating from bone, intestinal mucosa, and liver. Thus it reflects activity of hepatic and extra-hepatic conditions, and high values are found in rickets, osteomalacia, hyperparathyroidism, Paget's disease, and in the last trimester of pregnancy, in addition to the high values traditionally found in post-hepatic jaundice. The level of serum alkaline phosphatase is the resultant of intestinal, bony, and hepatobiliary phosphatase activity, together with the ability of the liver to excrete these phosphatases in the bile (*Fig.* 265). However, it is widely believed that values over 30 King-Armstrong units per 100 ml. plasma favour post-hepatic jaundice. This is certainly true in most cases, but, unfortunately, equally high values are found in hepatocanalicular jaundice, and in some instances of hepatocellular jaundice (*Fig.* 266). Increased serum alkaline phosphatase may be found in 'dissociated' jaundice when the serum bilirubin is normal or only slightly elevated in patients with hepatic metastases and others with bile-duct obstruction due to stone. Serum alkaline phosphatase estimation is normally considered with other tests for diagnostic purposes and has a definite but limited value. It may be combined with the following test:—

b. Serum Transaminase.—Serum glutamic oxalacetic transaminase (SGOT) and serum glutamic pyruvic transaminase (SGPT) are used for diagnostic aids as elevated values occur in hepatic jaundice. SGPT is more specifically related to the liver, as SGOT is usually raised in myocardial infarction and in a wide variety of extra-hepatic diseases, thus limiting its usefulness. However, in viral

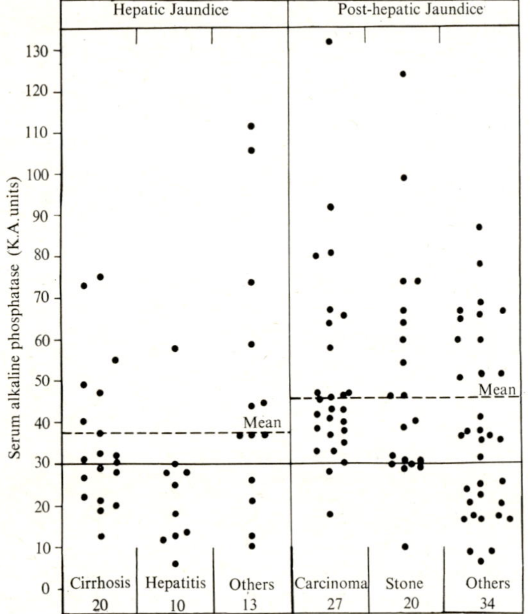

Fig. 266.—Scattergram showing levels of serum alkaline phosphatase in hepatic and post-hepatic jaundice. Although practically all cases of carcinoma of the biliary tree and stone in the bile-duct have values over 30 KA units, high values are found in individual cases of hepatic and post-hepatic jaundice. There is no significant difference between the mean value found in hepatic and post-hepatic jaundice.

Fig. 267.—The transaminase/alkaline phosphatase ratios of 106 jaundiced patients, 50 of whom were proved by other methods to be suffering from hepatocellular damage and 56 from obstructive jaundice. Values between 3 and 7 are equivocal. Values above 7 are extremely likely to be due to hepatocellular damage. Values below 3 are pathognomonic of obstructive jaundice. ● = patients with hepatitis; ○ = patients with obstructive jaundice.

hepatitis and cytolytic necrosis of the liver, both SGOT and SGPT can reach the very high level of 3000 Karmen units per ml. The ratio of transaminase to alkaline phosphatase has been used to sharpen the diagnostic ability of both tests (*Fig.* 267). A ratio above 7 indicates that the jaundice is extremely likely to be due to hepatocellular damage, whereas a ratio of under 3 is pathognomonic of post-hepatic jaundice.

TESTS OF EXCRETION.—The bromsulphthalein (BSP) excretion test is of little value in differentiating hepatic from post-hepatic jaundice. Recently ^{131}I-labelled rose bengal has been used to differentiate these two types of jaundice by the rate of disappearance of radio-activity from the liver. Cobalt-60 labelled vitamin B_{12} has also been used with scanning of the liver to pick up metastases which tend to show a lower uptake than normal.

Technique.—The BSP is given intravenously in 10 ml. of fluid into a vein in the *left* antecubital fossa; the dose is 5 mg. per kg. body-weight. After 30 min. 5 ml. blood are withdrawn from the *right* arm. Normally there should be less than 10 per cent of the BSP remaining in the circulation.

COMBINATION OF TESTS.—Recently a strong movement has emerged to limit the number of tests used in the differential diagnosis of jaundice and to restrict the sampling to one syringeful of blood. The group of tests shown in *Table X* are the most favoured and the most useful. A correct diagnosis should be made in 90–95 per cent of jaundiced patients if a careful assessment is made of both clinical and laboratory information. It has been suggested that a therapeutic trial with ACTH or cortisone should be undertaken where the diagnosis of jaundice remains uncertain and a hepatic type of jaundice is suspected. Such a trial is *not* recommended, as spurious improvement in jaundice may mask an underlying stone or carcinoma. It is wiser to carry out a laparotomy and so come directly to an exact diagnosis.

Pruritus.—The itch of unrelieved jaundice may be eased by giving norethandrolone 30 mg. or methyl testosterone 25 mg. sublingually daily, or else cholestyramine 5 G. orally per day.

THE MANAGEMENT OF PATIENTS WITH PORTAL HYPERTENSION

Portal hypertension most commonly occurs in association with hepatic cirrhosis. It is generally believed that the hypertension results from increased hepatic resistance to portal blood-flow due to the development of regenerating nodules together with the presence of intrahepatic arterioportal connexions. Other factors may be involved—for example, increased amounts of adrenaline and noradrenaline in the portal blood. Less commonly, portal hypertension is due to extrahepatic portal vein thrombosis; this usually occurs in infants or children following dehydration or infection, either manifest or presumed. Ascites may also appear early in these affected children and later remit in the continuing presence of portal hypertension. Portal vein thrombosis with hypertension may also occur in adults, probably associated with the blocking of other channels, as the main portal vein can sometimes be ligated with impunity. Occasionally cancer of the body of the pancreas may occlude the portal vein and cause hypertension.

CLINICAL PRESENTATION OF PORTAL HYPERTENSION

Increased portal pressure can probably exist for many years without becoming manifest. However, the following clinical presentations may occur:—
1. Symptomless splenomegaly.
2. Hypersplenism.
3. Acute or chronic bleeding from gastro-œsophageal varices.
4. Jaundice and other signs of cirrhosis or liver failure.
5. Œsophageal varices may be a surprise finding at a barium-meal examination.
It is with the management of varices that this section is principally concerned.

Bleeding Varices.—Blood-loss may be of any degree from a slight ooze to a catastrophic bleed, and may present as hæmatemesis or melæna. A particular feature of the hæmorrhage is that the blood may be bright red in colour, either when vomited or even when passed per rectum. This is puzzling, but might well be due to connexions between the œsophageal varices and the pulmonary veins. Portal hypertension is a relatively rare cause of upper gastro-intestinal tract hæmorrhage, occurring much less often than bleeding from peptic ulceration or gastric erosions. It accounts for less than 10 per cent of such hæmorrhages, the incidence varying with the locality. There is often no apparent precipitating cause for the hæmorrhage. The patient may have had portal hypertension for years, and then suddenly bleed from his varices. Injury from ingested rough food or peptic œsophagitis have been evoked as precipitating factors, but often neither is present. In children portal thrombosis may be suspected, but portal cirrhosis can occur in childhood; portal thrombosis can also arise in adult life. However, if cirrhosis is present, there may be a history of hepatitis or alcoholism, and the various stigmata of liver failure may be obvious clinically—jaundice, ascites, spider nævi, red palms, and porta-systemic encephalopathy. Gynæcomastia, loss of axillary hair, and testicular atrophy may be found in the male cirrhotic. It is important to differentiate (1) the patient with good liver function and portal thrombosis who tolerates well blood-loss and its replacement, and is a candidate for later surgical portal decompression, and (2) the cirrhotic in an advanced state of hepatic failure, where a severe bleed may be the forerunner of hepatic coma.

THE MANAGEMENT OF BLEEDING VARICES

It is essential to replace the blood-volume lost and to stop the bleeding, otherwise severe blood-loss may continue, owing to the high portal venous pressure. Further difficulties may arise from aspiration of vomited blood into the lung, or from the alimentary breakdown of blood into ammonia (and possibly other products) with the later development of hepatic coma. The measures available for treatment are as follows:—

1. Posture.—A comatose patient is best nursed on his side and, if the systemic blood-pressure is very low, the foot of the bed should be raised on blocks until resuscitation has raised the blood-pressure.

2. Sedation.—All sedation is potentially dangerous, but the patient must be given as much physical and mental rest as possible. Morphine should be avoided as adequate dosage may result in the patient going into coma. Paraldehyde or chloral hydrate by tube are safe drugs, but it will be found necessary in some cases to give a small dose of phenobarbitone or some other barbiturate. Barbiturates, however, should be given with the greatest care in this condition.

3. Blood Transfusion.—Early on the patient may not have lost much blood and blood transfusion may not appear to be urgent. However, alarming hæmorrhage may come on at any time, so that 3 or 4 pints (2000 ml.) of compatible blood should be available at immediate notice during a bleeding phase. When taking blood for cross-matching, the house-surgeon should also obtain specimens for the determination of liver function (*see* p. 369) and blood ammonia levels (in heparinized flask, kept cold and rapidly transported).

An intravenous infusion of 5 per cent glucose should be set up at the start of the illness before any blood is cross-matched, and the infusion of glucose continued until blood transfusion becomes necessary. The volume of blood to be transfused is deduced from the usual clinical indices of pulse, blood-pressure, hæmoglobin, mixed venous hæmatocrit, CVP (p. 24), and repeated assessment of the patient's general condition. If the technique is available, blood-volume estimation is very useful.

4. Intravenous Pitressin (Vasopressin).—This has been shown to bring about a pronounced lowering of the portal venous pressure without lowering the systemic blood-pressure. Twenty units of pitressin are given intravenously over a period of 10 minutes in 100 ml. of 5 per cent glucose solution. The patient may become pale, since pitressin is a powerful arterial vasoconstrictor, and he may experience some abdominal colic and possibly pass a stool, which is actually a desirable effect since it evacuates blood from the bowel. Pitressin should not

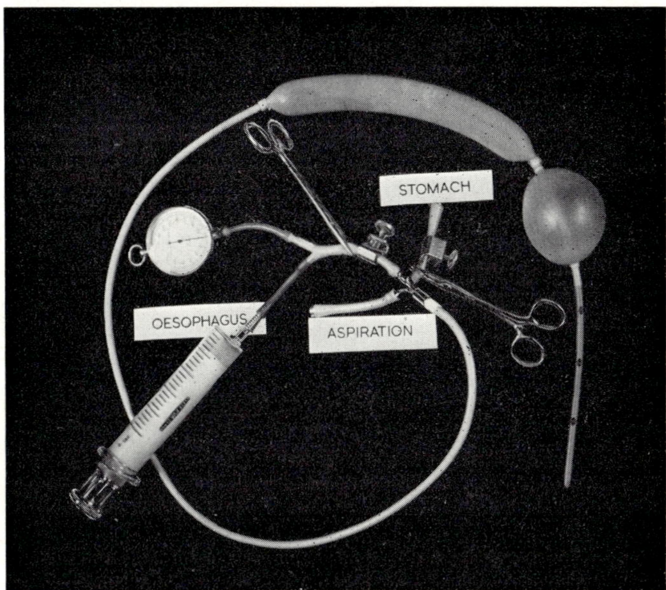

Fig. 268.—The Sengstaken triple-lumen tube for œsophageal tamponade, together with the necessary fitments for its successful use in compressing bleeding gastro-œsophageal varices.

be used in patients with a history of myocardial ischæmia, although in extreme cases, when very active bleeding is going on, careful use of pitressin may be indicated in a desperate situation. If pitressin is to be successful, it presumably acts by lowering the portal pressure in the region of the bleeding point in the œsophageal varix, thus allowing hæmostasis to occur. Unfortunately, recurrence of bleeding is common and repeated dosage of pitressin eventually fails to control the situation.

5. Tamponade.—The three-channel Sengstaken tube is used (*Fig.* 268).* One lumen leads to a spherical balloon which is distended with 150 ml. of water and remains in the stomach. The purpose of this balloon is so to position the tube

---

* Sengstaken tube (J. G. Franklin & Sons Ltd., London; Davol Rubber Co., Providence, Rhode Island, U.S.A.).

that vomiting of blood is prevented; if gentle traction is applied to the tube, via an overhead Balkan beam with a 1-lb. weight, it will also compress varices of the cardio-œsophageal wall (*Fig.* 269). It is important that the two balloons be mounted close together so as to avoid failure to exert pressure on the lower 2 in. of the œsophagus—the area where varices most commonly bleed. The third lumen leads to holes near the tip of the tube which are used for gastric aspiration. Suction will show whether or not bleeding is still occurring. This section of the tube can also be used for the giving of drugs and liquids below the site of compression.

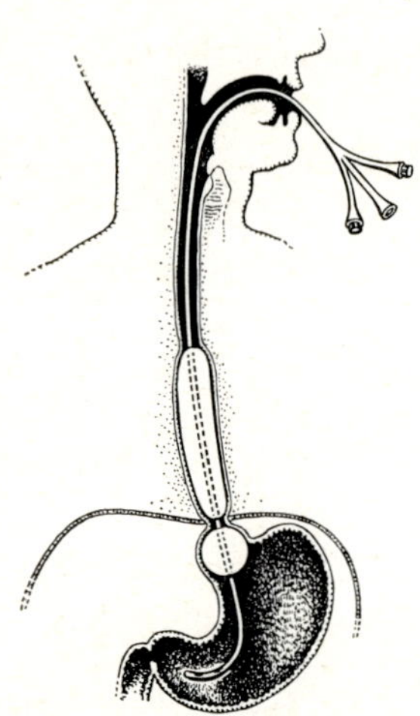

Fig. 269.—Showing the distended gastric and œsophageal balloons of the Sengstaken triple-lumen tube in position.

Indications for the Use of the Sengstaken Tube.—Continuing or recurring bleeding in hospital from known or suspected œsophageal varices especially when this happens despite adequate transfusion and all other recognized measures.

Some recommend the use of pitressin before the Sengstaken tube, because of difficulties with it due to a displaced balloon or pressure necrosis in stomach or œsophagus. The longer the balloon remains inflated in situ, the greater is the possibility of the development of pressure necrosis. It should not be left in position for more than 24 hours.

Important Points regarding the Use of the Sengstaken Tube.—

1. The apparatus must be tested under water to make sure that there are no leaks, and the three expanded proximal ends of the three channels should be correctly labelled.

2. The patient is given a series of local anæsthetic lozenges to suck during the hour prior to passing the tube. If he cannot co-operate, a local anæsthetic spray is used as an alternative.

3. Pass the well-lubricated tube orally. It is easier to pass if cooled beforehand, so as to make the tube firm. The patient's eyes are covered so that he does not see details of the procedure which might disturb him.

4. Distend the gastric balloon with water until it contains 150 ml. It is useful to add 20 ml. of 70 per cent diodone so that the position of the tube can be checked radiologically. It may even be possible to palpate the balloon in the epigastrium through the abdominal wall, although this must be very rare. The expanded end of this channel should be clamped (*Fig.* 268). The tube is then pulled gently up until the gastric balloon is felt to impinge at the cardia, and the tube is then fixed to the patient's cheek with adhesive strapping.

5. Inflate the œsophageal balloon with air, using a 50-ml. syringe and a Y-glass connexion to the sphygmomanometer until the pressure is 25–30 mm. Hg. Doubly clamp the expanded end of this channel.

6. Aspirate the contents of the stomach frequently with a 20- or a 50-ml. syringe in order to ascertain whether bleeding is continuing or not. If it has not stopped, apply gentle traction to the tube and refix it to the side of the patient's face and forehead in such a way as to maintain traction, and so hold the distended balloon against the cardiac orifice. This is often difficult to maintain

and, if so, the tube should be connected over a pulley to a 1-lb. (450-G.) traction suspended from a Balkan beam.

7. Remove saliva and other secretions from the pharynx by suction as often as is necessary in each individual case. This is especially necessary in the stuporose patient to prevent inhalation of pharyngeal contents into the bronchial tree.

8. Deflate the œsophageal balloon after 24 hours, but leave the tube in position. If bleeding occurs, reinflate the tube. If there is no further hæmorrhage during the next 24 hours, remove the water filling the gastric balloon and deflate the œsophageal balloon. The Sengstaken tube is then slowly and carefully removed.

SURGERY OF PORTAL HYPERTENSION

Emergency Surgery for Bleeding Varices.—This may become necessary if a patient has uncontrollable bleeding or recurrence of bleeding after initial success in arresting the bleeding by pitressin or tamponade. The operation of choice is portacaval shunt and the other procedures described below of necessity carry a high risk, but on occasion, offer the only chance of securing survival of the patient. As far as practicable, the routine investigations should first be performed.

Routine Pre-operative Investigation.—

1. Full blood-count.
2. Liver-function tests.
3. Barium swallow and meal.
4. Splenoportography.
5. Chest radiograph.
6. Prothrombin time.
7. Blood group and cross-match 4 pints of blood.

The patient must be prepared as well as possible for this severe operation. The hæmoglobin should be raised to at least 12 G. per cent. Protein intake in the diet should be reduced to 25 G. daily in the days immediately before operation. Oral neomycin is given in a dose of 6 G. daily, starting the day before operation and continuing for the first 3 days postoperatively.

Anæsthetic.—Morphine should be avoided in premedication and intravenous barbiturates given only in minimal doses as these drugs can be detoxicated only very slowly by a damaged liver. Some anæsthetic agents have to be avoided altogether, and a combination of nitrous oxide, oxygen, and relaxants is probably the safest in these difficult circumstances.

Selection of Patients for Surgery.—The indication for a shunt is hæmorrhage from œsophageal and gastric varices; portal hypertension must be confirmed at pre-operative splenoportography. Liver function must be satisfactory, and this should also be established in the pre-operative investigation. Serum albumin should be more than 3 G. per cent and the patient should not be jaundiced. Exceptions can be made to this in the individual patient when other criteria are met. Ascites is generally regarded as being a contra-indication to the procedure, although successful shunts have been performed in its presence. In general, younger patients are preferred as portasystemic encephalopathy tends to be commoner in middle-aged and older patients.

Types of Shunt.—Portacaval anastomosis probably gives the most satisfactory result as the veins are larger, and therefore the fall in the pressure in the portal system is greater than is possible using other shunts. On occasion, it may not be technically possible to perform the operation owing to the presence of portal thrombosis or to extensive collaterals surrounding the portal vein. Splenorenal anastomosis may then be considered or an anastomosis from the superior mesenteric vein to the inferior vena cava. This has been particularly successful in cases of portal thrombosis in children. For portacaval anastomosis the operation is performed through a thoraco-abdominal approach, and an end-to-side or a side-to-side anastomosis is made between the portal vein and the inferior vena cava.

Post-operative Management.—A drainage tube is left in the peritoneal cavity and an underwater thoracotomy drainage tube is also inserted. A chest radiograph is taken on the evening of operation to exclude the presence of a hæmothorax and to make sure that the lung has completely expanded. The peritoneal drainage tube may be removed on the second day unless there is free drainage from it. Glucose drinks are given from the first post-operative day, but protein is not allowed until the third day, and then only in small amounts of up to 25 G. daily for the first week. This is increased to 50 G. if there is no evidence of porta-systemic encephalopathy during this second week. If the patient has mild or moderate cirrhosis, he has a good chance of surviving for several years or more after portacaval anastomosis, but if there is advanced cirrhosis and parenchymal cell failure, a sustained remission is rarely possible.

Other Operations: Portasystemic Disconnexion.—If the patient's portal vein has been shown to be thrombosed or if he has poor liver function, and if he is too old or otherwise unfit for portacaval anastomosis, it may be possible to carry out a more minor procedure designed to disconnect the œsophageal varices from the high-pressure portal collaterals. The œsophageal veins can be attacked and tied directly at thoracotomy, and this procedure may be of value in an emergency. However, it is not possible to tie all the varices in the œsophageal region. Furthermore, gastric vessels are not seen, so that the operation has only a very limited application. A very high gastric transection provides a subcardiac porta-azygos disconnexion, which is of more general use in these particular circumstances. The left gastric and short gastric veins are divided, thus disconnecting the high portal pressure from the bleeding œsophageal and upper gastric varices. The stomach is also completely transected and immediately resutured. Even after this method, however, bleeding has been known to recur.

HEPATIC COMA

This condition is a neuropsychiatric disturbance with certain characteristic features—an often disordered consciousness, altered personality, noisy delirium, flapping tremor, rigidity, increased reflexes, and many other neurological features. Although patients may suddenly emerge from a deep coma and survive unexpectedly, hepatic coma should always be regarded as a grave condition with a grim prognosis.

Precipitating Factors.—Common among these is upper gastro-intestinal hæmorrhage in a patient with cirrhosis and portal hypertension. Here, the effect is due to ammonia or other products of bacterial breakdown of blood in the intestine, acting on a cirrhotic liver whose oxygen supply is further impaired by the anoxia following the hæmorrhage. Other precipitating factors are sepsis, an alcoholic bout, surgical operation, or the use of diuretics which may be related to a fall in serum potassium.

Treatment of Hepatic Coma.—

1. *No Protein.*—Calories are supplied by glucose drinks in the pre-comatose state or by 20 per cent glucose given in an intracaval drip if the patient is in coma. Full vitamin supplements are given parenterally, especially of vitamins B and K. After recovery from coma, protein may be recommenced but only in small amounts until the limit of the patient's tolerance is found. This may be between 25 and 50 G. daily.

2. *Blood Transfusion.*—The hæmoglobin level should be maintained above 10 G. per cent to enable an adequate supply of oxygen to reach the failing liver.

3. *Neomycin.*—Six grammes are given daily in divided doses. The purpose of neomycin is to decrease the formation of ammonia and other nitrogenous products during bacterial decomposition of blood and other proteins in the gut.

4. *Purges.*—Purgation with magnesium sulphate and the use of enemata are very important in clearing the bowel of protein.

5. *Other Therapy.*—Glutamic acid, arginine, ornithine, and choline have all been recommended in hepatic coma. None has proved of any real value. Cortico-steroids are worth using in acute coma associated with viral hepatitis.

6. *Fluid and Electrolyte Balance* must be maintained in the usual way. An accurate fluid chart is essential with daily serum-electrolytes and acid-base estimations.

7. *Avoid* morphine, barbiturates, and all sedation as far as is possible.

BILIARY CONDITIONS OF INFANCY: NEONATAL JAUNDICE
(*See* Chapter XL.)

DIAGNOSIS AND TREATMENT OF HYDATID DISEASE

Hydatid disease in man is caused by the ingestion of larval cysts of the worm *Echinococcus granulosus* (*Tinea echinococcus*). Hydatid disease is best known in the sheep-farming districts of Australia and New Zealand, but also occurs in Britain, particularly in Wales.

Prophylaxis.—Strict control is required over the disposal of sheep offal and the sale of horse meat in pet shops. All dog meat should be boiled and any infested dogs deinfested every few months. Adequate hygiene of dogs and their kennels should be practised, and dogs should be barred from kitchens. Children should be firmly instructed in personal hygiene and care taken in their access to infested dogs.

HYDATID LIVER

After ingestion, the wall of the ova is dissolved, the embryo reaching the liver by the portal vein. It is surrounded by lymphocytes and endothelial cells, and early cyst formation occurs, the cyst being visible after several weeks, becoming egg-sized after 3 months, but remaining symptomless at this time. Cysts grow very slowly, have a laminated wall and contain scolices and daughter cysts; they can eventually reach huge proportions after many years.

The great majority of liver hydatids are in the right lobe and some are symp-tomless. Later on, infection may supervene, or the cyst may rupture into the biliary tree, the peritoneum, or the blood-stream with resulting anaphylaxis. After a variable period of years the cyst may lose its blood-supply, the fluid get absorbed, and the cyst become calcified (*Fig.* 270).

Diagnosis.—This may be made from the various primary and secondary tumours of the liver, mucocele of the gall-bladder, and tumours of the colon or kidney. Radiology of the gastro-intestinal tract, biliary tree, or kidney may help in diagnosis, together with the demonstration of calcification in the liver or the presence of a raised irregular diaphragm. There are, in addition, certain immunity reactions to hydatid which vary in intensity according to the extent of absorption of hydatid antigen, which is treated by the body as a foreign protein.

1. *Eosinophilia* of 6 per cent or more is present in about one-third of cases.

2. *Casoni Intradermal Test.*—Sterile hydatid fluid, 0·2 ml., is injected intradermally, normal saline being used as a control. An immediate weal reaction occurs in positive cases. This reaction, which is seen within half an hour of the

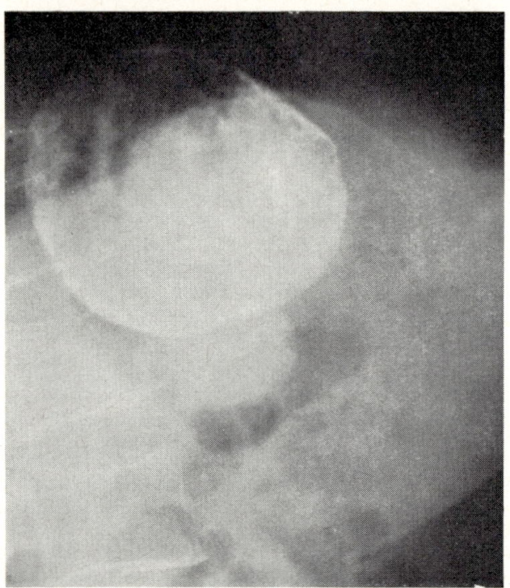

Fig. 270.—Large calcified hydatid in right lobe of liver.

injection, may be followed some 12 hours later by the development of a local area of induration and erythema. The results of the Casoni test are unreliable on occasion, as the Casoni antigen varies in its potency.

3. *Complement-fixation Test.*—A positive result of this test follows from the presence in the serum of specific antibodies to the hydatid antigen. It is rare in children, but is nearly always positive in those adults where the cyst contains viable parasites and leakage has occurred in the past.

Anaphylaxis.—This may occur after spontaneous rupture or leakage, but usually follows trauma, surgical puncture, etc. It may be confined to allergic skin manifestations such as urticaria, or a severe generalized effect may occur with pulmonary œdema and collapse.

Treatment.—This is, of necessity, surgical and is designed to remove the entire cyst with its contents without contaminating the field of operation by scolices, which would risk anaphylaxis and the possibility of further cyst formation. The liver is exposed by resecting a rib, if necessary, and the cyst area is packed off. The cyst is aspirated and immediately injected with up to 10 ml. of pure formalin, which should kill the parasite within a few minutes. The cyst can then be opened, sucked out, and the laminated membrane and its contents removed. After avulsion of complicated cysts, marsupialization has been advised, but as this technique gives rise to prolonged and usually infected drainage, recent preference has been for packing of the cyst cavity with omentum or partial hepatic lobectomy. Calcified cysts are not harmful and should be left alone.

PULMONARY HYDATID

This may be primary or secondary to a hepatic hydatid. The incidence of pulmonary hydatid is from 10 to 23 per cent of hydatid disease. It tends to give rise to symptoms in a younger age-group than liver hydatid, as the growth of a cyst in the lung is more rapid than a similar cyst in the liver. Symptoms are those of infection of the bronchi, lung, or pleura. Hæmoptysis is frequent and sometimes the hydatid material may be coughed up. A chest radiograph usually shows a clearly demarcated cyst cavity in the lung and the specific tests for hydatid discussed above may be positive. It is sometimes possible to remove the cyst in its laminated membrane after incising the adventitiæ, but where there has been infection, lobectomy may be required. Care should be taken not to rupture the cyst during anæsthesia. The use of formalin is not recommended for pulmonary hydatid.

BRAIN HYDATID

Hydatid cysts are rare but are usually single. They produce the symptoms and signs of increased intracranial pressure varying with their location. Diagnosis is by the usual neurosurgical methods and the treatment is surgical removal.

CHAPTER XXVIII

THE PANCREAS

By WILLIAM BURNETT

ACUTE PANCREATITIS

Diagnosis.—It is important to establish the diagnosis of acute pancreatitis from other acute abdominal conditions as conservative management is the treatment of choice in pancreatitis, whereas emergency operation is required in certain of the conditions which can be confused clinically with pancreatitis, such as perforated peptic ulcer, intestinal obstruction, acute cholecystitis, acute appendicitis, and mesenteric thrombosis. In many instances abdominal pain like that of pancreatitis is associated with nausea and vomiting, and there may also be tenderness and abdominal rigidity. However, chemical and radiological aids to diagnosis are available to reinforce the clinical diagnosis, which can be difficult to establish in some cases of acute pancreatitis.

The house-surgeon should arrange for the following investigations:—
1. Serum amylase.
2. Other enzyme and biliary tests where indicated.
3. Serum calcium.
4. Serum bilirubin.
5. Blood-sugar.
6. Straight radiograph of abdomen.

1. *Serum Amylase Estimation.*—Serum amylase can be elevated in a number of intra-abdominal disorders, but is characteristically very high in acute pancreatitis. The upper limit of normal is variously given as 150 or even up to 200 Somogyi units per 100 ml. serum. Any value above 300 units is regarded as pathological, but it is rare to find a level of under 500 units in early acute pancreatitis. Values of 1000, 2000, or even over 3000 units are regularly found. The highest levels are recorded within a few hours of the onset of the disease and these high levels usually return to near-normal levels within 48–72 hours of a patient's admission to hospital. It is often said that so much pancreatic exocrine

Table XII.—CONDITIONS ASSOCIATED WITH RAISED SERUM AMYLASE

1. Perforated peptic ulcer
2. Intestinal obstruction
3. Mesenteric thrombosis
4. Acute cholecystitis
5. Bronchial carcinoma
6. Mumps
7. Renal failure
8. The use of opiates

tissue is destroyed in extremely severe cases of pancreatic necrosis that the level of serum amylase cannot rise. However, this theoretical concept rarely occurs in clinical practice. The serum amylase estimation is a particularly valuable test since rapid methods for its estimation are now widely available; the result can be known within an hour of obtaining a blood sample. It is important to remember that a variety of conditions can result in elevation of the serum amylase, as shown in the table opposite (*Table XII*).

In this group it is extremely unusual for the serum amylase to rise above 500 Somogyi units, except in three conditions—perforated duodenal ulcer, intestinal obstruction, and mesenteric thrombosis. In perforated ulcer an escape of pancreatic juice from the duodenum into the general peritoneum results in rapid absorption of pancreatic enzymes with amylase values which can rise to 1000 or even 1500 Somogyi units. In intestinal obstruction, particularly when the bowel is strangulated, intestinal contents, including pancreatic juice, can pass through the damaged bowel wall, resulting in a rapid absorption of pancreatic amylase from the peritoneal cavity to give high serum levels.

2a. Other Serum Enzymes.—Serum levels of the other major pancreatic enzymes, lipase and trypsin, rise and fall in a manner roughly parallel with the serum level of pancreatic amylase. However, it is most convenient for the laboratory to monitor the degree of absorption of the various pancreatic enzymes by the level of serum amylase.

2b. Urinary Diastase.—This is often estimated in the diagnosis of acute pancreatitis. The enzyme concerned is precisely the same as that estimated in the serum amylase test, but for some obscure reason the term 'diastase' continues to be used—usually with different, and therefore confusing, units when this enzyme is estimated in the urine. An aliquot of early-morning urine, say 100 ml., is sent to the laboratory soon after admission. The normal range is 6–25 Wohlgemuth units per ml. If the level rises to over 100 units per ml. it indicates active pancreatitis. This test has no real advantages over the serum estimation, but, on rare occasions, may be positive after the serum level has returned to normal.

3. Serum Calcium (normal 5 mEq./l.) is not usually reduced in acute pancreatitis. Any fall in the calcium value is due to free fatty acids combining with serum calcium to form soaps in the areas of fatty necrosis, thus lowering the level of calcium in the serum. A fall in serum calcium is rarely observed clinically, but if it does occur, it may foreshadow the need for intravenous calcium gluconate (10 ml. of 10 per cent) to relieve tetany. It has also been stated that a high serum calcium might point to the diagnosis of parathyroid adenoma—a condition which, on rare occasions, is associated with acute pancreatitis.

4. Serum Bilirubin.—Mild degrees of hyperbilirubinæmia are quite commonly associated with acute pancreatitis.

5. Blood-sugar.—The fasting blood-sugar may be elevated in a small percentage of patients with pancreatitis.

6. Radiography.—A plain radiograph may show an isolated gas-filled coil or two of distended jejunum in the upper abdomen (*Fig.* 271). This appearance

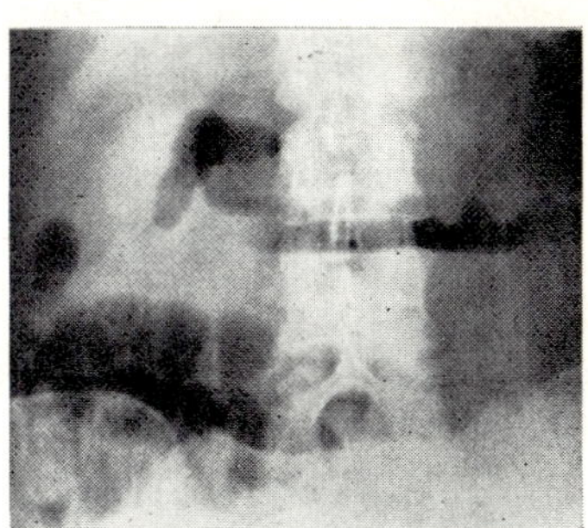

Fig. 271.—Isolated coils of distended gasfilled jejunum are displayed in this plain radiograph of a patient suffering from acute pancreatitis.

has been called the 'sentinel loop' and is thought to be pathognomonic of acute pancreatitis. A gastrografin meal on occasion shows widening of the C-curve of the duodenum and displacement of the stomach by an inflamed, swollen pancreas.

Diagnostic Paracentesis Peritonei.—If there is some doubt in regard to the diagnosis of acute pancreatitis, paracentesis peritonei may prove a valuable investigation, and possibly may spare the patient an operation which would not benefit him if the diagnosis is, in fact, pancreatitis. The following is a safe method of carrying out diagnostic paracentesis.

Technique.—A fine lumbar puncture needle is used—one that will just admit No. 6/0 polythene tubing. The needle, its stylet, and 18 in. (45 cm.) of the polythene tubing are first sterilized. The needle, with stylet in place, is introduced through the anæsthetized skin of the right iliac fossa at a point 1·2 in. (3 cm.) below the umbilicus and just lateral to the sheath of the rectus abdominis. The needle is steadily advanced and a characteristic sensation is felt as it enters the peritoneal cavity. The needle is advanced no further. The stylet is removed and aspiration attempted. If fluid is not obtained, the polythene tubing is threaded through the lumen of the needle and the needle is then withdrawn, leaving the tubing in place. Aspiration is performed with the patient in several positions. Unless all the intraperitoneal fluid is trapped in the lesser sac, a specimen will be obtained.

The peritoneal exudate in acute hæmorrhagic necrosis of the pancreas is prune-juice coloured and its amylase content is extremely high, a reading of many thousands being obtained. In the commoner, milder types of pancreatitis, only a little fluid is present, and this is pale, and serous in character, with no bacteria seen in the smear. The amylase concentration, however, is very high. Where there is gangrene of the bowel in the various conditions with strangulation, the peritoneal aspirate may be blood stained and foul smelling, and may contain many intestinal bacteria and can have a high amylase content.

Sequelæ of Acute Pancreatitis.—An initial acute attack may be the only one. However, repeated attacks of major or minor degree may occur after the primary attack. The term 'relapsing pancreatitis' is then used. Repeated attacks may be followed by the development of chronic pancreatitis.

MANAGEMENT OF ACUTE PANCREATITIS

Provided the diagnosis of acute pancreatitis is made with some assurance, a conservative régime is strongly advised. It is generally agreed that immediate operation has nothing to offer the patient and is against his best interests. Formerly held opinions that decompression of the biliary tree was of value have now been discarded. The main points to be observed in treatment are as follows:—

1. Nasogastric Aspiration should always be used. Continuous suction removes the gastric hydrochloric acid as soon as it has been secreted and so prevents it from entering the duodenum, thus suppressing the hormonal stimulation of the exocrine secretion of the pancreas. In addition to this important therapeutic function, nasogastric suction also brings relief from the persistent and very characteristic nausea and vomiting associated with pancreatitis, and so helps to alleviate the considerable pain found in this condition.

2. Relief of Pain.—Pethidine hydrochloride (B.P.) is the most appropriate drug to use, in a dosage of 50 to 100 mg. according to the degree of pain and the clinical condition of the patient. Morphine is contra-indicated because it increases spasm of the involuntary muscle of pye sphincter of Oddi and so, by impeding drainage from the pancreatic duct, results in increased pressure in pancreatic ducts and acini. Epidural anæsthesia and splanchnic block have been recommended for the relief of severe pain, but these procedures are very rarely required.

3. Inhibition of Pancreatic Secretion.—The vagal stimulation of pancreatic secretion can be inhibited by the use of anticholinergic drugs, of which the most commonly employed is propantheline bromide (pro-Banthine). This is given intravenously or, more commonly, intramuscularly in doses of 15 mg. up to a total of 60 or 90 mg. daily. This drug also causes a drying of the mouth and care should be taken therefore to prevent the development of parotitis. Propantheline bromide should not be used indiscriminately in older patients as retention of urine may also result. After nasogastric suction has been discontinued, it is possible to give pro-banthine orally.

4. Supportive Intravenous Therapy.—In acute pancreatitis there is often widespread intraperitoneal or retroperitoneal inflammatory exudate resulting in lowered blood-volume and hypovolæmic shock. There is an urgent need to restore an adequate blood-volume as soon as possible. Colloid infusions, such as albumin, plasma, or whole blood, are the most appropriate solutions to be used. The choice of the fluid to be used and the amount required are judged from blood-volume estimations, if these are available, or by changes in the hæmatocrit, and observations of pulse-rate, CVP, and blood-pressure. Shock is the principal cause of death in the first 48 hours and, although this can be entirely due to the loss of circulatory blood-volume, there is frequently an element of bacteriæmic shock due to bronchopneumonia, especially in those patients who have been given a large dose of morphine before being sent to hospital.

5. Water, Electrolytes, and Calories.—A careful daily and cumulative fluid-balance chart should be kept with appropriate allowance made for insensible loss. Daily serum-electrolyte studies are done, together with acid-base studies, as metabolic acidosis can readily develop in the course of the illness. Full water replacement is given by the intravenous route, calories are given as glucose, and sodium, potassium, and chloride are given in appropriate amounts to keep the serum levels within normal limits and to keep pace with any losses (*see* Chapter IV). Hypokalæmia can develop in the more severe cases and is treated by potassium chloride intravenously—given with care and only if the urinary flow is adequate. Calcium deficiency is uncommon, but, if it occurs, is treated by a calcium gluconate dose intravenously. If renal anuria develops, the full conservative management of anuria is instituted (*see* Chapter XXXI). If this is insufficient, dialysis may be required.

6. Antibiotic Therapy.—An antibiotic should always be prescribed in acute pancreatitis as a prophylactic against infection of the necrotic retroperitoneal (and possibly mediastinal) tissues and also against bronchopneumonia, so frequently the terminal event in severe pancreatitis. One of the broad-spectrum antibiotics is the drug of choice, and tetracycline may be given intravenously in doses of 1 G. daily in divided doses 6-hourly.

7. The Question of Trasylol.—The use of trasylol has been recommended for the first 3 or 4 days of the attack in a dosage of 50,000 units daily; even larger doses are preferred, up to 200,000 units run in slowly in a saline infusion over a 24-hour period. This drug has been advocated recently as being an anti-kallikrein factor—capable of preventing the severe systemic effects supposedly due to the absorption of the substance 'kallikrein' from the area of pancreatitis. The effectiveness of trasylol in acute pancreatitis is still disputed, but at present it should be tried in full dosage.

Recovery Phase.—As recovery proceeds, nasogastric suction and intravenous fluids can be gradually replaced by cautious oral feeding, and antibiotics and other drugs stopped as soon as possible. Early dietary requirements are met by

Pro-Banthine (G. D. Searle & Co. Ltd., High Wycombe, Bucks, and Chicago, 80, Illinois, U.S.A.).
Trasylol (F.B.A. Pharmaceuticals Ltd., Haywards Heath, Sussex).

a bland diet of high-calorie content; large meals are forbidden, to avoid major exocrine pancreatic activity. Although acute pancreatitis can be an isolated incident, it is regrettably the case that recurrences are quite common.

Indications for Surgery.—If a positive diagnosis of pancreatitis has been made, there is no need for laparotomy if the patient continues to improve on a conservative régime. If, however, (1) an upper abdominal mass appears associated with development of (2) high fever and (3) leucocytosis, the possibility of local *abscess* formation is obvious, and surgery may be required to drain the collection. Moderate *jaundice* persisting for some days is rare, but may justify biliary decompression. If at any stage of development of a pancreatic *pseudocyst* secondary septic infection occurs in it, a high white cell-count will be found, and drainage will be necessary to remove blood-clot, fibrin, and broken-down pancreatic residues.

Post-operative Management.—If operation has been performed, there will be a possibility of a pancreatic fistula developing; if so, digestion of the abdominal wall may occur, together with the distinct chance of wound dehiscence. It is advisable to apply continuous suction to any drain inserted in the wound, and the skin should be protected by the use of an aluminium paste.

INVESTIGATIONS AFTER ACUTE PANCREATITIS

In the later management after complete subsidence of the attack of acute pancreatitis, investigation should be carried out to establish the cause of acute pancreatitis. Cholecystography should be performed and, if a normal gall-bladder is found, intravenous cholangiography is then done in order to finally free the biliary tree from suspicion. This is of considerable importance, as pancreatitis is often associated with cholelithiasis and biliary-tract disease such as stone in the bile-duct or stenosis of the sphincter of Oddi. A plain radiograph of the abdomen discloses evidence of pseudocyst formation or calcification of the pancreatic area. Barium-meal examination can show up the distorting effects of a pseudocyst on the stomach and will also disclose the presence of any peptic ulcer. Blood-sugar estimation is valuable in order to establish whether diabetes is present or not. Analysis of duodenal contents and of the stool gives evidence of pancreatic deficiency. If gall-stones have been demonstrated, cholecystectomy should be carried out 4–6 months after the attack of acute pancreatitis. If a normal cholecystogram has been found in the post-pancreatitis investigations, there is no indication for cholecystectomy. Fæcal fat determinations may be advisable.

POST-OPERATIVE ACUTE PANCREATITIS

In recent years attention has been paid to the development of acute pancreatitis as a post-operative complication. It presents with symptoms which were formerly attributed to post-operative shock. The operations most liable to be followed by post-operative pancreatitis are gastrectomy and operations on the biliary tract. Pancreatitis usually presents within 2 or 3 days of operation with some upper abdominal pain and a circulatory collapse.

Treatment.—The treatment is as above for acute pancreatitis, and is conservative except in those instances where the post-operative pancreatitis is related to the leakage of a gastrojejunal anastomosis or a duodenal stump, both of which necessitate secondary relieving surgery. Steroids have also been used, but there is no satisfactory evidence of their efficiency in this condition.

CHRONIC PANCREATITIS AND STEATORRHOEA

With repeated attacks of pancreatitis, fibrosis of the gland occurs with loss of exocrine-secreting tissue. The most important defect in digestion is in fat absorption. In the absence of pancreatic lipase, the stools become bulky, foul smelling, and loose. Globules of fat are seen floating on the surface. The normal fat content of the fæces is about 20 per cent, but in chronic pancreatitis it may rise to 50 or even up to 90 per cent. The fæcal matter is measured in a 3-day pool of fæces and is expressed in grammes of fæcal fat per diem. Values above 7 G. are abnormal and in chronic pancreatitis levels of 10 to 20 G. or even higher may be found, depending on the fat intake. Pancreatin tablets may be given—400 mg. t.d.s. The serum amylase and lipase may be intermittently elevated if there is any obstruction to the pancreatic duct system.

Deficiency in pancreatic secretions may be estimated by the *secretin-pancreo-zymin test* in which a duodenal tube is passed, and the contents of the duodenal juices estimated for volume, bicarbonate, and pancreatic enzymes after the exhibition of secretin and pancreozymin.

Technique.—A double-lumen radio-opaque tube is passed transnasally into the stomach to the 60-cm. mark; its tip may be weighted with a small bag containing 1·5 ml. mercury. The patient then lies on his right side, the foot of the couch is raised and the tube slowly advanced to the 75-cm. mark. After 30 minutes the tip should have entered the duodenum, the more proximal openings still being in the stomach. The position is checked radiologically.

Two 10-minute samples are then aspirated by low pressure (-25 mm. Hg) and secretin given intravenously in a dose of 1·7 units per kg. body-weight. Three test specimens are then collected at 10-minute intervals; at 25 minutes pancreozymin is given in the same dose as secretin and three specimens collected between 30 and 60 minutes. Duodenal and gastric contents are kept on ice until analysed.

In normal subjects, after each injection the volume of duodenal juice rises to 40–60 ml. per 10 minutes, the trypsin output to 3500 (Gownelock) units, and amylase to 400 units. In chronic pancreatitis these values are halved.

Other Complications.—*Diabetes mellitus* sometimes develops and watch must be kept for it in patients with chronic pancreatitis. In patients suffering from severe and prolonged pain there is a very real risk of inducing *drug addiction*, and *suicide* may be attempted. If removal of stones and sphincterotomy have not eased the pain, a paravertebral block of the splanchnic nerves may be successful.

CANCER OF THE PANCREAS

Cancer causes deep jaundice and very careful preparation (p. 143) for operation is necessary. Diabetes may be present (p. 141). Relatives should be warned that the prognosis is poor. Radical resection is rarely justified for carcinoma of the head of the pancreas, but choledochoduodenostomy will relieve the jaundice (in 2–3 weeks) and the troublesome pruritus. Pancreaticoduodenectomy is practised for early ampullary carcinoma. Afterwards shock must be combated (p. 21) and watch kept for a pancreatic fistula. Serum amylase, blood-sugar, and electrolyte levels are determined daily.

Secretin, pancreozymin (Boots Pure Drug Co., Ltd., Nottingham).

CHAPTER XXIX

MANAGEMENT OF LOWER ABDOMINAL CASES

By JAMES KYLE

IN this chapter the intestinal complications of abdominal operations and their management are described. The care of patients having operations performed on the small or large intestine in general is similar to that outlined for gastro-duodenal cases in Chapter XXVI. Preparation of the colon for surgery is detailed in Chapter VI and rectal operations are considered in Chapter XXXVI. Acute appendicitis is the most common abdominal surgical emergency and consequently its management is described in detail below. Much care and repeated, detailed observation by the house-surgeon are required, particularly when immediate operation is not contemplated. Similar attention to detail is needed for the successful management of an ileostomy or colostomy.

INTESTINAL OBSTRUCTION

Intestinal obstruction may be the result of vascular occlusion or, much more commonly, it is caused by mechanical or neuromuscular factors. These latter two types can constitute the initial presentation of disease, e.g., carcinoma coli or strangulated hernia, or they may develop after an abdominal operation, e.g., paralytic ileus; in either case, their management is similar.

MESENTERIC VASCULAR OCCLUSION

Infarction of the bowel may result from stenosis or embolism of the superior mesenteric artery, or from thrombosis on the venous side.

Mid-gut ischæmia causes post-prandial upper abdominal pain, change in bowel habit, weight-loss, and eventually acute occlusion, resembling embolism.

Mesenteric embolism is sudden and occurs in patients with atrial fibrillation or atheromatous ulcers in their aorta. There is usually (but not always) severe abdominal pain. Shock and collapse may resemble acute pancreatitis or myocardial infarction; there may be evidence of embolism elsewhere. Signs of peritonitis (p. 346) are likely to be delayed for some hours, so that diagnosis may be difficult if there is no previous history of mid-gut ischæmia or fibrillation is absent. A straight radiograph of the abdomen is often unhelpful; an ECG should always be obtained, WBC count and serum amylase and transaminase levels, blood-urea, and electrolytes estimated.

If the patient's cardiovascular state after resuscitation permits laparotomy to be performed, re-establishment of arterial flow may be possible in the first 6 hours; resection will be necessary for older, localized infarcts; hence arrangements for blood transfusion (p. 43) must be made.

Mesenteric thrombosis can be even more difficult to diagnose. Often the patient is elderly, irrational, dehydrated, and uræmic, or suffering from cardiac or liver failure; this is the secondary type of thrombosis. Primary mesenteric thrombosis also occurs, usually in younger patients, some of whom have had earlier thrombotic episodes.

The onset is insidious. Abdominal pain, sometimes colicky and recurrent for days or even weeks, is the principal symptom. Localizing signs are few initially, but the house-surgeon must examine the abdomen repeatedly. There is sometimes shock particularly when the larger portal radicles are affected. Later there is gradual abdominal distension and paralytic ileus, and there may be melæna.

Treatment of secondary thrombosis is directed towards improving the patient's general condition, particularly by rehydration. Anticoagulants may be administered (p. 79) or rheomacrodex infused intravenously (1000 ml. per 24 hours); alternatively and especially if there is doubt about the diagnosis, laparotomy is undertaken. Resection is practised for primary mesenteric thrombosis and may be successful with smaller infarctions.

After mesenteric vascular operations the surgeon may order anticoagulants; watch must be kept on the fluid intake and output.

POST-OPERATIVE INTESTINAL OBSTRUCTION

A. PARALYTIC ILEUS

Most cases are the result of peritonitis paralysing the nerve plexuses in the intestinal wall, so preventing the propagation of peristalsis. Rarely, peristaltic activity may not recommence for many days (or even weeks) after an apparently successful operation, e.g., vagotomy plus pyloroplasty. Some of these latter cases may be the result of unsuspected electrolyte imbalance or fat necrosis.

Diagnosis.—

1. Absolute constipation; no flatus is passed.

2. Bowel-sounds absent—'the death-like stillness of paralytic ileus' (Hamilton Bailey). Sometimes respiratory sounds are heard; or there may be sounds like the bilge-water in a ship, caused by fluid being moved passively within dilated bowel.

3. Distension.—There is generalized distension, which if gross may embarrass respiration.

In many cases there are other signs of peritonitis (p. 346).

Management.—

1. Treat the cause.

2. Do *not* flog the bowel with so-called stimulants and purgatives.

3. Keep the stomach empty by aspiration. Miller-Abbott intestinal aspiration tubes are rarely used in Britain.

4. Maintain fluid balance by intravenous infusion (p. 32).

5. Check serum electrolytes daily.

6. Frequent re-examination of the abdomen.

7. Reassure the patient.

This régime may have to be kept up day after day, sometimes for weeks. Unremitting, cat-like vigilance is essential. Many patients with paralytic ileus already have had peritonitis and some may proceed to mechanical obstruction. By his management of such unfortunate patients the young doctor may make— or mar—his surgical reputation.

B. MECHANICAL INTESTINAL OBSTRUCTION

Developing a few days after operation, mechanical obstruction is mostly due to filmy adhesions. Many of these patients will settle on the non-operative régime outlined above for the treatment of paralytic ileus. But in some cases obstruction remains complete, or there may be strangulation, e.g., from an internal hernia—considerable experience is needed to diagnose these cases.

Rheomacrodex (Pharmacia (Great Britain) Ltd., The Avenue, West Ealing, London, W.13).

Diagnosis.—

1. Absolute constipation; no flatus passed.

2. Colicky abdominal pain. Frequent severe pains and shock suggest strangulation.

3. Vomiting or large gastric aspirates.

4. High-pitched frequent bowel-sounds accompanying the colic spasms.

5. Distension, except with very high intestinal obstruction.

6. Straight radiograph of abdomen, with patient erect (p. 704)—this reveals distended loops of bowel with multiple fluid levels.

Management.—Sometimes non-operative when there are thought to be multiple filmy adhesions or the patient has a well-scarred abdominal wall. But operative relief is advisable when mechanical complete obstruction persists for a day or two or when examination reveals:—

1. An abdominal lump;

2. Acute well-localized tenderness;

3. Sudden onset of shock.

Correction of fluid and electrolyte deficits and efficient nasogastric suction are just as essential in this type of obstruction as they are in paralytic ileus.

ACUTE APPENDICITIS

Early Cases.—The majority of patients with acute appendicitis reach hospital within 48 hours of the onset. They are treated by appendicectomy. When there is no perforation of the appendix and no peritonitis, antibiotics are not needed and oral fluids can commence 12–24 hours after operation. With a gridiron incision the stitches are removed and the patient allowed home in 7 days; with a paramedian incision even without complications, 2 or 3 extra days' stay in hospital are advisable.

If peritonitis has been found at laparotomy, it is treated as outlined on p. 347. While awaiting the bacteriological report on the intra-abdominal pus, an antibiotic is given systemically, e.g., tetracycline, 250 mg. per 24 hours given in the intravenous infusion. Oral fluids are withheld until there is clear evidence of the resumption of peristaltic activity. Watch must be kept for the development of residual abscesses in the iliac fossa, pelvis, or subphrenic regions.

Late Appendicitis.—Some patients only arrive at hospital after many days of abdominal symptoms; by this time a mass is mostly palpable in the iliac fossa, and sometimes per rectum. Often the patient is elderly and suffering from unrelated degenerative or infective conditions of the lungs, cardiovascular or urinary systems; these conditions require appropriate assessment and treatment.

The non-operative *Ochsner-Sherren regimen* is adopted for the management of late appendicitis. When no surgical facilities are available, it may have to be used in an early case. Modified forms of the regimen are also appropriate for the management of some other inflammatory lesions in the abdomen, e.g., cholecystitis, salpingitis, diverticulitis, pneumococcal peritonitis.

Ochsner-Sherren Regimen

1. *Position.—*The patient stays in bed, lying in whatever position he finds most comfortable.

2. *Recording Physical Signs.—*

a. Temperature and pulse-rate are initially measured and charted every 4 hours (*Fig.* 272).

b. The position and size of the mass are determined each day and marked on the patient's abdomen with a skin pencil (*Fig.* 273).

c. Rectal examination is performed on alternate days.

3. *Fluid and Food.*—If the attack is many days old when the patient is first seen and there is already a well-localized mass it is illogical to withhold oral fluids

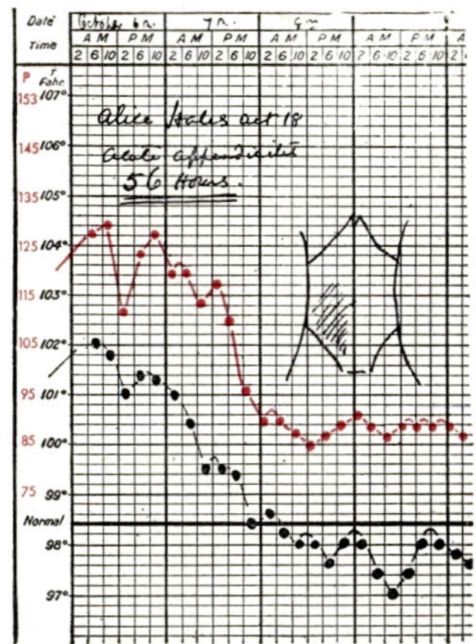

Fig. 272.—Chart of a case of acute appendicitis, first seen 52 hours after the onset of the attack, treated by the Ochsner-Sherren method.

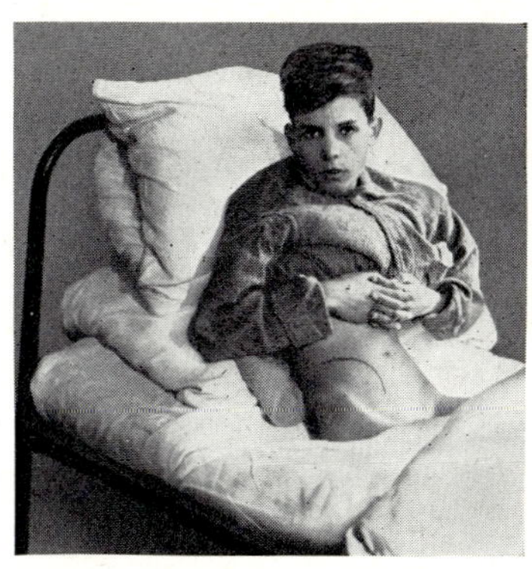

Fig. 273.—Appendix abscess. The extent of the lump has been marked on the skin.

completely—the patient will certainly have been taking some fluid at home without serious ill-effects. But to begin with the amount given in hospital should be small—60 ml. hourly. If this does not cause vomiting the amount given can rapidly be increased after 6–8 hours. Soft solids can be started in a day or two.

However, with an attack of only 48 hours' duration, when there is still acute tenderness or other reason for thinking that localization is not well advanced, e.g., rapid pulse and fever, then nothing should be given by mouth; only mouth-washes are permitted. Fluids are infused intravenously and may have to be continued for 2–3 days. Nasogastric aspiration is not usually necessary.

An accurately kept fluid balance chart is essential. Vomiting is a danger sign that the method may be failing and consequently it must be clearly marked.

4. *Drugs.*—

a. Purgatives are *never* given.

b. Pain-relieving drugs are not often needed when localization has occurred; morphine and its derivatives are best avoided on account of their nauseating effects.

c. Antibiotics are given in full doses, e.g., tetracycline 250 mg. per 6 hours i.m., or streptomycin 1 G. plus penicillin 1 mega unit twice daily. Remember they may render the diagnosis of residual abscesses more difficult.

5. *White Blood-cell Counts.*—A WBC count helps confirm the original diagnosis and repeated every one or two days it will indicate resolution or spread of the inflammatory process.

Warning Signs of Possible Failure.—The house-surgeon and nursing staff must be on constant lookout for evidence that the Ochsner-Sherren regimen may be failing, and give the surgeon timely warning. Signs suggesting possible failure are:—

a. Steadily rising pulse-rate;

b. Increasing pain and tenderness;

c. Persistently high (39° C., 102° F.) or swinging temperature for 2–3 days, or rigors;

d. Vomiting;

e. Increasing size of the mass in the iliac fossa;

f. WBC count rising progressively;

g. Diarrhœa, mucus per rectum, or bulging anterior rectal mass indicating the presence of an abscess.

To the discerning clinician, the signs of impending failure are often obvious in the worried patient's face. When careful reassessment indicates that the method has failed, operation must be resorted to—usually drainage of an abscess.

When the method succeeds, the patient before he leaves hospital should be advised to have an internal appendicectomy in 3 months' time.

PERITONITIS—See p. 346

RESIDUAL ABSCESSES

A. SUBPHRENIC ABSCESS

This may follow peritonitis from any cause; about one-third follow surgical disasters. The abscess becomes manifest in from 2 days to 2 months following laparotomy.

Localizing signs are minimal, and sometimes the patient may not feel particularly ill. The only evidence for some days is a rising evening pyrexia in the range 38°–40° C. (100°–104° F.). Most subphrenic abscesses are on the right side; there may be discomfort over or pain on compression of the right costal margin and loin. Sometimes shoulder-tip pain is experienced but it is strangely uncommon. Later there may be a pleural effusion.

Diagnosis.—(1) Four-hourly pulse chart reveals the swinging temperature; (2) WBC count over 15,000; the leucocytosis response may be modified by antibiotics or steroids; (3) No evidence of infection anywhere else; (4) Screening of the diaphragm—this is the most valuable investigation, but may need to be repeated. A high immobile diaphragm is revealed; there may be a pleural effusion above. Sometimes gas and a fluid level in the abscess cavity above the liver are seen—they can never be detected by percussion. The surgeon will want to know not only the side of the abscess but also whether it is anterior or posterior.

Treatment.—Extraperitoneal drainage, not as a midnight emergency but within a day or two of diagnosis.

Aftercare.—*Drainage tubes*: There are usually two large-bore tubes about 12 in. (30 cm.) long arching over the dome of the liver. These may be allowed to drain continuously or have suction applied to them. They are shortened very slowly over a period of 2–3 weeks. Sinogram pictures are taken every 3–4 days to make sure that the abscess cavity is obliterating itself satisfactorily.

Nutrition.—A blood transfusion, high calorie and protein diet, and anabolic steroids are valuable (*see* pp. 43, 46).

B. PELVIC ABSCESS

An abscess in the bottom of the pouch of Douglas may be a late result of peritonitis, e.g., from appendicitis or perforated duodenal ulcer. At first it has seemed that the inflammation has been subsiding. Then after a few days a swinging temperature develops. Irritation of adjacent bladder and rectum can give rise to frequency of micturition and diarrhœa. The WBC count is raised and, on rectal examination, the rectum feels decidedly hotter than usual. Its anterior wall is bulging and tender; later there may be fluctuation. The dome of a pelvic abscess is sometimes felt in one or other iliac fossa.

Treatment.—Drainage is necessary. Some abscesses will discharge spontaneously into the rectum. If not, once there is fluctuation, with the help of a large proctoscope, a pair of sinus forceps is plunged through the bulging anterior rectal wall into the abscess, and the blades opened. Alternatively, the abscess may be opened through the posterior fornix of the vagina.

While it is undoubtedly true that *early inflammation* in the pelvis, subphrenic space, or other localized areas of peritoneum will occasionally resolve with intensive, appropriate antibiotic therapy, when the manifestations outlined above are present it is always safer to assume that there is pus present which requires to be drained.

PYELEPHLEBITIS

This is a rare complication usually of gangrenous appendicitis and it still carries a high mortality. The appendix may have lain behind the ileum, in close relationship to the commencement of the superior mesenteric vein, and the diagnosis been delayed. Infected clot forms in the vein and emboli break off and pass to the liver, there to cause diffuse inflammation and multiple small abscesses.

Diagnosis.—There is a history of several days' duration and signs suggestive but not typical of appendicitis. The temperature is raised and usually swings between 38·5° and 41° C. (101°–106° F.). Rigors are the rule and the patient looks ill. In about half the cases the liver is enlarged and tender. Slight to moderate jaundice is often perceptible.

The serum bilirubin and transaminase levels are raised as is the WBC count. A blood-culture will usually reveal a Gram-negative organism.

Note.—Any patient developing a rigor after an abdominal operation must have a blood-culture taken.

Treatment.—Massive doses of tetracycline (250 mg. every 4 hours) or kanamycin in similar dosage are given intravenously. Later the antibiotic may have to be changed to one shown to be more appropriate as a result of tests on the organism obtained from the blood-culture. Total parenteral alimentation and fluid replacement are essential (p. 32). By the time the diagnosis is made the appendix will often have been removed. If not, appendicectomy is performed under antibiotic cover and the region drained; it is doubtful if it is worth tying the lower superior mesenteric vein at this late stage.

In the somewhat unlikely event of the patient surviving, one or more abscesses in or above the liver may require drainage.

FÆCAL FISTULA

When told that a patient has a fæcal fistula, the house-surgeon must first determine whether or not it is intestinal contents that are being discharged; a mixture of bile and old blood can often closely resemble these. If the discharge is coming from the intestine he must next decide if its origin is the small or large intestine, and then from the volume of the discharge whether the hole is small or large, e.g., breakdown of an anastomotic line. Fistula appearing within 2–3 days of operation may be associated with peritonitis, but after that time localization should have been achieved and contamination of the general peritoneal cavity is less likely (except for breakdown of anastomoses).

A. Large Intestine.—A fistula arising in the large intestine behaves in many ways like a temporary colostomy (*see* p. 400). Provided that the fistula is not arising from a carcinoma and that there is no obstruction in the distal colon, there is a strong tendency for it to close spontaneously. A disposable colostomy bag applied over the external opening keeps the patient clean and comfortable until closure is complete—often in 10–14 days, but sometimes only after many weeks.

B. Small Intestine.—While it is probable that many small intestinal fistulæ would eventually close if given enough time, the twin problems of skin digestion by the issuing intestinal juices and the frequently large losses of fluid and electrolytes (*Table II*, p. 35) demand much more active treatment than is necessary for a large intestine fistula.

That the fistula is arising in the small intestine can be proved by getting the patient to swallow 2–5 ml. of dye, e.g., indigo-carmine, and seeing it issue from the fistulous opening within 30 minutes. Alternatively, gastrografin can be injected down the fistulous tract and the patient then X-rayed; the characteristic mucosal pattern of small intestine is revealed, and sometimes an unsuspected abscess cavity as well.

Treatment.—(1) *The larger fistulæ.* The sudden outpouring of copious amounts of small intestinal contents within a few days of a laparotomy usually means that urgent re-exploration of the abdomen is necessary. The affected portion of intestine is short-circuited or resected; direct repair of the opening in the bowel wall is not often possible.

(2) *Small fistulæ.* Those that develop late, and most of the fistulæ that appear in Crohn's disease, do not require early operation and are treated as follows:—

a. Fluid and Electrolytes: Nothing is given by mouth. As with a malfunctioning ileostomy, up to 3 litres of fluid per day may be lost at first, and to this deficit must be added the patient's ordinary metabolic requirements of about 2 litres. Nutrition is particularly important in this group of patients; total parenteral alimentation is necessary and intravenous vitamins, amino-acid, and lipid preparations should be given from an early date (*see* p. 46) and blood transfusion is beneficial if the hæmoglobin level is subnormal after rehydration.

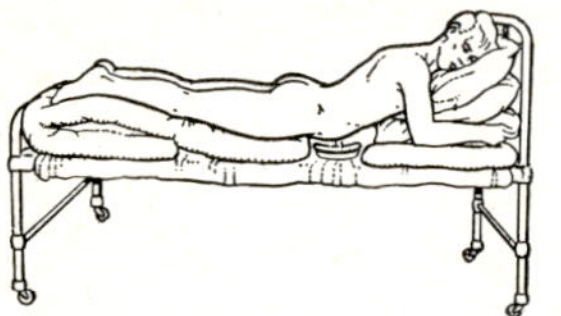

Fig. 274.—The prone position, showing the arrangement of the mattresses.

b. Skin Protection: As far as possible, the irritant digestive juices must be prevented from coming in contact with the skin or their enzymes must be inactivated. Considerable ingenuity and a great deal of patience may be needed to keep the abdominal wall dry.

Nursing the patient prone on a split mattress (*Fig.* 274) helps, but the position must occasionally be altered. It may be possible to apply a disposable ileostomy bag (p. 397) over the fistulous opening, and attach Paul's tubing to its distal end. To be successful the adhesive flange needs to be applied just as soon as the fistula is detected—before skin digestion begins. With large, irregular openings the skin around should be protected—again beginning early—with aluminium-zinc oxide paste. The preparations mentioned under Ileostomy Management (p. 399) may also be used. In addition, suction is applied to the fistula. Continuous suction with a Robert's type of pump is desirable and this means that the sucking end has to be of the sump suction type, with an air inlet. The tip of the Salem nasogastric tube (p. 348) may be introduced into the fistulous opening, or even a small sump suction tube. If no such tube is immediately available, one can be made by doubling back the distal third of a piece of tubing or 16 F catheter, tying it to the shaft and making some side-holes near the bend (*Fig.* 275). All these devices can be made to

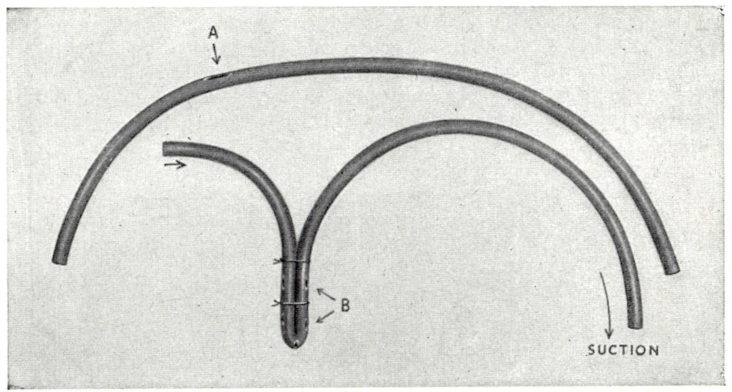

Fig. 275.—A simple rubber tube adapted for surface suction. An oval opening is cut at **A**, with its long axis in the line of the tube: this allows the lumen of the tube to be preserved when it is acutely bent at this point. The two limbs are held together by encircling ligatures, and additional holes (**B**) are cut on each side of the bend.

work well when the surgeon is standing beside them; the trouble is that as soon as they are left alone they tend to become dislodged and intestinal juice flows over the surrounding skin.

Persistence of the fistula for many weeks suggests that there is obstruction distally or that the fistulous tract has become partly lined by mucous membrane (operation will be needed in both circumstances) or that there is an underlying chronic inflammatory process, e.g., tuberculosis, actinomycosis, or regional enteritis.

ABDOMINAL DRAINS

Nowadays drainage of the peritoneal cavity is uncommon. Even if some purulent fluid is found, e.g., around an inflamed appendix, it is removed with the sucker during the operation and the inflammatory process controlled by systemic antibiotics—there can be little justification for inserting antibiotic powders or solutions into the peritoneal cavity. However, when an abscess has been opened or when leakage from the bowel may be expected, e.g., after intraperitoneal closure of a colostomy, a drain is inserted. Possible biliary or pancreatic leakage should also be anticipated and a drain is placed in any large cavity that cannot be obliterated at once, e.g., in the pelvis after excision of the rectum.

Types of Drain.—Sterile Sterivac latex tubing is the drain most used in Britain. It is relatively soft and supple and so unlikely to cause pressure necrosis of adjacent bowel, always the danger with more rigid tubes. The intraperitoneal

15

end may be split open for a distance of 10 cm.; the other end is led directly into a disposable bag beside the bed. When the diaphragm has been opened and only partially closed, e.g., in resection of carcinoma of the cardia, any drain left down to the tail of the pancreas should be of the under-water seal type (p. 310) to prevent the development of a pneumothorax.

Corrugated latex drains may be used when there is the possibility of leakage after extraperitoneal closure of a colostomy, or when oozing seems likely to continue from the subcutaneous tissues, e.g., after the repair of large ventral herniæ in obese patients. Such drains are usually cut about 2 cm. wide and project for about the same distance above the skin. They must be secured in position by a skin stitch and have a safety-pin through their outer end. Suction through a Sterivac drain or Surgivac apparatus (*Fig.* 276) may be used when there has been extensive subcutaneous dissection.

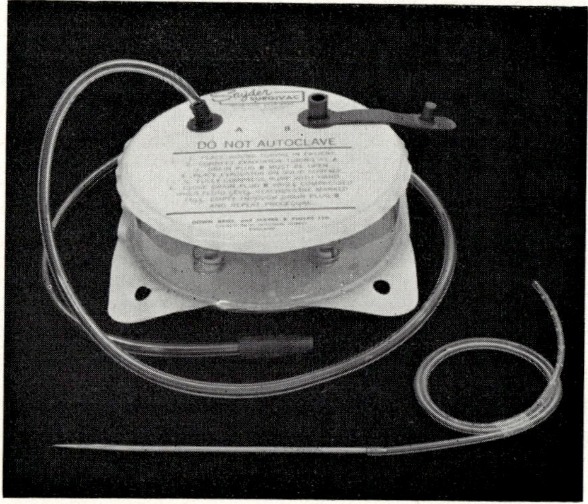

Fig. 276.—Surgivac suction drainage apparatus.

Management of Intraperitoneal Drains.—It is probable that after 48 hours bowel and omentum are so well matted around the drain that a good drainage track has been formed. Consequently the drain may generally be shortened, perhaps by 3–5 cm. per day, aiming to have it completely removed within 4–5 days of operation. But sometimes discharge is so copious that it is felt advisable to leave it longer since otherwise the discharge would pour over and macerate the surrounding skin. In this circumstance the drainage tube should be gently rotated each day to lessen the risk of its causing pressure necrosis of adjacent intestine.

Corrugated drains can nearly all be removed by the third post-operative day. When a drain is shortened or removed the fact should be recorded on the patient's temperature chart.

MANAGEMENT OF AN ILEOSTOMY

Most permanent ileostomies are constructed following total colectomy for ulcerative colitis. A much less common reason for fashioning an ileostomy is a prophylactic colectomy in a patient with familial polyposis coli. Temporary catheter ileostomies are occasionally made in the course of emergency abdominal operations but are now rare.

A permanent ileostomy should be sited 5 cm. away both from the anterior superior iliac spine and from the umbilicus; the skin around it should be flat and free from scars. A belt round the waist should be able to retain an appliance over the ileostomy opening comfortably and securely.

Pre-operative Counselling.—It is important to explain carefully to the patient before operation both the need for the ileostomy and what it will involve. In particular he must be reassured that an ileostomy is compatible with a normal life. He can do hard manual work afterwards and sports like golf and swimming can be indulged in. Reproductive activities are not interfered with in either sex. A former ileostomy patient is usually available and willing to come and talk to the patient, who can also obtain help, advice, and information from the Ileostomy Association* which now exists in many countries.

ILEOSTOMY APPLIANCES

Most ileostomies are fashioned so that after eversion of the ileal end there is a spout 3–4 cm. long projecting above the level of the skin; the mucosa is carefully stitched to the edges of the trephine hole in the skin. The projection is designed to allow irritant ileal contents to pass into an appliance, having had little or no contact with the surrounding skin.

Choice of Appliances.—Modern appliances have done much to make life easier for the patient with an ileostomy, and there is no doubt that whenever possible an adhesive appliance should be recommended. These have the enormous advantage that when used correctly they are virtually free from leakage and from odour, whereas non-adhesive appliances often fail in these respects, especially during the night.

A small number of patients are, or become, sensitive to the adhesive; a few others, for various reasons, find that they are unable to manage an adhesive appliance effectively, but all should give this form of apparatus a fair trial before changing to the non-adhesive variety.

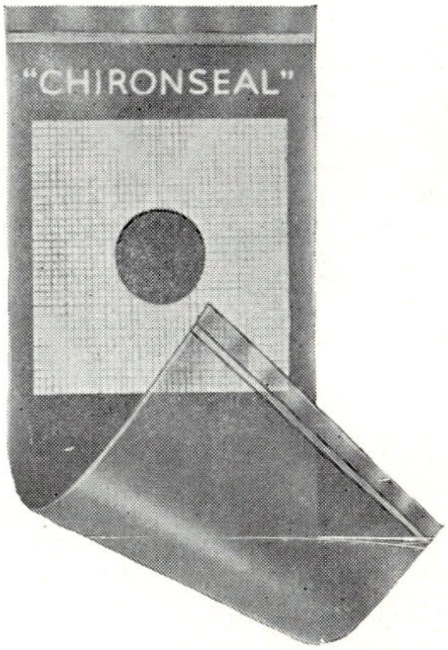

Available Appliances.—

1. The Chiron Disposable Plastic Bag is a narrow plastic bag attached to an adhesive-coated rectangular flange; in the centre of the flange is an opening into which the end of the ileostomy projects (*Fig.* 277). This type of bag is usually applied at the conclusion of the operation. Paul's

Fig. 277.—Disposable ileostomy bag, which is attached to the abdomen by the adhesive-coated rectangular flange.

---

* Ileostomy Association of Great Britain, 149 Harley Street, London, W.1.

tubing can be tied into a hole made in a corner of the bag. Otherwise the bags have to be changed frequently and the skin may become excoriated—something which must always be avoided if at all possible. Once regular ileostomy function has become established and œdema, etc., has subsided in 7–10 days, it is better for the patient to start using and become accustomed to the type of appliance that he will wear in the future.

2. Down Bros.' adhesive ileostomy appliance consists of a rubber or plastic disk with a central hole, around which is a grooved rim for the fitting of a detachable rubber bag (*Fig.* 278 A). The disk is fixed to the skin around the ileostomy with special double-sided adhesive plaster (*Fig.* 278 B).

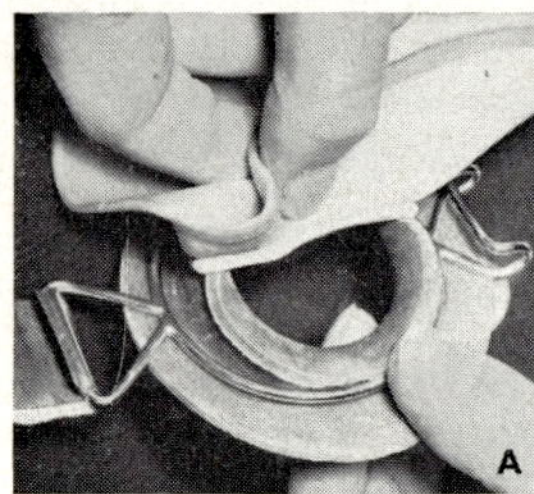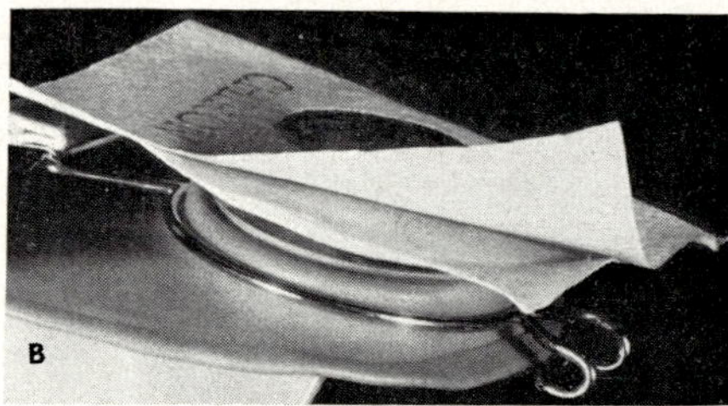

Fig. 278.—Down Bros.' ileostomy appliance. A, Placing the neck of the rubber bag over the rim of the rubber collar; B, Double-sided adhesive plaster applied to the rubber flange around the central hole. Showing the non-adhesive layer partially peeled off.

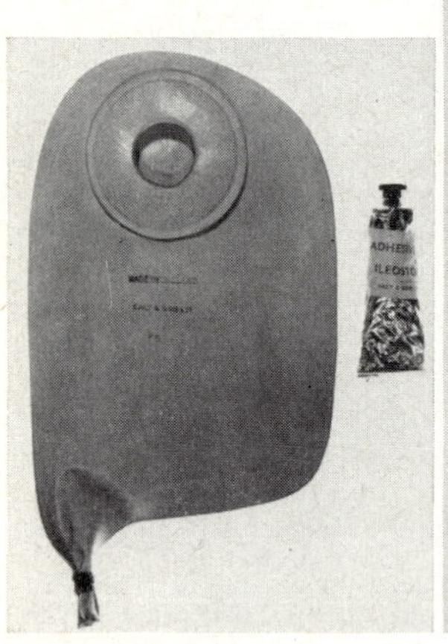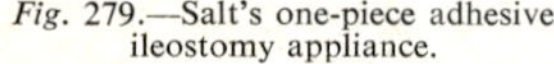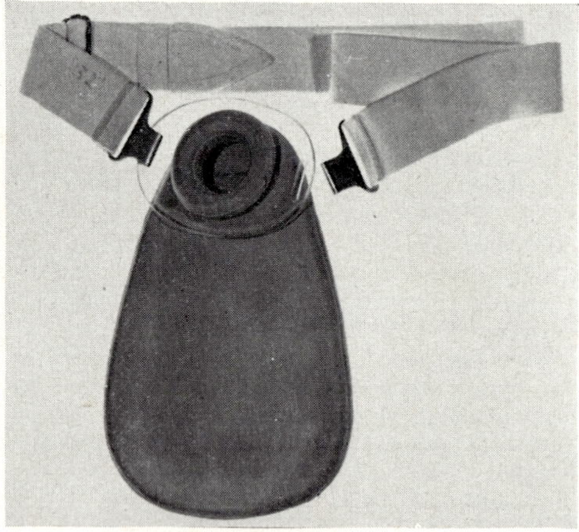

Fig. 279.—Salt's one-piece adhesive ileostomy appliance.

Fig. 280—Donald Rose's ileostomy appliance (non-adhesive).

3. Salt's adhesive ileostomy appliance consists of a flange and rubber bag made in one piece (*Fig.* 279), the flange being fixed to the skin around the ileostomy with a special sticky cement.

After a few weeks' use the rubber of these otherwise satisfactory appliances is inclined to become malodorous, in which event the apparatus should be discarded in favour of a new one.

4. The ileostomy belt made by Donald Rose is designed to give firm fitting without adherence. It consists of a rubber bag with a rolled rubber rim, the latter passing through a hole in a plastic flange to which the hooks of the belt are attached (*Fig.* 280). Although not quite so satisfactory as those just described, it is an efficient alternative for those patients who, for one of the reasons given already, are unable to tolerate the adhesive variety.

Management of Adhesive Appliances.—The bag should be emptied as necessary, and if the Down Bros.' appliance is being employed, it is best to change the bag 12-hourly, one of two bags being in use alternately. The rubber flange (or the whole apparatus in the case of the Salt appliance) should not be changed so often, as too frequent removal and reapplication of adhesive plaster tends to make the skin sore. Often it will be found that the flange will remain in position for 3–4 days.

Changing the Adhesive Flange.—The flange to be changed is removed with the aid of ether, zoff, or other solvent, and all traces of the previous adhesive are similarly removed from the skin, which is then washed with soap and water and dried gently. Hairs in the vicinity of the stoma should be shaved as necessary. The clean apparatus having been prepared, and the adhesive applied, it is pressed firmly into position around the ileostomy. The belt is then adjusted, and with the Down Bros.' appliance the bag is slipped on to the flange.

Management of Non-adhesive Appliances.—Some patients apply the apparatus direct to the skin, but usually it is best to have a small dressing around the ileostomy, on which the appliance is held by the belt. A satisfactory dressing, changed every 12 hours, consists of a 3-in. (7·5-cm.) square of lint (gauze is less satisfactory), with a central hole cut to the size of the stoma. Barrier creams or other ointments can be applied to the skin beneath the lint if desired.

Care of the Skin.—Provided the instructions are followed the skin beneath the adhesive rarely becomes sore except in those exceptional patients who are genuinely sensitive to the adhesive. Before assuming that a patient is allergic to adhesive, it is essential to ascertain whether the flange is being changed unnecessarily often; for most persons every 2–4 days is sufficient. Alternatively, the patient may not be changing it soon enough, thus allowing moist faecal matter to seep between flange and skin. These errors are liable to lead to excoriation of the epidermis, which should abate rapidly if a correct technique is employed. When a Down Bros.' flange has been applied, between this and the ileostomy there is an uncovered circle of skin which should be protected by tucking a small piece of cotton-wool in that groove, and renewing it every time the bag is changed.

Remember that the most potent cause of soreness is contact of ileostomy efflux with the skin. If this is prevented, the skin will remain healthy.

Treatment of Soreness of the Skin.—Karaya gum powder can be dusted on the sore areas of skin around the stoma; excess powder is wiped off, and the remainder forms a coagulum to which the adhesive appliance often coheres satisfactorily, and under which healing proceeds. An alternative measure is the application of siccolam cream, orabase, or, in mild cases, calamine lotion or calamine cream have proved effective.

Diet.—Dietetic restrictions should not be placed on patients with an ileostomy, for they will soon find out for themselves if there are any articles of diet

Zoff (Smith & Nephew Ltd., Hull and Welwyn Garden City, Herts).
Siccolam (British Drug Houses Ltd., London, N.1).
Orabase (E. R. Squibb & Sons, Liverpool).

that upset them. If desired, alcoholic beverages may be taken in reasonable quantities.

Complications.—'Ileostomy dysfunction' is the only common serious complication of the immediate post-operative period. It is the result of an incomplete obstruction and leads to a persistent looseness of the fæcal discharge, and frequently some abdominal colic. The patient becomes dehydrated, deficient in protein and electrolytes, loses weight, becomes very ill, and may die unless the condition is corrected—rehydration must be pursued energetically.

As a rule, dysfunction can be prevented by mucocutaneous suture at the time the ileostomy is constructed. Should this syndrome develop it is corrected by overcoming the stomal obstruction. The insertion of a short tube, dilatation, or nicking any granulation tissue may suffice, but if these simple measures do not correct it, refashioning of the ileostomy is necessary.

MANAGEMENT OF A COLOSTOMY

There are two principal types of colostomies: (*a*) A permanent end colostomy; and (*b*) A temporary colostomy, usually a loop of colon supported on a glass rod or a double-barrelled Paul-Mikulicz colostomy. With most patients the idea of having even a temporary colostomy causes considerable psychological perturbation and feelings of revulsion. Therefore before operation it is always worth spending time explaining to the patient exactly what the colostomy entails and more particularly what it does not prevent—it does not stop manual work, social or sex life. It is better still if a former patient with a long-established colostomy will come and talk to the patient who, understandably, is more likely to be reassured by the voice of personal experience than by that of a surgeon.

TEMPORARY COLOSTOMY

A loop colostomy, either transverse or left inguinal, may either be opened at the conclusion of the operation, or opening may be deferred for 48 hours. In either case the projecting colon is wrapped in petroleum jelly gauze, which is wound round under the projecting ends of the glass rod after a retaining loop of rubber tubing has been pushed over either end. Ordinary gauze is placed over the impregnated layer and the whole mass covered with absorbent cellulose tissue held in place by strapping or a binder. Sometimes a disposable bag can be applied at once.

Occasionally a right-angle glass Paul's tube may be tied into the opened colon (*Fig*. 281). Wide (2-cm.) thin tubing leads to a bag at the side of the bed. If a de Martell's clamp has been placed on the distal sigmoid limb of a Paul-Mikulicz colostomy it will cut through and fall free itself in 4–5 days.

Opening a Colostomy Loop.—The house-surgeon may be asked to do this about the second post-operative day. First reassure the patient that he will feel nothing. No anæsthetic is required. The opening is made with a cutting diathermy needle. It need only be 1–2 cm. long and should *not* cut down to the glass rod—the latter is often preventing the bowel from falling back into the peritoneal cavity.

Normally the glass rod is removed about the tenth day. Adjacent skin stitches are taken out about the sixth or seventh day; if they are left longer, stitch abscesses may develop.

Crushing a Colostomy Spur.—Nowadays most Paul-Mikulicz type of colostomies are closed by a formal operation. It is possible to crush the spur with an enterotribe and the now single opening may gradually retract and disappear as the bowels start working *per vias naturales*. However, the failure rate is high. The blades of the enterotribe must have moderately long and sharp teeth otherwise as the approximating screw is tightened each day, the enterotribe will tend to extrude itself instead of cutting through the spur. There is always a

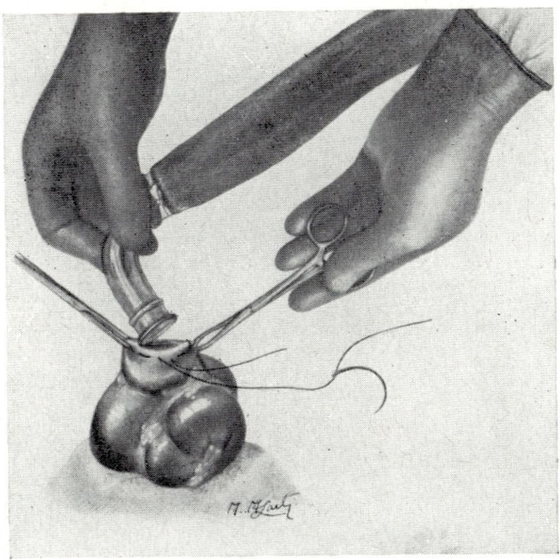

Fig. 281.—Method of inserting a Paul's tube.

chance of the enterotribe being thrown away in the mass of soiled cellulose and gamgee tissue, or vanishing down into the rectum. A long Kocher's forceps, with rat-teeth, may be used to crush the spur, but a turban of gamgee tissue must be built up around the handles, the ratchet on which is tightened one notch each day.

PERMANENT COLOSTOMY

Most permanent end-colostomy openings are in the left iliac fossa. They should be located on a flat area of skin, sufficiently far away from both the iliac spine and the umbilicus to prevent the flange of any colostomy appliance reaching either of these landmarks.

Usually the colonic mucosa has been stitched to the skin with catgut. A plastic disposable Chiron colostomy bag is applied at once, the opening in the adhesive rectangle of the bag overlying the colostomy orifice. The bowel is unlikely to act for 2–3 days. If the colostomy has not acted by the fourth day a glycerin or dulcolax suppository may be inserted into it or 100 ml. of olive oil run in; if possible avoid giving purgatives orally. During the patient's stay in hospital disposable adhesive bags may continue to be used. It is important that the patient should be taught how to attend to the colostomy himself before he leaves hospital. The house-surgeon should put a finger into the colostomy to ensure there is no stenosis before the patient goes home.

Regulating the Colostomy.—The patient will have no warning that the colostomy is going to function and no muscular control over this action. He must learn to regulate it either by: (1) diet, or (2) the wash-out technique. The former is preferred.

Diet.—As soon as his abdominal status permits, the patient is encouraged to take a mixed diet with plenty of roughage. He should experiment at home with different foods. Onions should be avoided, but most other vegetables can usually be taken. A little care should be exercised when starting to take fruits, but most types do not upset the colostomy. Normally the colostomy will act

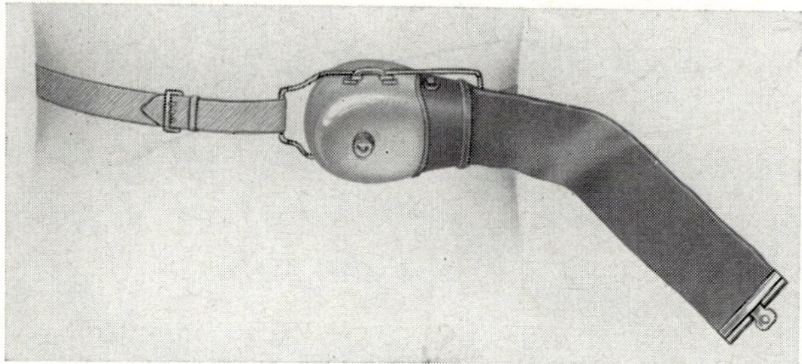

Fig. 282.—Plastic horn.

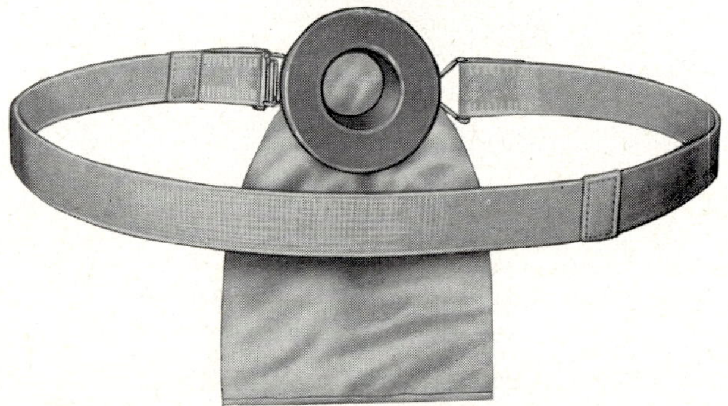

Fig. 283.—Dundas bag.

after an early morning cup of hot tea and perhaps a cigarette; often an evening movement will also follow a hot drink. The patient soon learns that the number and timing of motions are regulated by the type of food he eats.

If there is any difficulty in getting a satisfactory evacuation, a cellulose evacuant may be tried, e.g., celevac, one teaspoonful three times per day; this can be taken safely for months. Irritating loose stools are unusual; in hospital it is advisable to culture the fæces to exclude an infective enterocolitis before giving codeine phosphate, 30 mg., or diphenoxylate hydrochloride (lomotil), 5 mg. four times per day. At home the patient should first try cutting down the amount of fruit and green vegetables before resorting to drugs.

Wash-out Technique.—This is effective in securing one good bowel action each day but has certain disadvantages. The patient must always have the necessary apparatus with him; the procedure takes about 1 hour; there is a slight but real danger of perforating the colon with the rubber catheter.

The essential points in the technique are as follows. The patient sits or lies down beside a bucket or lavatory pan. A douche can holding 1 litre of tepid water is suspended from a hook 4 ft. (1·25 m.) up. A special plastic horn (*Fig.* 282) is then

Celevac (Harker Stagg Ltd., 6 Argall Ave., London, E.10).
Lomotil (G. B. Searle & Co. Ltd., Lane End Road, High Wycombe, Bucks).

placed with its bell end over the colostomy orifice; the narrower end is directed towards the bucket. Opposite the bell end is a valvular opening in the plastic horn through which a 16 F lubricated rubber catheter is very gently passed about 6 in. (15 cm.) into the colostomy. The catheter has already been connected to the douche can; the fluid is now allowed to run in quite rapidly. About 20 minutes later the colostomy works.

Appliances.—Some patients continue to use disposable Chiron adhesive bags. More satisfactory is the Dundas type of bag (*Fig.* 283). This has a firm plastic flange held in place on the colostomy by a belt; attached to this base flange is a disposable plastic bag. One difficulty with plastic bags as supplied is that they may become overdistended with flatus—a needle prick proximally will act as an escape valve. Disposing of disposable bags in a modern centrally heated home can be a problem.

When there is only one well-formed bowel movement per day some patients prefer a disk and colostomy belt (*Fig.* 284). A piece of cellulose wadding lies between the disk or plate and the colostomy, over which a piece of soft toilet

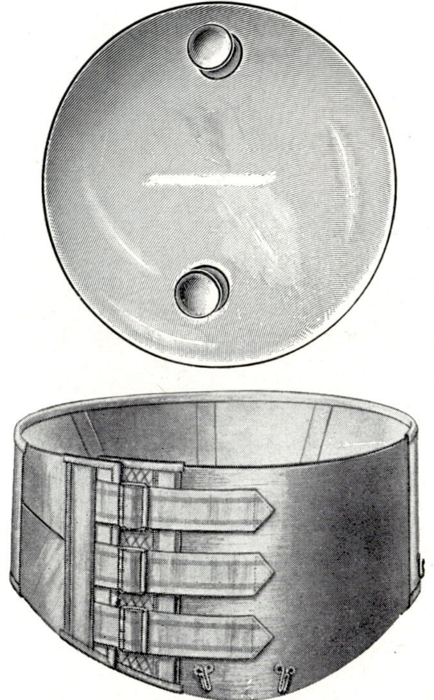

Fig. 284.—St. Mark's colostomy belt with disk.

paper may be placed to prevent the wadding sticking to the mucosa. The belt provides abdominal support and helps prevent herniation, particularly in those with a chronic cough or prostatism. An obese woman may prefer a colostomy cup built into a surgical corset.

CHAPTER XXX

THE ADMINISTRATION OF ENEMATA AND RECTAL SUPPOSITORIES

By Miriam A. Gough and D. L. Crosby

An enema may be defined as the introduction of fluid into the lower bowel. The term *evacuant enema* is used when the fluid is returned by the patient after a short interval, whilst a *retention enema* is one which must be retained by the patient in order to exert its effect. A *rectal suppository* is a cone-shaped mould which liquefies after insertion into the rectum.

Whilst the administration of enemata has few hazards in most patients, in the presence of ulcerative colitis there is a significant risk of perforation of the bowel wall, and enemata of any type should be avoided whenever possible in patients with this condition. When they are especially indicated they should be given by an experienced person and with the greatest caution.

INDICATIONS

The indications for the use of both enemata and rectal suppositories are similar and are as follows:—

A. EVACUATION OF THE LOWER BOWEL IN THE RELIEF OF CONSTIPATION OR AS A PRELIMINARY TO CERTAIN DIAGNOSTIC AND THERAPEUTIC PROCEDURES

1. Constipation.—It is usual to reserve the use of evacuant suppositories and enemata to those patients in whom:—

a. Oral aperients and dietary adjustments have been unsuccessful in causing a bowel movement.

b. Cleansing of the bowel is for some reason required to be more complete than is possible by the use of aperients.

c. The time available to achieve evacuation is limited.

Before resorting to the use of enemata and suppositories in patients complaining of constipation it is most important to exclude any underlying pathological cause and a digital examination of the rectum is mandatory. Sigmoidoscopic and radiological examination of the bowel should also be performed at some stage if there remains any doubt as to the underlying nature of the patient's condition. Digital examination is also important in order to exclude the presence of impacted scybala in the lower rectum, since these cannot usually be cleared by any procedure short of manual removal.

Simple constipation will in most patients respond to the insertion of evacuant suppositories, and enemata are only necessary in resistant cases. Whenever possible, treatment should also include instruction of the patient in how to regain a normal bowel habit.

2. Sigmoidoscopy.—Sigmoidoscopic examination of the rectum and lower sigmoid colon cannot be performed satisfactorily unless the bowel lumen is reasonably free from fæces. An adequate examination is usually possible for several hours following normal defæcation, but insertion of an evacuant suppository on the morning of the procedure may be necessary in some patients. Occasionally an evacuant enema may also be required in order to obtain conditions optimal to the examination; unfortunately it may alter mucosal appearances.

3. Preliminary to Barium Enema and Intravenous Pyelography.—Radiological visualization of the large bowel by barium enema (*see* p. 710), and of the urinary tract by intravenous pyelography (p. 714), are considerably hampered by the presence of fæcal masses and intestinal gas. These may either obscure normal appearances, or cause confusion by mimicking a pathological lesion. Oral aperients, dietary restriction, and evacuant suppositories are usually ordered as a routine before these examinations, but if preliminary radiographs suggest that the colon remains loaded with fæces, further examination should be deferred until evacuant enemata have been given.

4. Preliminary to Abdominal Surgery.—Most patients do not require a preoperative enema. However, it is undesirable that any patient should undergo planned major abdominal surgery in the presence of excessive colonic retention of fæces and it is of particular importance in surgery of the large bowel that the rectum and colon should be empty and reasonably free from pathogenic organisms. This may be difficult to achieve in the presence of disease of the sigmoid colon or rectum—particularly if low-grade intestinal obstruction also exists. In such situations, repeated rectal and colonic lavage may be a necessary supplement to other evacuant measures in ensuring that the maximum possible degree of cleansing is achieved. It is also the practice in many hospitals with such patients to sterilize the bowel contents pre-operatively with chemotherapeutic agents. (*See below*—Therapeutic enemata and suppositories.)

5. Preliminary to Rectal Administration of Chemotherapeutic Agents.—Prior to the rectal administration of chemotherapeutic agents, a normal bowel action should be encouraged if there is a marked degree of fæcal retention. However, the administration of evacuant suppositories or enemata may be occasionally necessary in some patients.

B. ENEMATA FOR DIAGNOSTIC PURPOSES

1. Barium enema examination is a common radiological investigation of the large bowel and terminal ileum in the diagnosis of pathological lesions of this segment of the alimentary tract. It is performed by administration of barium sulphate suspended in water into the rectum during radiographic screening (*see* p. 710). It is important that following this procedure patients should be encouraged to return the enema as soon as possible, since retained barium soon becomes inspissated following absorption of water. This leads to the formation of particularly hard scybala that may sometimes precipitate intestinal obstruction when there is a pathological narrowing of the bowel lumen.

2. Two-enema Test.—This is occasionally of value in the diagnosis of colonic obstruction but is much less used than formerly, due to the increasing use of other diagnostic techniques. Two consecutive evacuant enemata are given with an interval between them of 20 minutes to half an hour. The first enema will produce evacuation of the rectum. If the second enema is retained or returned without fæces or the passage of flatus, then it is suggestive that intestinal obstruction is present.

3. Cytology.—Repeated rectal and colonic lavage is used in some hospitals as an aid to the diagnosis of malignant lesions of the large bowel by the detection of malignant cells in the returned fluid.

C. RECTAL ADMINISTRATION OF THERAPEUTIC AGENTS

These may be divided into those acting locally on the lower bowel and those producing a systemic effect.

1. Local Action.—There are many varieties of rectal suppositories available which have a *local anæsthetic* and *lubricant* action in the relief of painful ano-rectal conditions such as anal fissure. When repeated medication of this type is necessary, patients should be instructed in the correct technique of self-administration.

Steroids in the form of suppositories and retention enemata (available in disposable packs, 20 mg. hydrocortisone in 100 ml. of fluid) are sometimes employed in the treatment of ulcerative colitis and other inflammatory disorders of the lower bowel.

Pre-operative sterilization of the bowel can usually be achieved by the oral administration of poorly absorbed *chemotherapeutic agents* such as neomycin and a number of sulphonamide derivatives. In some instances, however, as when a proximal defunctioning colostomy is present, or in the presence of a low-grade intestinal obstruction, sterilization of the distal bowel must be obtained either by retention enemata containing these agents, or by their administration through a colostomy stoma.

2. Systemic Action.—Rectal administration of *sedatives* is sometimes useful when oral administration is difficult and systemic injections are best avoided, e.g., mentally disturbed patients and children. *Bronchodilators* such as amino-phylline are also occasionally given in this way.

Rectal *magnesium sulphate* solution is still used in the alleviation of raised intracranial tension, this effect being achieved by its osmotic action in causing dehydration; 180 ml. (6 fl. oz.) of a 30 per cent solution are given by rectal tube and repeated at 6-hourly intervals. It is now, however, largely superseded by the intravenous infusion of potent osmotic diuretics.

Cation exchange resins are a particularly effective measure in the control of hyperkalæmia in patients with advanced renal failure, and are frequently given per rectum; 15–30 G. of sodium polystyrene sulphonate in 60–100 ml. water are usually given three or four times daily per rectum.

REQUIREMENTS AND PROCEDURES

1. Evacuant Suppositories.—The most familiar of these is the glycerin suppository consisting of glycerin solidified in gelatin, and acting by virtue of its hygroscopic and lubricant qualities. Bisacodyl (dulcolax) suppositories are also effective, causing a direct chemical stimulation of the rectum. A more recently developed suppository, anhydrous sodium acid phosphate and sodium bicarbonate in an inert base (beogex), utilizes a different principle in stimulating defæcation by distension of the rectum with carbon dioxide.

a. Requirements (*Fig.* 285).—A tray on which has been assembled:—
Suppository.
Hot water.
Disposable glove or finger cot.
Talc powder in a sprinkler.
Macintosh.
Paper towel.
Swabs.
Receiver.

Dulcolax (Boehringer Ingelheim Ltd., Isleworth, Middlesex).
Beogex (Pharmax Ltd., Crayford, Dartford, Kent).

A urinal, bed-pan, or commode should be readily available. Protective clothing should be worn by the person administering a suppository or an enema.

b. Procedure.—A clear explanation is given to the patient, privacy is ensured, and draughts are excluded. A bed-pan or urinal should be offered as an empty bladder lessens discomfort. The left lateral position is usual with the buttocks towards the edge of the bed although if movement is difficult the suppository can be inserted with the patient supine. The bedclothes are folded back and unnecessary exposure of the patient is avoided. The macintosh and towel are

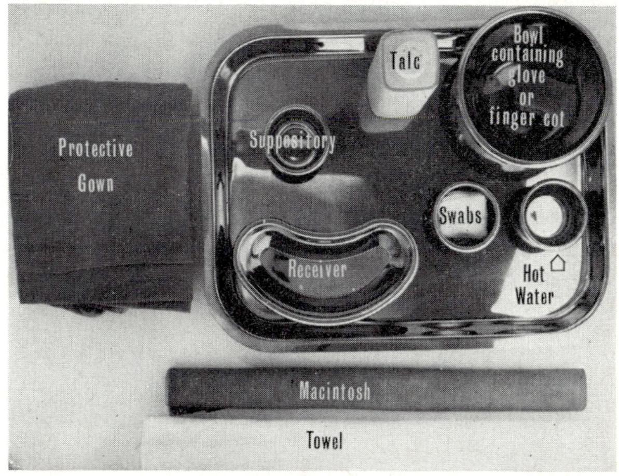

Fig. 285.—Photograph of tray with requirements for administration of an evacuant suppository.

placed under the buttocks. A nervous patient will relax more easily if told to breathe through the mouth. The glove or finger cot is worn, the suppository is taken out of its wrapper, dipped in hot water and gently inserted into the rectum for 5 cm. (2 in.). Pressure on the anus is required until the desire to expel the suppository has passed. The patient is left comfortable and encouraged to retain the suppository for as long as possible but is told to ask for a bed-pan or to be assisted to the commode when ready. Afterwards the bed-pan or commode is removed, covered, and taken to the sluice. The contents are noted and recorded. The patient who is able to do so may wish to cleanse himself, otherwise assistance is given. An opportunity is given for the patient to wash his hands, after which the bedclothes are re-arranged and a comfortable position ensured. Finally the equipment is cleared away.

2. Evacuant Enemata.—

a. Enema Saponis.—This consists of a soap-and-water solution which, by its bulk, stimulates emptying of the rectum. It remains the most commonly used variety of cleansing enema, though it is being rapidly replaced by more effective evacuant suppositories and disposable enemata. It is of considerable importance to remember that the soap-and-water enema is hypotonic and tends to be rapidly absorbed by the large bowel. Thus, when frequently repeated, water intoxication can occasionally occur. This is a particular hazard in infants and young children with megacolon. Isotonic enemata are now frequently used in order to avoid this danger, but are not entirely free from risk in that excessive absorption of electrolytes as well as water may occur and produce untoward side-effects in some patients.

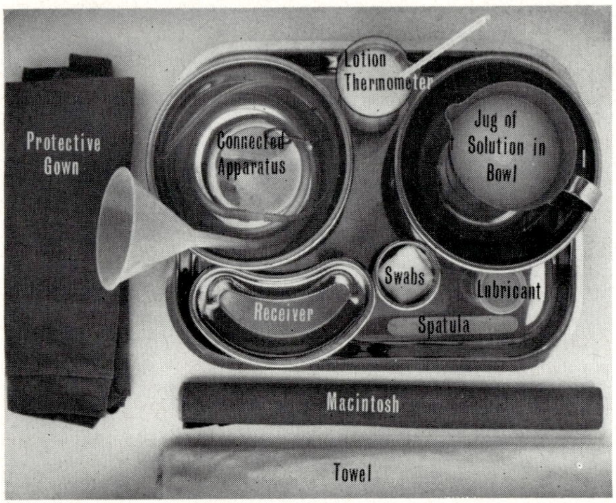

Fig. 286.—Photograph of tray with requirements for administration of an evacuant enema.

i. *Requirements.* (*Fig.* 286).—As assembled on tray for evacuant suppositories, with following differences:—

Enema soap solution, i.e., soap enema B.P.C. (enem. sap.). It contains 30 G. (1 oz.) soft soap in water to 600 ml. (20 fl. oz.).

Amount.—

Child	5 years of age	150 ml. (5 fl. oz.)
	10 years of age	300 ml. (10 fl. oz.)
	15 years of age	450 ml. (15 fl. oz.)
Adult		900 ml. (30 fl. oz.)
Elderly patient		600 ml. (20 fl. oz.)

The solution is prepared by mixing the soap and water thoroughly and straining it before use. It is given at 38° C. (100° F.).

Receptacle containing a funnel.

Length of tubing about 60 cm. (24 in.).

Long connexion.

Spring clip.

Soft catheter, size 22 or 24 French gauge, i.e., approximately 8 mm. in diameter.

Lubricant—e.g., yellow petroleum jelly.

Spatula.

Lotion thermometer.

ii. *Procedure.*—The preparation, management, and after-care of the patient are similar to those described in the procedure for administration of evacuant suppositories. The apparatus is connected and the end of the catheter is lubricated. The solution is poured through to expel the air. The tubing is then compressed with either the clip or the fingers whilst the catheter is gently inserted

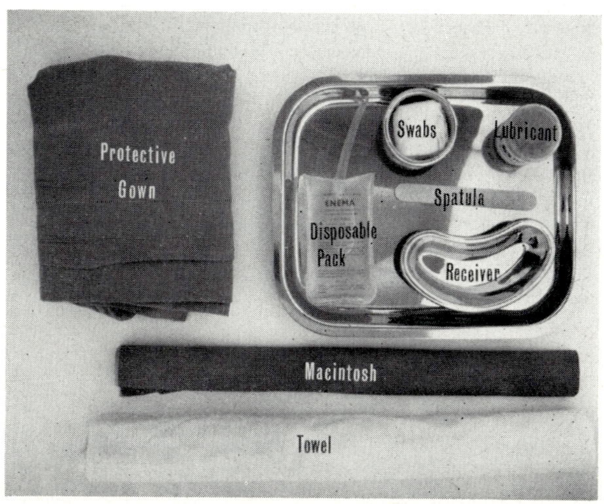

Fig. 287.—Photograph of tray with requirements for administration of disposable enema.

7–10 cm. (3–4 in.) into the rectum. The funnel is filled, care being taken to prevent entry of air, and it is raised 30 cm. (3 ft.) so that the required amount of fluid runs through steadily; 900 ml. (30 fl. oz.) should take approximately 3 minutes. The procedure should be discontinued if the patient complains of excessive discomfort or pain. The catheter is pinched and carefully withdrawn. The apparatus is disconnected and placed in the receiver. As the patient might feel faint when using the bed-pan or commode, the person who has administered the enema should remain within call. The equipment is cleared away, and each part is carefully rinsed and washed, particular attention being paid to the catheter which, with other contaminated articles, is sterilized by boiling for 5 minutes; disposable catheters are now widely used. Observations are as previously described.

b. DISPOSABLE EVACUANT ENEMATA.—These are being increasingly used both in hospital and general practice, because of their convenience and simplicity of administration. A common variety consists of 128 ml. of a sodium phosphate and diphosphate solution contained in a plastic bag to which is attached a nozzle for insertion into the rectum. The solution is hypertonic and increases the bulk of the rectal contents by osmotic attraction of fluid into its lumen.

i. *Requirements (Fig. 287).*—

Disposable enema (this may be warmed to body temperature by immersion in warm water).

Lubricant.
Swabs.
Macintosh.
Towel.
Receiver.

ii. *Procedure.*—The preparation, management, and after-care of the patient are similar to those described in the procedure for a simple soap-and-water enema. The cap of the disposable pack is removed. The end of the nozzle is lubricated and inserted into the rectum. The container is squeezed gently until all the fluid has been expelled, when the tube is removed and the pack discarded.

The dosage and directions for administration are clearly printed on the pack.

c. OLIVE-OIL RETENTION ENEMATA.—These are often used to soften the fæces in severe constipation and to facilitate painless defæcation following certain gynæcological and surgical procedures; 200–300 ml. (6½–10 fl. oz.) of oil are usually given. A disposable pack is commercially available.

i. *Requirements.*—As for evacuant enema, but a shorter piece of tubing and smaller catheter (size 8 or 10 English gauge, i.e., 5 or 6 mm. in diameter) are used.

ii. *Procedure.*—The warm oil is administered slowly, and to aid its retention the foot of the bed may be elevated. After a prescribed period, it is usual to follow it with a small 300-ml. (10-fl. oz.) soap-and-water enema. Directions for administration are given on the disposable pack.

Administration of any Retention Enema.—If it is found that the fluid is not being retained, it may be necessary to infuse the fluid more slowly using an intravenous administration set connected to the rectal tube.

d. TURPENTINE OR OX BILE ENEMATA.—These were formerly given as a remedy for abdominal distension due to flatus. They are of doubtful value, not without risk, and no longer advised.

3. Rectal and Colonic Lavage.—As already mentioned, this procedure is usually indicated when the maximum possible degree of large-bowel cleanliness must be obtained, e.g., prior to large-bowel surgery in which resection or anastomosis may be necessary. Isotonic fluid should always be used.

i. *Requirements.*—As for an evacuant enema with the substitution of a large quantity of isotonic saline (0·9 per cent solution) in place of the enema soap solution at 38° C.

Bucket.
Protection for the floor.

ii. *Procedure.*—The patient is prepared as for an enema, and up to 600 ml. (1 pint approximately) of fluid is introduced at one time and siphoned back by lowering the funnel and inverting it over the bucket. This operation is repeated until the fluid returns clear. The patient needs constant reassurance as the treatment can be tedious. If time permits, this can be obviated by using smaller quantities of fluid and repeating the procedure at intervals over a 2–3-day period. In this way the patient experiences less distress. It is essential that the returned fluid is observed, measured, and recorded to ensure that excessive fluid retention by the patient has not occurred.

CHAPTER XXXI

URINE EXAMINATION, TESTS OF RENAL FUNCTION, AND MANAGEMENT OF SOME RENAL DISORDERS

By John G. G. Ledingham

EXAMINATION OF THE URINE

THE testing of a sample of urine for sugar, protein, ketones, spun deposit, and specific gravity is an essential part of the full examination of any patient, whatever the presenting symptoms. In addition, in hospital it is often of value to have a record of the patient's 24-hour urine volume from day to day, even although the figures are normally at best rough estimates. Other tests of renal function may be performed as indicated by the clinical findings.

URINE VOLUME

The volume of urine passed in 24 hours depends upon many factors, including:
1. Fluid and electrolyte balance.
2. Rates of fluid loss from lungs, skin, and bowel.
3. The presence or absence of sugar in the urine.
4. The rate of secretion of antidiuretic hormone.
5. The action of diuretic drugs.
6. The integrity of function of the heart, liver, and kidneys.

In health there is a diurnal variation in renal function with relative retention of water and solute by night. Normal adults excrete between 1 and 2 litres of urine per 24 hours, with an average of 1500 ml., of which 60–80 per cent is passed by day. The diurnal rhythm may be abolished or even reversed in œdematous states, chronic renal disease, malabsorption, adrenal insufficiency, and in some cases of head injury. It may be of value therefore to record day and night urine volumes separately.

Polyuria.—Consistent increases in 24-hour urine volumes above 3 litres constitute polyuria which is most commonly caused by psychological overdrinking, by the glycosuria of diabetes mellitus, or by chronic renal failure. Less common causes include diabetes insipidus, potassium depletion, hypercalcæmia, and acromegaly. Patients suffering from frequency of micturition may complain of passing excessive amounts of urine, and it is important to distinguish polyuria from frequency in such cases.

Nocturia may be defined as the passing of more than one-third of the 24-hour urine volume at night. This symptom must also be distinguished from nocturnal frequency, with which it is often confused.

Oliguria is traditionally defined as the production by an adult of less than 400 ml. urine per 24 hours. The causes of oliguria are discussed in a later section (*see* p. 430).

URINE COLOUR

The yellow colour of normal urine is derived largely from *urochrome*, a pigment of unknown origin. In health the depth of the colour is related to the rate of urine flow, and in part to the urine *p*H, more acid and concentrated specimens being deeper in colour.

Abnormal Coloured Urine may be seen in a number of conditions, most of which are rare and of little significance—but important colour changes may also be observed. The presence of excess *bilirubin* in the urine, as may occur in obstructive or hepatocellular jaundice, produces an orange-yellow colour which tends on standing to change to green-brown. *Hæmoglobin* in the urine following severe exercise, burns, prolonged exposure to cold, in severe hæmolytic anæmias or paroxysmal hæmoglobinuria, or after incompatible blood transfusion colours the urine a clear red, which becomes darker on standing. *Myoglobinuria* produces a similar colour change. Smoky-red urine is characteristically associated with the loss of unhæmolysed red cells from the kidney or lower urinary tract. The urine of patients taking *dindevan* (phenindione), if alkaline, is often coloured orange-red and this colour can be dispersed by the addition of acid.

In *porphyria* excessive amounts of porphyrins may be excreted, some of which turn urine a dark purple or port-wine colour. Porphobilinogen is itself a colourless compound, but it may, on breaking down in urine allowed to stand, give rise to products which are dark orange in colour.

In conditions in which large amounts of *urobilinogen* are present, urobilin may accumulate on standing, with resultant colour change to deep orange. The urine of patients with *alkaptonuria* on standing becomes black with the formation of homogentisic acid. In rare cases of widespread malignant melanoma *melanin* pigment may be excreted in the urine, colouring it a deep brown-black.

Clarity of Appearance.—Fresh samples of urine are not always clear. A visible cloudiness may be caused by mucus in both acid and alkaline urines. Amorphous phosphates or carbonates may form an opalescence in neutral or alkaline urine, but dissolve with the addition of acid.

In acid urines, especially if concentrated, urate deposits forming a white or pink cloud may be seen. These characteristically disappear on heating or with the addition of strong nitric acid.

The presence of phosphate, carbonate, or urate deposits is of no pathological significance. Large numbers of pus cells may also cause clouding, which in contrast to that of phosphate deposits does not disappear, but increases with the addition of acid.

URINE SPECIFIC GRAVITY

The concentration of solute in urine is usually and most simply assessed by measurement of urine specific gravity, using a hydrometer. This procedure estimates the total weight of the various particles in solution in the urine. There is usually good correlation between specific gravity and total solute concentration or osmolarity, and in most circumstances measurement of the former will give adequate clinical information. Osmolarity can be calculated from observation of the freezing-point of urine samples, but this determination requires costly apparatus and is little used outside specialized units.

Factors altering Specific Gravity.—In the presence of glycosuria the specific gravity of urine is high in relation to the solute concentration, and the same is true when urine contains the dyes used in intravenous pyelography. A low specific gravity in relation to osmolarity is observed when there are more than normal amounts of urea present. Protein in the urine has little effect upon specific gravity unless present in large amounts. If proteinuria is greater than

5 G. per litre, however, a correction may be made by subtracting 0·001 from the reading for every 5 G. per litre of protein present.

Readings of Urine Specific Gravity.—These should always be made at room temperature (15°–20° C.; 59°–68° F.). Considerable errors may be introduced if this rule is not observed, since for every 3° C. (5° F.) rise in temperature above 16° C. (60° F.) there will be a decrease of 0·001 in the hydrometer reading. Detergents should not be used in washing urine-testing vessels since, by alteration of surface tension, they may distort hydrometer readings.

The use of specific-gravity measurements in the assessment of renal function is discussed in a later section (*see* p. 425).

URINE REACTION

Individual samples of urine taken at random may be acid, neutral, or alkaline. Under exceptional circumstances the human kidney is able to excrete urine as acid as pH 4·5 or as alkaline as pH 8·0, but most random samples range between 5·3 and 7·5. Urine is most acid at night and in the early morning, but there are usually increases in pH in the mid-morning, early afternoon, and evening.

The recording of urine reaction is a traditional part of the routine ward test, but is usually of little or no value. In certain situations, however, it may be desirable to alter urine pH for therapeutic reasons, and in such it is important to ensure that the desired changes are achieved by night as well as by day.

Indications to Alkalinize the Urine.—

1. *Sulphonamide Therapy.*—The incidence of crystalluria has fallen recently with the introduction of sulphonamide mixtures (e.g., sulphatriad) and of more soluble individual compounds. Crystalluria can still occur in acid urines, however, and the solubilities of nearly all drugs of this group, particularly of sulphadiazine and its methylated derivatives sulphamerazine and sulphamethazine, are increased in alkaline urine. The risk of crystalluria can therefore be reduced by therapy with sufficient alkali (sodium or potassium bicarbonate or citrate 6–10 G. per day) to increase urine pH throughout the period of treatment to 7·5 or higher. Alkali therapy may, however, be contra-indicated (potassium salts are particularly dangerous in the presence of renal damage) and many prefer to rely upon a high fluid intake to reduce the risk of crystalluria.

2. *Streptomycin Therapy.*—When streptomycin is used in the treatment of urinary infections, the best results are obtained if the urine is kept alkaline. Antibacterial activity diminishes in direct proportion to urine acidity, and *in vitro* there is a twenty- to eighty-fold decrease in streptomycin bacteriostasis as the pH is reduced from 8·0 to 5·6. Sodium bicarbonate or citrate 6–10 G. daily may be necessary to maintain urine pH at the desirable level of 7·5 or higher.

3. *Gout.*—Renal deposition of urates may occur in chronic gout and in such circumstances, especially when uricosuric drugs (e.g., probenecid, anturan, aspirin, phenylbutazone) are used, it is important to maintain a high urine volume and to alkalinize the urine day and night to reduce the risk of further deposits.

4. *Cystinuria.*—In cystinuria excessive amounts of cystine (and of arginine, lysine, and ornithine) are excreted in urine. Cystine stones form easily in acid urine, and a high fluid intake and alkalinization of the urine may help to prevent continued nephrolithiasis in these patients. Alkali therapy in cystinuria remains an important aspect of management even since the successful introduction of treatment with penicillamine.

5. *Hæmoglobinuria.*—Alkalinization of the urine may help to prevent precipitation of hæmoglobin in the renal tubules.

6. *Urine Infection.*—The practice of rendering the urine alkaline in urinary-tract infections is of doubtful value, and may be dangerous if potassium salts are used in patients with severe impairment of renal function.

Indications to Acidify the Urine.—There is sound evidence that maintenance of an acid urine is of value in preventing urine infection in the presence of an indwelling catheter, and acid therapy may also be used in the prevention of recurrence of phosphatic calculi.

Oral ammonium chloride 2 G. t.d.s. is an effective drug, but patients are easily nauseated by this, and it should be particularly avoided in patients with advanced hepatic or renal disease.

URINE ACID EXCRETION

The renal tubules secrete hydrogen ions at a rate of about 40–80 mEq. per day. The secreted ions have three possible fates:—

1. The largest portion reacts with filtered bicarbonate to form carbon dioxide and water.

2. Some combine with monohydrogen phosphate and sulphate to form the dihydrogen salts (titratable acid).

3. Some combine with ammonia (NH_3) to form ammonium (NH_4).

Urinary pH is only a rough guide to the ability of the kidney to excrete acid. Measurement of total hydrogen-ion excretion can be made only when the titratable acid, ammonium, and bicarbonate content of the urine are known.

Failure of normal acid excretion occurs in rare renal tubular disorders (e.g., renal tubular acidosis, Fanconi syndrome) and in some cases of chronic renal disease. If one of these conditions is suspected, the maximal hydrogen-ion excretion may be tested in the following way:—

Maximum Acid Excretion Test.—Ammonium chloride, 0·1 G. per kg. body-weight, is given by mouth, and the urine is collected over the next 8 hours. Normal subjects produce urines of pH less than 5·3 and excrete hydrogen ion at rates exceeding 60 μEq. per minute, of which approximately equal amounts derive from ammonium and titratable acid. In *renal tubular acidosis* urine pH does not fall below 5·3, and hydrogen-ion excretion, of which most is ammonium, is less than 40 μEq. per minute. In *chronic renal disease* changes in urine pH and total urinary hydrogen ions after ammonium chloride are often less than normal, and excretion of ammonium is particularly reduced.

Measurement of pH.—Urine pH as tested by ordinary litmus paper has little value. More precise information can be gained by the use of BDH narrow-range indicator papers. Accurate measurements can only be made by the use of pH meters.

PROTEINURIA

Normal persons may excrete between 40 and 80 mg. of protein in the urine in 24 hours, and random samples contain 4–8 mg. per 100 ml. Proteinuria in excess of 150 mg. per 24 hours is abnormal, but does not always signify the presence of renal disease.

Benign Proteinuria.—

1. POSTURAL.—Three to five per cent of young adults, males more commonly than females, are found to have abnormal proteinuria when up and about, but not after a period of rest in bed. Standing in a position of exaggerated lordosis can induce significant proteinuria in a substantial proportion of young normal males, who do not otherwise show it. Postural proteinuria is usually small in

amount (less than 1 G. per day), but protein concentrations have been recorded as high as 1000 mg. per 100 ml. Proteinuria is not the only urinary abnormality that can be induced by lordotic posture—excessive numbers of red cells, white cells, and casts may also be excreted.

2. FUNCTIONAL.—Abnormal proteinuria may also be observed in patients without renal disease after severe exercise, in fever, in emotional stress, and after exposure to extremes of heat or cold. Patients with cardiac failure may also have proteinuria without structural renal disease. After severe exercise, proteinuria, cylinduria, and hæmaturia may persist for as long as 24 hours.

CAUSE AND SIGNIFICANCE OF BENIGN PROTEINURIA.—There is no generally accepted cause of this condition. Follow-up studies of patients originally diagnosed as having benign proteinuria have revealed that as many as 30 per cent ultimately develop persistent proteinuria.

Proteinuria in Renal Disease.—Persistent proteinuria, whether symptomatic or not, always indicates underlying renal disease, but is not incompatible with continued good health for many years. Protein loss is usually greater by day than by night, and is increased by erect posture, exercise, and fever.

HEAVY PROTEINURIA.—Excretion of more than 4 G. of protein per 24 hours in urine is usually associated with the nephrotic syndromes: for example in glomerulonephritis, 'lipoid nephrosis', intercapillary glomerulosclerosis, amyloidosis, systemic lupus erythematosus, or renal vein congestion (renal vein thrombosis, or constrictive pericarditis).

MODERATE PROTEINURIA (0·5–4 G.) may occur in any of the above conditions, but is commonly associated with chronic glomerulonephritis, nephrosclerosis, pyelonephritis, or polycystic kidneys.

Tests with Urinary Protein.—The concentration of protein in a random sample of urine depends upon the rate of urine flow. Minor degrees of proteinuria may be missed therefore if the tests are performed on dilute urine, and it is good practice to correlate the result of the test with the urine specific gravity. Critical tests should be performed only on concentrated urine samples.

QUALITATIVE TESTS.—Tests should be performed on clear urine. Filtering or centrifuging will usually remove turbidity.

1. *Boiling Test.*—This test is reliable and detects protein concentrations as low as 5–10 mg. per 100 ml.

About 5 ml. urine are poured into each of two test-tubes and one is then boiled. A cloud may appear in the boiled tube, which could be caused either by protein or by phosphates. A phosphate cloud is dispersed by addition to the boiled tube of a few drops of 5 per cent acetic acid.

2. *Salicylsulphonic Acid.*—Five ml. of urine are taken in each of two test-tubes, and to one is added a few drops of a saturated solution of salicylsulphonic acid. Clouding indicates protein or proteose: that due to proteose disappears on heating and reappears on cooling.

QUANTITATIVE TESTS.—

1. *Grading in Quantitative Tests.*—With experience and care, the degree of opalescence elicited by the heat test or by the salicylsulphonic acid test can be graded, and an estimate of the quantity of protein may be made as follows:—

Minimal cloud	Trace	5–10 mg. per 100 ml.
Light cloud	1 plus	100 mg. per 100 ml.
Heavy cloud	2 plus	300 mg. per 100 ml.
Light coagulum	3 plus	500 mg. per 100 ml.
Heavy coagulum	4 plus	1000 mg. per 100 ml. or more

2. *Esbach's Test.*—An aliquot of the 24-hour urine is acidified. Special test-tubes are provided with the Esbach albuminometer and these are filled with urine to the mark 'U' and Esbach reagent (a mixture of 10 G. per litre picric acid and 20 G. per litre citric acid) is added up to the mark 'R'. The contents are then mixed and allowed to stand vertical for 24 hours. The volume of the protein precipitated is then read off the scale on the tube, which is calibrated to give grammes of albumin per litre of urine.

This test is extremely inaccurate and probably gives no better results than the simpler test described above.

3. *Twenty-four-hour Urinary Protein.*—An estimate of the protein content of a 24-hour sample of urine can be made by comparing the turbidity produced by the addition of salicylsulphonic acid against a set of standards made from dilutions of gelatin in formalin. This method is probably the best quantitative one available, and should be used when the progress of renal disease, such as nephrotic syndrome, is being followed in response to therapy.

4. *Albustix.*—Paper sticks impregnated with dye indicators change colour in urines containing protein, and may be used in detecting or estimating the degree of proteinuria present. Interpretation of colour change can be difficult and this test is less accurate than the older methods.

Bence-Jones Protein.—The protein present in urine in most renal disease is 60–90 per cent albumin, most of the remainder being globulin. Abnormal low molecular weight globulins (Bence-Jones protein) may be excreted in multiple myeloma, in primary amyloidosis, in macroglobulinæmia, and rarely in chronic leukæmia, or other malignant diseases involving bone. These proteins coagulate between 45° and 55° C. (113° and 131° F.) and partially or totally redissolve at higher temperatures. They may therefore be detected by a simple boiling test in which a cloud appears and then fades as urine is heated to boiling-point in a test-tube. If there is albuminuria in addition to Bence-Jones proteinuria, the latter can be detected if albumin precipitated by boiling is first filtered off and the supernatant then heated to 45°–55° C. (113°–131° F.). Only 50–60 per cent of patients with myeloma excrete Bence-Jones protein.

GLYCOSURIA

The presence of glucose in the urine is easily detected and is most commonly caused by diabetes mellitus. Every patient with glycosuria, however, does not have diabetes mellitus. Glucose may reach the urine also in renal glycosuria (reduced renal threshold for glucose), in alimentary glycosuria (when blood-sugars above 180 mg. per 100 ml. may transiently follow large carbohydrate meals), and in the course of intravenous infusions with dextrose solutions. Transient glycosuria associated with hyperglycæmia may occur without indicating true diabetes in patients with cerebrovascular accidents, after myocardial infarcts, and rarely in hyperthyroidism.

Tests.—If *Benedict's solution* is used to test urine for glucose, other reducing substances (e.g., lactose, pentose, homogentisic acid, streptomycin, salicylates) may be detected and cause confusion. This problem can best be solved by abandoning the use of Benedict's solution and using, as a screening test for glucose, clinistix (impregnated paper sticks containing glucose oxidase) which turn blue in the presence of true glucose only. Clinistix detect only the presence or absence of glucose and the amount present can then be determined by the use of clinitest.

Albustix, Clinistix, Clinitest (Ames Company, Stoke Poges, Slough, Bucks).

Clinitest Reagent.—The tablets used are self-heating and dissolve rapidly. Five drops of urine and 10 drops of water are mixed in a test-tube, and one clinitest tablet is added. The solution boils rapidly and 15 seconds after boiling the colour present compared with the colour scale provided with the reagent will indicate the concentration of glucose present. Clinitest is no less accurate and is more convenient than the old tests for the presence of reducing substances in urine, and can now be recommended for routine use.

URINARY KETONES

In poorly controlled insulin-deficient diabetes and in conditions of deficient carbohydrate intake (e.g., prolonged vomiting, diarrhœa, or fasting) acetone, aceto-acetic acid, and β-hydroxybutyric acid may be excreted in urine. Pregnant women and young children with diabetes or with deficient intake of carbohydrate become ketotic particularly easily.

Tests for Ketonuria.—

1. *Ferric Chloride Test* (*Gerhardt's Test*).—Dilute ferric chloride is added to a test-tube of urine drop by drop until all ferric phosphate is precipitated. The precipitate, if heavy, is filtered and the supernatant is brown-red in the presence of considerable amounts of aceto-acetic acid. Salicylates also give a positive reaction, but prolonged boiling prior to the test will distinguish since aceto-acetic acid is volatile and is thus driven off.

The ferric chloride test is a relatively insensitive test for ketonuria.

2. *Rothera's Test.*—Enough ammonium sulphate crystals to fill a test-tube for half an inch are mixed with a pinch of powdered sodium nitroprusside. The tube is then half filled with urine and is thoroughly shaken. Then 3 ml. concentrated ammonia are added. In the presence of aceto-acetic acid or acetone, a purple colour develops.

Rothera's test is very sensitive and detects minimal degrees of ketonuria.

3. *Acetest.*—The acetest reagent tablets contain sodium nitroprusside, disodium phosphate, and amino-acetic acid. One drop of urine is placed on the tablet and the colour observed after 30 seconds, compared with the standard chart, indicates the presence and amount of ketone in the specimen.

Acetest tablets are now widely used. They are reliable and have largely replaced the Gerhardt and Rothera tests.

TESTS FOR BLOOD

The distinction between hæmaturia (red cells in urine) and hæmoglobinuria (pigment in the urine), both of which colour the urine pink, must be made by microscopic examination of the urine (*see* p. 419). Hæmaturia is easily detected by microscopy, but red cells are rapidly destroyed in alkaline or dilute urine, and it is of great importance to examine only fresh specimens. Mild degrees of hæmoglobinuria may result in doubtful colour changes in the urine, and in such a situation chemical tests for blood may be useful. The benzidine test is highly sensitive, but gives false positive results, and the guiac test is insensitive. The simplest confirmatory tests for the presence of hæmoglobin in urine is the use of occultest tablets, which contain orthotolidine, a substance which turns blue in the presence of hæmoglobin. Alternatively, spectroscopic examination of the urine (*Fig.* 288) can be undertaken in the laboratory.

Significance of Hæmaturia.—Blood intimately mixed with urine suggests loss of red cells from the kidney. Bladder lesions usually cause bleeding at the end of, and urethral lesions at the beginning of, micturition. Hæmaturia is always

---

Acetest (Ames Company, Stoke Poges, Slough, Bucks).

of pathological significance and the following may be mentioned as possible causes.

1. *Renal Parenchymal Diseases.*—Acute glomerulonephritis, focal glomerulonephritis, pyelonephritis, polycystic kidneys, nephrosclerosis, renal tuberculosis, systemic lupus erythematosus, polyarteritis nodosa, Henoch-Schönlein purpura, and hypernephroma.

2. *Renal-tract Disorders.*—Papillomata, carcinomata, renal calculi, sulphonamide crystalluria, cystitis, prostatic hypertrophy, stricture, angioma of renal pelvis, schistosomiasis, and trauma.

3. *Systemic Disorders.*—Bleeding diseases (e.g., leukæmia, thrombocytopenic purpura, scurvy, hæmophilia), subacute bacterial endocarditis, and anticoagulant therapy.

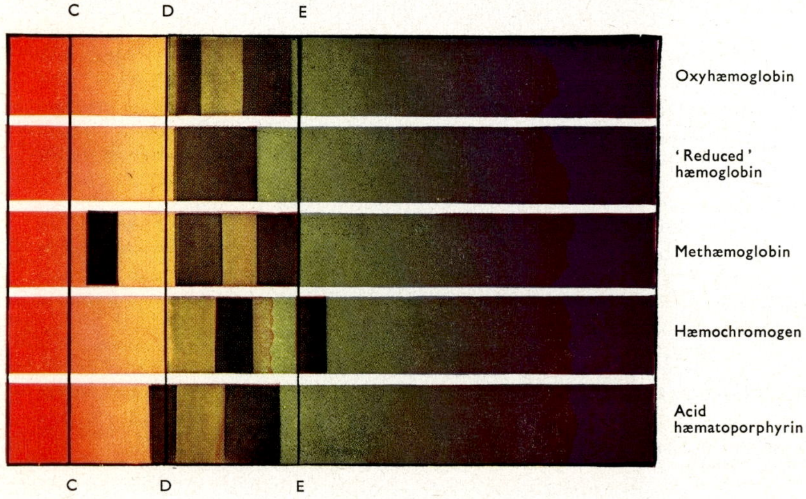

Fig. 288.—Spectra of hæmoglobin and hæmoglobin derivatives.

BILE PIGMENTS IN URINE

Bile pigments may appear in the urine in patients with obstructive or hepatocellular jaundice, but are not present in hæmolytic jaundice.

Fouchet's Test.—Five ml. of urine are mixed with 10 ml. of 10 per cent barium chloride. The precipitate, which contains bilirubin, is filtered off and to it are added 1–2 drops Fouchet's reagent (25 G. trichloracetic acid in 100 ml. water and 10 ml. 10 per cent aqueous ferric chloride). A green colour confirms the presence of bilirubin.

Urobilinogen.—The normal 24-hour excretion of urobilinogen in urine in healthy adults is said to be between 0·5 and 4 mg., but recent work has shown that the amount is dependent upon urine pH. Increased amounts of urobilinogen may be present in the urine in hepatocellular damage or in hæmolytic diseases. It is absent in obstructive jaundice if obstruction is complete, but may be present in excess in incomplete obstruction.

Ehrlich's Aldehyde Test for Urobilinogen.—Two drops of newly made Ehrlich's reagent (a 3 per cent solution of dimethyl aminobenzaldehyde in 50 per cent hydrochloric acid) are added to 5 ml. of fresh urine. A bright red colour, of depth dependent upon the amount of urobilinogen present, develops in 1 minute (or longer if the urine is cold).

A closely similar red pigment forms when urine containing porphobilinogen is mixed with the reagent. This pigment, in contrast to that formed by urobilinogen, is not soluble in chloroform.

Ehrlich's test can be roughly quantitated by preparing serial dilutions of urine for testing and expressing results in terms of the highest dilution giving the characteristic pink colour. In random specimens normal urines do not give a positive reaction at dilutions greater than 1 : 10.

ELECTROLYTES IN URINE

In the presence of healthy kidneys the urinary contents of sodium and chloride usually reflect the state of sodium balance, and therefore of extracellular fluid volume at the time. Urinary sodium and potassium can now be simply and rapidly measured with the flame photometer, and urinary chloride by titration with silver nitrate. If facilities for these measurements are not available, Fantus test for urinary chlorides may be useful to indicate the rate of urinary salt excretion.

Fantus Test.—Ten drops of urine and 1 drop of 20 per cent potassium chromate are placed in a test-tube, using clean glass-droppers. Silver nitrate, 2·9 per cent, is then added drop by drop until the indicator changes from yellow to red. The number of drops required is roughly equivalent to the number of grammes of chloride present per litre of urine.

URINE MICROSCOPY

Microscopic examination of fresh urine is probably the most useful single test of the overall health of the kidneys and renal tract. It is an investigation easily performed in ward side-rooms.

Microscopy.—A fresh, early-morning, clean specimen of urine should be taken and, ideally, 15 ml. is centrifuged for 5 minutes (at about 2000–3000 rev. per minute). The supernatant urine is decanted and 1 drop of the unstained sediment is then examined under the microscope. The sediment may contain the following elements:—

1. CELLS.—These may arise from the glomeruli, from the renal tubules, from the lining of the renal tract, and, in women, from the vulva or vagina.

a. Epithelial Cells.—These are normally present and are increased in amount in renal diseases, especially in the diuretic phase of acute tubular necrosis.

b. Red and White Cells.—These are present in relatively small numbers in health and are often increased in disease of the kidney or renal tract (*vide infra*). Only when they are incorporated into casts can it be certain that these cells arise from the kidney.

2. CASTS.—Casts are cylindrical structures formed from coagulated material in the distal nephron. Their width may be taken as evidence of their origin, the largest being derived from the collecting ducts. Casts are most easily formed in the presence of acid urine containing increased amounts of protein. Casts may contain red cells, white cells, epithelial cells, or a mixture of these elements.

Granular casts appear homogeneous and colourless with a coarse granular texture. Their origin is uncertain, but may be from degeneration of cellular casts.

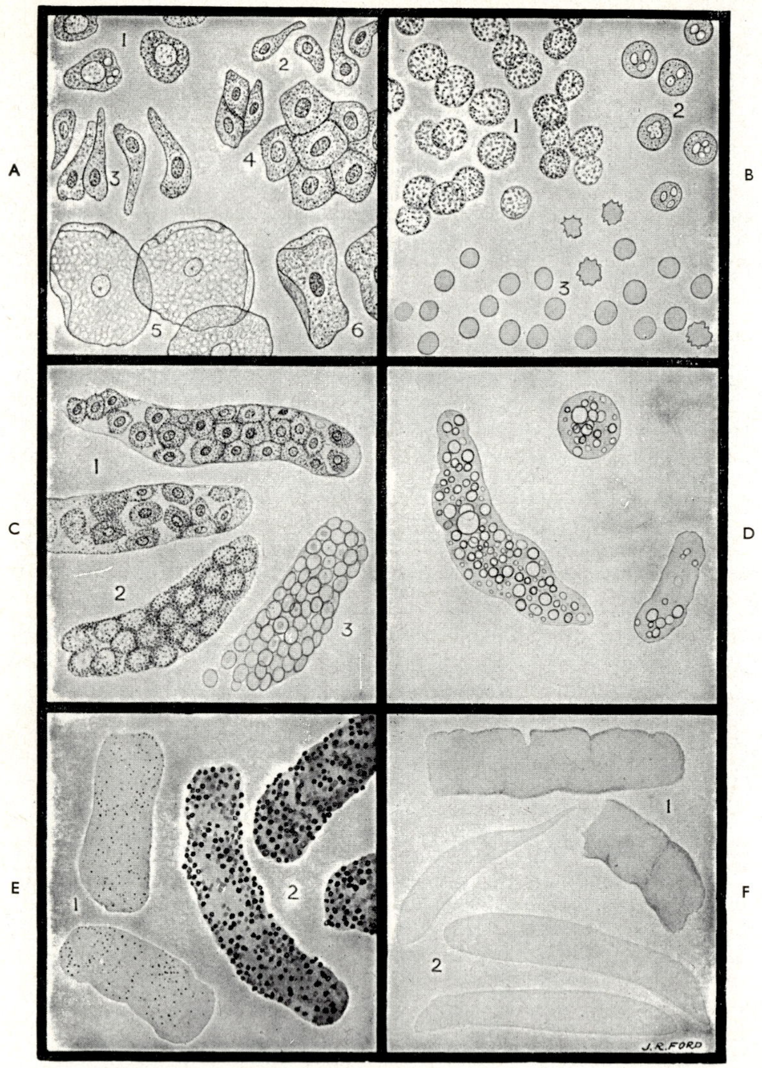

Fig. 289.—Microscopical characters of organized urinary deposits. A, Epithelium from: (1) Renal tubules; (2) Bladder (deep); (3) Renal pelvis; (4) Bladder (superficial); (5) Vagina; (6) Urethra. B, (1) Pus cells; (2) The same treated with acetic acid; (3) Red blood-corpuscles. C, Casts: (1) Epithelial; (2) Pus; (3) Blood. D, Casts, fatty. E, Casts: (1) Finely granular; (2) Coarsely granular. F, Casts: (1) Waxy; (2) Hyaline.

Fatty casts also have a granular appearance, but are seen to contain fat globules staining well with Sudan III. Waxy casts probably represent the ultimate in degeneration of cellular casts, while hyaline casts (clear colourless structures with a faint outline) are precipitates of protein. The appearances of the cells and casts which may be seen in urine sediment are illustrated in *Fig.* 289.

Significance of Cells and Casts.—Most normal urine sediments are found to contain one to two red cells and one to two white cells per high-power field. Granular and hyaline casts occur in normal urine and may be seen in one in every ten or so high-power fields. Increased numbers of any of these three elements may be found in the urines of normal persons after exercise, standing in a lordotic posture, or after periods of fever.

Red Cells.—The causes of hæmaturia are many (*see* p. 436), but red cell casts or casts stained brown with hæmoglobin indicate renal parenchymal damage, and may be seen in glomerulonephritis, lupus erythematosus, polyarteritis nodosa, tubular necrosis, Henoch-Schönlein purpura, or in renal trauma.

White Cells.—Increased numbers of white cells in the urine are also seen in many diseases, and the only way to be sure that pus cells come from the kidney and not from the lower urinary tract is to identify them in casts. Such casts are a valuable sign of pyelonephritis and may be seen in the absence of bacteriuria or pyuria. They are also seen occasionally in acute glomerulonephritis.

Casts.—Increased numbers of granular, hyaline, and epithelial casts may be seen in any renal parenchymal disease, but are found in most profusion, sometimes accompanied by fatty debris, in the nephrotic syndrome.

Quantitative Assessment of Urine Deposit.—The techniques of quantitative assessment depend upon accurate timing of collections for periods varying between 2 and 12 hours. An aliquot of the fresh sample is centrifuged, and the sediment resuspended in 0·5 ml. urine. One drop is transferred with a pipette to the standard counting chamber of the hæmocytometer. The total number of casts, red cells, and white cells may then be counted and the rate of excretion calculated. The errors of this procedure are obviously considerable, but it nevertheless has value in the diagnosis of minor degrees of abnormality, and serial examinations may provide information of the progress of renal disease. In recent years short-timed collections have been preferred to the overnight periods originally used, because, with time, casts and cells may degenerate and become unrecognizable.

Normal Rates of Excretion.—Up to 1 million red cells, 2 million white cells, and 10,000 casts may be excreted by a normal adult in 24 hours, but mean rates are considerably lower. A convenient short-period technique has been described in which 4-hour urine samples are analysed. Normal subjects are found to excrete both red and white cells at an average rate of 50,000 per hour, and not exceeding 400,000 per hour.

White-cell Excretion in Pyelonephritis.—The diagnosis of chronic pyelonephritis in life may be difficult, and urine microscopy, bacterial counts, and culture of the urine may give persistently normal results. In recent years a provocation test for the excretion of white cells in urine has been used.

Technique.—After a 2-hour or 4-hour control collection of urine, prednisolone 21-phosphate, 5 mg., is given intravenously. Urine is collected 1 and 2 hours after the injection. The control and test urine samples are examined and a quantitative estimate is made of the rate of white-cell excretion in each period. In normal persons the rate may rise after injection, but does not exceed 400,000 cells per hour. In most patients with chronic pyelonephritis this rate is exceeded.

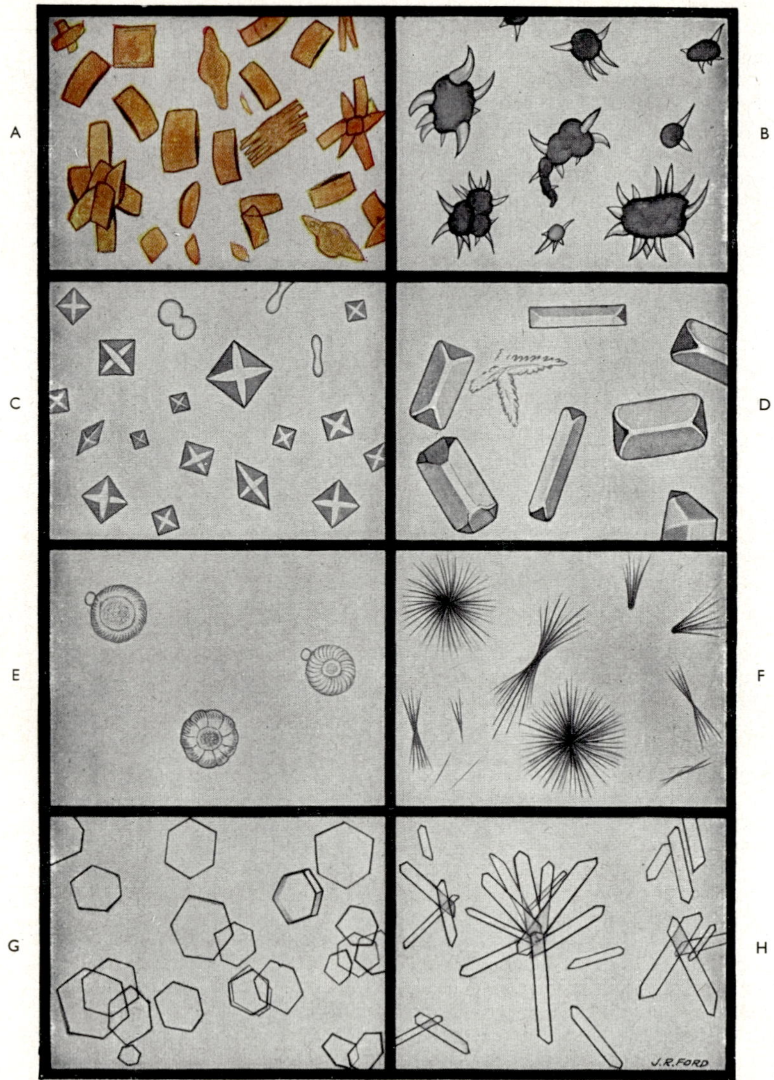

Fig. 290.—Microscopical characters of crystalline urinary deposits. A, Uric acid. B, Ammonium urate. C, Calcium oxalate. D, Ammonium-magnesium phosphate. E, Leucin. F, Tyrosin. G, Cystin. H, Stellar phosphates.

High rates may also occur in patients with acute glomerulonephritis. The cause of this strange phenomenon is unknown.

Unorganized Deposits in Urine Sediment.—Various crystalline and amorphous deposits may be found in the urine sediment (*Fig.* 290). Few are of any clinical importance and they will not be further discussed.

RENAL FUNCTION TESTS

The decision to carry out special tests of renal function, designed to confirm or exclude renal damage, must be based upon the clinical findings and upon the results of urine microscopy and the routine ward tests. The presence of protein-uria, of increased numbers of cells or casts in the urine, or evidence of impaired urine concentration demand further investigation whether or not there are symptoms of renal disease.

TESTS OF GLOMERULAR FILTRATION

In any progressive disease involving destruction of renal parenchyma there may be a decrease in the glomerular filtration rate (GFR) which can be used as one index of the degree of damage. Urea and creatinine of the endogenous waste products are excreted by the kidney at rates dependent in part upon the GFR. If the rates of formation of these substances were constant, their blood concentration would be dependent only on renal function. Unfortunately this is not the case. Urea is a product of protein catabolism and is synthesized by the liver. Its rate of formation is raised by a high-protein diet, by absorption of digested blood from gastro-intestinal hæmorrhage, by trauma, whether surgical or otherwise, and by conditions associated with increased tissue destruction (e.g., fever, diabetic ketosis, steroid therapy). Decreased rates of formation occur in starvation or in severe liver disease.

Creatinine derives from muscle creatine and in normal subjects its rate of excretion may be taken as an index of total body-muscle mass. Creatinine formation is independent of diet or of hepatic disease. Measurement of creatinine in blood may therefore provide a better index of renal function than does urea. It is technically difficult to measure creatinine, however, while measurement of urea is both simple and accurate, and, unless there is severe liver disease or a wide deviation from normal in protein intake, it is quite adequate to measure blood-urea.

Blood-urea.—In normal persons the concentration of urea in blood lies between 15 and 40 mg. per 100 ml. This concentration is not affected by moderate falls in the GFR and, with rates as low as 50 per cent of normal, blood-urea is only a little increased to 40–50 mg. per 100 ml. Further small reductions in the GFR are then associated with rapidly increasing urea retention. The finding of a small rise in blood-urea with other evidence of renal disease may be taken to indicate a loss of 50 per cent at least of functioning renal tissue. A normal blood-urea conversely cannot be taken as evidence of intact kidneys, and clearance studies or a concentration test must be used to reveal more minor damage.

Urea concentration is also dependent upon changes of volume in body-fluid compartments and considerable rises may occur in the absence of renal disease. Contractions of the extracellular fluid volume *per se* results in an increased blood-urea which may be further raised by functional impairment of the kidneys as the blood-pressure and GFR fall. Extracellular fluid volume is closely dependent upon sodium balance, and most cases of 'extrarenal' (contraction) uræmia are related to excessive losses of sodium from the gastro-intestinal tract or the kidneys.

Causes of a Raised Blood-urea.—

1. *Renal Disease.*—Any condition in which destruction of renal tissue occurs may be associated with retention of urea in the blood.

2. *Post-renal Causes.*—Obstruction of urethra or bladder, or bilateral ureteric obstruction from whatever cause.

3. *Extrarenal Fluid Losses.*—

a. *Gastro-intestinal*: Loss of electrolytes and fluid may be profound after prolonged vomiting, in intestinal obstruction, and with profuse diarrhœa.

b. *Renal*: Chronically damaged kidneys are unable to conserve sodium and, unless dietary intake is well maintained, renal and extrarenal uræmia may summate in their effects with dangerous or fatal results, especially if vomiting becomes a complicating factor. Sodium should therefore not be restricted in the diet of patients with chronic renal failure, unless the indication (e.g., cardiac failure resistant to digitalis therapy) is overwhelming.

Excessive losses of sodium from the kidneys may also occur in the diuretic phase of acute tubular necrosis, in diabetic pre-coma, in the course of prolonged diuretic therapy, and in adrenocortical insufficiency.

Serum Creatinine.—If dietary protein is normal and there is no serious liver-cell damage, estimations of serum creatinine are not of greater value than those of urea. Large changes in protein intake may have profound effects on blood-urea without a change in the GFR, however, and in selected patients blood-creatinine levels are of value. Normal serum creatinine concentrations lie between 0·4 and 1·2 mg. per cent per 100 ml., and increases occur, in parallel with increases in blood-urea, in renal, extrarenal, and post-renal uræmia.

CLEARANCE TESTS

The clearance of a substance is defined as the volume of plasma which would theoretically be completely cleared of the substance by its excretion in the urine in 1 minute. The concept is an artificial one and is simply one way of looking at the relation between the plasma concentration of the substance and its rate of excretion by the kidney.

In order to determine the clearance of substance X it is necessary to know accurately the rate of urine flow in ml. per minute and the concentration of X in both urine and plasma. The clearance is then given by:

$$\text{Clearance of X (ml. per min.)} = \frac{\text{Amount of X excreted in the urine in mg./1 min.}}{\text{Plasma X in mg./ml.}}$$

As discussed above, urea or endogenous creatinine clearance determinations may be useful in assessing degrees of renal damage, when because the glomerular filtration rate is more than 50 per cent of normal, blood-urea or creatinine concentrations remain normal. Clearances of inulin and PAH for accurate determination of rates of glomerular filtration and renal blood-flow will not be discussed here. *In neither urea nor creatinine clearance studies is it necessary or desirable to catheterize the patient.*

Endogenous Creatinine Clearance.—The clearance of endogenous creatinine correlates better with glomerular filtration rate, measured by inulin clearance, than does urea clearance. A disadvantage is that techniques for measuring plasma creatinine tend also to measure non-creatinine chromogens; this source of error is offset, however, by the small amount of creatinine normally secreted by the renal tubules. Considerable errors may result from inaccurate timing of urine collections or from incomplete bladder emptying in any clearance study over a short period. These errors may be minimized by using a 24-hour period of collection and taking one blood sample in the day, since plasma concentrations of creatinine do not fluctuate greatly in 24 hours.

Normal Results.—Endogenous creatinine clearances range from 95 to 140 ml. per minute in males and from 85 to 125 in females.

Urea Clearance.—Urea clearance is still widely used in the assessment of minor degrees of renal damage. The source of error in this technique is that the fraction of filtered urea diffusing back from the tubular fluid is inversely proportional to the rate of urine flow. However, at rates of flow exceeding 2 ml. per minute, urea clearance remains nearly constant. Short periods of collection (20–60 minutes) in fasting hydrated patients are normally used because blood-urea concentrations may rise after food. One blood sample is taken in the middle of each period.

Normal Clearances are 60–75 ml. per minute in males and 50–60 in females.

If rates of urine flow do not exceed 2 ml. per minute, the clearance can still be calculated, using a correction factor. The normal clearance may be calculated from the expression UV/P (where U is urine-urea in mg. per ml., V is urine volume in ml. per minute, and P is plasma urea in mg. per ml.). Corrected clearance $= U\sqrt{(V)}/P$.

CONCENTRATION AND DILUTION TESTS

Tests of the kidney's ability to concentrate or dilute urine are useful in detecting relatively small deteriorations in renal function. Reduced concentrating capacity may be found before there is a measurable fall in the GFR, and certainly before proteinuria or elevations of blood-urea or creatinine are observed. At rates of filtration between normal and 25 per cent of normal there is a progressive impairment of concentrating and diluting function, so that at about 25 per cent of normal GFR, urine specific gravity is fixed at 1·010 (isosthenuria). Subsequent deterioration of renal function cannot be further reflected by concentration tests. Only in patients with normal or near normal blood-ureas therefore is the concentration test of value. This test should never be performed in patients with more serious degrees of renal failure, not only because it gives no useful information, but also because fluid restriction (or loading) may be dangerous in such patients.

Concentration Test.—If random early-morning specimens of urine have a specific gravity of 1·023 or more, there is no need to perform the test.

Technique.—Maximal concentration in subjects of average hydration studied in temperate climates is not achieved for 30 hours, but 90 per cent maximal values are observed after 20 hours of fluid restriction. In any serious attempt to assess renal powers of concentration therefore, 20 hours or more of fluid deprivation may be necessary. It is convenient to start the test at 12 noon and continue it until 8 a.m. the following day.

As an alternative procedure, fluid restriction can be avoided if an intramuscular injection of pitressin in oil, 5 units, is given. All specimens of urine passed over the succeeding 24 hours are tested for specific gravity. The pitressin test is less unpleasant for the patients and gives reliable results, but pitressin must be avoided in patients with a history of ischæmic heart disease.

Interpretation.—In interpreting the results of a concentration test there are one or two points of importance to be considered:—

1. At high rates of solute excretion, intact kidneys cannot concentrate urine normally.

2. In patients accustomed to a high fluid intake there may be gross defects in urine concentrating powers for several days of water restriction, before normal function is restored.

3. Non-renal diseases may impair urinary concentration—e.g., diabetes insipidus, compulsive water drinking, potassium deficiency, hypercalcæmia.

Normal patients up to the age of 65 years should be able to concentrate urine to 1·026 or more. Even at the age of 90 a concentration of 1·023 should be attainable.

Dilution Test.—Although part of the dilution of urine occurs in the distal nephron at sites not directly involved in the concentration processes, concentration and dilution functions are usually jointly involved in renal disease. Therefore little can be gained in theory from the use of a dilution test and, since emotion, nausea, and fear may inhibit water diuresis in normal subjects, the results of the test are often unreliable.

Procedure.—One litre of fluid (or 20 ml. per kg. body-weight) is given by mouth over a 30-minute period in the morning. One of the hourly urine samples collected over the next 3 hours should have a specific gravity of 1·003 or less.

Interpretation.—Non-renal diseases may impair urinary dilution—e.g., cardiac failure, cirrhosis of the liver, adrenal insufficiency, steatorrhœa.

PHENOLSULPHONPHTHALEIN (PSP) EXCRETION

Phenolsulphonphthalein is both filtered at the glomerulus and secreted by the renal tubules. Only if the transport mechanisms in the tubules are grossly damaged in the presence of a normal renal blood-flow (a situation which must be extremely rare) does PSP excretion (at the blood concentrations used) measure tubular secretory function. Rather does it measure rate of delivery of PSP to the tubules in the renal circulation—that is, renal blood-flow.

The test, if critically used, may be helpful in detecting early renal disease before there is a change in the clearance of urea or creatinine. It is always abnormal in the presence of urea retention.

Technique.—The test depends upon accuracy in the collection of urine samples and is not suitable for study of patients unable to empty their bladders normally.

The patient drinks 200–300 ml. of water and is instructed to drink further similar amounts at ½-hourly intervals for 2 hours to ensure an adequate urine flow. PSP, 6 mg., is given intravenously 30 minutes after the first water load, and the bladder is emptied 15, 30, 60, and 120 minutes later. An aliquot of each sample is then alkalinized with 25 per cent NaOH. The depth of the red colour formed is compared with standard solutions of PSP by eye or using a colorimeter. The amount of dye in the urine can then be calculated.

Interpretation.—The 15-minute sample is the most important in detecting mild degrees of renal damage. Normally about 35 per cent (30–50 per cent) of the injected dose is excreted in the first 15 minutes, and a further 20 per cent in the succeeding 15 minutes. At 2 hours 70 per cent of the dose has been excreted unless renal damage is gross. (The 2-hour figure may be normal in patients who have lost about 50 per cent of their functioning renal tissue.)

INTRAVENOUS PYELOGRAPHY AS A TEST OF RENAL FUNCTION

The contrast media used in intravenous pyelography are iodine-containing compounds (opaque to X-rays), which are both filtered by the glomeruli and secreted by the renal tubules. The concentration of medium in the glomerular filtrate is the same as that in blood, but the reabsorption of water and the secretion of medium by the tubules results in a concentration increase of more than a hundredfold by the time the renal pelvis is reached. At this stage in fluid-deprived normal subjects given conventional doses, the contrast is easily detectable on radiographs, and the position, shape, size, and symmetry of the kidneys and renal tract can be seen (*see* p. 714).

While the main use of an intravenous pyelogram is to demonstrate renal and renal-tract anatomy, the appearance of normal amounts of contrast medium in the 5-minute radiograph may be taken as evidence that there is no major disturbance of renal function. On the other hand, poor pictures, or even absence of contrast, is not always indicative of renal damage.

RENAL BIOPSY

Percutaneous biopsy of the kidneys has been practised since 1954, but the technique is not easy and may be hazardous in inexperienced hands. The objects of biopsying a kidney are first to obtain a diagnosis and prognosis, and second to assess accurately the results of treatment in the nephrotic syndrome. The main danger is of hæmorrhage resulting from trauma to the kidney.

Contra-indications to the procedure are:—

1. The presence of only one kidney.
2. A bleeding tendency.
3. Malignant hypertension.
4. Renal tuberculosis.
5. Renal carcinoma.

It is also undesirable to attempt biopsy in patients unable to co-operate with the procedure.

Indications.—The principal indications for biopsy are:—

1. In the diagnosis of the type and degree of disease in the nephrotic syndrome, and in following the response to therapy.

2. To make the diagnosis and assess prognosis in patients with acute renal failure of unknown origin.

Technique.—Routine checks of bleeding and clotting times, platelet counts, and prothrombin times must be performed, and the biopsy abandoned unless these are normal. It is wise also to group and cross-match 2 pints (1000 ml.) of blood. An intravenous pyelogram is taken to confirm the presence of two functioning kidneys, and special radiographs are taken (with the patient prone) on full inspiration and expiration to determine the position and movement of the kidneys.

For the biopsy itself the patient lies prone on a firm table with a small sandbag under the abdomen. The positions of the iliac crests, spinal processes, the 12th rib, and the lateral edge of the sacrospinalis muscle are marked out with a skin-marking pencil. From these landmarks and the special pyelograms, the point lying over the outer aspect of the lower pole of the kidney to be biopsied can be found (*Fig.* 291). Local anæsthetic is injected and an 8-in. (20-cm.) long fine exploring needle (*Fig.* 292 B) is inserted vertically through the selected point and is pushed towards the kidney in small increments while the patient holds his breath. After each increment any movement of the needle with respiration is observed. A characteristic swing of the needle is seen when the kidney has been pierced. The depth of the organ beneath the skin is then known, and the same exploring procedure is repeated with the biopsy needle (usually a long

17

Vim-Silverman needle with Franklin modification, *Fig.* 292 A) and the biopsy is taken while the patient holds his breath. The use of the needle is not easy and requires practice.

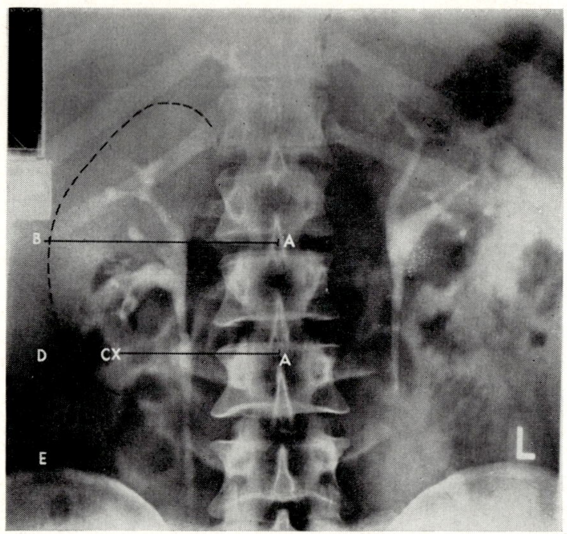

Fig. 291.—Location of kidney for biopsy. The iliac crest, the spines of the vertebrae, and the 12th rib are palpated in the patient and marked out with a skin pencil. The distance of the lateral border of the kidney from the midline (A–B) and of the point selected for puncture from the midline (A–CX) or from the lateral border of the kidney (D–CX) can be measured on the radiograph. D–E represents the distance of the lower pole of the kidney from the iliac crest. From these measurements a point on the skin can be selected which approximately overlies the lower pole of the kidney. Through this point the kidney is located by vertical introduction of the guide needle.

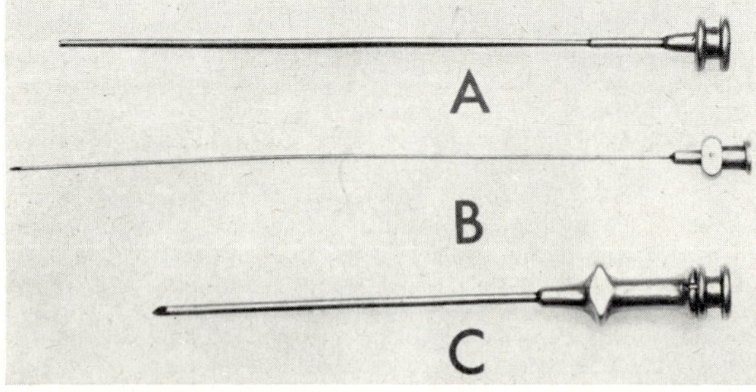

Fig. 292.—Vim-Silverman biopsy needle. A, The special insert with divided prongs designed to grip a plug of tissue within the lumen. B, The fine guide needle used to locate the kidney. C, The needle cannula with obturator in place.

After the biopsy, microscopic hæmaturia is invariable, and macroscopic is not uncommon. The patient should be kept in bed for 24 hours and pulse-rate and blood-pressure should be checked 2- or 4-hourly.

MANAGEMENT OF SOME RENAL DISORDERS
1. ACUTE URINARY TRACT INFECTIONS

Infections of the urinary tract may be confined to the bladder and urethra, or may involve the interstitial tissues of the kidneys (pyelonephritis). Urinary infections are common, particularly in women, and occur with increasing frequency with advancing years in both sexes. There are a number of predisposing factors of which obstructive lesions are the most important. Patients who have been catheterized are at risk and with indwelling catheters infection is inevitable. Approximately 2 per cent of women develop urinary infections in the last half of pregnancy or early in the puerperium (p. 437).

Causative Organisms.—Most infections arising outside hospital are caused by coliform organisms, but *Bacillus proteus*, *Pseudomonas pyocyaneus*, staphylococci, and fæcal streptococci may be more common causes in patients in wards, in those who have been treated previously by antibiotics, or who have obstructive lesions of the urinary tract.

Asymptomatic Bacteriuria.—Excretion of urine containing more than 100,000 bacteria per ml., without increase in pus cells, in patients who have no symptoms or other signs of infection, has been termed 'asymptomatic bacteriuria'. It occurs quite commonly in hospital in-patients and some have doubted its significance. Most authorities believe, however, that bacteriuria is a valuable sign of renal infection and that it should be treated as such.

Infections of the Lower Urinary Tract.—*Cystitis* is usually a mild disorder with little systemic disturbance and fever, if present, is small (38°–39° C.; 99°–101° F.). The diagnosis is easily made in most cases on clinical grounds—marked frequency and dysuria, sometimes strangury and hæmaturia—and can be confirmed by the detection of increased numbers of pus cells and bacteria in freshly voided clean specimens of urine. Sometimes, particularly in the very old, the only symptoms may be enuresis or incontinence associated commonly with a deterioration in mental function. A mid-stream specimen of urine is sent for examination and determination of bacterial sensitivities.

A course of the appropriate antibiotic together with a high fluid intake will usually clear up the infection within a few days. In women there is rarely any indication to investigate matters further, unless the disease persists or recurs frequently. In men, however, proven urinary infections without obvious cause demand investigation of the renal tract with pyelography.

Acute Pyelonephritis.—Acute pyelonephritis is characterized by a sudden onset of fever (39°–40° C.; 102°–104° F.), often with rigors, associated with headache, vomiting, and malaise, and usually, but not always, with loin pain and tenderness, dysuria, and frequency. Typical cases are easily recognized and the diagnosis can be confirmed by the presence of a polymorph leucocytosis in the blood, and large numbers of pus cells and organisms in a clean specimen of urine. In some patients atypical pains may cause difficulty, and fever and dysuria do not always occur. The urine may even be free of pus cells and organisms for short periods early in the disease, but repeated urine examinations will ultimately reveal the diagnosis.

Even without treatment acute pyelonephritis may clear up spontaneously, but bacteriuria often persists and relapses are common.

DIAGNOSIS AND TREATMENT OF ACUTE RENAL INFECTION

Confirmation of the clinical diagnosis depends upon the demonstration of excessive numbers of organisms and pus cells in the urine. Urine culture is desirable in planning treatment.

Bacterial Counts.—Bacilli found as contaminants in properly taken clean specimens of urine are usually only present in small numbers. In true infections the organisms may amount to hundreds of thousands per ml. of urine. Quantitative bacterial counts are therefore of great value in diagnosis. The simplest test is performed on freshly obtained uncentrifuged urine. A smear is made on a glass slide with a wire loop and is stained with methylene blue. If bacteria are easily seen there are probably more than 100,000 bacteria per ml. of urine, and infection can be diagnosed. In a more accurate test the number of colonies obtained from streaking one loopful of uncentrifuged urine on an agar plate is counted. If 100 or more colonies develop, infection is confirmed.

White-cell Excretion.—This subject has already been considered (*see* p. 421).

Treatment.—Sulphonamide drugs (*see* p. 72) are often given before the results of urine culture are available—usually with good results, even if the organisms cultured are found *in vitro* to be insensitive to these drugs. Other commonly effective antibiotics include tetracycline, ampicillin, nitrofurantoin (furadantin), and cephaloridine. The choice of which to use is dependent upon the organism isolated and its sensitivities. Antibiotics, when given, should be continued for several days after the results of urine examination have returned to normal. Resistant patients, or those in whom repeated attacks occur, may do well on courses of rotating antibiotics, with 7–10 days on each drug, e.g., sulphadimidine, furadantin, and ampicillin.

2. ACUTE RENAL INSUFFICIENCY

Whatever its cause, the first clinical sign of impairment of acute renal function is a substantial reduction in urine volume. In patients at risk from renal failure therefore, whether or not known to have preceding renal disease, it is of the utmost importance to keep accurate *input–output fluid charts* and, if possible, records of *daily weights*. Urine volumes below 400 ml. per 24 hours constitute oliguria and the term 'anuria' should be restricted to conditions in which urine secretion is reduced to a few ml. a day or to nil.

Causes of Acute Renal Failure.—There are many causes of this syndrome which may be classified as follows:—

1. Circulatory Causes.—

a. Extrarenal Uræmia.—The causes of this condition have already been discussed (*see* p. 423). Normal renal function is restored by prompt infusion of plasma-expanding fluids (*see* pp. 30 and 43).

b. Tubular Necrosis.—If renal vascular shutdown occurs, as a result of shock or hypotension for some hours, or if renal poisons (e.g., carbon tetrachloride, di-ethylene glycol, potassium chlorate) have been ingested, structural damage of tubule cells may occur. Probably because of deficient renal cortical blood flow there is an increased risk of renal structural damage in patients with impaired hepatic function (hepatorenal syndrome).

The causes of acute tubular necrosis are similar to those of extrarenal uræmia, but the condition is particularly common after abortion, concealed accidental hæmorrhage, crush injuries, or major surgery associated with unreplaced blood-losses and hypotension.

Oliguria is usual in this condition and complete anuria suggests the possibility of a complicating post-renal obstructive lesion. Urine specific gravity in acu·e tubular necrosis is near or at 1·010.

The prognosis in cases of acute tubular necrosis, given good conservative management and, if necessary, dialysis, depends upon the underlying cause. In the presence of widespread traumatic tissue damage (whether due to accident or major surgery), mortality is about 50 per cent. On the other hand, in most medical or obstetric cases, 80 per cent of patients may be expected to recover.

c. Cortical Necrosis of the Kidney.—If hypotension and shock are sufficiently prolonged, the damage to the tubules may be irrecoverable and total necrosis of the renal cortex ensues. This condition, which is invariably fatal, is fortunately rare. The commonest causes are abortion and concealed accidental hæmorrhage.

2. OBSTRUCTIVE CAUSES.—Obstruction of the lower (post-renal) urinary tract is an obvious cause of acute renal failure which is sometimes overlooked with serious or fatal consequences. In the presence of obstruction anuria rather than oliguria is the rule and, if acute renal failure develops, obstructive causes should be immediately excluded by cystoscopy and retrograde catheterization of the ureters. If the obstruction is not immediately remediable, nephrostomy may be life-saving.

3. CAUSES DUE TO PRIMARY RENAL DISEASE.—These causes include acute glomerulonephritis, acute necrotizing papillitis, malignant hypertension, poly-arteritis nodosa, eclampsia of pregnancy, systemic sclerosis, and leptospirosis. Oliguria rather than anuria is the rule, but anuria may be seen in acute glomerulonephritis. When urine is passed, the specific gravity is likely to be at or near 1·010.

1. Management of Extrarenal Cases.—Prevention is better than a cure, and adequate electrolyte and fluid, or blood, replacement in most of the conditions liable to cause circulatory renal damage will prevent tubular necrosis. Recently evidence has accumulated that the intravenous infusion of 200–500 ml. of 10 or 20 per cent mannitol may have a favourable effect in preventing tubular necrosis in patients at risk. Difficulties arise when pre-existing renal disease is compli-cated by extrarenal uræmia, or when it is not certain whether or not true renal damage has been caused. Nice judgement is required in these cases to steer between the Scylla of over-enthusiastic salt and water replacement with resultant water intoxication or œdema, and the Charybdis of under replace-ment of requirements with resultant continued inadequate renal perfusion. In judging deficits of fluid and electrolytes, it is obviously ideal to know the volume and electrolyte composition of the fluids, the loss of which have caused the problem. Such information is rarely available for the period preceding renal failure, but should always be followed in the period following establishment of the diagnosis.

The amount of salt and water best replaced depends upon the availability of dialysis facilities. If these are readily available, then overloading with saline in an attempt to treat the extrarenal factor adequately is a more pardonable offence than under-infusing, since in the former situation the excess can be dialysed out, while in the latter further renal damage, perhaps impairing the ultimate prog-nosis, may result. If there are no available dialysis facilities, under-replacement is preferable.

2. Management of Acute Renal Failure.—If extrarenal factors have been treated, post-renal obstruction excluded, and oliguria persists, the problem becomes one of management of a patient with acute and potentially recoverable renal damage. The treatment indicated is the same whether the cause is acute tubular necrosis (as it most commonly is) or some other form of acute damage.

OLIGURIC PHASE.—During this phase the patient may pass 50–400 ml. of urine per 24 hours. Following the suppression of urine, urea, creatinine, potassium, phosphate, sulphate, unidentified anions, and hydrogen ions accumulate in the blood. Acidosis, with a fall in serum bicarbonate, hyperkalæmia, and hyper-phosphatæmia with hypocalcæmia result. Anæmia, due to bone-marrow depres-sion, and leucocytosis are common.

There is unusual susceptibility to infection which remains the commonest cause of death in these patients. The most harmful of the changes is as follows:—

Hyperkalæmia.—The toxic effects of high concentrations of serum potas-sium on the heart are potentiated by hypocalcæmia and death from cardiac arrest becomes increasingly likely as the serum potassium rises above 7 mEq./l. The rate of rise of serum potassium, even with ideal treatment, is related to the rate of protein catabolism. It is highest in surgical and traumatic cases, especially if there is infection. Blood transfusion is hazardous because stored blood contains high concentrations of potassium.

Estimations of the serum potassium are of course indispensable, but are not always a sure guide to the imminence of cardiac abnormalities. Electrocardio-grams should be taken in patients with serum concentrations higher than 6·5 mEq./l., especially if there is clinical evidence of arrhythmia. The signs of hyperkalæmia on the ECG are peaked T waves, ST segment depression, broadening of the QRS, and flattening of P waves. (*See Fig*. 17 D, p. 34.)

Treatment: Total exclusion of potassium from the diet is essential; with a rising serum concentration, ion exchange resins may be used (e.g., katonium 'A', 15 G. t.d.s.), but take 24–72 hours to act. Emergency treatments of value are:—

i. Intravenous injection of 10 per cent calcium gluconate, 10–30 ml., to antagonize the cardiotoxic effects of hyperkalæmia.

ii. Injection of 100–200 ml. of 50 per cent dextrose intravenously with soluble insulin, 20–30 units.

iii. Infusion of molar sodium lactate, 200 ml. over 2–3 hours.

The latter two manœuvres both facilitate entry of potassium into the cells.

These emergency treatments are of short-term value and should be used only to tide patients over a dangerous few hours while they are transferred to a dialysis unit.

MANAGEMENT OF THE OLIGURIC PHASE.—

1. The patient should be weighed accurately in the same clothes every 12–24 hours. Excessive or inadequate fluid replacement is then easily detected. The patient should be allowed to lose weight at the rate of 0·25–0·5 kg. daily (this is the inevitable endogenous tissue weight-loss).

2. Water intake should be limited to about 500 ml. per 24 hours, with addi-tional amounts equal to the amount of urine passed in the preceding 24 hours. These figures should not be adhered to slavishly without consideration of the daily weight changes. The amounts of fluid required depend considerably upon variations in rates of loss from lungs and skin.

3. In the oliguric phase no electrolytes should be given.

4. Protein foods must be avoided and 100–200 G. carbohydrate are given, with the water allowance, either as an intravenous infusion, if vomiting is a problem, or orally. Many patients tolerate oral lactose better than oral glucose.

Katonium (Bayer Products Co., Surbiton-upon-Thames, Surrey).

5. Anabolic steroids (durabolin, adroyd, or nilevar) are sometimes given in an attempt to reduce endogenous protein catabolism. They are of doubtful value.

6. Nausea is often prominent and vomiting upsets electrolyte balance. Both should be prevented if possible by the use of phenothiazine drugs, e.g., chlorpromazine 25–50 mg. t.d.s.

7. Control of infection is extremely important. Patients should be barrier-nursed. Prophylactic antibiotics are of no proven value and may favour the growth of resistant organisms, but appropriate chemotherapy must be prescribed early and in full doses as soon as infection is detected.

8. Dialysis—*see below*.

9. The uses of steroids or agents to induce diarrhœa or vomiting as have been advocated in the past are actively dangerous. Bladder catheters should be avoided whenever possible.

Indications for Dialysis.—These include:—

1. A blood-urea of over 400 mg. per cent per 100 ml.
2. A rise in serum potassium above 7·0 mEq./l.
3. ECG changes of potassium intoxication.
4. A fall in serum bicarbonate below 12 mEq./l.
5. Uræmic coma or deterioration in general condition.

It should be remembered that in the presence of fever or trauma, dialysis should be given earlier rather than later.

MANAGEMENT OF THE DIURETIC PHASE.—When urine flow is re-established, excretion of fluid and electrolytes usually increases gradually. If losses of urine exceed 3 litres per day, as they may, it is important to measure the urine sodium content and to replace loss of salt as well as of water. Potassium losses should not be replaced until the serum concentration falls below normal.

PERITONEAL DIALYSIS

In recent years there has been a revival of interest in the technique of peritoneal dialysis. Solutions introduced into the abdomen equilibrate with body fluids across the semipermeable peritoneal membrane along osmotic, concentration, and electrochemical gradients. Sterile solutions of appropriate composition can therefore be used to adjust towards normal disturbances in the concentrations of dialysable substance in body fluids.

Indications.—Peritoneal dialysis is a simple procedure of value in the treatment of the following conditions:—

1. *Acute Renal Failure.*—An acceptable alternative to hæmodialysis while recovery of renal function is awaited.

2. *Chronic Renal Failure.*—In selected patients, especially those in whom there has been an acute potentially reversible deterioration, or those with totally inadequate function who are awaiting definitive treatment by renal transplantation.

3. Rare cases of *intractable cardiac failure*, in whom œdema is not responsive to full doses of potent diuretics.

4. As an alternative (less effective) to hæmodialysis in the treatment of severe *poisoning* by dialysable drugs, e.g., salicylates, barbiturates, glutethemide (doriden), and phenothiazine derivatives.

Technique.—Peritoneal dialysis is best carried out in a side ward. Strict aseptic techniques are mandatory.

Durabolin (Organon Laboratories Ltd., Staines Road, Morden, Surrey).
Adroyd (Parke, Davis & Co., Hounslow, Middlesex).
Nilevar (G. D. Searle & Co. Ltd., High Wycombe, Bucks, and Chicago, 80, Illinois, U.S.A.).
Doriden (Ciba Laboratories Ltd., Horsham, Sussex).

Apparatus.—

Sterile Pack Requirements.—Trocar and obturator size 17F for paracentesis; scalpel blade (Bard Parker No. 11); syringes; needles; forceps; needle holder; scissors; silk sutures; sterile towels

Drugs.—Heparin 5000 units per ml., 5 ml.; local anæsthetic, 20 ml.

*Disposable Equipment.**—

1. Plastic peritoneal catheter—about 30 cm. long, curved at the tip, with multiple small perforations in the terminal 8 cm.

2. Plastic tubing: Y-shaped to connect two 1-litre bottles of dialysing fluid with the peritoneal catheter; side-arm to connect the system with a 2-litre drainage bottle.

Dialysis Fluid.—Manufacturers supply dialysis fluid of the composition shown in *Table XII.* Two different osmolar strengths are available, depending on the concentration of dextrose included, one at 372 mOsmols per litre (1·5 per cent dextrose) and one at 677 mOsmols per litre (7 per cent dextrose). The stronger solution may be used alone, or more commonly mixed with the weaker, in those patients in whom there is overhydration or œdema. Neither solution contains any potassium, which must therefore be added in physiological concentrations when dialysis is performed on patients with near normal, normal, or low concentrations of serum potassium. Some 30–50 litres of fluid are required for a single dialysis.

Table XII.—DIALYSIS FLUID COMPOSITION

	1. 372 *mOsmols/l.*	2. 677 *mOsmols/l.*
Sodium	140 mEq./l.	140 mEq./l.
Calcium	3·6 mEq./l.	3·6 mEq./l.
Magnesium	1·5 mEq./l.	1·5 mEq./l.
Chloride	100 mEq./l.	100 mEq./l.
Lactate	45 mEq./l.	45 mEq./l.
Dextrose	15 G./l.	70 G./l.

Procedure.—A *premedication* of pethidine 100 mg. or phenergan 50 mg. may be given ½–1 hour before dialysis. Some patients experience abdominal pain with 1·5 per cent dextrose and nearly all do so with the very hypertonic 7 per cent solution. This pain is best controlled with pethidine 50–100 mg., or by the addition of 10 ml. of 0·5 per cent procaine to each 2 litres of dialysis fluid.

Insertion of Catheter.—A good site for insertion is in the midline, one-third of the distance down from the umbilicus to the symphysis pubis. The bladder must be emptied in those patients producing urine. The skin and subcutaneous tissues are infiltrated with local anæsthetic and a stab-wound is made with the scalpel. The trocar, with obturator in place, is pushed vertically into the peritoneal cavity. This step is most easily achieved when the muscles of the abdominal wall are contracted by the patient lifting his head from the pillow. The trocar should be held like a screwdriver and introduced in a series of rapid twisting movements. When the peritoneum has been punctured (there is usually a characteristic 'give') the obturator is removed and the instrument directed towards the left side of the pelvis. The catheter is then introduced down the trocar deep into the pelvis, and the trocar is withdrawn over the catheter and discarded. The skin is closed and the catheter secured by a purse-string suture.

---

* These disposable items are commercially available from Abbott Laboratories Ltd., Queenborough, Kent, Allen & Hanbury Ltd., London, E.2, or from Baxter Laboratories, Thetford, Norfolk.

Fluid Exchange.—Dialysis fluid is warmed in a water bath to 40° C. (104° F.) before infusion, and heparin, 1000 units, is added to each 2 litres to prevent the formation of fibrin clots in the catheter. In a single exchange 2 litres are run into the peritoneum in 10–15 minutes. After equilibration for 30–60 minutes, the dialysate is siphoned through the side-arm of the plastic tubing into the drainage bottle which lies on the floor by the patient's bed. A further 2 litres of fresh warmed dialysis fluid are then run into the peritoneum and the cycle is repeated 15–20 times over 36–48 hours.

Fluid Balance.—Patients should be weighed before and after the procedure. Accurate records *must* be kept of the volume of dialysate recovered with each 2-litre cycle. In the first two or three exchanges there may not be recovery of all the fluid infused, but the total amount unrecovered should never be allowed to exceed 600 ml., unless the patient is as obviously dehydrated as at the start. As the procedure progresses, the volume of recovered fluid should exceed that given by an amount dependent on the osmolarity of the dialysis fluid. A solution containing 1·5 per cent dextrose is a little hypertonic to plasma and 100–200 ml. more fluid is recovered than introduced in each exchange. A mixture of equal parts of 1·5 and 7 per cent removes 500–700 ml. in each 2-litre exchange. Use of 7 per cent dextrose alone is not recommended, since removal of body fluids may then be dangerously rapid.

Problems and Complications.—

1. *Failure to empty the Peritoneum.*—This may be caused by kinking in the tubing, malposition of the peritoneal catheter, or blockage of the latter by fibrin clot. It is often worth washing out the catheter with sterile saline, using a 50-ml. syringe.

2. *Protein Loss.*—There may be considerable loss of plasma proteins in the dialysate. It is therefore good practice to estimate the protein content of the recovered dialysate and to infuse reconstituted plasma if loss exceeds a total of 10–20 G.

3. *Infection.*—Peritonitis is a rare complication and should be prevented by good aseptic technique. When it occurs, prompt therapy with an antibiotic appropriate to the causative organism is indicated.

4. *Bleeding.*—Minor bleeding into the peritoneum during dialysis is not uncommon and needs no particular treatment.

5. *Loss of Dialysis Fluid into Tissues.*—If the catheter is incorrectly placed, so that its tip lies outside the peritoneal cavity, fluid leaks locally into the tissues.

Other rare complications recorded include perforation of a loop of bowel adherent to the abdominal wall and shock in some œdematous patients from whom fluid has been removed too rapidly with the 7 per cent dextrose solution.

CHAPTER XXXII

THE UPPER URINARY TRACT

By J. D. FERGUSSON and J. P. WILLIAMS

EMERGENCIES

CHIEF among the conditions requiring urgent attention are renal injuries, acute infection (pyelitis), and renal or ureteric colic. The common symptom is pain, varying in quality and severity according to the cause, accompanied in many instances by overt clinical evidence of urinary disease (frequency, dysuria, hæmaturia, etc.). A presumptive diagnosis can generally be reached from a consideration of the history and symptoms, supplemented by careful clinical examination. It is obligatory that this latter should include readings recorded on a chart of the pulse-rate, temperature, and blood-pressure in addition to inspection of the urine (if any can be voided). At the same time attention should be directed towards the exclusion of injury or disease of other systems.

HÆMATURIA

Hæmaturia is a sign of cardinal importance and must never be ignored. The first step is to ensure that the urine does in fact contain blood (*see* p. 419). Remember also that anticoagulants can cause a pink discoloration of the urine quite apart from true bleeding. It is necessary therefore in all cases of doubt to examine a specimen of urine under the microscope so that the presence of red blood-cells may be confirmed. At the same time the spun deposit should be examined for other abnormal constituents, i.e., hyaline, granular tubular casts, and fragments of papillæ. In appropriate cases the urinary deposit should be stained by the Papanicolaou method for malignant cells.

The presence of more than two or three white cells per high-power field will suggest an infective process and, if pyogenic organisms are absent and the diagnosis remains obscure, should lead to a search for tubercle bacilli. The line of further investigation will be suggested by consideration of the history and physical examination. If fresh blood is seen in a specimen voided in the casualty department or clinic, early cystoscopy may be invaluable in revealing its source.

TRAUMA TO THE KIDNEY

Injury to the kidney varies from mild contusion to complete splitting or avulsion. The former may give rise to little more than slight loin pain and microscopical hæmaturia, while with the latter there is all the general evidence of hæmorrhagic shock, often with an increasing hæmatoma in the flank and an absent psoas shadow on plain radiography of the abdomen. Associated injuries frequently complicate the clinical picture. It is evident that in all cases of abdominal injury repeated examination of *all* the body systems is the surest guide to correct management, since injuries both above and below the diaphragm may reveal themselves but slowly. A CVP monitor (p. 24) is useful.

Management.—Provided there is no other indication for laparotomy, current opinion favours conservative management. In cases of suspected renal or ureteric damage an intravenous pyelogram is mandatory. There may be no concentration of dye at all in the pelvis or ureter if the kidney is avulsed and lacerated, or if the pelvis is full of clot. This examination may at least give assurance that there is a functioning normal kidney on the other side.

Indications for Urgent Operation.—If there is an increasing mass in the loin or if the general signs of hæmorrhagic shock develop or increase in spite of rapid blood tranfusion, no time should be lost in undertaking exploration. Whatever the mode of injury an abdominal approach is advisable so that a proper inspection of all potentially damaged viscera may be performed. Whilst the patient is under observation it is important to keep all the urine that is passed in separate jars so that the amount of bleeding may be compared. The great majority of cases will respond to conservative management and it is remarkable to what extent a seemingly seriously damaged kidney will recover its function, at any rate so far as pyelographic appearances are concerned. 'Delayed rupture' of a subcapsular hæmatoma is fortunately rare (unlike the spleen) but no firm guidance can be given as to how long a patient should be kept under observation on this account.

Even if surgery is undertaken nephrectomy should only be performed if absolutely necessary to control hæmorrhage. There have been many cases reported where suture of partial lacerations has been carried out with good results. If following this procedure no function returns, secondary nephrectomy can always be carried out at a later date. Little information is available concerning the late results of conservative surgery (residual pathology, development of hypertension, etc.) and all cases should be entered for long-term follow-up.

ACUTE PYELONEPHRITIS

This condition is most commonly seen in the first trimester of pregnancy and also in children, when it is frequently associated with vesico-ureteric reflux. In both types of patient treatment has in the past often been inadequate and recurrence common. Pyelitis is also a complication of ureteric obstruction, be it due to calculus or other obstructive pathology of the lower tract (e.g., disease of the prostate or urethra). It is likewise commonly encountered as a complication of recurrent cystitis (ascending infection) in women in whom the predisposing cause remains obscure. Symptoms vary between a mild backache with discomfort in the loin and low-grade pyrexia to a fulminating infection with severe pain, violent rigors, and vomiting. The differential diagnosis is lengthy, but the commoner conditions are acute appendicitis, mesenteric adenitis, cholecystitis, and acute adnexal pathology. In few of these acute abdominal emergencies does the patient complain of headache, whereas it is an almost invariable accompaniment of acute pyelitis and may be very severe.

Investigation.—In all cases of acute abdominal pain the urine must be examined as a routine (Chapter XXXI), and in cases of pyelitis pus cells, if not organisms, will nearly always be seen. An important exception to this is obstructive pyelitis in its early stages.

Treatment.—If the presence of many pus cells and motile organisms in a hanging drop preparation confirms the clinical diagnosis, immediate chemotherapy should be started whilst awaiting the bacteriological report on the midstream urine (*see below*). For cases of moderate severity sulphadimidine 2 G. at once and 1 G. q.i.d. should be given or nitrofurantoin 200 mg. q.i.d. (adult dosage). More severe infections are better treated with ampicillin 0·5 G. stat. and 0·25 G. q.i.d. The patient should be confined to bed and bland drinks encouraged. Within 48 hours the *in vitro* sensitivities of the infecting organism to the standard antibacterial agents will be available and treatment can be modified if necessary. By then the acute episode should be subsiding and further investigation can be arranged. It is important that chemotherapy is adequate, and to ensure that the infection has indeed been eliminated examination of the mid-stream urine at repeated monthly intervals is advisable. In resistant cases, trimethoprim 80 mg. plus sulphamethoxazole 400-mg. tablets, four tablets daily, may be tried.

RENAL AND URETERIC COLIC

Renal colic is usually of sudden onset and unheralded by other symptoms. The pain may be felt in the renal angle or in the loin and flank. Ureteric colic felt in the flank and groin accompanied by a frequent desire to micturate suggests impaction of a stone in the intramural ureter. Renal and ureteric colic may be of such severity as to cause the patient to vomit and even collapse.

The characteristic of any colic is that the patient is unable to lie still (as he does in peritonitis) and tends to writhe about in pain. The temperature is often subnormal and shock may be present depending upon the severity of the pain.

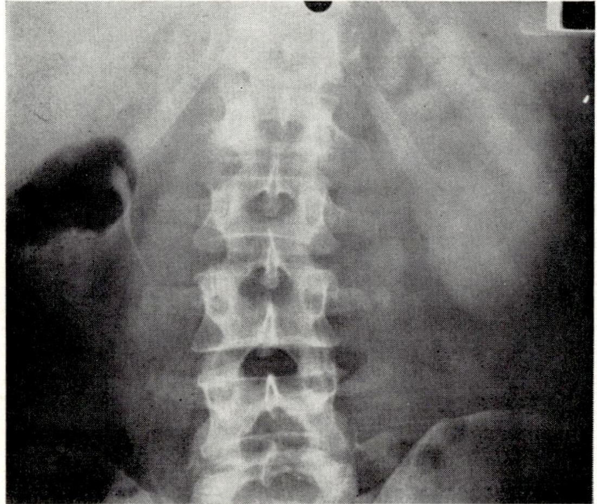

Fig. 293.—Nephrogram in a case of left ureteric calculus.

There is usually considerable tenderness in the renal angle with guarding in the appropriate quadrant of the abdomen. Rebound tenderness, although characteristic of peritoneal inflammation, may also be elicited in cases of ureteric colic. The severe pain usually ceases abruptly, leaving a residual ache in the affected loin and tenderness over the course of the obstructed ureter for several days. There is a great tendency for attacks to recur, particularly in the first 48 hours.

Management.—Blood in the urine detectable by the naked eye is seen in about 40 per cent of cases, microscopic hæmaturia in 80 per cent. In severe cases with a clear diagnosis pain must be relieved as quickly as possible and this is best done by giving pethidine 15–25 mg., or morphine 10–16 mg., intravenously, depending on the weight of the patient. This brings about dramatic relief in most cases but occasionally has to be repeated. It is helpful to have a plain radiograph of the renal tract as soon as possible, but if the patient is in severe pain this should be relieved first by an appropriate injection. Many cases of ureteric colic show no radio-opaque calculus and may be presumed due to the passage of oxalate or uric acid crystals, often brought about by inadequate fluid replacement following periods of prolonged exertion. Lack of visualization of a calculus in the plain radiograph, however, may be due to its superimposition on a bony shadow or to the fact that the stone is non-opaque. Some support

for the diagnosis may be gained when the patient is known to have passed gravel or a stone during a previous attack. In cases of metabolic stone disease a family history may often be obtained.

Pyelography.—In cases of colic an intravenous pyelogram should be carried out as soon as convenient (Chapter XLVII). This may show a nephrogram effect which indicates an obstructed kidney (*Fig.* 293), confirm the site of obstruction, or reveal it in the case of non-opaque calculus (*Fig.* 294).

As a rough guide it may be stated that one-third of stones seen in the upper ureter and two-thirds of those seen in the lower will pass spontaneously provided their diameter is less than 4 mm. Unless a solitary kidney is obstructed no immediate measures to dislodge or remove the calculus need be undertaken.

As soon as acute symptoms have subsided the patient should be encouraged to take abundant fluids and

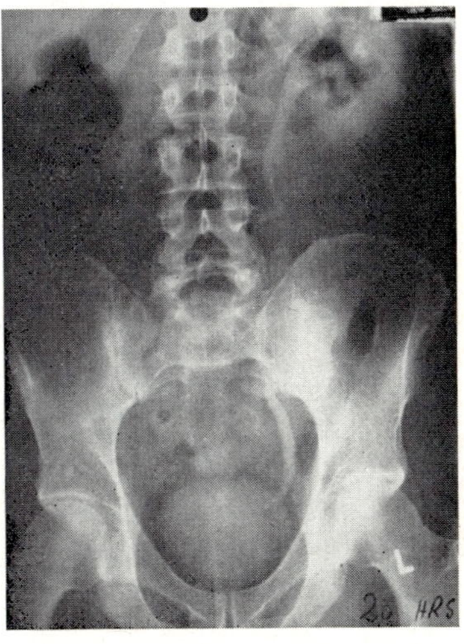

Fig. 294.—Twenty-hour film following intravenous pyelography in a case of calculus at the lower end of the left ureter.

to be as active as possible. Very often the onward progress of a small ureteric calculus seems to be brought about by ensuring a few good actions of the bowel. Fasting serum calcium levels should be checked on three occasions.

PREPARATION FOR OPERATION

Except in the direst emergency no operation should ever be performed on the kidney or upper urinary tract without prior X-ray examination. It is the house-surgeon's duty to check that the radiographs are correctly orientated and labelled, and to ensure that they accompany the patient to the theatre.

As soon as a decision on surgery has been taken, clear instructions should be given to the nursing staff as to the scope of the operation and the area to be prepared. It is strongly advisable, particularly in a busy hospital, that at the time of preparation the site of operation should be distinguished either by an indelible skin marking or by a label attached to the patient.

In other respects pre-operative management conforms to the usual routine (p. 133) including general clinical assessment, shaving and preparation of the skin, supportive measures to counteract dehydration and electrolyte imbalances (p. 32), and blood grouping with preparation for transfusion as necessary. Pre-operative breathing exercises are taught as a routine to all patients undergoing major surgery and, of course, are continued post-operatively with the help and encouragement of the same physiotherapist (p. 164). Suitable premedication should be arranged in consultation with the anæsthetist (p. 103).

Be sure to warn the radiology department if X-rays will be required during the operation.

POSITION ON THE TABLE

The position of the patient on the operating table naturally varies with the surgical approach to be employed. In the conventional approach to the kidney and upper ureter via an oblique incision in the flank, the patient lies with the affected side uppermost on the 'break' of the operating table (*Fig*. 295). Stability

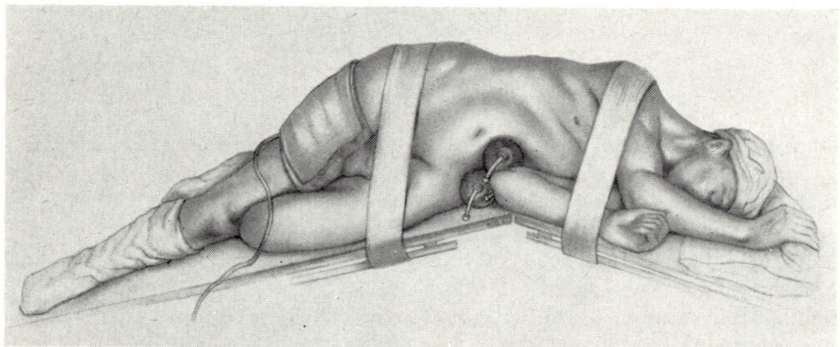

Fig. 295.—Position on operating table for right kidney exploration. The upper arm may be supported on a raised arm-rest.

is achieved by flexing the lowermost thigh and knee, and by drawing the uppermost arm forward on a support. Improved access may also be gained by rotating the pelvis backwards and securing it by a band of wide adhesive strapping attached to the table. Obvious modifications will be required if other approaches are employed, and provision for turning the patient into a supine position must be made if separate exposure of the lower end of the ureter may be needed.

POST-OPERATIVE CARE

Position.—Unless contra-indicated by shock or other general considerations, most patients recovering from kidney or ureter operations are best treated in a sitting-up position following return to consciousness.

Sedation.—During the immediate post-operative period adequate sedation should be provided, e.g., pethidine 50 mg.

Fluid and Electrolytes.—Close attention is paid throughout to fluid and electrolyte requirements. In straightforward cases of nephrectomy or operation for stone, oral fluids are to be preferred, supplemented if necessary by drip infusion up to a daily intake of about 2000 ml. Some limitation, however may be called for in the presence of previous overhydration or impending cardiac failure.

In operations involving the bowel (e.g., ureterocolic anastomosis) or when post-operative ileus develops, oral fluids should be stopped and the daily requirement given by the intravenous route for 36–48 hours. Normal saline is a dangerous solution: 4·3 per cent dextrose in 0·1 per cent saline is safer and should be used in metabolically uncomplicated cases.

Mannitol.—Many surgeons favour the intravenous infusion of 200 ml. 15 per cent mannitol at the conclusion of operations on the urinary tract to promote an osmotic diuresis. For detailed management of intravenous fluid and electrolyte therapy *see* Chapter IV.

Records.—A fluid intake and output chart specifying the routes, quantities, and character of all fluids administered and discharged is indispensable. The metric system only is used. Uncomplicated cases should be encouraged to sit out of bed during bedmaking on the second post-operative day. Thereafter progressive ambulant activity may be enjoined subject to the limitations imposed by indwelling catheters, drip infusions, and drainage-tubes.

Bowels.—Following difficult kidney operations it is not uncommon for some degree of flatulent abdominal disturbances to occur by the second day. A mild aperient (milpar 15 ml.) on the second or third evening followed by an evacuant suppository (dulcolax) the next morning will generally suffice to bring relief, failing which an enema may be given.

MANAGEMENT OF A PYELOSTOMY OR A NEPHROSTOMY

Temporary nephrostomy drainage may be established after certain operations upon the kidney, particularly after nephrolithotomy. The catheter in the renal pelvis allows irrigation of the calices. Saline solution is employed for the irrigation during the first 24 hours. It is best to use only a few millilitres of fluid, intermittently, i.e., just enough to make certain that the catheter does not become blocked. A nephrostomy tube used purely for temporary drainage is generally retained for about 10 days. At the end of this time the retaining stitch is cut and the tube removed. In other circumstances, as when solutions are employed for the dissolution of calculi, the period may have to be extended.

Nephrostomy (or pyelostomy) tubes should be not only stitched to the skin but also taped. If there is considerable drainage of urine along these tubes a satisfactory collecting apparatus may be made by sticking a Chiron bag (p. 397) over the emerging tube, having first painted the skin well with Tinct. Benz. Co. If by mischance or design a nephrostomy tube should come out and require replacement, a fresh sterile tube must be introduced forthwith: the track can close with embarrassing speed.

Removing the Tube.—When pyelostomy or nephrostomy has been employed to relieve ureteric obstruction the need to continue with this form of drainage can be gauged by clamping the tube. If obstruction still prevails, clamping the tube will invoke pain in the loin, followed by leakage of urine around the tube. In order to demonstrate the exact site of such obstruction, hypaque (as used for intravenous urography) can be instilled down the tube. It should be remembered that the normal renal pelvis has a comparatively small capacity (about 7 ml.) and therefore the medium should be injected slowly and a radiograph taken when about 10 ml. (or less if the patient experiences pain) have been injected. Too much contrast medium will lead to perirenal extravasation and obscure the radiographic outline of the ureter and renal pelvis.

Reactionary Hæmorrhage.—Following nephrostomy, and especially in cases where the operation has been performed on an obstructed and engorged kidney,

Milpar (Phillips, Scott, & Turner, St. Mark's Hill, Surbiton, Surrey).
Dulcolax (Boehringer Ingelheim Ltd., Isleworth, Middlesex).

reactionary or secondary hæmorrhage is to be feared. Therefore always be fore-armed by having the patient grouped and making provisional arrangements for blood transfusion.

MANAGEMENT OF DRAINAGE-TUBES IN THE PERINEPHRIC SPACE

The house-surgeon should be viligant that a drainage-tube designed to drain the perinephric space is not removed too early. A drainage-tube in this situation can do little harm and it should be left in place (although it can be turned and, in certain cases, shortened) for several days after it has apparently ceased to function. Especially after conservative operations upon the kidney and ureter such as for the removal of calculi, late leakage of urine is liable to occur. Following these operations the saying, 'It is better to leave a tube in the perinephric tissues a week too long than remove it a day too early' should be remembered.

THE MANAGEMENT OF ADRENAL CASES

By F. Dudley Hart

Before the advent of cortisone Addison's disease was the only condition in which pure hypoadrenalism was encountered, and Addison's disease is, and always has been, a comparatively rare disorder. At the present time patients whose adrenal glands have been rendered incapable of reacting to the body's needs in times of stress (such as a surgical operation or severe infection) are numerous. This is because the administration of cortisone or one of its ana-logues—hydrocortisone, triamcinolone, prednisone, prednisolone, methyl-prednisolone, betamethasone, or dexamethasone—for rheumatoid arthritis, ulcerative colitis, asthma, and many other general and dermatological conditions is customary, and because the administration of cortisone for any length of time subdues the output of adrenocortical hormones from the adrenal glands for some months. On this account, so common has the state of subfunctioning adrenal glands become that while taking the history of a patient admitted for a major operation the house-surgeon should always ask: "Do you know if you have ever had a course of cortisone, ACTH, or any similar drug?"

Subnormal Adrenocortical Function in relation to any Surgical Operation.— Before an operation, on no account discontinue or reduce the dose of steroid (cortisone) of a patient who is receiving this form of therapy.

What is much less obvious, and of equal importance, is to know that patients who have received cortisone therapy for periods of more than a few days during the 12 months prior to admission for operation must be placed in the same category, to wit that of subnormal adrenocortical function. To perform an operation upon a patient with subfunctioning adrenal glands without first supplementing the circulating adrenocortical hormone is to invite post-adrenal exhaustion that may end fatally in spite of belated treatment. Cortisone can be given by mouth, when its effects are apparent within 12 hours; or by intra-muscular injection, when its effects are more delayed. *Cortisone cannot be given by the intravenous route.* Intravenous medication is by hydrocortisone hemi-succinate or by sterile alcoholic hydrocortisone solution (B.P.), either of which must be given well diluted in an intravenous drip infusion. In an emergency hydrocortisone hemisuccinate may be given directly into a vein without setting up a drip infusion (*see* p. 29).

To combat the stress of an operation (or a severe infection) the following plan should be adopted:—

1. For an Elective Operation.—

If the Accustomed Dose is known increase that dose at least three- or four-fold, according to the severity of the operation the patient is about to undergo. When in doubt, high dosage is to be preferred to low.

If the Dose the Patient received is not known follow the dose-scale given in the section on Total Adrenalectomy (*see below*).

2. For an Emergency Operation.—When there is little time for pre-operative preparation intravenous hydrocortisone hemisuccinate, 100–200 mg., should be given intravenously immediately before operation, and again during, preceded (if sufficient time permits) by 200–300 mg. of hydrocortisone intramuscularly. Alternatively prednisolone-21-phosphate may be given intravenously in equivalent dosage.

In all cases remember that the threat of delayed wound healing as a result of cortisone therapy is dwarfed by the probable impending catastrophe of sudden collapse due to adrenal exhaustion.

After the operation continue with the increased dosage for 2–3 days, after which gradually reduce it to the usual maintenance dose which is reached in from 8 to 14 post-operative days.

3. When Infection is Present, or supervenes, an appropriate antibiotic must always be given in addition to the cortisone therapy. It must be noted especially that high cortisone dosage frequently masks the classic signs of inflammation while leaving the infecting organisms unaffected; it also initiates and aggravates peptic ulceration.

MANAGEMENT FOLLOWING BILATERAL TOTAL ADRENALECTOMY

The following plan of management is applicable whether one or both adrenal glands are removed at the same operation. Sometimes total adrenalectomy is performed in two stages: at the first operation one adrenal gland is removed, and subsequently, at another operation, the second adrenal. In the case of a unilateral adrenal tumour the affected adrenal only is removed.

Pre-operative Management.—At 72, 48, 24, and 1 hours before operation cortisone 100 mg. is given by intramuscular injection. Matched blood should be in readiness, for almost certainly blood transfusion will be required (p. 43).

Post-operatively.—

On the Evening of the Day of Operation cortisone 100 mg. is given intramuscularly. Although the adrenal medulla is also removed in adrenalectomy pressor agents, e.g., noradrenaline or methedrine, are only rarely necessary during or after the operation to restore or maintain the blood-pressure provided cortisone *and blood* replacements are adequate. If post-operative hypotension does not respond immediately to supplementary hydrocortisone administration (when in doubt always employ hydrocortisone intravenously) almost always the fault lies in inadequate blood replacement. The rapid transfusion of 1–2 units (500–1000 ml.) of blood will restore the blood-pressure to safe levels.

*First Post-operative Day.—*In the morning, cortisone 100 mg.; in the evening, cortisone 50 mg.

Subsequently the patient should be able to take cortisone by mouth, in which event the dosage is as follows:—

*Second Post-operative Day.—*Cortisone, 50 mg., 8-hourly by mouth.

*Third Post-operative Day.—*Total dose 100 mg. in divided doses.

The drug is then reduced gradually to the usual maintenance dose of 25 mg. a.m. and 25 mg. p.m., which must be continued for the rest of the patient's life.

ADRENALECTOMY FOR CUSHING'S SYNDROME

As hypercortisonism has been present for months or years because of adrenal hyperplasia or neoplasm, it is more than probable that higher post-operative doses than those given above will be required and in the event of the dosage being insufficient, crises of hypocortisonism are more likely to occur than when normal adrenal glands have been removed.

Signs of Hypocortisonism (adrenal deficiency) are weakness, apnœa, anorexia, nausea and vomiting, low blood-pressure, and rapid pulse. In some cases tachycardia alone is present. Such signs call for higher dosage and the post-operative doses given above must be increased by 50 per cent or more. If rapid therapeutic results are required hydrocortisone hemisuccinate 100–200 mg. can be given by intravenous injection during the operation, or subsequently.

Rarely a patient adrenalectomized for Cushing's syndrome requires a maintenance dose of cortisone 25 mg. thrice, instead of the usual twice, daily. Hydrocortisone may be given throughout, instead of cortisone, both by intramuscular injection and by mouth, the dose ratio being 25 : 20, cortisone : hydrocortisone.

POSSIBLE NECESSARY VARIATIONS IN POST-OPERATIVE TREATMENT IN ALL CASES OF ADRENALECTOMY

Aldosterone, the sodium-retaining hormone, is also sacrificed when the adrenal glands are completely removed and in many cases cortisone (or hydrocortisone) alone is insufficient to maintain balance.

Signs of Aldosterone Deficiency are those of a sodium-deficient state characterized by symptoms of nausea and anorexia, leading, if untreated, to vomiting. The serum-sodium is low and the serum-potassium high.

In such cases deoxycortone can be given by intramuscular injection in 2–8 mg. doses, or in mild cases under the tongue (linguettes), but as a rule fludrocortisone is preferable, as it is given orally in doses of 0·1 to 1 mg. Fludrocortisone is a most potent substance having powerful cortisone-like as well as sodium-holding effects. For maintenance therapy 0·1–0·2 mg. can be given daily, or more commonly every few days, in addition to the usual maintenance 50-mg. daily dose of cortisone.

In a Salt-deficiency Crisis fludrocortisone 1 mg. is given by mouth. Too high dosage will cause intra- and extracellular retention of water, with pitting œdema, a rise in the blood-pressure, and, in the course of time, a Cushing-like facies.

Warning: Any patient who is on maintenance therapy with adrenocortical hormones should always carry on him a card which clearly states the nature of his illness and the type and dosage of hormone being taken.

CORTISONE THERAPY AFTER HYPOPHYSECTOMY

Adrenal replacement therapy with cortisone is required, usually in somewhat smaller doses than after adrenalectomy. Salt-retaining hormones (deoxycortone or fludrocortisone) are required but rarely. When diabetes insipidus develops pituitary snuff may be used. Patients with hypopituitarism (Simmonds's disease; Sheehan's syndrome) should, if submitted to operation, be treated as adrenal-deficient cases, but subsequent maintenance therapy is, as after hypophysectomy for other conditions, carried out with cortisone on the lower dosage scale.

PATIENTS WITH ADDISON'S DISEASE

When it is necessary to operate for some other condition on a patient who is suffering from Addison's disease the patient must receive pre- and post-operative therapy in exactly the same manner as that recommended for patients undergoing adrenalectomy.

CONN'S SYNDROME

This condition results from a hypersecretion of aldosterone. It is characterized by hypertension, weakness, hypokalæmia, and sometimes alkalosis. Frequent electrolyte investigations (including serum calcium and magnesium) and ECG are necessary. Intravenous pyelography and selective renal arteriograms are used to exclude renal artery stenosis.

ADRENALECTOMY FOR PHÆOCHROMOCYTOMA

Phæochromocytomata are tumours of the adrenal medulla, usually benign, but about 10 per cent prove to be malignant. As a rule they are unilateral, but occasionally bilateral tumours occur. The symptoms are those of adrenaline overdosage, viz., headache, palpitation, vomiting, sweating, dyspnœa, weakness, and pallor. Typical attacks are associated with hypertension. Ten per cent of the patients have diabetes mellitus.

Pre-operative Preparation.—For an adult 20–40 mg. of phentolamine (rogitine) should be given by mouth after meals three times a day for one or two days prior to operation. Phenoxybenzamine may also be used but causes tachycardia. The latter can be controlled by propanalol, 20 mg. by mouth. Adequate pre-operative sedation is important.

Recently α-methyl-para-tyrosine, in doses of 600–4000 mg. daily, has been used successfully in the treatment of patients with, and in preparation for operation for, a phæochromocytoma. The drug markedly reduces the excretion of catecholamines in the urine.

Anæsthesia.—Anæsthetic agents likely to cause serious cardiac arrhythmia in the presence of high adrenaline values, such as ethyl chloride or cyclopropane, should not be employed.

During the Operation.—The hazardous phases in the operation are during the induction of anæsthesia, positioning of the patient on the operating table, when the tumour is manipulated, and immediately after the removal of the tumour; 5 mg. of phentolamine is given intravenously prior to commencing the anæsthetic. With an intravenous drip infusion of dextrose-saline running, the operation is commenced. The blood-pressure rises sharply when the adrenal gland is handled, and to counteract this rise another 5 mg. of phentolamine is given into the tube of the intravenous drip. Should it be necessary, yet another dose is given. As soon as the adrenal gland has been extirpated a considerable fall in blood-pressure is to be expected and is to be combated by giving an injection of noradrenaline.

Post-operatively.—Blood-pressure should be charted every 15 minutes for the first 6 hours, then every 1 or 2 hours for the next week. During the week following the operation noradrenaline always should be at hand for immediate injection in case of need; some patients will only respond to blood transfusion.

Rogitine (Ciba Laboratories Ltd., Horsham, Sussex).

CHAPTER XXXIII

THE LOWER URINARY TRACT

By J. D. Fergusson and J. P. Williams

URINE SAMPLES FOR DIAGNOSTIC PURPOSES

If a specimen of bladder urine is required only for diagnostic purposes urethral catheterization should, wherever possible, be avoided; alternative techniques are available.

1. The Mid-stream Specimen should preferably be obtained first thing in the morning since any bacteria present will have been multiplying in the urine overnight. The genitalia are carefully cleaned with an aqueous solution of chlorhexidine (1 per cent), the prepuce being retracted and the penis held in one hand so that the stream of urine is directed into a receptacle placed on a stool. A sterile jar is held in the patient's right hand, and the patient told to count up to four once the stream of urine has started and then to half fill the sterile container, passing the rest of the urine into the receptacle on the stool. The sterile container has a screw cap which is then applied and the correctly labelled jar sent to the laboratory, along with a request form giving details of the clinical condition and drugs administered.

In the female the genitalia are likewise carefully cleaned with chlorhexidine solution and the patient is instructed to sit on the lavatory seat as far back as possible with the legs widely apart and the labia minora separated with the fingers of the left hand. The patient is then instructed to pass urine in the same

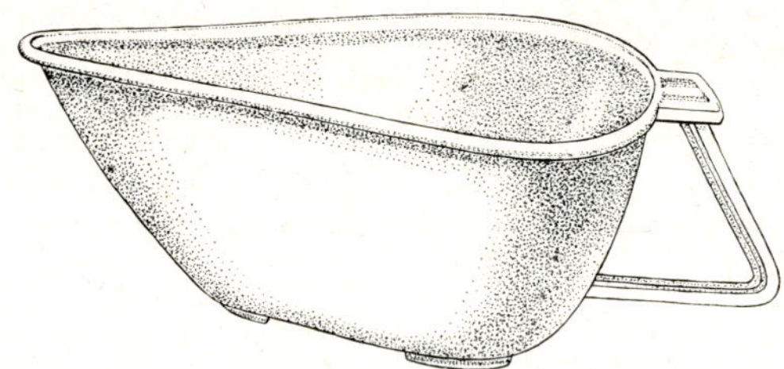

Fig. 296.—St. Peter's boat.

way as the male, but the mid-stream urine should be directed into a sterile St. Peter's boat (*Fig.* 296) and the specimen thus obtained transferred to a sterile container similar to that used for the male.

2. In infants the simplest method is to fit a Chiron ileostomy bag (p. 397) over the genitalia in either sex.

3. Suprapubic Aspiration of the distended bladder affords an occasional method of obtaining uncontaminated urine and may be appropriate if the patient's co-operation cannot otherwise be obtained. When the bladder is full a weal of local anæsthetic is raised in the skin two fingerbreadths above the symphysis

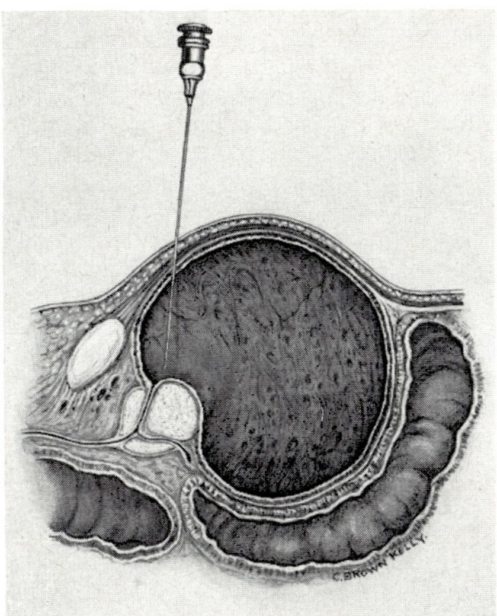

Fig. 297.—Suprapubic puncture of the full bladder, using a lumbar-puncture needle.

pubis and a 20 S.W.G. lumbar-puncture needle is directed downwards and slightly forwards (*Fig.* 297). The 'give' as the bladder is entered is unmistakable. The urine may then be aspirated into a 20-ml. syringe. No dressing is necessary. The patient is then instructed to empty the bladder normally.

RADIOLOGICAL ESTIMATION OF RESIDUAL URINE

A final radiograph taken after micturition during routine intravenous urography (p. 714) gives a valuable guide (*Fig.* 298). If only such information is required and the integrity of the upper renal tract is not in question, radiological evidence may simply be obtained by asking the patient not to drink for 6 hours, emptying the bladder as much as possible and then taking 18 G. of hippuran by mouth. One hour later the bladder is radiographed in the anteroposterior plane and the patient asked to void, a further radiograph then being taken in the erect position to estimate the residue. In fat patients where the soft part shadow

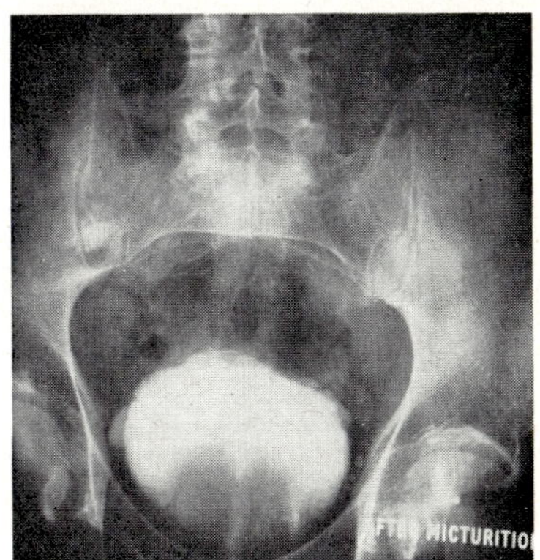

Fig. 298.—Residual urine.

of the bladder may be difficult to define an intravenous injection of 20 ml. of 45 per cent hypaque will usually provide adequate contrast.

URETHRAL CATHETERIZATION

The proper use of the urethral catheter is the most important single factor in the successful management of bladder and prostatic cases: misuse can cause disaster. In the male a brusque forcing of the catheter may bruise the urethra and cause copious bleeding, while cruder effort will tear a false passage and result in failure to enter the bladder. Both misdemeanours may leave the patient a legacy of stricture which is a life sentence. This mechanical disaster is only equalled by the introduction of infection. The bladder is especially liable to infection if it has been a long time distended or if an indwelling catheter has to be replaced. In any event imperfect aseptic technique is inexcusable.

Types of Catheter.—The introduction of the plastic catheter has brought many advantages. The old-fashioned red-rubber catheters were irritant to the urethra and strength was obtained at the expense of internal diameter.

Gibbon Catheter.—The modern Gibbon catheter, constructed of polyvinyl chloride, is relatively small, has a wide bore in relation to its external diameter, and causes minimal irritation (*Fig.* 299). In our opinion it is ideal for the relief

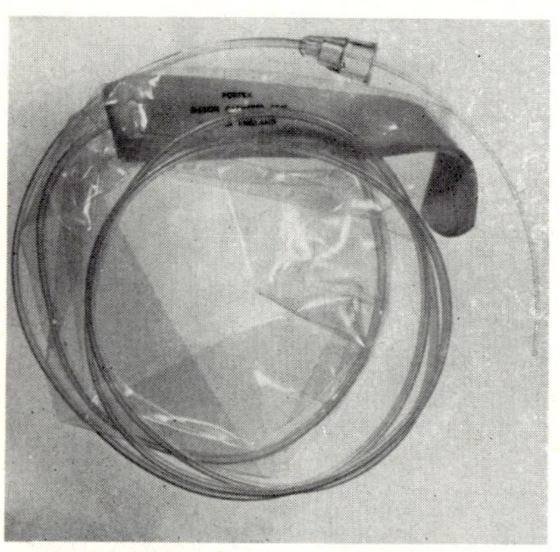

Fig. 299.—Gamma-ray sterilized Gibbon catheter.

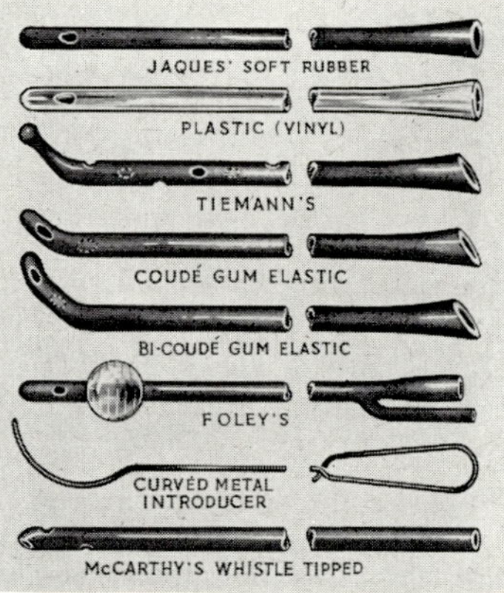

Fig. 300.—Various types of urethral catheters.

of long-standing urinary retention. The proximal or urethral component is now made continuous with a long drainage length so that only one connexion need exist between the bladder and the drainage bag or bottle. To facilitate introduction the catheter is stiffened by a plastic stylet which is subsequently withdrawn by holding the entire length of tubing straight and exerting a steady pull.

Tiemann Neoplex Catheter.—Where a Gibbon catheter cannot be introduced a Tiemann neoplex catheter is recommended (*Fig.* 300). This catheter has a slightly curved extremity which is tapered. Plastic catheters of the Porges or neoplex variety have the advantage of being relatively rigid so that they may be used to negotiate a urethra rendered narrow by prostatic disease or urethral stricture.

Foley Catheter.—The latex Foley catheter (*Fig.* 301) is of softer material and has an inflatable bag near its end so that on distension (with water) the latter is held within the internal meatus. The bag capacity varies from 5 to 30 ml. and is clearly marked on each catheter. The disadvantages of the Foley catheter are that its lumen is relatively small and, despite the thickness of its wall (in which the inflation channel is fully incorporated), it remains only semi-rigid.

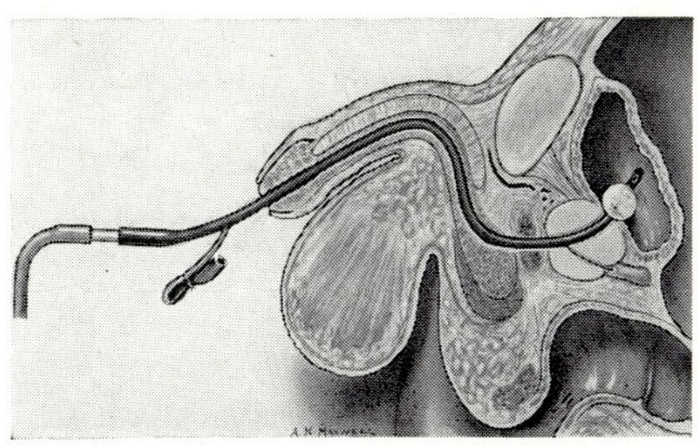

Fig. 301.—Foley's balloon-ended self-retaining catheter in place.

It cannot therefore be used to overcome serious urethral obstruction without the aid of a metal introducer. When using the latter it is important to be sure that *both* are well lubricated! By nature of its softness the Foley catheter will collapse if firm suction is applied, so its use is not recommended if much bleeding and clot obstruction are likely. Uneven distension of the balloon with consequent angulation of the tip may likewise sometimes interfere with drainage, but, nevertheless, this type of catheter is often extremely valuable, especially in female cases, and is widely used. Further advances in plastic engineering have now led to a Gibbon catheter with a Foley bag incorporated in it.

Gum-elastic Catheters.—Before the advent of plastics gum-elastic catheters constructed in the form of a woven silk tube impregnated with resin were widely used. Such catheters had the advantage of being semi-rigid and were made either straight, or with one bend (coudé) or two (bicoudé) to negotiate the prostatic urethra (*Fig.* 300). Although nowadays outmoded, they can still be used for relieving retention due to prostatic obstruction, but are not suitable as indwelling catheters since they are irritant to the mucosa and not easy to fix in position. Moreover, their surface tends to become roughened with age and their method of sterilization is also a drawback (*see below*).

Sizes of Catheters.—Catheters and bougies are calibrated according to two main scales. The widely used French (or Charrière) scale is a direct indication of the external circumference in millimetres. An 18F catheter will usually rest comfortably in the normal adult male urethra. The English scale is an arbitrary one and is rapidly becoming merely of historical interest (10E corresponds roughly in size with 18F).

Sterilization of Catheters.—The immense advantage enjoyed by the modern catheter is its method of sterilization. Plastic catheters are packed in a series of sealed envelopes at the factory and then submitted to sterilization by gamma irradiation. There is thus no handling between manufacture and time of use. The outer envelope is cut by an assistant and the inner envelope containing the catheter shaken out on to the dressing trolley. After cutting or tearing this inner envelope the catheter itself is made to protrude and is then introduced into the urethra from within the envelope, being at no time touched by the house-surgeon's hands. Prepacked Gibbon catheters are disposed of after use, but the larger Porges catheters may be resterilized by boiling or by immersion in chlorhexidine for 20 minutes. Gum-elastic catheters may be boiled for 3 minutes in protective gauze wrapping but usually emerge soft and sticky. Sterilization in formalin vapour for 24 hours is not entirely reliable and demands, moreover, that the catheter be carefully washed prior to introduction.

CATHETERIZATION FOR RETENTION

In cases of acute (painful) retention of urine or where difficulty in catheterization is expected there is every reason to relieve the patient's anxiety and discomfort by suitable sedation. If the patient is much distressed give an injection of morphine 15 mg. intramuscularly, otherwise chlorpromazine 25 mg. intramuscularly should be prescribed (dosage for men of average build). In the male the glans penis should be carefully cleansed, the foreskin being withdrawn and all smegma wiped away. Aqueous chlorhexidine (strength 1 per cent) is preferred for this purpose. Holding the penis in the left hand the anterior urethra is anæsthetized and lubricated by injecting a gel of 1 per cent lignocaine and 0·25 per cent chlorhexidine (lidothesin) via the external meatus. A suitable preparation in a collapsible tube fitted with a boilable nozzle should be laid out immersed in a kidney dish containing 1 per cent chlorhexidine on the catheterization trolley (*Fig.* 302).

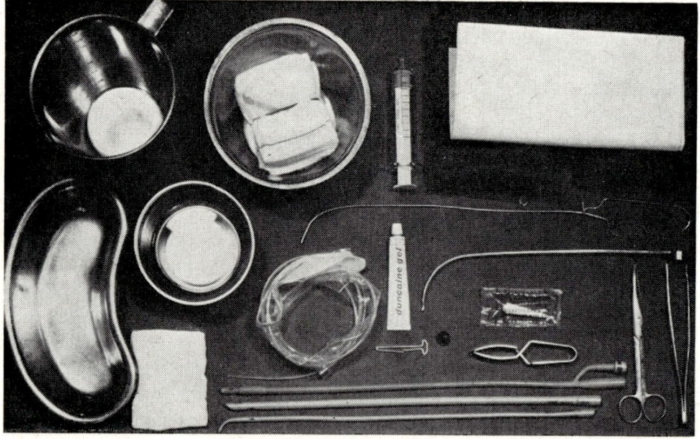

Fig. 302.—Catheterization trolley. On the left are receptacles and galley pots containing swabs and chlorhexidine. A variety of catheters are at the bottom; above them is a tube of local anæsthetic, penile clip, spigot, metal urethral bougie, and catheter introducer. On the right are sterile glove packet (top), scissors, and forceps for no-touch technique.

After the lubricant has been injected it should be massaged well down the urethra for a few moments before a penile clamp is applied. The latter should be left in place for 2 minutes to allow the anæsthetic to act and the house-surgeon should use the time to wash his hands again. In some units the use of sterile disposable gloves has become routine and there is much to recommend this practice. The penis is then wrapped in a sterile swab and held in the left hand,

Lidothesin 1 per cent (Willows Francis Ltd., Ashley Road, Epsom, Surrey).

while the tip of the catheter, lubricated and held vertically in its envelope in the right hand, is gently introduced down the urethra. As the bulb of the urethra is reached the penis should be rotated down into the line of the patient's body and the catheter further introduced towards the bladder. This manœuvre is only necessary with the more rigid catheters. If a stylet is present it should now be removed and a sample of the urine collected into a sterile bottle for laboratory analysis.

In difficult cases it is often helpful to place a sandbag under the patient's buttocks so that the curvature of the bulbous urethra is diminished. Once the catheter has been introduced into the bladder and a specimen of urine taken it should immediately be connected to the drainage bag or bottle. In cases of acute retention due to prostatic hypertrophy or stricture and where there is no bleeding, the use of a uri-bag with the Gibbon-type catheter is advised. This has but one junction so that the risk of introducing infection is minimized. The bag is light, may be hooked on to the side of the bed, and is easily handled by the nursing staff during bed making. Moreover, on account of its lightness the ambulant patient can carry the bag about with him so that his activity is in no way curtailed. It is important, however, that it should be carried well below the level of the bladder!

Securing the Catheter.—The usual Gibbon catheter has two flaps attached to the tubing, some 8 in. (20 cm.) from its tip. These flaps are secured to the shaft of the penis by strapping, or in the female to the inner side of the thigh (*Fig.* 303).

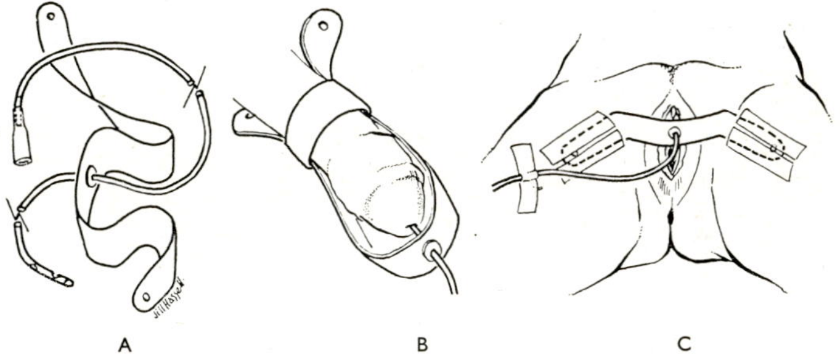

Fig. 303.—A, Gibbon's catheter. B, In use in the male. C, In use in the female.

If a Foley catheter has been introduced the bag should immediately be distended to the requisite volume, thus rendering it self-retaining. At this stage it is imperative to replace the prepuce over the glans penis otherwise paraphimosis may develop. A small protective dressing of ribbon gauze or lint smeared with a greasy antiseptic preparation (sulphanilamide ointment or flavine and paraffin) is then applied to the external meatus.

Methods of securing other indwelling catheters rely mainly on the use of adhesive strapping applied longitudinally along the exposed portion of the catheter and continued proximally over the shaft of the penis: the surface of the catheter should be cleansed of lubricant and carefully dried and the pubis shaved. Three 6-in. lengths of ½-in. (1·25 cm.) adhesive tape will suffice (with some overlapping) to enclose the circumference of the catheter. A further 8-in. (20-cm.) length of ½-in. strapping wound spirally upwards around the catheter and continued on to the penis will complete the fixation. Tight circumferential strapping around the penis should be avoided as it is likely to lead to œdema.

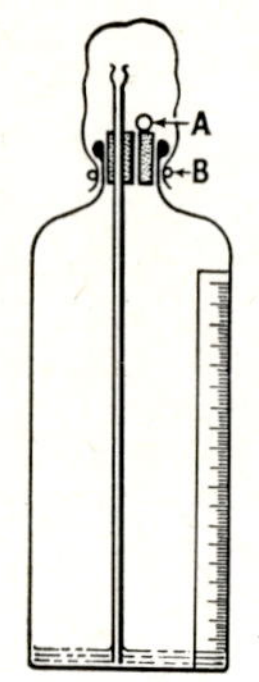

Fig. 304.—The Bristol pattern of infection-preventing urine-collecting bottle. **A**, Tablet of formagene; **B**, rubber band.

Collecting Apparatus.—Bacteriological studies have demonstrated that infection may readily occur via the lumen of the drainage-tube attached to the catheter. A closed system of drainage such as that provided by the Gibbon catheter connected with a uri-bag or ending under a measured quantity of antiseptic solution in a sterile bottle is thus to be recommended (*Fig.* 304). When a separate drainage-tube has to be attached to an ordinary catheter the choice may lie between rubber or transparent plastic tubing. Rubber tubing is heavier and may drag on the catheter, but has the advantage of being more easily 'milked' to free the system of debris or clots. The tubing should of course be sterile and a glass connexion of suitable size will be required to link it with the catheter. Care should be taken to ensure that the lumen of the latter is adequate and small-bore glass nozzles are to be avoided. Plastic tubing can usually be directly inserted into the end of the catheter, and in the collecting apparatus supplied by Messrs. Bard Davol* the end of the tubing is shaped for this purpose. This equipment also incorporates a plastic 'trap' at its distal end to avoid bacterial contamination when changing the collecting bag (*Figs.* 305, 306).

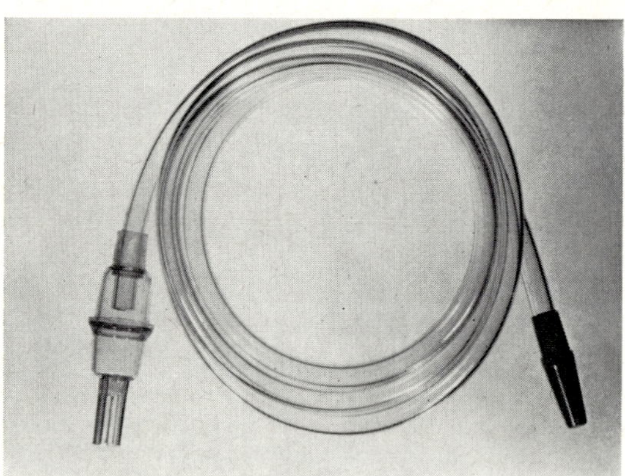

Fig. 305.—Bard Davol drainage-tube with 'trap'.

Sterile disposable collecting bags for urine vary in their efficiency and cost. The following features are important:—

1. They should preferably be made of transparent material so that the quality and quantity of drainage can readily be observed.

2. The incorporation of a printed scale to register the approximate amount is an advantage.

---

* Bard Davol Ltd., Clacton-on-Sea, Essex.

3. They should be so constructed as to avoid seams which may leak when the bag becomes distended.

4. Provision should be made for a carrying handle which can either be used by the patient (if ambulant) or attached to the side of the bed.

5. The junction of the collecting tubing with the bag should be reinforced or capable of support in such a way as to avoid angulation with consequent obstruction of drainage.

6. An adequate length of collecting tubing of sufficient calibre should be attached.

DECOMPRESSION OF THE BLADDER

Although the merits of slow decompression of the distended bladder remain debatable, there may still be occasional justification for its use.

1. Hypodermic Needle Method. — The simplest, if least scientific, method is to introduce a hypodermic needle into the lumen of the spigoted catheter and allow the urine to discharge slowly drop by drop.

2. Drip Chamber.—Alternatively, the incorporation of a screw clip and drip chamber in the drainage system distal to the catheter

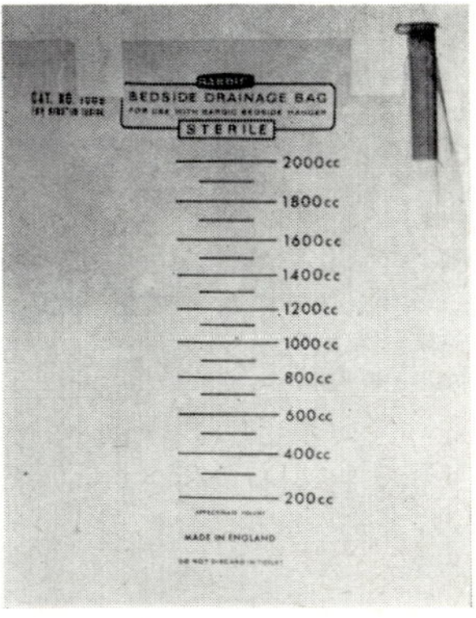

Fig. 306.—Disposable drainage bag.

will allow the outflow to be regulated. Frequent adjustment will be necessary to compensate for changes in bladder pressure.

3. Gravimetric Decompression.—The same applies to gravimetric decompression where the drainage tubing is connected with an inverted U-tube (as in cystometry) positioned at such a height, and gradually lowered, so as to regulate the overflow. Constant supervision is required in all cases since failure to adjust the rate of drainage to variations in bladder tone will defeat the purpose of the procedure.

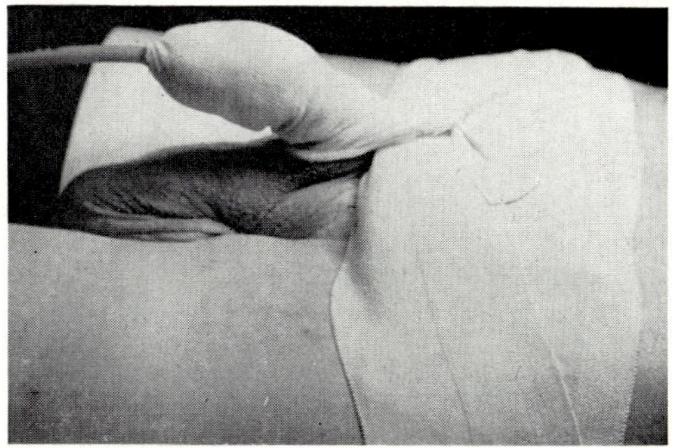

Fig. 307.—Tubegauz penile dressing and catheter.

CATHETERIZATION AT OPERATION

After prostatectomy or operations on the bladder it is usually necessary to drain the bladder for some days. In these circumstances a firm wide-bore catheter that will withstand the suction of a Wardill syringe must be used. A 22F neoplex catheter with an open 'whistle tip' end is favoured. This should be secured either by a nylon stitch through the eye of the catheter, which is then knotted as a loop and the ends brought out and anchored to the anterior abdominal wall, or by a stitch embracing the catheter as it issues from the external meatus and securing it to the frenum. In either case tubegauz No. 12 forms a simple and effective penile dressing (*Fig.* 307).

Some surgeons favour the use of a wide-bore plastic Y connexion placed between the catheter and the drainage-tube. One limb of the Y is normally left occluded but is available for suction as required. It has the merit that no disconnexion of the drainage system is needed.

FAILED CATHETERIZATION

When catheterization fails to relieve retention the bladder must be drained suprapubically. As a temporary measure suprapubic aspiration may be performed (*see* p. 446) or a fine catheter introduced by the Supracath technique.

SUPRAPUBIC CATHETERIZATION

1. Suprapubic Stab Cystotomy.—If it is thought that several days' drainage will be needed a Riches suprapubic catheter may be used. This consists of a self-retaining rubber catheter (*Fig.* 308) which is introduced through a small

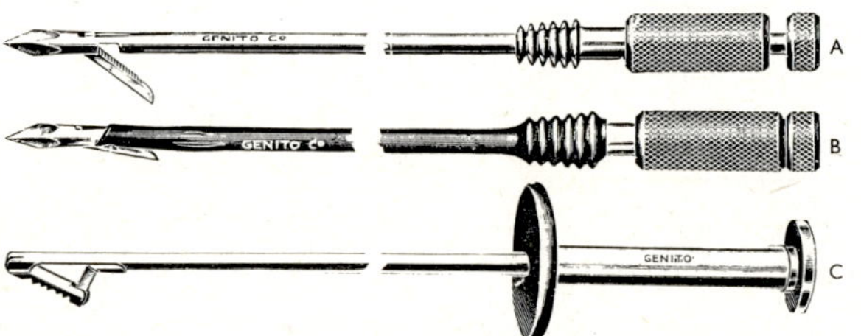

Fig. 308.—A, The suprapubic catheter introducer; B, The catheter stretched on the introducer; C, The advancer.

stab wound in the midline two fingerbreadths above the pubis under local anæsthesia. The trocar-pointed introducer over which the catheter is stretched is plunged into the distended bladder and the retaining screw unwound so that the introducer may be withdrawn. After appropriate advancement a retaining flange is placed over the emerging catheter and taped on to the abdominal wall. Be sure that the catheter is introduced well into the bladder so that as the bladder vault falls away during emptying the catheter remains at the correct depth (*Fig.* 311).

2. Formal Suprapubic Cystotomy.—Owing to improvement in the quality of urethral catheters, and to the better control of infection by chemotherapy, the need for permanent suprapubic cystotomy drainage has nowadays greatly diminished. In most cases where corrective surgery is excluded by senility or intercurrent disease, continuous drainage with an indwelling urethral catheter of the latex Foley type is generally to be preferred. When, however, catheterization is impracticable for mechanical reasons, or fails to provide free drainage on account of debris or clot in the bladder, formal suprapubic drainage may be called for.

Supracath (Bard Davol Ltd., Clacton-on-Sea, Essex).
Tubegauz (The Scholl Manufacturing Co. Ltd., 182–204 St. John's Street, London, E.C.1).

Technique.—The procedure, which should be carried out in the operating theatre, consists of the introduction of a large self-retaining catheter, at least 32F, of the De Pezzer or Malecot type (*Fig.* 309). These catheters are nowadays made

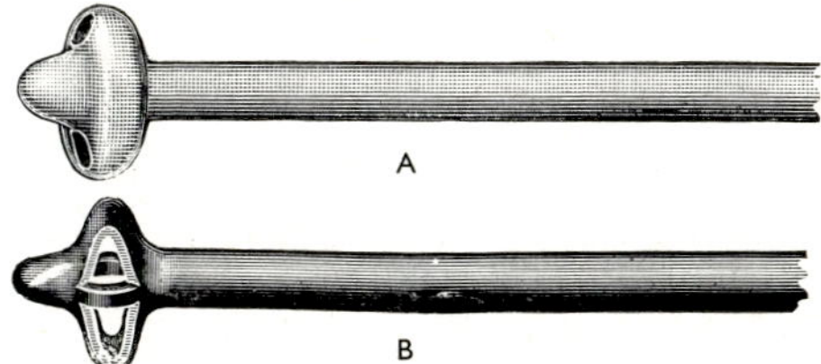

Fig. 309.—A, De Pezzer catheter; B, Malecot catheter.

of latex rubber which retains its resilience and is less irritant than the old-fashioned red-rubber variety. Encrustation is minimal and the risk of the material perishing and the expanded head breaking off in the bladder when the catheter is changed has all but been eliminated.

Formal suprapubic cystotomy should always be carried out well away from the symphysis pubis and preferably at a point at least half-way between the latter and the umbilicus. If a retaining belt is going to be worn it will 'sit' more comfortably at this level, while if drainage is only to be temporary the obliquity of the track will encourage more rapid closure after the catheter is withdrawn.

The formal operation may be performed under either general anæsthesia or local anæsthesia, infiltrating 1 per cent lignocaine subcutaneously and into the abdominal wall at the above-mentioned site. The bladder is distended. A 4-cm. vertical incision is then made through the skin and between the recti muscles.

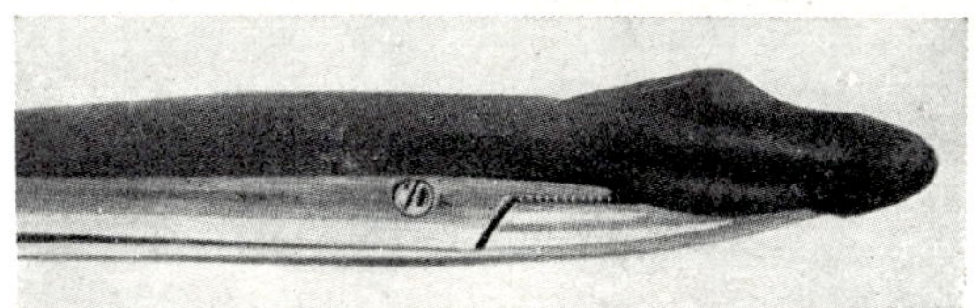

Fig. 310.—Method of stretching a de Pezzer catheter with a hæmostat.

The peritoneum is swept cranially with a swab, the recti being gently retracted laterally. Two catgut stay stitches are inserted into the bladder wall and, using a scalpel, a small stab incision is made between them. Excess bladder fluid is sucked away.

For purposes of introduction the tip of the catheter is grasped by a long hæmostat and the shaft pulled up tightly between the handles of the forceps so as to reduce the calibre of the expanded end. Alternatively, when introducing a Malecot catheter the end of the forceps may be inserted into the lumen of the catheter via one of the drainage openings in the 'butterfly' portion (*Fig.* 310).

Care should be taken to advance the catheter sufficiently within the cavity of the bladder to avoid extrusion as the latter contracts (*Fig.* 311). On the other hand, the expanded end should not be allowed to dangle like the clapper of a bell, as intermittent contact with the sensitive trigone may cause considerable discomfort.

The stay stitches may then be crossed and tied to ensure a snug fit for the emerging tube. A few interrupted stitches complete the closure of the small abdominal incision; a skin stitch may help secure the tube.

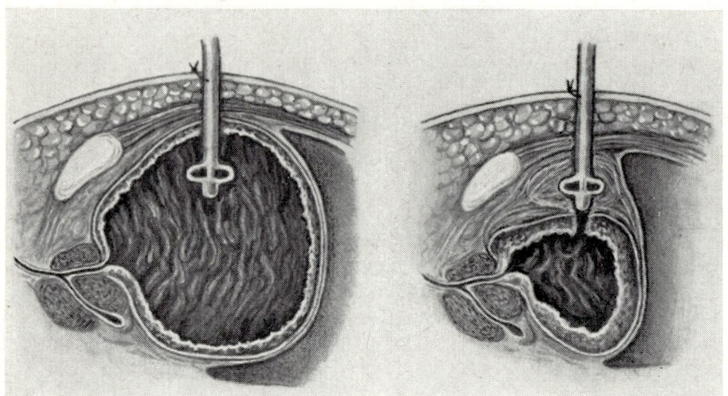

Fig. 311.—Unless the expanded end of the catheter is pushed well into the bladder it will be dragged out as the bladder contracts, for the catheter is fixed to the skin by a stitch.

Changing the Tube.—When permanent suprapubic drainage has been established it becomes necessary to change the tube from time to time. If latex catheters are used an interval of between 3 and 4 weeks is usually sufficient and a gentle wash-out with sterile saline (using a tube and funnel or a 50-ml. disposable syringe) should be given through the new catheter to ensure that drainage is satisfactory.

To remove the tube a blunt-ended introducer is inserted into the lumen and advanced as far as it will go. The catheter is pulled up tightly over the introducer so as to straighten out the expanded end and then withdrawn from the bladder. A sterile replacement should be immediately available and is introduced in similar manner.

Difficulty may sometimes occur when the previous catheter has fallen out and the fistulous track has contracted. In such an event gentle dilatation with graduated uterine dilators (Hegar's) will often facilitate reintroduction.

INSTRUMENTATION OF URETHRAL STRICTURE

Method.—The secret of success in relieving acute retention due to urethral stricture is gentleness. After appropriate sedation and anæsthetization of the

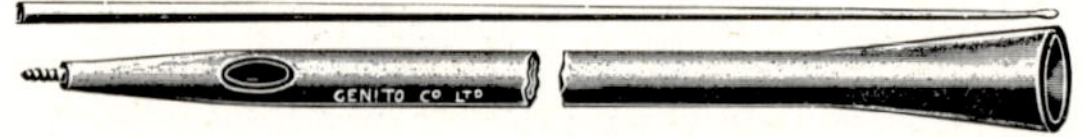

Fig. 312.—Phillips' catheter. The guide is inserted through the stricture, after which the catheter is screwed on to the guide.

urethra a small sound or bougie (14F) should be cautiously introduced down the urethra using an aseptic technique. If after careful manipulation this fails to negotiate the stricture, filiform bougies should be tried. The possession of a set of graduated screw-on bougies offers an incalculable advantage in such circumstances, since if a small filiform can be induced to pass, further 'followers' of increasing size can be attached in sequence and the stricture thus enlarged (*Fig.* 312).

Should a filiform bougie fail to negotiate the stricture the method of 'faggoting' should be tried, several filiforms being introduced at the face of the stricture so that one may be induced to pass through the stretched face of the obstruction (*Fig.* 313). Once a fine bougie has entered the bladder urine will trickle alongside it and it is often wise at this stage to leave the instrument indwelling for the time being. As the œdema subsides the flow will usually increase and in 48 hours further dilatation may be attempted with a greater prospect of success.

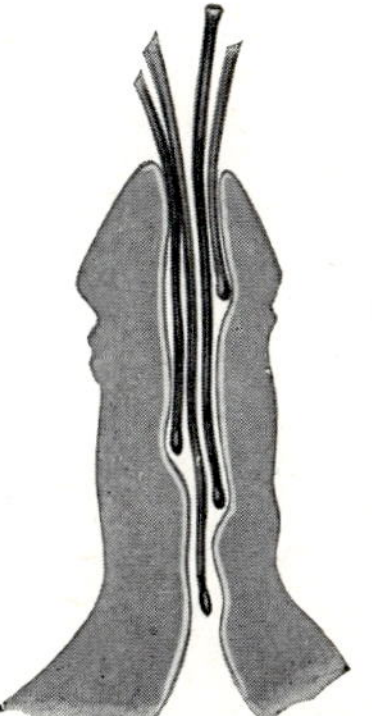

Fig. 313.—Finding the lumen of a strictured urethra by means of multiple filiform guides.

MEATAL STENOSIS

Narrowing of the external meatus may be either congenital or acquired and prevent the passage of a catheter (or cystoscope). Where the opening cannot be enlarged sufficiently by gentle dilatation meatotomy will be required.

Technique.—A short ($\frac{1}{4}$-in.; 6-mm.) incision is made either with a small bladed scalpel or with the tip of a pair of scissors inserted into the meatus in a downward direction.

Meatal stricture may result from the forcible instrumentation of a small meatus or from indwelling catheterization with too large a catheter. The condition will generally yield to regular dilatation, and once a reasonable size has been achieved the patient can be provided with a short glass rod or similar blunt instrument to continue self-treatment as necessary. Better than these, however (and more economical), are the tapering plastic sheaths in which disposable intravenous needles are now contained (provided that any slight roughness on their surface is carefully filed down beforehand).

MANAGEMENT OF CLOT RETENTION

Bleeding into the bladder of such severity as to cause clot retention may occur with vesical tumour, after irradiation (telangiectasia), in benign prostatic hypertrophy, and as a complication of bladder and prostatic surgery. When

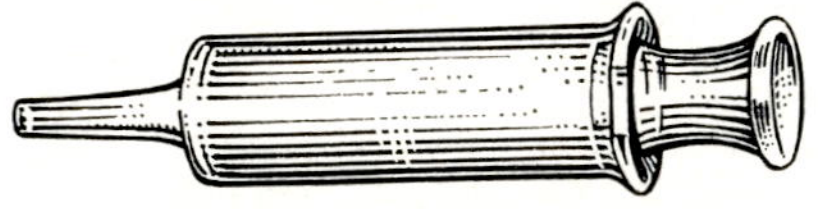

Fig. 314.—Wardill's all-glass bladder syringe.

acute, the patient is often severely shocked and urgent transfusion may be required.

1. Aspiration and Wash-out.—If an indwelling catheter is already in place (failing which a wide-bore plastic catheter should be passed), suction applied with a Wardill syringe (*Fig.* 314) will sometimes suffice to clear the obstruction;

a glass syringe is more effective than a plastic one. The bladder should be washed out with sterile normal saline until the fluid is returned clear. It is wise then to leave the catheter in situ until all evidence of further bleeding has ceased.

2. Bigelow's Evacuator.—Should suction with a Wardill syringe fail the patient must be taken to theatre and more forceful irrigation and suction applied using an evacuating cannula attached to a Bigelow evacuator. In resistant cases the secret of success often lies in introducing the cannula and then rapidly and repeatedly withdrawing the obturator until the clot follows through.

Suprapubic Drainage.—When catheterization and evacuation fail the bladder must be drained suprapubically.

IRRIGATION AND INSTILLATIONS INTO THE BLADDER

Bladder irrigations to combat infection have been largely given up and replaced by systemic chemotherapy. However, small quantities of chlorhexidine 1–5000 or acriflavine 1–10,000 solutions may be instilled into the bladder for prophylactic purposes after instrumentation.

The Mechanical Removal of Debris is often best achieved by forceful irrigations of sterile normal saline. In particular, the removal of phosphatic debris may be facilitated by the prior instillation of a 1 per cent solution of acetic acid.

Clorpactin 0·5 per cent may be instilled into the bladder immediately prior to the removal of *vesical tumours* to reduce the risk of implantation with viable cells at operation. Clorpactin is, however, sometimes irritant, causing intense frequency and dysuria, and some surgeons prefer the use of a 5 per cent solution of silver nitrate.

Therapeutic Bladder Installations include the use of silver nitrate for the treatment of Hunner's ulcer and of oncolytic agents such as epodyl or thiotepa for the treatment of superficial tumours. Both the latter, in addition to being lethal to cancer cells, are depressant to the bone-marrow and repeated checks on all formed elements in the peripheral blood must be undertaken during treatment. It is imperative that the strength of all solutions instilled into the bladder (and the period for which they can be safely retained) should be checked beforehand.

ACUTE RETENTION OF URINE

Paramount among the commoner urological emergencies requiring immediate attention is acute urinary retention. The combination of a painfully distended bladder with inability to void distinguishes the condition from:—

1. Chronic retention in which the distension, though often greater, is painless and associated with ineffectual frequency or overflow incontinence.

2. Oliguria or anuria when little or no urine is passed but the bladder remains empty.

Except in unconscious patients or in traumatic cases with severe shock, acute retention is unlikely to be overlooked. Even in such circumstances routine clinical examination should immediately reveal the distended viscus. Uncertainty may yet occasionally arise on account of obesity, abdominal distension from other causes, or where the bladder has become displaced, as following previous surgical excision of the rectum. In a majority of cases, however, the condition is self-evident and some idea of the more usual causes (excluding post-operative retention) may be gleaned from *Table XIII*.

Careful attention to the history, particularly of antecedent urinary symptoms or disease and recent use of drugs, as well as to the age of the patient and the

Hibitane, Clorpactin, Epodyl (I.C.I. Ltd., Pharmaceuticals Division, Macclesfield, Cheshire).
Thiotepa (Lederle Laboratories Ltd., Bush House, Aldwych, London, W.C.2).

circumstances in which retention has occurred, will often suggest the cause. Further evidence must be sought by clinical methods, always including thorough inspection and palpation of the external genitals and rectal examination. The information thus gained will in most cases reveal the diagnosis and indicate the appropriate means of relief.

As will be seen from *Table XIII* a majority of cases stem from some form of prostatic obstruction which, even where drugs or neurological disorders are

Table XIII.—Analysis of 300 Consecutive Cases of Acute Retention in a General Hospital

	No. of Cases
Benign prostatic hyperplasia	193
Malignant disease of the prostate	39
Urethral stricture	23
Phimosis	14
Vesical tumour (clot retention)	9
Inflammation (cyst-prostatitis)	4
Impacted urethral calculus	3
Rupture of urethra	2
Papilloma of urethra	1
Spinal injury	4
Neurological disease	4
Miscellaneous (drugs, constipation, etc.)	4

implicated, often coexists as an essential component. Stricture has nowadays become less common because of the better treatment of urethral inflammation and trauma. Among the elderly uncircumcised, however, inflammatory phimosis (particularly in diabetics) remains a not unusual cause of obstruction.

MANAGEMENT OF ACUTE RETENTION

Irrespective of the cause, the presence of a painfully distended bladder calls for early relief. Except in obvious cases of hysteria and occasionally others where no obstructive cause is immediately apparent, attempts to induce voluntary voiding are generally a waste of time. Traditional remedies such as sedation or sitting in a hot bath are rarely effective and even if successful seldom bring more than temporary relief. Similar objections apply to the use of parasympathetico-mimetic drugs such as carbachol which, in addition to carrying certain risks, may only increase discomfort.

It should be clearly recognized that with few exceptions the onset of retention reflects the presence of an underlying obstructive lesion for which admission to hospital and further investigations will be required. The practice of relieving the condition by catheterization in the casualty department and then discharging the patient to await events is only mentioned to be condemned.

1. Outside Hospital.—Nowadays, except in isolated areas, transfer to hospital is generally practicable within a few hours and it is unlikely that the patient will come to any harm during this period if adequately sedated. Such a course is strongly to be recommended as avoiding the risk of infection, etc., contingent on an immediate attempt to decompress the bladder in unfavourable surroundings. In adverse circumstances, however, the latter may have to be considered, the choice lying between catheterization and suprapubic aspiration. Briefly, the factors influencing a decision will be (*a*) the presumed nature of the obstruction, (*b*) the availability of suitable equipment (catheters, aspirating needles, etc.), and (*c*) the period likely to elapse before hospitalization can be effected. Generally speaking catheterization is to be preferred and is more readily accepted by the patient as a logical method of relief. The risk of infection can be reduced by appropriate chemotherapy and when, as for example at sea, some delay can be foreseen before further assistance is obtainable, the catheter should be left indwelling. Continued or repeated suprapubic aspiration, on the other hand, is fraught with the hazard of extravasation and can only be condoned as a short-term expedient or as a forced alternative where attempts at urethral instrumentation have failed. In the latter case, if circumstances permit, the deliberate performance of open cystostomy drainage may well prove preferable (*see* p. 455).

2. Inside Hospital.—On arrival at hospital management becomes more clearly defined. All cases with acute retention should be admitted forthwith and any thought of relieving the condition in the casualty department must be rigorously excluded. Once in bed and following suitable sedation the conditions are favourable for an attempt at catheterization. Strict attention to asepsis is obligatory and, if successful, closed drainage to a sterile receptacle combined with chemotherapy will minimize the risk of infection. Unless there is good reason to believe that the cause is purely temporary (e.g., drugs, alcoholic excess) the catheter should be left indwelling while further investigations are being undertaken.

If catheterization fails, either through apprehension and resistance on the part of the patient or on account of obstinate obstruction (e.g., stricture), preparation should be made for a further attempt under general anæsthesia. Suprapubic aspiration as an alternative has little or no place in hospital practice save when an anæsthetic is precluded or in occasional cases of acute urethral inflammation.

Subsequent Investigation.—Once the distended bladder has been relieved the emergency is over. Continued catheter drainage combined with prophylactic chemotherapy affords an opportunity for further study and the planning of definitive treatment. Three factors affect the latter:—

1. The nature of the obstruction.
2. The condition of the remainder of the urinary tract (including renal function).
3. The overall clinical status of the patient.

The pattern of investigation should thus be arranged accordingly.

The essential urological requirements include:—

1. *Urine.*—Full laboratory investigation (including bacteriology).
2. *Radiography.*—Appropriate radiological examination (excretion urography).
3. *Electrolyte Block.*—Estimation of the blood-urea and renal-function tests are usually redundant if pyelography shows good concentration.
4. *Serum Acid Phosphatase.*—Where cancer of the prostate is suspected the serum acid phosphatase should be determined, bearing in mind that raised values may follow recent palpation of the gland.
5. *Hæmoglobin Estimation and Blood Grouping.*—Cross-matching will be required if surgery is intended.
6. *Cardiorespiratory Assessment.*—With regard to other systems simultaneous investigation and restorative therapy should be carried out as indicated.

CHRONIC RETENTION OF URINE

As the name implies, this condition carries little of the urgency associated with the acute variety. Nevertheless, the effect of long-standing incomplete obstruction is to produce more severe damage to the upper urinary tract. Impaired renal function and an added susceptibility to infection render it vital that such cases should be investigated and treated with extra caution. Although, as in the acute variety, benign prostatic enlargement remains the commonest cause, the relative frequency both of urethral stricture and prostatic cancer is somewhat increased. The possibility of neurogenic dysfunction should also be considered.

Investigation.—Time given to preliminary investigation is generally well spent and any attempt to relieve the distended bladder better postponed until the diagnosis is reasonably assured. In addition to full clinical examination, urine studies and excretion urography are essential, while owing to the likelihood of renal impairment estimation of the blood-urea and serum electrolytes will usually be required. Any accompanying anæmia should likewise receive attention. It is important that the programme of initial investigation and management should be so planned as not to prejudice the success of ultimate treatment.

1. Benign Prostatic Enlargement.—As well as treatment of any aetiological factor (drugs, diabetes, etc.) free catheter drainage should be instituted under full aseptic precautions. The need for slow decompression has been overstressed and, indeed, as most methods are erratic and require constant supervision, its purpose is apt to be defeated. The potential hazards of hæmorrhage and suppression following the rapid release of long-standing tension are generally more than counterbalanced by the benefits of unobstructed drainage and early mobility. Nevertheless, some caution is merited in cases with obvious clinical uræmia and those in which urography shows poor concentration. Close attention should be paid to the fluid balance and electrolyte requirements, and failure to respond by diuresis after free drainage has been instituted calls for expert medical supervision. Appropriate chemotherapy should be maintained throughout the period of catheter drainage.

2. Urethral Stricture.—When not already established from the previous history, the diagnosis may only come to light during attempted catheterization. If unsuccessful, a second smaller catheter may be tried, failing which resort must be made to filiform bougies. Prolonged efforts to negotiate a difficult stricture with the patient in bed are not justifiable and the case should be taken to the theatre for further instrumentation.

3. Prostatic Cancer.—The susceptibility of this condition to endocrine therapy may sometimes render catheterization avoidable. Except where a major element of benign obstruction coexists, an initial trial with œstrogens will often induce a dramatic response. Before commencing treatment the clinical diagnosis must be reasonably assured, and preferably supported by a raised serum acid phosphatase value or radiological evidence of secondary spread. Adequate dosage is important and oral stilbœstrol 50 mg. b.d. is recommended (25-mg. tablets are obtainable). If a more rapid effect is required soluble stilbœstrol diphosphate (honvan) may be administered daily (up to 7 days) in doses of 250 mg. by the intravenous route. Transient subjective disturbances commonly follow the injections, which should be given slowly. Prolonged parenteral therapy is contra-indicated in patients with signs of cardiac decompensation or hepatic disease.

<h3 style="text-align:center">HÆMORRHAGE</h3>

Bleeding from the lower urinary tract is usually unmistakable and is readily confirmed if clots are present. Where the urine is doubtfully discoloured or recent hæmorrhage appears to have ceased, microscopic confirmation may be called for (p. 419). In a majority of cases the source lies above the external urinary sphincter and blood is voided intermittently with the urine (hæmaturia). Spontaneous bleeding from the external meatus is far less common and generally implies a urethral lesion.

Honvan (Ward, Blenkinsop & Co. Ltd., Wembley, Middlesex).

Hæmaturia.—Relative to the age of the patient, the quality and pattern will often suggest the probable cause. Painless profuse hæmaturia in the middle-aged or elderly is characteristic of vesical neoplasm, while in younger subjects the painful passage of cloudy, blood-tinged urine generally denotes infection. Accompanying difficulty may be due to either clots or prostatic obstruction, but the latter (the decoy prostate) should never be accepted as the cause until other more sinister lesions have been excluded. Careful inquiry should be made into the circumstances in which the hæmaturia has occurred with due regard for trauma or factors influencing local congestion (hypertension, alcohol, etc.), and special note taken of any previous hæmorrhagic tendency or the use of anti-coagulants.

Immediate Treatment.—Except in cases of severe exsanguination following injury or repeated bleeding from other causes, the first requirement is to reassure the patient that a catastrophic outcome is unlikely. Among the more intelligent and introspective the appearance of blood in the urine is apt to induce extreme apprehension which at this stage it is usually reasonable to allay. Most attacks subside spontaneously and give respite for further investigation, and it is only when accompanied by retention or profound anæmia that urgent action is demanded. In these circumstances immediate admission is obligatory pending catheterization, clot evacuation, and transfusion as indicated.

Subsequent Investigations.—The scope of subsequent investigation will depend largely on the clinical features of the case:—

1. Full laboratory examination of the urine (p. 411), including bacteriology.

2. Excretion urography (p. 714).

3. Serum electrolyte and urea levels. (When indicated, steps are taken to deal with fluid requirements, continued blood-loss, and infection.)

4. Hæmoglobin level.

5. Blood group.

6. Cystoscopy. Whenever the urine has been totally blood-stained, cystoscopy is indicated and, unless the view is likely to be obscured by profuse bleeding or clots, early arrangements should be made. In younger patients where the circumstances strongly point to inflammation and the infected urine is merely streaked with blood, instrumental examination can sometimes be deferred. Subject to satisfactory clinical and radiological findings and an appropriate response to chemotherapy (confirmed by subsequent urine examination) the need for cystoscopy can be decided later. Recurrent bleeding (or infection) will in any event demand full reassessment.

Hæmorrhage from the Urethra.—Compared with hæmaturia, independent urethral bleeding is uncommon. Except when due to trauma (*see below*) the immediate consequences are unlikely to be serious and investigation can be planned at leisure. Possible causes include neoplasms and local 'inflammatory' polypi, and it should be remembered that recurrent lesions sometimes arise in the urethral remnant following cystoprostatectomy for bladder tumours.

Investigation.—

1. Urine culture.

2. Blood tests for venereal diseases.

3. Urethroscopy.

4. Radiography. In obscure cases of bleeding accompanied by pain or difficulty on voiding a stone or foreign body may have to be considered and a plain radiograph will often prove helpful.

Hæmospermia.—The alarm generated by the appearance of blood in the seminal fluid is generally out of all proportion to its significance. Practically all cases are due to simple congestion—sometimes aggravated by a hypertensive element. When recurrent, the remote chance of a urethral or prostatic neoplasm or of tuberculous vesiculitis may have to be excluded by urethroscopy and bacteriological investigation of the urine (or semen).

INFECTION OF THE LOWER URINARY TRACT

Ascending infection of the urethra and bladder is particularly common in women, and the presenting symptoms of frequency and painful micturition may be so intense as to call for early relief. Coliform infections predominate, but other organisms are often present, and the urine ranges between cloudy and turbid and may be tinged with blood.

Management.—A representative sample should be sent to the laboratory for bacteriological investigation *before* instituting treatment. Catheterization is to be avoided and a clean mid-stream specimen obtained by the method outlined above (p. 446) will suffice. If any urethral or vaginal discharge is present a swab should be taken (p. 500). Pending the results, treatment should be commenced with a suitable sulphonamide (e.g., gantrisin 1 G. every 6 hours) supplemented by copious fluids and an alkalinizing diuretic (e.g., Mist. Pot. Citrate et Hyoscyamus 15 ml. every 6 hours). Antibiotics have little place at this stage and except where allergy or previous failure have been reported sulphonamides are to be preferred on account of their general effectiveness, freedom from side-effects, and relative cheapness.

Similar management applies in the male where comparable infection (cystoprostatitis) is more likely to be hæmatogenous. Cases associated with urethritis or a urethral discharge should be referred to the venereologist without delay.

Prolonged Infection.—All cases of resistant or recurrent lower urinary tract infection require further investigation. Failure to respond to simple chemotherapy implies either specific infection (e.g., tuberculosis) or the presence of some underlying pathological cause (e.g., congenital anomaly, tumour, calculus, obstruction, etc.). Primary lesions in the upper tract should be excluded and, likewise, inflammation of adjacent organs (e.g., cervicitis, diverticulitis) must be considered. Apart from any particular studies demanded by the latter, full laboratory investigation and radiological examination should preferably precede cystoscopy.

TRAUMATIC CASES

Internal Violence.—The commonest cause of injury to the lower urinary tract is unskilled or injudicious instrumentation (*see* Catheterization, p. 448). Bleeding from mucosal abrasion may be profuse at the time but usually ceases spontaneously. Deeper penetration may, in addition, result in a false passage or ultimate stricture. Extreme care is thus incumbent on all those responsible for the passage of urethral instruments.

External Violence.—Of greater immediate concern is the effect of external trauma where the degree of damage is often more difficult to assess.

Rupture of the Bladder may be suspected when as a sequel to local injury pain is experienced in the lower abdomen and attempts to void are inhibited or ineffectual. In some cases a little blood-stained urine may be passed. Damage may be limited to contusion (in which case the bladder fills with blood-stained urine) or result in actual rupture with intra- or extraperitoneal extravasation (or both). Clinically the presence of superficial bruising and tenderness often obscures the underlying condition and the possibility of associated internal injuries must also be taken into account. (*Fig.* 315.)

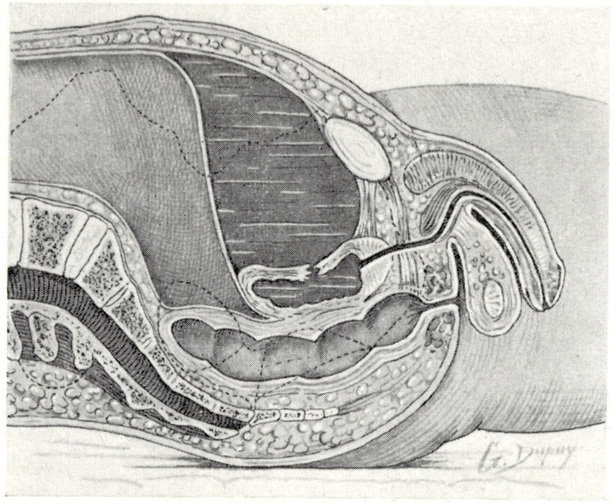

Fig. 315.—Extraperitoneal rupture of the bladder. The bladder is empty or practically so.

The immediate danger, however, lies in continuing hæmorrhage which may call for transfusion. Following treatment for shock (p. 23), as soon as the blood-pressure is restored excretion urography may clarify the issue by demonstrating whether or not the bladder remains intact. Failing this and in the face of continuing symptoms, further advice should be sought and arrangements made for early exploration.

Rupture of the Urethra may be associated with fracture of the pelvis or result from a perineal injury. A plain radiograph will reveal the former and often add substance to a presumptive diagnosis. Bleeding per urethram following injury is highly suggestive and the immediate risks are those of extravasation and retention. The relative importance of any associated injuries must again be considered.

Management.—Whenever rupture is suspected, and particularly if the bladder is distended or ingravescent bruising is noted in the perineum, the need for immediate treatment is urgent. No attempt should be made either by the patient to pass urine or by the house-surgeon to pass a catheter. It is essential that instrumentation should be performed by an expert in the operating theatre so that, if urinary diversion and drainage are required, suitable facilities will be to hand. The house-surgeon should ensure that adequate supplies of blood are available for transfusion and that the patient has no other injuries; if there are fractures the orthopædic department should be informed, so that any necessary reductions can be performed under the one anæsthetic.

PROSTATECTOMY

Investigation.—Patients admitted to hospital for elective prostatectomy will usually have had the following tests:—

1. Full blood-count.
2. Plasma electrolyte.
3. Blood-urea.
4. Serum acid phosphatase.
5. Intravenous pyelography.
6. Urinalysis and culture.

The house-surgeon must ensure that the results of these investigations performed in the out-patient department are in the patient's notes. A fresh sample of the patient's blood is sent to the laboratory for grouping and cross-matching. If there has been a long interval between out-patient visit and hospital admission the blood chemistry tests and urine culture should be repeated.

A full medical history must be taken and a careful physical examination of all the body systems performed, paying particular attention to the cardiorespiratory systems. As in all branches of surgery, time spent in bringing these systems to their optimum state prior to operation is time well spent.

The management of acute retention of urine due to benign prostatic hypertrophy has already been discussed (*see* p. 458). Suffice it to say that prostatectomy in these cases should be undertaken as soon as the above-mentioned investigations have been completed and have revealed no contra-indication to immediate surgery.

Associated Conditions.—If a catheter specimen (in cases of retention) or the mid-stream urine reveals urinary infection, appropriate chemotherapy should be prescribed pre-operatively and continued after operation for about 10 days. The presence of associated pathology (e.g., bladder diverticula, calculi, neoplasms), as well as other conditions (e.g., hernia, hydrocele), may affect the type and scope of surgical treatment and the operating-theatre staff should be warned accordingly.

Post-operative Treatment.—

Pulse-rate and Blood-pressure.—Post-operatively pulse-rate and blood-pressure are recorded at hourly intervals.

Drainage.—Careful watch is kept on the drainage from the bladder to ensure that it is free and that no clots are forming. Should there be any doubt on this score a very gentle irrigation of not more than 20–30 ml. of sterile saline should be performed. This must of course be carried out with full aseptic technique. In retropubic prostatectomy (and in transvesical prostatectomy with closure of the bladder) reliance is placed on urethral catheter drainage. Depending on the type of operation the catheter should remain in situ until all risk of extravasation has ceased and the urine has become clear and drains freely.

Removal of Catheter.—As a rough guide, the time for removal of the catheter varies between 2 and 5 days after retropubic prostatectomy, and up to 10 days if the bladder has been opened.

Prevesical Drain.—It is customary likewise for the main wound to be drained by a small rubber dam down to the prevesical space. This can be shortened on the second post-operative day and finally removed at 5 days.

Ambulation.—The patient should be encouraged to sit out of bed for bed-making on the second post-operative day and thereafter his activity is gradually increased.

Fluids.—Mannitol, 250–500 ml. of 15 per cent, will often have been given at the end of the operation by intravenous drip. It is followed by 5 per cent dextrose. By the day following operation no further intravenous therapy should be required and the patient is encouraged to drink bland fluids. An accurate intake-output chart is kept.

Food.—Light diet can be taken on the second day and is rapidly increased. An aperient may be given on the third or fourth evening.

Post-operative Complications.—

Incontinence.—After removal of the catheter a slight degree of urinary incontinence may worry patients in the early days, but they may be assured that as they become more active full control will be restored.

Late Temporary Blood-staining.—Slight blood-staining of the urine may reappear between the sixth and tenth post-operative days and should not be allowed to alarm the patient. Occasionally more serious secondary hæmorrhage occurs, in which case blood transfusion is required. Clot retention has been discussed (*see* p. 457).

Suprapubic Leakage of Urine may sometimes occur, particularly if the urethral catheter becomes obstructed or surgical closure of the bladder or prostatic capsule has been insecure. In such cases it may be necessary to change the catheter and to continue free drainage for a further period. Persistent urinary leakage thereafter usually denotes residual obstruction at the operation site and calls for endoscopy. Any urinary infection should be treated.

Post-prostatectomy Urethral Stricture may be either at the meatus (usually owing to too large a catheter having been employed) or at the apex of the prostatic cavity. It is likewise prone to occur following the repeated movement of large instruments in the urethra, as during a prolonged session of perurethral resection.

HAZARDS OF ENDOSCOPIC RESECTION OF THE PROSTATE

The house-surgeon should be aware of the hazards peculiar to this form of prostatic surgery.

Hæmolysis.—This may occur through the entry of irrigating fluid into the blood-stream via the venous channels exposed during the operation. It is important therefore that the fluid used should not only be sterile but isotonic and free from injurious electrolytes. Solutions of glycine (1·1 per cent) or glucose (5 per cent) are commonly employed and an ample supply (up to 20 litres) should be available.

Hæmorrhage.—Post-operative hæmorrhage may be troublesome if due care is not taken to achieve hæmostasis at the conclusion of perurethral resection. The malignant prostate seems particularly prone to this complication. In a small controlled trial it has been shown that ϵ-amino caproic acid (EACA) significantly reduces blood-loss in (retropubic) prostatectomy, and the drug may therefore be particularly useful in perurethral surgery. It appears to cause no thrombo-embolic complications.

EACA is given in an intravenous drip, starting at the time of operation with 0·5 G. per hour and rising to a total of 6 G., i.e., 12 hours' duration.

Extravasation.—Perforation of the prostatic capsule leading to extravasation may occasionally take place in cases of radical or difficult resection. The injury may be noted at the time or only become apparent later. The onset of lower abdominal pain accompanied by collapse and local tenderness or swelling will indicate the need for suprapubic drainage.

HYPOTENSIVE ANÆSTHESIA

This technique is recommended in cases of prostatectomy and cystectomy, the authors having an experience of more than 500 cases without complications. The operation is then carried out in a virtually bloodless field.

Technique.—Hexamethonium, 20 mg., is given intravenously after induction of anæsthesia and the systolic blood-pressure kept at between 50 and 60 mm. Hg. Intravenous methedrine is given as required in 4-mg. doses to maintain this level. The time taken for the blood-pressure to return to its normal level varies between 1 and 5 hours and the patient is kept recumbent until it has reverted to a satisfactory level. Using this technique the average blood-loss in our cases was 135 ml., but if it should exceed 200 ml. it is imperative to restore the deficit by transfusion, since the effective capacity of the vascular bed is reduced and a loss of this amount becomes highly significant.

It is the practice of some surgeons to give 250 ml. of 15 per cent mannitol at the conclusion of these operations to induce a diuresis.

BLADDER CANCER

Industrial Hazards.—In all cases of suspected cancer of the urothelium inquiry should be made as to whether the patient has at any time been employed in the chemical, rubber, plastic, or gas industries. There is a clear association between the use of certain chemicals used as anti-oxides and the development of bladder cancer. In the British dyeing industry the use or production of β-naphthylamine is now prohibited. Xenylamine is even more carcinogenic and may be produced in a variety of chemical processes. Benzidine is less carcinogenic,

Table XIV.—Summary of TNM Classification of Epithelial Tumours
of the Bladder

T = Primary Tumour
    Requires histological examination of biopsy specimens and bimanual palpation of empty bladder under general anæsthesia

    T1   Tumour with biopsy evidence of subepithelial infiltration only

    T2   Tumour with infiltration of superficial muscle: induration felt on bimanual examination

    T3   Tumour with deep muscle infiltration: hard, nodular bladder wall. Still mobile

    T4   Tumour fixed or invading adjoining organs

N = Regional Nodes
    Specimens from laparotomy

    N−   (negative histologically)

    N+   (positive histologically)

M = Distant Metastases
    Includes involved nodes above common iliac arteries, but not locally invaded organs

    M   Metastases

    MO No metastases present

but its use probably continues, though illegally, in the rubber and printing trades. Thus a detailed history of industrial exposure, however long ago, should be obtained in the interests of the patient or his family, since such an association affords grounds for compensation. If the surgeon is of opinion in such a case that there has indeed been industrial exposure he should provide the patient or relative with a certificate to that effect, bladder cancer now being a notifiable industrial disease (No. 39). This certificate is then taken to the pension authorities who will initiate a full inquiry into the case.

Methedrine (Burroughs, Wellcome & Co., Euston Road, London, N.W.1).

Records.—In cases of tumour of the bladder, not only must the cystoscopic appearances be recorded, but biopsy should be performed and a careful bimanual examination carried out with the bladder empty while the patient is still relaxed under the anæsthetic.

These findings should be recorded, preferably in code form (TNM), as recommended by the *Union Internationale contre le Cancer* (*Table XIV*). By the adoption of this nomenclature for clinical staging and pathological grading, not only is time saved, but the uniformity of description will lead to a more ready assessment of treatment and prognosis.

MANAGEMENT OF A CASE OF URETEROCOLOSTOMY

The patient should be admitted 5 days prior to surgery.

1. Pre-operative.—

a. A General Assessment should be made, including a chest radiograph, ECG (if indicated), and IVP. Anæmia must be corrected by pre-operative transfusion.

b. Bowel Preparation.—The colon must be rendered sterile and as empty as possible. Four days prior to operation the patient is placed on a high-calorie, low-residue diet. Phthalylsulphathiazole 2·5 G. 6-hourly sterilizes the bowel and also has a slight laxative effect. Alternatively, neomycin 1 G. 6-hourly may be given. Forty-eight hours prior to surgery streptomycin 1 G. is given intramuscularly and this is continued for 7 days.

Two days prior to operation an enema saponis is given and this is followed by a rectal wash-out. Two tablets of senokot are given that evening. On the day before operation a further rectal wash-out is given and only glucose drinks and complan are allowed.

2. Post-operative.—At the conclusion of the operation a firm wide-bore tube is introduced into the rectum and held by a stitch. This tube is removed on the seventh day, but should be reintroduced every night for the succeeding 5 nights. Thereafter the patient should be encouraged to void per rectum every 2 hours and twice during the night.

It is our custom to place all patients on sodium bicarbonate 1 G. every 6 hours before they leave hospital.

The serum electrolytes should be checked frequently whilst the patient is in hospital, again 2 weeks after discharge, and at suitable intervals thereafter so that hyperchloræmic acidosis may be detected early and treated by augmentation of the alkali. With modern techniques of ureterocolic anastomosis this complication is diminishing, and it seems likely that it is mainly in those cases where renal function is already impaired at the time of surgery that further deterioration takes place, with consequent metabolic imbalance. It is sound policy to explain to the patient and his family how there may arise an alteration in the biochemical state and what symptoms may be looked for. The use of salt at table should be discouraged and the importance of regular voiding of urine by day and night stressed. Occasionally hypokalæmia may develop; this is easily remedied by oral potassium supplements.

MANAGEMENT OF A CASE OF INTESTINAL URINARY CONDUIT

This form of urinary diversion is becoming increasingly popular. The house-surgeon should arrange for a surgical fitter to measure the patient for a suitable appliance *before* operation.

Senokot (Westminster Laboratories Ltd., Hull, Yorks).
Complan (Glaxo Laboratories Ltd., Greenford, Middlesex).

The house-surgeon should be present at this interview so that he may mark on the patient's abdomen the exact site for the stoma (*Fig.* 316). The site must allow the belt to ride comfortably when the patient is in any position without

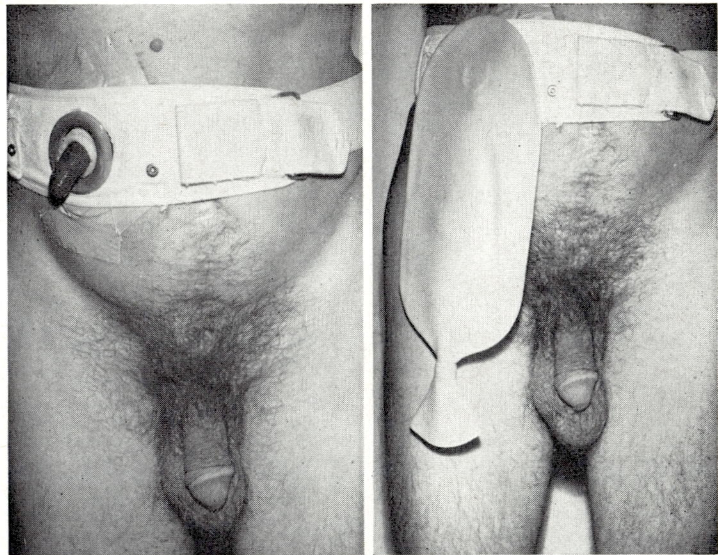

Fig. 316.—Management of a case of intestinal urinary conduit. On the left the belt helps to secure the flange over the ileostomy spout; on the right the bag is shown attached.

the flange impinging either on the costal margin or the iliac crest. It is usually possible to arrange for the patient who is to undergo this procedure to meet and be reassured by a patient who has accommodated himself or herself well to the same operation.

CIRCUMCISION
1. IN INFANTS

Circumcision (other than for religious reasons) should only be performed if there is a true surgical indication.

Parents should be reminded that the normal adhesions between prepuce and glans disappear spontaneously during the early years of life. Only gentle attempts at retraction of the foreskin should be made when the child is bathed.

If recurrent balanitis is a problem, or if it has led to preputial fibrosis and stenosis, then operation may properly be advised.

Operation.—The operation should be performed under general anæsthesia. The parts are cleaned with cetavlon 1 per cent, the foreskin freed by gently passing a probe between the glans and inner surface of prepuce, the foreskin fully retracted (if possible), and all smegma wiped away. The foreskin is then replaced and grasped in three fine hæmostats which are held by an assistant. These should be held so that the foreskin is only slightly extended; excessive

Cetavlon (I.C.I. Ltd., Pharmaceuticals Division, Macclesfield, Cheshire).

tension will lead to an undue amount of shaft skin being pulled forward and removed. The dorsum of the prepuce is then divided to within 2 mm. of the corona and a circumferential incision at right-angles to this made on each side with Mayo's scissors until the frenum is reached. Bleeding vessels are picked up in fine artery forceps as they are met. A horizontal mattress suture is carefully placed to control the frenal vessels (*Fig.* 317). Hæmostatic sutures are then placed under the artery forceps and additional sutures inserted as required to unite the two layers of the remaining prepuce. Fine 00 chromic catgut on a straight atraumatic needle is suitable for this operation.

A few turns of ½-in. gauze roll soaked in paraflavine emulsion are then applied to the wound and held in place by a stitch (through the gauze only!). The child may be allowed home after 24 hours in hospital and the dressing soaked off in the bath 5 days later.

Complications.—Reactionary hæmorrhage should not occur if due care is taken with hæmostasis. A proportion of infants develop a small meatal ulcer due to the unprotected glans being bathed in an acid urine. Simple boracic

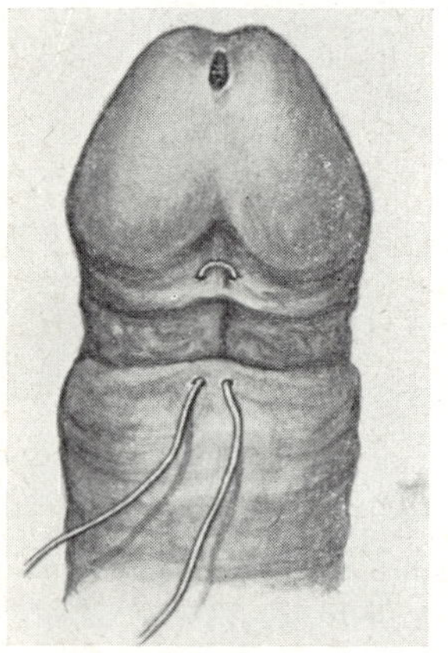

Fig. 317.—The three-in-one frenal stitch.

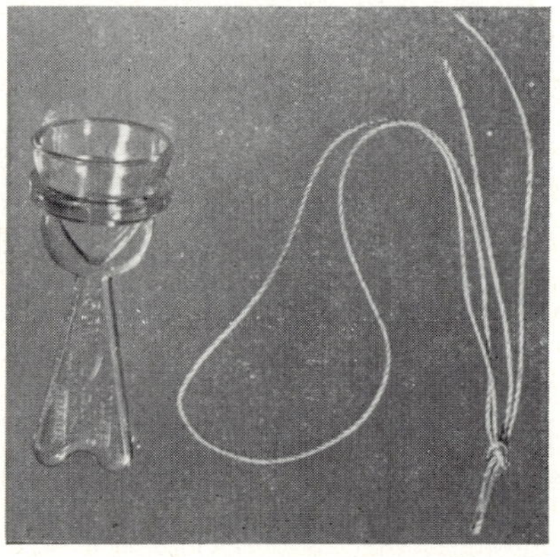

Fig. 318.—The Plastibell.

powder and frequent changes of nappies will deal with this, but rarely a meatotomy is needed because of subsequent fibrosis.

Plastibell Technique.—An alternative technique is the Plastibell procedure. For use in neonates this technique has much to commend it. The apparatus consists of a conical plastic device which fits over the glans penis. It is made in three sizes: 11-mm., 13-mm., and 15-mm. diameter (*Fig.* 318).

A 1-cm. dorsal incision is made in the prepuce and any underlying adhesions gently freed. A Plastibell of suitable size is then placed over the glans and the foreskin drawn forward over it. A firm linen ligature is then tied on the ridge of the Plastibell and the redundant (distal) foreskin trimmed away. The handle of the instrument is broken off and the Plastibell remains as a protective collar over the glans. The skin under the ligature becomes dry and separates with the Plastibell between 5 and 7 days after the operation.

No dressing is required at the end of the procedure.

Plastibell (Messrs. Charles Thackray, Leeds, agents for Messrs. Hollister, U.S.A.).

2. IN ADULTS

The indications here are recurrent balanitis (sometimes associated with diabetes mellitus), phimosis, and following the relief of paraphimosis by dorsal slit (*see below*). The technique is similar to that outlined above but it is wiser to keep the patient in hospital for 4 or 5 days.

It is helpful to prescribe stilbœstrol 5 mg. b.d. over the operative period to prevent painful erections.

PARAPHIMOSIS

Usually this condition is already far advanced when the patient is first seen and efforts to reduce the constricting band by the injection of hyaluronidase or the application of a 1–1000 adrenaline compress are doomed to failure.

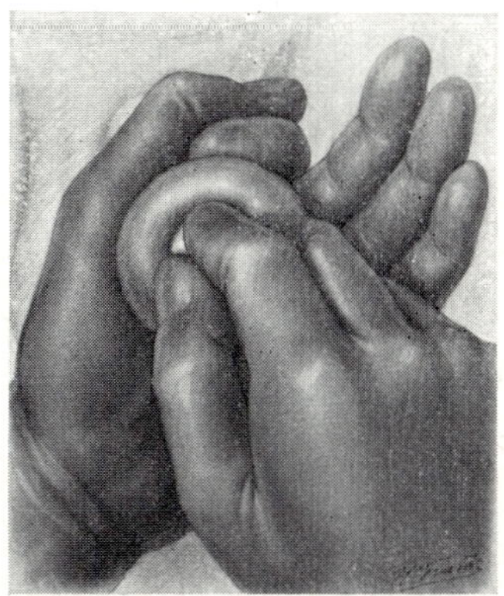

Fig. 319.—A method of forcible reduction of a paraphimosis.

Reduction.—A short-acting anæsthetic should be given and a gentle but firm attempt made to reduce the paraphimosis (*Fig.* 319).

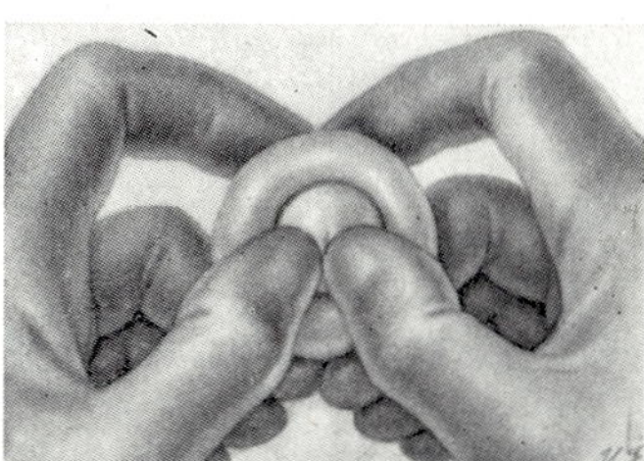

Fig. 320.—Alternative method of forcible reduction of a paraphimosis.

The tyre-like swelling of foreskin is firmly compressed for 2–3 minutes; then, with the index and middle fingers of each hand behind the swelling and the thumbs giving counterpressure on the tip of the glans, an attempt is made slowly and steadily to draw the foreskin forward (*Fig.* 320).

If this fails and the local condition is not too unfavourable an immediate circumcision may be performed. Alternatively, and in all long-standing cases, it is better merely to perform a dorsal slit and carry out an elective circumcision at a later date when all œdema and inflammation have subsided.

ASPIRATION OF HYDROCELE

A prerequisite to successful treatment is to establish the position of the normal scrotal contents as far as possible and to define the extent of the hydrocele. The latter can generally be distinguished by transillumination, which will also demonstrate the distribution of any superficial vessels to be avoided.

Technique.—The scrotum is firmly grasped with the left hand so as to render the hydrocele tense and a convenient area selected for aspiration. After swabbing the skin with a suitable antiseptic (chlorhexidine 1 per cent, cetavlon 0·5 per cent), a sterile No. 1 (intravenous) needle is advanced sharply into the cavity of the hydrocele. As soon as the fluid commences to drip from the needle, the latter is attached to a 20-ml. syringe and evacuation continued by aspiration. It is essential to maintain firm pressure on the hydrocele throughout so that the sac is emptied completely. The needle is then withdrawn and the skin puncture sealed by application of a small collodion dressing.

Using this method it is possible to dispense with the preliminary hypodermic injection of local anæsthetic required when a larger trocar and blunt cannula are employed, but care must be taken that the sharp end of the needle is not allowed to penetrate beyond the hydrocele cavity. By observing the above precautions complications such as hæmorrhage (hæmatocele) and infection should be avoidable.

Following aspiration it is important that the residual scrotal contents should be carefully palpated so that no underlying abnormality is overlooked.

SEMEN ANALYSIS

Semen analysis is required in the investigation of male infertility. The ejaculate should be examined within 2 hours. The normal volume is between 2 and 4 ml. In the laboratory the ejaculate is diluted with 4 per cent bicarbonate in 1 per cent phenol, and a 1–10 or 1–20 dilution made according to the initial sperm count. A normal specimen shows 60 per cent of sperms to have good motility 2 hours after ejaculation and 70 per cent of 200 counted sperms should be normal in form. The normal sperm count is 40×10^6 per ml.: oligospermia may be suspected with a count of less than 20×10^6 ml.

Semen analysis is a skilled technique and should only be undertaken by laboratories regularly practising this examination.

CHAPTER XXXIV

PRINCIPLES OF MINOR SURGERY

By G. B. ONG

THERE are many minor surgical procedures which can be performed by junior hospital staff or in a doctor's surgery. However, the occasional operator should beware of lesions which may be much more extensive than at first appears. For example, a lipoma in the neck may have prolongations, even into the axilla; a cervical abscess in fact may be a deep-seated branchial cyst.

EXTENT OF SKIN CLEANSING AND TOWELLING

Before any minor operative procedure is undertaken, the patient's skin should be prepared carefully. The operative field is shaved of any hair. The area that is to be shaved is liberally smeared with soap solution and a safety razor is used. Extreme care must be exercised in shaving in order to prevent any scratch or cut on the skin. Any cut on the skin will serve as an entry for bacteria and thus give rise to infection. In cases requiring emergency operation, this part of the preparation can be carried out in the operating theatre and is best done when the patient has been anæsthetized.

Skin Antiseptics.—After the operative field has been shaved and cleansed, the surgeon paints the whole area with an antiseptic solution. The following antiseptic agents are currently used before minor surgery.

1. *Tincture of Iodine* (2·5 *per cent*).—This is one of the most effective and widely used bactericidal agents. Unfortunately in sensitive persons it tends to cause a skin rash and its use should be avoided in areas like the scrotum and vulva. The tincture, after application, should be left to dry off before any excess is removed by cleansing with 70 per cent alcohol.

2. *pHisohex.*—This contains 3 per cent hexachlorophane in a detergent cream. As an antiseptic it is relatively mild but repeated use will produce a cumulative effect against bacteria, particularly staphylococci. It is a popular antiseptic in skin preparation prior to surgery.

3. *Savlon Liquid Antiseptic* is made up of 0·3 per cent chlorhexidine and 3 per cent cetrimide (cetavlon). Savlon hospital concentrate is five times the strength of the liquid antiseptic and is used as a soap concentrate for scrubbing the hands and for skin preparation.

4. *Merthiolate* is thiomersal tincture. It is used in preparing sensitive areas like the vulva and scrotum.

All skin antiseptics should be allowed to act for 3–4 minutes.

The extent of skin preparation depends on the type of operation to be performed. For small tumours of the *scalp*, an area of 2–3 in. (5–7·5 cm.) around the tumour is normally sufficient. In operation on the *neck* the preparation should extend from the jaw in front and mastoid process behind to the upper part of the chest as far as the nipple. After cleansing this area the head is draped with two towels over a waterproof sheet. The top towel is folded over the head, covering the face and head from the jaw upwards. The towel is now held in

pHisohex (Bayer Products Co., Surbiton-on-Thames, Surrey).
Savlon and cetavlon (Imperial Chemical Industries, Macclesfield, Cheshire).
Merthiolate (Eli Lilly & Co. Ltd., Basingstoke, Hants).

place with towel clips. The lower part of the neck at the level of the suprasternal notch is now covered with more towels. A large abdominal sheet is then spread over the whole field.

For operation on the *chest wall* the extent of preparation should be as far as the nipple line of the contralateral side of the chest. Above, the preparation should be as high as the axilla which should have been shaved of any hair, and below it should be down to the level of the umbilicus. Towels are then draped over this area. It should be wide enough to expose a sufficiently wide field. Once the towels have been applied they should not be moved.

TECHNIQUES OF SIMPLE SUTURES

General Principles.—Many of the principles given for the emergency treatment of inflicted wounds (p. 51) are also applicable to clean surgical wounds. Before sutures are applied to a wound, all bleeding points must be caught and ligated with fine plain catgut or touched with coagulating diathermy. The approximation of the skin should be accurate. All dead spaces in the subcutaneous tissue should be obliterated either by an extra layer of interrupted sutures or by interrupted deep cutaneous sutures. They should only approximate the edges of the wound and should not be so tight as to cut through or devitalize the skin.

Types of Sutures.—

1. *Interrupted sutures* are most commonly applied and are suitable for almost all wound closures. The knots are tied with a reef knot (*Fig.* 321). In cutting

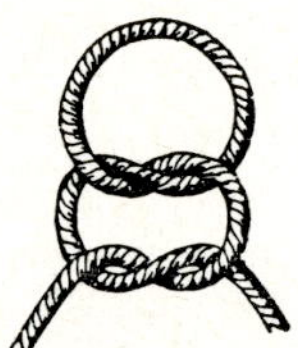

Fig. 321.—Reef knot.

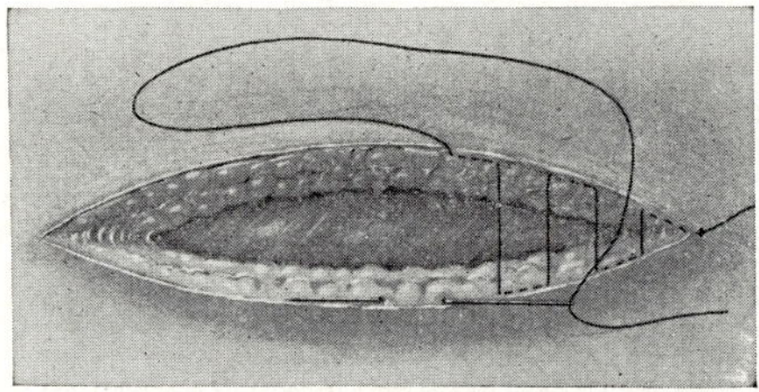

Fig. 322.—The subcuticular suture.

these ties, about $\frac{1}{2}$ in. (1 cm.) should be left behind, for this extra length of the sutures will prevent the knots from slipping and also facilitate the removal of the sutures.

2. *Continuous sutures* are frequently used in wound closure. In applying this suture care must be taken not to pull it too tight as this will cause ischæmia and thus interfere with proper healing. A continuous subcuticular suture of nylon monofilament gives a very neat scar (*Fig.* 322).

3. *Everting sutures* are usually applied in vascular anastomoses but may be used to secure accurate apposition of skin edges. In blood-vessels the endothelial surfaces of the edges are brought together so that there is no rough surface. This will prevent clots being formed at the suture line and thus obliterating the lumen. These sutures may be either interrupted or continuous (p. 59).

PATHOLOGICAL AND BACTERIOLOGICAL SPECIMENS

Most specimens excised should be sent for histological examination. Even the most ordinary and innocent-looking lesion sometimes provides a surprise.

Pus or caseous material should be submitted for culture and determination of the sensitivities of any organisms present.

EXCISION OF CYSTS

1. Sebaceous Cysts.—A sebaceous cyst arising from the sebaceous glands of the skin has a definite line of cleavage. Excision in an uncomplicated case usually presents no difficulty and, provided the correct plane is found, the cyst can be removed intact. Local anæsthesia (0·5 per cent lignocaine with 1–200,000 adrenaline) is infiltrated around and beneath the cyst; cysts on the face may require a general anæsthetic. An elliptical incision to include the punctum is made over the cyst. The skin edges are then held apart using skin hooks or a pair of Allis forceps. The incision is deepened until the correct line of cleavage is reached. By dissecting it with a pair of fine scissors, the cyst can be shelled out. Any small bleeders are caught and diathermized or ligated. The gap in the subcutaneous tissue is then approximated with 0 catgut sutures and the skin closed. This technique is applicable particularly to small cysts and to those on the face. Drainage is not necessary except when the cyst is very large and after excision an extensive raw area is left.

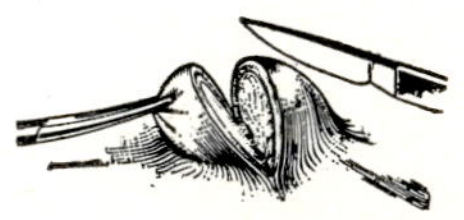

Fig. 323.—Excision of a sebaceous cyst: the cyst has been bisected.

Alternatively—and especially with large scalp cysts—the technique of slicing the cyst boldly in two may be employed (*Fig.* 323). Each half of the cyst capsule is seized in turn with artery forceps and avulsed.

2. Dermoid Cyst.—This occurs frequently over the external angular process lateral to the orbit. Although congenital it may first appear some years after birth. It is freely movable and not attached to the skin. Excision is carried out under local anæsthesia of 0·5 per cent lignocaine with 1–200,000 adrenaline.

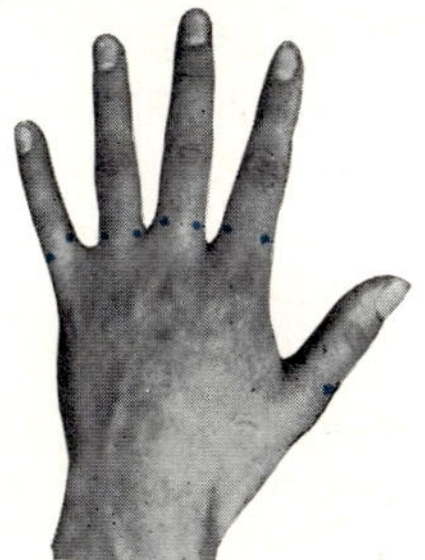

Fig. 324.—Points of puncture for anæsthetizing a digit.

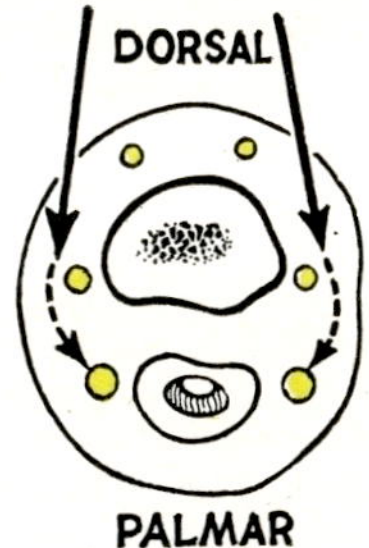

Fig. 325.—Anæsthetic solution should always be introduced from the dorsal surface.

An incision is made over the cyst which is easily removed when the correct line of cleavage is reached. *Meticulous care is needed in controlling any bleeding.* Due to the looseness of the scalp over the cranium, any oozing that takes place will cause the blood to track extensively and this gives rise to marked swelling and bruising.

19

Warning.—Occasionally an intracranial extension of an angular dermoid may take place. It communicates with the intracranial portion by a narrow neck. An impulse may be felt on coughing. Here excision will require an osteoplastic flap and if possible a neurosurgeon should be consulted first.

3. Implantation Dermoids.—Among other types of cysts that will require excision are implantation dermoids. They frequently appear over the palms and soles. These cysts are caused by sequestration of the epithelium as the result of trauma. They are most common among seamstresses who frequently sustain needle pricks. In the soles, they are usually met with among people who do not wear shoes.

Excision is done under local anæsthesia; digits may be blocked with 0·5 per cent lignocaine without adrenaline as shown in *Figs.* 324, 325. An incision is made over the cyst along the skin crease. If it is situated over the digits, a lateral skin incision is made. Incisions over the palmar surface of the terminal portion of the digits should not be made.

EXCISION OF A GANGLION

The common site is on the dorsum of the wrist. Many ganglia disappear spontaneously after trauma or may rupture following digital pressure. This is often followed by a cure. However, they may recur and will require excision.

Operation.—If the ganglion is large and is attached to an important tendon, the operation may be facilitated by exsanguinating the limb with an Esmarch bandage (p. 56) and applying a tourniquet of the sphygmomanometer cuff type. Here general anæsthesia or a brachial plexus block (p. 131) is necessary for the use of a tourniquet.

Using a skin crease incision and small hooks or retractors, the neck of the ganglion is followed down to the joint capsule or tendon-sheath and there divided. If solid tissue is removed histological examination is advisable to exclude synovioma.

MANAGEMENT OF INGROWING TOENAIL

Ingrowing toenails are the result of wearing shoes that are too tight and the erroneous method of trimming toenails down below the skin edge. Due to repeated trauma the nail edge will cut into the soft lateral tissue which ultimately becomes infected.

Non-operative Treatment.—It is an extremely painful condition and treatment at this stage can be carried out by non-operative measures. Tight shoes are avoided and it may be necessary to soak the foot in warm water in order to soften the nail. A pledget of gauze soaked in antiseptic (e.g., cetavlon) is then introduced beneath the sharp corner of the nail where it bites into the toe. The infection can be controlled after several applications and further trouble is prevented by not wearing tight shoes and by cutting the nail straight across or only slightly curved so that it projects beyond the skin.

Wedge Resection.—In intractable cases operative treatment will be necessary. Local digital nerve-block is employed. The digital nerves are situated just beneath the apex of the crease made by the next toe and the sole on the medial side and a corresponding point on the opposite side. A subcutaneous ring of anæsthetic solution around the base of the digit is usually required for complete anæsthesia. When full anæsthesia has developed, a longitudinal wedge of tissue including the affected one-third of the nail, its bed, and nail fold is excised

(*Fig.* 326). The latter must be removed to prevent regeneration of that part of the nail. Bleeding can be controlled by means of pressure. The raw area can usually be approximated with two stitches at each end (proximal and distal)

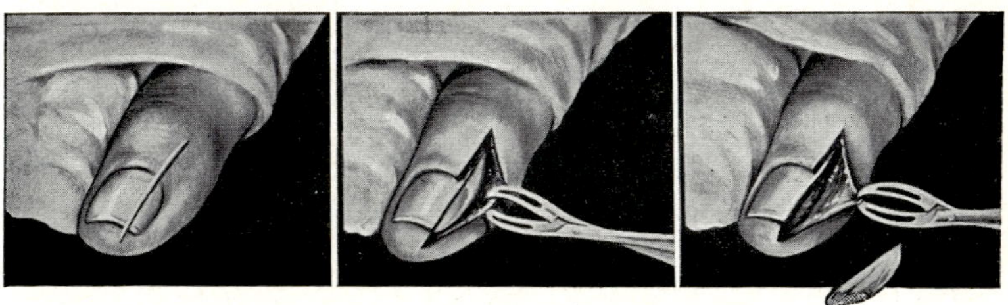

Fig. 326.—Wedge resection operation for ingrowing toe-nail.

of the wound to obtain primary healing. If infection is present, the wound must be allowed to granulate and daily eusol dressing is given until it heals.

Hibb's Operation.—Recurrence following this operation occasionally arises and radical operative treatment (Hibb's operation) may be required (*Fig.* 327). This is better carried out under general anæsthesia; a small piece of rubber

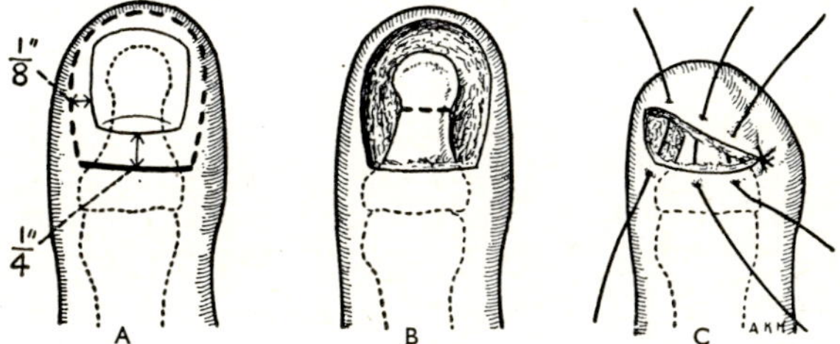

Fig. 327.—Hibb's operation: Excision of the nail, nail bed, and part of distal phalanx.

tubing may be used as a tourniquet around the base of the big toe. A hexagonal incision is made over the skin surrounding the nail. The nail is now removed and the whole of the nail bed is excised. It is important not to leave any nail bed behind as subsequent regeneration of this is the cause of failure in most cases. The periosteum of the phalanx must be pared bare of all cartilage-like tissue, especially at the proximal lateral corners. The terminal phalanx is now exposed, and the portion distal to the insertion of the extensor tendon is trimmed off with a pair of bone-cutting forceps. After the bleeding has been controlled the distal edge of the skin incision is stitched to the proximal one. The incision is covered by petroleum-jelly gauge and a pad of wool. The stitches are removed after 10–14 days. This leaves a good functioning toe but the cosmetic result is poor.

BED-SORES

The development of bed-sores may occur with great rapidity and unless energetic treatment is instituted bed-sores will contribute to the morbidity and mortality of bedridden patients, particularly the aged, the paralysed, and the debilitated.

Prophylactic care of the skin should be carried out in any patient who is confined to bed. Good nursing care is the key to prevention. The skin over the sacrum and the heels is particularly susceptible. Pressure on the skin over these areas causes impairment of its blood-supply and necrosis eventually takes place. This can be avoided by frequent change of position. A 2-hourly ward routine for such changes should be established. The area is kept clean by rubbing with alcohol if dry, and by repeated application of eusol dressings if infected. Paralysed patients may be nursed on a bed with an alternating pressure pad. Infra-red light treatment increases the local blood-supply and promotes healing. Control of incontinence—fæcal and urinary—is most important. Measures to build up the general health and resistance of the body are also valuable (p. 46). These include a high-protein diet, vitamin C, and iron, and sometimes anabolic steroids (e.g., adroyd) and blood transfusion are advisable.

It cannot be emphasized too strongly that: (*a*) 2-hourly changes of position and (*b*) keeping the skin dry are the most important measures in the prevention of bed-sores, and they must never be neglected.

When a large area of the skin has sloughed with exposure of bony prominences, operative treatment is required. This is carried out only when the general condition of the patient is good. A general anæsthetic and preparations by blood transfusion are necessary. The bed-sore and all adjacent avascular tissue are widely excised. Diseased bone may need to be chiselled away; this is often the case with trochanteric bed-sores. Hæmostasis can be obtained by individual ligature of bleeders with plain catgut.

A rotational skin-flap should then be carried out either at the time of the operation or delayed if the area is badly infected. This flap must have a broad base, preferably as broad as it is long, to ensure good blood-supply. The skin incision for the flap is first marked out. A cut is then made right down to the underlying muscle or periosteum. The flap is then undermined in this plane towards its base. The subcutaneous fat must not be trimmed away. Meticulous hæmostasis is necessary and the flap must be sutured without tension.

A firm pressure dressing and drainage, preferably of vacuum type (p. 65), for 48 hours are recommended. The original site from which the flap is taken can be covered with a Thiersch graft (p. 486) as it is not at a pressure point. When there is no infection the dressing can be left intact for 7–10 days. At this time healing will have occurred. However, pressure on it should be avoided and the patient is allowed to lie on the affected area only when healing is solid.

PROTECTING THE SKIN OF INCONTINENT PATIENTS

Incontinence of urine and/or fæces is a potent predisposing factor in bed-sores.

Causes.—As well as from senility and mental deficiency, incontinence may result from a variety of nervous diseases and operative damage to the sphincters. The house-officer should perform a rectal examination to ensure there is no fæcal impaction or rectal prolapse.

Treatment.—For what is believed to be temporary urinary incontinence in a man, a length of wide colostomy tubing fixed by adhesive strapping to the penis and shaved pubes is led to a receptacle at the bedside (*Fig.* 328). When the urinary incontinence is likely to be of long standing, a No. 14 F latex catheter of the Foley's type, passed aseptically and connected by sterile tubing to a sterile bottle (the system being closed, apart from the air vent in the stopper of the bottle), is the most practical solution of a difficult problem. A daily

Alternating pressure pad (Talley Anæsthetic Equipment, London, N.7).
Adroyd (Parke, Davis & Co., Staines Road, Hounslow, Middlesex).

bladder-wash is advisable when mucus or phosphate debris is detected in the urine. A high fluid intake should be insisted upon and any urinary infection treated appropriately. Whenever practicable, the patient should sit out of bed for as many hours a day as possible.

Urinary incontinence in a female is difficult to treat as leakage around a Foley catheter is common. A gynæcological lesion, such as prolapse, should be looked for and a gynæcologist consulted if necessary. Again, any urinary infection will require energetic treatment.

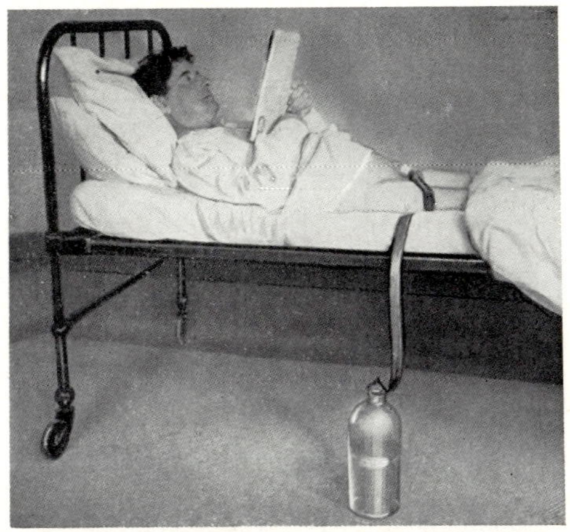

Fig. 328.—Patient with incontinence of urine treated by Paul's tubing attached to the penis.

For incontinence of fæces little can be done, except regular rectal wash-outs. The successful prevention of bed-sores in this instance is, indeed, a tribute to excellent nursing. The lubricant group of laxatives should be avoided, but bulk-forming preparations (e.g., celevac) may enable the patient to regain some control. A Thiersch steel wire inserted subcutaneously around the anus and knotted so that the anus only admits the index finger will control a rectal prolapse. Only in exceptional circumstances is it necessary for the surgeon to divert the urinary or fæcal outflows to the anterior abdominal wall.

MANAGEMENT OF ABSCESSES

When inflammation is proceeding to the stage of abscess formation, it is a general rule that to await fluctuation is to wait too long. Pus should be released as soon as possible, taking care of adjacent anatomical structures. Intravenous anæsthesia is mostly necessary and properly controlled antibiotic therapy and analgesics may be given afterwards.

ABSCESS OF THE NECK

In drainage of abscesses situated in the neck it is most important that the collar-stud variety should be recognized. Simple drainage of the superficial part of the abscess produces inadequate drainage and is a cause of persistent sinus.

Celevac (Harker Stogg Ltd., 6 Argall Ave., London, E.10).

Operation.—An incision should be made along the skin crease. It is most desirable that the operation be carried out under general anæsthesia. When the incision is made, pus will drain out but the investing fascia must be incised along the line of incision to reveal deeper extensions and/or granulation tissue. These need to be removed by dissection or curettage, otherwise a persistent sinus will result. The pus or caseous material must be cultured for pyogenic and acid-fast bacteria. Histological examination of the excised lymph-node is also useful. When tuberculous lymphadenitis is confirmed, antituberculous chemotherapy is commenced. Streptomycin, 1 G. three times per week by injection, and PAS, 4 G. four times per day, and INH, 100 mg. twice daily, either together or on alternate weeks are given for up to 3 months.

The drainage wound is lightly approximated with a few stitches around a soft rubber drain which can be removed after 24–48 hours. A primary focus of infection must be looked for and treated, e.g., septic teeth, tonsils, and very occasionally spinal tuberculosis.

AXILLARY ABSCESS

Abscesses of the axilla must be opened promptly, for the pus tends to extend along the path of the nerve-trunks into the neck. The site of the incision will depend upon the situation of the pus. *In acute abscesses pus usually lies under the pectoralis major.*

Operation.—Abduct the arm fully. Make an incision quite 2 in. (5 cm.) long ust below the fold of the pectoralis major (*Fig.* 329).

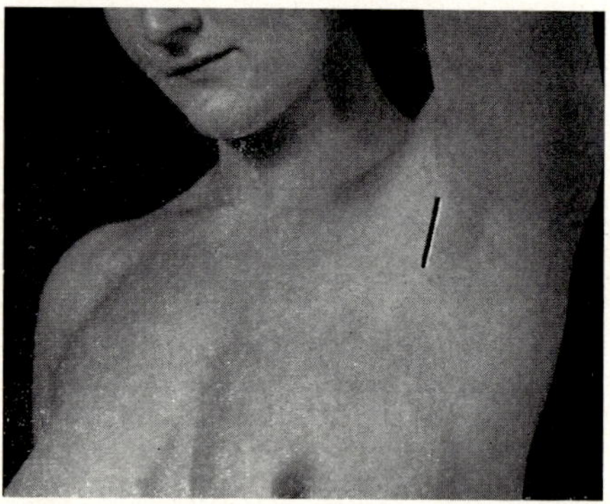

Fig. 329.—An incision for opening a deep-seated axillary abscess.

Hilton's Directions for Opening a Deep Abscess in the Axilla.—Cut through the skin, cellular tissue, and fascia of the axilla about ½ in. (1·3 cm.) behind the axillary edge of the great pectoral muscle. At that part we meet with no large blood-vessel. Then push a grooved director upwards into the swelling in the axilla; if you watch the groove in the director, a little stream of pus will show itself. Take a blunt pair of forceps and run the closed blades along the groove in the director into the swelling. Now open the handles and so tear open the abscess.

In late cases, when the whole axilla is merely a bag of pus, an incision into the lower part of the middle of the space will be found convenient.

BREAST ABSCESS

In dealing with mastitis at the stage of cellulitis a conservative approach is adopted. The patient is confined to bed and a broad-spectrum antibiotic, e.g., tetracycline 250 mg. every 6 hours, is given for 7 days. Locally the breast is supported by a firm bandage and local heat is given to relieve pain. The milk is expressed by the patient. If the infant has been breast-fed for a considerable length of time weaning should be carried out. Stilbœstrol, 10 mg. three times a day, will suppress secretion of milk.

Antibiotics without drainage should not be given if pus is already present (*Fig.* 330). Antibiotics may sterilize the pus in the abscess and a discrete indurated mass may form. It is then not possible to differentiate it from carcinoma. Such a mass has been designated 'antibioma'. When such a condition is met with, exploration with a needle may reveal pus which should be completely removed.

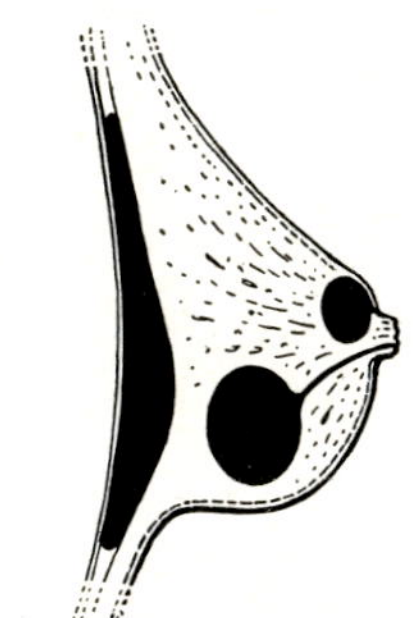

Fig. 330—Subcutaneous, intramammary, and retromammary abscesses of the breast. Intramammary is the common variety.

Operation.—

a. Incision and Drainage.—Drainage is indicated when on emptying the breast of milk an area of tense induration persists. Operation is carried out under general anæsthesia. A radial incision, or a curved one at the areolar-cutaneous junction, is made. A hæmostat is introduced into the breast abscess. On opening the jaws of the hæmostat, pus will ooze out. A specimen is taken for culture. A finger is then introduced (*Fig.* 331) as the hæmostat is withdrawn. All loculi are broken by the finger so that there is now only one large abscess cavity. If the point of entry is not the most dependent one, a counter-incision is made and a drainage-tube is inserted (*Fig.* 332). The dressing is changed on the second day when the drainage-tube is removed. Subsequent daily dressings are carried out until it is completely healed. Antibiotics are given for about 7 days.

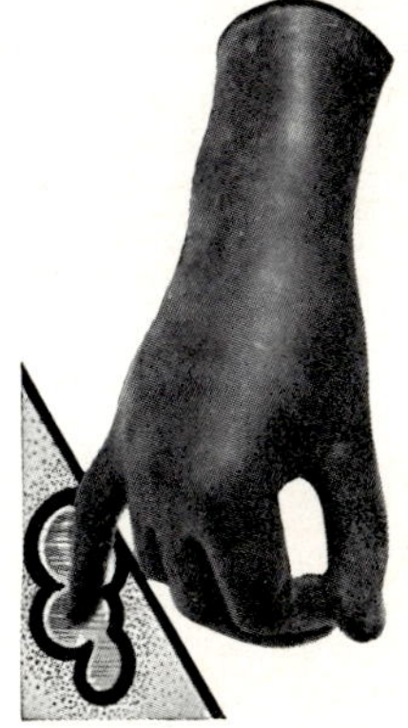

Fig. 331.—A finger is introduced into the abscess cavity in order to search for loculi.

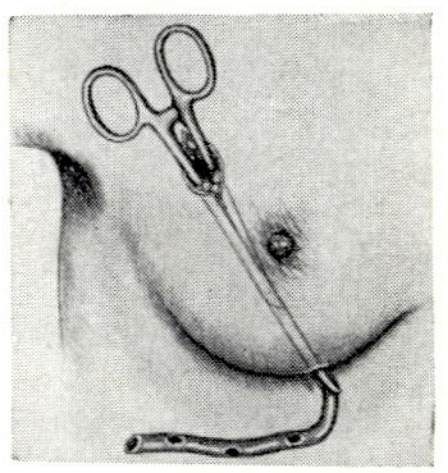

Fig. 332.—If a counter-incision is required the original incision can be closed.

b. Excision and Obliteration.—Complete removal of all dead tissue and obliteration of the resulting cavity are possible with an abscess not extending beyond one quadrant of the breast or behind the nipple. The main abscess cavity and all loculi are opened widely, all dead tissue is removed by sharp dissection, and the cavity obliterated by interrupted stitches. A broad-spectrum antibiotic such as tetracycline is given. The incision is dressed on the third day and stitches are removed on the seventh day. This treatment can be employed in 75 per cent of cases of breast abscess and more than halves the time for complete healing.

ACUTE SUPPURATIVE PAROTITIS

Conservative Treatment.—If infective parotitis threatens, no effort should be spared to cleanse the mouth. In addition to mouthwashes, boroglycerol, applied on a small swab held by forceps, is efficacious. A sialogogue in the form of chewing-gum is a useful adjunct. Before these measures are applied, a specimen of the infected saliva should, if possible, be expressed from Stensen's duct in order that the sensitivity of the organisms can be tested against antibiotics. While awaiting the pathological reports, a course of penicillin should be commenced forthwith. In many instances the principal organism is a staphylococcus. The patient's general condition, especially his fluid and electrolyte status, often requires urgent attention (*see* p. 32).

Operative Treatment.—*Do not wait for fluctuation.* The fascia that surrounds the parotid gland is tense and unyielding. If, after 48 hours, the symptoms show no signs of abating, or before that time in very acute cases, adequate incision is indicated. Blair's method of exposing the parotid gland cannot be bettered. The incision is made in front of the ear. It is a long incision, extending from the zygoma to the angle of the jaw. It passes down to the parotid fascia. The anterior edge of the skin is undercut and pulled forward, thereby exposing practically the whole of the parotid gland (*Fig.* 333). The capsule is incised *transversely*, if necessary in two or three places. Special care is taken not to injure the two main divisions of the 7th nerve. If pus does not flow, a hæmostat is passed into the transverse incision and its jaws opened. This method spares the facial nerve, and allows a virulently inflamed parotid room to expand. A small piece of soft corrugated rubber is laid along the length of the wound. The skin edges are approximated loosely, the drainage material having its exit at the most dependent point.

If necessary, the operation can be performed satisfactorily under local infiltration anæsthesia.

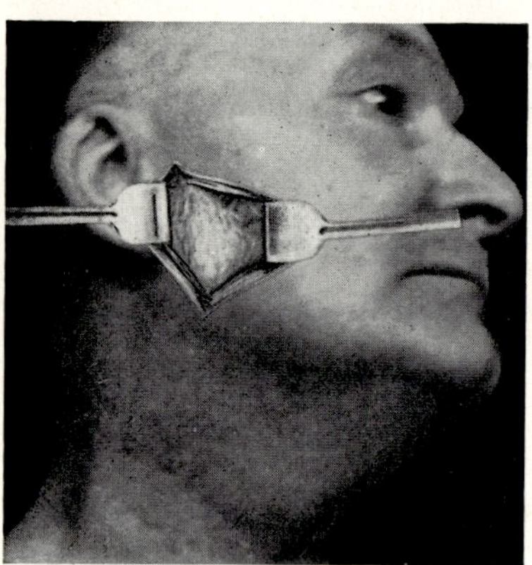

Fig. 333.—The parotid gland exposed through Blair's incision.

TROPICAL ULCERS OR TROPICAL PHAGEDÆNIC ULCERS

Tropical ulcers are some of the most common conditions met with in tropical regions. These ulcers are due to minor trauma and subsequent bacterial infection. They are commonly seen in individuals who are suffering from malnutrition and chronic debilitating diseases, e.g., malaria. They are especially prevalent in countries with a hot and damp climate. Although common among natives, they are occasionally seen in Europeans who do not suffer from any dietetic deficiency.

Pathology.—The ulcer begins with the formation of a bleb or scab. This soon ruptures with discharge of serosanguineous material. With the rupture of this bleb, a slough is exposed. This sloughing process extends in all directions until a well-defined ulcer several inches in diameter is left. The base of the ulcer is formed of necrotic subcutaneous tissue, muscles, or tendons. As most of these ulcers are neglected, they become chronic with marked scarring. The surrounding skin becomes atrophic. In time these ulcers may heal leaving behind paper-thin scars with pigmented edges. These may break down at any time and ulcers with pale bases and devoid of granulations result. Marked deformity with contracture eventually occurs. A small proportion of these long-standing ulcers may eventually undergo malignant change.

Other types of tropical ulcers may be due to specific bacterial, protozoal, fungoidal, and helminthic infections.

Veld Sore.—One of these tropical lesions is the Veld sore. From these ulcers the Klebs-Lœffler bacillus may be grown. Clinically these sores start spontaneously or are superimposed on some abrasions. At first the vesicle is filled with straw-coloured fluid but it soon ruptures leaving a shallow ulcer covered with a thin grey pellicle. There is severe pain and the raw ulcerated area may spread peripherally. In a few weeks it becomes chronic. This lesion now takes a characteristic appearance of a punched-out ulcer with undermined edges.

In a proportion of cases diphtheritic paralysis has been observed with these ulcers. There may be ataxia with loss of knee-jerks, anæsthesia, and inco-ordination.

Guinea Worm.—Parasitic infestations may manifest themselves as sores. The guinea worm may produce a chronic lesion in the skin. This infection is transmitted by an intermediate vector, *Cyclops*, which is a water flea. This water flea is swallowed in contaminated water. In parts of the tropics, water from shallow wells and pools is drunk without boiling and thus infection takes place. The adult worm lodges itself in the subcutaneous tissue. The female adult appears beneath the skin as an inflamed area and, penetrating the surface for the purpose of ovulating, sets up a blister which ruptures. Occasionally the head of the worm emerges. The ulcer causes an intense burning sensation and is relieved by immersion in water. This is due to the discharge of embryos into the water. The embryos are swallowed by the *Cyclops*, so completing the cycle.

Leprosy.—Indolent ulcers in the soles and palms may be due to trophic changes as the result of neural leprosy. These sites are particularly susceptible as the anæsthetic foot is frequently subjected to pressure. There may be other evidence of leprosy. The great auricular nerves are frequently thickened and so are the ulnar nerves. In the latter cases claw hands may be present. The *Mycobacterium lepræ* can be demonstrated from culture of the nasal swab.

Mycetoma (Madura Foot) is caused by a variety of fungi and associated organisms. The disease is common in parts of India and Africa. It is a chronic granulomatous disease of the connective tissue of the foot. The organisms are introduced by a break in the skin and hence are usually found in individuals who go about bare-footed.

The infection begins as a nodule which grows slowly and over periods of years may break down to produce typical sinuses. Serosanguineous discharge with characteristic granules containing the fungi can be produced. The multiple sinuses extend into the deeper structures of the foot and ultimately even the bones may be involved in the destructive process. As the foot enlarges, the long bones undergo atrophy from disuse. X-ray shows expansion of the bone with periosteal reaction and areas of osteoporosis.

Yaws or Frambœsia is caused by a specific spirochætal infection. It is common in South-east Asia, the Pacific Islands, India, and Africa. The disease is transmitted by a species of flies (*Hippelates pallipes*). The organisms are deposited on cuts and abrasions. A papule first develops which later becomes covered by yellowish secretion or scab. Subsequently it becomes ulcerated. In the beginning it is usually single, but crops of papular lesions may appear over the whole body. However, the scalp and the external genitalia usually escape. In the primary lesion, the organisms are best demonstrated by dark-ground illumination using scrapings of an incised papule.

Management of Tropical Ulcers.—In the *investigations* of ulcers the following lines should be taken:—

1. Examination of local discharges. Microscopy of these may reveal the specific organisms. Should suspicion of yaws be aroused a dark-ground illumination may reveal *Treponema pertenue*. If the ulcers are trophic in nature, the palpation of thickened nerves will lead to a diagnosis of leprosy. This can be confirmed by demonstrating the mycobacterium from the nasal secretions. Straining of the secretion with methylene blue may reveal the diphtheroid bacilli, indicating the ulcer is Veld sore. Microscopic examination of the dark granules from discharge of the Madura foot will reveal the causative fungus and thus confirm the diagnosis.

2. Blood examination sometimes may reveal pancytopenia characteristic of hypersplenism which has been found to be associated with some of the cases of tropical ulcers. Such ulcers will heal with splenectomy. Sickle-cell trait has been known to be associated with tropical ulcers in 50 per cent of the cases.

3. Biopsy of the ulcer edge in chronic tropical ulcers may reveal malignant change in such a lesion and hence will influence the treatment.

Treatment of Tropical Ulcers.—

1. *Improvement of General Health.*—General treatment directed towards the improvement of the patient's health should be carried out in every case. Nutritious food rich in vitamins should be given. Most of the inhabitants in the tropics are suffering from chronic protein deficiency. Many never have milk in their diet. Skimmed milk is a valuable source of protein and should be given when available.

2. *Specific Treatment.*—When the diagnosis is established, specific treatment is instituted. Most of the known causes of tropical sores can be treated with the specific antibiotics or by chemotherapy. Yaws respond well to penicillin and tetracycline (p. 74), while Veld sore will heal with antidiphtheritic serum. In guinea worm infestation, the worm can be killed by injecting 1–1000 mercury dichloride solution into it. Under local anæsthesia an incision is made in the skin about the middle of the worm. The dead worm is then extracted with a small strabismus hook.

In tropical phagedænic ulcer, which is by far the commonest of the tropical sores, the organisms are usually sensitive to one of the antibiotics. The benefit derived from the administration of penicillin is most evident in the acute stage of the disease. Within 48 hours the discharge is reduced and granulation tissue begins to form. When the area is large, Thiersch skin-graft will produce rapid healing.

When the ulcer is indolent, an antibiotic is less beneficial. A period of bed-rest and clean dressings with zinc paste will cause healing in a large proportion of cases. If the ulcer breaks down or fails to heal with conservative treatment, the fibrotic ulcer base is excised and full-thickness skin-graft, either by a cross-leg flap or pedicle graft, is done. This is especially applicable when the ulcer is over the tibial region.

SKIN-GRAFTING BY THIERSCH'S METHOD

Skin-grafting by Thiersch's method has a great field of usefulness, and comparatively small granulating areas can be covered with satisfactory grafts without hospitalization. The technique shown pictorially in *Figs.* 334–339 is useful. A really sharp razor (preferably not hollow-ground), a pair of ordinary wooden butter pats, and a probe are the only instruments required.

SURGERY IN PATIENTS WITH HÆMOSTATIC DEFECTS

Investigation of the Patient reported to be a 'Bleeder'.—Although it is true that most patients alleged to have a bleeding tendency, after full investigation, have no discoverable abnormality of hæmostasis, investigation of all suspects is advisable, whether they are for minor or major operations. The patient's history is extremely important and may be practically diagnostic.

In the personal medical history, ask particularly about previous hæmorrhage after tooth extraction, epistaxes, episodes of joint pain and swelling, and major bruising. Contrary to popular belief, most patients with major coagulation defects do not bleed excessively after a minor cut, for instance while shaving. Women almost always overestimate their ease of bruising, men underestimate theirs. A family history of excessive bleeding is sought, especially among siblings and the maternal family, since the major coagulation defects (hæmophilia and Christmas disease) are transmitted as sex-linked recessives.

On physical examination, large bruises, muscle or subcutaneous hæmatomas, and evidence of old, usually multiple joint damage are common in a coagulation disorder, petechiæ and splenomegaly in platelet abnormalities.

The absence of a convincing history or corroborative physical signs does *not* exclude completely a hæmostatic defect, and if elective minor surgery is contemplated, it is wise to have the patient screened hæmatologically, as the problem will almost certainly recur, possibly under more urgent circumstances. If any suspicious finding has emerged, the patient must be referred for hæmatological testing. It is often recommended that some screening tests, e.g., bleeding time and clotting time, be performed by the house-surgeon, but (*a*) the tests may be normal in severe hæmorrhagic disease, and (*b*) the results are rather unreliable except in experienced hands. Markedly abnormal results call for a full investigation. Simple methods for the tests are:—

Bleeding Time (Duke's Method).—The ear-lobe is cleansed, then dried with ether, and pricked with a sterile disposable blood lancet (e.g., hemolet). A stop-watch is started, the drop of blood removed every half-minute with filter paper which does not touch the skin. The time till bleeding stops is noted. Up to 5 minutes is normal; the time is prolonged in capillary or platelet disorders.

Whole-blood Clotting Time (Lee and White method).—This is performed in clean, dry glass tubes of standard size (3 in. $\times$ $\frac{3}{8}$ in. (7·6 cm. $\times$ 1 cm.)), and is done in triplicate. Three ml. of blood are taken by clean venepuncture and a stop-watch started when 1 in. (2·5 cm.) of blood is placed in the first tube. The tubes are kept at 37° C., in a tumbler or beaker if necessary, and gently tilted to the horizontal position at half-minute intervals, till clotting occurs. Vigorous shaking

THIERSCH AND PARTIAL-THICKNESS SKIN-GRAFTING

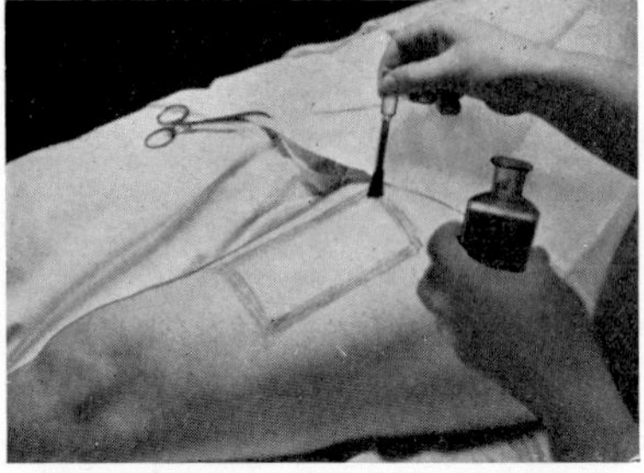

Fig. 334.—The first step is to map out the area from which the graft is to be taken. The edges are outlined with iodine.

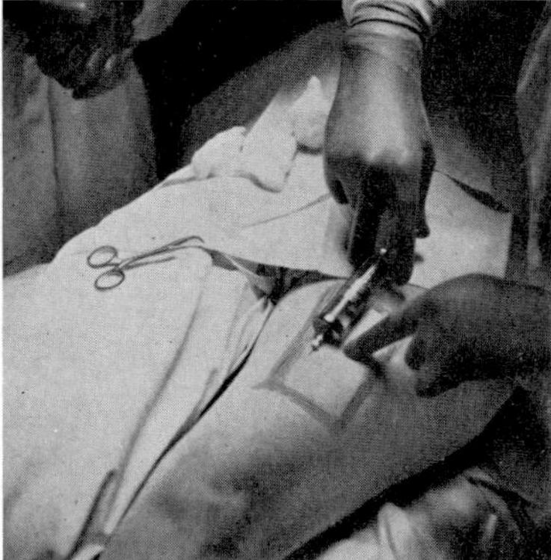

Fig. 335.—The marked area is infiltrated with local anæsthetic. Had it not been mapped out, it would be difficult to tell which part was anæsthetized and which was not.

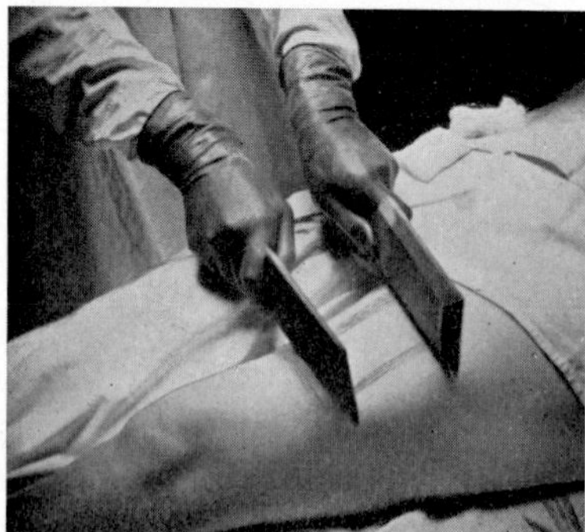

Fig. 336.—The anæsthetized area of skin is stretched forcibly. A pair of ordinary butter pats, which have been sterilized by boiling, are drawn apart steadily and then held firmly in place.

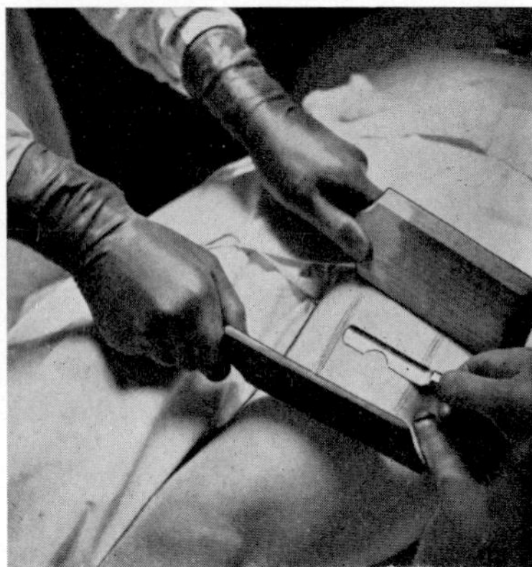

Fig. 337.—With the skin stretched to the fullest degree, the graft is cut with a very sharp razor, moist with saline solution. A sawing movement is used and care is taken that only skin is removed.

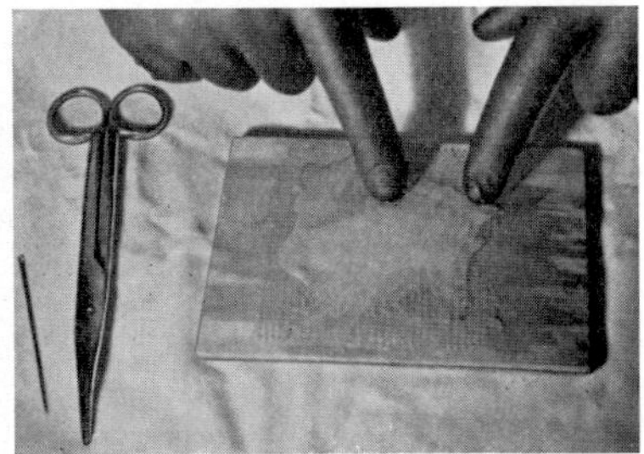

Fig. 338.—Each graft is about 1 in. (2·5 cm.) square, and one by one they are transferred to the surface of a piece of tulle gras, which has been cut to the shape of the area to be grafted. The grafts, as they lie on the tulle gras, must have their raw surfaces uppermost.

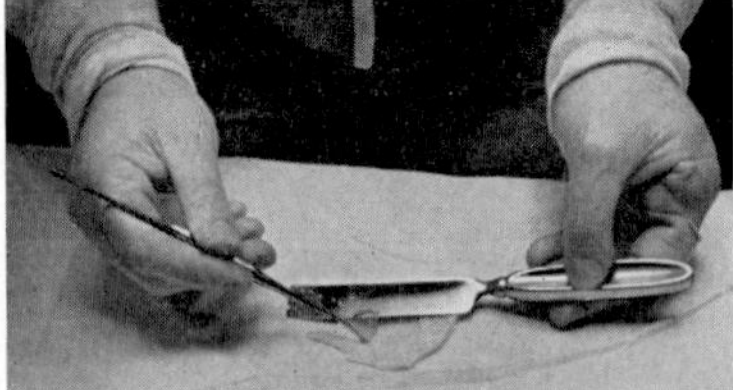

Fig. 339.—The piece of tulle gras covered with the grafts is laid skilfully on the area to be grafted. A few layers of dry gauze are placed over the tulle gras, which in turn are covered firmly with flexible adhesive plaster. The area from which the graft was taken is covered with tulle gras and a dry dressing. The dressings are not disturbed for a week.

vitiates the results. Up to 10 minutes is normal; a prolonged time indicates a severe coagulation defect.

Lastly, patients with previously proved major hæmorrhagic diseases are issued with, and should carry, a small diagnostic card or book, giving details of their disease and the consultant to be contacted.

MANAGEMENT OF A 'BLEEDER' DURING SURGERY

1. Wounds and Minor Surgery.—The commonest cause of excessive bleeding after minor surgery is surgical failure to secure hæmostasis. If the patient has a generalized hæmorrhagic disease, temporary control may be obtained in suitable sites by local pressure, e.g., in a tooth socket or limb incision. Local coagulant therapy should be tried if the wound is small and accessible. Tubegauz or oxycel soaked with thrombin, or stypven (Russell viper venom) mixed with dilute adrenaline for vasoconstriction, has the advantage of not obscuring a hæmato-logical diagnosis. It is, however, essential not to persist with repeated local applications where hæmorrhage is continuing and a hæmostatic defect is likely, as much tissue bruising and damage will result.

In a patient known to have a major hæmostatic defect, e.g., hæmophilia or thrombocytopenia, no surgery should be undertaken without help from the hæmatology and blood transfusion services. In hæmophilia, pre-operative infusion of a blood product containing antihæmophilic factor (Factor VIII, AHF), such as fresh-frozen plasma, cryoprecipitate, or Factor VIII concentrate, is required, and this will usually be followed by a daily dose of the product for several days. Such patients must be kept under surveillance for many days post-operatively. The bleeding in a coagulation disorder is characterized not so much by its severity as by its persistence; in a badly managed patient, severe anæmia results from even minor surgery. Never give an injection intramuscularly to a hæmophiliac.

Patients on oral anticoagulant therapy having elective minor surgery are usually advised to miss 24 hours' therapy before and 24 hours' therapy after the operation. In thrombocytopenia, elective minor surgery is avoided in the acute condition, or if the platelet count is less than 40,000 per c.mm. in the chronic disease. A patient with idiopathic thrombocytopenic purpura is very likely to be on corticosteroid therapy (*see* Chapter XXXII) which requires dose adjustment over the time of surgery.

2. Hæmatoma and Hæmarthrosis.—Patients with hæmophilia may present with large hæmatomas or hæmarthroses. These lesions usually require intravenous Factor VIII therapy, and aspiration of a hæmarthrosis, rarely required except for severe pain, should be performed *only* under such cover, with hæmatological supervision and with full aseptic precautions.

3. Major Surgery.—Major emergency surgery in a 'bleeder' is a daunting prospect, but some measures can reduce the risks. In idiopathic thrombo-cytopenic purpura (the usual operation being splenectomy), corticosteroids with or without ACTH may reduce the bleeding time, and fresh blood in plastic bags (therefore platelet-rich) immediately pre-operatively may make operation safer. The effects of oral anticoagulant therapy can be quickly reversed by intravenous synthetic vitamin K—the prothrombin time returns to normal in half an hour—but there is a definite risk of new thrombosis in the originally affected blood-vessel. The management of a hæmophiliac requiring major emergency surgery follows the lines mentioned previously, but daily replacement Factor VIII therapy must be continued for some weeks.

Tubegauz (The Scholl Manufacturing Co., 182–204 St. John's Street, London, E.C.1).
Oxycel (Parke, Davis & Co., Staines Road, Hounslow, Middlesex).

CHAPTER XXXV

THE MANAGEMENT OF THE GYNÆCOLOGICAL PATIENT

By C. E. B. RICKARDS

Fixing the Date for the Performance of a Gynæcological Operation.—During the reproductive phase of life the planning of a gynæcological operation is to a large extent influenced by the menstrual cycle (*Fig.* 340). As a rule operations upon the uterus, and particularly those involving a considerable loss of blood

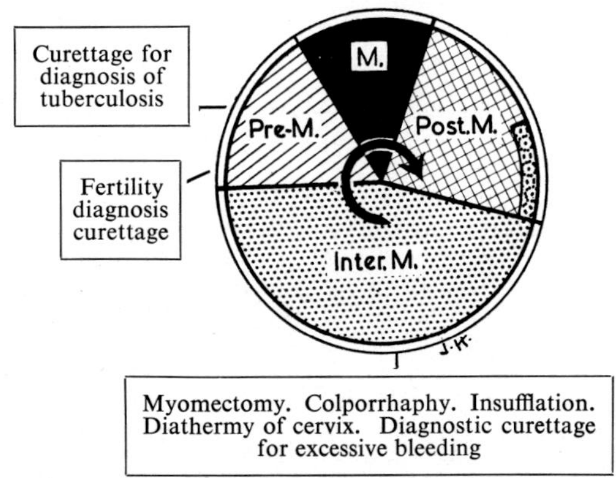

Fig. 340.—The phases of the menstrual cycle and their important bearing on the dates on which certain operations should be arranged. There is some difference of opinion regarding the best time to carry out diagnostic curettage.

such as myomectomy, are best performed during the intermenstrual phase. In cases of protracted menstrual loss this precept cannot always be observed, but at least the full flush of the monthly period can be avoided. It is most inadvisable to perform any plastic operation upon the vagina during menstruation because the menstrual blood, the congestion, and the increased coagulation time all contribute to obscuring the field, thereby rendering the operation unnecessarily difficult. Diagnostic curettage carried out during the reproductive phase of life with the object of ascertaining the cause of irregular or excessive menstruation should *not* be carried out when the patient is menstruating, because at this time usually very little endometrium is obtained. In cases where curettage is to be carried out as one step in the investigation of infertility it should always be performed during the secretory stage because only at this time can histological evidence be obtained that ovulation is proceeding. In investigations of infertility it should be known that subclinical tuberculosis is an important causative factor, and the typical giant-cell systems are most likely to be discovered during the premenstrual phase of a cycle; at this time, too, better specimens can be obtained for guinea-pig inoculation. A detailed inquiry as to the dates of the last menstrual period must be made in all patients upon whom curettage is proposed. To perform curettage on a patient whose period is overdue may be tantamount to procuring abortion. Deep radial diathermy coagulation of the cervix uteri must never be carried out when the patient is menstruating, because of the risk of incurring serious post-operative hæmorrhage. Because of the danger of producing air embolism, tubal insufflation must never be performed in the presence of uterine bleeding, however slight.

Admission to Hospital.—In many gynæcological departments it is the practice to admit patients for hysterectomy, colporrhaphy, or for more minor procedures, on the day prior to operation. Inasmuch as patients are spared the anxiety of a protracted pre-operative wait, this tradition has something to recommend it. On the other hand, the disadvantages of the system are that an 18–24-hour pre-operative stay in hospital barely gives sufficient time for laboratory investigations, a radiograph of the chest, and, should it be required, a physician's assessment of the patient's general condition. Moreover, if other problems have arisen since the patient's name was entered on the waiting-list for a particular operation, it is possible that the extent, or even the nature, of that particular operation will have to be revised, in which event there is but little time to discuss the matter with the patient and her relatives.

History.—It must be remembered that the house-surgeon's own recorded history of the newly admitted patient, coupled with his findings on physical examination—always important—are doubly so when the interval between the patient's last attendance at the out-patient department and her admission is longer than one would have wished. Should the history or physical signs elicited by the house-surgeon be in any way at variance with those recorded in the out-patient notes, the surgeon-in-charge should be notified as soon as possible. At this juncture it will be helpful to remind the newly appointed house-surgeon of some special points in taking the history of a gynæcological patient.

Marital Status and Religion of the Patient are factors that must be taken into consideration in decisions concerning some gynæcological conditions. While no doubt these entries will have been made already on the patient's case-history sheet by the clerical or nursing staff, the house-surgeon will do well to note them.

The Menstrual History must include: (*a*) age of onset; (*b*) usual duration of the flow; (*c*) amount of the loss—scanty, moderate, or profuse; (*d*) presence or absence of dysmenorrhœa—if present, its relation to the menstrual cycle, its duration, and the age at which it commenced must be ascertained; (*e*) absence or presence of intermenstrual discharge—if present, the amount, the colour, and whether or not there is an unpleasant odour must be recorded.

Previous Obstetrical History.—In relevant cases an account of pregnancies, confinements, and puerperia must be ascertained and recorded.

Previous Operations.—Details of any previous pelvic operation are very important. For instance, when adhesions from a previous pelvic operation are likely to be present hysterectomy by the vaginal route would be a most unwise choice.

It should be noted that although these special points are of cardinal importance, they must not monopolize the clinician's entire attention. On the contrary, it is just as necessary to interrogate the patient concerning her family history (especially in regard to tuberculosis) and previous illnesses as it is before a patient undergoes an operation on any other part of the body. While the house-surgeon's notes naturally will disclose his findings of an examination of the pelvic viscera and related parts, they should also bring out in strong relief the result of his:—

General Examination of the Patient, which will include the findings on examination of the heart and the lungs, the abdomen, and gross reflexes. Because thrombophlebitis is a common complication after pelvic operations, it is most necessary to find out if any venous abnormality is present. The urine is examined, and when the patient has lost much blood as a result of abnormal menstruation, or looks anæmic, a red-cell count is carried out. Should the red-cell count be low and/or the operation is likely to entail a considerable loss of blood, arrangements for the provision of matched blood should be made in good time. In this connexion the house-surgeon is reminded that all Rh-negative female patients *must* be transfused with Rh-negative blood, and, because of the demand, this is sometimes in short supply.

Thus it is evident that it is upon the result of the house-surgeon's findings that an up-to-date assessment of the patient's fitness to undergo the proposed operation is made; it is also possible that as a result of his general examination certain post-operative complications can be anticipated. If, in his opinion, the house-surgeon feels that the operation should be postponed until certain aspects of the case are clarified or remedied, he should lose no time in letting his chief know what seems to him (the house-surgeon) to be the safer course.

Consent for Operation.—A fuller account of this extremely important matter will be found on p. 102. Attention will be directed here to those special aspects of what constitutes consent for the performance of a gynæcological operation that may jeopardize reproductive activity or interfere with the patient's capacity to have intercourse. In such cases, in addition to the written consent of the patient, it is advisable to obtain the *written consent of her husband.* It is also highly important that the house-surgeon should realize that in event of litigation the mere possession of a stereotyped consent form bearing signatures may be ruled as insufficient evidence that the patient and her husband did, in fact, understand the nature of the operation which the patient was to undergo. On the other hand, to be able to produce in Court a brief handwritten statement to the effect that the whole matter was explained by the house-surgeon, signed by the patient and her husband, and witnessed by a state registered nurse will quash allegations that the plaintiffs did not understand. These pre-operative discussions and preparation of documentary evidence are time-consuming and this is another good reason why the patient should be admitted early enough to obviate the plea that the parties concerned were 'rushed' into giving their permission for the operation to be performed.

Significance of a Coincidental Vaginal Discharge.—While a patient is sometimes admitted solely for an investigation of the cause of a vaginal discharge, attention is directed here to a vaginal discharge not obviously linked with the condition for which the patient was admitted.

A certain amount of vaginal discharge is normal. The branching glands of the healthy cervix secrete mucus, the amount and viscosity of which vary with the phase of the menstrual cycle. In addition there is constant desquamation to cells from the multilayered vaginal epithelium. When the œstrin content of the circulating blood is within normal limits these desquamated cells give rise to a white, curdy substance, the amount of which also varies according to the phase of the menstrual cycle as well as from woman to woman. Whether such a discharge is noticed or complained of depends upon the sensitivity and standard of personal hygiene of the woman herself. Discharges other than these require investigation (*see* p. 500).

Like normal discharges, pathological discharges can arise from the cervical canal or from the vaginal walls, or both. Also it must be remembered that the urethra may be the primary seat of an infection giving rise to a vaginal discharge.

An Excessive Discharge of Colourless Mucus is due to over-activity of the glands of the cervix uteri. The contraceptive pill may cause it.

A Semipurulent or Purulent Discharge resulting from infections of the cervix is slimy, opaque, and yellow in colour, or tinged with yellow.

The presence of either of these discharges may be the reason why the patient has been admitted to hospital.

Usually the cervicitis that gives rise to these discharges is treated by deep radial diathermy coagulation of the walls of the cervical canal. On the other hand, when a purulent or mucopurulent vaginal discharge is discovered in a patient who has been admitted for some procedure designed to overcome sterility, such as tubal insufflation, the surgeon must be informed. Doubtless he will order that the proposed operation be postponed, because if it is undertaken in the presence of cervical infection there is a possibility that infected material will be transported from the lower to the upper genital tract, and give rise to salpingitis.

Of the pathological discharges that come from the vaginal walls the most common are those due to *Trichomonas vaginalis*, *Candida albicans*, a fungus, undetermined infections, or to senile changes in the vaginal epithelium.

A Discharge due to Trichomonas vaginalis, which is extremely common, is usually profuse, watery, and pale yellow in colour; sometimes it contains small bubbles, believed to be due to an associated gas-forming micrococcus. In addition to the discharge, the patient complains of local discomfort and often of intense pruritus vulvæ. On examination with a speculum the vaginitis is found to be most pronounced in the upper part of the vagina, and particularly in the posterior fornix. In these regions the vaginal epithelium is patchily reddened.

A Discharge due to Candida albicans (thrush) tends to occur in patients who are pregnant and those who suffer from glycosuria, but there are many exceptions to both these predisposing factors. Usually no sign of discharge is seen when the vulva is inspected, but on digital examination of the vagina thick cheesy material will be discovered on withdrawal of the finger.

An Indeterminate Infection may be due to *Streptococcus*, *Staphylococcus aureus*, or other organisms, and on examination with a speculum a general reddening of the vaginal walls will be observed.

A Discharge consequent upon Atrophic Vaginitis is common in elderly women in whom the ovaries have ceased to function adequately. The layers of the vaginal epithelium are much reduced in number and the canal becomes vulnerable to infection. The vaginal walls are smooth and fragile, and small hæmorrhages into the epithelium are often present, particularly in the region of the external urinary meatus. The desquamated vaginal epithelial cells are small, contain little glycogen, and have irregular, crenated edges. It is on these, and not on the bacteriological findings, that the diagnosis is confirmed.

Microscopical Examination of a Vaginal Discharge.—In all cases where a profuse discharge exists a specimen should be examined under the microscope and sent for culture. The *Trichomonas vaginalis* (*Fig.* 341) can be seen in a high-power field, and this investigation can be carried out by the house-surgeon.

20

The mycelial threads of a *Candida albicans* (syn. *Monilia*; thrush) infection can be seen after staining (*Fig.* 342) and being grown on suitable culture media.

Acute or subacute *Trichomonas vaginalis* should be treated with arsenical pessaries or flagyl before an elective operation is undertaken. In all but urgent

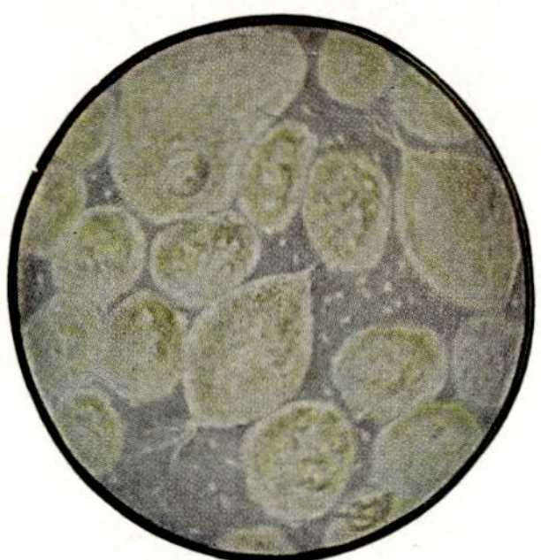

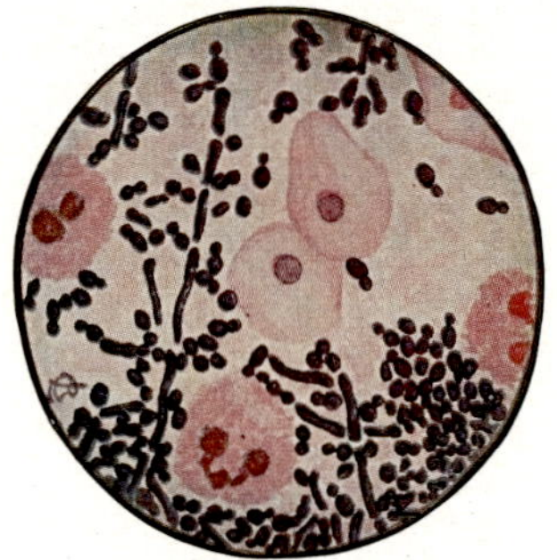

Fig. 341.—*Trichomonas* from a vaginal discharge (unstained).

Fig. 342.—*Candida albicans* (Gram's stain).

cases severe vaginal moniliasis must be controlled with topical applications of gentian violet or, better, mycostatin (nystatin) vaginal pessaries before operation is carried out.

Women with a discharge due to senile vaginitis are often admitted to hospital for investigation of post-menopausal bleeding, and whether an operation is delayed or not on account of vaginitis depends very much on the circumstances of the individual case.

A Gonococcal Discharge.—Comparatively rarely, and usually in a younger woman, an infection due to the *Neisseria gonorrhœæ* will be discovered, in which event pus can be expressed from the urethra and/or purulent material will be seen on the cervix. The method of obtaining specimens from each of these sites is described on p. 501, and the method of staining and recognition of the causative diplococcus in Chapter XLVI. Unless an emergency exists, the gonorrhœa must be treated before the operation is undertaken.

It is necessary to keep the question of a vaginal discharge in a gynæcological patient awaiting operation in proper perspective. Often it is a part of the condition for which the patient has been admitted, and operation must only be postponed when the reasons for such postponement are valid.

Procidentia Ulcer (known formerly as a 'decubitus ulcer') is not due to friction or pressure on the prolapsed portion of the vagina while the patient lies in bed (decubitus), but to inadequacy of the blood-supply to the most dependent part of the procidentia. Such an ulcer is nearly always benign, clear-cut, and is seldom infected. There are two facts to remember about such an ulcer. The first is that it is not invariably benign, and careful histological scrutiny must be carried out on the excised specimen. The second is that if the ulcer is clean and well within the area it is proposed to excise in the course of a plastic operation, the presence of such an ulcer predisposes neither to infection nor to delayed healing. Therefore there is no necessity to cancel, or even to postpone, the operation when the ulcer lies within the excision zone. On the other hand, should the ulcer be large or infected, then the procidentia must be reduced and antiseptic pessaries and douches given until signs of gross infection have abated and until the ulcer has diminished to such a size that it no longer impinges upon the limits

Flagyl (May & Baker Ltd., Dagenham, Essex).
Nystatin (E. R. Squibb & Sons, Twickenham, Middlesex).

of the proposed excision. It is thought by many that œstrogens taken by mouth or applied locally improve the blood-supply to the part and accelerate healing of the ulcer.

Points in investigating Gynæcological Patients who also complain of Urinary Symptoms.—Some form of urinary trouble is complained of in a large proportion of gynæcological patients. The most common of these symptoms are increased frequency, dysuria, urgency, or stress incontinence. Except for the last, such symptoms can be wholly or partially functional.

Increased Frequency.—It is important to find out whether this is nocturnal as well as diurnal. When the patient is compelled to rise from her bed more than once during the night the cause is likely to be physical. In all cases where there is even a suspicion of infection a mid-stream specimen (*see* p. 446) or, failing that, a catheter specimen of urine must be obtained and examined bacteriologically before operation.

Stress Incontinence.—In cases of stress incontinence the degree of the disability must be assessed. In the minor forms a small amount of urine escapes only in the presence of a full bladder and a cough, sneeze, hearty laugh, or heavy lifting, all of which cause a sudden rise in intra-abdominal pressure. In the worst cases, even when but little urine is present in the bladder, there is almost constant dribbling.

When stress incontinence occurs in the absence of laxity of the anterior vaginal wall cysto-urethrography should be carried out in order to assess the efficiency of the internal vesical sphincter. In such cases, if there is radiological evidence of poor internal sphincteric control, one of many operations to create an effective urethral sphincter may well offer the best prospect of a cure.

Before any operation for stress incontinence is even contemplated, the house-surgeon is reminded that it is his duty to make sure that the patient's incontinence is a mechanical one, and not due to an underlying neurological lesion.

PRE-OPERATIVE CARE

Bowels.—Patients for colporrhaphy or for vaginal hysterectomy may be given an enema on the night before operation. Many hospital patients scheduled for abdominal hysterectomy or another intra-abdominal gynæcological operation are subjected to the same routine, but in some hospitals the pre-operative administration of an enema has been given up in favour of the insertion of a suppository (*see* p. 406).

Vagina.—Patients for abdominal hysterectomy or a vaginal plastic repair receive a douche on the night before operation. This is followed by the insertion of an antiseptic or an antibiotic vaginal pessary as high as the finger will reach. By rendering the vagina as clean as possible the incidence of post-operative infection and secondary hæmorrhage is diminished.

Sedation.—It is important that anxiety should be allayed and sleep ensured; consequently a sedative, usually a barbiturate, is prescribed (p. 104).

Skin Preparation.—In some hospitals it is still the practice to shave the pubic hair, wash and paint the skin, and cover the abdomen with a sterile towel on the night before the operation (p. 135). In cases of emergency this preparation is carried out in the anæsthetic room or in the operating theatre after the patient has been anæsthetized.

Special Preparation for Cases of Rectovaginal Fistula.—A course of antibiotic or sulphonamide effective against bowel organisms is commenced five days prior to operation (p. 77). It is essential that the lower bowel should be empty at the time of operation; consequently a rectal washout is given before the patient is conveyed to the operating theatre.

Special Preparation for a Case of Vesicovaginal Fistula.—Success in the treatment of this condition is most frequent following the first attempt. Failure is sometimes due to undertaking operative repair in the presence of a urinary infection. Therefore if on laboratory examination the urine is found to be infected the operation must be postponed until the urine is sterile. It is also necessary for the vagina to be well nourished and free from infection. Low-pressure vaginal douches (the pressure must be low to avoid forcing fluid into the bladder) are helpful in this respect. Even if the urine is sterile, it is advisable to commence a course of a suitable sulphonamide (*see* Chapter VI) before operation.

Pre-operative Routine in the Operating Theatre.—
Lithotomy Position.—During the preliminary measures about to be described the lithotomy position is adopted. If it is possible that the operation will be performed via the abdomen the legs are held in abduction by nurses, and the foot of the table is lowered. Should it be certain that the operation will take place via the vaginal route the leg supports are fixed to the table and the lithotomy position is maintained mechanically. In either event it is important that the thighs should be raised gently and simultaneously and that excessive abduction be avoided (*see* p. 149).

Catheterization.—Whether the patient is for abdominal section or for a vaginal operation, she must be catheterized on the operating table. A silver or a plastic catheter should be used for this purpose, and all the precautions to prevent transmitting infection into or along the urethra described in Chapter XXXIII must be taken. The house-surgeon should remember that in the fully anæsthetized patient the bladder wall is likely to be atonic and the organ cannot be emptied completely unless suprapubic pressure is applied. Especially when abdominal panhysterectomy is to be performed, it is essential to express every millilitre of urine, otherwise the avoidance of wounding the bladder when dissecting that organ from the cervix uteri will be rendered more difficult.

Bimanual Examination.—After catheterization it is imperative for the surgeon to carry out a thorough bimanual examination. This must be performed even in the most obvious cases of prolapse because, as a result of the relaxation of the abdominal musculature afforded by anæsthesia, palpation of the internal generative organs is greatly facilitated, and consequently the findings may differ from those recorded in the patient's notes. In this connexion it should be recalled that sometimes prolapse of the uterus or the vagina is associated with other pelvic pathological conditions.

After the examination, if the patient is for abdominal hysterectomy the vagina must be cleansed thoroughly, and most operators like to have the vaginal walls painted with an efficient coloured antiseptic such as merthiolate solution, or Bonney's blue.

Special Precautions when a Vaginal Operation is to be performed.—The vagina and pudendal regions are douched thoroughly with a non-irritating antiseptic solution. The parts are then dried and painted with a coloured antiseptic. If the case to be operated upon is one of rectovaginal fistula, the anal canal and the lower rectum are douched with 5 per cent dettol solution before the operation is commenced.

POST-OPERATIVE CARE

Occasions when a Vaginal or a Uterine Pack is inserted after the Operation has been concluded.—
Vaginal Pack (*Fig.* 343).—It is still the practice of many surgeons to insert a light gauze pack moistened with flavine emulsion into the vagina following colporrhaphy, vaginal hysterectomy, and diathermy coagulation of the cervix. The gauze absorbs much of the early post-operative oozing. Twenty-four hours after insertion the pack is removed with due gentleness.

Uterine Pack.—An intra-uterine pack is employed only to control excessive uterine hæmorrhage, such as occurs occasionally after abortion or removal of

Dettol (Reckitt & Colman Ltd., Hull, Yorks).

a hydatidiform mole. The pack is left in situ for 24 hours; sometimes it is advisable to give 0·5 mg. ergometrine intramuscularly before its removal.

Post-operative Care: All Cases.—

Stage of Recovery from a General Anæsthetic.—During the stage of recovery from a general anæsthetic the care which must be bestowed on a patient who has undergone a gynæcological operation is no less (or more) than that which is necessary for a patient who has undergone any other lower abdominal or pelvic operation of a similar magnitude (p. 106).

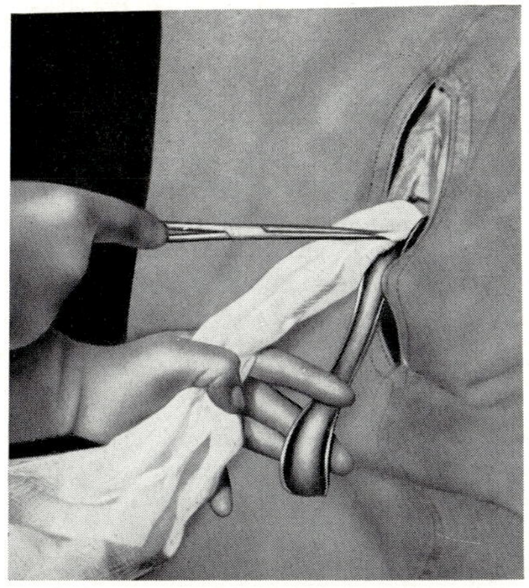

Fig. 343.—Insertion of a vaginal pack following diathermy coagulation of the cervix uteri.

Post-operative Sedation is also similar to that described in other chapters.

Posture; Leg Exercises; Early Ambulation.—After the patient has regained consciousness she is placed in a comfortable sitting posture. Movements in bed are not restricted except in exceptional circumstances, notably when a plastic operation has been performed and it is feared that non-restriction of certain movements will result in undue tension on the suture line. With this exception, early movements of the legs are especially important, for they aid in the prevention of pelvic and femoral thrombosis. Early rising is the rule, and most gynæcological patients are assisted out of bed for a short period on the 2nd or 3rd post-operative day, and thereafter are allowed up for an increasingly longer time. In nearly all gynæcological services routine exercises under the supervision of a physiotherapist are carried out. Gynæcological operations are followed by a higher incidence of thrombophlebitis than that which might be expected in some of the other surgical wards. For these reasons the gynæcological house-surgeon must be vigilant in organizing preventative measures and in conducting frequent careful examinations of the patient's legs, especially the groins and calves.

Post-operative Care of the Bladder.—Following an abdominal gynæcological operation it is rare for the patient to have difficulty in passing urine. On the other hand, as a result of reflex causes or local bruising, post-operative retention of urine is extremely common after a vaginal operation such as anterior or posterior colporrhaphy. All gynæcological surgeons agree that on no account should overdistension of the bladder be allowed to occur. They are, however, divided in the matter of how best to deal with the problem. Many insert a self-retaining urethral catheter at the close of the operation. Others, arguing that retention of urine is not invariable, instruct their house-surgeon to insert a self-retaining catheter if the hoped-for spontaneous micturition does not materialize. The management of the self-retaining catheter does not differ from that described in Chapter XXXIII, except perhaps in one particular. Because so often in gynæco-logical patients a functional element exists (they are convinced that they will not be able to pass urine lying down) it is a good plan to prescribe a tranquillizer such as chlorpromazine (largactil) 25 mg. t.d.s. on the day before and on the day on which it is proposed to remove the indwelling catheter.

When an operation for a vesicovaginal fistula has been carried out an indwell-ing catheter must be left in place for 7–10 days, and in these cases active suction drainage (which will evacuate every drop of urine as soon as it enters the repaired bladder) and the administration of a suitable antibiotic are likely to help in preventing breakdown of the bladder suture line and reformation of the fistula.

Care of the Bowels.—Enemata are unpleasant for the patient and their admini-stration is time-consuming and disagreeable for the nurse; also it is possible that they are a source of cross-infection by enterococci and other pathogens. Although they are given in the obstetric wards to patients who have undergone Cæsarean section, because patients who have been delivered in this way are particularly prone to distension, post-operative enemata now are hardly ever needed in the gynæcological wards, where reliance is placed on the administration of liquid paraffin or agarol, and if the bowels have not been opened by the evening of the third day, an evacuant suppository is inserted (p. 406).

Care of the Vagina.—

1. *Special Cases.*—In patients who have undergone colporrhaphy or diathermy coagulation of the cervix, in order to reduce post-operative odour and discharge it is advisable to instil a paste containing sulphonamide (sultrin (triple sulfa) cream) high into the vaginal canal on the second day following operation. Special plastic applicators are used for placing the paste into position.

2. *Routine Care of the Vagina and Vulva.*—In most cases, and particularly when sulphonamide paste has been inserted into the vagina, douching during the post-operative period is contra-indicated. The vulva should be swabbed gently night and morning, and dried with a sterile swab. The application of alcohol-containing antiseptics is unnecessary and painful. In cases where infection supervenes, usually the patient will complain of tenderness, and more often than not the recorded temperature will show at least some irregularity. In relatively virulent infections reddening, œdema in the vicinity of the wound, and a discharge, often, but not necessarily, offensive, will occur. A swab from the upper part of the vagina must be obtained for full bacteriological investigation, including culture and sensitivity of the organisms to antibiotics, which are then prescribed.

Care of the Abdominal Wound.—Among gynæcological surgeons it is tradi-tional to use Michel's clips for closing the skin incision. In many services, tension sutures have been discontinued. After closure the wound can be sprayed with nobecutane, which on drying forms a transparent waterproof veneer, in

Largactil (May & Baker Ltd., Dagenham, Essex).
Agarol (William R. Warner & Co. Ltd., Eastleigh, Hants).
Sultrin (Triple Sulfa) Cream (Ortho Pharmaceutical Ltd., Saunderton, High Wycombe, Bucks).
Nobecutane (Duncan, Flockhart, & Evans Ltd., Birkbeck Street, London, E.2).

which event no other dressing whatsoever is applied. Patients do not object to this practice, which has the advantage that no abdominal bandage is required, and the upper abdomen and the thorax are left completely free. Patients breathe better and move more freely when this method is employed.

Michel's clips are removed with a special instrument on the sixth or seventh day. The practice of removing alternate clips on one day and the remainder on the next is to be deprecated, as women are often apprehensive about the procedure and there is no necessity for them to be subjected to it twice. In a nervous patient a tranquillizer, or pethidine 100 mg., should be given intramuscularly one hour before the removal of the clips. Tension sutures are removed on the tenth day, or sooner if they are cutting into the skin.

Post-operative Hæmorrhage can either be (*a*) reactionary or (*b*) secondary.

a. Reactionary Hæmorrhage occurs during the first 24 hours following operation, and is due to the blood-pressure rising to its pre-operative level after a fall that occurred during the operation and continued for some time afterwards.

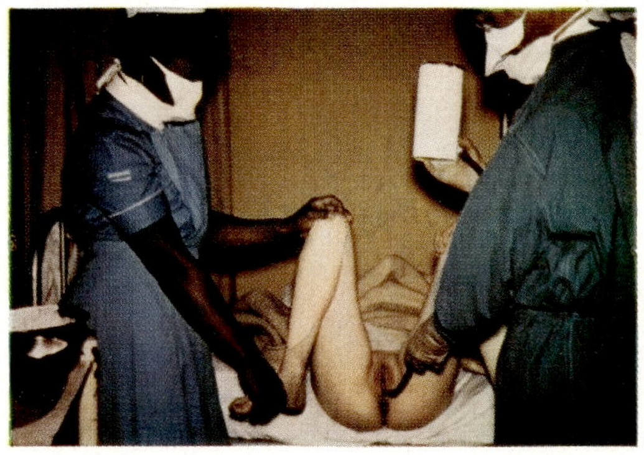

Fig. 344.—Reactionary hæmorrhage. Giving a hot douche to a patient in bed.

If the reactionary loss is not severe, the patient is placed under the close supervision of a special nurse who records the pulse-rate and the blood-pressure every half-hour. Morphine 15 mg. is also administered. If the hæmorrhage is severe, it is always wise to return the patient to the operating theatre and search for the bleeding point. In some cases it may be considered that the loss can be controlled by vaginal douching and plugging. The douche at 47·2° C. (117° F.) is given with the patient in her bed as soon as the morphine has taken effect. To give this douche the patient is placed across the bed, her thighs being held in the lithotomy position by two assistants (*Fig.* 344). A right-angled vaginal retractor is then slipped along the posterior vaginal wall, and blood and clot are washed out with the hot solution. Following this, sterile gauze from a 6-in. (15-cm.) roll is packed into the vagina (*see Fig.* 343), the pack being inserted along the tongue of the retractor otherwise pain and shock will be produced. This procedure is followed by a pad being placed over the vulva and kept in position with a T-bandage.

b. Secondary Hæmorrhage is a result of infection of the wound, and occurs between the seventh and tenth post-operative days. The bleeding occurs suddenly

Pethidine (Roche Products Ltd., 15 Manchester Square, London, W.1).

and usually is brisk, although it may be heralded by a slight warning hæmorrhage. Prompt active measures are imperative. Morphine is administered *statim*. Arrangements for blood transfusion are made. Before giving the vaginal douche, a specimen is secured by passing a swab on a holder high into the vagina. The swab is sent for a full bacteriological examination. If, as is usually the case. the hot douche controls the hæmorrhage, the vagina is packed fairly firmly. Occasionally bleeding is due to a spurting artery, and it is then necessary to take the patient to the operating theatre and to ligate the bleeding vessel. In all cases, while awaiting the bacteriological report antibiotic therapy is given.

Examination prior to Discharge from Hospital.—The house-surgeon must examine the patient before permitting her to leave hospital. If hysterectomy has been performed a vaginal examination must be carried out, and any undue thickening or tenderness recorded in the notes. It is also necessary to perform a vaginal examination on patients who have had colporrhaphy performed. In this instance often adhesions have formed between the anterior and posterior walls of the vagina; these can be broken down digitally. Another important consideration is that occasionally a swab or a pack has not been removed from the vagina, and this will be detected and removed, thus sparing a lot of trouble for all parties concerned.

ARRANGEMENTS FOR FOLLOW-UP

All patients who have been operated upon in the gynæcological department should receive instructions to report in four to six weeks after they leave hospital. On the occasion of their post-convalescence attendance, the vaginæ of those who have undergone abdominal total hysterectomy must be palpated with especial care. The vagina should feel soft and pliable at its upper end. A speculum is then inserted. In many cases small red granulations will be discovered running transversely across the roof of the canal. These give rise to a dark blood-stained discharge. Such granulations can be removed with a sharp curette in the out-patient department. In examining patients who have undergone colporrhaphy, attention is again directed to the fine adhesions that may occur between the anterior and posterior vaginal walls. This may be the last opportunity to break down these still friable adhesions digitally, for eventually they become too tough so to do.

GYNÆCOLOGICAL PROCEDURES AND MINOR OPERATIONS

Speculum Examination.—Familiarity with the use of the vaginal speculum is indispensable for gynæcological examination and treatment. It can only rarely be used with an intact hymen. The rules to remember are:—

1. It must be warmed and lubricated, but, if cultures are required, no antiseptic must be used.

2. The anterior or urethral aspect of the introitus is very sensitive, so during introduction press the speculum backwards against the posterior or perineal aspect, or first pull the perineum backwards with a finger in the vagina.

3. Good light must be available.

Sims's Speculum.—This can only be used in the lithotomy or lateral position with the legs well flexed.

It is introduced as shown in *Fig.* 345, and then rotated as in *Fig.* 346. With backward traction on the perineum, a good view is obtained of the cervix and anterior vaginal wall. The posterior vaginal wall can be viewed during withdrawal. It has the disadvantage, however, that in the lateral position, especially in obese patients, the upper buttock has to be lifted out of the way (*Figs.* 345, 346), and if a cystocele is present it obstructs the view and a vaginal depressor has, rarely, to be used to keep it out of the way (*Fig.* 347).

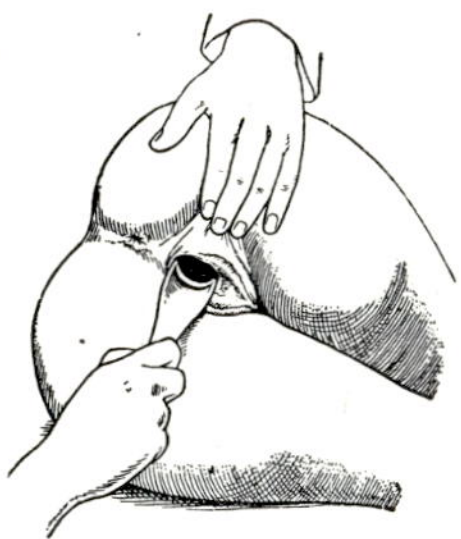

Fig. 345.—Introducing a Sims's speculum.

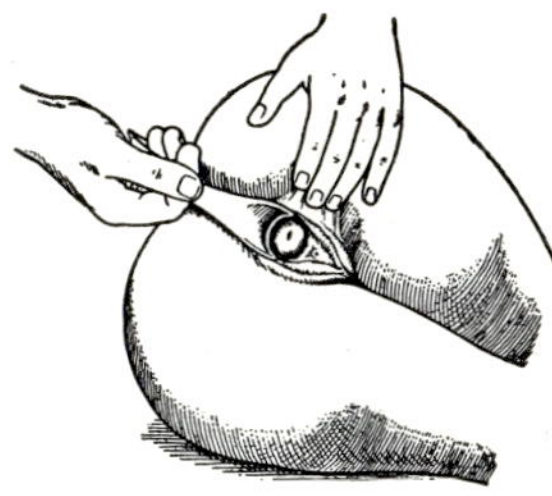

Fig. 346.—Showing Sims's speculum in place and the cervix exposed.

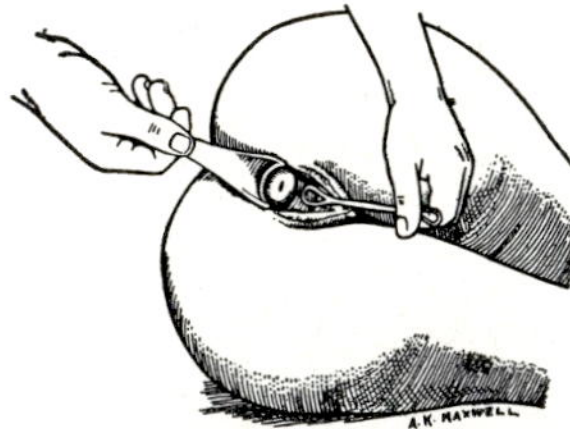

Fig. 347.—When the anterior vaginal wall bulges forwards a vaginal depressor aids in obtaining a good view of the cervix.

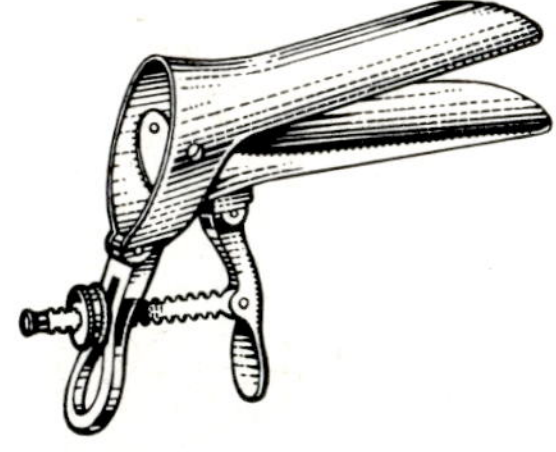

Fig. 348.—Bivalve speculum.

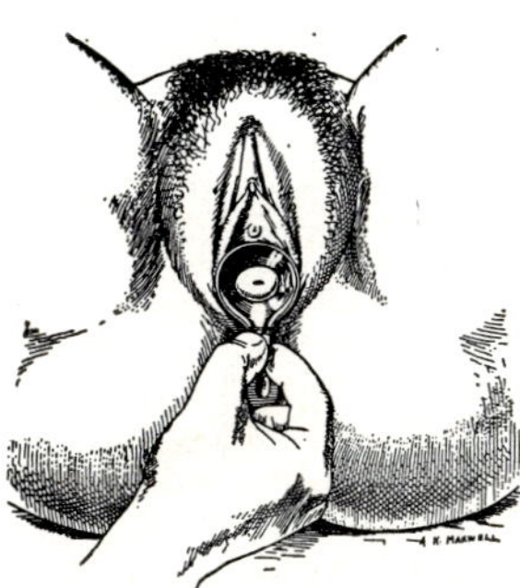

Fig. 349.—Cusco's bivalve speculum in use.

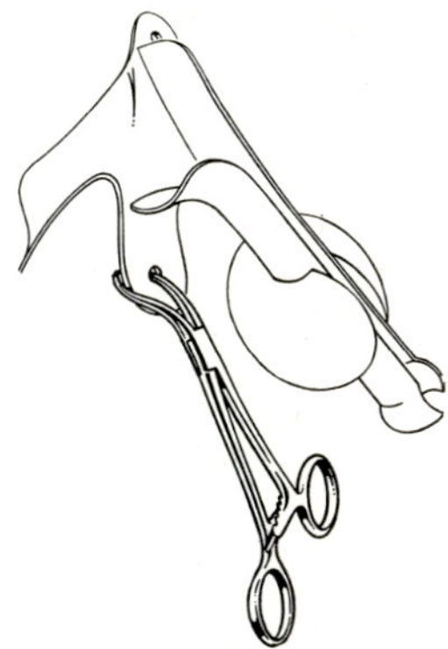

Fig. 350.—Auvard's speculum, modified.

Bivalve Speculum (*Fig.* 348).—This is perhaps the most useful speculum for routine investigation.

It is easier to introduce than Sims's speculum, gives a better view of the vagina and cervix, and can be used with the patient in the dorsal as well as the lateral and lithotomy positions. It is introduced with the closed blades parallel to the labia, and when fully inserted, the handle is rotated backwards and the blades opened (*Fig.* 349). In the dorsal position the handle can be rotated anteriorly if it is more convenient for the operator. By slowly withdrawing the speculum, a view of the whole vagina can be obtained.

Auvard's Speculum (*Fig.* 350).—This is, as a rule, only suitable for use in operative gynæcology, with the patient anæsthetized. A useful minor modification is to have a hole drilled in each wing. On each side one prong of a towel clip can be passed through this hole and secured to towels to prevent it falling out (*Fig.* 350).

PURULENT VAGINAL DISCHARGE: OBTAINING SPECIMENS FOR BACTERIAL EXAMINATION

Equipment.—Useful equipment is shown in *Fig.* 351. Two sterile swabs on sticks are required, one for the cervix and one for the urethra. If they are not long enough to reach the cervix, they can be held in a sponge-holder (*Fig.* 352).

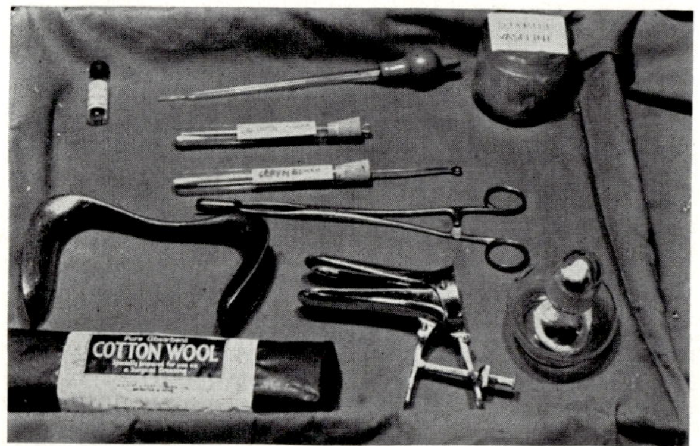

Fig. 351.—In addition to specula, the equipment for obtaining specimens of vaginal discharges is shown.

Other equipment is a pipette, a small bottle of sterile normal saline solution, a jar of sterile petroleum jelly (many water-soluble lubricants are unsuitable as they contain antiseptic or are not isotonic with the vaginal secretion), and some cotton-wool.

Technique.—The external genitalia are inspected; any redness or excoriation suggests either *Trichomonas vaginalis* or thrush. If the latter is suspected glycosuria must be excluded, as thrush tends to occur in the presence of sugar. The speculum is then lubricated with petroleum jelly and introduced.

Vaginal Discharge: Macroscopical Appearance.—*See* p. 490. A blood-stained discharge suggests cervical erosion, polyp, cervical carcinoma in the woman who has borne children, or senile vaginitis in the post-menopausal patient.

Method of obtaining Specimens of Discharge.—In *Trichomonas vaginalis*, if the discharge is copious, it will collect in the hollow of the speculum. The latter is withdrawn and the discharge dropped on to a slide. If less copious, 0·5 ml. of saline is squirted from the pipette into the posterior fornix, mixed with the discharge with the end of the pipette and then drawn up and transferred to a slide. A cover-slip is then applied and the specimen examined microscopically immediately or within half an hour. The *Trichomonas* organism is larger than a pus cell, is actively motile, and should be easily recognized (*Fig.* 341, p. 492). Warming the slide a little increases this motility.

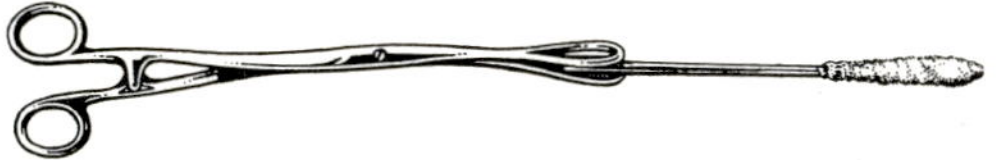

Fig. 352.—Method of using a throat swab to obtain a specimen of discharge from the cervix.

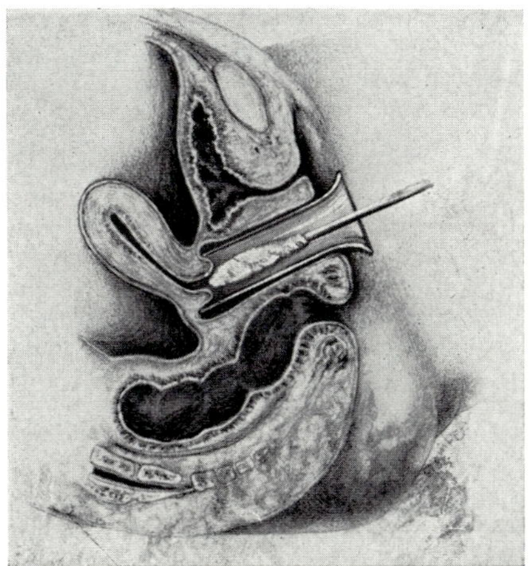

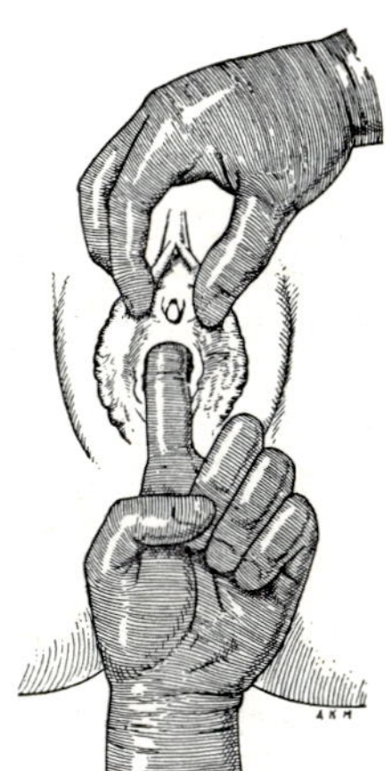

Fig. 353.—Taking an *endo*cervical specimen of discharge.

Fig. 354.—Expressing pus from the urethra.

When the discharge is mucopurulent and comes from the endocervix it is advisable to exclude gonorrhœa, a condition much less common than previously in gynæcological practice. A vaginal smear is useless for this purpose. Such a smear must be taken from the endocervix. The cervix is wiped clean and a throat swab inserted into the cervical canal, rotated, and withdrawn (*Fig.* 353). Care must be taken not to contaminate it with the vaginal wall. It is then smeared on a glass slide and sent to the laboratory for staining. If a culture is required, the swab itself is sent to the laboratory. When gonorrhœa is suspected, a smear should also be taken from the urethra. The latter is wiped clean and milked downwards with the gloved finger (*Fig.* 354). Any discharge will then appear at the orifice, and a smear is taken with another swab.

TREATMENT OF VAGINAL DISCHARGES

Gonorrhœa.—Gonorrhœa is diagnosed by the demonstration of Gram-negative diplococci in smears of urethral and cervical discharges, and by a gonococcal complement-fixation test. Concomitant syphilis should be excluded by appropriate serological tests.

Treatment.—While the resistance of gonococci to penicillin has increased in many parts of the world, a single injection of 600,000 units procaine penicillin G is still generally effective. Alternatively, oxytetracycline, 250 mg. four times a day for 4 days, may be given.

No local treatment is necessary, but diagnostic tests should be repeated before and after the next menstrual period.

Trichomonas Vaginalis.—Pessaries such as S.V.C. or penotrane are very effective; one pessary is inserted night and morning as high in the vagina as possible. There is usually symptomatic relief within two or three days, but treatment should be continued for four weeks. Even so, recurrence is common, and the reason for this is not known. It may be that the *Trichomonas* is harboured in some inaccessible place, like the endocervix, urethra, or even rectum, or that reinfection is taking place during coitus. All these hypotheses are speculative. In recent cases a course of treatment lasting for a month or six weeks, and continued during menstruation, may be tried. Flagyl (metronidazole) given for 8 consecutive days to the patient *and* her consort, in a dose of one 200-mg. tablet t.d.s., has been found to be highly effective. In most departments this has now become the standard treatment. For resistant cases antiseptic pessaries containing chloramphenicol, in addition to other ingredients, may be tried.

Thrush.—This condition quickly responds to painting the vaginal canal with 1 per cent aqueous solution of gentian violet. This treatment should be carried out on alternate days. It is effective but inconvenient, and stains the patient's clothing. The condition also responds to pessaries such as nystatin or penotrane. One is inserted night and morning for a week. Again recurrence is common, and it is particularly liable to occur when glycosuria is present. It is a frequent concomitant of diabetes and occurs often in pregnancy.

Senile Vaginitis.—This occurs post-menopausally or after the ovaries have been removed surgically. It is due to thinning and atrophy of the vaginal epithelium. Stilbœstrol, 0·5 mg. b.d. for 12 days, cornifies the epithelium, but it may also hypertrophy the endometrium and very occasionally give rise to uterine hæmorrhage. Œstrogen pessaries, one inserted into the vagina at night for 12 days, or œstrogen creams, are equally effective and do not usually cause endometrial bleeding. It is a good plan to keep these patients on maintenance doses of œstrogen administered locally in the form of pessaries. One pessary used every week indefinitely usually keeps the vaginal canal healthy.

Prepubertal Vaginitis.—Like the senile vagina, the prepubertal vagina is not markedly cornified and therefore not resistant to infection. A smear should always be taken to find the causative organism. This can be obtained by doing a rectal examination and massaging the vagina downwards. Pus will then appear at the vaginal orifice and a smear can be taken with a throat swab. Any foreign body, like a small bead, which the child may have introduced into the vagina, may also be felt by rectal examination. Stilbœstrol, 0·25 mg. b.d. for 10–12 days, with penicillin, usually results in a cure. Local treatment is not necessary and should be avoided.

Cervical Erosion.—Here the portio of the cervix is covered with a single layer of columnar epithelium indistinguishable from that which is normally present

---

S.V.C. (Stovarsol Vaginal Compound) and flagyl (May & Baker Ltd., Dagenham, Essex).
Nystatin (E. R. Squibb & Sons, Twickenham, Middlesex, and New Brunswick, New Jersey, U.S.A.).
Penotrane (Ward, Blenkinsop & Co. Ltd., Wembley, Middlesex).
Œstroform Pessaries (British Drug Houses Ltd., Graham Street, London, N.1).

in the canal itself. The affected area presents as a bright red, velvety patch. The lesion can occur in the virgin, but is commoner in parous patients and may coexist with lacerations (ectropion) or a mucous polyp. Biopsy of the cervix should precede treatment to exclude early carcinoma or carcinoma in situ. Either multiple wedges or a cone biopsy can be taken.

CAUTERIZATION OF THE CERVIX

The most efficient method of treating an erosion is by cautery or by a diathermy needle. In all but the most superficial cases (which can be treated by cauterization), a general anæsthetic is required. Having passed a speculum and applied a vulsellum to the cervix, cauterization is carried out either by radial incisions about $\frac{1}{8}$ in. (3 mm.) deep, starting at the external os and extending to the edge of the erosion, or by a series of local pin-point applications. Occasionally cauterization with silver nitrate or copper sulphate will effect a cure in a small erosion. Cauterization leaves a sloughing ulcer which takes about 6 weeks to heal, during which time a discharge is present. There is a slight risk of ascending infection and, to avoid this, the safest time for cauterization is 5–6 days after menstruation has ceased. At least 3–4 months must be allowed for a post-partum erosion to heal spontaneously before considering cauterization. It must be borne in mind that many erosions occurring in the early weeks following childbirth are physiological and do not call for any special treatment.

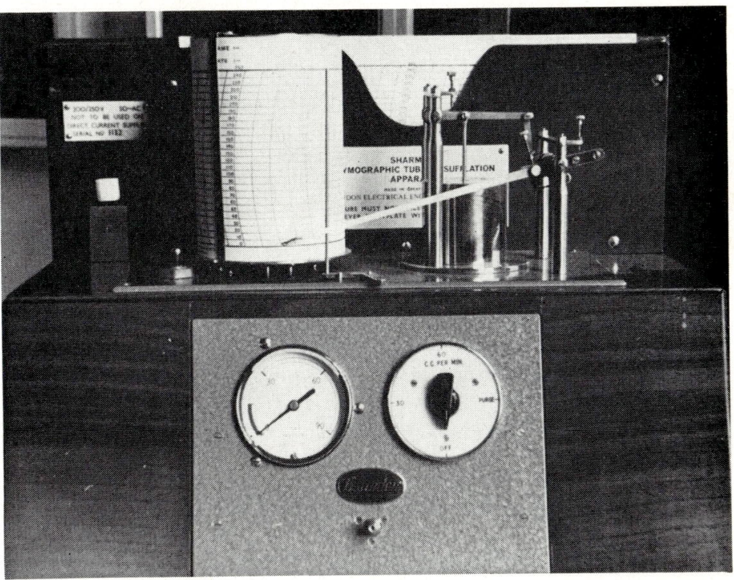

Fig. 355.—Rubin's apparatus for tubal insufflation.

INVESTIGATION OF A CASE OF STERILITY

Either husband or wife, or both, may be at fault in these cases and it is probably wisest to examine a specimen of the husband's semen before subjecting the wife to any investigation. It is collected in a sterile test-tube (not a condom) and examined within 2 hours. If it contains adequate numbers of actively motile sperms, the wife is then examined.

In the wife it is necessary to know: (1) if the tubes are patent; (2) if not patent, where the blockage occurs; (3) if ovulation is occurring; (4) the activity of spermatozoa after coitus—Hühner's test.

1. Insufflation.—The American worker Rubin has claimed much for the therapeutic value of this test, but it is being regarded with less enthusiasm than formerly in many gynæcological departments. The optimum time for carrying it out is about 7 days after a period. Cervical sepsis should be cleared up before it is undertaken.

The patency of the Fallopian tubes may be tested by passing carbon-dioxide gas through them. Rubin's apparatus (*Fig.* 355), or a modification of it, is easy to use.

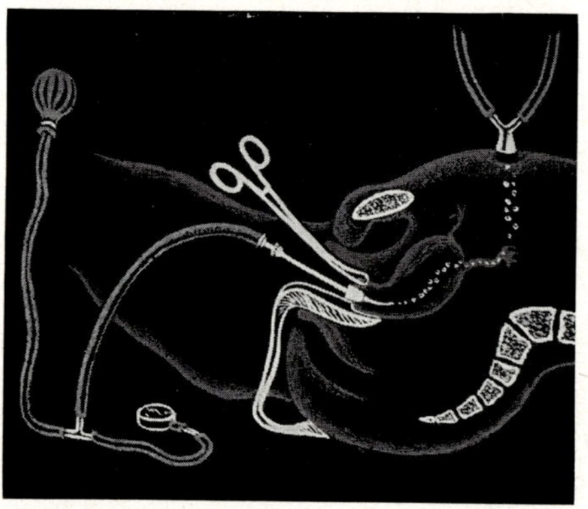

Fig. 356.—The principles involved in insufflation for testing the patency of the Fallopian tubes.

Technique.—Before starting it is wise to test the apparatus and see that there are no leaking connexions. With the patient in the lithotomy position, the vagina is swabbed out with cetavlon or dettol, and a lubricated Sims's speculum then passed. The cervix is seized with a vulsellum, swabbed clear of mucus, and again painted with an antiseptic. A uterine sound may now be passed to note the size and position of the uterus, and a suitable nozzle then introduced. The flange is pressed firmly against the cervix to ensure an air-tight connexion, and the apparatus turned on. If the tubes are patent, gas should pass through at a pressure of about 80 mm. Hg and can be heard as a soft hissing sound by an assistant auscultating with a stethoscope in each iliac fossa (*Fig.* 356). When gas passes through the Fallopian end of the tubes into the peritoneal cavity, the pressure in the manometer ceases to rise. To the inexperienced, a leak at the cervix may be mistaken for gas passing through the tubes. If this is suspected, the head of the table can be tilted down and the vagina filled with sterile saline. Any leak through the cervix will then produce obvious bubbling.

Usually gas passes through at a pressure of about 80 mm. Hg, but occasionally there is spasm of the tube walls or it is just possible that the sides of the tubes

Cetavlon (I.C.I. Ltd., Pharmaceuticals Division, Macclesfield, Cheshire).
Dettol (Reckitt & Sons Ltd., Hull, Yorks).

may be lightly adherent. In such cases the operator may raise the pressure very gradually up to 200 mm. Hg.

At high pressure, however, there is a risk of introducing a considerable quantity of gas into the peritoneal cavity if the tubes do eventually open and there is said to be a slight risk of embolus. Shoulder-tip pain indicates that gas has collected under the diaphragm, but this symptom is not serious and soon disappears.

2. Hysterosalpingography.—Injection of a radio-opaque solution into the uterus usually gives a very good idea of its size and shape, and shows if the tubes are patent or blocked. Should such blockage occur a good indication of its site can be obtained.

Lipiodol gives a satisfactory shadow, but it may remain in the peritoneal cavity for several months. Newer preparations such as endografin are preferable, as they are absorbed much more rapidly. The syringe and nozzle shown in *Fig.* 357 will be found satisfactory in most cases, and the technique of introduction is similar to that used in insufflation. It is essential to get a tight

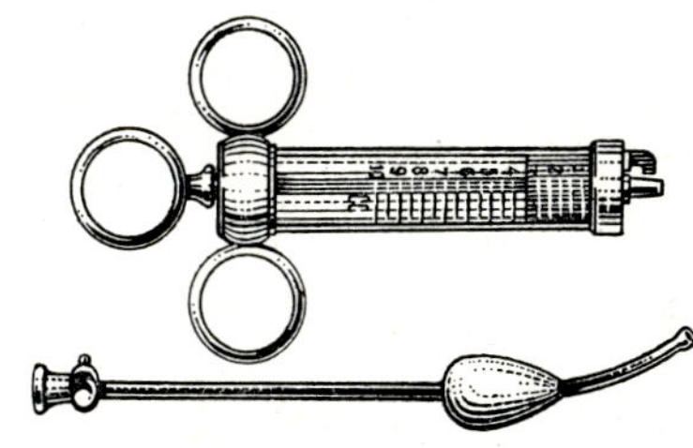

Fig. 357.—McCurrich's modification of Everard Williams's hysterosalpingography syringe.

seal between the nozzle and the cervix, as only small quantities of the medium are injected, and it easily escapes back through the cervix. For this reason, the operator may prefer to use Leech-Wilkinson's cannula (*Fig.* 358), which is

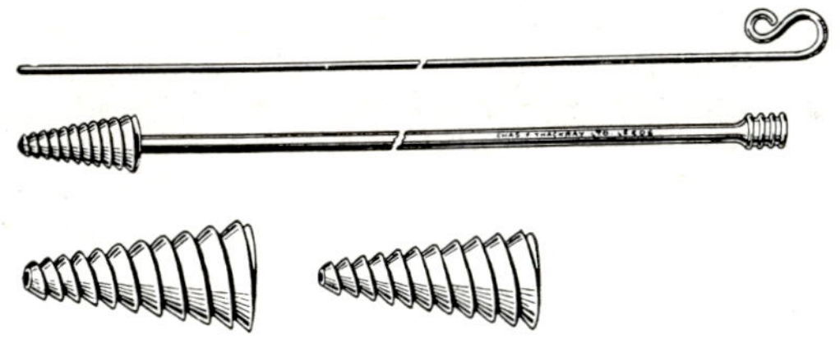

Fig. 358.—Leech-Wilkinson's cannula.

screwed into the cervical canal and ensures a tight seal. This can be used with a Record syringe. The procedure is best carried out on the X-ray table and viewed under the fluorescent screen. It is advisable to have a torch handy when working in the dark. An anæsthetic is not essential, but most operators still find it desirable to use one. A suitable cannula is introduced, and then connected to a 10 ml. syringe containing the medium. A firm hold is kept on both the cannula and the vulsellum while the patient is being placed in position under the fluorescent screen.

The medium is then slowly injected and, if the seal is satisfactory, not more than 10 ml. need be used. The radio-opaque solution should be seen filling the uterine cavity and tubes if they are patent, and in normal cases the solution spills over into the peritoneal cavity. If the uterus is retroverted, an oblique or lateral view may have to be taken in order to see the tubes. When the view

Endografin (Pharmethicals (London) Ltd., Burgess Hill, Sussex).

is satisfactory, a film is taken, and it must be developed before the nozzle is disconnected in case more medium has to be injected. (*Figs.* 359, 360.)

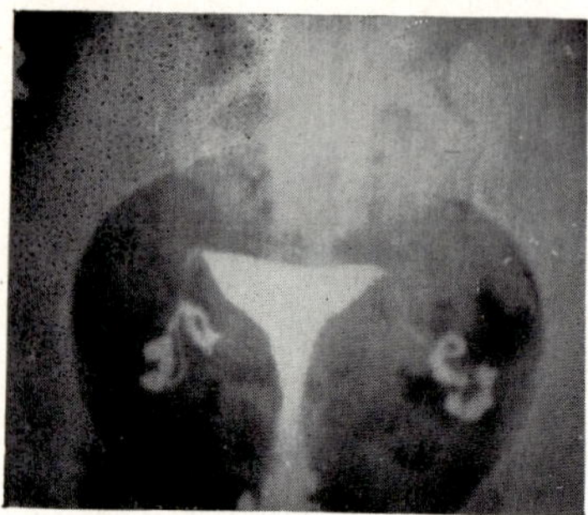

Fig. 359.—Normal hysterosalpingograph.

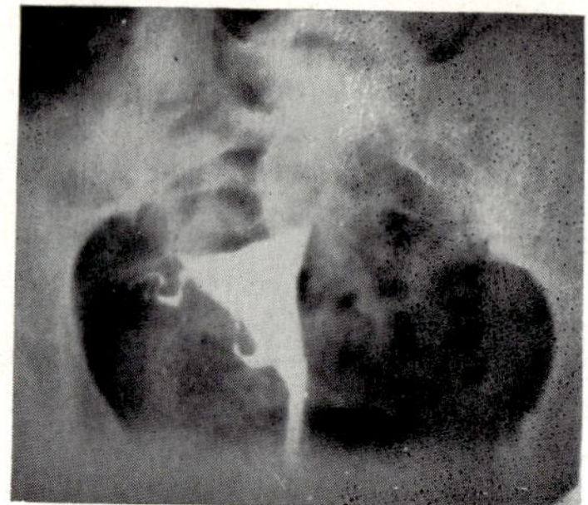

Fig. 360.—Left Fallopian tube blocked and right Fallopian tube patent.

Difficulties and Dangers associated with Insufflation and Uterosalpingography.—

Shock.—Occasionally when an instrument is passed into the uterus and the patient is unanæsthetized, collapse may occur.

Sepsis.—Latent infection may be reactivated or introduced during the procedure, resulting in salpingitis or peritonitis.

Air and Lipiodol Embolus.—This is most likely to occur when high pressure is used and when the endometrium is not intact, e.g., after curettage, and in the immediate pre- and post-menstrual periods. (*Air Embolus, see* p. 8.)

3. Biopsy of Endometrium.—

a. Ovulation Test.—A biopsy of the endometrium carried out as an out-patient or office procedure may be done, with proper antiseptic precaution, in order to find out whether the patient has ovulated during the present menstrual cycle. No anæsthetic is required. A biopsy curette such as Randall's (*Fig.* 361)

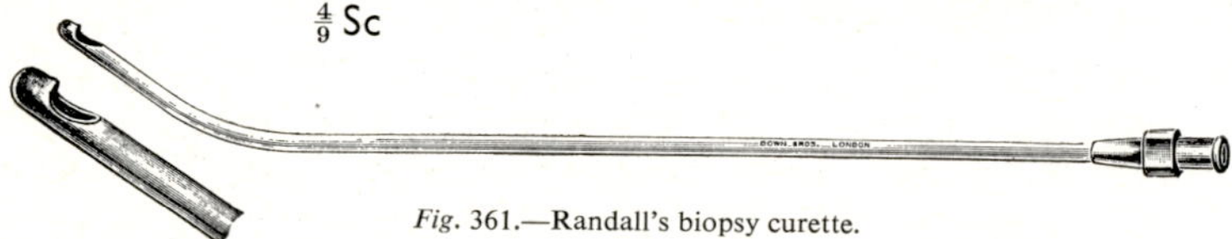

Fig. 361.—Randall's biopsy curette.

is introduced through the cervix to the fundus of the uterus and drawn down sharply. The curette is then withdrawn, and a syringe containing normal saline attached. The strip of endometrium in the lumen is then injected into formol saline and sent for histological examination. When the specimen reveals a secretory or progestational pattern of endometrium, it indicates that a corpus luteum is present and therefore that ovulation has taken place.

b. Rough Test for Carcinoma of the Endometrium.—A Randall's curette may also be used to recover a biopsy of the endometrium in cases of suspected carcinoma. A positive finding is of great value, but it must be remembered that only one small slice of endometrium has been removed and that a cancer elsewhere may have been missed. If the biopsy is negative and cancer is suspected, a thorough curettage must be performed.

c. In cases of *suspected metropathia* a specimen of endometrium can be obtained in this manner and sent to the laboratory for examination. It must be remembered, however, that specimens of endometrium obtained from different parts of the uterus at the same time may show differing histological patterns and too rapid conclusions must not be drawn from examination of a single specimen.

4. Hühner's Test.—This investigation is designed to show the presence or absence of sperms in the vagina and cervix after intercourse. The patient is instructed to report within 2 hours of intercourse. She is placed in the lithotomy position and a Sims's or bivalve speculum is inserted without lubrication or antiseptics. Using pipettes, as for vaginal discharge, specimens are obtained from the posterior fornix and from the cervical canal. Separate pipettes are used and a drop from each examined under the microscope. The spermatozoa collected from the posterior fornix are frequently dead, but there should be 5–10 actively motile sperms per high-power field in the specimen derived from the endo-cervical canal.

POPULATION CONTROL WITH INTRA-UTERINE DEVICES

Intra-uterine contraception theoretically meets a need not available with other methods since it requires only initial motivation and a few minutes of

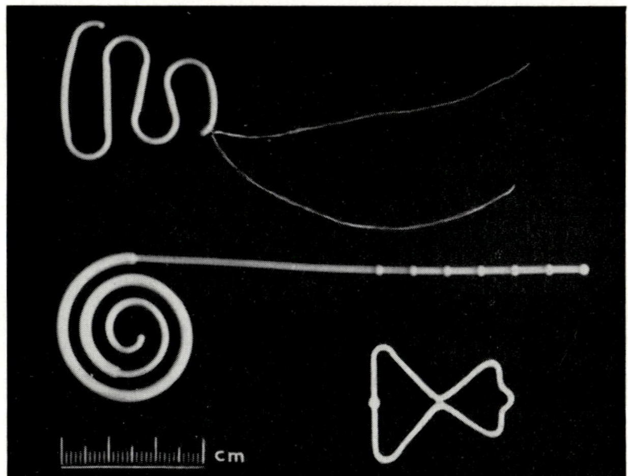

Fig. 362.—Intra-uterine contraceptive devices: plastic loop (*above*), spiral, and bow (*below*).

medical time to provide years of effective, reversible birth control at low cost. The availability of synthetic materials with low tissue reactivity has eliminated the need to remove and replace intra-uterine devices at frequent intervals.

Complications such as sepsis, intra-uterine perforation, abnormal bleeding, pain, and ectopic pregnancies have been reported. These are mainly related to those devices with a transcervical stem, serious complications being rare with a completely intra-uterine device inserted by a person trained in the technique and who can recognize contra-indications to their use.

Contra-indications.—Rigid exclusion of patients with pelvic inflammatory disease or even with a history of pelvic inflammation is important. Abnormal bleeding should be investigated and corrected before insertion of an intra-uterine contraceptive device (IUCD).

The Timing of Insertion.—This is disputed, but probably insertion shortly after menstruation would avoid insertion during an early pregnancy; following pregnancy insertion at the post-partum visit six weeks after delivery is reasonable.

Technique of Insertion.—A number of different designs are available. The spiral, or loop, and the bow (*Fig.* 362) are made of linear polyethylene and are inserted into the uterine cavity through a thin tube less than 4 mm. diameter. The position of the uterus is determined by pelvic examination. The size and direction of the uterine cavity can be assessed with a uterine sound. The tubular insertor containing the spiral, loop, or bow is inserted along the cervical canal through the internal os and the device is pushed from the insertor tube into the uterine cavity by means of a plunger. The use of a tenaculum on the cervix is usually unnecessary. Very occasionally slight dilatation of the cervical canal to 4 mm. may be required.

Removal.—Devices with cervical extensions (e.g., spiral and loop) are easily removed, even by the patient. A completely intra-uterine device (e.g., bow) is removed by the operator inserting a hook-shaped instrument into the uterus. This requires more skill than insertion. Attention should always be paid to the manufacturer's detailed instructions.

CHAPTER XXXVI

MANAGEMENT OF ANORECTAL CASES

By H. E. LOCKHART-MUMMERY

MANY anorectal lesions are both extremely painful and very embarrassing. In this chapter advice is given to the junior hospital doctor on their investigation and management. The comfort and speed of recovery of patients with such lesions are greatly increased by attention to detail. Guidance is also provided for the lone practitioner working far from a main hospital who may have to perform operations on the anorectal region.

RECTAL EXAMINATION

Before proceeding to rectal examination of any patient it is essential that the patient should have been examined lying on his back, so that the general condition can be assessed and the abdomen and groins can be carefully examined and palpated. Rectal examination should then be carried out with the patient in the left lateral position; the patient's head and shoulders should be on the opposite side of the couch and his spine obliquely across the couch with the buttocks supported on a sandbag or soft pillow on the near edge of the couch, and the knees drawn up. Time is well spent in getting the patient into the correct position before starting the examination, for a faulty position leads to a difficult and therefore inadequate examination. Throughout the examination the surgeon must be gentle and must explain to the patient exactly what he is doing and going to do, so that the patient is neither hurt nor frightened. The order of examination should be:—

1. Inspection.
2. Palpation with a finger.
3. Sigmoidoscopy.
4. Proctoscopy.

If a patient is complaining of severe anal pain careful inspection alone will often suffice to make a diagnosis, for instance in a case of acute anal fissure or an anal abscess. Further examination should then be deferred until the patient is anæsthetized or the local condition has been cured.

Occult Blood.—If the stool is to be tested for the presence of occult blood, the test should be performed at this stage, wiping the finger of the glove after rectal examination on a piece of filter-paper (*see* p. 701).

Once an instrument has been passed a false positive result may be obtained. Menstruation and internal hæmorrhoids may give similar misleading results.

SIGMOIDOSCOPY

This is invariably required as part of a complete rectal examination and is best performed, for the first time anyway, without any preparatory enema or suppository. The best preparation for sigmoidoscopy is a normal bowel action, but in a persistently constipated subject where a sigmoidoscopy is impossible, an enema or a glycerin suppository may be given to induce an evacuation of the rectum immediately before sigmoidoscopy.

A sigmoidoscope with proximal lighting has many advantages because the lighting is even and does not become obscured if there are fæces or fluid in the bowel. A most useful and popular instrument is the Lloyd-Davies pattern sigmoidoscope which is made in two diameters ($\frac{1}{2}$ and $\frac{3}{4}$ in. outside diameter; 14 and 19 mm.) and the larger one is made in three lengths (8, 10, and 12 in.; 20, 25, and 30 cm.); all these instruments fit the same lighting system (*Fig.* 363).

The instrument, with the obturator in position, is lubricated and passed gently into the anal canal, which runs in a slightly forward direction towards the patient's umbilicus. As soon as the tip of the instrument is through the

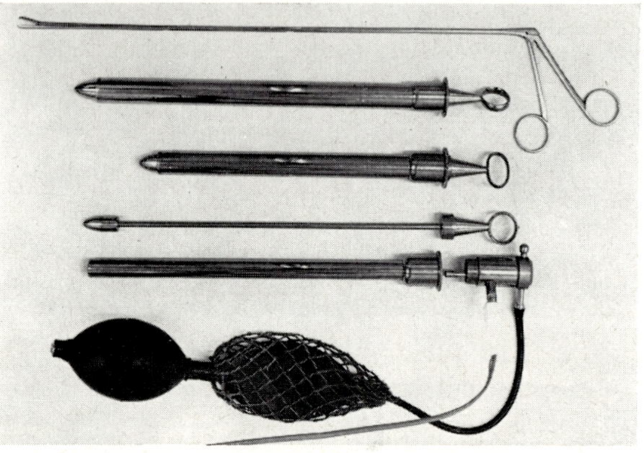

Fig. 363.—Lloyd-Davies pattern sigmoidoscopes, all fitting the same lighting system. Biopsy forceps for use through the instrument are also shown.

anal canal the obturator is removed and the eye-piece, light, and bellows are attached. The rest of the examination is carried out under direct vision and no attempt should be made to pass the instrument blindly into the upper part of the rectum. The rectum follows the curve of the sacrum and the instrument must therefore be directed more posteriorly. The bowel is gently inflated with air in order to separate the walls and the instrument is passed under direct vision, noting the appearance of the mucous membrane and any abnormality. When the upper rectum is reached at about 13 cm. from the anal verge, the direction of the bowel forwards and to the left must be followed. However, there is frequently some spasm at this rectosigmoid angle, which may be difficult to pass. Force or forcible distension of the bowel with air should never be used, but with patience and gentle insufflation the spasm will frequently relax and allow the instrument to be passed further up the bowel into the lower sigmoid. If the spasm does not relax, or attempts to negotiate the rectosigmoid cause pain, the examination should be abandoned. On withdrawing the instrument, however high it has been passed, withdrawal should be slow, with careful inspection of the wall; it is all too easy to miss a small lesion such as a polyp on the way in and one should take the opportunity of a second look on withdrawal.

The normal mucous membrane of the rectum is pale pink, with capillaries and sometimes small veins visible in the submucosa; this is called the normal vascular pattern and any departure from it, i.e., inflammation, ulceration, or neoplastic formation, will be observed. The presence of blood and mucus should be noted and any organic lesion, such as a polyp or a carcinoma, must be recognized. The total distance visualized should be recorded, and also the distance from the anus of a polyp or other abnormality and the quadrant affected.

Biopsy.—If an ulcerating lesion, such as a possible carcinoma, is seen a biopsy should be taken. This is a perfectly safe procedure provided a good view of the lesion to be biopsied is seen with the sigmoidoscope, and it is usually preferable and wiser to use the larger size sigmoidoscope for obtaining a biopsy.

Following a rectal or sigmoid biopsy, a barium-enema examination should not be attempted for 48 hours on account of the risk of perforation.

PROCTOSCOPY

An ordinary tubular proctoscope is the most useful pattern and these are made in varying sizes and can be had with a built-in light attachment, or, alternatively, an Anglepoise type light behind the operator's head will give adequate

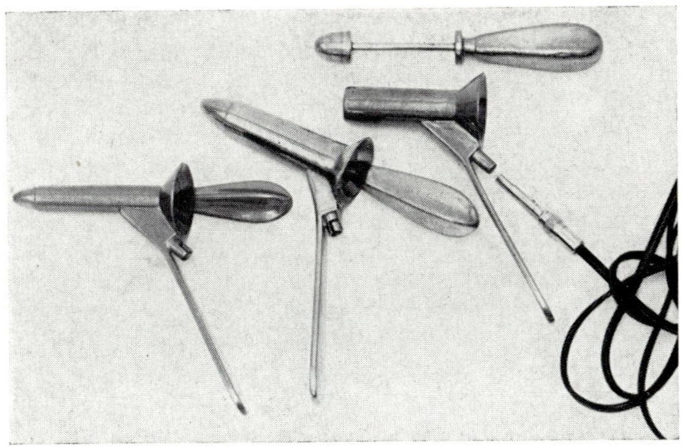

Fig. 364.—Tubular proctoscopes, with interchangeable illumination. The longest one shown is that normally used for the examination of adults.

illumination (*Fig.* 364). A proctoscope is designed for inspecting the rectal ampulla and the anal canal only, higher lesions being detected by sigmoidoscopy.

The proctoscope is inserted up to the full distance allowed by the flange; the obturator is withdrawn and the light directed in. The patient is asked to relax, and the lumen of the lower rectum and particularly the anterior rectal wall will be clearly seen. As the proctoscope is withdrawn the mucous membrane begins to close in and this marks the level of the anorectal ring. Prolapsing internal hæmorrhoids will become apparent as they bulge into the lumen of the instrument and, as it is withdrawn further, lesions in the anal canal, e.g., papillæ or a fissure, will become apparent. The proctoscope is then reinserted with its obturator; on withdrawing the proctoscope the second time the patient is asked to strain down, and the size and severity of the internal hæmorrhoids can then

Anglepoise lamp (Herbert Terry & Sons, Ltd., Redditch).

be more accurately assessed. They will sometimes be seen to bleed on straining in this way, or some other bleeding point in the anal canal may become apparent. Long forceps and small bits of cotton-wool are very valuable during proctoscopy for swabbing away mucus or small traces of blood.

RECORDS OF RECTAL EXAMINATION

The results of a rectal examination are conveniently recorded by the use of a rubber stamp (*Fig.* 365). The outer circle represents the anal margin; the inner circle represents the upper end of the anal canal. Local lesions such as piles, fissures, fistulæ, etc., can be shown in a graphic manner. The same system is used for recording operative procedures in this region.

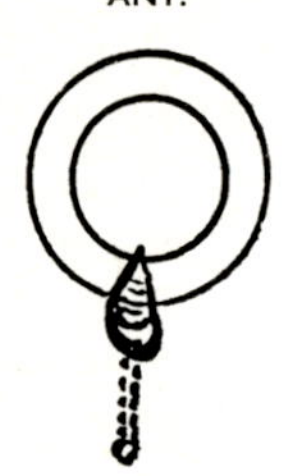

Fig. 365. — Fac-simile record of the findings in a case of a chronic posterior fissure with a short direct fistula.

MINOR ANORECTAL PROCEDURES

PRE-OPERATIVE MANAGEMENT FOR OPERATIONS ON THE ANAL REGION

It is desirable to have the rectum empty and clean before any operation on the anal region, but it is not essential and for patients admitted with severe anal pain, i.e., with an acute ischiorectal abscess, it is kinder to dispense with all local pre-operative preparation. Once the patient is anæs-thetized the anal area can be shaved as necessary and the rectum evacuated manually if there is any fæcal impaction.

For routine cases, i.e., operative treatment for hæmor-rhoids, anal fissures, or fistulæ, the patients are best admitted to hospital the day before operation, when the anal area can be shaved and a soap-and-water enema given. On the day of operation and not less than 2 hours pre-operatively, the rectum is best washed out with about half a pint (250 ml.) of plain water. Following this wash-out the patient is kept ambulant for about a quarter of an hour so that any fluid in the bowel gravitates into the rectum, and the patient is asked to evacuate any such fluid.

OPENING ABSCESSES

The large and deeper abscesses around the anal canal, i.e., in the ischiorectal fossæ, require in-patient treatment and general anæsthetic for laying open. Small perianal abscesses, however, can be opened in the out-patient or casualty department with a local anæsthetic.

Perianal Abscess.—The area is cleaned and gently shaved if possible, though sometimes this may cause undue pain and can then be omitted. The area of central softening is infiltrated with local anæsthetic, e.g., lignocaine 1 per cent, and, after allowing 2 or 3 minutes for this to work, a small incision radiating from the anal canal into the softest part of the swelling is made and pus is let out. The edges of the incision are then gently removed with scissors, leaving an elliptical hole through which the abscess can drain freely. A flat dressing is applied and held in place with a T-bandage. The patient is advised to sit in a warm bath twice daily, and particularly after any bowel action, and to keep a clean gauze dressing over the wound until the discharge stops.

To detect the possible cause of chronic anorectal suppuration such as tubercu-losis and Crohn's disease, any tissue excised should be submitted to the Patho-logy Department.

Ischiorectal Abscess.—It is always desirable to (*a*) open the abscess *before* fluctuation develops; (*b*) exclude the presence of a fistula-in-ano; and (*c*) ensure that the cavity granulates from the bottom outwards.

Under general anæsthesia, with the patient in the lithotomy position, a cruciate incision is made boldly over the most tense, tender part of the swelling. Pus is immediately released, and a sample is sent for bacteriological culture. The edges of the skin-flaps are then excised so as to allow adequate drainage. The floor of the cavity is wiped clean and carefully inspected and probed for any deep communication which would require to be opened up. Oozing from the cut edges abates after a few minutes. The cavity is packed with gauze impregnated with petroleum jelly, and a sterile dressing and T-bandage are then applied.

ANAL HÆMATOMA

These follow the rupture of a small perianal vein and present as painful rounded dusky lumps at the anal verge, usually of sudden onset. If seen within a day or two of onset, evacuation of the hæmatoma with a local anæsthetic is the best treatment and results in dramatic relief of pain. The patient is placed on his left or right side so that the hæmatoma will lie on the lower buttock. About 5 ml. of 1 per cent lignocaine are injected under the swelling. When this has become effective the swelling is incised and the clot evacuated and enough skin excised to leave a small pear-shaped wound which will remain flat and heal by granulation (*Fig.* 366). A small piece of oxycel gauze laid flat on the wound is the best immediate dressing and a twice-daily warm bath the best after-treatment. The wound should be inspected from time to time to make sure that it is healing without pocketing and usually heals within a week.

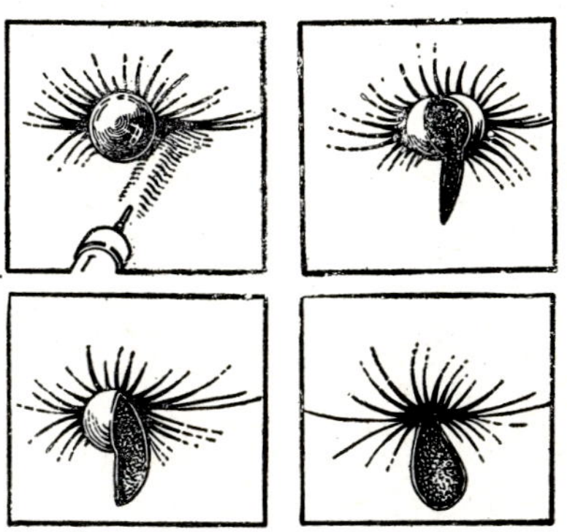

Fig. 366.—Excision of an anal hæmatoma. The drawings show the successive stages from the superficial injection of lignocaine to the splitting of the swelling into two portions and their excision. Adequate external drainage by a pear-shaped wound is effected.

More extensive and œdematous swellings at the anal verge occur as a result of thrombosis in the external plexus of perianal veins and these swellings are best treated by conservative measures rather than by evacuation. A few days' rest in bed with the application of compresses of evaporating lead lotion are very soothing and the acute stage usually settles within a few days.

ANAL FISSURE

An anal fissure is one of the most painful anal conditions, and consequently the patient is most grateful for gentle examination and expeditious treatment. Pain is felt particularly at and after defæcation, but in the more severe cases it may last most of the day. The diagnosis is usually suggested by the history and can be confirmed by examination. The fissure is nearly always dorsal in position and can be seen on gentle eversion of the anal verge, particularly if

Oxycel (Parke, Davis & Co., Hounslow, Middlesex, and Detroit, Michigan, U.S.A.).

the patient strains down gently. There is usually much anal spasm and any attempt to pass a finger or instrument causes pain and further spasm, and is greatly resented.

Treatment.—Some anal fissures will respond to treatment by softening of the stool with the aid of a suitable mild laxative and the local use of a St. Mark's dilator (*Fig.* 367). But if these measures do not work or in the more painful and severe fissures other measures are necessary. Most acute anal fissures will respond to full anal dilatation which is best carried out under a short general anæsthetic. The anus is gently dilated until the tips of four fingers can be inserted into the anal canal, which is then gently stretched with these four fingers. *Forcible disruption should not be attempted.*

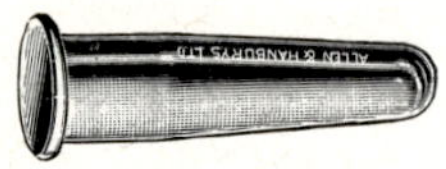

Fig. 367.—St. Mark's Hospital dilator.

As an alternative to dilatation of the anal canal a lateral sphincterotomy may be performed for painful chronic fissures, excising a small triangle of smooth muscle from the lower internal anal sphincter.

Technique of Lateral Sphincterotomy.—With the patient in the lithotomy position, an anal retractor is inserted to expose the side of the anal canal. A circumferential incision about 2 cm. long is made in the lower anal mucosa (*Fig.* 368). The circular fibres of the internal sphincter are seen below the mucosal flap and a triangular portion of the muscle is excised, extending from the anal margin to the mucocutaneous junction. Longitudinal muscle fibres are revealed, separating the internal from the external anal sphincter, which is not damaged. After securing hæmostasis, the mucosa is repaired with a few interrupted catgut stitches.

After-care is as for internal hæmorrhoids (*see* p. 517).

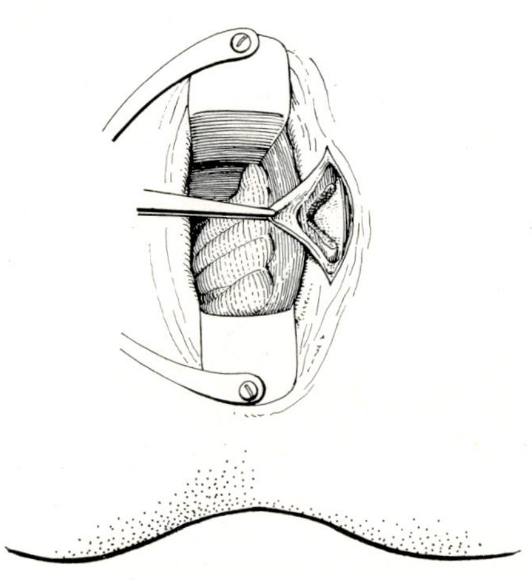

Fig. 368.—Lateral sphincterotomy for fissure-in-ano. A lateral wedge of the lower internal sphincter is excised between the anal margin and the mucocutaneous junction.

LOCAL ANÆSTHESIA

Many anal operations, including dilatation and sphincterotomy, can be performed under local anæsthesia if for any reason a general anæsthetic is considered impracticable. For effective local anæsthesia of the anal region about 15 ml. of 1 per cent of lignocaine are required. A small subcutaneous bleb of local anæsthetic is raised about 1½ in. (3 cm.) behind the anal verge in the mid-line, and through this a 2-in. needle is inserted into the ischiorectal fossa of each side, putting about 5–7 ml. of local anæsthetic into each. This will result in anæsthesia of the inferior hæmorrhoidal nerve and will lead to complete anal relaxation and anæsthesia. A further ½–1 ml. of anæsthetic can be put under the base of the fissure or under any associated skin tag. After allowing a few minutes for the anæsthetic to work, minor anal operations can usually be carried out without any discomfort to the patient.

INTERNAL HÆMORRHOIDS

Acute Attack: Palliative Treatment.—If a patient is seen in an acute attack with prolapsed thrombosed hæmorrhoids an attempt at manual reduction is usually valueless and causes extreme pain. Immediate hæmorrhoidectomy is occasionally indicated and possible, provided the patient can be admitted to hospital and the operation carried out under perfect conditions.

For most cases seen, however, the condition is best treated by bed-rest and the application of local soothing compresses. Lead lotion, containing spirit as a 1 in 8 solution, is an effective local application. Gentle aperients should be given orally in order to soften the stool and make defæcation less painful, and suitable analgesics such as aspirin or para-cetamol can be given as required. Stronger analgesics may be needed for the first 48 hours or so.

Injection Treatment of Hæmorrhoids.—The injection treatment of internal hæmorrhoids is indicated particularly in the early stages when bleeding rather than prolapse is the chief symptom. However, even with rather larger piles which tend to prolapse, good palliation can often be achieved by injections.

The solution used is 5 per cent phenol in arachis oil. A 10-ml. Gabriel syringe is required, with a three-finger grip and a bayonet lock for attaching the needle to the syringe (*Fig.* 369).

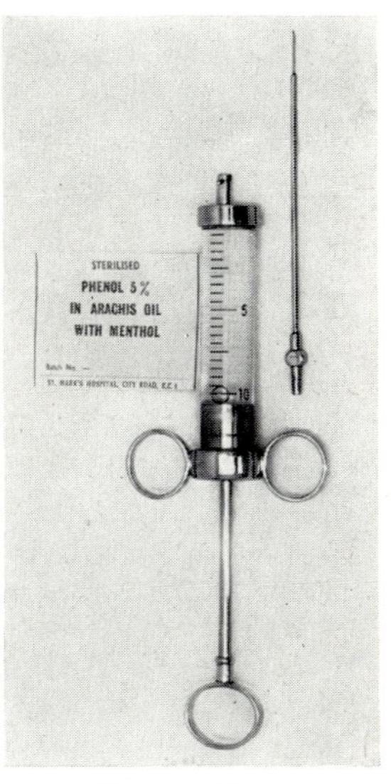

Fig. 369.—A 10-ml. Gabriel syringe with bayonet lock, for injection treatment of internal hæmorrhoids.

Technique.—One should aim at the first visit to inject the solution into the three primary hæmorrhoidal areas, that is the right posterior, right anterior, and left lateral positions. The needle should be inserted at the upper end of the hæmorrhoid at about the level of the anorectal ring (*Fig.* 370) and as the injection is given the proctoscope is withdrawn slightly so that the injection solution can run down into the hæmorrhoid proper. The solution is injected slowly into perivenous, submucous space. The amount injected into any quadrant is usually 2–3 ml.; occasionally a larger amount, up to 5 ml., may be required in a large hæmorrhoid, but it is probably wise not to give more than about 10 ml. as a total dose at any one attendance.

Bearing in mind that the object of the treatment is to produce a chemical sclerosis, the following practical hints may be of use:—

1. Inject fairly high up into the pedicle of the hæmorrhoid or into the hæmorrhoid proper. If the injection is made too low severe pain will be produced.

2. The needle must be gently and correctly inserted into the submucous layer and the mucosa must be seen to expand slowly as the injection is given. If the needle point is too superficial a white spot will be observed as soon as the injection is started. In this case the needle should be passed deeper or removed and inserted at a different place. If the needle is too deep, so that it reaches the muscle of the rectal wall, no mucosal swelling will be seen as the injection starts, and pain or other trouble may well be caused.

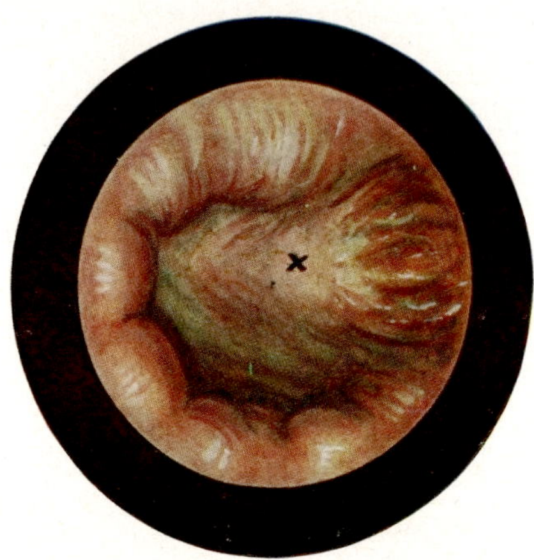

Fig. 370.—Correct site for injecting a hæmorrhoid.

3. Injection of too large amounts must be avoided or there will be some risk of necrosis and sloughing. This applies particularly when reinjecting a pile previously treated, as the submucous fibrosis produced by the previous injection will to some extent prevent diffusion of the solution.

4. The dose, and the distribution of the dose between the hæmorrhoids, must be varied according to the individual requirements. It is usually best to try to give an adequate dose into each hæmorrhoid at the first attendance and to see the patient again in 6 weeks' time. By then all palpable sclerosis should have settled and a further, usually smaller, injection can be given into any hæmorrhoidal tissue that remains.

A diagrammatic record should be made in the notes of the amount of the solution injected at each site.

Complications after Injection.—These are all rare, as this is a remarkably safe form of treatment. Occasionally a superficial ulcer is produced, which is usually symptomless but may occasionally lead to bleeding. It heals quickly and usually requires no treatment. Hæmaturia is occasionally reported, but this is due to an error in technique and the insertion of a needle through into the prostate. No treatment is usually required. Abscess formation is very rarely produced and again is due to an error in technique, with excessive pooling of the solution at one place.

Ligature Operation for Internal Hæmorrhoids.—General anæsthesia is mostly employed. The patient is placed in the lithotomy position; in the male, the scrotum is strapped up on to the lower abdominal wall. Before hæmorrhoid-ectomy is carried out, all patients should have a preliminary sigmoidoscopy.

The three primary hæmorrhoids—right anterior, right posterior, and left lateral—are grasped with Kocher artery forceps. Dealing with the hæmor-rhoids in the reverse order, gentle traction is applied to the left artery forceps. With the operator's left index finger in the anal canal, an equilateral triangular incision, of side 2 cm., is made with a scalpel or sharp scissors (*Fig.* 371); the apex surrounds the pedicle of the hæmorrhoid. The small skin-flap is dissected medially off the internal sphincter muscle; a few small bleeding points may

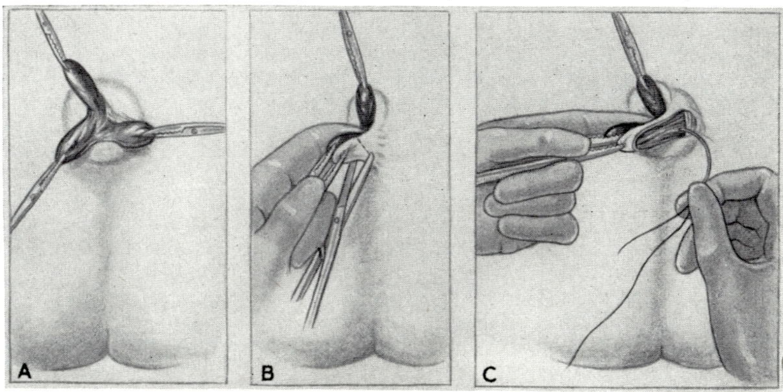

Fig. 371.—Ligature of hæmorrhoids: A, The 'triangle of exposure'; B, The skin cut for the left lateral hæmorrhoid; C, Transfixion of the pedicle. The muscle exposed at the centre of the cut is the lower border of the internal sphincter.

require ligation. With the hæmorrhoid pulled well down its pedicle is clearly defined, then transfixed and ligated with No. 1 chromic catgut, and the hæmor-rhoid excised. The two other primary hæmorrhoids are dealt with in similar fashion. Secondary piles may have to be left as it is important to leave adequate mucocutaneous bridges between the three raw areas. Three pieces of jelonet are then tucked into the lower rectum and spread over the three triangular areas. Only if bleeding has been very troublesome is it necessary to insert a large-bore rectal tube, with jelonet wound around it. Gauze dressings and wool are then put on and held in place by a T-bandage.

POST-OPERATIVE CARE

When the patient is returned to bed the nursing staff should check that the dressings have not moved during the journey back from the operating theatre and that the T-bandage is tight enough to hold them firmly in position over the anal region. Post-operative analgesics are given as required, but usually only small doses are necessary.

Micturition.—After 12 hours check whether or not the patient is passing urine normally. If the patient has any difficulty in passing urine he should be encour-aged to get out of bed to use a bottle.

Dressings.—Anal wounds do well if they are covered with a firm moist dress-ing held in place by a T-bandage. Such dressings are comforting to the patient

Jelonet (Smith & Nephew Ltd., Hull & Welwyn Garden City, Herts).

and also help to minimize local œdema. A suitable lotion to use on the dressings is 1–200,000 domiphen bromide B.P. (bradosol) lotion or 2½ per cent milton (1 per cent hypochlorite). Occasionally patients will be seen whose skin becomes sensitive to such lotions and then normal saline can best be used for the dressings. After the first week when the wounds are granulating cleanly, lotio rubra can be substituted as a dressing solution, though it sometimes causes quite severe stinging when first applied.

The dressings are first changed on the evening of the operation and again the following morning. The gauze is moistened and folded so that it lies in the anal groove and firmly against the perianal skin, but it is not necessary in most cases to try to tuck a corner of gauze into the anal canal, as this procedure frequently causes a good deal of pain. Relaxing in a warm bath is both very soothing to the patient and good local treatment to the anal wounds; such baths should be given twice daily, starting the morning after operation, and the routine should be for the patient to relax in the bath for a quarter of an hour or so and then return to bed where a clean dressing is applied. Once the bowels start to act a bath should follow every bowel action and then a fresh dressing follow the bath. After a week or so when the wounds are clean and small, all moist dressings can be stopped and after the twice-daily bath the anal area should be dabbed dry with gauze or a clean towel and a very small dressing of dry cotton-wool applied; this is all that is necessary and the T-bandage can be dispensed with.

The technique of dressings is rather different for the large anal wounds that may follow the operative treatment of an extensive anal fistula. The dressing technique for these wounds should aim to ensure that the wounds heal from the bottom and that the superficial parts do not heal together prematurely. These wounds are therefore best treated by dressings that are gently tucked in towards the top of the wound, which requires skilled nursing technique and a good light if this is to be done properly and without causing the patient undue pain.

Irrigation.—These more extensive wounds also benefit usually from twice-daily irrigation as well as the bath and dressing routine described above. For an irrigation the patient is placed on his or her left side with the buttocks lifted out over the edge of the bed; a macintosh sheet is placed underneath and is laid over the side of the bed into a bucket. The wound is irrigated gently with 2 pints (1 litre) of a suitable solution, either dilute (1–10) hydrogen peroxide if there is blood-clot or local sepsis, or normal saline or 1–200,000 bradosol. Following the irrigation the surrounding area is carefully dried and the moist dressing tucked gently into the depths of the wound.

In ensuring satisfactory healing of these large fistula wounds it is best to return the patient to the operating theatre once weekly, where under anæsthesia the wound can be suitably explored and trimmed as necessary, and satisfactory healing thus ensured.

Post-operative Rectal Examination.—Following *hæmorrhoidectomy* it is not usually necessary to pass a finger into the anal canal until the sixth or seventh post-operative day. There is still some tenderness and spasm at that time, but this usually subsides within the next week. A finger should be passed again when healing appears complete in order to ensure that everything is satisfactory, but routine daily dilatation is not necessary; the best dilator for the anal canal is a normal daily bowel action.

Following operations for *anal fissure* and particularly in those patients who have had a good deal of spasm pre-operatively, it is probably wise to start

Bradosol (Ciba Laboratories Ltd., Horsham, Sussex).
Milton (Milton Antiseptics Ltd., London, W.1).

passing a finger about the fourth day and then to get the patient to pass a St. Mark's dilator daily themselves. This helps to overcome spasm and gives the patients confidence that their anal canal is of normal calibre; though its passage often causes some discomfort at first, the patients soon learn to do it themselves with little trouble.

Care of the Bowels.—There is no one routine that will always suit every patient, as patients vary in their normal bowel habits. On the whole it is wise not to attempt to confine the bowel for too long after operations on the anal region as a hard fæcal mass is then likely to form in the rectum, the evacuation of which will cause more pain and probably more damage to the healing wounds than an earlier but softer bowel action. It is better to try to get the bowel moving from the third day onwards, and to try to keep the motions soft for the first week so that they cause little pain, but thereafter to become normally formed so that adequate anal dilatation is produced by the motion.

The patients should be asked on admission what aperient, if any, he is in the habit of taking as this gives one some idea as to whether large or small doses of aperients will be needed in the post-operative phase. The patient can be started on a normal diet from the day following operation and a mild laxative with some paraffin is given from the day following operation. A suitable preparation is milpar, but simple liquid paraffin or one of the emulsions of paraffin may be given if preferred. The dose should be 15 ml., twice daily to start with, but reducing to once daily as soon as the bowels begin to act. For patients who are habitually constipated or who habitually take stronger aperients senokot granules or tablets may be given in the evening as well. After the first week it is best to stop all preparations containing paraffin and to try to produce a normal formed motion by giving preparations such as normacol or isogel, i.e., hydrophilic colloids that act by retaining water in the bowel lumen. As before, senokot or stronger aperients may also be continued for patients who require this.

Management of Post-operative Hæmorrhage.—

Reactionary Hæmorrhage.—This usually occurs within 24 hours of operation and is most commonly from a small artery in the perianal tissues and seldom from the pedicle of a ligated hæmorrhoid. Treatment should be tried first with a firm local dressing, elevation of the foot of the bed, and sedation, all the time

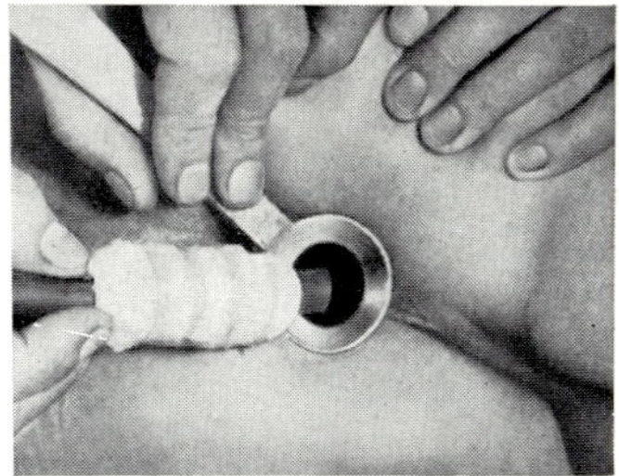

Fig. 372.—Post-operative hæmorrhage from the rectum. Method of introducing a tube surrounded by gauze into the rectum through a proctoscope.

keeping a careful watch on the patient's pulse-rate and blood-pressure. If these measures do not suffice to stop the hæmorrhage or there is evidence of bleeding into the rectum as shown by a rising pulse-rate, the patient should be returned to the theatre and anæsthetized. The bleeding vessel can then be identified and ligated.

Secondary Hæmorrhage.—This occurs from one of the ligated pedicles after hæmorrhoidectomy, usually between the fifth and tenth post-operative days, though rarely as late as the twelfth day. It occurs in about 1–2 per cent of hæmorrhoidectomies. The bleeding can be quite severe and usually requires plugging of the rectum in order to stop it.

Milpar (Charles H. Phillips Chemical Co., Ltd., London, W.3).
Senokot (Westminster Laboratories Ltd., London, N.W.1).
Normacol (Norgine Ltd., London, W.C.1).
Isogel (Allen & Hanburys Ltd., London, E.2).

Methods of Plugging the Rectum.—An injection of omnopon 20 mg. or equivalent should be given and the patient placed on his left side with buttocks well over the edge of the bed. A tubular proctoscope is passed and a large amount of blood and clot will be evacuated, and the rectum is then irrigated with plain water to remove most of the clot. With the proctoscope still in position a stout-walled rubber tube of ½ in. (1·25 cm.) outside diameter, with a gauze 'surround' wrapped about it and smeared with petroleum jelly, is pushed into the rectum through the proctoscope (*Fig.* 372). As soon as the tube and surround are felt to slip into the rectum the proctoscope is withdrawn over the outer free end of the tube. Traction on the tube now brings the gauze up against the anal canal and in this position effective pressure is exerted against the bleeding point in the internal hæmorrhoidal region. A stout safety-pin is passed through the tube just external to the anus and several pieces of dry dressing gauze are placed on each side between the anus and the safety-pin. In this way traction and pressure against the hæmorrhoidal bleeding point are maintained. A firm pad of gauze and wool is applied. The foot of the bed is raised on blocks and the usual general treatment of hæmorrhage is adopted, including blood transfusion if there has been serious loss of blood.

A close watch is kept on the patient and his anal area to make sure that no further hæmorrhage is taking place. This rarely happens and the tube and surround are removed by gentle traction 48 hours later, following a rectal instillation of olive oil which will help the patient's subsequent bowel action.

Alternative method: A somewhat simpler method is to pass into the rectum without the need of a proctoscope a rather large Foley catheter with a 30-ml. balloon. Once the catheter is through the anal canal the balloon is blown up to its full capacity and gentle traction on the catheter will then bring the balloon against the bleeding point. As in the other method this traction can be maintained by passing a large safety-pin through the catheter (taking great care not to puncture the side-tube leading to the balloon) and wrapping gauze between the anal verge and the big safety-pin. However, though rather easier for the patient than the tube with gauze surround, these Foley catheters are more liable to slip out of the anus than the tube and surround of the previous method and therefore may not be so effective in controlling the hæmorrhage.

MAJOR RECTAL SURGERY

PRE-OPERATIVE TREATMENT

Patients about to undergo major rectal surgery such as excision or anterior resection of the rectum for carcinoma are best admitted to hospital 4 days or so before the operation. A full general physical examination should be carried out and essential investigations include:—

1. Radiograph of the chest.
2. ECG.
3. Full blood-count.
4. Hæmoglobin estimation.
5. Determination of blood group and preparations for transfusion.
6. Blood-urea.

If the growth is a large one and rather fixed in the pelvis or if the blood-urea is raised an intravenous pyelogram is advisable.

Preparation of the Bowel.—If the operation planned is an excision of the rectum and no untoward difficulty is anticipated, no particular preparation of the bowel

Omnopon (Roche Products Ltd., 15 Manchester Square, London, W.1).

is needed other than the administration of an enema the night before operation. However, for more difficult cases where the rectum might be damaged during the dissection or when any resection with anastomosis might be the operation to be carried out, pre-operative preparation of the bowel with anti-bacterial drugs in order to reduce the bacterial activity within the bowel is advisable. The following schedules can be used:—

First Schedule.—Oral phthalylsulphathiazole (sulphathalidine) is given for 5 days pre-operatively; the dose should be about 10 G. in 24 hours and the drug is best given 4-hourly, i.e., 1·5 G. 4-hourly day and night. During these 5 days the diet should be light and of low-residue character, and an enema should be given 2 days before operation and again the evening before operation.

Second Schedule.—Give castor oil 30 ml. 3 days before operation, and then start sulphathalidine 1·5 G. and neomycin 1 G., given together at 4-hourly intervals until 4 hours before operation. During these 3 days a strictly fluids-only diet is given, but no wash-outs or enemata should be administered.

Third Schedule.—Give castor oil 30–40 ml. 24 hours before operation. Then give sulphathalidine 1·5 G. and neomycin 1 G. together, hourly for 4 hours, and then 4-hourly until 4 hours before operation. No wash-outs or enemata are administered.

The first schedule will give a good reduction in bacterial content of the bowel, but will not produce a sterile bowel. The second schedule, requiring a 3-day preparation, should produce a bowel that is clean and sterile at the time of operation and should probably be administered if an anterior resection is planned. The third schedule is that for quick preparation of the bowel and is only used where there is little time to prepare the patient for surgery, i.e., where the operation is of a semi-emergency character.

MANAGEMENT AFTER EXCISION OF THE RECTUM

Posture and Supervision.—When the patient is returned to bed after an excision of the rectum he should be placed on his back for some hours with the foot of the bed raised on 6-in. (21-cm.) blocks. There will probably be both an intra-venous drip and a catheter in position, and the nursing staff should check that these are satisfactory and not obstructed. The pulse-rate and blood-pressure should be taken on return to bed and thereafter half-hourly for the first 2 hours and then hourly for 6-8 hours. After a few hours, if the general condition is satisfactory, the bed can be taken off the blocks and the patient gradually sat up on pillows and turned partly on one or the other side; his position should be changed a little every few hours so that no pressure necrosis on the perineal wound is produced.

On the evening of operation the perineal wound should be inspected to make sure that there is no undue bleeding and the abdominal dressing should be taken down so that the colostomy can be inspected, to ensure particularly that it is of good colour and has an adequate blood-supply.

General Management.—In the first few days after operation the patient should be encouraged to move about in bed and to breathe deeply and cough up any sputum that he can. If a trained physiotherapist is available to help him with breathing exercises this is a great advantage. Patients should be encouraged to start getting out of bed on the first or second post-operative day and to exercise the muscles of the legs and feet even when in bed.

The intravenous drip is usually required for about 36 hours post-operatively, but may then be taken down if the patient's abdominal condition is satisfactory,

---

Sulphathalidine (Merck, Sharp, and Dohme Ltd., Hoddesdon, Herts).

i.e., the abdomen is soft and flat with normal peristaltic sounds. The colostomy will frequently not start to act until the fourth or fifth post-operative day, though it is usual for flatus to be passed on the second or third day. No aperients are usually needed, but if the colostomy has not worked by the fourth day a mild aperient (15 ml.) of milk of magnesia may be given with advantage.

If the patient's abdominal condition is unsatisfactory, as shown by abdominal colic, distension, nausea or vomiting, or a drop in urinary output, a nasogastric tube should be passed and the stomach aspirated, and the intravenous drip should be restarted. The wound should be inspected and the abdomen examined to try to determine the cause, and a plain radiograph of the abdomen may be of great value in differentiating between an ileus and a post-operative mechanical intestinal obstruction.

Management of the Bladder.—Male patients are usually returned from the theatre with an indwelling Gibbon catheter and female patients with a small Foley catheter. These catheters are best left on open drainage for 4 days and they should be removed on the morning of the fifth day if the patient's condition is otherwise satisfactory. Even if the patient thereafter appears to pass urine satisfactorily, a check on the amount of urine remaining in the bladder should be made by passing a catheter after evacuation; if the amount of residual urine is more than about (120 ml.) it is probably wise to replace the indwelling catheter for a few more days and then try again to remove it. A specimen of urine should be cultured for organisms. On the other hand, if after removal of the catheter the patient is unable to pass urine on his own, the catheter should be replaced within 6–8 hours; it is wrong to allow the bladder to become over-distended with urine as this will certainly delay the return of normal micturition. Most patients will pass urine after removal of the catheter on either the first or second occasion, but if a return to normal micturition is unduly delayed skilled urological advice should be sought as there may well be some bladder-neck obstruction which may require surgical treatment.

Management of the Perineal Wound.—The perineal wound after excision of the rectum heals better if it is adequately drained, that is, with a central opening at least 2 in. (5 cm.) long. A drain is usually inserted at the time of operation and this should be removed after 48 hours. For dressing of the perineal wound the patient should be laid on his side with the buttocks over the edge of the bed and the wound inspected in a good light. The daily routine should be the passage of a finger, in a sterile glove and dipped in 1–200,000 bradosol solution, into the depths of the wound so that any loculi can be broken down and drainage thereby encouraged. If there is much blood-clot in the depths of the wound it may be irrigated as previously illustrated by hydrogen peroxide or bradosol solution. One end of a fairly large gauze dressing should then be dipped into the solution and tucked into the depths of the wound.

Warning.—Neither small pieces of gauze nor ribbon gauze should ever be used in these perineal wounds as it is all too easy for a small gauze slip to be lost in the depths of the wounds and to cause indefinite delay in healing.

The sutures should be removed on the seventh to the ninth day, depending on their appearance, and, once the wound is clean and granulating, a twice-daily bath and the occasional passage of a finger into the depths are all that are needed to ensure satisfactory healing.

Occasionally a patient will return from the theatre with packing in the perineal wound; this is sometimes necessary where there has been difficulty in controlling bleeding at the time of operation. The packing is usually removed

48 hours after operation and is best removed under anæsthesia, either in the patient's bed or in the operating theatre. Provided bleeding does not recur, the further management of the perineal wound is as above.

MANAGEMENT AFTER ANTERIOR RESECTION OF THE RECTUM

The management of these cases is that of any major abdominal operation. No rectal treatment is called for and indeed no suppositories or enemata should be given. If a patient is having difficulty in passing wind or in having his bowels open following such an operation, a flatus tube may be passed for an inch or so into the lower rectum or a well-lubricated finger may be passed gently to determine whether any fæcal matter has come into the rectum. After about a week a glycerin suppository may be used to aid rectal evacuation if all the signs suggest that the anastomosis has healed satisfactorily.

CHAPTER XXXVII

PERIPHERAL VASCULAR SURGERY

By H. H. G. Eastcott

In diseases of the peripheral vascular system the common problems are those of pain, swelling, and ulceration of the lower limb. The causes for these troublesome symptoms may arise from disease in each of the three main systems—venous, arterial, or lymphatic, in this order of frequency.

EXAMINATION OF A PATIENT WITH PERIPHERAL VASCULAR DISEASE

History.—

Pain from venous insufficiency is worse on standing and in hot weather, and is usually relieved by walking or elevating the limb. Ischæmic pain is brought on by walking; ask how far the patient can walk before pain starts. In the later stages there is pain in the toes or forefoot when the patient rests with the limb horizontal. Standing or sitting with the leg down gives relief. Warm weather is preferred and complications are commoner in a cold spell.

Swelling suggests venous and sometimes lymphatic obstruction, though it is also present in some patients with severe chronic ischæmia owing to peripheral stagnation and the continual hanging down of the foot because of pain.

Ulceration in vein cases tends to be slow in developing, with a long history of pain and tenderness at the affected site, which is nearly always to one side of the ankle. Arterial disease causes ulceration and gangrene at pressure areas mostly on the foot, and its development is often rapid and without previous local symptoms.

Physical Signs.—A good light is essential, preferably daylight, and there must be free access to both sides of the limb. The patient should have been comfortably warm for at least 20 minutes before the examination.

On Inspection the following should be noted: wasting, deformity, swelling, pallor, or congestion; prominence, inflammation, or collapse of superficial veins; or undue pulsation over the course of the main artery; ulceration, cellulitis, bruising, blistering, or fungous infection of the skin.

Palpation.—

1. Skin warmth or coolness and its distribution.

2. Pulsation of main, named arteries (*Fig.* 373). A system of notation is suggested.

3. Cough impulse or percussion thrill over large veins.

4. Tenderness over or near any vessel or in its distribution.

Auscultation.—

1. Systolic bruits whose loudness and pitch depend upon the degree of the narrowing in the main artery which produces them. The 'seagull's cry' murmur is one typical example over a tight arteriosclerotic stenosis, and may often be heard at the common femoral or the carotid bifurcation.

2. A full-cycle continuous machinery murmur is heard over an arteriovenous fistula and is loudest near the communication.

3. A double murmur, not continuous, but to and fro, is heard over some large aneurysms with a relatively normal-sized proximal artery, and is probably due to recoil and regurgitation of blood in diastole.

General Assessment.—It is important for the house-surgeon to remember that the peripheral arteries are only a small part of the complex cardiorespiratory

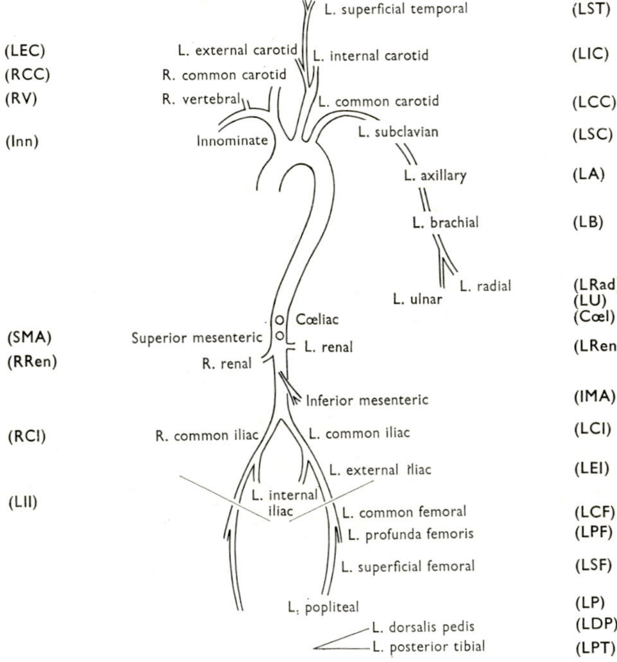

Fig. 373.—Arteries of surgical importance and a system for their clinical notation.

oxygen transport system. There is no point in correcting a defect of a peripheral part if the central mechanism is, and is allowed to remain, defective. Consequently after checking the pulse and blood-pressure, the house-surgeon should order: (1) Radiography of chest; (2) ECG; and (3) Full blood-picture.

SPECIAL ARTERIAL INVESTIGATIONS

Oscillometry.—This test can be of considerable value when pulsations are reduced or obscured by soft-tissue swelling, or if a measured comparison is required with the healthy limb or serial readings for progress assessment.

Clinical records which contain such observations are much more useful than those which record only the presence or absence of palpable pulses, which must be liable to observer error.

Blood-pressure readings in the lower limbs can be obtained by this method, using the change in the degree of deflexions as visible end-points of systolic and diastolic pressures in exactly the same way as Korotkoff's sounds.

Oscillations may be increased in acute venous insufficiency.

Arteriography.—This forms an essential part of the investigation of a patient with severe symptoms of occlusive disease (*see* p. 721). Two techniques are in general use: needle puncture and arterial catheterization. The following notes indicate the appropriate investigation to order.

1. *Direct Needle Puncture of a Limb Artery* is used for most patients requiring femoral arteriography, with delayed films to show the tibial and pedal arteries. Some patients with upper-limb occlusions are suitable for subclavian or brachial puncture, though only if these puncture sites are clinically free from disease. Puncture of the limb arteries is the only method suitable for investigation of the smaller arteries of the extremity, e.g., in Raynaud's phenomenon. General anæsthesia improves the distal filling and facilitates the puncture. For carotid and vertebral arteriography pictures are clearest with the puncture method.

A simple method of obtaining a femoral arteriogram is to inject 15–20 ml. of 45 per cent hypaque into the common femoral artery with a long film cassette beneath the thigh and another beneath the calf and foot. The upper exposure is made at the end of the injection and the lower exposure two or three seconds later, or longer if the limb is severely ischæmic. Either two portable X-ray tubes can be used or the tube of a fixed set can be moved quickly down its runners to make the lower exposure.

2. *Direct Puncture of the Lumbar Aorta* is safe for its routine examination and shows up all its main branches, though poor contrast values may be obtained in the lower limbs beyond the popliteal bifurcation; also within the abdomen shadows of the main visceral arteries may obscure one another.

3. *Transfemoral Catheterization* allows selective contrast study of the individual aortic branches from the bifurcation upwards. It should not be employed in patients with occlusive disease at or near the point of entry of the catheter. Kinking or looping of the iliac artery, or thrombus in an aneurysm, may hold up the catheter.

4. *Arch Aortography* via a catheter in the common femoral or axillary artery provides a full view of the proximal aorta and the coronaries and the main trunks to the neck and upper limbs. If access via a limb artery is impossible intravenous injection may show the aortic arch and its branches reasonably well.

ACUTE ISCHÆMIA

Recognition and Assessment.—The clinical appearances of acute ischæmia are unmistakable, no matter what the cause. The application of an Esmarch's tourniquet is a typical example producing complete and sudden arrest of the blood circulation, with all pulses absent. The extremity is waxy white and soon becomes cooler to the touch as its heat is lost.

If stagnant blood is present in sufficient quantity, diffuse cyanosis may partly mask the pallor. This is seen when a sphygmomanometer cuff is inflated to well above systolic pressure without first raising the limb. The same effect is produced when venous occlusion complicates an acute ischæmia.

In the conscious patient these colour and temperature changes are accompanied by numbness of the digits, appearing within 15 minutes of the arrest of the circulation in the limb and spreading upwards at 1–2 in. (2·5–5 cm.) per minute, along with weakness of the intrinsic muscles of the hand or foot.

It cannot be too strongly emphasized that these same features of acute ischæmia always appear with any sudden, complete obstruction to the main arterial
circulation, whether from arterial embolism, thrombosis, or injury.

Only where some large alternative artery of supply is spared will acute ischæmia be less clearly recognizable, the differences then being chiefly in the degree
and extent of the effects, and not in their character. For example, in traumatic
brachial arterial spasm the hand is recognizably affected, and the foot in popliteal embolism. In *Volkmann's ischæmic contracture* collateral arteries in the
middle portion of the limb suffice to keep its skin alive, though the muscles
beneath are already suffering subacute ischæmic damage, made worse by any
swelling, bruising, or hæmatoma inside their fascial compartment; within 6
hours irreversible damage will have occurred.

Sudden arrest of the flow in the main artery above its large proximal limb
branches is even more serious and usually causes acute, massive ischæmia
followed in most cases by extensive *moist gangrene*. Typical examples of this
disaster follow obstruction of the common iliac or common femoral artery by
surgical ligation or acute embolism.

Exceptionally, in some young subjects such a limb may survive without
surgical correction of the obstruction, but never if there is hypovolæmia or
damage to potential collaterals from concomitant limb injury.

Surgical or Traumatic Shock is significant in both the diagnosis of acute
ischæmia and its outcome. Peripheral vasoconstriction favours the closure of
the remaining blood-vessels and is accentuated by local traumatic stimuli within
the injured limb. It is therefore of practical importance to examine all four
extremities for skin warmth and to compare their pulses when uninjured peripheral
areas are obviously vasoconstricted and all distal arterial pulses are reduced.
Hypovolæmia must be corrected before any valid assessment can be made of the
circulation in the injured limb (*see* p. 21). This is perhaps the only permissible
reason for delay in undertaking arterial repair.

Central Circulatory Failure from cardiorespiratory disease acts in the same
way in patients with peripheral arterial embolism, by accentuating the ischæmic
features before and after operation, the results of which are highly dependent
upon the patient's general condition.

Ischæmic muscle contracture, though diagnostic and serious in itself, does not
mean that it is too late for surgery to save the limb. However, once the pale
anæsthetic skin of the distal part of the limb has become patchily cyanosed and
the tips of the digits are stained a dark plum colour, irreversible changes are
present and revascularization at this stage cannot succeed. Much harm can be
caused by such late intervention due to the transfer of grossly damaged tissue
products into the general circulation. There may be cardiac arrest.

TREATMENT OF ACUTE ISCHÆMIA

Conservative Measures only apply to a few cases in which definite early spontaneous improvement is already taking place, or in whom a 2–3-hour period of
observation can be justified by the need for resuscitation or other general supportive treatment during the interval. *Such patients should never be left overnight* unless the ischæmia is already hopelessly irreversible. In these cases the
problem has become less urgent; in fact, delay may allow time for improvement
in the collateral circulation and later the amputation, though inevitable, may
be made at a more distal level.

Traditional remedies such as vasodilators, lumbar paravertebral or epidural sympathetic block, cooling the extremity with an electric fan, and over-vigorous body heating have very little to recommend them even in the late case, and nothing at all in the early, still viable ischæmic limb whose prime need is the restoration of the main artery. At best these measures are of doubtful effectiveness; at their worst they are made the excuse for procrastination and delay.

Essential steps include:—

1. Placing the fully exposed ischæmic limb lower than the rest of the body (sitting the patient up and raising the bed-head for lower limb ischæmia; in the upper limb raising the legs has been shown to increase blood-flow).

2. Gentle warming of the patient and exclusion of draughts will avoid additional vasoconstriction. Overheating will exhaust him and may shunt blood away from the high-resistance zone of the obstructed limb. The limb should be placed comfortably on a soft pillow to prevent pressure upon its extremities by the bedclothes. A bed-cradle should be employed.

3. Relief of pain by the injection of morphine or pethidine, together with alcohol by mouth which offsets vasoconstriction.

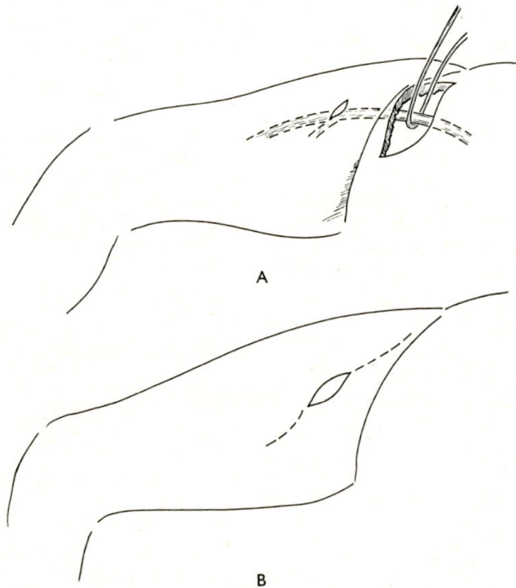

Fig. 374.—A, Temporary control of external iliac artery before exploring a stab wound of the groin. B, The stab wound is extended along the line of the femoral artery before attempting to expose the lesion.

4. Heparin is given intravenously immediately in any case of occlusive acute ischæmia other than those due to soft-tissue injury or complications of saccular or dissecting aneurysm (*see* p. 79). At least 50 mg.* as a loading dose is followed by a maintenance schedule of 100 mg. 6-hourly by intermittent intravenous

---

* Heparin: 100 mg. equal approximately 10,000 units.

injection, which can be given by the nursing staff via a Gordh needle (*see Fig.* 45, p. 80) or combined with a continuous intravenous infusion (*see* p. 36).

5. Continuous infusion intravenously of low molecular weight dextran (LMDX) improves the peripheral circulation in most forms of ischæmia probably by reducing blood viscosity, though its mode of action is not yet fully agreed. It is convenient to combine the heparin and LMDX solutions in the proportions 100 mg. to each 500 ml. given at the rate of 1 litre each 24 hours.

Operation.—Any surgeon should be prepared to expose and repair a main limb artery or to remove an embolus from it. The vascular dissection is little more exacting than that of careful varicose vein surgery. The suturing technique is simple and can soon be learned on the cadaver.

Anæsthesia.—Local infiltration is well suited to the cardiac patient requiring common femoral embolectomy, and the use of the Fogarty balloon catheter gives access to popliteal or even aortic emboli and associated thrombus through this same incision.

Injured patients, most of whom were previously fit, require general anæsthesia for more extensive soft-tissue or bone surgery.

Repair of an Arterial Injury.—The following simple principles should be followed:—

1. First the artery is exposed above the site of damage (*Fig.* 374), placing a tape sling beneath it to ensure control. The traumatic wound can then be enlarged along the line of the artery. The arterial wound is then explored.

2. A formal arteriotomy will nearly always be necessary. Though the artery may appear intact exploration of the lumen, at the point at which pulsations can be felt to cease, usually reveals an occluding plug consisting of loose arterial wall and pale friable thrombus (*Fig.* 375).

3. The artery should be mobilized above and below the wounded portion sufficiently to permit the application of bull-dog clips (*Fig.* 376) as soon as the thrombus is removed and free bleeding has been obtained from the distal as well as the proximal ends. Heparin is then given.

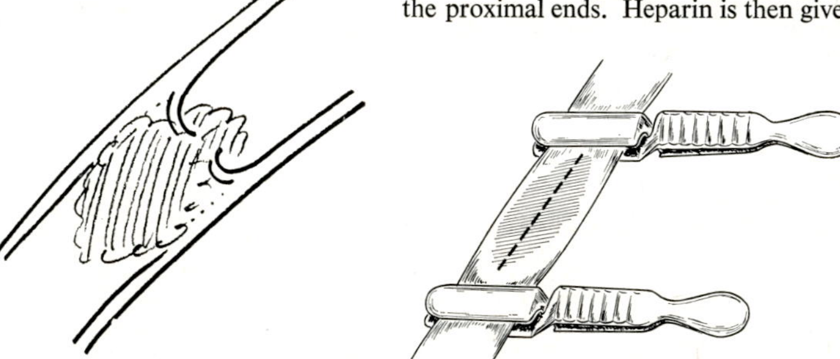

Fig. 375.—Artery occluded by contusion: curled-up inner coat and platelet thrombus require surgical removal.

Fig. 376.—Incision over contusion.

4. Lateral repair of a small wound is sometimes possible, provided the artery is not narrowed by the sutures. A continuous arterial silk (5/0 gauge) suture mounted on a small atraumatic needle is suitable for most cases.

5. End-to-end anastomosis is not difficult and is nearly always better than lateral repair. *Fig.* 377 shows the steps of the procedure.

6. Replacement of a segment is necessary if tension is too great after excision of the damaged portion. For peripheral arterial grafts the saphenous vein is preferable to any of the plastic cloth tubes, which should only be used if no suitable vein is available. The same applies to patch grafting of a simple arteriotomy.

7. Shortly before the clamps are removed the action of the heparin is reversed by giving intravenous protamine, 100 mg. protamine for every 5000 units of heparin.

8. A vacuum drain is inserted (p. 65).

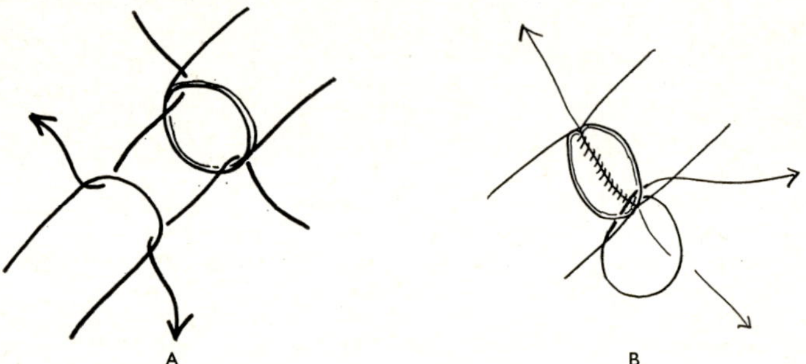

Fig. 377.—A, End-to-end anastomosis—slinging sutures. B, Continuous suture. For posterior layer either rotate the anastomosis or suture from within the lumen.

Embolectomy.—

1. The artery is exposed, centring the incision on the lowest point of palpable pulsation.

2. When it has been fully mobilized at and on both sides of the obstruction, a short longitudinal incision is made over the block with a No. 15 blade, *without applying any arterial clamps.* This is important, for there is seldom any bleeding from the cut into the lumen; premature clamping will break up the occluding material which may then be much more difficult to remove.

3. Inserting a Watson Cheyne dissector between the thrombus and the intima the obstruction is easily freed, and begins to be pumped down and out through the arteriotomy. A gush of arterial blood from the upper end is anticipated and the proximal clamp is applied.

4. Heparin should now be given in full systemic dosage, if it was not given before operation.

5. The distal thrombus may now be gently drawn out, or helped by vigorous squeezing of the lower and middle thigh between the two fists.

6. Various instrumental aids may be tried, including suction with a long polythene catheter, retrograde flushing from a more distal branch, or gentle curettage with a long endarterectomy loop. The best method, however, is to use the Fogarty balloon (p. 542) which is passed beyond the thrombus and is inflated, and with gentle traction the obstructing material is brought out.

7. Closure is then carried out as described above.

After-care.—Close watch is kept upon the pulse-rate and blood-pressure, and upon the state of the operated extremity.

The conservative measures adopted pre-operatively should be continued.

It is best to give no anticoagulants once the circulation has been restored, for they encourage bleeding which in turn leads to general deterioration and hypovolæmia, and the peripheral circulation once again may fail. Moreover, platelet thrombus formation is not prevented by heparin.

Reoperation may be required for an early recurrence of ischæmia after initial improvement.

CHRONIC ISCHÆMIA

Intermittent Claudication is the usual complaint. In two-thirds of all cases femoropopliteal occlusive disease is the cause, the calf muscles being chiefly affected. Most patients are over 60 years old and in about half the condition is bilateral, though not actually disabling. In a minority, aorto-iliac obstruction is responsible; such patients are on the average 10 years younger and their pain is more severe and it involves the whole limb.

Diagnosis is from:—
1. Lumbosacral root irritation (pain from buttock to outer calf).
2. Osteo-arthritis of hip (stiffness and pain on rising).
3. Venous insufficiency (pain on standing; better with walking).

Typically the pulses are reduced or absent beyond the groin, and after exercise the foot becomes pale, with loss of pulses previously present. Bruits are common at the groin and along the course of the femoral canal.

In patients with aorto-iliac occlusive disease one or both common femoral pulses will be absent or small in volume, with a bruit.

SEVERE ISCHÆMIA

Wasting and fasciculation are present in the muscles within the area of the reduced circulation. Distally the effects are more striking, the toes becoming atrophic with thick coarse nails. The whole foot shows rubor in dependency and pallor in elevation, and later develops pressure sores or dry gangrene of one or more toes.

Infection between the toes may expose the sides of the flexor tendons, or spreading into the web then reaches the sole or the dorsum of the foot, a typical sequence in diabetic patients.

DIABETIC GANGRENE

This takes two main forms:—
1. Ischæmic gangrene, which is common, premature, and severe in diabetic patients, with absent peripheral pulses and a cold extremity. The limb prognosis is bad.
2. Infective neuropathic gangrene with normal peripheral pulses and a warm dry skin, but absent pain and vibratory sense, plus impaired deep reflexes. With correct treatment of the diabetes and free surgical drainage of any spreading sepsis the limb prognosis should be good.

TREATMENT OF CHRONIC ISCHÆMIA OF THE LOWER LIMB

Conservative.—Most cases should be treated conservatively.

Rest, abstinence from smoking, and a low-calorie diet are advised. Vasodilators are of very doubtful value and may shunt the blood away from the high-resistance obstructed zones. Anæmia if present is corrected.

Claudication tends in cases with an acute or recent onset to show early spontaneous improvement.

Operation.—Arterial reconstruction is indicated in approximately 10 per cent of patients attending hospital with intermittent claudication due to femoropopliteal occlusion. In the smaller group with limited aorto-iliac disease the operability rate is much higher, though with extensive aortic occlusion approaching the renal arteries the bias should again be towards conservatism unless symptoms are crippling.

Deterioration or Relapse is often due to recent extension of the arterial thrombosis or to added infection at the periphery, or both. Control of these factors will help to limit further damage. As in primary acute ischæmia, heparin and low molecular weight dextran infusion (*see* pp. 30 and 79) are often used to conserve the remaining circulation, and if sepsis is present, appropriate antibiotics should also be given locally and systemically.

Lumbar Sympathectomy.—This valuable operation acts by ensuring the maximal blood-flow through the affected limb at all times, removing the adverse effects of periods of vasoconstriction which are inseparable from normal conditions of life in temperate or cool climates. Its selective property explains its superiority over generally acting vasodilator drugs or body heating, both of which may have the opposite effect from that which is intended.

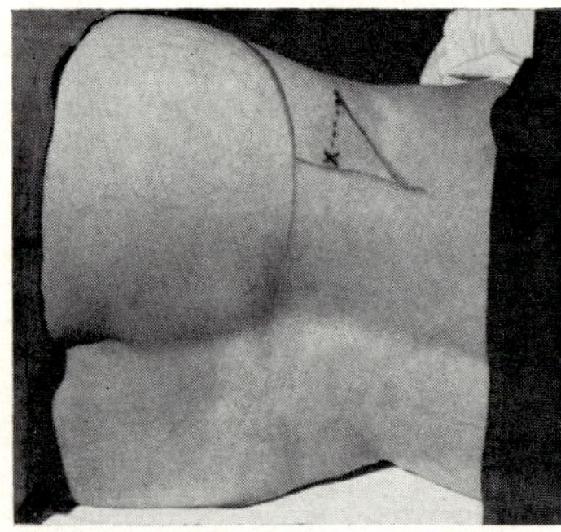

Fig. 378.—Site for insertion of the needle in lumbar paravertebral block. The needle is inserted at **X**.

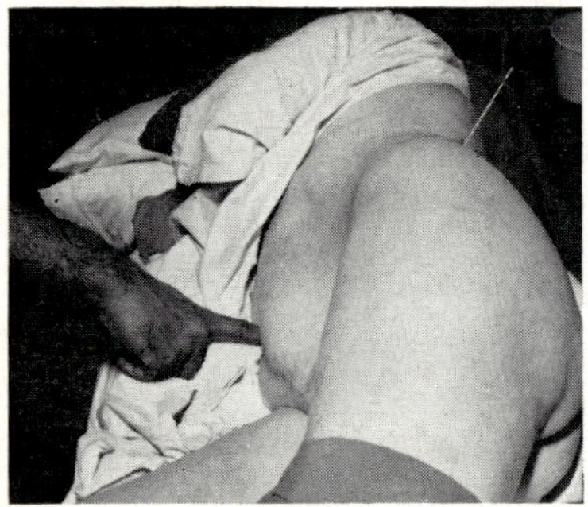

Fig. 379.—Direction for advancing the needle— towards the patient's umbilicus, marked by an assistant's finger.

Used preventively it should limit the tendency to progressive occlusion during such periods of stagnation. When rest pain or minor gangrene are already established sympathectomy gives good relief in about 50 per cent of cases, though for more severe acute deterioration, as in primary acute ischæmia, it has little value because of limited arterial inflow which cannot respond to vasodilatation.

Phenol (10 per cent) paravertebral block may give the same lasting benefits as operative sympathectomy in elderly, unfit patients. Between 10 and 20 ml. of phenol are injected near the lumbar chain using a long fine needle similar to that employed for lumbar puncture, but about twice as long.

Technique of Lumbar Paravertebral Block.—The patient lies in the lateral position on the operating table, the side to be injected being uppermost. The tip of the 12th rib is located and an imaginary line drawn vertically downwards to the lateral edge of sacrospinalis muscle and the point of intersection is marked **X** (*Fig.* 378). An assistant's finger marks the umbilicus (*Fig.* 379).

With full aseptic precautions, a 22-gauge 15-cm. long needle is introduced through a skin weal raised by local anæsthetic at point **X**. The needle is advanced towards the patient's umbilicus.

Lignocaine 2 per cent is infiltrated along the needle track, which runs inwards and forwards (*see Fig*. 379), advancing the needle until either the lumbar vertebral body is encountered or the aorta or vena cava. The needle position should be adjusted to lie between these vascular structures and the bone, and then a test dose of 10 ml. of the lignocaine solution is injected. There should be a warming of the affected lower limb and loss of goose-flesh reaction. Between 10 and 20 ml. of 10 per cent phenol may then be safely injected.

Arterial Reconstruction.—Case selection and management are critically important and, whereas in acute ischæmia operation is so urgent that often a relatively inexperienced surgeon must be prepared to undertake it, in chronic ischæmia if there is any doubt even the most expert operator should desist from an intervention which could worsen the condition of the limb if the restoration should fail. Unfortunately early and late failures are both common, familiar occurrences in this work.

It is safe to say that in the limbs autogenous repair methods have given the best late results, i.e., endarterectomy or autogenous vein by-pass grafting according to the length of the occlusion.

Plastic cloth grafts, of which knitted dacron is the best, are preferable for by-passing the aorta to the iliac or femoral arteries.

Major Amputations of the Lower Limb.—Not all cases are suitable for arterial reconstruction. Advanced or infected cases are better managed by primary amputation.

Mid-thigh.—Equal D-shaped anteroposterior flaps are made so as to reach well beyond the proposed line of bone section which should be well beyond the mid-shaft of the femur. No tourniquet is necessary in ischæmic cases. The flaps should be cut boldly and without undermining the skin or fascia. An oblique line of muscle section is made leading down to the bone at the point where it is proposed to divide it. The two flaps are then held together with only the bone remaining so that the exact place of section can be judged. The commonest mistake is to cut the flaps too short and the bone too long. No tension in the flaps will be tolerated or the bone will make its way through the centre of the wound. The flaps should be handled with the fingers rather than with dissecting forceps. The fascial layer of the closure should be with strong catgut with the knots inverted. The skin is best closed with 36-gauge stainless-steel wire with 'steri-strip' applications to any gaping points between the sutures.

Aftercare is described on p. 267.

Below Knee.—The same method is followed. The important points here are, first, to divide the fibula well above the proposed line of tibial section, and, second, to bevel the front of the tibia with an initial oblique saw cut at 45° running back to about half-way through the shaft. The bone is then divided opposite the lower point of this cut in the transverse line. It is wise to drain all major amputation wounds for the first 2 days. One more dressing is necessary after the removal of the drains and before suture removal. Steel sutures can be left in for several weeks if necessary. Stump movements should be started early and weight-bearing on crutches as soon as possible.

ARTERIAL SURGERY FOR PERIPHERAL ANEURYSM

Operation is required for established complications of an aneurysm or to prevent them. The majority of arteriosclerotic aneurysms are symptomless, and most occur in the patient whose whole main arterial system is somewhat widened with redundant curved portions, particularly the abdominal aorta and, in women, the right common carotid, an appearance which may suggest localized aneurysm, but this should only be diagnosed if the diameter of the segment can be felt to be locally expanded and with an expansile impulse between the fingers of the two hands.

Small aneurysms often thrombose, sometimes giving rise to peripheral emboli before they do so; in such patients a fairly severe ischæmia is caused. If, however, the aneurysm thromboses without previously having compromised its future collateral circulation in this way, the effects are mild and the process can be regarded as a spontaneous cure. A popliteal aneurysm may behave in either of these ways. It is a very common condition which is often missed both before and after it has become occluded.

Large aneurysms thrombose less often. As their diameter widens the strain on the thinned-out wall increases. Rupture is possible in any aneurysm from local disease or injury, but most of those which do give way are over 3 in. (7·5 cm.) in diameter. This will include many abdominal aortic aneurysms and some popliteal and femoral ones. Warning pains are usually experienced beforehand, either from the lesion, or its pressure upon nearby nerves or the main vein which accompanies it.

Ligation is safe and satisfactory for a painful or leaking popliteal aneurysm. The Hunterian (proximal) operation in the thigh is ideal in the elderly patient who is unfit for a long reconstructive procedure in the prone position.

Technique.—A short-mid-femoral incision is made along the line of the sartorius muscle which is displaced backwards to reveal the fascia over the adductor canal. This is incised and the saphenous nerve will be seen. Close beneath this is the femoral artery. The ligature is passed around it using a cholecystectomy forceps and taking care to avoid injury to the underlying femoral vein.

Reconstruction is the accepted modern operation. When undertaken before complications have occurred the results are good, and the mortality and morbidity are low in the hands of an experienced operator. Ruptured, leaking, or acutely ischæmic thrombosed cases do less well, yet the urgency of their condition may require them to be operated upon by any general surgeon. Transfer to a special unit usually means more delay and danger than an early operation undertaken in the peripheral hospital.

The Abdominal Aortic Aneurysm is partly or completely excised and a knitted dacron cloth tube is substituted. For leaking cases woven teflon is better; it bleeds less when the clamps are removed.

Peripheral Aneurysms are best replaced by reversed saphenous vein, though in the emergency case a dacron tube is quicker; the latter is also used in some subjects whose veins are all too small to use as grafts.

Heparin should be used in most interval cases during the clamping period, but in operations for leakage or rupture it causes dangerous oozing and is best avoided.

POST-OPERATIVE CARE AFTER ARTERIAL RECONSTRUCTION

The management of patients after arterial reconstruction is as for acute ischæmia, except that heparin should now be avoided because of the serious risk of reactionary hæmorrhage. Otherwise, the management is that appropriate to other operations in the part of the body concerned.

Operative Blood-loss should always be measured: swab weighing is simple and sufficiently accurate as a guide to blood replacement. In major cases such as those involving the abdominal aorta at least 8 pints (4000 ml.) of blood should be cross-matched, though this amount will not often be used if the operator is thoroughly experienced in this work, and if the use of heparin during operation can be dispensed with. Routine arterial surgery in the limbs other than for a large aneurysm or arteriovenous fistula should need no blood replacement, though it is wise to have 2 pints cross-matched in most cases.

Preventive Antibiotic Treatment should not be given as a routine for it increases the risk of establishing a resistant strain. If, however, an essential operation must be conducted in a contaminated case, the risk of secondary hæmorrhage may be averted by giving the two most suitable antibiotics as judged by the result of sensitivity tests.

When the ankle-pulses are first noted, often not until the day after operation, their position is marked upon the skin, to be regularly checked thereafter.

Fluid-balance Records are important as a guide to replacement. Limb cases need no infusion unless there has been undue blood-loss or a temporary improving post-operative ischæmia which would be helped by low molecular weight dextran.

All abdominal cases at first require intravenous fluids and a nasogastric tube should be passed; there may be a post-operative ileus for same days (*see* p. 343).

Abdominal arterial operations may be followed by either (i) retention of urine, (ii) oliguria from fluid loss with insufficient replacement, or (iii) anuria due to tubular necrosis following serious difficulties in the theatre. A fine Gibbon catheter should be inserted into the bladder and the rate at which urine replaces that which is initially drawn off, and the urine's specific gravity and urea content will distinguish between these three causes, and will guide the rate of fluid administration.

Ambulation.—In favourable cases both the catheter and the intravenous infusion can be dispensed with in two or three days and the patient can begin to move about out of bed. Those with an arterial anastomosis at the groin or knee should not walk more than necessary until the end of the first week.

Sutures.—Tension sutures are advisable in most patients with a long abdominal incision to prevent strain from coughing or gas distension. They should not be removed until the tenth to fourteenth day, according to the build of the patient and his general progress (p. 343).

THE SURGERY OF THE VEINS

Venous insufficiency is commoner in women, and causes congestive pain and swelling, often with localized tissue damage, where the venous pressure is high either as a result of loss of valvular competency or occlusion of the lumen, successively or at the same time in different veins. An inflammatory response (thrombophlebitis) is due in acute cases to altered blood products in the thrombus, and in the chronic stage to stagnant tissue fluids and metabolites in the drainage area of the vein. Less often is it due to bacterial invasion which in the limbs is probably almost always a complication of established ulceration or other loss of skin cover, for example, after minor trauma.

The damaging effects of venous insufficiency are highly variable in practice; this may be explained by a cumulative effect with reduction of venous reserve as the condition advances with the passage of time. Other factors such as above-average height and body-weight tend to increase the hydrostatic pressure head upon the lowest points of venous stasis. All these considerations apply both to superficial varicose veins and to failure of the deep venous channels.

VARICOSE VEINS

The exact causation of this common conditions is not yet known. Heredity, standing, childbearing, a hot climate, hyperthyroidism, alcohol, and congenital and acquired arteriovenous fistula may be associated. Possibly as a result of valve incompetence near the saphenofemoral opening, the inner calf tributaries of the internal saphenous vein are first affected in most cases, and some authorities believe that secondary incompetence of communicating channels to the deep veins may thus be caused.

Clinical Assessment.—Useful tests include the presence of a *cough impulse* down the main course of the internal saphenous and its larger varicosities, checked by compression at the groin or along the upper course; also the transmission with percussion of a sharp *fluid thrill* up or down the vein between the varices and the main trunk.

The short saphenous rarely shows a cough impulse, because the valves of the deep veins of the thigh prevent this. A percussion thrill, however, can usually be elicited between varices over the outer posterior surface of the calf or ankle, and the upper end of the vein behind the knee.

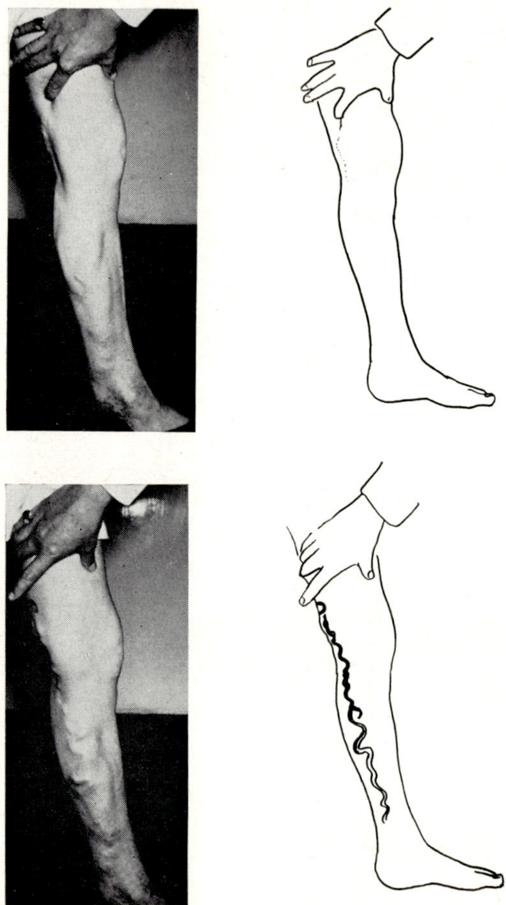

Fig. 380.—Trendelenburg's test. Digital compression of the main saphenous vein in the thigh, after elevation: *above*, no early refilling, *below*, release of compression allows incompetent downward filling. Compression site is marked with a circle before operation.

Trendelenburg's Test (*Fig.* 380) may be used to show up the main sites of incompetence. The leg is raised above body level in order to drain the varicose vein, and then with the suspected incompetent proximal vein compressed with one finger, the patient is asked to stand up. If the site of leakage has been correctly identified the varices should remain comparatively empty, though they may fill slowly from below through secondary incompetent communications. On removing the compression the varices at once refill, the blood can be seen to be running down within the affected vein, and often felt as a fluid thrill at the point previously compressed.

Locating Perforating Veins.—In performing the Trendelenburg test, when the patient stands up, before the tourniquet is released, it may be noticed that the leg veins are filling relatively quickly (within 30 sec.) from below. This is because blood is leaking out superficially from the deep veins through incompetent connecting perforator veins. Their exact location may be determined by repeating the test, having pairs of thin rubber tubing tourniquets 5 cm. apart placed progressively distally on the limb till the leak is isolated between them.

Perthes's Test (*Fig.* 381) is the reverse of the above: a light venous tourniquet is applied just above the main varices and the patient is instructed to walk several times up and down the room. Being prevented by the constriction from refilling from above, and with the muscle pump emptying the deep veins if these are normally competent, the blood in the varices in turn empties into the deep compartment and the varices disappear. This proves not only that the

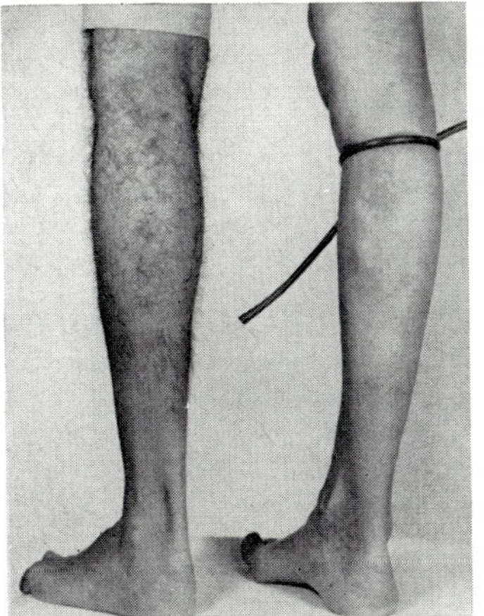

Fig. 381.—Perthes's test: walking with a light tourniquet in position allows emptying of the calf varices to take place via the patent deep veins. Varices remain full and pain is marked if deep channels are non-functioning.

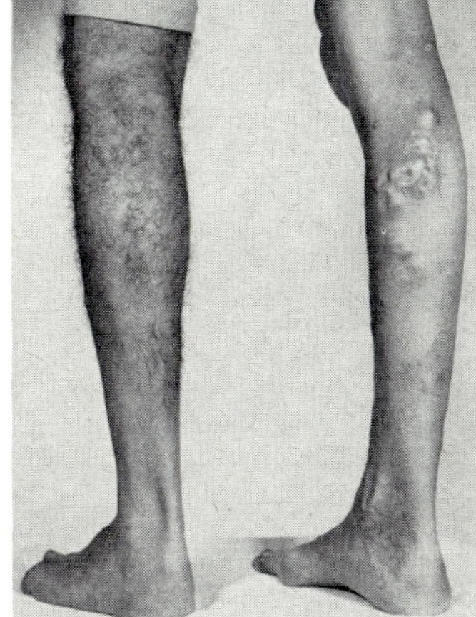

Fig. 382.—Positive Trendelenburg's test in short saphenous vein. The calf veins are empty after elevation and application of tourniquet below the knee (*left*). Refilling from the popliteal fossa is rapid when the tubing is removed (*right*).

veins fill from their own incompetent proximal course, but also that the deep venous drainage is normal, both points being important. When the deep veins are occluded pain in the leg becomes acute after a short walk.

Short Saphenous Vein.—Testing of incompetence is shown in *Fig.* 382.

Increased Local Heat is present over varices and incompetent perforators, due to warmed blood coming out from within the deep compartments of the limb.

Œdema is often present in the more extensive cases, especially in heavy people or late in pregnancy.

Eczema is commoner in men, and is probably started by irritation and scratching. It is typically seen in the lower anterior tibial region.

Ulceration is sometimes produced in the same place and in the same way. The true *varicose ulcer* is uncommon; it is well localized, superficial, and causes no great distress; quite unlike the *gravitational ulcer* of deep venous insufficiency which is almost always post-tibial, deeply based, and very painful, yet the leg shows no visible varicose veins. It is clearly wrong to term the latter ulcer 'varicose'; a venous ulcer is a better description.

OPERATION FOR VARICOSE VEINS

Indication.—Small isolated varices may be treated by injection (p. 540). An unfit patient may have to wear supporting elastic stockings permanently. But most cases benefit from operation. It is wrong to promise that every minor blemish will disappear; many small varices away from the main saphenous vein and the 'sunburst' venular type of lesion are likely to persist, as will prominent veins below ankle-joint level. However, they should not progress and ulceration is prevented. Vague leg pains not related to the main vein are unlikely to be cured by operation.

Pre-operative Preparation.—After the patient has had a shave and hot bath the evening before operation he is stood up on a low stool in a good light and the main varices are marked using a throat swab and 1 per cent gentian violet solution, or a fibre ink writer. The main veins are lined in and the suspected sites of perforators are marked with a circle (*see Fig.* 380).

Anæsthesia.—General anæsthesia is mostly preferred and is necessary if the veins are to be stripped. Local anæsthetic can be employed when only a flush saphenofemoral ligation is proposed. About 15 ml. of 1 per cent lignocaine are injected in the line of the skin incision, with small amounts infiltrated more deeply downwards or in a triangular pattern around the saphenous opening. Care is taken by preliminary aspiration to ensure that a vessel is not entered.

Preparation.—The legs and pubes are shaved. Skin preparation must be thorough. The entire leg (except toes and sole of foot) and the groin and lower abdomen must be painted with the chosen skin antiseptic. A small sterile gauze sock is placed over the foot; the genitalia are covered. Sterile drapes are then applied so that the legs are abducted, the heels resting comfortably on a board placed transversely across the lower end of the table.

High Ligation.—This consists of tying and dividing the long saphenous vein (and all its tributaries) at its junction with the femoral vein. To avoid injury to the femoral artery its pulsation is first noted. A 2-in. (5-cm.) incision in the line of the groin fold is made medial to it, and 1 in. (2·5 cm.) below the pubic tubercle. It is deepened through fat and superficial fascia, and small double hooks or a mastoid self-retaining retractor inserted to improve the exposure. Identification of the saphenous vein is aided by its being dilated or having a frank varix on it, and by the tributaries which enter it.

Classically there are three main tributaries—the superficial epigastric and circumflex iliac running downwards, and the superficial pudendal joining medially (*Fig.* 383). In practice there are many variations and the operator must dissect carefully to discover the arrangement in any individual case. Often the two sides

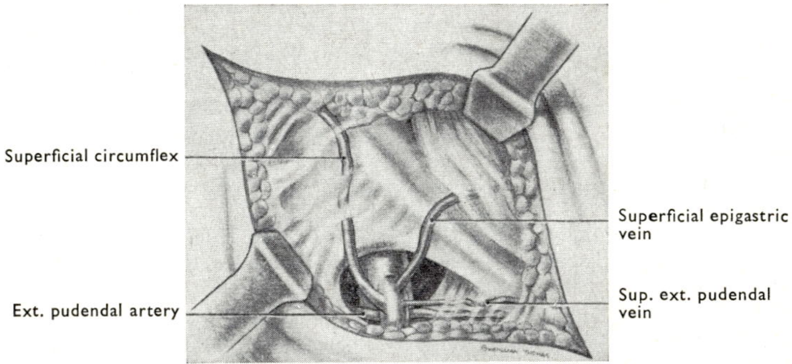

Fig. 383.—Termination of the right long saphenous vein. Ligation must be made above all its branches.

are mirror images of each other. The small veins are clipped, divided, and tied with No. 0 plain catgut. The long saphenous vein is clipped and divided 1 in. (2·5 cm.) below its termination; using small gauze pledgets mounted on Mayo's artery forceps for dissection, its confluence with the femoral vein is displayed all round. Often the small pudendal artery running transversely distal to the junction has to be divided and tied. A strong catgut ligature is then tied round the saphenous vein flush with, but not encroaching on, the wall of the femoral vein. The distal end of the saphenous vein is tied off or dealt with as described below under Stripping.

Finally, the fascia is sutured across the saphenous opening and then the subcutaneous fatty tissue approximated with fine plain catgut. The skin is then sutured, the sutures remaining for 5–7 days.

Previously marked incompetent perforating veins may have to be ligated through a 2-in. (5-cm.) vertical incision medial to the lower tibia.

Stripping Veins.—If a Myer's vein stripper (*Fig.* 384) is to be used the artery forceps on the distal end of the main vein in the groin is left in position and a ligature is placed loosely round the vein. The operator then makes a 0·5 in.

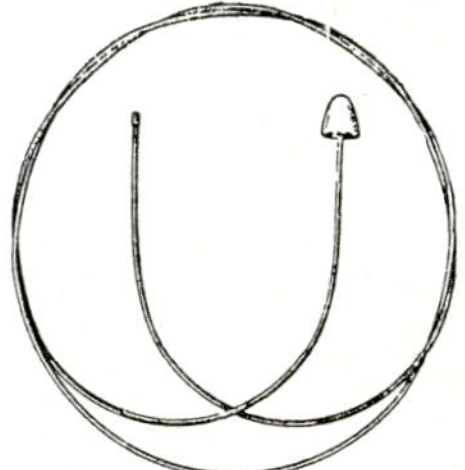

Fig. 384.—Myer's vein stripper.

(1·2 cm.) transverse incision about 0·5 in. (1·2 cm.) above and in front of the tip of the medial malleolus. The saphenous vein is lifted up and a fine plain catgut ligature threaded below it and tied on the distal side. A similar ligature is put loosely round the proximal part and its ends held in an artery forceps. Using the forceps to steady the vein, the vein is cut half-way through with a sharp scalpel so that the lumen is seen. Back-flow of blood is controlled by elevating the forceps.

The probe end of the vein stripper is passed into the lumen, then up the saphenous vein to the groin. A small cut in the side of the vein there enables it to emerge, bleeding then being stopped by tightening the ligature previously placed there. If upward progress is arrested, withdrawing the stripper 2 in. (5 cm.) and rotating it on its long axis may help it follow the lumen upwards; external pressure over the end of the stripper also assists it in negotiating any obstruction. The acorn is screwed on to the distal end of the stripper, which is then pulled upwards till the acorn lies in the subcutaneous tissues, the vein having been divided. The foot of the operating table is raised to check venous bleeding.

The ankle incision is then stitched, a dressing applied, the leg elevated, and a 4-in. or 6-in. (10–15-cm.) crêpe bandage applied from the base of the toes upwards. As the bandaging advances proximally the stripper is pulled steadily towards the groin, stripping out the vein.

Post-operative Care.—As well as the firmly applied operative 6-in. bandages of sterile crêpe, the patient is next day shown how to apply the 'blue line' or Bisgaard type elastic bandages from toes to patellar tubercle and for at least 3 weeks must always wear these whenever the leg is to be lowered below the horizontal.

The foot of the bed is raised on blocks during the patient's stay in hospital. Many patients (without ulcers) can return home after 36 hours. Stitches are removed at the end of 1 week.

Walking is encouraged as soon as possible and as far as is reasonably comfortable, but standing should be avoided. Marking time lessens the harmful congestive effect.

Injection-compression (Fegan's technique).—Either as primary treatment or in the completion of the operative cure this method is finding increasing use in the British Isles.

The Principles which distinguish it from earlier injection methods are:—

1. Confining the injection (sotradecyl 1–2 ml.) to a short segment on either side of the puncture by digital compression.

2. Applying and maintaining firm and secure compression by bandages evenly applied and held in place by strips of elastoplast and held up if necessary by suspenders. These bandages remain in place for 6 weeks.

3. The patient is instructed to walk at least 3 miles each day. With ordinary injection methods and without continuous support the newly formed thrombus often becomes separated from the vein wall along one side for a considerable distance, thus early recanalization may occur and initiate the recurrence of the varices. This tendency for occluded veins to reopen is well established, though often forgotten. It may be a result of the abundant fibrinolytic activity present in all veins, and necessary to their continued normal function.

SUPERFICIAL THROMBOPHLEBITIS

When a large varicose vein becomes thrombosed, as in some heavy middle-aged men, and in women in their puerperium, a tender raised rounded nodular cord is formed usually along the line of the main saphenous vein, somewhere near the knee; the overlying skin becomes reddened and slightly œdematous, though there is no general swelling of the limb nor any more ankle œdema than may have already been present before the complication.

The treatment of this common, temporarily disabling condition is firm elastic support, and continued normal activity. Pain and local reaction may be reduced by giving phenylbutazone, 100 mg. four times a day for 5 days. No anticoagulants

Sotradecyl (Philadelphia Laboratories Inc., Philadelphia, U.S.A.).
Elastoplast (Smith & Nephew Ltd., Hull and Welwyn Garden City, Herts).

are normally needed, though if a patient is considered to be in special risk of spreading thrombosis, for example, after operation or confinement, a week's course of phenindione or other oral prothrombin depressor drug is advisable (*see* p. 81).

The tender lump formed by a thrombosed large varix may take many weeks to diminish in size: and so it is worth considering excising it locally in order to shorten the disability.

Another indication for early operation exists when in an elderly patient a prominent varicose internal saphenous vein, present for many years without symptoms, then develops a spreading thrombosis which daily extends a little more proximally up the thigh, and is clearly destined to involve the sapheno-femoral opening in time. A preventive ligation at this site is advisable before the deep femoral is reached. A tongue of thrombus may in fact have to be extracted from the main vein (*see also* Thrombectomy for iliofemoral thrombosis, *below*).

DEEP-VEIN THROMBOSIS (PHLEBOTHROMBOSIS)

Prevention.—This dangerous complication of old age, serious disease, hospitalization, and major operations of all kinds can be lessened in incidence and severity by keeping patients up and about, prescribing deep-breathing exercises, and ensuring adequate hydration when necessary (*see* p. 166). At operation a clean and expeditious technique is desirable, so shortening the time under anæsthesia and the amount of tissue trauma which appears to be responsible for the thrombotic tendency. Where this is inevitable, as in the case of major fractures of the lower limb in the elderly, a course of oral anticoagulants should be given, for this has been shown to reduce strikingly the incidence of pulmonary embolism in these patients and in those who are overweight.

Diagnosis.—The diagnosis of acute deep-vein thrombosis should be suspected when at the end of a week the patient shows a low pyrexia and increased pulse-rate, with some tenderness in the calf or along the course of the main vein. Swelling of the calf and ankle suggests femoropopliteal thrombosis, while if the thigh is mainly involved the block is probably iliofemoral. Homans's sign (pain in the calf on passive dorsiflexion of the ankle) is useful in detecting the early case.

Later the swelling may diminish to some extent, as collateral venous channels open up to help bridge the occlusion. Some of these enlarged veins can be seen crossing the groin or extending up towards the costal margin if the occlusion has reached the inferior vena cava. Swelling in this instance is usually unequal on the two sides, perhaps because the thrombus has spread upwards from the more involved limb.

Massive spreading thrombosis of deep and superficial veins produces a hot, swollen, cyanosed and even blistered limb which may then develop venous gangrene.

Treatment.—Heparin, rather than the oral agents, is advisable for this serious condition, The common practice of giving heparin only to 'cover' the first 24 hours during which an oral drug is gaining effective levels, while perhaps suitable for mild cases, is open to the objection that once the heparin is stopped a complete arrest of fibrin deposition is no longer ensured; also any spontaneous and beneficial fibrinolytic activity in the heparinized system is lost with the return of renewed normal or abnormal levels of intravascular fibrin formation. It is therefore recommended that heparin should be continued for several days, or at least until clinical resolution has taken place; after this time the oral agent may be introduced, mainly to prevent recurrence.

A contra-indication to heparin is of course any early post-operative state, when reactionary bleeding may be due to fibrinolysis. After 3–4 days it is usually safe, though not if there is any evidence of infection.

THROMBECTOMY FOR ILIOFEMORAL THROMBOSIS

Patients with iliofemoral venous thrombosis may now have early operative removal of the obstruction.

One technique involves a limited exploration of the saphenofemoral opening, followed by a sutured repair of the deep femoral once a free flow of blood has been obtained from distal and proximal ends. The approach is as for displaying the saphenofemoral junction (*see* p. 538) and then freeing the femoral vein for 0·5 in. (1·2 cm.) above and below, passing tapes around it temporarily. Thrombus is sucked out through a small phlebotomy incision. Heparin and low molecular weight dextran should be given at once and for some days after operation.

An alternative and preferred technique is to use a Fogarty balloon catheter. Thrombosis in the iliofemoral venous segment can be located exactly by ascending venography, injecting 10–15 ml. of 25 per cent hypaque or 60 per cent urografin

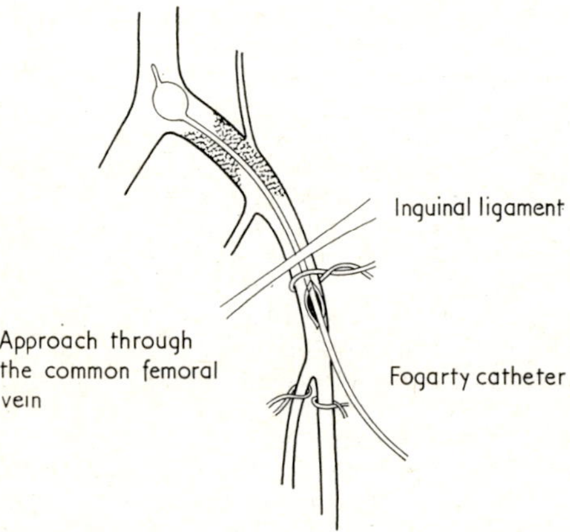

Fig. 385.—Thrombectomy by insertion of a Fogarty catheter into the femoral vein just below the inguinal ligament, advancing its tip beyond the thrombus and then withdrawing the inflated balloon.

intravenously at a distal point. A 3-in. (7·5 cm.) vertical incision is made over the femoral vein, starting just above the inguinal ligament. The common femoral vein and saphenofemoral junction are cleared and tapes passed around the principal veins to control them (*Fig.* 385). A 1-cm. long incision is made in the common femoral vein just below the inguinal ligament. The tip of a Fogarty catheter is inserted and pushed up till it is judged to be well clear of the upper limits of the thrombus. The balloon is then inflated with 2–5 ml. of fluid and the catheter withdrawn, bringing the thrombus in front of it. Further venograms through a polythene catheter show if all the thrombus has been removed. The phlebotomy incision is then sutured, the tapes removed, and the skin closed.

An early and dramatic resolution of pain and swelling are usual, and late post-phlebitic complications appear to be lessened. The success rate with the Fogarty catheter is now approaching 80 per cent; rethromboses may eventually be treated by infusion of fibrinolytic agents, e.g., streptokinase.

LIGATION OF THE DEEP VEIN

For many years it has been thought necessary sometimes to ligate the femoral or iliac vein in some patients with repeated pulmonary embolism. Usually in such cases a continued course of heparin has not been tried; ligation should not be considered unless it has. Unfortunately late thrombectomy (after the first 3–5 days) has not given as good results as in cases operated upon early.

Ligation of the inferior vena cava has been advocated. Like iliofemoral ligation it carries an inevitable penalty of obstructive sequelæ, often severe in the older, heavier types of patient. Operative narrowing of the vena cava by a mesh of sutures or a serrated clip aims at maintaining patency while preventing the onward passage of an embolus.

Pulmonary Embolectomy.—Once thought to be heroic and fruitless, this was largely abandoned until the recent introduction of small ready-sterilized pump oxygenator circuits not requiring blood to prime them. A subacute deteriorating case of pulmonary arterial obstruction in an otherwise good-risk patient should now be considered for the operation whether or not the apparatus is available, provided a surgeon with vascular or thoracic experience is available in the emergency.

LATE POST-PHLEBITIC COMPLICATIONS

Pain, swelling, and ulceration are the effects of an insufficient venous return over months or years, and the brunt of the condition is borne by the tissues over the ankle perforating veins.

For a long while there is pain, tenderness, induration, and pigmentation at these sites, with fibrosis and fat necrosis beneath the thinned and unhealthy skin.

Some small injury opens up these pathological tissues and spontaneous healing is seldom possible. The result is a chronic venous ulcer.

TREATMENT OF VENOUS ULCER

Local Applications.—These are of little use except as palliatives and for the control of skin eruption. Antibiotic and other creams and ointments tend to set up sensitivity states which are often part of the presenting syndrome.

Support.—Reversal of the local congestion and chronic inflammation and sepsis can only be achieved by firm support in ambulant patients or by elevation, preferably in hospital.

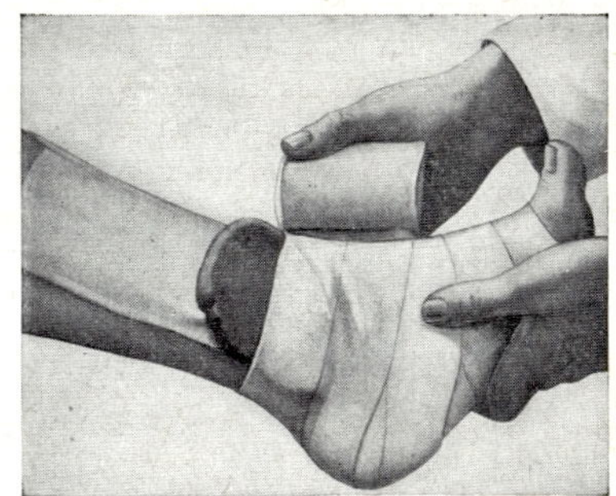

Fig. 386.—Showing pad of cellulose sponge used near the internal malleolus. In women it is better to apply the adhesive plaster from above downwards.

A non-stick dressing, a sterile foam plastic pressure pad, and a Bisgaard bandage, however, are effective in most early cases (*Fig.* 386). Other proprietary bandages such as viscopaste, dalzoband, or cereband are useful for the control of minor cases and those with skin sensitivity to adhesive or rubber (*see* p. 194).

Elevation.—Raising the foot of the bed at night gives the ambulant outpatient the advantage of several hours of continuous relief of venous hypertension and augments the good effects of the support by day.

Viscopaste, Dalzoband, Cereband (Smith & Nephew Ltd., Hull and Welwyn Garden City, Herts).

In-patient treatment is essential in the severe, resistant type of ulcer with such severe pain and tenderness that support can no longer be tolerated. Provided that the ankle pulses are present very high elevation is advisable using an inverted chair backed with pillows (*Fig.* 387), as well as the tilted bed.

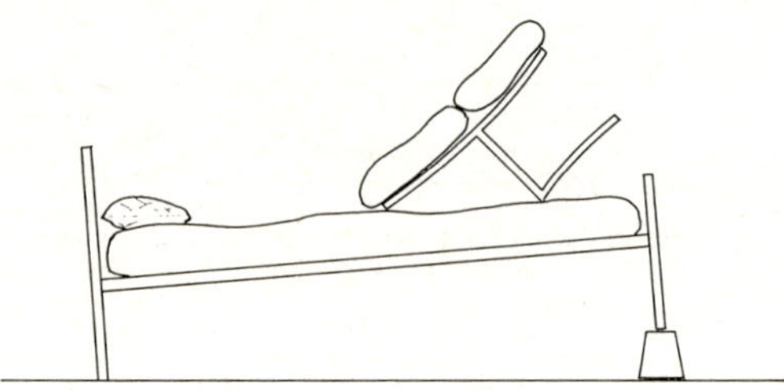

Fig. 387.—A simple method of providing for high elevation of the congested lower limb.

Skin-grafting.—This hastens healing in the milder cases, pinch grafts being very easy to apply under local anæsthesia in the ward by the junior surgical resident (*see* p. 485). Any necessary larger plastic procedure should be combined with ligation of the perforating veins, a major undertaking for it opens up the deep fascial layer and approaches the posterior tibial vessels and nerve. Results are excellent, however, providing that the incompetent communications have been fully identified and interrupted.

Post-operative Care.—This is as for the conservative in-patient régime. After leaving hospital support should be continually worn, though in these patients an elastic stocking may after one month replace the unsightly Bisgaard bandage.

Requests to inject remaining visible veins should be resisted unless these are grossly and obviously incompetent, and therefore adding to the impairment of total venous return.

Weight reduction is one important contribution which the patient can make towards future control of his condition.

CHAPTER XXXVIII

INJURIES OF THE HAND AND FINGERS

By Eric L. Farquharson

"It is more important to save the injured finger of a young worker, than to operate on an extensive carcinoma in an old patient." (Böhler.)

INJURIES of the hand and fingers are the most common of all domestic and industrial accidents. A critical appreciation of their severity is therefore essential to the general practitioner and to the factory surgeon, both of whom should be prepared either to carry out correct treatment or to refer the case without delay to a hospital.

In the present state of shortage of hospital beds in large industrial cities, it is a counsel of perfection to urge that all hand injuries except those of a trivial character should be admitted to hospital. Most cases must perforce be dealt with as out-patients, and a serious responsibility rests upon the house-surgeon or casualty officer who is required to undertake their treatment. It should always be remembered that in most cases it is the *initial* treatment that determines the final result.

1. All aseptic precautions are essential. The initial treatment should not be carried out in a casualty department unless a well-equipped operating theatre is attached.

2. Full anæsthesia of the part must be provided. For injuries of the distal two-thirds of a finger, local anæsthesia is usually entirely satisfactory. For injuries of the proximal segment of a finger, or of the palm or dorsum of the hand, a general anæsthetic is desirable.

3. All except the most superficial wounds must be explored carefully, in order that all foreign matter can be removed and the full extent of the injury determined.

4. Except in clean-cut wounds, débridement should be performed with meticulous care and with the aid of a tourniquet.

5. Primary suture is permissible only in circumstances detailed on p. 548.

Preparation of the Part.—All traumatic wounds of the hand are contaminated to a varying degree, and thorough cleansing is essential. Soap (preferably ether soap) and water are among the best cleansing agents. The entire hand is placed in a basin and is lathered energetically. A handful of wool or gauze is used in preference to a nailbrush, as this latter may liberate latent organisms from the deeper layers of the skin or may traumatize exposed tissues in the wound. When all possible dirt has been removed, the soap is washed away with sterile water or with some solution such as cetavlon. The skin around the wound may be painted with a stronger antiseptic such as iodine, but this should not be allowed to enter the wound.

Local Anæsthesia of a Finger or Thumb (*see* p. 561).

Tourniquets.—When possible, a tourniquet should be employed during the repair of hand injuries, in order that the operation can be conducted in a bloodless field, and that delicate tissues may be spared the trauma of repeated swabbing. A simple tourniquet for a finger is provided by a rubber band applied tightly around its base.

Cetavlon (I.C.I. Ltd., Pharmaceuticals Division, Macclesfield, Cheshire).

For operations on the hand the tourniquet must be applied to the upper arm. Owing to the risks of nerve injury in this situation, a tourniquet of rubber tubing is *absolutely forbidden*. The safest and most satisfactory tourniquet for the arm is a pneumatic tourniquet or the arm-band of a sphygmomanometer. This can be retained for periods of 1–1½ hours with perfect safety.

The limb should first be emptied of blood by means of an Esmarch's rubber bandage (*Fig.* 388), which is applied tightly from the finger-tips upwards to a level just above the elbow. The sphygmomanometer arm-band is then applied and is inflated to a pressure of 20–30 mm. Hg above the systolic, after which the rubber bandage is removed. The rubber tubing connecting the arm-band to the sphygmomanometer bulb should be clamped with a hæmostat close to the arm-band, otherwise slow leakage of air may occur at the valve.

A baking-tray type of wire grid (*Fig.* 389) is an effective device for steadying the hand during operation.

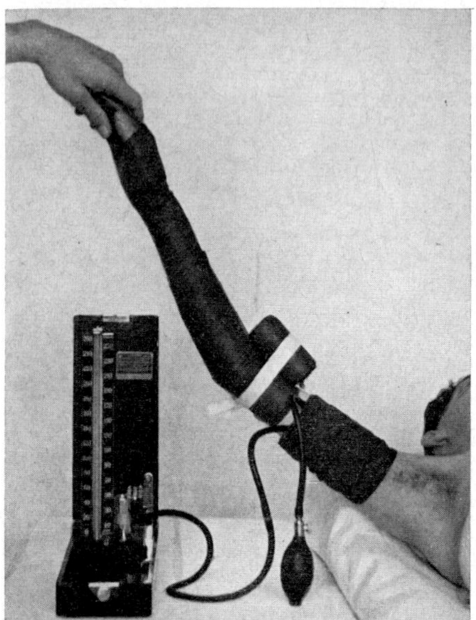

Fig. 388.—Method of obtaining a bloodless field in operations on the hand or fingers. Before the sphygmomanometer arm-band is inflated, the limb is emptied of blood by means of an Esmarch's rubber bandage applied from the finger-tips upwards.

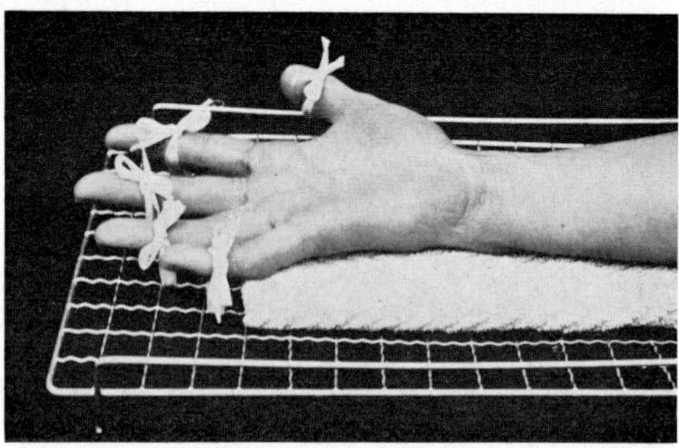

Fig. 389.—A wire grid ('baking-tray'), which is easily sterilized, makes an excellent support for the hand during operations. The digits are held in extension by separate tapes tied to the grid.

Excision or Débridement.—Formal *excision* of the wound (in the strict sense of the term) is rarely practicable in the case of the hand and fingers, since there is so little tissue to spare, but as thorough *débridement* as is possible must be carried out. Any ragged, devitalized, or grossly contaminated skin edges are excised, so as to leave the wound margins as healthy as possible. It is better to accept a slight deficiency of skin than to leave in situ skin that is almost certain to become infected. Equally important is the subcutaneous fatty tissue, which on the palmar surface often prolapses through the skin wound; this tissue has little resistance to infection, and, if bruised or contaminated, should be excised widely.

The wound is explored thoroughly to ensure the removal of all foreign material and devitalized tissue, and to investigate possible damage to the deeper structures. If the wound requires to be enlarged, any incisions used for this purpose must be made with care and forethought. No such incision should be made to cross a major crease; it should lie either *in* a crease or be placed in an area where creases are absent. Thus, a transverse wound on the flexor surface of a finger must not be enlarged by cutting up or down from its centre, for a crippling keloid scar will then result. Instead, an incision should be made distally from one end of the wound and, if necessary, another incision made proximally from its other end (*Fig.* 390). If necessary, the transverse wound is extended so that both the longitudinal incisions will lie beyond the flexion creases. The double flaps which are raised give excellent exposure. Incisions used to enlarge wounds of the palm or wrist region should be placed with similar regard to the principles involved.

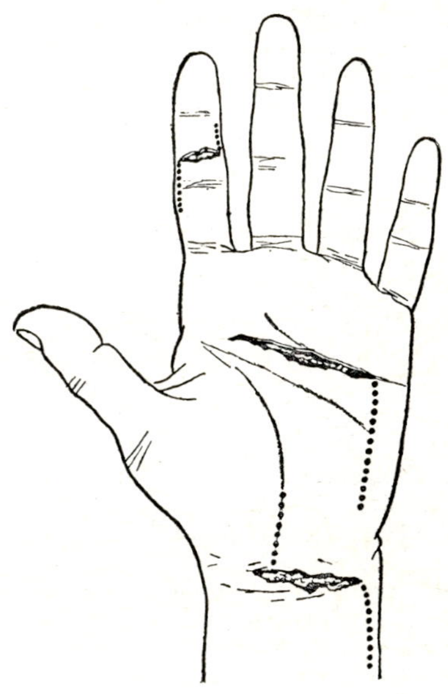

Fig. 390.—Incisions that are permissible for enlarging wounds of the hand and fingers. An incision should never cross a crease; it should lie either *in* a crease or in an area where creases are absent.

Hæmorrhage should be arrested if possible by forci-pressure. Buried ligatures are best avoided, but, if a vessel requires ligation, fine silk should be used in preference to catgut, since the latter forms a favourable nidus for bacterial growth.

Primary Suture.—The first aim in treatment is to avoid infection, which is particularly disastrous in the hand and fingers since it may spread to tendon-sheaths or to deep fascial spaces. Even if it is confined to the skin, suppuration may cause permanent disability owing to the formation of an indurated scar.

Chemotherapy has done much to reduce the incidence of infection, but it in no way obviates the necessity for correct surgical technique.

Primary suture is permissible only when the wound is recent, when contamination is minimal, and when the skin edges can be brought together without tension.

Fine non-absorbent suture material threaded on a slender needle should be used. The minimum number of stitches are inserted, and they are tied without tension. No attempt is made to secure a 'neat' wound by accurate coaptation of the skin edges, since the serous exudate, which is potentially infected, should be allowed free exit. It should

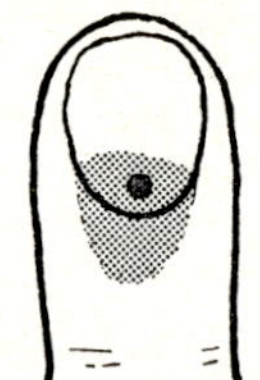

Fig. 392.—Trephining the nail in order to evacuate a subungual hæmatoma.

be noted that the superficial horny layer of the palmar skin does not unite by first intention, but is always desquamated.

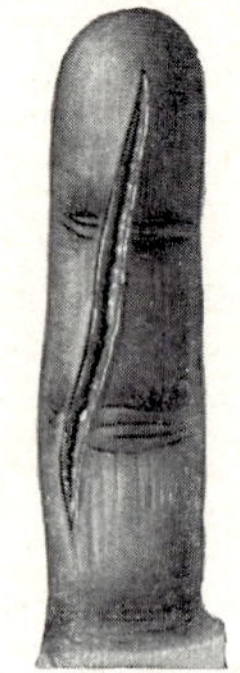

Fig. 391.—A clean-cut linear wound on the palmar surface of a finger does not gape, because of the attachment of skin to deep fascia. Stitches are therefore unnecessary, and may predispose to infection.

In cases where the above conditions do not pertain, *the skin should not be sutured*. Adequate apposition can often be obtained by the pressure of dressings alone; if not, the wound must be left open and allowed to heal by granulation. With such treatment healing may be expected to occur without suppuration and with the formation of a supple scar—a result far superior to that obtained when primary suture has been followed by even a mild degree of infection.

Linear Cuts and Lacerations.—The wound should be explored carefully, but, if it is a relatively clean-cut one, débridement is not required. On the palmar surface of the hand or finger linear wounds do not gape (*Fig.* 391), unless there is tension in the subcutaneous tissues, so that stitches are unnecessary and may predispose to infection.

Subungual Hæmatoma.—This causes pain and may become infected, and should be evacuated. Under digital ring block, a sharp scalpel blade is used as a drill to trephine a small hole just above the quick (*Fig.* 392). By gently squeezing all the blood can be evacuated.

'Burst Finger' is the result of severe compression. The skin literally bursts open, and tendons, bones, or joints may be exposed. Because of swelling of the subcutaneous tissues, it is usually impossible to close the wound without tension (*Fig.* 393). Stitches should therefore be avoided as far as possible, and, after careful débridement (which includes the removal of all devitalized fatty tissue), the wound edges are approximated by the pressure of dressings alone. A few stitches may be necessary to secure a covering for exposed tendons and bones, but these must be tied loosely.

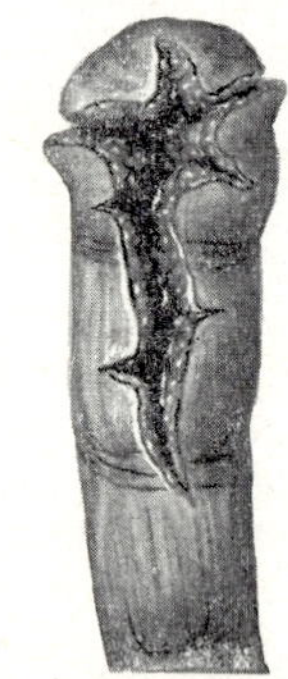

Fig. 393.— In an irregularly lacerated or 'bursting' wound, gaping is due mainly to swelling and oedema, so that the skin cannot be closed without tension. Stitches are therefore dangerous.

Wounds with Raised Skin-flaps.—It is most important to assess the viability of any raised skin-flap, as judged by its colour and by the presence of bleeding at its free edge. For this purpose it is necessary to remove the tourniquet as soon as the initial débridement has been completed. If the edges appear to be completely ischæmic, the flap must be trimmed down until bleeding occurs. All skin considered to be viable should be gently but thoroughly cleansed with saline, and any ragged edges excised.

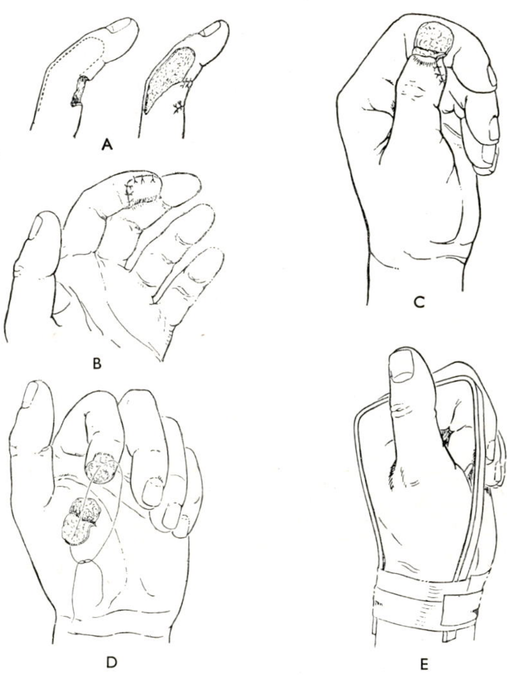

Fig. 394.—Methods of replacing skin-loss in the fingers by local flaps. A, Rotational flap from side of finger to palmar surface. B and C, Different types of 'cross-finger' flaps. D and E, Thenar flap applied to tip of index finger, and method of subsequent immobilization, by means of an aluminium splint.

As much as possible of the subcutaneous fat is cut away, as this tissue has very little vitality. The flap is then dusted with antibiotic powder, and is returned to position, where it is secured by the minimum number of fine stitches. One or two rubber tissue drains are placed beneath it, in order to prevent hæmatoma formation, and a compression dressing is applied. There must be no tension on the flap, or inevitably sloughing will occur; it is far better to leave a gap to heal by granulation, or to which a skin-graft can be applied. If the evidence suggests that the entire flap may be non-viable, it should be ruthlessly cut away and replaced by a skin-graft, since leaving it to necrose in situ can serve only to promote sepsis. It should be noted that flaps which are based distally are usually ischæmic, and therefore unlikely to survive.

Wounds with Loss of Skin.—All loss of skin in the hand and fingers should be made good by skin-grafting as soon as possible, since this not only hastens healing, but by preventing infection it obviates fibrosis and contracture.

Partial-thickness Grafts have the advantage that they are readily available, and 'take' successfully in a large proportion of cases, even in the presence of a mild degree of sepsis. Owing to their poor wearing qualities, they are less satisfactory on the palmar than on the dorsal surfaces, but as a temporary expedient they may be excellent (*see* p. 485).

Full-thickness Grafts should if possible be used for replacing skin lost from the finger pulps or from the palm. Free grafts are the more easily applied: they involve only one operation, and do not require the patient's admission to hospital—but they are less certain to 'take' in conditions where complete asepsis cannot be assured. They may be taken from the post-auricular region or from the forearm. They should be cut accurately to the shape required, without subcutaneous fat, and stitched under normal tension. A severed finger-tip may sometimes be stitched back in position, with a successful result.

Small defects on the palmar or dorsal surface of a finger can be covered by swinging over a flap of skin from the lateral surface, where it can be better spared (*Fig.* 394 A). The donor area is then covered with a split-skin graft. Alternative methods are by the use of *cross-finger* and *thenar* flaps. These are illustrated in *Fig.* 394 B–E. Such flaps must be planned with meticulous care, so that they can be stitched in position without tension, and immobilization must be maintained until a successful 'take' is assured. The donor area is covered with a split-skin graft. It should be noted that such methods of treatment carry a slight but inescapable risk of damaging healthy structures in the rest of the hand, either by spread of infection or as the result of the immobilization. They should not be undertaken, therefore, by the inexperienced, or in the presence of gross contamination. The application of a split-skin graft as a purely temporary expedient is often to be preferred.

When a large area of skin has been lost or is considered to be non-viable, conservative treatment presents considerable problems. In cases where a single finger (but not, of course, the thumb) has been seriously denuded ('skinned or degloved finger'), amputation is usually the best treatment, the bone being divided at a level at which an adequate covering of healthy skin can be obtained. The more complicated skin-grafting procedures necessitated by such injuries involve a prolonged period of incapacity, which the patient can seldom afford, and the end-result, as regards either function or appearance, is by no means assured. Such treatment should be attempted only in those patients who voluntarily demand it, and in whom there is evidence of the ability to co-operate.

Loss of skin from the thumb or from the body of the hand invariably demands some method of skin-grafting, since amputation is never justifiable on this account. Occasionally, the skin of an injured finger which requires to be amputated may be used to cover a defect in the hand. The finger is split longitudinally, and the bones and nail are removed. The skin is then opened out, trimmed as required, and sutured in position over the raw area.

Pedicle Grafting from Distant Sites.—Grafts to replace skin-loss from the body of the hand may be taken from the thigh, the abdominal wall, or the opposite forearm. When the loss affects the palm of the hand, a broad-based flap, cut to the exact size required, may be raised from the abdominal wall, and sutured accurately to the edges of the defect (*Fig.* 395). The bed from which the flap has been raised is then covered with split-skin grafts. Careful fixation of the hand against the donor site is of course essential. When much contamination has occurred it may be desirable to delay skin-grafting until sepsis has been overcome, and the denuded area is covered with healthy granulations.

Foreign Bodies in the Hand or Fingers.—Unless the foreign body can be identified easily by palpation, its removal is usually much more difficult than would appear. If it is radio-opaque, radiographs in at least two planes must be taken immediately before operation. To assist in the localization, various devices may be employed—e.g., crossed wires strapped to the skin. When the foreign body has been localized as accurately as possible, a corresponding mark is made on the skin surface. If a needle or other elongated object is being sought, the incision should be made across its long axis. Wooden foreign bodies are always contaminated, so that after their removal the wound should not be sutured.

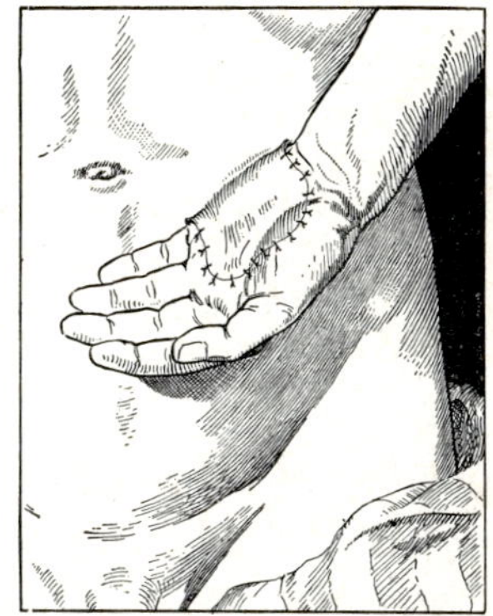

Fig. 395.—Direct pedicle flap from abdominal wall for replacement of skin loss in palm.

Grease-gun Injuries to the hand and fingers result from the misuse of high-pressure equipment in the garage trade. The jet of grease expelled from the fine nozzles in use may penetrate the tissues for a considerable distance. Distension of the tissue planes with grease may lead first to numbness, and then to gangrene, so that amputation is not infrequently required. Treatment consists in immediate exploration of the part, with removal of as much of the grease as is possible. The wound is then left widely open to granulate.

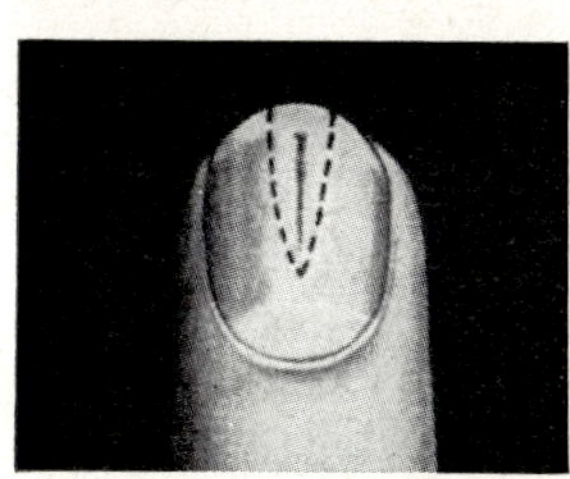

Fig. 396.—A wedge-shaped piece of nail should be removed to give access to a foreign body beneath the nail.

Splinter below the Nail.—Failure to remove all or part of the foreign body causes infection. Under a digital ring block a wedge of nail overlying the splinter is excised (*Fig.* 396). The foreign body is removed and the wound thoroughly cleaned and dressed.

Wounds with Division of Nerves.—The median and ulnar nerves are commonly severed in transverse wounds across the front of the wrist region (*Fig.* 401), and, unless special care is taken, such nerve injuries may be overlooked. Lesions of these nerves can be detected by the methods illustrated in *Figs.* 397–400. Where doubt exists as to the possibility of nerve injury, the nerves should be exposed and examined carefully during the surgical toilet of the wound.

The digital nerves are frequently divided in wounds involving the sides of a finger. Since anæsthesia of a finger is no small handicap, they should be sought for carefully, and, if at all possible, repaired by *primary suture*. These nerves are structures of appreciable size, and their repair is not so difficult as might be supposed. Since they are unmixed sensory nerves, the results of repair are most gratifying.

A severed median or ulnar nerve may be repaired also by primary suture, provided that conditions are ideal—i.e., in a recent clean-cut wound, and where the operator has experience and all necessary facilities. When such conditions do not pertain, it is often better to make no attempt at primary repair, but

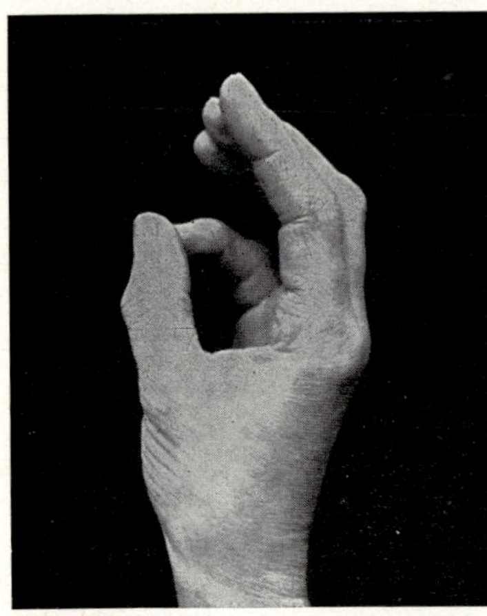

Fig. 397.—Test for median nerve injury. Approximation of thumb to little finger (thenar muscles).

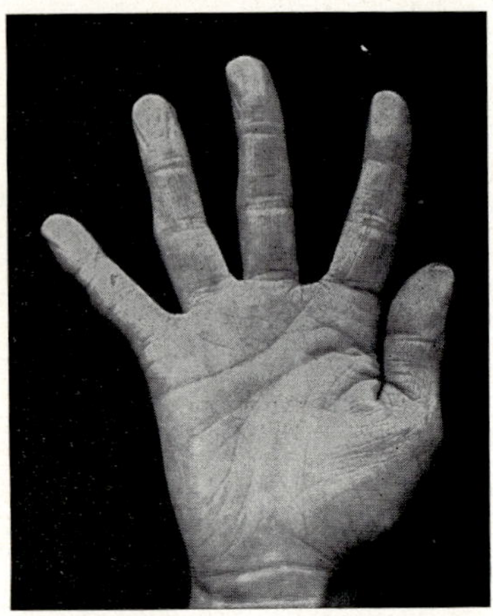

Fig. 398.—Test for ulnar nerve injury. The patient is asked to spread his fingers widely (posterior interossei).

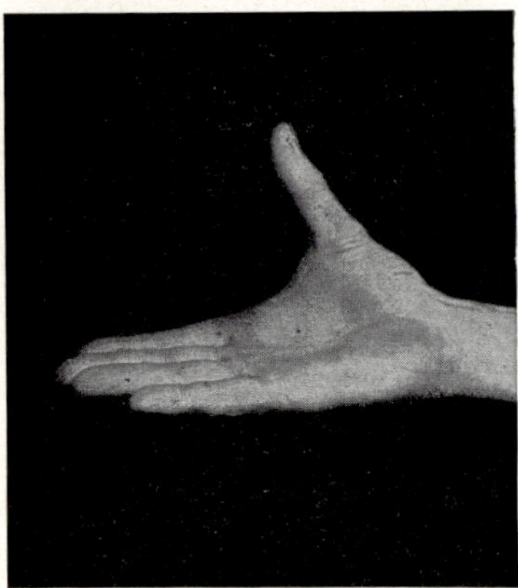

Fig. 399.—Another test for median nerve injury. Simple abduction of the thumb —raising it towards the vertical when the plane of the hand is horizontal (abductor pollicis brevis).

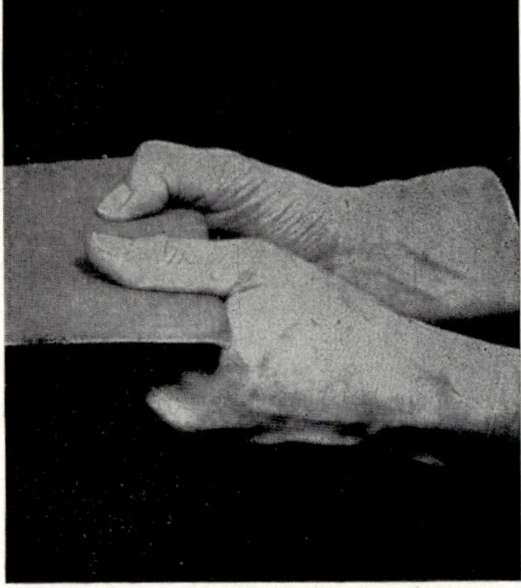

Fig. 400.—A constant sign (Froment's) in ulnar paresis. When gripping a thin board the affected thumb is bent at terminal joint by the long flexor, since the adductor is paralysed.

simply to place the nerve-ends under adjacent structures for protection. Secondary suture is carried out, if possible, between 2 and 5 weeks after the injury. This has the advantage that the difficult and delicate operation of nerve suture can be carried out under the most favourable conditions. Also, the nerve-sheath will have thickened appreciably during the first few weeks after division and should be the better able to hold sutures. On the other hand, a considerable gap may have developed between the nerve-ends, and this may greatly increase the difficulties of repair.

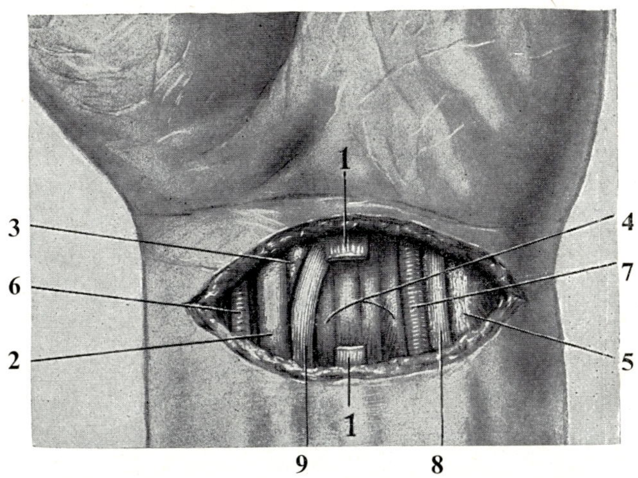

Fig. 401.—Anatomy of the nerves and tendons at a level just above the wrist-joint—a common site of injury. In this case the tendon of the palmaris longus (1) alone has been severed. 1, Palmaris longus. 2, Flexor carpi radialis. 3, Flexor pollicis longus. 4, Flexor digitorum sublimis. 5, Flexor carpi ulnaris. 6, Radial artery. 7, Ulnar artery. 8, Ulnar nerve. 9, Median nerve.

Wounds with Division of Tendons.—Division of tendons is a frequent complication of incised wounds of the hands and fingers. The function of any tendons underlying a wound should therefore be investigated by careful examination. Sometimes the first glance at the hand will lead one to suspect that a tendon has been severed (*Fig.* 402), so constant is the position of the fingers at rest, owing to the delicate balance between flexor and extensor tendons.

It is now generally agreed that the treatment of tendon injuries, like that of nerve injuries, depends on the conditions present, and on the experience of the operator. The results of tendon repair as a whole are liable to be very disappointing—especially when this is attempted by the inexperienced, and under conditions which are not ideal. Now that the risks of sepsis have been reduced by antibiotics, the commonest cause of failure is the development of adhesions between the tendon at the point of suture and the surrounding tissues. The choice of treatment should depend on the site of tendon division, and on whether flexor or extensor tendons are involved.

Flexor tendons in the fingers (i.e., between the metacarpophalangeal and distal interphalangeal joints) are enclosed within a relatively rigid sheath, and the adhesions which occur are liable to cause absolute fixation of the tendon. When a sublimis tendon *alone* is divided it should be disregarded, lest its repair should jeopardize the function of the more important profundus tendon; this latter tendon, acting alone, can do all that is normally required in finger flexion, and the loss of the sublimis will usually cause no demonstrable disability. When *both* flexor tendons are cut in a finger and are repaired side by side, cross-union

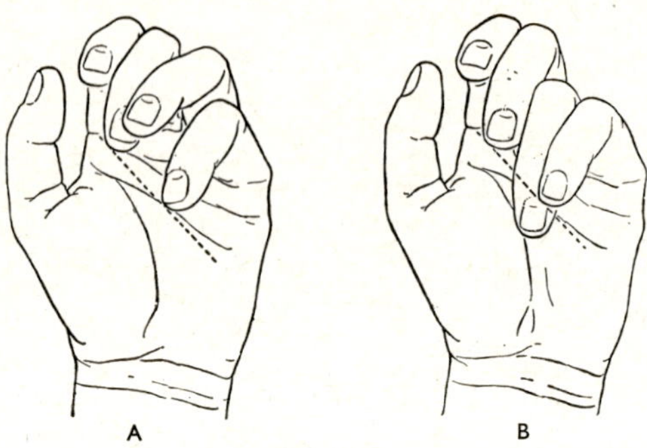

Fig. 402.—'Spot' diagnosis of tendon injury. The abnormal position of the ring finger in A suggests a severed flexor tendon; that in B a severed extensor tendon.

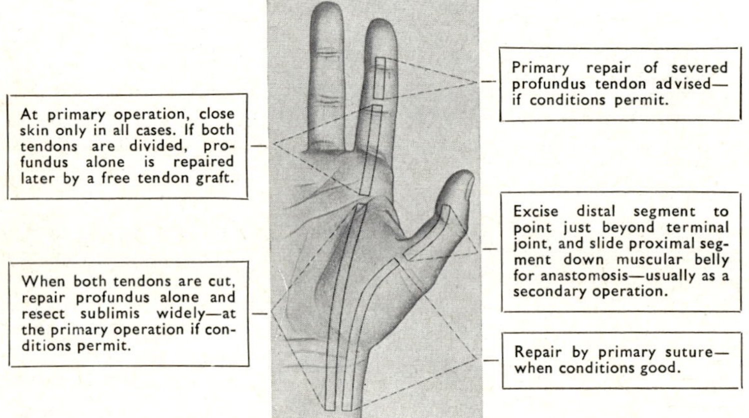

Fig. 403.—Drawing to indicate the treatment of divided flexor tendons—according to the site of division.

almost invariably occurs, together with adhesion to the surrounding sheath, so that complete fixation of both tendons is liable to result.

Bunnell and others have shown that, in such cases, the best results are obtained by a secondary operation, at which the profundus tendon is reconstituted by a free tendon-graft, and the sublimis is resected widely. The graft is obtained from the tendon of the palmaris longus, or, if this is not available, from the long extensor to the second toe. It is used to replace the profundus tendon from a point well proximal in the palm to a point just beyond the distal interphalangeal joint. In this way the point of tendon suture is transferred to a situation where the surrounding tissues are more elastic and where adhesions are less important.

When, therefore, both sublimis and profundus tendons are severed distal to the level of the metacarpophalangeal joint, the skin only should be sutured in the first instance.

Flexor tendons in the palm or at the wrist are surrounded by loose synovium or paratenon, so that adhesions are of less importance. Primary repair gives fairly satisfactory results, and should therefore be attempted if conditions are suitable. If both sublimis and profundus tendons are divided within the constricted region of the carpal tunnel, the profundus alone should be repaired; the cut sublimis tendons are resected widely, in order to allow more space for functional recovery of the more important profundus tendons.

When the flexor pollicis longus tendon is divided in the thumb beyond the level of the metacarpophalangeal joint, the distal segment (except for its terminal $\frac{1}{4}$ in. (6–7 mm.)) is excised. The proximal segment is detached from its muscular belly, pulled downwards for anastomosis to the remaining stump of the distal segment, and then re-attached to the muscle belly. This should usually be done as a secondary operation, the skin alone having been closed in the first instance.

Extensor tendons are generally believed to be more amenable to repair than flexor tendons, but this is not always borne out in practice. There is no rigid sheath enclosing the tendons, and since the degree of excursion required is less than that in the case of flexor tendons, the disability resulting from adhesions is much less severe. On the other hand, because the extensor tendons are flattened, it is difficult to obtain accurate end-to-end apposition without bunching up or overlapping, which militates against a successful result. Furthermore, extensor tendons are frequently divided over a finger-joint where they form the posterior capsule; in such cases the joint is usually opened, and its function may thereby be impaired. It is usually advised that primary repair should be attempted when conditions are suitable.

Extensor tendon division over the proximal interphalangeal joint is usually confined to the central slip of the tendon inserting into the second phalanx, and the injury is very liable to be missed since no immediate disability is apparent. As, however, the ends of the severed central slip separate, the two lateral slips slide forwards around the sides of the joint and come to act more as flexors, with the result that progressive flexion of this joint and hyper-extension at the terminal joint (*boutonnière* deformity) are produced. Such deformity can be prevented only by primary or *early* repair of the divided segment.

Compound Fractures of the Fingers.—Careful débridement is essential. Completely detached fragments of bone are removed, and bone ends which are grossly contaminated are trimmed with bone shears. Buried ligatures should be avoided. The minimum number of stitches should be inserted, so that there will be no obstruction to the escape of exudate.

For fractures of the proximal two phalanges of a finger it is essential, in order to secure correct alinement, that the finger should be immobilized in the flexed position; in the case of an individual finger, its tip should point towards the tubercle of the scaphoid. There are many different methods of securing a finger in this position; wire or plaster splints may be used, or the finger may simply be strapped over a roller bandage placed in the palm (*see Fig.* 407).

When, in the case of the finger, the fracture is comminuted, and is associated with considerable damage to the soft parts, amputation should be considered, since a stiffened and painful finger is likely to result. This applies particularly

22

in the case of artisans, to whom an early return to work and an immediate and final settlement of compensation claims are most important—from both economic and psychological viewpoints.

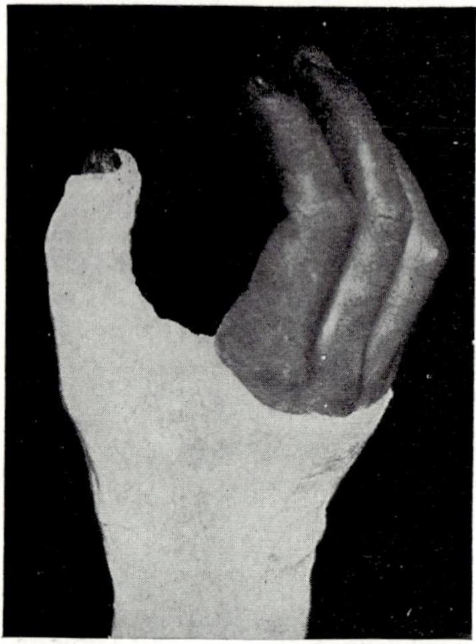

Fig. 404.—A plaster cast applied to immobilize the thumb in the position of function.

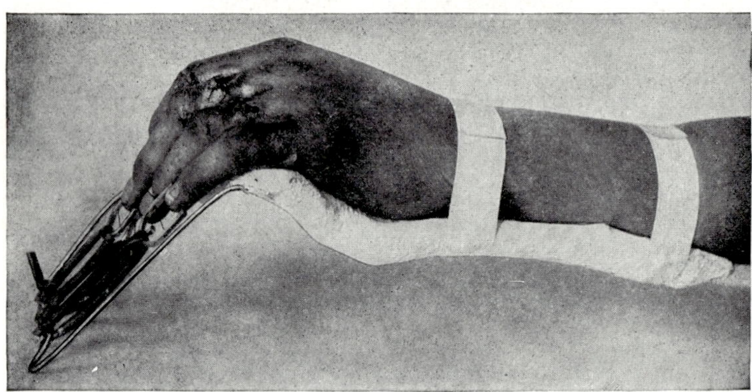

Fig. 405.—Method of applying continuous traction to the fingers. The plaster splint supports the fingers in flexion. Each finger pulp is transfixed with a silkworm gut or wire stitch. Traction is applied to a wire loop incorporated in the plaster.

In the thumb, the most rigid conservatism is essential. After thorough débridement, the wound is covered with gauze, and a plaster cast is applied with the thumb in the position of function (*Fig.* 404).

Continuous traction is desirable when the fracture involves a joint surface, or when there is overriding of the fragments which cannot otherwise be corrected.

Pulp traction is the most efficient method. If a special stirrup is available, its pin is passed through the finger-tip immediately in front of the phalanx. Failing this, stout silkworm gut or stainless-steel wire may be used. Traction is applied

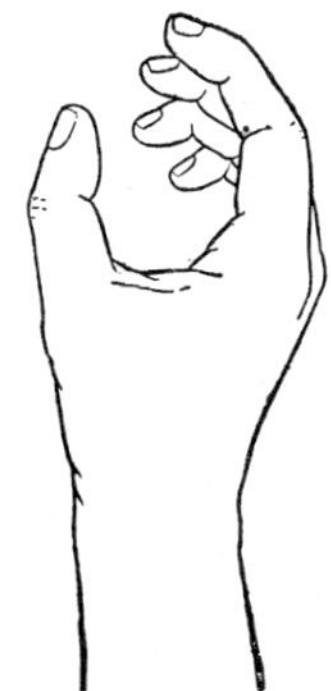
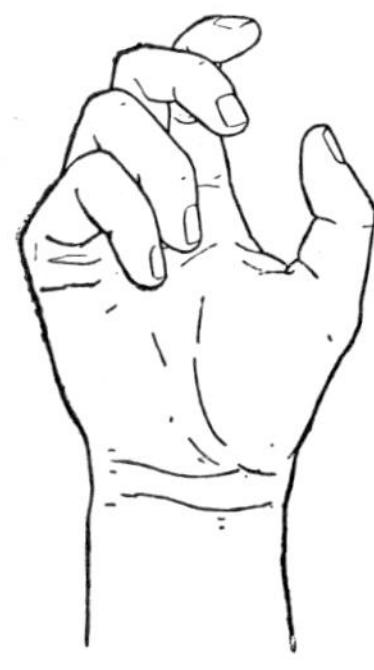

Fig. 406.—The 'position of function'. Note that all fingers are flexed—the little finger the most, and the index the least. The thumb is well forward in the opposed position, lying directly in front of the index. The wrist is in slight dorsiflexion.

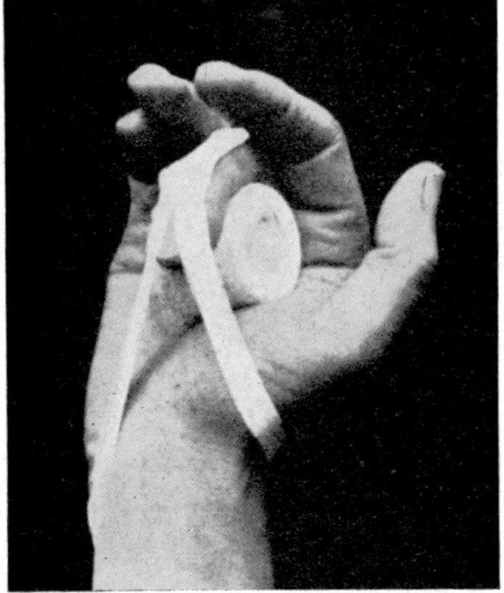
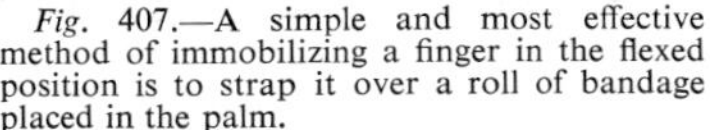
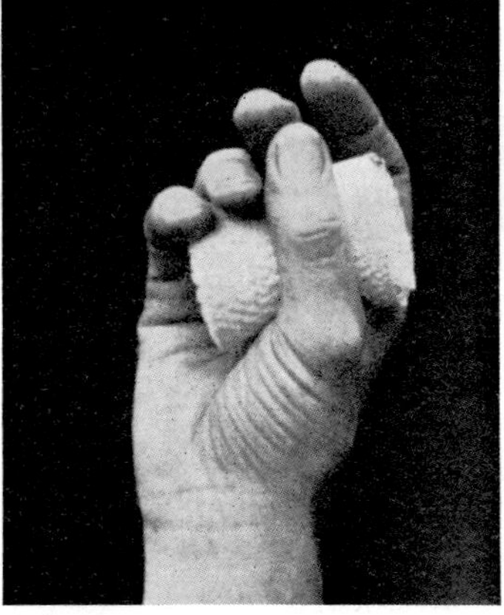

Fig. 407.—A simple and most effective method of immobilizing a finger in the flexed position is to strap it over a roll of bandage placed in the palm.

Fig. 408.—The thumb should be kept well forward in the opposed position by means of a roll of wool or gauze placed between it and the palm.

by means of tape or fine rubber tubing to a wire loop incorporated in the plaster cast. *The traction must be so arranged that the digit is in the 'position of function'* —flexion in the case of a finger (*Fig.* 405), opposition in the case of the thumb.

Internal Fixation.—The difficulties of effective immobilization by conservative treatment and the risk of subsequent stiffness of the fingers have led some surgeons to develop methods of internal fixation—by small screws, by intramedullary or interosseous wiring, or by intramedullary bone pegs. These methods are not recommended, however, except for those who have special experience.

Bites and Allied Injuries.—All wounds sustained from contact with teeth are potentially serious, owing to the risks of infection. Human bites are much more dangerous than dog bites because of the unusual virulence of the organisms concerned.

Bites of all description, and any wound of the knuckles sustained from contact with an adversary's teeth, should be treated with great respect.

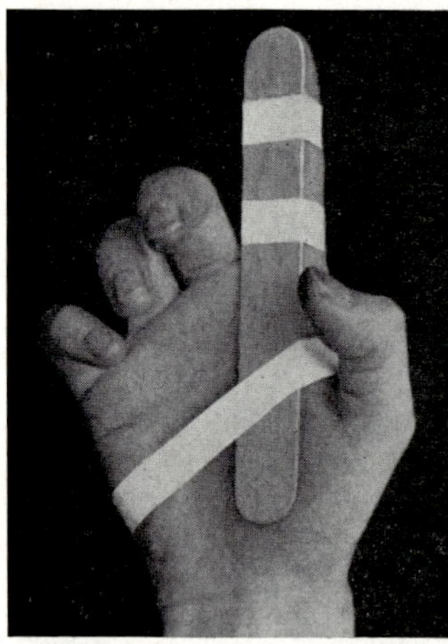

Fig. 409.—". . . the evil straight wooden splint, which tends to cause a series of ankyloses in extension." (*Iselin.*)

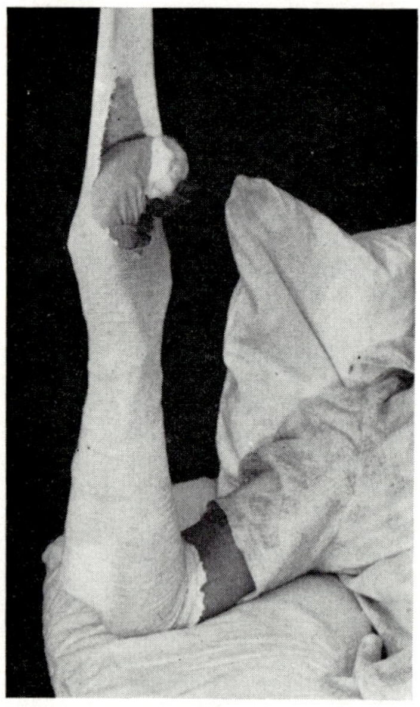

Fig. 410.—Method of elevating the hand. The position of function is maintained by a plaster splint.

Exploration and débridement should be particularly thorough, and should be carried out, if necessary, under general anæsthesia. The number of stitches should be reduced to a minimum. If a joint has been involved, it should be thoroughly irrigated with saline and left widely open. The part is then immobilized in the position of function, and intensive chemotherapy is prescribed.

After-treatment.—'*Position of Function.*'—Following upon the initial treatment of a wound of the hand or fingers, there is inevitably some degree of immobilization—from the presence of dressings, and from the patient's natural disinclination to use the part. Such immobilization should be in the 'position of function' as described by Kanavel (*Fig.* 406). This is the position in which stiffness is least likely to occur, and it should be in our mind's eye every time we apply a dressing to an injured hand or finger. The metacarpophalangeal joints, owing to the special arrangement of their collateral ligaments, are particularly liable to become stiffened in extension. For this reason, if a wound is situated near the base of a finger, it is desirable that the finger should be bandaged or otherwise immobilized in flexion (*Fig.* 407). If one finger only is affected, the remaining fingers must not be included in the dressing, but should be left with a full range of movement. When several fingers are involved, the hand should be bandaged in the 'closed-fist' position. A thumb which becomes stiffened in the plane of the palm is practically useless, since it cannot be brought into opposition with any of the fingers. Whenever a bandage is applied to enclose the hand or the base of the thumb, a roll of wool should be placed between the thumb and the palm, so that the thumb lies well forward in the opposed position (*Fig.* 408). "It is essential to forbid the use of the evil straight wooden splint, which tends to cause a series of ankyloses in extension." (Iselin.) (*Fig.* 409.)

After most hand injuries of any severity it is advisable that the patient should be confined to bed for a few days, with the forearm suspended vertically, in order to reduce congestion and œdema (*Fig.* 410). Thereafter, active movements of the fingers should be commenced as soon as is practicable.

The average patient has a touching faith in the surgeon's ability to restore function, and all too frequently he fails to realize the necessity for co-operation on his own part. Active use of the hand during convalescence must be insisted upon, and the patient should be encouraged to return to work as soon as possible after his wounds have healed. Finger-stalls should be prohibited, since they serve only to prevent active use of the part. A cut finger which has healed does not require 'protection'; it has greater need of being hardened up by exposure to the air, and by the minor traumata of normal use.

CHAPTER XXXIX

ACUTE INFECTIONS OF THE HAND AND FINGERS

By David Bailey

The use of antibiotics has improved the prognosis in infections of the fingers and hand, but these infections remain common and are responsible for much time lost from work. It is unfortunately true that discredited methods of treatment are still used—methods which not only lead to unnecessary prolongation of disability but which are sometimes responsible for crippling and deformity.

A description will be given of modern methods of treatment which have been found to give good results in practice. Although simple, these methods require meticulous attention to detail and much patience in their execution. Anyone who has the responsibility of treating these infections must give them the time and attention they merit; there is no place for casual methods of treatment.

THE GENERAL PRINCIPLES

These are best stated in the form of five rules and a 'rider':—

1. Rest is required during the diffuse stage of infection.
2. Elevation is required to reduce œdema.
3. Spreading infection must be controlled by antibiotics.
4. No operation until localized pus has formed.
5. Established abscesses are drained by small incisions sited to provide direct drainage and designed to preserve function.

There are no standard incisions in the surgery of the infected hand.

The student may be relieved to know that it is no longer necessary for him to memorize the standard incisions which used to be illustrated, but he should not be tempted to think that treatment is any easier.

Fomentations and 'hot soaks' are not used. They make the skin soggy and often are responsible for delay in instituting effective treatment. They may encourage unnecessary pointing, with needless soft-tissue destruction. 'Drawing' ointments and magnesium sulphate paste are similarly contra-indicated.

The Practical Application of these Principles.—Operation is required for the drainage of localized pus and for this purpose only. No incision should be made until there is definite evidence of abscess formation. Recognition of abscess formation is therefore all-important, and is suggested by change of symptoms, viz. a diffuse ache is replaced by a more severe throbbing pain. The presence of pus is also confirmed by the signs of (*a*) visible subcuticular pus, (*b*) well-localized tenderness found by pressing on the suspected area with the closed points of a pair of fine forceps, or (*c*) the appearance of a dusky cyanotic spot in the centre of a reddened area of cellulitis.

In the Diffuse Stage of Infection, before localization has occurred (the stage of cellulitis), three methods, *and three only*, are employed. These methods, which are designed to abort the infection if it is early, or to localize it if it is more advanced, are as follows:—

Rest is obtained by splinting the hand in the position of function by means of a plaster-of-Paris slab (*Fig.* 411).

Elevation is needed to reduce œdema, and usually is carried out by placing the patient's arm in a sling which retains the arm in front of the opposite shoulder. In more severe cases elevation above the head is required and the arm is secured in this position by suspending it from an overhead support, such as a drip apparatus stand.

Antibiotic Therapy has resulted in an increase in the number of infections aborted completely, and also in the control of spreading cellulitis, lymphangitis,

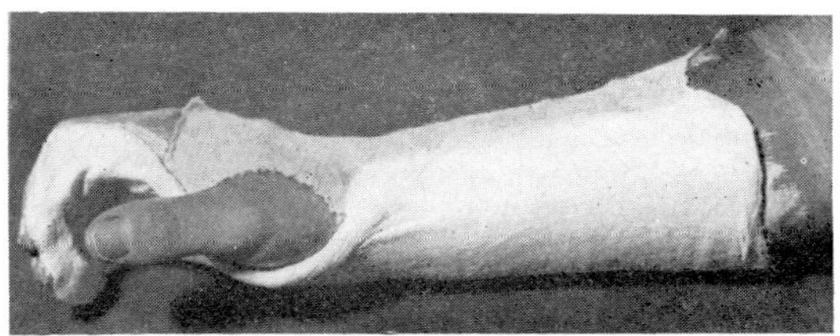

Fig. 411.—Hand immobilized in the position of function with a plaster-of-Paris slab.

and bacteriæmia, but it is unnecessary in the treatment of small, well-localized abscesses (unless these are complicated by systemic infections such as diabetes). Penicillin (600,000 units of procaine penicillin intramuscularly each day in moderate infections; 500,000 units of aqueous solution b.d. or 6-hourly, if more severe) is the antibiotic used most frequently. Oral penicillin may also be used especially for the treatment of children. Before penicillin is given inquiry must be made for previous sensitivity; neglect of this precaution may lead to disaster. When such a history is obtained another antibiotic should be used; tetracycline (250 mg. orally every 6 hours for adults) is usually preferred, and it may also be given if the infective organisms are thought to be resistant to penicillin. It is also a useful antibiotic if for any reason repeated injections are inadvisable. In hospital personnel, in whom bacteriological tests so frequently show a penicillinase-producing staphylococcus, cloxacillin (orbenin) should be used.

In the Stage of Localization, where a definite abscess is present, operation is the main method of treatment. This may be necessary either when the patient is first seen or after some days of conservative treatment. In the former instance, if the infection

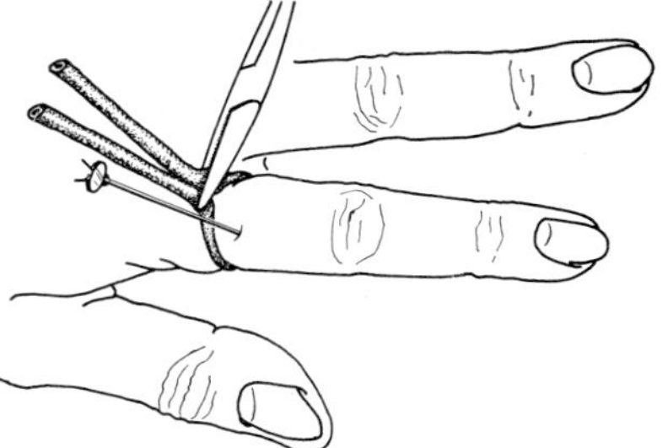

Fig. 412.—Site of injection for digital nerve-block following the application of the tourniquet.

is even moderately severe, an intramuscular injection of penicillin (500,000 units) should be given about half an hour before the proposed operation.

Anæsthesia can be either local or general, but it is important that no matter how superficial the infection may appear, no incision should be undertaken without complete anæsthesia. Local anæsthesia is preferable for ambulant patients; it is also convenient for a surgeon who is working single-handed. If general anæsthesia is employed, it must give full relaxation; there is no place for

Orbenin (Beecham Research Laboratories, Brentford, Middlesex).

a 'whiff of gas', which so often results in a struggling patient and does not permit the meticulous, unhurried technique that is essential for success. 'Freezing' with an ethyl chloride spray is useless.

For infections of the distal segments of the fingers digital nerve-block (ring-block) is used. After sterilizing the skin, 1 ml. of 2 per cent procaine or lignocaine (xylocaine; duncaine), *without adrenaline*, is injected around each digital nerve at the base of the finger, using a No. 17 hypodermic needle (*Fig.* 412). Anæsthesia is complete in 10 minutes. If the infection is more proximal, a wrist-block may be carried out. Five ml. of 1 per cent lignocaine (with 1–100,000 adrenaline) are injected around both the ulnar nerve and the median nerve (*see Fig.* 397) at the level of the distal flexor crease of the wrist. (In some cases blocking of the branches of the radial nerve is also required.) A longer wait is necessary before anæsthesia is complete: about half an hour must be allowed.

The Operation.—It is essential that a clear view is obtained into the depths of the abscess cavity and, for this reason, the operation must be carried out in a bloodless field. In the case of a finger this is secured by applying a fine rubber catheter tightly around the base of the finger and clipping it in place with a hæmostat (*see Fig.* 412). This tourniquet is best applied before injecting the local anæsthetic. In the case of more proximal infections, the patient's arm is elevated above the patient's head for a minute, and is rendered ischæmic by inflating a sphygmomanometer cuff around the upper arm to a pressure above the systolic level. Because this soon causes pain it should be deferred until anæsthesia is complete and the operation is about to commence.

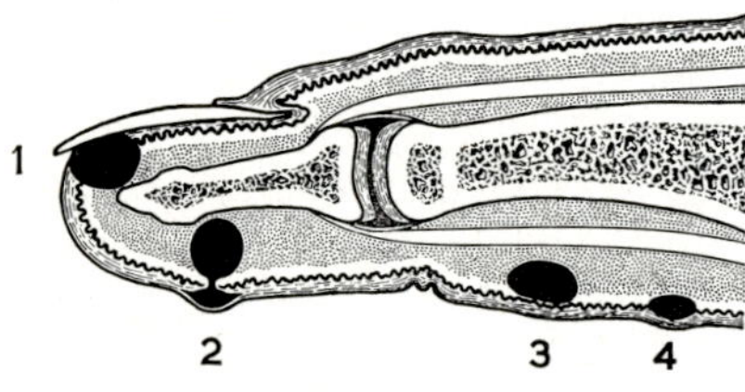

Fig. 413.—Diagram of finger to show various types of abscess. 1, Apical abscess; 2, Pulp abscess with collar-stud extensions; 3, Subcutaneous abscess; 4, Intracutaneous abscess.

The skin of the affected part is cleaned with a solution of 1 per cent hibitane in spirit or cetrimide, and the operation is planned. The aim is to provide drainage by the most direct route by an incision which will heal with the least possible scarring. The site of incision should be chosen before anæsthetizing the part, as the position of maximum tenderness often has a good deal to do with the choice, and its direction should correspond with the tension lines (Langer's lines) of the skin. An incision which crosses the flexor creases is particularly to be avoided.

The instruments used in operating on the infected hand must be delicate, and a meticulous no-touch technique is followed. The operator's hands are gloved for the protection of his skin, but as they are not sterile they must not be allowed to come into contact with any part of the infected hand or any of the sterile dressings, and only the handles of the instruments are touched.

If *subcuticular pus is visible*, this may represent the superficial component of a collar-stud abscess (*Fig.* 413) and the operation is commenced by uncapping the superficial abscess, using a fine scalpel (No. 11 Bard-Parker). This accomplished, a deep extension is sought, and if such is present it is probed to determine its extent. The sinus is then enlarged by an incision through the dermis (in the direction of Langer's lines) to permit inspection of the walls of the deeper cavity. The edges of the incision are parted, and pus is mopped out with a pledget of

Xylocaine (Astra-Hewlett Ltd., Watford, Herts); Duncaine (Duncan, Flockhart, & Evans Ltd., Birkbeck Street, London, E.2).
Hibitane (I.C.I. Ltd., Pharmaceuticals Division, Macclesfield, Cheshire).

cotton-wool. Any loose slough is picked out with fine forceps and obviously dead subcutaneous fat is cut away, care being taken not to remove any healthy tissue. During the removal of dead tissue the depths of the cavity are inspected frequently, to make sure that important adjacent structures, such as tendon-sheaths or digital nerves, are not damaged.

If *subcuticular pus is not visible*, the abscess is opened by an incision 0·5 cm. in length placed immediately over it. When pus is located, if necessary the incision is extended to make it long enough to provide adequate drainage. The subsequent toilet of the abscess cavity is precisely similar to that described in the preceding paragraph.

Irrespective as to whether the abscess is superficial or deep, the edges of the skin incision are cut back with fine pointed scissors to form a narrow diamond-shaped opening (*see Fig.* 419), the wound is dusted lightly with chloramphenicol-lactose powder (5 per cent), and a dry gauze dressing is applied. No drains of any sort are used and the wound should never be plugged with a gauze wick. The dressing is bandaged into place (tubegauz is most satisfactory for the fingers, *see* p. 193), the tourniquet is then removed, and the arm elevated in a sling.

After-care.—The patient is instructed to keep the dressings dry and not to interfere with them in any way. If drainage is efficient, relief will be immediate and no analgesics are required. The first dressing should be carried out on the day following operation; as a rule the gauze dressing can be removed easily, but when it is stuck fast it must be soaked off in a 1 per cent solution of cetrimide.

The wound edges should be gently separated and the abscess cavity probed carefully to make certain that drainage remains adequate; if there is any doubt about this, the opening must be enlarged under anæsthesia. Whether this step is necessary or not, a fresh dry gauze dressing is applied, and the part is bandaged. Subsequent dressings are carried out at intervals of one to three days until healing is complete. Antibiotics are not usually required after the first 24 hours unless (*a*) the abscess is very large, (*b*) there are signs of bone infection, or (*c*) there is evidence of spreading infection. When there is much œdema or surrounding cellulitis, it is necessary to continue splinting and elevation of the hand for several days.

SPECIFIC TYPES OF INFECTION

Paronychia, the commonest infection of the hand, occurs at the sides of the nail or superficial to its base. It begins as a cellulitis, but pus rapidly forms, and if left untreated it may discharge spontaneously by separation of the cuticle from the surface of the nail, or, more often, extension occurs beneath the base of the nail so that the nail floats on a pool of pus (*Fig.* 414).

Treatment.—Antibiotic therapy is employed only if the infection is seen at a very early stage when there is a prospect of it being aborted com-

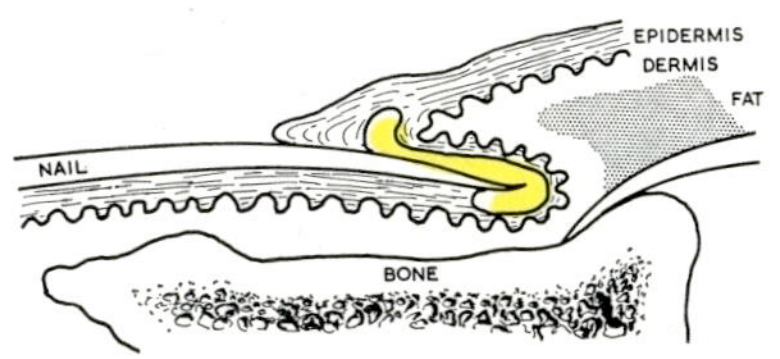

Fig. 414.—Diagram showing situation and extension of pus in paronychia. (Sagittal section.)

pletely. When pus has formed operation is required, and, as a rule, antibiotics are then unnecessary. It is important to realize that the pus is subcuticular and not

Tubegauz (The Scholl Manufacturing Co. Ltd., 182–204 St. John's Street, London, E.C.1).

subcutaneous (*see Fig.* 414): incision into the deep layers is therefore unnecessary and harmful. To release the pus, all that is necessary is to strip back the cuticle and lateral nail folds from the surface of the nail. This is carried out with the closed points of fine dissecting forceps (*Fig.* 415), and no cutting is required except to trim away loose portions of cuticle. No drains are used and it is unnecessary to tuck gauze between the edge of the nail fold and the nail. The base of the nail is resected (*Fig.* 416) only if it is undermined by pus, when it will be obviously loose and lacking its normal lustre. Care must be taken that no small fragments of dead nail remain, or infection will be prolonged.

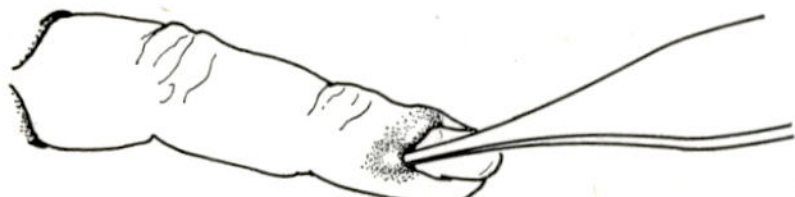

Fig. 415.—Elevation of nail fold to drain a paronychia.

In after-care it is important to make sure that the stripped cuticle does not become adherent to the nail prematurely.

Pulp Abscess.—Infection of the terminal pulp space is common and serious. When the patient is first seen pus may not be localized and it is a bad mistake to incise too early.

Treatment.—In the stage of cellulitis, pulp infections are treated conservatively with rest and antibiotics. When there is clear evidence of localized pus, operation is required forthwith. The old 'hockey-stick' incision should not be used. Incisions must be placed directly over the abscess and should correspond in direction to Langer's lines (*Fig.* 417). A collar-stud abscess is common in the pulp, and the sinus communicating with the deeper pocket must not be overlooked. Failure to recognize this deep extension is the commonest mistake made in the treatment of this condition.

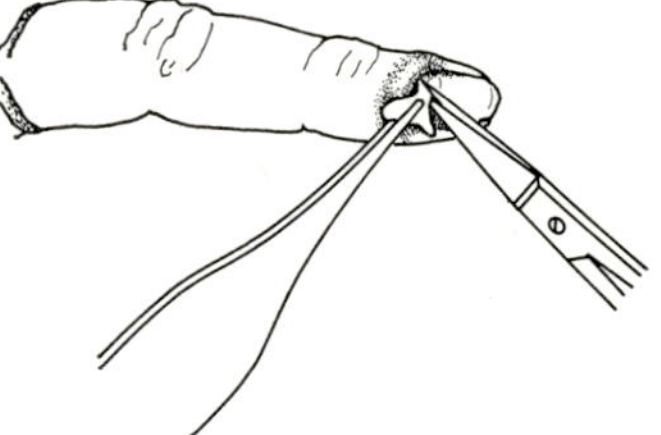

Fig. 416.—Resection of base of nail when it is undermined by pus.

If treatment has been delayed pulp abscesses are often complicated by sloughing of soft tissue or by bone infection. Necrosis of the terminal phalanx (a result of infective thrombosis and not of tension ischæmia) is best recognized by probing at the time of operation; the grating sensation of bare bone is characteristic. X-ray changes do not appear for at least 10 days. Recognition of bone infection

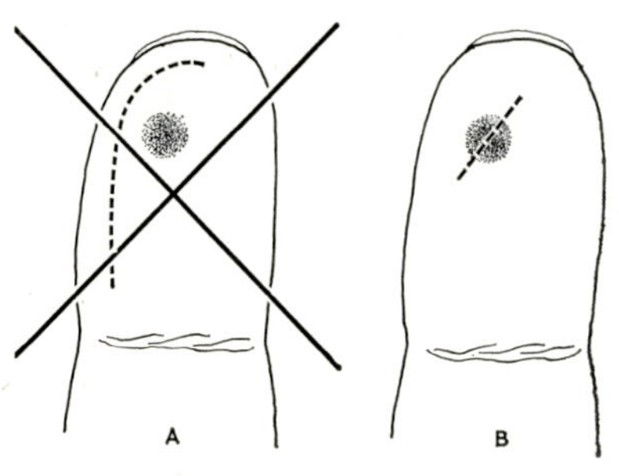

Fig. 417.—Incision for pulp abscess. A, Wrong; B, Correct.

is important, as it is a very strong indication for antibiotic therapy (which is not required in small uncomplicated pulp abscesses). Early osteitis may resolve with antibiotic treatment but, in more severe cases, sequestration occurs which may involve the whole of the distal three-quarters of the terminal phalanx; the wound will not heal until the sequestrum has separated, which may take several weeks. Bone infection not only leads to prolonged disability but is responsible for scarring and deformity. It can be avoided only by adequate drainage at the right time.

Apical Abscess.—The pus is situated at the extreme tip of the finger distal to the phalanx or just dorsal to its tip (*see Fig.* 413). The main pulp space is not involved and the abscess points under the free edge of the nail. Tenderness is localized to the finger-tip.

Treatment.—Localized pus is nearly always present when the patient is first seen, and it should be drained by a short transverse incision situated dorsally at the tip of the finger (*Fig.* 418 A). In most cases a V-wedge of nail is removed (*Fig.* 418 B) to permit free drainage of the cavity, which extends down to the periosteum. Bone infection is rare and the prognosis is good.

Web Abscess.—Infection of the web spaces commonly follows blistering of the palmar skin. When first seen the patient's hand is often grossly

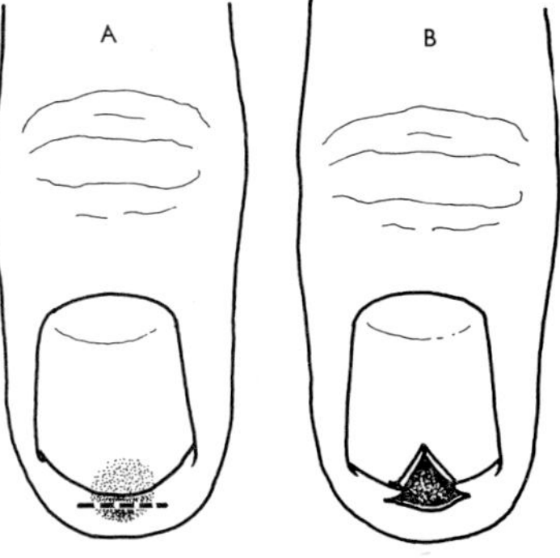

Fig. 418.—Apical abscess. A, Site for initial incision; B, Excision of V-wedge of nail.

œdematous, particularly on the dorsum, and exact localization of the pus may be difficult. A characteristic separation of the adjacent fingers is seen at a later stage.

Treatment.—In nearly all cases 24 hours spent in conservative treatment is worth while. The hand is immobilized in a dorsal plaster-of-Paris splint, and is elevated. Antibiotics are given in full dosage to control spreading infection. When swelling has been reduced, the abscess is opened by a transverse incision on the palmar aspect, opposite the interdigital space and about 1 cm. proximal to the free edge of the web (*Fig.* 419). Initially the skin only is incised, to avoid damage to adjacent digital nerves. The abscess cavity is entered by blunt probing, and its extent determined. Subcutaneous tissue is incised carefully to unroof the abscess and to provide free drainage. Rarely a dorsal counter-incision is required, but a vertical web-splitting incision is to be avoided because this leads to a bridle scar. Through-and-through drains can only cause harm, and are not used. Splintage and antibiotics are continued until œdema has subsided (which it will do rapidly if drainage is adequate). These abscesses are most satisfactory ones to treat because almost always rapid and sustained improvement follows the evacuation of the pus.

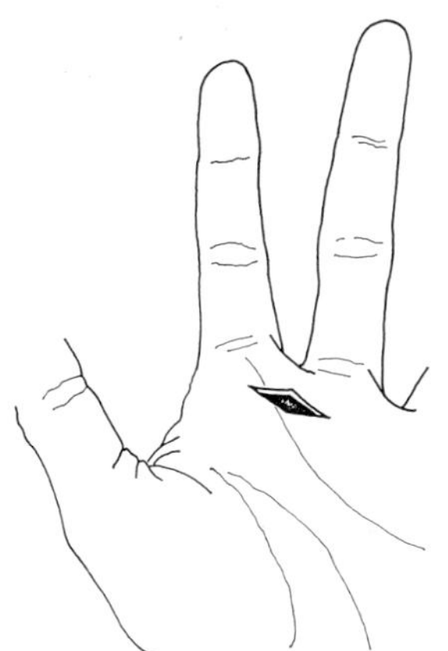

Fig. 419.—Site of incision for drainage of a web space. Edges cut back to form a diamond-shaped opening.

Subcutaneous and Intracutaneous Abscesses (*see Fig.* 413, p. 562).—Subcutaneous infections, similar in many respects to pulp abscesses, occur in the more proximal parts of the fingers or in the palm. They are treated along the same lines as a pulp abscess and no special comment is needed, except to give a warning that, in the case of a subcutaneous abscess on the anterior aspect of the finger, the floor of the abscess cavity lies very close to the flexor tendon-sheath. If the depths of the abscess cavity are not clearly seen, the tendon-sheath may be opened with serious results.

Intracutaneous Abscesses (*see Fig.* 413, p. 562), in which the pus lies actually *within* the dermis, are comparatively uncommon and even less commonly recognized. They are small, but very painful. They are only certainly recognized at operation, when care must be taken not to trespass into the subcutaneous tissue.

Deep Palmar Abscess, in which the pus is situated deep to the thick palmar fascia, is very uncommon, and usually the infection follows a penetrating injury. Extension along the path of the penetration to the subcutaneous plane often occurs, in which event a collar-stud abscess (*Fig.* 420) results.

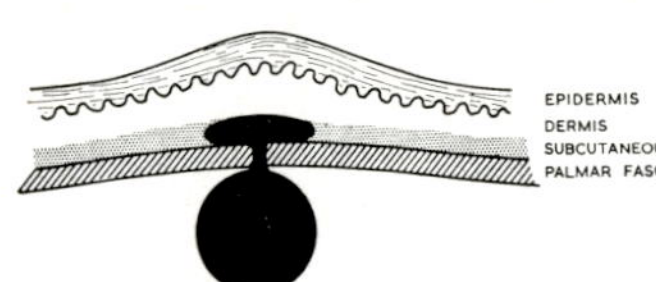

Fig. 420.—Deep palmar abscess with collar-stud extension through the palmar fascia.

Swelling of the dorsum of the hand is pronounced; the paradox of dorsal œdema when the pus lies anteriorly is now well known, and on this score mistakes should not occur. The concavity of the palm may be obliterated in the region of the abscess.

Treatment.—A short period of conservative treatment is often needed to limit the spread of infection and to reduce œdema. Once localization of the pus has occurred, the abscess should be opened by the method used for subcutaneous abscesses, but it must be remembered that the pus lies more deeply and the palmar fascia must be incised to permit free drainage. The skin is opened in the direction of the tension lines *but the fascia should be incised vertically* and particular care is needed to avoid damage to nerves and tendon-sheaths.

A Carbuncle on the dorsal surface of a digit or the hand is not uncommon, and like a carbuncle elsewhere, it commences as a furuncle resulting from infection of a hair follicle. Invariably treatment should be conservative; antibiotic therapy is particularly helpful in localizing the infection and keeping it localized. After a few days a core of slough separates and can be lifted out, leaving a surprisingly large hole, which rapidly heals.

Erysipeloid.—Infection with the *Erysipelothrix rhusiopathiæ* (of Rosenbach) usually follows minor injuries caused by fish scales or meat bones, and most often occurs in housewives, fishmongers, and butchers. To the inexperienced it resembles cellulitis, but the colour of the affected part is more dusky, itching is common, and pain is absent. The treatment is conservative and the response to penicillin almost pathognomonic.

ACUTE SUPPURATIVE TENOSYNOVITIS AND ARTHRITIS

Patients with these serious infections must be treated as in-patients with facilities for frequent inspection, the regular administration of antibiotics, and full facilities for operative treatment when required. Only a bare outline of treatment is given here.

Suppurative Tenosynovitis usually results from a penetrating injury on the palmar surface of a digit, often near a flexor crease. It is recognized by the rapid appearance of a fusiform swelling of the finger which is held in flexion. Attempts at passive extension are extremely painful and tenderness is present along the line of the affected sheath, particularly at its extremities. Constitutional signs of infection are usually present.

Treatment.—If seen early, treatment may be conservative, but should not be persisted in for more than 24 hours if there is no obvious improvement. Surgical treatment is difficult and requires a detailed knowledge of the surgical anatomy of the tendon-sheaths (*Fig.* 421). Briefly the essential is to expose and drain the affected sheath at the site of the causative injury, and also at its proximal and distal extremities. The sheath is exposed by short transverse incisions (*Fig.* 422). In the case of the thumb and little finger this may entail an incision in front of the wrist to expose and drain the radial and ulnar bursæ. After drainage, the

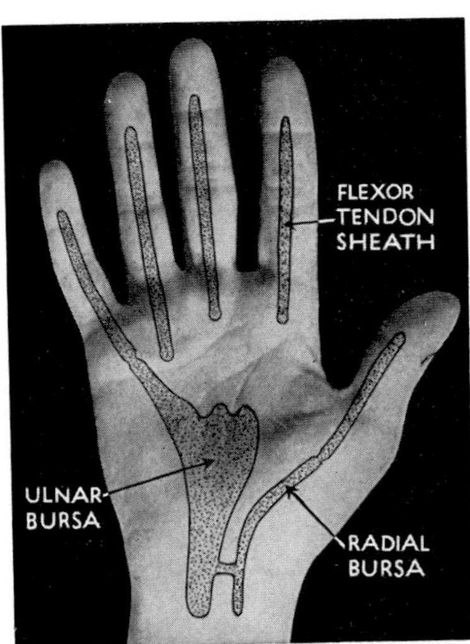

Fig. 421.—The flexor tendon-sheaths of the hand.

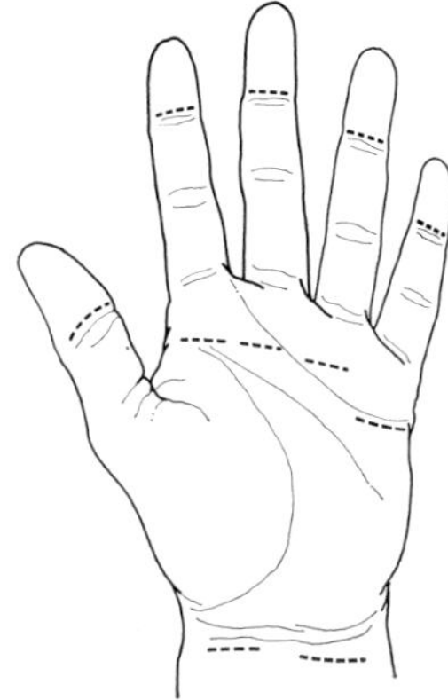

Fig. 422.—The sites of incision for treating suppurative tenosynovitis. The sheath is also exposed at the site of initial trauma.

sheath is washed through with a solution of penicillin (10,000 units per ml.) introduced by means of a whistle-tipped ureteric catheter, and the wounds are left open. Rest, elevation, and antibiotics are continued until healing is complete and physiotherapy is usually required later to mobilize the fingers. Long lateral incisions are unnecessary, and may be crippling; they should not be used.

Suppurative Arthritis.—Infection of the joints usually results from a deep abrasion of the knuckles, and the results are serious.

Treatment.—This may be initially conservative, but exploration and débridement of the joint cavity under antibiotic cover are often required. The results of treatment still leave a lot to be desired, principally because the condition often goes unrecognized until late.

RECORD KEEPING

Accurate notes should be kept of all cases, including details of the condition of the hand when first seen and all treatment given. A standard form is desirable, as this permits easy assessment of the efficacy of various methods. In describing a finger, its name (and not its number) should be given.

CHAPTER XL

SURGICAL PÆDIATRICS

By F. H. ROBARTS

DURING the past ten years the physical and psychological needs of infants and children in hospital have received far more consideration than ever in the past. Developments in these fields range from the almost general encouragement of free and frequent daily visiting, 'play ladies', occupational therapy and educational facilities for older children to the quite considerable utilization of parents in assisting with the general daily care of feeding and bathing of small children. In addition, consideration is being given to an increase in the amount of clinical investigation and even operative treatment which may be conducted on a 'day-bed' or out-patient basis. Quite a considerable proportion of the simpler operative load—herniæ, circumcisions, and excisions—have been managed for many years on an out-patient basis; it was found safer for the child to avoid the respiratory and gastro-enteric infections acquired so often as an in-patient. Out-patient management is now advantageous from the psychological needs of the infant and small child and of its parents; this has also important implications with regard to the financial aspects of the hospital service, the time factor of waiting lists, and the undesirability of these lists from the patient's point of view. There will, however, always be the need for the admission of children and infants to hospital for the conduct of many procedures and treatments and sometimes this may be for protracted periods. When it is possible, small and larger children should be prepared for the uncertainties and unpleasantnesses of this period, and most children's hospitals issue to parents leaflets which they may use for this purpose.

THE COLLECTION OF SPECIMENS

Blood.—The '*heel stab*' usually will provide sufficient blood for the performance of several biochemical estimations.

Venepuncture.—In order to obtain sufficient blood (2 ml.) for culture and serological tests, venepuncture is necessary. In a small, fat baby this procedure frequently presents difficulties. The cubital fossæ, the wrists and ankles, and the scalp are first examined, both visually and by palpation, for a suitable vein. When the search proves fruitless, recourse must be made to puncture of a larger and more deeply situated vein, the choice in successive order being:—

1. *The external jugular vein*, where it crosses the belly of the sternomastoid muscle, is rendered visible (*a*) by securing the body of the child firmly as it lies on a table or a person's lap; (*b*) by the lowering of the head, and (*c*) by turning it to one or other side. Straining and crying distend the vein and, provided movement is controlled, are distinctly advantageous. The vein, which is somewhat mobile, is steadied between the fingers of the free hand, and punctured in the line of the blood-flow towards the thorax (*Fig.* 423).

2. *The femoral vein*, where it lies medial to the femoral artery just below the inguinal ligament, is capable of yielding an ample quantity of blood for all procedures. After

thorough cleaning, the contaminated state of the area in the infant is no deterrent to the choice of this site. The child is held securely with the legs abducted and extended and that on the side chosen for puncture externally rotated. The right-handed operator will find the right femoral vein more easily approached and vice versa. The index finger of the left hand palpates the right femoral artery just below the inguinal ligament. With

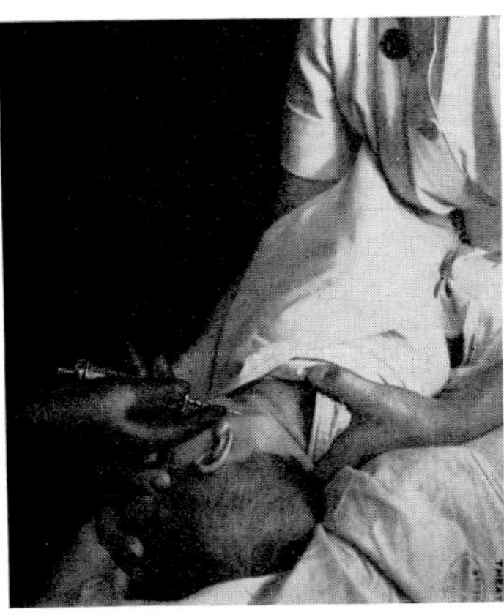

Fig. 423.—Venepuncture in an infant. The external jugular vein is a good site if the child is held in this position.

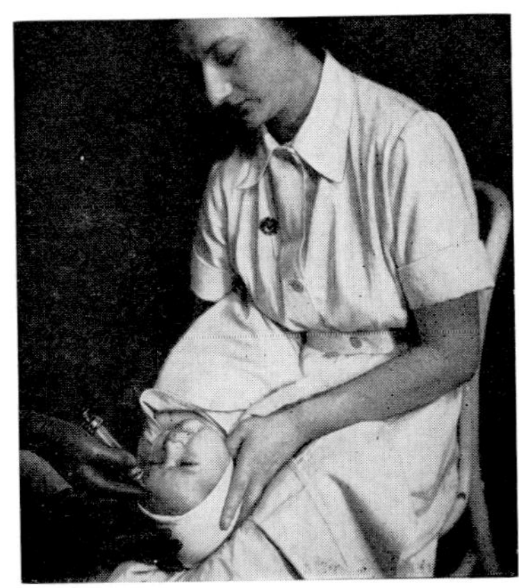

Fig. 424.—Puncture of the superior longitudinal venous sinus.

an intramuscular type of short-bevelled needle already affixed to the syringe, puncture is made over the vein just medial to the artery, the puncture being at right angles to the skin surface. The needle is advanced until the resistance of the superior ramus of the pubis is encountered. Slight withdrawal of the needle with suction applied to the syringe will result in the rapid aspiration of blood. Pressure over the site of puncture prevents the extravasation of blood on the final withdrawal of the needle, the area thereafter being sealed and bandaged.

3. *The superior longitudinal sinus* may be punctured with a short and short-bevelled needle close to the posterior angle of the anterior fontanelle. The head of the infant is steadied in the mid-supine position by an assistant. The needle is advanced obliquely, strictly in the sagittal plane, and is directed towards the external occipital protuberance (*Fig.* 424). The resistance of the aponeurosis and of the membrane of the fontanelle can be appreciated as these structures are perforated. If blood is not obtained immediately the procedure should be abandoned; persistence in the endeavour may lead to the extravasation of blood or the more serious intracranial complications of infection and thrombosis of the sinus; this procedure is now rather to be discouraged.

Urine.—In older children, both in hospital wards and out-patient departments, there is usually little difficulty in obtaining urine for routine chemical and for bacteriological examinations. For the latter 'clean-catch' specimens can be got after adequate cleaning of the genitalia with soap and water followed by the proper drying of the parts with a clean towel, care being taken in the female always to swab and dry from before back towards the perineum.

A final swab with methylated ether, but not with any antiseptic preparation, may be permitted. In very small children who cannot or will not micturate to order a sterile plastic and adhesive bag of which there are several types available may be carefully applied to the genital area (*Fig.* 425). In older children of both sexes the standing position, in the female with the legs apart, is better than squatting. The first part of the specimen may be discarded. For the results to be valid all urine specimens for bacteriological examination should be transported in a refrigerated container to the laboratory with the minimum of delay. In very particular situations careful catheterization may be performed: even midline suprapubic puncture with a fine lumbar puncture needle is permissible, the palpably full bladder being steadied against lateral mobility with the fingers

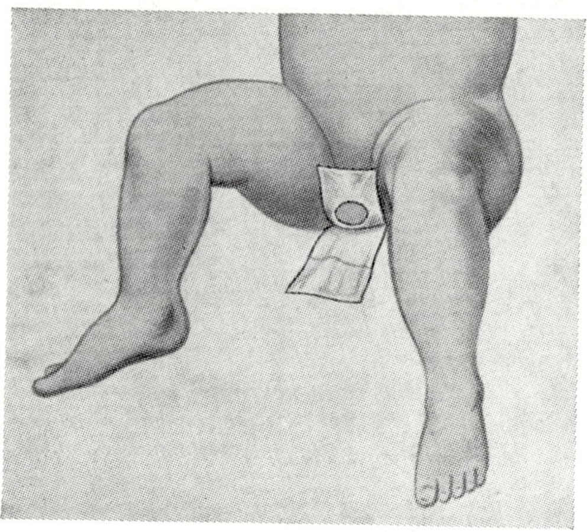

Fig. 425.—Adhesive plastic bag for the collection of urine in infants. Great Ormond Street pattern in situ.

of the other hand (*see* p. 446). There is very seldom any subsequent trouble from bleeding or extravasation.

Fæces.—There is no difficulty in obtaining adequate specimens of fæces, but those for testing for the presence of occult blood may require for accurate assessment the dietetic restriction of red meats in older children. Routine rectal swabbing on admission for bacteriological purposes is a useful practice in a children's hospital; it ensures prompt control of endemic dysenteric infections.

Collection of Sputum.—Young children are rarely able to provide sputum. Tubercle bacilli, when present, are most easily found in early morning stomach washings. A No. 10 catheter is used, joined by a glass connexion and a piece of rubber tubing to a glass funnel. The tip is lubricated with sterile glycerin, passed into the mouth, and swallowed. Sterile water is poured into the funnel and at once siphoned back into a sterile bowl; this is repeated several times until about 200 ml. of water have been used. The whole of the washings is sent to the laboratory.

CEREBROSPINAL FLUID COLLECTION

Lumbar Puncture.—For lumbar puncture, infants can be restrained adequately and safely in the flexed, left lateral position. Over the age of 1 year general anæsthesia may be necessary; even in later childhood reliable co-operation of the patient cannot be assured. The patient's temperament must then influence the decision whether or not an anæsthetic should be used. With infants and young children shorter needles and of finer calibre than for the adult are required. The technique of puncture is the same as for the adult (*see* p. 673), except that the space between the second and third lumbar vertebræ should never be used in infants whose spinal medulla may still lie at this level. Obviously the distance of the theca from the surface is less than in the adult and the less resistant tissues may fail to give the warning sensation of penetration of the dura. On this account as the needle is advanced withdrawal of the stylet at intervals is sometimes advisable. Accurate manometric readings are difficult to obtain because of the wide fluctuations in the fluid level produced by quite small movements on the part of the child.

Cisternal Puncture.—This procedure should only be performed by a skilled clinician. Methods of restraint, the type of needle, and variations in technique on account of the smaller and more resilient structures are similar to those advocated for lumbar puncture in the younger age-groups.

Lateral Ventricular Puncture.—This valuable procedure is possible without the making of a bur-hole only as long as the anterior fontanelle is open, and can be used in infants under the age of 1 year and in some hydrocephalics. Diagnostically, this technique is of value for air or dye ventriculography in cases of hydrocephalus or suspected cerebral tumour, and therapeutically for the reduction of intracranial pressure before and after neurosurgical procedures or in basal meningitic infections with subarachnoid block, and for the introduction of antibiotic agents.

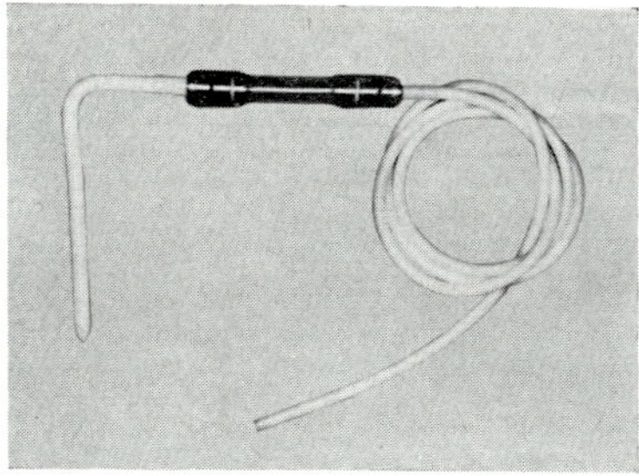

Fig. 426.—Holter valve.

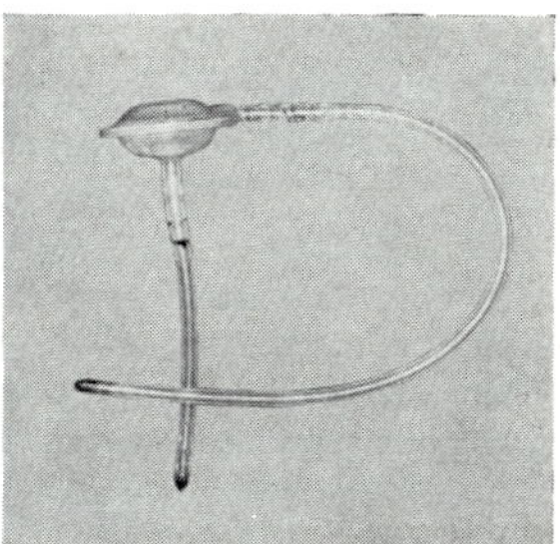

Fig. 427.—Pudenz pump system for shunting CSF.

The infant's head is restrained in the supine attitude. A lumbar puncture needle, or preferably a brain needle with trocar for the initial cranial puncture and blunt stylet for use within the brain substance, is introduced through the lateral angle of the anterior fontanelle and is directed towards the base of the skull with a slight inclination from the midline. Depending upon the degree of ventricular dilatation, cerebrospinal fluid should be obtained at a varying depth up to 3 cm. from the surface. In order to avoid cerebral damage a 'dry tap' requires the complete withdrawal of the needle before a puncture in another plane is made. On withdrawal of the needle the skin punctures are sealed with collodion.

Lateral ventricular puncture can be employed for continuous decompression over a period of time, the cerebrospinal fluid being permitted to drain into a water-seal flask. Firm fixation of the needle and full restraint and sedation of the child, if not comatose, are essential.

At the present time the much more energetic treatment of the spina bifida-hydrocephalus complex stems in large measure from the development of apparatus and procedures for the controlled shunting of excess or obstructed cerebrospinal fluid from the ventricular spaces of the brain either to the sub-arachnoid cisternæ (Torkildsen operation) or more usually to the blood circulation in the right atrium of the heart or to the peritoneal cavity by the use of either the Holter valve or the Pudenz pump system (*Figs.* 426 and 427). The use of these expensive plastic and metal gadgets requires absolute asepsis in their operative insertion and also the sterility of the cerebrospinal fluid and relative normality of its protein levels in order to avoid infection and blockage of the flow. In preparation for the use of these shunts, but perhaps before the lumbar wound of repair is healed or in the presence of meningitis or ventriculitis, fluid-pressure control may require frequent cranial tapping. The insertion of the very simple Rickham reservoir (*Fig.* 428) is a prelude to the use of the Holter or Pudenz systems and helps to avoid damage to cortical tissues from repeated punctures, and both simplifies and ensures the success of these repetitive processes.

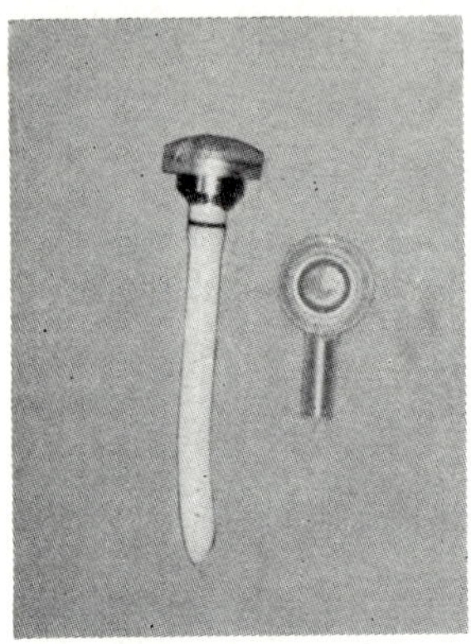

Fig. 428.—Rickham reservoir for repeated CSF tapping.

Subdural Tap is indicated as a diagnostic procedure in an infant in whom increasing intracranial pressure as a sequel to previous intracranial hæmorrhage is thought to be due to a chronic subdural hæmatoma. The anterior fontanelle usually is still patent; moreover, as a result of increased intracranial tension, the sutures of the skull may be separated sufficiently to permit puncture through them. The child is restrained with the head in the mid-supine position. With a shortened lumbar puncture needle orientated strictly at right angles to the surface of the skull, punctures are made at the lateral angles to the anterior fontanelle and the coronal sutures. After the sensation of dural puncture has been experienced, a protracted pause should be made because the fluid contents of the hæmatoma may be too viscid to issue immediately. The colour of the fluid varies according to its age, being frankly hæmorrhagic or more commonly yellow. A 'dry tap' is an indication for puncture at another site. Puncture on both sides of the skull should always be made, as the lesions are not infrequently bilateral.

RESUSCITATION

(*See also* Chapters I, II, and III)

Resuscitation of the newborn infant and young child demands the immediate establishment of an adequate and free airway. Often this may be simply achieved by the effective suction of mucus and fluid from the pharynx and laryngeal aperture but at other times may require intubation with an endotracheal tube and endoscope. An adequate supply and range of suitable tubes and endoscope blades must always be readily to hand on the resuscitation tray or in the emergency box. Some may prefer relatively soft Portex tubes, others firmer or even

armoured tubes. Oxygen should be available for delivery by mask or for connexion to the endotracheal tube; incubators or tents may be necessary for more
prolonged therapy and periodic control of the oxygen concentration by oximetric
estimation may be necessary as a precaution against retrolental fibroplasia

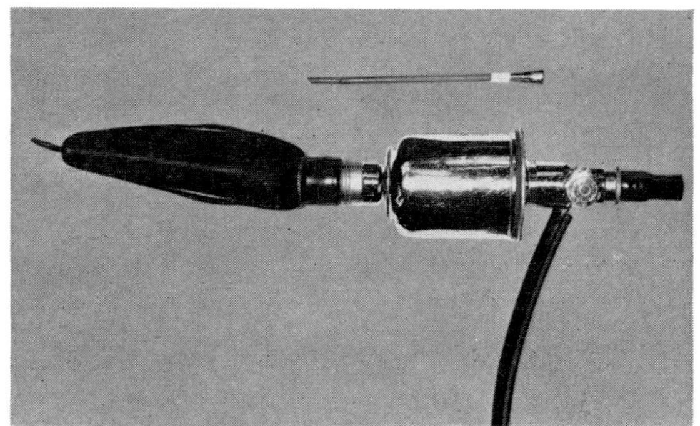

Fig. 429.—Artificial ventilation of the lungs by squeezing the bag of a Waters's canister
apparatus.

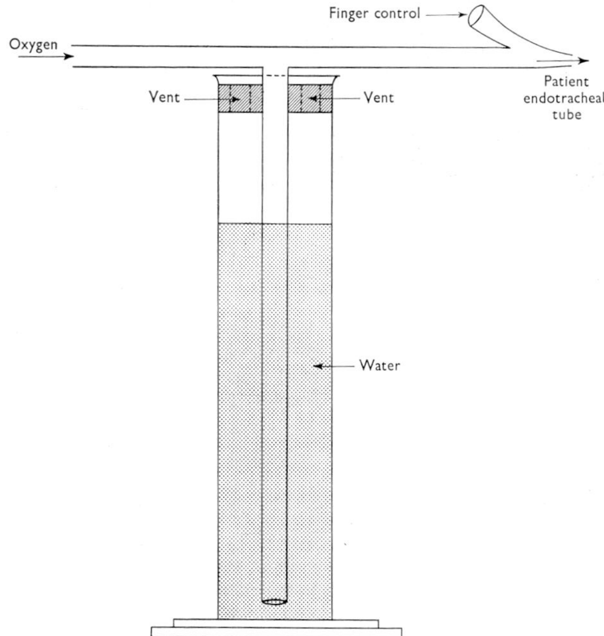

Fig. 430.—Water manometer for controlling the pressure used during artificial ventilation.

which oxygen concentrations of over 40 per cent tend to induce in the newborn and premature baby.

Simple control of respiration may be obtained by very gentle mouth-to-mouth or mouth-to-tube breathing once the airway has been established or more satisfactorily by the gentle squeezing of the bag of a Waters's canister apparatus coupled to compressed air or oxygen (*Fig.* 429). A simple water manometer apparatus can be used and adjusted so as to avoid the delivery at too great a pressure (*Fig.* 430). More sophisticated positive-pressure ventilating machinery, such as the Bird, the Barnet, or the Engström, all require much more skilled control and work on a variety of principles of volume, pressure, and time cycling.

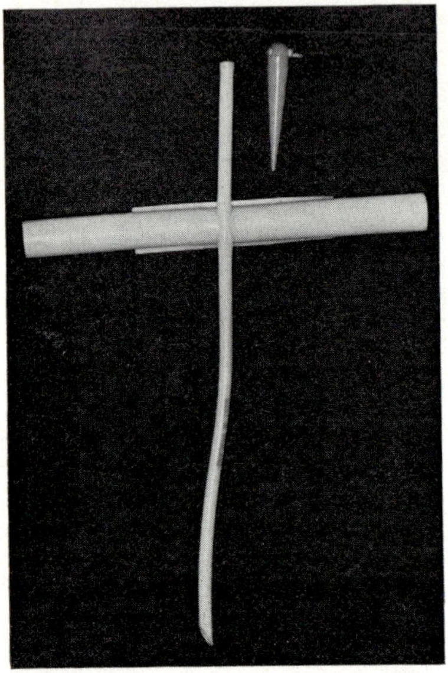

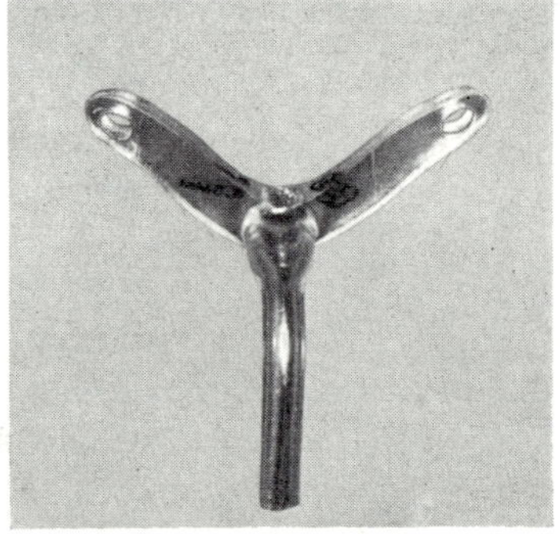

Fig. 431.—Jackson Rees endotracheal tube.

Fig. 432.—Plastic tracheostomy tubes for infants.

They are useful for more prolonged respiratory control when they may be employed in conjunction either with the Jackson Rees endotracheal tube or with an established tracheostomy. The Jackson Rees tube (*Fig.* 431) permits fixation to the face and direct access for tracheal toilet and suction. It is comparatively non-irritating to the mucous membrane even when used for several days, but thereafter subglottic stenosis may ultimately ensue. For tracheostomy plastic tubes of the Great Ormond Street pattern are preferable because of their pliability and their ability to conform and for the adequate range in which they are manufactured (*Fig.* 432). It is important to remember in the use of flexible tubes of small calibre that further narrowing may occur in the lumen by bending or twisting even to quite a slight degree.

Continuing respiratory obstruction is very exhausting to a small child; its presence is readily indicated by inspiratory intercostal indrawing, and by restlessness and tachycardia. Continuous nursing is essential when a small child is maintained with a tracheostomy. The head must be in the extended position and adequate suction with a sterile catheter must always be available; humidification of the atmosphere or gases is desirable and regular instillation of small amounts of sterile 0·9 per cent sodium chloride solution is necessary. A spare tracheostomy tube of the right size must always be available.

The use of excessive pressure, either with or without intubation, can cause pulmonary damage, pneumothorax, surgical emphysema, or even rupture of the stomach. There is no place for the administration of oxygen by intragastric tube, a procedure recommended in certain quarters some years ago. It is ineffective and dangerous.

The administration of analeptic respiratory stimulants such as lobeline or of morphine antagonists such as nalorphan into the umbilical vein in the cord has its dangers; erroneously retrograde injection in an umbilical artery may have a permanent neurotoxic effect upon a sciatic nerve.

Cardiac Arrest (*see* Chapter I).—In an infant or child cardiac arrest seldom requires opening of the chest; because of the compressibility of the soft thoracic cage external massage is adequate and effective. Care is essential in applying pressure; this should be done with two fingers over the lower sternum and a sharp 'jab' inwards made at regular intervals of about a second. More forceful application over a wider area may cause damage to the liver, stomach, or lung. Defibrillation may necessitate direct access to the heart and small electrodes are available for use in young children.

Hypothermia in infants and small children occurs readily after long journeys or protracted operations. In transit it may be avoided by the careful use of hot-water bottles for the warming of incubators which are not heated by the electrical system of the ambulance or helicopter. In the operating theatre thermostatically controlled water-heated or electrical blankets may be used, or warmed Gamgee around all parts to which access is not necessary is safe and effective. In incubators servo-control systems permit the constant maintenance of pre-set temperatures in situations of undue thermal instability, but haste in any rewarming process is to be avoided.

THE TREATMENT OF SHOCK

In the young the effects of shock are liable to be more rapid and more profound than those produced by similar noxious stimuli in an adult. The reason for this is the greatly increased metabolic demand for fluid in the infant and young child in whom the total blood-volume is much less in quantity but is greater in proportion to weight than it is in the adult. The following tables of *basic metabolic fluid requirements* for each 24 hours will be of service:—

24-HOURLY BASIC FLUID REQUIREMENTS

Birth to 2nd birthday	- 160 ml. per kg.	5 years to 7 years	- 80 ml. per kg.
2 years to 4 years -	- 100 ml. per kg.	8 years to adult years	- 60 ml. per kg.

It should be appreciated that in the first few days of life, often nursed in an atmosphere of high humidity and before renal function is fully established, a considerable reduction in the fluid requirement per kg. per diem of such an infant may occur; care also in the supply of Na ion, especially after an operation, is accordingly important. The daily fluid requirement of such a case could be as low as 45–50 ml. per kg.

Having appreciated how relatively great is the daily requirement of fluid in the very young, it will be understood that loss of body fluid from manifest or occult hæmorrhage, from the surface of burns and scalds and into the tissues adjacent to such injuries, from vomiting, and the reactionary effusion of generalized peritonitis can produce a state of profound shock with great rapidity.

Posture.—The elevation of the limbs and trunk and the 'head-low' position are generally applicable, and when there is any possibility of vomiting this position gives an additional safeguard against the aspiration of vomitus which is such a very real danger in infancy.

Sedation.—The avoidance of overdosage or of inadequate dosage through ignorance or enthusiasm is important. Heroin is still the most satisfactory drug for infants and children because its effects are certain, but without the depressant features upon respiration and the alimentary tract which accompany the use of morphine. A suitable scale of dosage is as follows:—

HEROIN
0·6 mg. up to 2 yr. of age 1·25 mg. up to 6 yr. of age 2·5 mg. up to 12 yr. of age

The avoidance of the application of heat in any form. As in the adult, warming of the body surface only embarrasses the body's natural reactions to shock.

Pressor drugs are seldom, if ever, indicated in the young child. *The availability of suction is essential*; respiratory obstruction potentiates the state of shock.

Oxygen therapy can be of considerable value, and is administered most suitably by mask when indicated with a flow of 3 l. per minute. For babies an incubator with controlled oxygen supply is essential.

Fluid Therapy.—Provided there is no contra-indication to its use, the oral route is the safest for the administration of saline and dextrose. In babies subcutaneous infusion of normal saline or half-strength normal saline, combined with 5 per cent dextrose, can be given and absorption aided by the addition of hyaluronidase. Both of these are, however, slow, somewhat limited, and uncontrolled. The intravenous route may, however, be necessary for speed of effect or from the nature of the substance required. At an approximate estimate, 30 ml. of crystalloid solution or 20 ml. of plasma or blood per kg. of body-weight may be given safely and the effect then carefully assessed before any more fluid is added to the circulation. Facilities for radio-isotope techniques in the estimation of blood-volumes and the response to therapy are available, but reticence in the use of such agents as iodine isotopes in small children is the restrictive factor. Rate of replacement can be checked by CVP measurements (p. 24).

Charts.—For drip infusions careful recording of the rate of flow and the amount given is of vital importance. Recording of the passage of urine and if possible of the amount passed (obtained by indwelling catheter, if necessary) is the best method of assessing the adequacy of the circulation.

Clinical Assessment of Progress.—The efficiency of the capillary circulation, the respiratory rate and rhythm, the mental state and behaviour, and the urinary flow (*see Table V*, p. 93) are the best criteria upon which to judge clinical improvement. The features of the pulse and the blood-pressure are useful but less indicative of the actual clinical state of the child.

INFUSIONS

The restoration and maintenance of a normal fluid and electrolyte balance are of vital importance in the care of sick children, and especially of infants, in whom dehydration and loss of electrolytes can occur with rapidity. Conversely, overhydration is produced in them more readily than in adults; for this reason constant vigilance in the administration is required (*see also* p. 32).

When it is to be given parenterally, it is a wise precaution to divide the daily maintenance fluid requirement (*see Table*, p. 575) into two or three equal parts, to ensure that these 12-hour or 8-hour estimates are met as accurately as possible. Obviously additional amounts are required for the correction of dehydration, and when water and electrolytes are being lost from the body's economy. In small infants the loss of weight which has occurred is usually known or can be calculated and, on the basis of 1 pint (568 ml.) of water weighing $1\frac{1}{4}$ lb. (570 G.), this loss can be used to obtain a rough estimate of the amount of additional fluid that can be administered safely and quite rapidly. In older

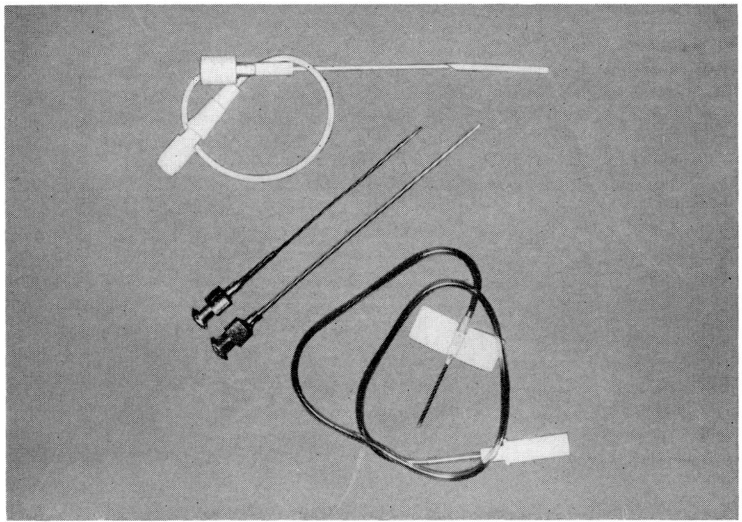

Fig. 433.—Intravenous cannulæ. *Top*, Intracath (Bardic); *middle*, Intracath (Jelco); *bottom*, Scalp vein needle with butterfly holder.

children, where the higher degree of accuracy in these computations is not so imperative, empirical amounts can be added to the basic requirement. The clinical effect produced provides an indication of the total quantity to be administered in the current 24 hours.

Routes of Administration:—

1. Subcutaneous Infusion is given in the form of isotonic saline or half-normal saline solution with 5 per cent dextrose. The latter, however, sometimes causes a mild tissue reaction. Absorption of larger amounts of fluid is aided by the administration of hyaluronidase, one ampoule (1500 IU) per litre of fluid.

Injection with a syringe provides rapid administration; the preliminary injection of hyaluronidase and massage of the area after the injection hasten absorption. Drip administration with a Y-connexion to the two needle sites is a more usual practice but is slower. Sixty to 90 ml. of the chosen solution can be given by the first method, and larger amounts over a longer period by the second. This is quite a good method for correcting less severe degrees of dehydration, and for maintaining the immediate needs of the newborn during the early post-operative period, but is less in favour and less used than formerly. It should be recalled that persistence or occurrence of minor degrees of dehydration simulate the physiological state during the first few days of life (i.e., before full feeding is established); *slight subhydration is infinitely preferable to overhydration*, but milk feeding is best both for adequate hydration and for the metabolic needs of the rapidly growing child.

2. Intravenous Infusion.—*Percutaneous venepuncture* is often practicable, even in quite small children, with a flanged scalp vein needle or intracath or Braunula cannula in older children (*Fig.* 433). There are several types on the market which have now been improved for ease of puncture and for the prevention of breaking off at the connexion and the subsequent danger of becoming free in the venous circulation. A vein of the dorsum of the hand or foot, the cubital fossa, or the scalp is the most serviceable (*Figs.* 434, 435). A light splint and firm strapping should be employed to immobilize a limb. Embedding of the needle or catheter in plaster-of-Paris moulded to the scalp is also very effective (*Fig.* 436).

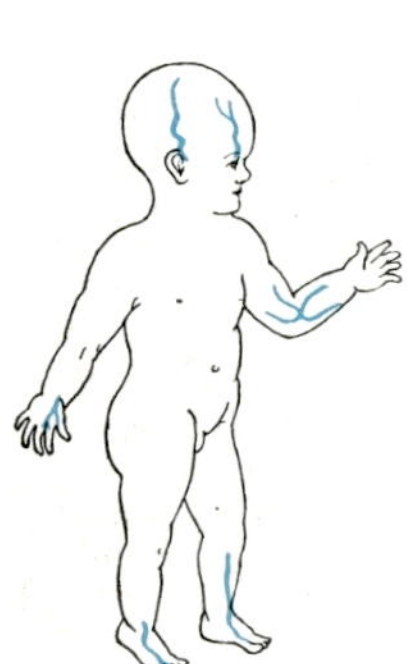

Fig. 434.—Veins usually accessible for intravenous therapy in infants and young children.

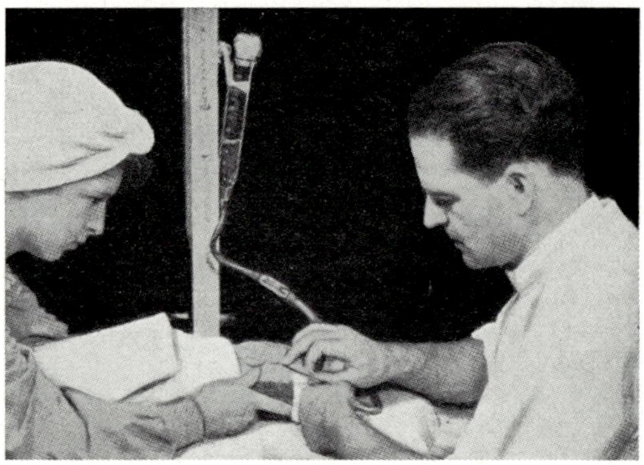

Fig. 435.—Note the method whereby the nurse holds the head steady. The arms, legs, and body have been wrapped in a blanket so that the patient cannot move during the procedure. The nurse's forearms and elbows stabilize the infant's body. The position of the right and left thumbs of the nurse holding the infant's head is important. The patient should be on a firm table, never held in the nurse's lap. The surgeon administering the fluid has both hands practically free, but can exert additional steadying pressure on the infant's head with the 3rd and 4th fingers of his right hand. The temporal vein is the best.

Cutting down on a vein under local anæsthesia or under general anæsthesia immediately prior to operation is necessary when the veins are collapsed, the baby is fat, or percutaneous puncture has failed. The internal saphenous vein just above and anterior to the medial malleolus (*Fig.* 434), or a vein of the cubital fossa, is suitable for the purpose. The vein is cannulized with a polythene tube of suitable calibre. Within the first 2 weeks of life the umbilical vein can be readily exposed in the attachment of the umbilical cord to the baby or in its passage through the linea alba to the falciform ligament. It may be necessary to wash out thrombus before cannulization is achieved and infusion established.

Continuous intravenous drip infusion: Not uncommonly difficulty is encountered in establishing a satisfactory flow. This may be due to venospasm induced by the cannulization, the shocked condition of the child, or to mechanical obstruction. First ascertain that the line of the vein is not compressed by strapping. Next, apply warmth to the limb proximal to the cannula. If unsuccessful, alteration in the position of the limb or the cannula will be required to establish the flow.

The amount of fluid to be given hourly must be stated in writing, and the rate of flow adjusted accordingly. In infants this amount may be as low as 10–15 ml. or less per hour, and the standard flask is far too large to observe accurately the

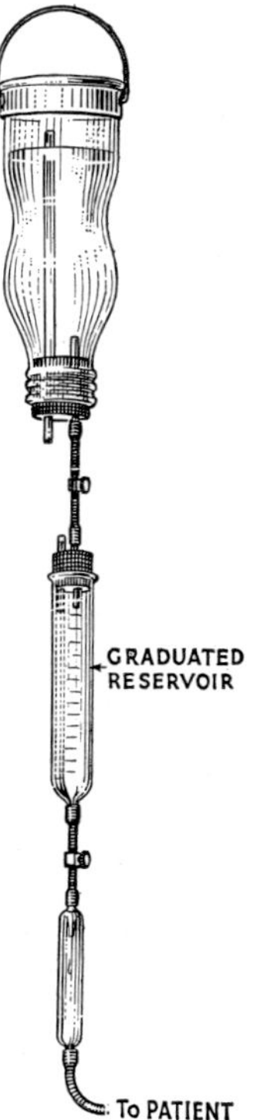

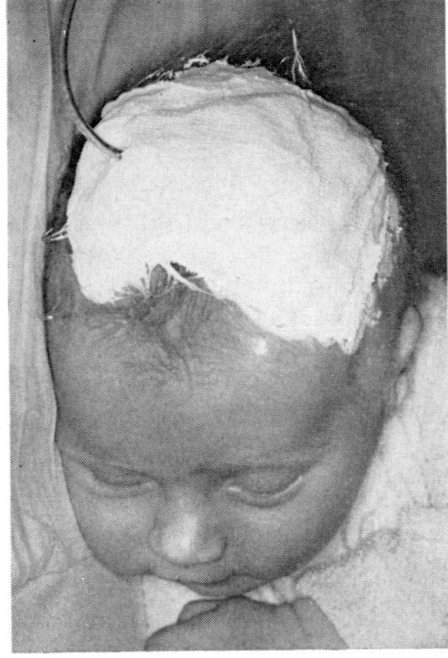

Fig. 436.—Plaster embedding for scalp-vein infusion.

Fig. 437.—The interposition of a small, closely calibrated reservoir in the infusion set permits slow and accurate drip infusion.

decrease of so small an amount. The interposition of a smaller and more closely calibrated reservoir (*Fig.* 437), which is filled as required from the standard container, is a safeguard against the dangers of overloading the circulation.

The type and amount of fluid to be given are dictated by the clinical deficiencies (*see* p. 32); guidance is obtained by electrolyte estimations performed initially and subsequently for the full control of therapy. The body-weight of the young patient is another important factor in these calculations, and account must be taken of the special losses of vomiting, diarrhœa, ileostomy, renal failure, fever, etc. Normal 0·9 per cent saline or at half-strength with 5 per cent glucose may be given in alkalotic states, Ringer-Lactate or Hartmann's solution in acidosis, 10 per cent fructose for additional calories. Potassium increments should be given orally if possible or added in carefully controlled amounts to the parenteral solution. Care with saline is necessary in the immediate post-operative period. Maintenance of intravenous infusion can be continued with daily increments of protein hydrolysate (aminosol-vitrum) 3·3 per cent in 5 per cent glucose or with 15 per cent fructose combined with a fat emulsion preparation (intralipid-vitrum) 10–20 per cent solution in amounts of 20 ml. per kg. Care in their use is essential because of vein reaction to the hydrolysate, although the fat emulsion tends to offset this effect when given concurrently. Because the solutions are good culture media anything that may be left and not required at that administration must be discarded. In the malabsorptive states of infancy prolonged use of intravenous therapy is sometimes forced upon the clinician. The dangers of *Esch. coli* septicæmia may be offset by an appropriate antibiotic such as colomycin and by the frequent changing of the sites of infusion, difficult though this may sometimes be in practice.

BLEEDING AND BLOOD REPLACEMENT

THE CONTROL OF HÆMORRHAGE IN THE NEWBORN

During the first week of life, usually between the third and fourth days, spontaneous hæmorrhage sometimes occurs into the alimentary canal, when it is evidenced by melæna or the passage of fresh blood per rectum, or by hæmatemesis; from the umbilicus (when it is likely to be due to insecure ligation of the cord); from the nose and mouth; or into the skin and subcutaneous tissues at points of pressure and on the scalp. Bearing in mind the small blood-volume of the infant, the amount of blood lost may be considerable and the immediate effects alarming. Spontaneous hæmorrhage arises from the low level of blood-prothrombin, which, in the first week of life, is approximately 25 per cent of the adult value; in prematurity sometimes it is even lower.

Treatment.—Hypoprothrombinæmia can be countered rapidly by the administration of a water-soluble analogue of vitamin K★ in an intramuscular dose of 1 mg. This dose should not be repeated because of hæmolytic and possible neurotoxic effects through hyperbilirubinæmia. In addition, blood transfusion should be carried out as soon as possible in necessary cases. In bleeding from the umbilicus local treatment, apart from the placebo use of styptic, is seldom necessary.

BLOOD TRANSFUSION

The principles and technique of blood transfusion in the adult (p. 43) are applicable to those belonging to the younger age-groups. For the female child Rhesus compatibility should be assured. If time does not permit the necessary tests to be performed, Rhesus-negative blood must be used. The amount of blood to be transfused and the rate of its administration will depend upon the clinical condition; in infants the avoidance of overtransfusion is especially important. Below the age of 2 years the formula, 20 ml. per kg. of body-weight gives some indication of the quantity that can be given safely, but the degree of anæmia and (if known) the amount of blood lost will assist in computing necessary modifications of this arbitrarily contrived estimation.

★ Konakion (Roche Products Ltd., 15 Manchester Square, London, W.1).

Aminosol-Vitrum and Intralipid-Vitrum (Paines & Byrne Ltd., Pabyrn Laboratories, Greenford, Middlesex).
Colomycin (Pharmax Ltd., Crayford, Dartford, Kent).

In order to help in calculating how much blood will be required for a transfusion in a child, it is helpful to be able to refer to the normal total blood-volume at various ages:—

TOTAL BLOOD-VOLUME

Birth	..	300 ml.	6 years	..	1500 ml.
6 months	..	500 ml.	7 years	..	1700 ml.
1 year	..	600 ml.	8 years	..	1900 ml.
2 years	..	850 ml.	9 years	..	2100 ml.
3 years	..	1000 ml.	10 years	..	2300 ml.
4 years	..	1150 ml.	11 years	..	2500 ml.
5 years	..	1350 ml.	12 years	..	2700 ml.

In neonatal surgery accurate blood replacement during operation is essential and this implies an accurate assessment of the amount of the blood-loss. This estimation is achieved either by a swab-weighing process using sensitive scales or colorimetrically by a machine of the Perometer type which gives a direct and continuing reading of great accuracy. The temptation to over-transfuse must be avoided. Checks of the CVP are useful.

In general whole blood is best, but freshly drawn blood is better in infective processes and in clotting-deficiency conditions such as hæmophilia when specific globulin fractions are not available. Packed-cell transfusion is appropriate in anæmia and platelet transfusion in thrombocytopenic states. Even marrow transfusion is possible in aplastic anæmia.

Exchange Transfusion.—Replacement transfusion is now the accepted treatment of erythroblastosis fœtalis caused by Rhesus incompatibility of the mother and fœtus. Possibly there is also a place for this procedure in older children as a means of effecting extrarenal depuration in cases of anuric or other forms of intoxication. In cases of erythroblastosis fœtalis an *exchange* transfusion, given as soon after birth as possible, not only eliminates the necessity of repeated small transfusions, with their attendant difficulties, but usually prevents the development of disturbing neurological sequelæ caused by intensification of the coincident kernicterus with fixation of bile-pigments in the basal ganglia.

Increasing hyperbilirubinæmia to the indirect level of 20 mg. per 100 ml. is the best criterion for deciding when an exchange transfusion is necessary, the objectives of this form of therapy being: (*a*) correction of anæmia; (*b*) lowering of excessive serum-bilirubin and circulating antibodies; and (*c*) replacement of fragile by more stable erythrocytes.

For exchange transfusion in infants heparinized blood is much safer than citrated blood. The donor blood should be fresh and warm, in order to avoid hyperkalæmia, the manifestations of which are irritability and tachycardia—signs which call for the administration of calcium gluconate.

Technique (*Fig.* 438).—A length of polythene tubing or special umbilical vein catheter is inserted into the open mouth of the umbilical vein in the upper portion of the stump of the umbilical cord, which has been cut across ½ in. (1·25 cm.) from its attachment to the abdominal wall. The cannula is passed into the vein in an upward direction, almost parallel to the abdominal wall. During its passage an assistant applies syringe suction to the end of the tubing, to free the lumen of the vein of newly formed clot. When venous blood is withdrawn and after recording the central venous pressure, the transfusion is begun in aliquots of 20 ml. The baby's blood-volume is estimated at 40 ml. per lb. (80 ml. per kg.) of body-weight and it requires 80 ml. per lb. of body-weight to effect a 90 per cent replacement. In small babies aliquots of 10 ml. are more suitable and manometric adjustment for the avoidance of excessive central venous pressure at the end of the procedure is essential. A slight deficit is better than a slight surfeit and about 1½ hours should be taken to accomplish the exchange. The type of blood used is also important—packed cells are appropriate in the presence of hydrops and whole blood binds in its albumin more bilirubin when this is in marked excess.

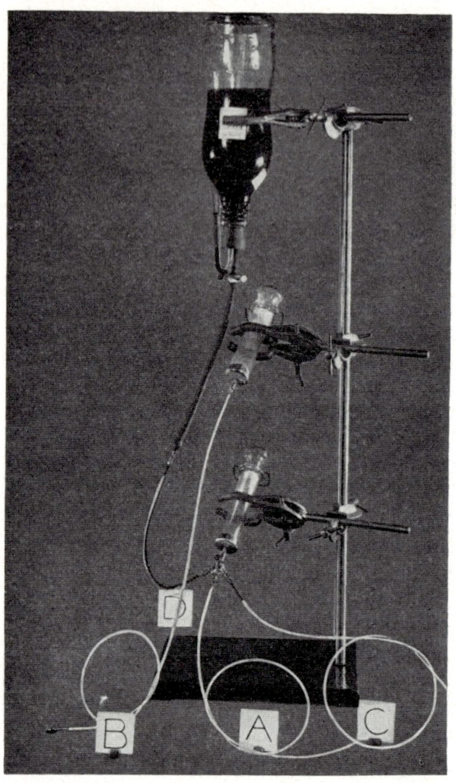

Fig. 438.—Basic apparatus for exchange transfusion. A, To patient; B, Heparin syringe to connect periodically at 'D' on three-way syringe for flushing purposes; C, To discard; D, From donor blood.

PRE-OPERATIVE PREPARATION AND MEDICATION

Increasing efforts are made to admit children to hospital less and less even for operative intervention. Many operations—incisions and biopsies, excisions, circumcisions, and herniotomies—can be done on an out-patient basis. In Britain the almost ubiquitous car allows many young patients to be brought and taken home over quite long distances. To do this on a completely empty stomach for the infants and young children with whom this routine is more usually practised is harmful, and a light meal of milk and bread and butter without crust or biscuit may be permitted no later than 4 hours before the intended operation. If the general anæsthesia has been of relatively short duration and the operation uneventfully accomplished feeding is also permissible soon after the return of full consciousness. A ready decision to retain the child in hospital must be taken if there has been any difficulty either with the operation or the anæsthetic. This is essential to the safety and the success of an out-patient routine.

A Pre-operative Antisialogogic Drug is given to all who are to receive a general anæsthetic, irrespective of age and whether or not a pre-operative sedative drug is given. Atropine, which is extremely well tolerated in both infants and children, not only reduces the amount of saliva secreted, but prevents over-secretion of the tracheobronchial glands, which otherwise occurs in response to the stimulus produced by anæsthetic vapours. Atropine also protects the heart from the effects of vagal stimulation.

Atropine is given by subcutaneous injection 30 minutes before operation. The following doses can be employed with safety:—

ATROPINE	
Up to 1 year	0·3 mg.
1 to 5 years	0·4 mg.
5 years and over	0·6 mg.

Disadvantages.—By reducing sweating, Nature's chief method of adjusting body temperature is impaired, and this is a possible cause of anæsthetic convulsions. Atropine also is inclined to accelerate the rate of the heart-beat.

In an emergency, atropine can be given intramuscularly or intravenously.

Pre-operative Sedative Drugs.—

In Infants, and especially in neonates, in whom any form of physical depression must be avoided, pre-operative sedative drugs should not be given up to the age of one year, for little, if any, memory of an incident such as the induction of an anæsthetic is retained. A possible exception to this rule is when the effect of pre-operative sedation is desirable in the immediate post-operative period, e.g., to prevent crying when consciousness returns following a cleft palate operation (p. 298).

In Children.—Varying opinions are held as to which drug, or combination of drugs, is the best. Often those who have decided views on this matter acclaim as best the one with which they are most familiar. Actually the search for a safe, pleasant, and *reliable* pre-operative sedative suitable for children is still proceeding. All the following have their advocates:—

1. Barbiturates.—

Phenobarbitone may be given 60 to 90 minutes before operations upon the respiratory passages in children. Consciousness with slight drowsiness and active reflexes are retained.

PHENOBARBITONE	
1 to 2 years	60 mg.
3 to 6 years	90 mg.
6 years and over	120 mg.

Seconal can be given to children who are to receive a general inhalation anæsthetic when it is desirable to have the child asleep but capable of response to stimuli.

SECONAL
1 to 3 years...................... 50 mg.
3 to 6 years......................100 mg.
6 years and over.................150 mg.

Thiopentone can be administered in the form of a suppository or gravitated into the rectum as a 5 per cent solution in a dosage of 20 mg. per lb. Because of the depth of unconsciousness produced within 15 minutes *continuous nursing supervision of the patient is essential* until the anæsthetist takes charge.

Disadvantages of Barbiturates.—The rate of absorption from the alimentary canal is uncertain due, in part, to the capsule. This disadvantage and the difficulty of persuading any child to swallow a capsule can be obviated by cutting the capsule, emptying the powder therefrom, and admixing it with a spoonful of jam or ice-cream.

2. Opiates may be given to older children. Usually one of these drugs is prescribed prior to the intravenous induction of anæsthesia in order to render the child conscious but drowsy.

Omnopon (Papaveretum, B.P.C.) in doses of 0·6 mg. per kilo is a satisfactory premedicant for children of all ages.

3. Phenothiazine derivatives do not provide satisfactory sedation, but their value lies in their properties of preventing bronchoconstriction during anæsthesia and in allaying post-operative restlessness and post-operative vomiting. The most popular drug of this group for children is vallergan, trimeprazine tartrate, 2 mg. per kg. administered 1 hour before operation.

Disadvantages of Opiates.—Morphine (and to a lesser extent other opiates) has a reputation of causing respiratory depression, which may render 'open' methods of inducing anæsthesia difficult. Another disadvantage is that all these drugs delay the return of consciousness following the conclusion of the anæsthetic.

PRE-OPERATIVE PREPARATION

Bowel and Urine Sterilization.—Pre-operative treatment is also required in large-bowel surgery and in operations for urinary diversion. The established preparation with the non-absorbable sulphonamides is still current practice, but more specific control can be obtained by bacteriological stool analysis with the construction of a sensitivity antibiogram. This details the antibiotic agents especially indicated for a particular patient and for the greatest clinical security. Neomycin is very often the basis for this sort of prophylaxis. In urinary diversion similar bowel preparation may be necessary as also may be the continuation of therapy for the control of chronic urinary tract infection. Antibiotic umbrella cover may be desirable for operations in areas of previous or continuing low-grade infection, as for interval appendicectomy after drainage of an appendix abscess, or curettage of bone in chronic osteomyelitis of either pyogenic or tuberculous origin (*see also* p. 72).

Covering and Position in Theatre.—The practice of swaddling in Gamgee or cotton-wool and of splinting a baby on a board or crucifix is seldom followed now, but loss of body heat while in the operating theatre and exposed upon the table

Vallergan (May & Baker Ltd., Dagenham, Essex).

is prevented by the avoidance of undue exposure and by the maintenance of an environmental temperature of 27° C. (80° F.) and a humidity of about 70 per cent and by the use of water-heated or electric blankets, thermostatically controlled. It must be appreciated that positioning and the use of polystyrene foam rests and wedges may render these methods of heat control much less effective through reduced contact. It is also important to remember that in neonates it is difficult to make a safe contact with the standard diathermy pad. Two smaller pads of equal total area, provided they are both used and correctly wired, can be more effective and efficient, and avoid the poor contact which causes a diathermy burn usually over such an awkward area as the sacrum. Better still, do not use diathermy with neonates. Closed-circuit anæsthesia also helps to conserve body heat.

POST-OPERATIVE CARE AND SEDATION

The principles of care of the airway until consciousness and the cough reflex return are at least as important in young children and infants as in the adult (p. 106). The majority of anæsthetists retain the child in their immediate care until consciousness returns. All apparatus for suction, endoscopic intubation, and delivery of oxygen must be to hand as well as the drugs of the resuscitation tray.

Speaking generally, the relief of pain and its associated restlessness following an operation upon a child is dependent still upon the use of opium derivatives.

Morphine is not well tolerated by infants and young children, in whom it tends to produce undesirable depression of respiration, and perhaps vomiting, both of which are a great danger to babies in the post-operative period. Also it is inclined to have a depressant effect upon intestinal activity. Nevertheless, in many hospitals morphine is the standard post-operative sedative drug for use in children aged 5 years and over, and an indication of the dose required is afforded by calculating the dose as:—

$$(\text{age in years}/2) \text{ mg.,}$$

i.e., 6 years = 3 mg., 10 years = 5 mg.

For a child below the age of 5 years, and for infants, post-operative sedation may still in some parts of the world be best supplied in the form of:—

Tincture of Opium (Nepenthe), of which *one minim is given for each year of age.* The effect of nepenthe (which is the preparation usually prescribed) is more moderate and more prolonged than that of morphine. The following table shows *approximate* equivalents:—

NEPENTHE		
1 year requires 1 minim (0·06 ml.) = 0·66 mg.	morphine	
2 years require 2 minims (0·12 ml.) = 1·33 mg.	,,	
3 years ,, 3 minims (0·18 ml.) = 2·00 mg.	,,	
4 years ,, 4 minims (0·24 ml.) = 2·66 mg.	,,	
5 years ,, 5 minims (0·3 ml.) = 3·33 mg.	,,	

Heroin.—In spite of its reputation for inducing drug addiction that some years ago almost forfeited its place in the *British Pharmacopœia*, heroin is of very great value in children of all ages. Given subcutaneously, it is almost immediately effective and is very well tolerated, even by babies, and is to a great extent free from the undesirable side-effects of morphine. The dosage is as follows:—

<table>
<tr><td colspan="2" align="center">HEROIN</td></tr>
<tr><td>Up to 2 years.....................</td><td>0·6 mg.</td></tr>
<tr><td>2 to 6 years......................</td><td>1·25 mg.</td></tr>
<tr><td>6 years and over..................</td><td>2·5 mg.</td></tr>
</table>

The very short period of need for this drug post-operatively and the far greater control that can be exercised over children, as compared with adults, practically eliminates all risk of the development of addiction to this valuable drug in children. Heroin is banned in many countries.

SPECIAL POINTS IN THE SURGICAL CARE OF CERTAIN PÆDIATRIC CONDITIONS

In the neonatal period the greatest urgency may attend two surgical causes of the **Respiratory Distress Syndrome** (R.D.S.)—congenital diaphragmatic hernia and the pulmonary tension syndrome. Simple clinical and radiological examinations will reveal a marked mediastinal shift and, in addition, in the former the irregular opacities of bowel and viscera usually in the left chest, or in the latter an area of gross emphysema and rib spreading. Maintenance of adequate pulmonary ventilation, especially in the latter, may be difficult or even be made worse by artificial ventilation. Reduction in intrapleural and/or intrapulmonary tension by the introduction of an intercostal needle or catheter may be necessary, but in that case early operative intervention is indicated. Ambulance transfer will require to be speedy and even a police escort may be justified at certain times of the day in many cities. Medical supervision and all the necessary resuscitation apparatus should travel with the child. In diaphragmatic hernia respiratory problems may embarrass the post-operative state; they are due to pulmonary hypoplasia or agenesis and to raised intra-abdominal pressure as well as circulatory and feeding difficulties.

In **œsophageal atresia** tracheo-œsophageal fistula usually coexists and contamination of the lungs may occur either through overspill into the trachea through the laryngeal aperture from the blind upper pouch when the baby is in the 'head-up' position, or else by reflux from the stomach of acid content along the lower œsophageal segment and through the fistula when the baby is in the 'head-low' position. The latter effect is the more undesirable. When the inability to pass a stiff No. 8 F catheter beyond the 10-cm. mark in the œsophagus raises the suspicion of this condition, the child should be transferred in the 'head-up' position (about 45°) and oro-pharyngeal suction be performed at least every 15 minutes or as indicated. Obviously nothing must be given by mouth and antibiotics of a broad-spectrum type—ampicillin or cloxacillin—should be administered if pulmonary contamination has occurred. Radiography—*see* p. 722.

In œsophageal atresia, premature babies and those with other associated anomalies such as congenital heart disease or bowel atresia there is a high risk from rushed definitive operative procedures, and deferment from these for some weeks is desirable. Gastrostomy for feeding (and deflation of the stomach sometimes) is essential and the care of this has problems of its own (*vide infra*). Even the intrathoracic ligation of the fistula may be postponed. Continuous nursing has then to be provided to ensure safe positioning of the child, for aspiration at frequent intervals and in an emergency, and for supervision of the gastrostomy tube and its feeding reservoir. Inhalation and regurgitation have obviously to be avoided at all costs.

Complications.—Post-operatively, apart from the general problems of incubator care, difficulties may be remarkably few. Any leak at the anastomosis within the chest will soon be appreciated clinically and radiologically. In these circumstances temporization is usually regretted later. If it is not already present a gastrostomy must be made and all oral feeding stopped if it has been started. At the least drainage to the site of the anastomosis or, alternatively, a formal exploration of the chest and discontinuation of the anastomosis, with exteriorization of the proximal œsophagus in the left neck and ligation of the distal portion, are required. In ordinary circumstances oral feeding, after gastrografin examination has given proof of œsophageal integrity, is permitted from the seventh day post-operatively.

Gastrostomy, either of the Kader-Senn or Witzel type, is best made through a right or midline vertical incision and the Pezzer catheter, or small bile-duct T-tube with 1-in. limbs brought out through a separate stab incision high on the left side.

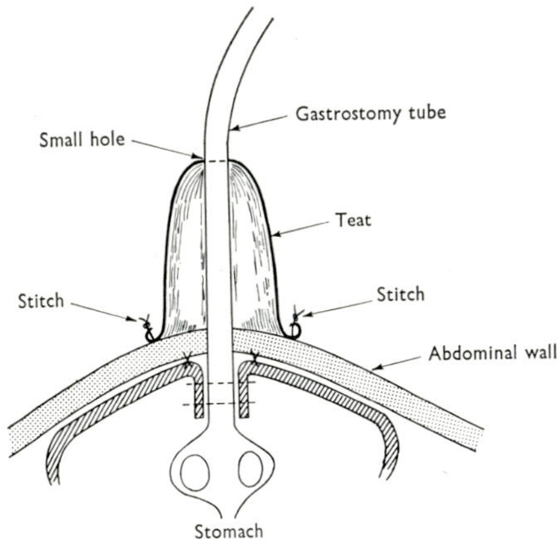

Fig. 439.—Teat used to secure a gastrostomy tube.

Mobility of the tube at the point of entry (which leads to enlargement of the hole and increasing mobility of the tube and difficulties in its retention and of leakage of feeds) is best prevented by threading on to it a teat, the base of which can then be easily affixed to the abdominal wall (*Fig.* 439). The free end should not be spigoted, but a raised reservoir will provide a small head of pressure to prevent siphoning while still allowing eructation and regurgitation of feed. If the tube does come out, another, no smaller but if anything larger, should be available for immediate reinsertion.

Congenital Intestinal Obstruction is seldom in doubt on clinical and radiological grounds (*see* p. 723) though its cause may only be revealed at laparotomy. In

23

high atresia of the duodenum anastomotic procedures are the rule, often in association with gastrostomy without or with transanastomotic intubation. The intubation may be of the 'double-lumen' type, with limbs proximal and distal to the anastomosis, thus permitting fluid returned proximally to be fed back into the distal loop; early institution of feeding is essential to the processes of rapid growth of the neonate.

Lower intestinal obstructive states, whether due to atresia or to the muco-viscoid state of meconium ileus, are probably more safely managed by some form of enterostomy, either double-barrelled or of the Bishop end-to-side variety. In this situation care of the skin against digestive excoriation, and the use of oral enzyme preparations, such as pancrex or cotazym, to aid digestion, and the use of mucolytic agents, such as acetylcystine, to liquefy residual inspissated bowel content, will be needed. As a result of infarction of the foetal bowel gross inadequacy of secretory and absorptive gut may render alimentation a very difficult problem, which even parenteral feeding with amino-acid solution and fat emulsion preparations may not help to circumvent. Aminosol-vitrum and intralipid-vitrum and plasma are all useful towards this end. The spur of a

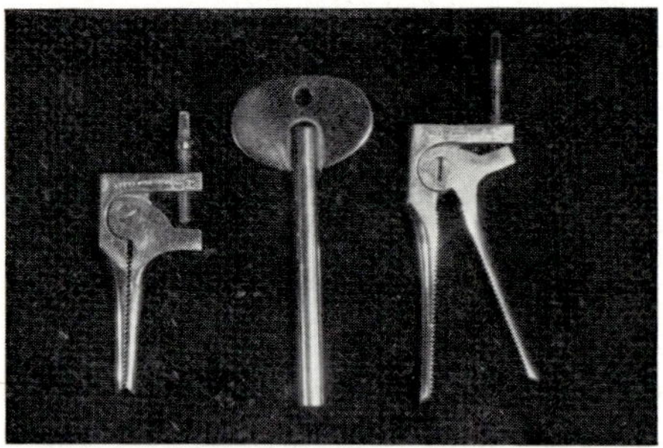

Fig. 440.—Enterotribe for crushing the spur of a double-barrelled enterostomy.

double-barrelled enterostomy should be crushed as soon as possible in order to encourage onward passage of intestinal content; special enterotribes are available for this purpose (*Fig.* 440). More formal operative closure is often required if spontaneous closure is unduly delayed.

Anorectal Atresia (Imperforate anus) and **Hirschsprung's Disease** (Congenital megacolon) may each appropriately demand colostomy, usually left iliac and preferably of a defunctioning type with a skin bridge. Loop colostomies, besides being less efficient, are accompanied in infancy by the complications of prolapse, intussusception, and bleeding. In general their care is similar to that for colostomy in the adult (p. 400), but it is wise to remember that unless made sufficiently proximal to the aganglionic segment, preferably with frozen-section control at the time of its manufacture, the colostomy may not work well. Also it is important to remember that closure of a colostomy can be associated with considerable blood-loss and transfusion facilities should be available for small children.

Congenital Hypertrophic Pyloric Stenosis.—Provided the diagnosis has been clinched by the palpation of a pyloric tumour, there is seldom any need for medical treatment of hypertrophic pyloric stenosis of infants. The adequate

Pancrex (Paines & Byrne Ltd., Pabyrn Laboratories, Greenford, Middlesex).
Cotazym (Organon Laboratories Ltd., Staines Road, Morden, Surrey).
Aminosol-Vitrum and Intralipid-Vitrum (Paines & Byrne Ltd., Pabyrn Laboratories, Greenford, Middlesex).

correction of dehydration and alkalosis, modern anæsthetic agents administered by those skilled in their application to the infant, the more effective control of infections—both respiratory and gastro-enteric—by antibiotics, and isolation facilities in cubicles, have reduced the operative mortality-rate to a very low figure. Ramstedt's operation of pyloric myotomy is decisive, and almost immediately curative.

Pre-operative Treatment.—Dehydration calls for correction by the administration of subcutaneous saline infusions, unless it is very severe, when intravenous infusion, or even blood transfusion, should be substituted. Subcutaneous infusions are given into the axillæ or interscapular areas, and it is important to direct such infusions away from the operative area, especially during the final 24–48-hour period occupied in preparing the child for operation. All established cases of pyloric stenosis have gastritis in varying degrees of severity, and in order to minimize the risk of post-operative gastro-enteritis this must be controlled as far as possible by gastric lavage. For this purpose normal saline should always be employed; sodium bicarbonate solution must be rigorously avoided, as it is prone to precipitate or exaggerate a state of alkalosis. According to the severity of the gastritis, evidenced by the amount and nature of the gastric residue obtained just prior to feeding time, lavage may be required on several occasions. It must always be performed $1\frac{1}{2}$ hours before operating, leaving the tube in situ so that the stomach can be emptied immediately before and, if necessary, during the operation. Feeds containing milk should be discontinued at least four hours before operation. Synthetic vitamin K analogue* in a dose of 1 mg. should be given intramuscularly in order to counter the hæmorrhagic tendency associated with the hypoprothrombinæmia of the starvation state. No preparation of the operative area is necessary, but umbilical infection associated with a polyp of granulation tissue should receive attention. Unless local anæsthesia alone is employed there is no necessity for the bandaging of the infant to a cruciform splint or for its fixation on a 'pyloric board'.

Pre-operative sedation is undesirable. Immediate recovery from the general anæsthetic is essential for the avoidance of the risk of asphyxia from the aspiration of vomit. Atropine 0·3 mg. may be given half an hour before operation if the anæsthetist so desires.

Post-operative Treatment.—Sedation is very seldom indicated, and antibiotics are only required for the treatment of associated or developed infection. The bowels usually function normally after the second or third day, when the infant, especially if it is being breast-fed, may often be discharged to its mother's care or, if arrangements can be made for the mother to reside in or near the hospital, she can suckle the infant until the stitches are removed on the tenth post-operative day.

Feeding.—Pædiatric units vary in the details of the schedules for the post-operative feeding of infants submitted to Ramstedt's operation. Some infants tolerate quite a rapid increase in the quality and quantity of their food; others progress more slowly. Provided the infant was prepared adequately for operation, it is seldom necessary to supplement oral feeding by parenteral infusion at this stage. (*See* Table, p. 590.)

Acute Appendicitis.—In 60 per cent of younger children under 4 years of age and 40 per cent of older children appendicitis is already complicated on admission

---

* Konakion (Roche Products Ltd., 15 Manchester Square, London, W.1).

by perforation and by some degree of peritonitis. Accordingly paralytic ileus (*see* p. 389) is frequently encountered after appendicectomy and drainage. The principles of gastro-intestinal rest and deflation by aspiration, hydration, and electrolytic control by parenteral infusion, broad-spectrum antibiotic dosage, or

SCHEDULE OF FEEDING AFTER RAMSTEDT'S OPERATION		
HOURS AFTER OPERATION	TYPE OF FEED	AMOUNT OF FEED (FL. OZ.)
2	Isotonic saline plus 10 per cent dextrose in equal parts	$\frac{1}{2}$
4	" " "	1
6	" " "	$1\frac{1}{2}$
8	" " "	$1\frac{1}{2}$
10	Normal feed, half-strength, diluted with 5 per cent dextrose	
12	Expressed milk if breast-fed	$1\frac{1}{2}$
15	" " "	2
18	" " "	2
21	" " "	2
24 hours and 3-hourly thereafter until midnight of second day	Normal feed, three-quarter strength, with 5 per cent dextrose	$2\frac{1}{2}$
		$2\frac{1}{2}$
		—
		17 (510 ml.)
		—
Third day 7 × 3-hourly feeds	Normal feeds, full strength	
Fourth day 6 × 3-hourly feeds	Return to breast if breast-fed	

specific antibiotic if bacteriologically indicated, and adequate sedation control this situation effectively. Residual abscess and mechanical adhesive intestinal obstruction can complicate and delay recovery. Further surgical intervention may be necessary more promptly than in the adult if conservative management of these complications fail. Generally drains are shortened daily and removed in 4–6 days; stitches are removed by the seventh day. Early ambulation is desirable if the clinical progress permits.

Intussusception.—Conservative reduction by barium enema (*see* p. 710) is possible when the diagnosis is made relatively early and before the appearance of blood and mucus in the bowel on rectal examination. When well established the obstructive and strangulating effects of intussusception should be fully appreciated and gastric aspiration immediately instituted and the availability of blood at operation arranged. The post-operative period after a difficult reduction may be complicated by a brisk general febrile reaction and toxæmia; generally progress is smooth and many infants may be allowed home in 2 or 3 days after feeding has been fully resumed and bowel action has returned to normal. Stitches in a paramedian wound should be removed on the tenth post-operative day.

Obstructive Urinary Conditions may, especially in baby boys, present as acute emergencies requiring urinary tract decompression by either unilateral or bilateral nephrostomy or ureterostomy. The retention of tubes and catheters in these situations sometimes tries the ingenuity of the most inventive house-surgeon. Urinary diversion is now performed more often into an ileal or colonic conduit than into the colon in continuity, but transplantation into an isolated rectum has its advocates. The care of the ileo-ureterostomy spout is similar to that for ileostomy for ulcerative colitis (*see* p. 397), but leakages and displacements of the flange are more troublesome in children. An appliance with fluid content should be applied to the abdominal wall for a day or two before operation in order to find where it adheres most securely. The site for the spout should then be indelibly marked on the skin.

Abdominal Intubation.—There are a number of procedures both in the alimentary tract and in the genito-urinary system which require intubation for a variable period of time—gastrostomy, enterostomy, nephrostomy, urethrostomy, tracheostomy, etc. Each of these procedures has its own special points in management, but all have one basic characteristic—if they are to be satisfactorily maintained any dislodgement or dysfunction must be immediately remedied by correct replacement. Delay in reinsertion of the tube may precipitate the creation of a false passage or lead to failure to re-establish the former one.

BILIARY AND PANCREATIC CONDITIONS MET WITH DURING INFANCY

Investigation of Neonatal Jaundice.—The persistence of jaundice, especially when it has appeared after the first few days of life, soon raises the question of cause and the possibility of its remedy by surgical means. Congenital atresia of the bile-ducts and choledochus cyst of the common bile-duct are two conditions that may be amenable to surgical correction, the former, however, at the best in only about 20 per cent of cases.

Erythroblastosis Fœtalis.—Especially amongst the causes of neonatal jaundice which must be eliminated is erythroblastosis fœtalis. Rh-factor and blood-group incompatibility of the parents and thereby of the baby and its mother in whom antibodies develop is shown by blood-group testing and the Coombs test. The maternal history of more than one pregnancy or of previous blood transfusion is obtained. Jaundice in a neonate suffering from erythroblastosis fœtalis develops and deepens and the serum-bilirubin concentration rises very rapidly. The stools become acholic only in the presence of blockage of the biliary ducts by the inspissation of bile. Urobilinogen is present in the urine. Nucleated red blood-cells and reticulocytes may be found in the peripheral blood.

Other Causes of Jaundice requiring elimination are bacterial sepsis, spirochætal infections of congenital syphilis or leptospirosis, viral infections causing hepatitis and cytomegalic inclusion disease, and the protozoal infection of toxoplasmosis. Metabolic causes of jaundice are found in galactosæmia and with the immaturity of the liver cells which may cause the fleeting physiological jaundice of the first few days of life or the more persistent type of 'familial non-hæmolytic jaundice'. Other and rare forms of hæmolytic anæmia may require to be excluded. For these and the other foregoing conditions reference to text-books of pædiatric medicine will detail the specific investigations that should be performed.

For Treatment of Erythroblastosis Fœtalis by Exchange Transfusions, see p. 581.

Congenital Atresia of the Bile-ducts.—In this condition regurgitation of bile into the blood-stream is unremitting. The depth of clinical jaundice and the bilirubin content of the serum increase gradually and constantly, the initial yellow colour of the skin changing to a greenish bronze as bilirubin oxidizes to biliverdin in the tissues. The stools are colourless until the deepening jaundice may tinge their surface from the desquamation of yellow-tinted mucous membrane cells and the yellowness of the mucus secreted by them. The urine is dark and contains bile-salts, but no urobilinogen. The van den Bergh reaction gives the 'direct' response and the alkaline phosphatase level of the blood is raised. Bile is absent from specimens obtained by duodenal intubation both before and after the use of

25 per cent magnesium sulphate and other cholagogues. With the passage of time (and consequent advancing liver damage) definite findings become increasingly obscured. The specific tests of liver damage—the thymol turbidity test, the cephalin-cholesterol flocculation test, and increases of serum glutamic oxalo-acetic transaminase (SGOT) and serum glutamic pyruvic transaminase (SGPT) (in order of increasing sensitivity)—will render positive results which complicate the diagnosis.

When congenital atresia of the bile-ducts is strongly suspected, even although some of the signs and specific tests are equivocal, at the age of 4 to 6 weeks a limited laparotomy of the upper right abdomen is indicated. Polythene-tubing catheterization of the collapsed gall-bladder is performed, the organ often being hidden in a deep cleft of the enlarged liver. After irrigating the bile-ducts with normal saline solution injected through the tubing, 10 ml. of 30 per cent diodrast is injected through the tubing and per-operative cholangiography is carried out. A biopsy specimen from the edge of the liver is taken, also. When a normal cholangiograph is not obtained the laparotomy wound should be extended so that the actual state of the biliary ductal system can be ascertained. By this procedure inspissation of bile within the ducts may be observed and cleared; usually such inspissation is a complication of jaundice resulting from erythroblastosis foetalis (hæmolytic disease of the newborn) or viral hepatitis Type B.

Choledochus Cyst causes jaundice of the regurgitation type, but some inter-mittency of the obstruction is not unusual. Infection of the biliary tract is liable to occur with pain and fever, and the cyst, which usually is large before symptoms and signs develop, will be palpable below the liver. The child is usually of the female sex. The indications for surgical exploration of the abdomen are obvious.

Mucoviscidosis is a congenital abnormality affecting mucus-secreting glands of the alimentary and respiratory tracts. Inspissation of the secretions of these glands causes secondary dilatation of the ducts and acini of exocrine glands, and ultimately fibrosis and increased ductal and acinar obstruction, especially evident in the pancreas. Secondary changes are also produced by the retention of secre-tions within the mucous membrane linings of the greater part of the alimentary tract, the gall-bladder, and the trachea and bronchi. In addition, the salivary glands are involved and the sweat-glands produce an abnormal secretion. These changes, and especially those in the pancreas, cause at the least impaired intestinal digestion of the cœliac type; at the most (fortunately not common) the state of neonatal intestinal obstruction known as meconium ileus results. The pathologi-cal condition of the respiratory tract permits frequent staphylococcal infections of the lungs, and these are particularly damaging to these tissues of the baby, with the production of patches of bronchopneumonia, abscess formation, and pleural infections, not infrequently complicated by pneumothorax, which may be of the tension type. The condition is genetically determined in a recessive manner and once the disease, in one or other of its forms, has become manifest in a family it is probable that many of the offspring will be affected similarly.

Surgical interest focuses especially upon the obstructive condition of meconium ileus and upon the complications of pulmonary infection.

Meconium Ileus.—The diagnosis of meconium ileus rests upon obtaining a familial history of significance in the case of a neonate exhibiting acute intestinal obstructive manifestations with a considerable degree of abdominal distension. On percussing the abdomen, areas of tympany and others of dullness are found; there is also a 'doughy' sensation on palpation. These findings are reflected in the radiological picture (*see* p. 724) of considerable jejunal distension and a mottled 'ground glass' opacity of the lower abdominal field. Areas of calcification sometimes accompany these appearances and indicate the previous occurrence of a fœtal peritonitis resulting from the rupture of a dilated jejunal loop. In these urgent circumstances there is no place for proof of the suspected condition by laboratory investigation. The great difficulties of the relief and cure by operation of this type of obstruction will not be discussed here.

Investigation of a Case of Suspected Fibrocystic Disease of the Pancreas.—In the infrequent event of recovery from meconium ileus, and in other infants less seriously afflicted in whom chronic intestinal indigestion develops with recurrent staphylococcal pulmonary infections, proof of the existence of fibrocystic disease of the pancreas and of mucoviscidosis can be obtained by the following investigations:—

1. *Examination of the Duodenal Juice.*—The passage of a tube into the duodenum requires the use of a radio-opaque tube and radiological verification that the tip of the tube is within the duodenum before aspiration of a specimen is performed; alkalinity and a yellow colour characterize satisfactory siting of the tube. The aspirated fluid is likely to be small in amount and viscid; enzymatic evaluations show reduced activity, but usually it is the tryptic activity alone that is estimated. Hormonal stimulation by the injection of secretin does not produce any increase in enzymatic activity. Little reliance should be placed upon the estimation of the tryptic activity of the stools, although this test may be used to reinforce suspicions prior to more detailed investigation.

2. *Estimation of the Sodium Chloride Content of the Sweat—'Sweat Test'.*—In mucoviscidosis the sweat is found to contain a considerably increased concentration of sodium and chloride. Sweat can be collected by securing to the lumbar region a well-washed, dried, and weighed cotton swab, covered by a piece of plastic sheeting and held in place by waterproof adhesive strapping. The swab is kept in place for 4 to 6 hours, if possible. It is then removed and reweighed immediately. A biochemical estimation of the sodium and chloride content is then carried out, the normal value for each factor being approximately 21·5 mEq. per ml. These values may be quadrupled in mucoviscidosis, but even double values are strong evidence of the disease. The method of obtaining a specimen by enveloping the child's body in a large plastic bag is fraught with danger, as 'heat stroke' and exhaustion may supervene, and fatalities have occurred during the performance of the test carried out in this manner. Iontophoresis with pilocarpine is being developed as a safe method of stimulating the secretion of sweat in a limited area of the body surface, but this method necessitates the use of special apparatus.

CHAPTER XLI

EMERGENCY DENTAL TREATMENT

By H. S. M. CRABB

THE main reasons for which persons seek emergency dental treatment are **pain,** either on its own as 'toothache' or associated with swelling or ulceration, **hæmorrhage,** and **traumatic injuries** of the teeth or jaws.

A brief description of the anatomy of dental structures (*Fig.* 441) is relevant to the problems of diagnosis and treatment. The main mass of a tooth consists of *dentine*, which has a similar consistency to bone. The crown of the tooth is covered with enamel, a hard insensitive substance almost entirely inorganic in composition. In the centre of the tooth, the *pulp*, a vascular tissue well supplied with nerve-fibres, sends cellular prolongations into the dentine and contributes to the sensitivity of that tissue. The root dentine is covered with a thin layer of *cementum* in which are embedded the *periodontal fibres* which suspend the tooth in a sling from the surrounding *alveolar bone*. (This bone constitutes the wall of the socket which remains for some time after a tooth is extracted.) The alveolar bone is covered by *gingival tissue* or *gum*.

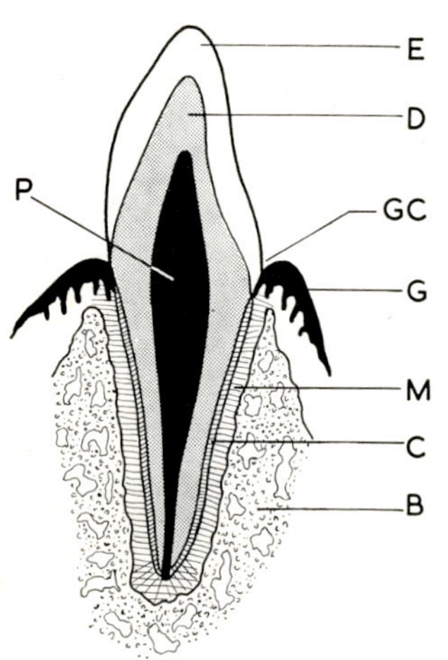

Fig. 441. — Longitudinal section of tooth in situ. E, Enamel; D, dentine; G, gingiva; GC, gingival crevice; M, periodontal membrane; C, cementum; B, alveolar bone; P, Pulp.

THE ORIGINS OF DENTAL PAIN

Because the pulp is a tissue confined within a hard-walled chamber it is evident that any inflammatory reaction to injury of this tissue cannot produce the swelling usually associated with inflammatory reaction in soft tissues. Instead, pressure within the virtually closed pulp chamber rises with resulting spasms of pain with every pulsation of the circulation. The commonest cause of such an inflammatory reaction (pulpitis) is dental caries, which progresses from the enamel through the dentine to reach the pulp.

Dental Caries starts as a limited breakdown of the enamel, no obvious cavity being apparent on visual examination. As the lesion progresses the enamel is undermined and breaks down, exposing the carious dentine. Limited sensitivity of the tooth at this stage may be treated by breaking away weak enamel with a fine chisel to expose the softened carious dentine and excavating this soft material. After washing away debris with warm saline the cavity may be dressed with a stiff paste of zinc oxide and oil of cloves. Severe and continued pain usually requires treatment by extraction unless specialized dental advice is available.

In the early stages of pulpitis the patient experiences momentary pain following cold and hot drinks or the eating of sweet substances. Later, there are bouts of stabbing pain for several minutes. Ultimately, the pain comes on spontaneously and continues for increasingly longer periods, which drives the patient to seek relief. This is **toothache of pulpal type.**

Table XV.—DIFFERENTIATION BETWEEN PULPAL AND PERIODONTAL PAIN

CHARACTERISTIC	PULPAL PAIN	PERIODONTAL PAIN
History	Usually history of past 'twinges' of pain of increasing duration	May be a history of bout of sharp pain or occasional dull pain
Type	Stabbing	Dull ache
Duration	A few minutes to half an hour	Several hours or more
Intermittency	Occasional attack increasing in frequency	Continuous
Distribution	Frequently referred to other teeth or structures along pathway of 5th nerve, particularly the same division	Usually localized, may be referred to tissue areas in proximity
Severity	Will drive patient to seek relief, but pain may suddenly have stopped	Will drive patient to seek relief as pain steadily increases
Aetiology	Usually the result of dental caries. Can result from recurrent caries or pulp pathology under existing restoration of tooth. Can result from a blow on a tooth (not necessarily recent) which may otherwise appear sound	Usually the terminal result of pulp necrosis. Can result from any damage to periodontal tissues such as trauma or foreign body forced into periodontal tissues (giving localized soft-tissue abscess in gingivae)
Special problems	Pain may be difficult to localize if referred from one jaw to the other. Block anæsthesia to eliminate pain may assist diagnosis. The application of cold, using a cotton-wool pledget sprayed with ethyl chloride, may provoke a response in the affected tooth	With a periapical abscess local infiltration of anæsthetic is unwise and anæsthesia may be poor. Block anæsthesia is preferable. An abscess may sometimes be swiftly incised under local application of ethyl chloride spray

As the pressure in the pulp chamber rises with the inflammatory response the venous return is obstructed and necrosis of the pulp supervenes, with the relief of the pain. From this point onwards progress depends upon the virulence of the invading organisms and the resistance of the patient. The whole situation may remain in balance for years and give rise to no symptoms. At any time there may be acute abscess formation in the periodontal tissues beyond the root apex. The tooth then becomes tender to bite on or to touch and, as the acute reaction increases, the patient becomes affected with continuous pain which is made excruciating by touching the tooth. This is **toothache of periodontal type.** The abscess may then extend through the bone in one of several directions, following the lines of least resistance to the soft tissues and giving rise to the classic swollen face associated with the dental abscess.

It is important to recognize that limited pulpal pain may arise from any irritant to the pulp, such as cold drinks, which can produce momentary pain in open tooth cavities or by seepage around old broken-down restorations. Recession of the gum at the neck of a tooth may also be associated with momentary pain from cold stimuli or from sweet drinks and foods, and the exposed neck of the tooth may be sensitive to touch. Also, 'periodontal pain' may not necessarily be associated with a tooth abscess but can arise from any form of injury to the periodontal tissues and investing bone. Pain of dental origin may also be associated with infected buried roots of teeth, cysts, or unerupted teeth. Radiographic examination may be necessary to exclude these.

The significant features of pulpal and periodontal pain are summarized in *Table XV*.

Differential Diagnosis.—Pain in the face and jaws is not necessarily of dental origin. It is therefore important to consider pain of non-dental origin. For example, tenderness to percussion and a continuous dull pain in a number of premolar and molar teeth of the upper jaw should arouse suspicion of a maxillary sinusitis which may be totally without dental origin and for which dental extractions would be futile.

NEURALGIAS

Primary neuralgias, such as trigeminal neuralgia, may be eliminated inasmuch as the pain is distinctive: the pain is stabbing and excruciating, of short duration with complete remission between spasms, always follows the same pathways at the same tempo, and has a refractory period. Trigger zones may be identified. In mandibular neuralgias there is usually accompanying pain in the tongue.

In patients complaining of pain radiating over the face from the temporal region, associated with the pain or clicking in the temporomandibular joint or limitation of joint movement, joint dysfunction may be related to abnormal tooth relationships; treatment by bite equilibration may be of value and dental advice should be sought.

PERICORONITIS

Localized inflammation of the soft tissues surrounding an erupting tooth, particularly a lower third molar, may give rise to considerable pain and be associated with ulceration of the gum around the erupting tooth, secondary infection, and difficulty in opening the mouth. Frequently the upper third molar may be biting the gum tissue overlying the erupting lower third molar. In such cases removal of the upper third molar and irrigation of the soft-tissue flap around the lower erupting tooth with hypertonic saline may afford temporary relief. Local application of trichloracetic acid using dressing tweezers beneath the gum pocket around the erupting tooth, immediately followed by glycerin, gives some relief from pain and may be repeated daily for a few days. In swelling around the lower third molar region care must be taken to exclude abscess formation and spread of infection arising from any of the lower molars. With spreading infection and pyrexia systemic antibiotics should be administered.

DENTAL ABSCESS

As a general rule extraction of the tooth involved in a dental abscess is desirable, in order to remove the cause of the condition and if possible to effect drainage of pus. Where dental attention is available, pus may sometimes be drained by opening into the pulp chamber of the tooth and it may not be necessary then to remove the tooth which can afterwards be treated. Sometimes extraction may not immediately be possible or drainage may not follow extraction. Where an abscess is present as a swelling in the mouth, incision will usually effect drainage of pus and give relief. The fluctuant subperiosteal abscess may be incised (*Fig.* 442) after local application of an ethyl chloride spray or a general anæsthetic. Local infiltration anæsthesia is contra-indicated. When an abscess presents as a fluctuant swelling in the soft tissues of the face there is a risk of damage to the facial nerve in incising the cheek tissues. It is better for the inexperienced operator to wait until the abscess is almost pointing through the skin before incising. With intra-oral or extra-oral swelling, with or without incision, systemic antibiotic therapy should be administered if drainage is not obtained. Systemic antibiotic therapy may be of value when extraction or incision is not possible and in such cases should be given prophylactically.

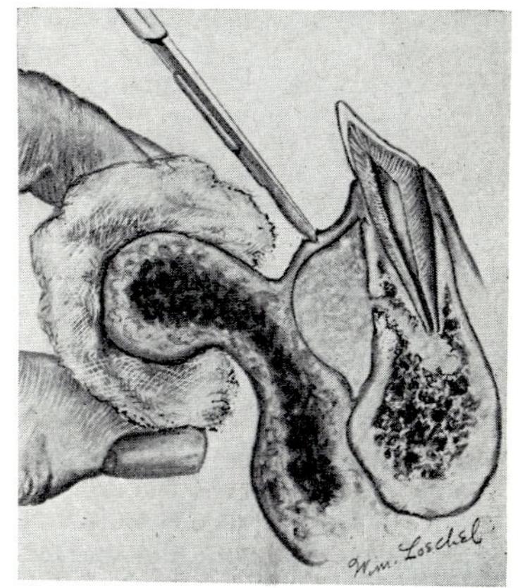

Fig. 442.—Method of incising a dento-alveolar abscess.

GINGIVAL ULCERATION

Inflammation of the gingivæ may arise from local irritation or be superimposed on an underlying systemic disorder. Apart from swollen and bleeding gums associated with endocrine changes, which may arise in pregnancy, and the gingival detachment and bleeding which in elderly persons on a poor diet may be symptomatic of ascorbic-acid deficiency, the principal condition for which relief is likely to be sought is ulceropseudomembranous gingivitis (Vincent's infection). The classic features of this condition are gums which bleed readily on slight trauma such as toothbrushing, a complaint of soreness, ulceration of the crest of the gums between the teeth at various points, and a characteristic foul halitosis. The ulcers may be covered with a greyish pseudomembrane, removal of which discloses a raw bleeding surface. There may be associated lymph-gland enlargement and pyrexia. Microscopical examination of smears taken from the ulcers reveals large numbers of *Borrelia vincenti* and *Fusobacterium plauti-vincenti*.

Treatment.—For local treatment the gums may be swabbed with cotton-wool soaked in hydrogen peroxide 10 v/v and the mouth should be cleaned of debris and dental scaling of calculus deposits undertaken as soon as possible. A single application of a 15 per cent solution of chromic acid to the interdental ulcerated areas, followed by a 2 per cent hydrogen peroxide mouthwash, will help to reduce discomfort. The chromic acid should be applied with care to the interdental spaces and gingival crevice, using dressing forceps. Chromic acid application to the gingivæ should not be repeated because of risk of damage to healthy tissue. The patient's toothbrush should be destroyed and the patient urged to use a mouthwash vigorously—hot saline (a teaspoon of salt to a tablespoon of water) three to four times a day, after meals, and last thing at night, is appropriate. Smoking should be discouraged. Systemic treatment, advisable where there is general malaise, lymph-gland enlargement, or pyrexia, is as follows: penicillin, preferably by the intramuscular route, is given as 2 ml. procaine penicillin, fortified, or 200,000 units benzyl penicillin with 600,000 units procaine penicillin daily for 3 to 5 days. Alternatively, oral administration of phenoxymethyl penicillin V may be used, the dosage being 1 tablet of 250 mg. four times a day, half an hour before meals, for 5 days. Treatment with metronidazole, 200 mg., three times a day for 7 days, is extremely effective, but should not be given in pregnancy or to nursing mothers. Prolonged dosage in males may also affect spermatogenesis. Systemic antibiotic therapy or treatment with metronidazole should give considerable improvement within 48 hours. Failing such improvement the diagnosis should be suspected. Non-specific gingivitis, herpetic gingivitis, or erythema multiforme may have to be considered. Care must be taken to exclude blood dyscrasias to which gingival ulceration may be a manifestation of secondary infection; this possibility should always be considered where there is history of malaise, lassitude, and headaches.

Tooth extraction should not be performed in the presence of acute Vincent's infection because of the risk of a rapidly spreading soft-tissue involvement.

Recurrence of Vincent's infection is likely if there is any source of bacterial stagnation throughout the mouth, and early dental treatment should be sought to deal with potential sites of stagnation.

Some patients may ask advice on account of ulceration beneath a denture. They should be advised to leave the dentures out for one week and should be referred for dental advice. Persistent ulcerative lesions in relation to dentures should arouse suspicion of neoplasia.

LOCAL ANÆSTHESIA

Provided there is no general medical contra-indication to the use of adrenaline, the use of standard local anæsthetic cartridges containing one of the synthetic materials, such as lignocaine hydrochloride 2 per cent with adrenaline 1–80,000, is appropriate for both local infiltration and block anæsthesia for dental purposes. Initial discomfort can be much reduced by the use of a surface anæsthetic on the mucous membrane of the site of injection and by using the anæsthetic at blood temperature.

Anæsthesia for dental extraction may be achieved by infiltration of 1 ml. of solution into the soft tissues, stretched tightly to facilitate easy penetration, over the apex of the tooth concerned on its buccal and also in its palatal or lingual aspect. This is particularly so in children and young adults where the surrounding bone is not dense. For molar teeth, however, a block anæsthetic is usually indicated. General anæsthesia can be used if an anæsthetist is available and special care must be taken to pack off the throat during the extraction, as well as taking the usual anæsthetic precautions.

For Extraction of Lower Teeth, all of the lower teeth on one side of the jaw can be anæsthetized with the *inferior dental block* injection which will provide anæsthesia of the teeth and supporting bone, while the buccal soft tissues need a separate local infiltration or, in the case of lower molars, an infiltration around the long buccal nerve. The lingual tissues are dealt with by anæsthesia of the lingual nerve.

Technique.—A long needle (42 mm.) is used. With the patient's mouth wide open, place the forefinger on the triangle of soft tissue immediately behind the last molar tooth (*Fig.* 443); the finger should be placed so that its upper border is

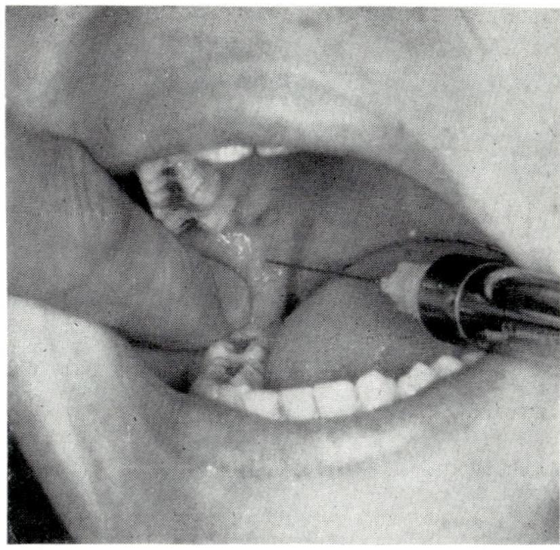

Fig. 443.—Photograph showing technique for inferior dental block injection for right side. Note that the barrel of the syringe rests over the premolar/molar region of the left side. (For injection of the left side the operator stands behind the patient so that his left arm is around the head giving support, with the index finger placed in the retromolar region as for the right side.)

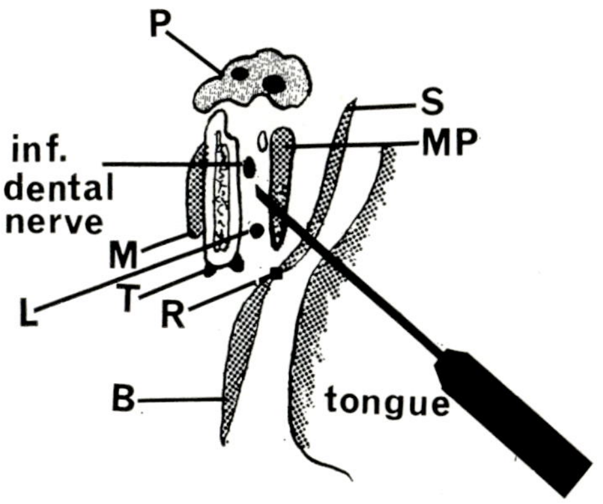

Fig. 444.—Diagram of oblique section illustrating relationship of needle and syringe in an inferior dental block injection (direct technique). B, Buccinator muscle; MP, medial pterygoid muscle; S, superior constrictor muscle; T, insertions of temporal muscle; M, masseter muscle; R, pterygomandibular raphe; L, lingual nerve; P, parotid gland.

in line with the occlusal surface of the lower teeth. The mucous membrane over the site of injection is dried and cleaned with alcohol on cotton-wool and the point of the needle inserted into the mucous membrane just over 1 cm. behind the finger-nail and level with it. The barrel of the syringe should lie over the pre-molar teeth of the opposite side. After depositing a few drops of anæsthetic solution submucously, the needle is then advanced through the tissues, piercing the medial pterygoid muscle (*Fig.* 444), until bone is felt. The anæsthetic solution is then deposited above the inferior dental nerve as it enters the canal on the internal surface of the ramus of the mandible. If the mouth is kept wide open, then the 'S' shape of the inferior dental nerve is straightened out and it lies in close approximation to the medial surface of the ramus. As the needle is withdrawn some anæsthetic solution is injected so as to be deposited around the lingual nerve (*Fig.* 444). (Dental textbooks describe also an indirect technique of injection which avoids the pterygoid muscle, but the direct approach described here is the simplest and most straightforward method.) Immediately after injection or within 10 minutes the patient should experience tingling and numbness of the lower lip and, as the more central nerve-fibres are reached, the teeth will begin to feel 'wooden' to the patient. The long buccal nerve is anæsthetized by depositing 0·5 ml. of anæsthetic solution in the tissues of the buccal sulcus alongside but slightly above the last lower molar tooth.

Anæsthesia is tested before extraction by pushing a blunt probe down the gingival crevice alongside the root of the tooth on both buccal and lingual sides.

For Extraction of Upper Teeth infiltration anæsthesia buccally and palatally can be used. For molar teeth the *posterior superior dental* block may be necessary. The aim of this injection is to reach the posterior superior dental branch

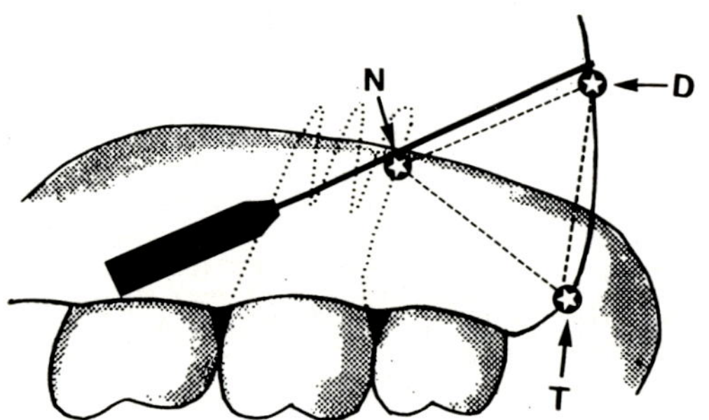

Fig. 445.—Diagram illustrating relationships in posterior superior dental block injection. N, Point of insertion of needle in buccal sulcus; T, corner of tuberosity; D, point to be reached on posterior surface of maxilla. ND = DT = NT. Needle must be passed close to bone *upwards*, *backwards*, and *inwards*.

of the second division of the 5th nerve where it enters the posterior surface of the maxilla. The point of injection is the reflection of the buccal mucosa above the distal part of the second upper molar tooth (or first molar if no third molar is present). A long needle (42 mm.) is used and it is directed upwards, backwards, and inwards for approximately half of its length and the anæsthetic solution deposited. Care must be taken to keep the needle in close proximity to the maxilla to avoid damaging the pterygoid venous plexus (a large hæmatoma may otherwise result; for this reason scrupulous care in the drying and cleansing of the injection site is necessary to avoid the risk of a possible hæmatoma becoming infected). It is worth remembering that the point of insertion of the needle, the back of the tuberosity, and the point to be reached approximately form an equilateral triangle (*Fig.* 445). This injection will anæsthetize the upper second and third molars and part of the first molar, an additional infiltration being needed over the anterior root of the first molar. Infiltration of anæsthetic into the palatal mucosa is necessary for extraction and for molar and premolar teeth can be given with least discomfort by injecting into the soft tissue over-lying the anterior palatine foramen.

THE EXTRACTION OF TEETH

The basis of successful extraction procedures lies in the recognition of the fact that the removal of a tooth is not achieved by the simple use of force and that its effectiveness is conditioned by:—
1. The root anatomy of the tooth concerned.
2. The nature of the bony architecture surrounding the tooth.
3. The direction in which the force is applied.

As the principal aim is to dilate the socket of the tooth to enable the tooth to be freely removed, a gentle easing and rocking movement is generally used,

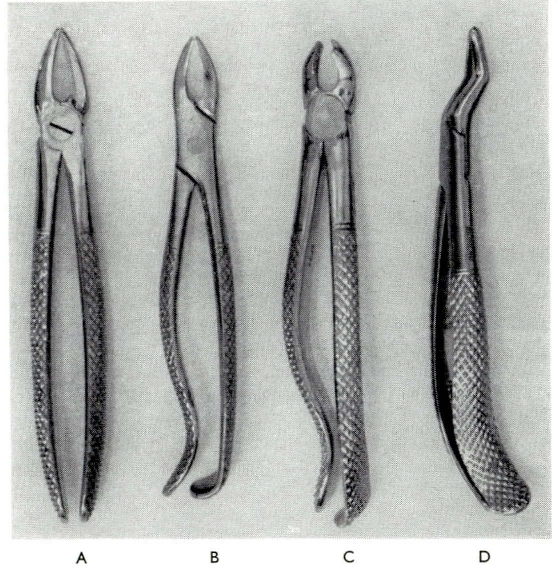

A   B   C   D

Fig. 446.—Dental forceps for upper teeth. A, Straight forceps; B, curved forceps for premolar teeth; C, molar forceps (left side illustrated here); D, bayonet forceps, the angulation of which assists access, particularly with some upper third molars.

with certain reservations. Bulbous or excessively curved roots or dense sur-rounding bone may lead to breakage of the crown of the tooth; without pre-operative radiographs this eventuality cannot always be foreseen. Simple extractions may be achieved by the use of dental forceps. For single-rooted

upper anterior teeth a pair of straight forceps (*Fig.* 446) is employed, and for
upper premolars a pair of forceps with curved blades and with curved handles
(*Fig.* 446), designed to give clearance of the lower lip, are used. For lower
incisors, canines, and premolars lower-root forceps (*Fig.* 447) are used, these
having blades at right angles to the handles. For upper molars, beaked forceps
(*Fig.* 446) to accommodate the root anatomy are employed and are designed for

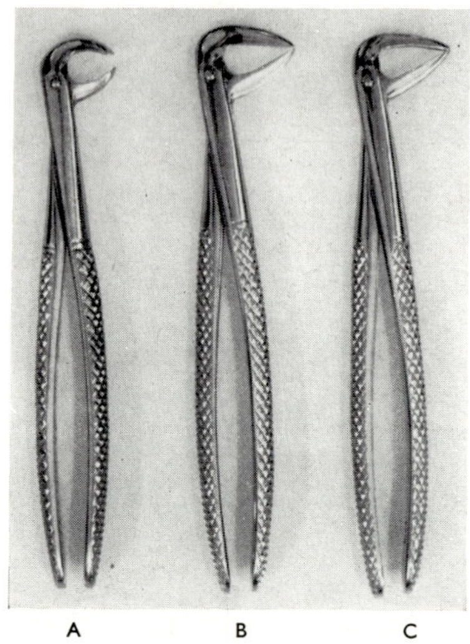

Fig. 447.—Dental forceps for lower teeth. A, Full molar forceps; B, root forceps; C, fine
root forceps, suitable for lower incisors and small roots.

right and left sides separately. For lower molars, beaked forceps with blades at
right angles to the handles (*Fig.* 447) are used.

For the right-handed operator, the lower teeth on the patient's right side are
extracted standing behind the patient. All other teeth are extracted standing
in front of the patient.

If forceps are placed haphazardly over the tooth the soft tissues are easily
damaged and the crown of the tooth may break off. The forceps *must* be applied
so that the blades slide along the side of the root surface and are pushed up as far
as they will go, thus dilating the surrounding alveolar bone and displacing the
soft tissues.

While the forceps are held in the right hand, the left hand should be placed
(*Fig.* 448) so that:—

1. The lips or cheek are not crushed against other teeth by the handles of
the forceps.

2. Movements of the investing bone are appreciated by the fingers.

3. In the case of lower teeth the jaw is supported.

4. The fingers are ready to compress the dilated walls of the socket immediately after extraction, a manœuvre designed to aid repair and reduce post-
operative discomfort.

When extracting upper teeth the patient's head should be supported by an assistant standing behind the patient.

After forcing the blades of the forceps well up the root, the tooth is gripped firmly and gently eased to and fro in a buccal–lingual direction, moving from buccal to lingual in the first movement. This procedure should not be carried

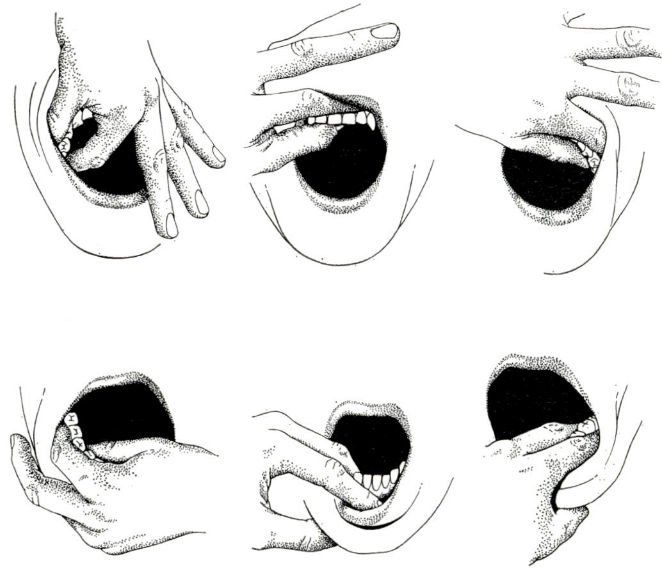

Fig. 448.—Diagram illustrating use of left hand for support and control during extraction procedures for various teeth.

out with jerky elbow or wrist movements, but by means of a 'persuasive movement' obtained from the movement of the whole of the upper part of the body of the operator. Care should be taken not to force each movement beyond a safe limit and the feeling transmitted to the hand holding the forceps and the fingers of the other hand will indicate when there is a sense of 'give'. As the lateral movements of the tooth are increased and the tooth begins to lift, slight rotation or figure-of-eight movements of the forceps may then assist the removal of the tooth. *Tables XVI* and *XVII* indicate the common variations in root anatomy which may be met and show how such variations may affect the permissible type of movement in extraction. Also tabulated are the type of forceps appropriate to the various teeth and some notes on possible hazards.

DECIDUOUS TEETH

The main point to remember in extracting deciduous teeth in children is that there is risk of damage to underlying developing permanent teeth if the extraction is too vigorous. The molar roots are well spread out and the developing permanent tooth lies beneath and between these.

Table XVI.—Common Variations in Root Anatomy of Upper Teeth

Tooth	Shape	Forceps	Notes
Central incisors	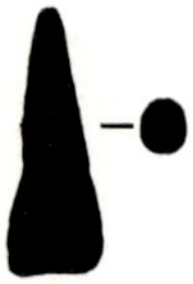	Straight	Have conical roots—usually easy to rotate, but roots can be triangular in section
Lateral incisors	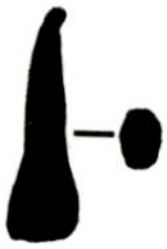	Straight	Roots flattened side to side and thin. Forceps must be well up the root. The root will break easily on sudden movement or rotation
Canine	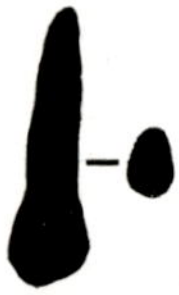	Straight	Root triangular in cross-section. This tooth is long-rooted—get forceps well up the root. Part of buccal bony plate often comes away on extraction, but healing is usually unaffected by this if rough bone edges are trimmed off
First premolar	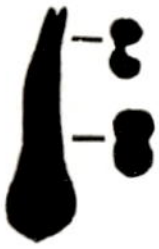	Premolar forceps, curved handles	This tooth has two divergent roots, sometimes curved, and fracture of buccal root often occurs during extraction. Movements should be primarily to the buccal side to ensure getting out the palatal root (buccal root can be dissected out later if need be). Once the tooth starts to 'give', pull downwards
Second premolar	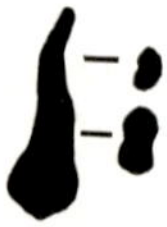	Premolar forceps, curved handles	Usually single rooted. No particular hazard unless the tooth has erupted in abnormal position

Table XVI.—Continued

TOOTH	SHAPE	FORCEPS	NOTES
First molar		Full molar upper forceps for right or left side as indicated	This tooth has three roots, well splayed out. One or more of these roots is easily broken if the extraction is hurried
Second molar		Full molar upper forceps for right or left side as indicated. Bayonet forceps may sometimes be used	This tooth is also three-rooted. The roots are not usually as splayed out as the first molars and the root mass may be at an angle to the crown
Third molar		Full molar or pre-molar forceps, depending on crown shape and angulation. Bayonet forceps may sometimes be used	This tooth is usually easily extracted although access may be difficult with the mouth wide open as the coronoid interferes. Get patient to half-close the mouth and to deviate the lower jaw to the same side

Note: The silhouettes of tooth shapes are intended to show the approximate shape of the roots and not relative sizes of teeth.

POST-OPERATIVE CARE

Once the tooth has been removed and the bony walls of the socket compressed between the fingers and thumb, the patient is permitted to wash out the mouth with a warm mouthwash, such as hypertonic saline or other bland solution. Then the patient is given a gauze pack and asked to bite on this for 10 minutes, after which a firm blood-clot should be present in the socket and bleeding from the socket should have been controlled. The pack must be placed so that the soft tissues surrounding the socket are compressed against the bony wall and are not pushed outwards. Persistent hæmorrhage is dealt with as described below.

The patient should be given suitable analgesic tablets to control post-operative pain. (Tab. Codeine Co. B.P., 2 tablets 4-hourly for the first day or two as required, is usually all that is needed.) Instructions should be given on the need to avoid violent exercise, alcohol, or hot food and drinks and excessive rinsing for the next 24 hours, to reduce the risk of bleeding.

Table XVII.—COMMON VARIATIONS IN ROOT ANATOMY OF LOWER TEETH

TOOTH	SHAPE	FORCEPS	NOTES
Central incisor		Lower root forceps	These teeth have very fine roots flattened from side to side and fracture easily on rapid movement. In older people, particularly, the roots may be brittle
Lateral incisor		Lower root forceps	
Canine		Lower root forceps	This is a fairly long-rooted tooth in which the root runs in a slightly posterior direction. Care must be taken to apply the forceps in line with the axis of the root and well up the root
First premolar		Lower root forceps	The root may taper and curve backwards and the root cross-section be triangular and therefore the tooth should not be rotated. Bone is often dense in this region
Second premolar		Lower root forceps	The investing bone is often dense. This tooth can be rotated, but if there is no 'give' do not force this movement but use a buccal-lingual movement, as the root may be triangular in cross-section, leading to root fracture

Table XVII.—Continued

TOOTH	SHAPE	FORCEPS	NOTES
First molar		Lower full molar forceps	There are usually two divergent roots situated mesially and distally, and flattened in a bucco-lingual direction. These teeth will usually yield to a bucco-lingual movement. The forceps must be well down the root or the crown will be crushed and broken, leaving root fragments behind which are difficult to remove
Second molar		Lower full molar forceps	
Third molar		Lower full molar forceps	The pattern of root formation of these teeth is variable. These teeth may sometimes be easily removed or may be quite impossible to remove without a planned surgical approach. In an attempted emergency extraction do not pursue forceful removal if there is no 'give', or fracture of the jaw may result

The patient should be advised that if bleeding should occur this may be controlled by biting firmly on a gauze pack (or a clean folded handkerchief) placed over the socket for 15 minutes. If bleeding persists then the patient should return for treatment. At bedtime the mouth may be cleaned with a mouthwash of warm salt water (1 teaspoonful of salt to a tumbler of water) and for 3 days thereafter the mouth should be rinsed after meals and last thing at night with a fairly hot salt mouthwash.

SOME COMMON COMPLICATIONS OF EXTRACTIONS

1. Fracture of the Tooth.—This may either be the result of a hurried extraction and improperly applied forceps, or result from unyielding dense bone and an unfavourably placed root mass. In the event of a small piece of root being left behind this may be left alone and the situation reviewed after the socket has healed. If, however, the crown breaks off, leaving the main root mass behind, this usually needs to be removed surgically, although sometimes individual roots may be grasped with root forceps and removed. No reference is made here to the accessory use of elevators and bone chisels, etc., the use of which should not be attempted by inexperienced operators. For the inexperienced operator under emergency circumstances treatment is then directed at preventing the pain which will ensue if the tooth pulp has been exposed in the remaining root mass. If so, the pulp should be cauterized, while the tooth is still anæsthetized, with a hot instrument. Calcium hydroxide paste can then be applied to the exposed pulp surface and the root mass covered with a stiff zinc-oxide–eugenol paste. The patient should be referred to a dental surgeon as soon as possible.

2. Fracture of the Alveolar Bone is a relatively common feature of extractions. If a piece of bone is fractured and lies only partly attached, it should be dissected out and removed. All loose bone fragments should be removed. In the extraction of upper second and third molars the maxillary tuberosity may fracture. This is particularly prone to occur with single-standing molars in old persons where the antrum has expanded and weakened the surrounding bone. During the molar extraction the bony tuberosity may be felt to 'give' as the tooth is moved. In this event it is better to postpone the extraction and have the matter dealt with surgically at a later date. If the extraction has already reached the stage where the tuberosity has partly torn away from the investing tissues, the bone segment and the tooth must be carefully dissected out from the soft tissue. The soft tissue must then be closely apposed and sutured at once, and the patient referred for specialist treatment in view of the risk of an oro-antral fistula. There is a risk of severe hæmorrhage with tuberosity fracture because of the close proximity of the large vessels of the infratemporal fossa. Bleeding may be difficult to control and it may be necessary to resort to packing with gauze soaked in Whitehead's varnish to control the hæmorrhage.

3. Fracture of the Mandible may occur during extraction of lower teeth, particularly molars. Unless the tooth is almost removed, it is better to stop the extraction.

4. Post-extraction Hæmorrhage.—Hæmorrhage from a tooth socket is rarely a major emergency and it is important to realize that there is plenty of time to take the necessary measures in a deliberate, unhurried way. The majority of patients with post-extraction bleeding suffer from reactionary hæmorrhage, occurring within 24 hours of extraction, and many are quite anxious and look ill from loss of sleep and from swallowing and vomiting blood. Initial cleansing of the mouth and reassurance will do much towards recovery. It is always necessary to take a history, with the aim of excluding a possible clotting disorder. The importance of this is because a bleeding socket may be treated by tight suturing and this could have fatal consequences in a hæmophiliac (*see* p. 485).

If local hæmorrhage persists after extraction, following the use of the gauze pack for 10 minutes, as already described, the socket should be inspected carefully to see that no fragments of bone are loose or partly attached to periosteum. If these are present they should be removed. The soft tissues around the socket should then be sutured across the socket using a horizontal mattress suture and gelatin foam sponge tucked under the sutures into the socket. The object of the suturing is to tighten the mucoperiosteum against the underlying bone, thus reducing the blood-flow in the tissue. When such measures fail to control the bleeding, then ribbon gauze soaked in Whitehead's varnish can be tucked under the sutures into the socket and the patient given a gauze pack to bite on. If the patient is apprehensive and uncooperative and is suffering from hæmorrhage which is difficult to control, the administration of morphine, with the patient being put to bed and the head being supported in an upright position, will permit the necessary treatment to be carried out more smoothly.

Secondary hæmorrhage may occur from 1 to 10 days after extraction due to infection. In such cases the problems of control of bleeding are the same as in reactionary hæmorrhage, but suturing may contribute to the sealing in of an infected blood-clot and therefore systemic antibiotics should be administered.

On very rare occasions a central hæmangioma gives rise to severe hæmorrhage with blood gushing from the socket. The socket must be immediately plugged. One useful way of plugging a socket in such circumstances is to replace the original tooth, ram it home, and hold it there under pressure until surgical assistance can be obtained.

5. Dry Socket.—If a patient presents in the days following an extraction with pain from the socket, he may be suffering from a 'dry socket', which is associated with an absence of blood-clot in the socket. The socket is infected and the pain is due to the stimulation of exposed nerve-endings in the sequestrating wall of the socket. Debris should be washed out of the socket by syringeing with warm saline solution and this should be repeated daily. A dressing of ribbon gauze soaked in Whitehead's varnish or gauze and oil of cloves may assist the control of pain by exclusion of food and other debris from the socket. An analgesic, such as Tab. Codeine Co. (two tablets, 4-hourly) should be given. It usually takes 7–14 days to overcome all discomfort, but the syringeing and dressing of the socket offer some relief. If there is persistent marked pain, a raised temperature, or anæsthesia of the lip, then an infected jaw fracture or osteomyelitis should be suspected.

TRAUMATIC INJURIES

INJURIES TO TEETH

If teeth are broken, loose fragments should be removed and torn soft tissues should be searched for embedded broken fragments before suturing. If wound contamination is likely then ATS or AT toxoid as appropriate should be given (*see* p. 67). Fracture or dislocation of anterior teeth is a common result of a blow on the face. There may be a fracture of the crown or roots of a tooth, or both. Root fracture, in the absence of radiographic evidence, may be suspected if the tooth is not displaced but is extremely mobile. Mobility of several upper anterior teeth should arouse suspicion of a fractured premaxilla. Fracture of the crown of a tooth may or may not expose the pulp. Such teeth can sometimes be preserved by specialized treatment. If the pulp is exposed emergency treatment consists of cautery of the pulp under local anæsthesia, dressing the surface with a calcium hydroxide paste, and protecting the broken surface of the tooth. Calcium hydroxide should also be applied to sensitive surfaces of fractured teeth where the pulp is not exposed. This dressing may then be covered with tin-foil (in an emergency milk bottle-tops will serve well) and this in turn is covered with a zinc-oxide pack or cold-cure acrylic resin to form a temporary splint. The patient should be referred as soon as possible for dental treatment and the provision of more robust splinting of the cast-metal or stainless-steel-banded type.

PARTLY DISLOCATED TEETH

These can be treated by manual reduction of the dislocation and splinting the tooth to its neighbours by wrapping tin-foil over the teeth and covering with a cold-cure resin as described above, referring as soon as possible for dental treatment.

TOTAL DISLOCATION OF TEETH

If the patient is seen immediately after the tooth has been knocked out, the tooth may be immersed in concentrated penicillin solution, washed well in isotonic saline, taking care not to handle the root more than necessary, and replaced in its socket. If seen after half an hour from the time of injury the root surface should be scraped free of remnants of soft tissue and, after immersing the tooth in penicillin solution, it is washed well in isotonic saline. The socket is cleaned of blood-clot and the tooth replaced and splinted as described for partial dislocation. The advice of a dental surgeon should be sought as soon as possible.

DISLOCATION OF THE TEMPOROMANDIBULAR JOINT

This may occur during extraction of a tooth, especially under general anæsthesia, or as the result of excessive yawning. Sometimes dislocation may be associated with injury. In the latter case care must be taken not to confuse the condition with fractured condyles. When a jaw is dislocated the condyles have slipped forward over the articular eminence and the patient is unable to close his mouth. The dislocation may usually be reduced early on as follows: the operator holds the patient's lower jaw so that his thumbs rest on the molars and his fingers are supporting the jaw underneath, covering his hands in a towel or thick gauze (so as to avoid damage to his fingers when the mandible snaps back into place under the pull of the masseters and medial pterygoid muscles). Pressing firmly downwards with the thumbs and upwards with the fingers, the head of the condyle is then depressed to clear the articular eminence and slips back into the articular fossa. If reduction of the dislocation is delayed it may be difficult to reduce it without general anæsthesia. After reduction the patient must be cautioned against opening the mouth too wide or yawning. A nonstretch supportive bandage may be worn to support the lower jaw until local discomfort has been overcome (p. 182).

FRACTURES OF THE JAWS

In the treatment of patients with jaw injuries it is assumed that every patient will be examined for injuries elsewhere in the body and that shock and hæmorrhage will be dealt with appropriately. Immediate attention must also be given to the control of respiration and the maintenance of an airway, particularly in the unconscious patient. The tongue must be pulled forward and the mouth and pharynx searched with the finger for any fragments, debris, broken teeth, or dentures. The tongue may be held forward by means of a suture or a safety-pin passed through the tongue and held externally. Where there is bleeding, the patient may need to be placed on his side or face downwards during transportation to drain blood and assist the maintenance of the airway. Where soft-tissue wounds accompany the fracture, the soft tissues should be preserved as much as possible, in spite of sometimes unpromising appearances, as the capacity to survive damage is considerable. Wounds inside the mouth should be closed, particularly if bone is exposed, so as to reduce the risk of infection. Otherwise, apart from the cleaning of debris and gentle débridement, it is more important in the early stages to retain fragments still attached to periosteum. Soft tissues should not be sutured under tension because of the risk of scarring and contraction, and in wounds perforating the face it is better to suture skin to mucous membrane and leave closure to later plastic surgery, rather than to attempt immediate closure of the wound. Systemically acting antibiotics should be given prophylactically. The patient should be referred to a maxillofacial centre for comprehensive treatment.

EMERGENCY FIXATION OF JAW FRACTURES

In fractures of the lower jaw where there is no obvious displacement, the mouth should be closed and held by means of a barrel bandage, designed to support the lower jaw. Bandaging which exerts pressure in such a way as to push the jaw backwards could have fatal consequences due to obstruction of the airway. Where the patient has dentures these should be used to aid the positioning and splinting of the jaws. Where there is displacement of fragments a barrel bandage is better than nothing if no other facilities are available, but it is preferable to use eyelet wiring (*Fig.* 449) to wire the jaws together in as normal a position as possible until full splinting, direct wiring, or pinning can be used to immobilize the fracture.

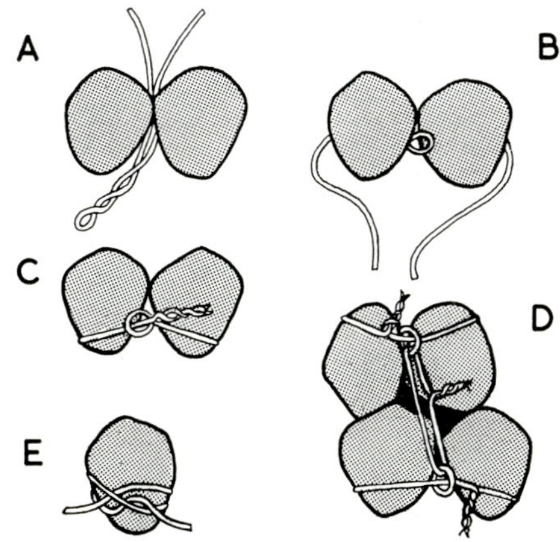

Fig. 449.—Diagram illustrating eyelet wiring. A, Eyelet with ends passed through interdental space; B, free ends brought back through neighbouring interdental spaces; C, one end passed through eyelet and joined with other free end; D, cross-wiring through opposite eyelets to obtain fixation; E, clove-hitch method of securing wire on an isolated tooth.

Wiring.—Soft stainless-steel wire of 0·35–0·5 mm. diameter is used for this purpose. Where lack of experience does not permit eyelet wiring, simple direct wiring may be used. The wires are passed around the teeth and twisted until tight (*Fig.* 450 B). The ends of the upper and lower wires are then twisted until tight and finally twisted together (*Fig.* 450 C). Care must be taken in twisting the wires or they may easily break. Eyelet wiring is more effective. An eyelet is made by wrapping the wire around the shank of a dental bur or other thin cylindrical object and twisting the wire to form the loop. The projecting lengths (about 5 in., 12·5 cm.) are passed between two teeth so that the loop is on the buccal side (*Fig.* 449 A); the ends are brought through the adjacent interdental spaces (*Fig.* 449 B) and then joined by twisting after passing one end through the eyelet (*Fig.* 449 C). Isolated teeth may be wired, if necessary, using a clove hitch (*Fig.* 449 E). After several points of anchorage are obtained the jaws are wired together by cross-wiring through the eyelets (*Fig.* 449 D). Care must be taken to cut short and turn in the ends of the wire so that they will not lacerate

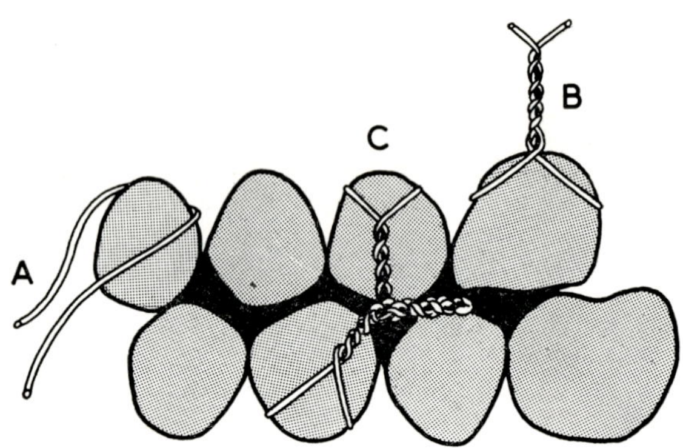

Fig. 450.—Diagram illustrating stages of simple wiring for jaw fixation. A, Loop of wire passed through interdental spaces; B, ends twisted together; C, ends of opposite wires joined together.

soft tissues or cause discomfort. *Wiring should only be attempted if the patient is fully conscious* and likely to remain so, and there is no risk of the airway becoming blocked. A person with wire cutters should accompany the patient in transport in readiness to free the jaw if there is any threatened obstruction of the airway as may occur from vomiting or hæmorrhage.

CHAPTER XLII

THE EYE

By the late F. A. WILLIAMSON-NOBLE

THE house-surgeon's duties fall into two categories: (*a*) those in the out-patient department; (*b*) those in the wards.

This chapter is written for the house-surgeon who is in charge of ophthalmic cases in a general hospital, and the general practitioner who may have to provide emergency treatment, rather than for the house-surgeon at a special eye hospital.

A. IN THE OUT-PATIENT DEPARTMENT

1. EYELIDS

The lashes, if misplaced and pointing inwards (*trichiasis*), may rub against the cornea and cause much discomfort. They can be permanently removed by electrolysis or more satis-factorily by diathermy. A fine needle is used as the active electrode and a current of 150 mA. is passed for 1–2 seconds after infiltration of the lid with lignocaine and

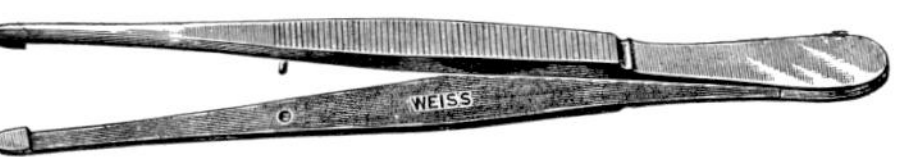

Fig. 451.—Epilation forceps for removal of lashes.

insertion of the needle to reach the root of the lash. If it resists gentle traction with forceps the coagulation should be repeated. Temporary removal is effected by flat-pointed epilation forceps (*Fig.* 451), a constant gentle pull bringing the lashes away with little pain. Removal of a lash from the centre of a stye (hordeolum) may aid materially in its resolution.

Entropion.—In the aged it is not un-common for spasm of the orbicularis to occur with resulting inversion of the lower lid, which turns the lashes in so that they irritate the conjunctiva and cornea. Such a condition is a frequent cause of intractable uni-ocular conjunctivitis, and is easily dealt with by the '*skin and muscle operation*' (*Fig.* 452). This opera-tion is condemned by some authors and a more complicated procedure involving displacement of a strip of the orbicu-laris is recommended. However, the skin and muscle operation has produced satisfactory results in a number of cases and has only twice needed repetition.

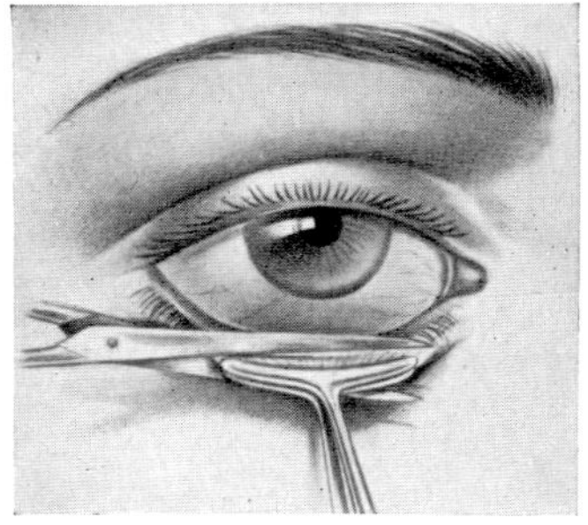

Fig. 452.—'Skin and muscle operation'; the fold of skin included in the grasp of the T-shaped forceps is being cut off with scissors. The forceps are rather smaller than those usually employed.

It is performed as follows:—

After cleaning the skin of the lids with spirit or tincture of iodine, infiltrate along the whole length of the lower lid with 4 per cent lignocaine. Apply a T-forceps (*Fig.* 453) to the skin of the lid, so that the upper arm is parallel with the margin and distant

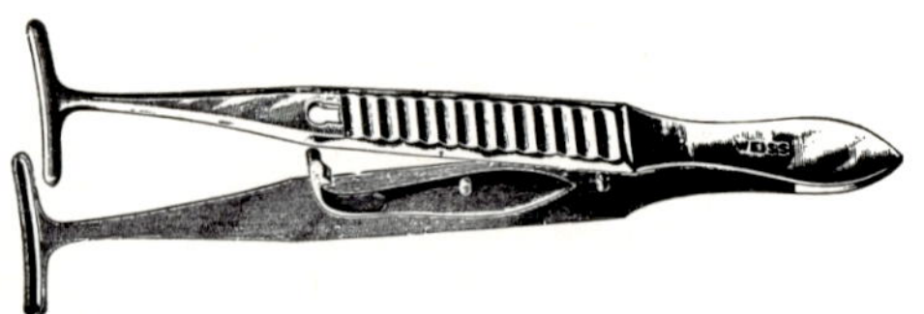

Fig. 453.—T-shaped forceps for skin and muscle operation.

about 1 mm. from the line of the lashes. The amount of skin included between the blades of the forceps has to be rather carefully estimated, so as to be sufficient to correct the defect—it is usually a strip about 6 mm. wide. This is then cut off with a straight pair of scissors, leaving a raw area in which lies the orbicularis, whose exposed portion is grasped with fixation forceps (*Fig.* 454) and cut away with scissors. Hæmorrhage is easily controlled by swabbing and touching the bleeding points with a heated probe or electro-cautery. The margins of the wound are united by three or four interrupted silk sutures, taking care to pass them deeply enough to include the muscle. No dressing is needed, but the line of incision is painted with tincture of iodine, a process which should be repeated daily until the stitches are removed on the sixth or seventh day. An immediate over-correction is not uncommon, but this usually remedies itself in the ensuing few weeks.

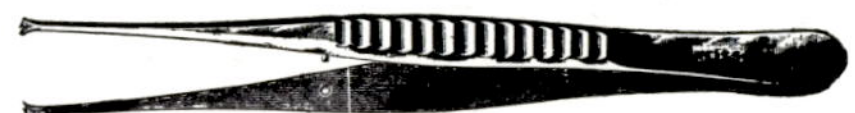

Fig. 454.—Fixation forceps, used for grasping the orbicularis fibres in the 'skin and muscle operation'. Also used for grasping the conjunctiva of the eyeball in intra-ocular operations.

Eversion of the Lids.—Examination of the lower conjunctival fornix is simple. The patient looks up, the lower lid is pulled downwards, and gentle pressure backwards will then reveal it in its whole extent. To get a similarly good view

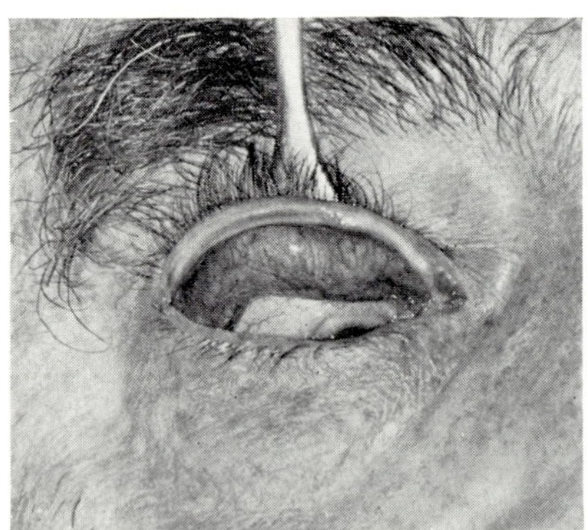

Fig. 455.—Desmarres' retractor inserted and turned back. The lower edge of the fornix is just visible.

of the upper tarsal conjunctiva requires the knowledge of a little manœuvre very readily acquired and yet very frequently bungled. The method advised requires the use of only one hand, leaving the other free for any purpose such as painting the lids. First of all persuade the patient to look steadily downwards at the floor or at his own hands, with the head thrown slightly backwards; then place the ulnar border of the index finger on the upper lid immediately above the margin of the tarsal plate; the thumb is placed on the lower lid, pressing gently backwards. The index finger then gently presses the margin of the eyelid down on to the thumb, and by a slight movement the thumb completes the eversion. Straight pressure backwards on the eyeball may then bring the folds of the upper fornix into view. If not, a Desmarres' retractor should be passed in behind the skin of the everted upper lid (*Fig.* 455). When the handle of the retractor is raised, the upper conjunctival fornix comes into view. Before carrying out this manœuvre it is advisable to instil a drop or two of 0·5 per cent amethocaine. Standing in front of the patient, use the right hand for the left eye, and vice versa.

Foreign bodies can usually be removed from the conjunctival surface of the lids by wiping them off with cotton-wool, moistened in boracic lotion and wound around the end of a glass rod (*Fig.* 456).

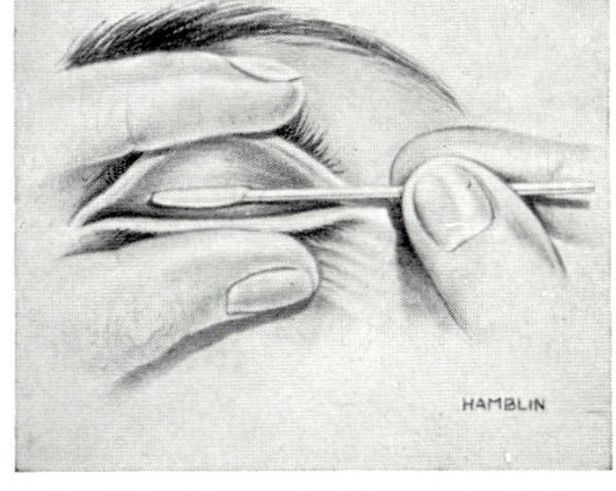

Fig. 456.—Removal of foreign body from the conjunctiva of everted upper lid (*see text*).

Conjunctival concretions are often the source of ocular discomfort and may act as foreign bodies. To remove them, the eye should be anæsthetized—instil 3 drops of 0·5 per cent amethocaine solution at 5-minute intervals—and then the lids are everted. The concretions are visible as small yellowish-white areas, and are readily picked out by the point of a Beer's knife (*Fig.* 457). A pair of fine straight iris forceps is sometimes helpful in freeing the concretion from a tag of conjunctiva.

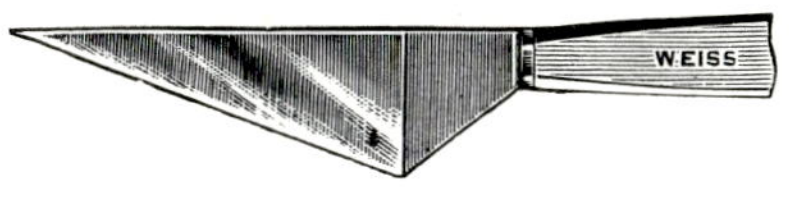

Fig. 457.—Beer's knife.

Expression of the Meibomian Glands.—This may often give relief in cases of chronic conjunctivitis and blepharitis, particularly when associated with thickening of the lids.

After anæsthetizing (*see above*), the lid is everted and pressure is made with a glass rod on its conjunctival surface, against the finger or thumb-nail held in contact with the skin surface of the lid. In this way, the contents of the Meibomian glands may be squeezed out and a mixture of fluid and sebaceous secretions accumulates at the gland orifice on the lid margin. The procedure should be continued until no more secretion can be expressed, and is usually carried out on both upper and lower lids. An alkaline lotion (as below) is employed afterwards for bathing the lid margins night and morning and an ointment of albucid 6 per cent is applied to the lid margins at night.

> ℞ Sodii Bicarb.   0·5 G.
> Liq. Carb. Det. (Wright)   0·40 ml.
> Aq.   ad 30·0 ml.
> Mix with an equal volume of warm water before use.

Meibomian Cysts (Tarsal Cyst, Chalazion).—When this affection occurs in the upper lid, the patient may complain of blurred vision owing to distortion of the cornea produced by pressure of the cyst on it, which results in a temporary astigmatism, sometimes amounting to as much as 3 D. In the early stages, when

Albucid (British Schering Ltd., Slough, Bucks).

the lid is swollen and inflamed, surgical interference is inadvisable owing to the danger of spreading the infection, and at this stage much relief can be obtained by hot bathing, which can be carried out by the patient as follows: wind some cotton-wool around the bowl of a wooden spoon and dip it into a bowl of hot lotion, e.g., 4 G. of boric acid in 600 ml. of hot water. Hold the wool up against the closed eyelids, having it as hot as can be comfortably tolerated. As soon as it cools, dip the wool again, and continue the treatment for 10 to 15 minutes. Care should be taken to keep the lotion hot during this period, and it may be necessary to warm it up once or twice. When finished, a little yellow oxide ointment (Ung. Hydrarg. Oxid. Flav., 1 per cent) should be rubbed gently into the

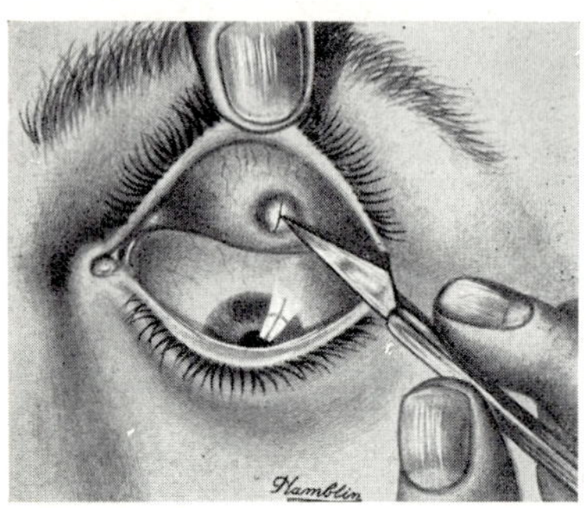

Fig. 458.—Incision of Meibomian cyst (chalazion) of upper lid. The lid has been everted and the cyst is being opened by a vertical incision with a Beer's knife.

lid, and a pad applied for an hour or so. Internal administration of penicillin or albucid (sulphacetamide), 2 tablets, three times daily, is useful in aiding resolution. As a result of these measures, or sometimes without any treatment at all, the cyst may disappear. Should it remain, however, it should be dealt with as follows:—

Evert the lid and apply one or two crystals of solid cocaine over the conjunctival surface of the swelling. Leave it to act for 2 minutes, then with a fine-needled hypodermic syringe inject *into the cyst* about 0·3 ml. of 2 per cent lignocaine in 1–10,000 adrenaline. Let this again act for 2 minutes. With a Beer's knife (*Fig.* 457), make a vertical incision through the wall of the conjunctiva (*Fig.* 458), and then thoroughly scrape away with a small curette all the gelatinous and diseased tissue from the walls of the cyst. It is best to apply a pad and bandage for a few hours, and to have the eye bathed frequently with boric lotion for some days. It sometimes happens in old cysts that most or all of the contents are fibrous and cannot be removed by curetting. In such cases, a fine-toothed pair of forceps should be introduced into the wound and made to grasp the small mass of tissue at the bottom of it. It is then possible to remove this with scissors and a Beer's knife. Hæmorrhage can be checked by application of a cautery or the point of a heated squint hook. In cysts

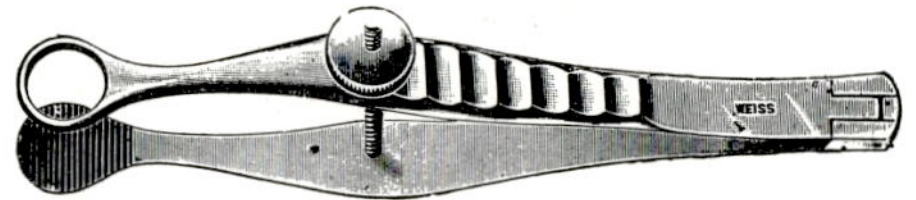

Fig. 459.—Blepharostat; used for grasping the lid and controlling hæmorrhage.

of the lower lid, the patient should be directed to look up towards the eyebrow, to protect the cornea from burning.

Should the cyst involve several glands, it is better to make an incision through the conjunctiva parallel with the lid margin and about 4 mm. distant from it, over the affected area. The edges of the conjunctiva are dissected up and the underlying mass of degenerate tarsal cartilage and glands grasped in the forceps and dissected out in a sausage-shaped mass. The edges of the conjunctiva can be brought together by a continuous suture, which can be left untied so as to avoid the irritation caused by knots. This is a procedure which requires previous infiltration of the lid from the skin surface with lignocaine and adrenaline. Hæmorrhage is usually slight, but should it be troublesome, a blepharostat (*Fig.* 459) may be applied to the lid. This is also a useful instrument when the cyst is near either end of the lid and difficult to expose by eversion.

Stye (Hordeolum).—Cases of orbital cellulitis have been reported from time to time as following the injudicious or too early opening of these small abscesses. It is therefore advisable, in the early stages, to limit surgical procedures to removal of the infected lash from the swelling and to order hot bathing, and perhaps some anti-staphylococcal treatment (p. 75). The abscess usually ruptures of its own accord, but if not, and it is definitely pointing, a small prick with a sterile Beer's knife will allow the contents to escape, especially if followed by hot bathing. Should there be a succession of styes, pulv. myristicæ (nutmeg) 0·6 G. in a capsule b.d. for 2 weeks is often effective.

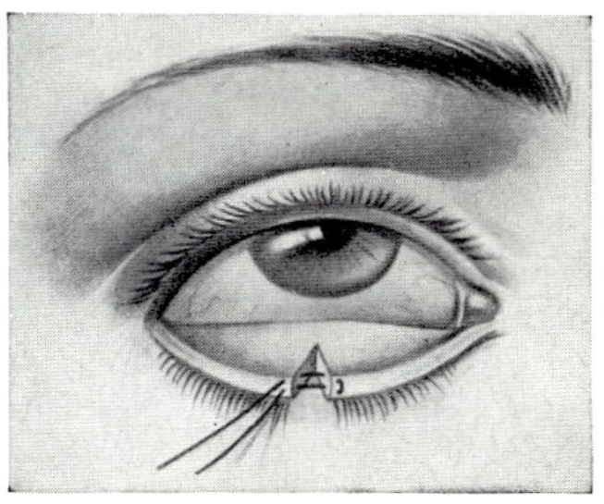

Fig. 460.—Method of passing a stitch to secure accurate co-aptation of a wound involving the lid margin.

Wounds of the Eyelid usually heal readily after cleaning and the insertion of fine silkworm-gut stitches. If the lid margin is involved, very careful co-aptation of the wound is needed or an unsightly gap will remain, with perhaps one or two ingrowing lashes. Such cases are best left to the visiting surgeon, but if this is not possible, an effort should be made to unite the edges of the wound by means of a stitch passed as shown in *Fig.* 460. The stitch used for this should be of very fine material, e.g., virgin silk, as used for corneoscleral sutures.

Tarsorrhaphy is an operation which is required in cases of **neuroparalytic keratitis**—a degenerative change of the cornea which is liable to occur when the eye is anæsthetic. The condition is most commonly seen following alcohol injection of the Gasserian ganglion for trigeminal neuralgia, or as a sequel of herpes zoster involving the ophthalmic division of the fifth nerve, though there are other causes. The operation is sometimes done in cases of exposure keratitis, to protect the cornea when the lids do not cover it, e.g., pronounced exophthalmos. It is performed as follows:—

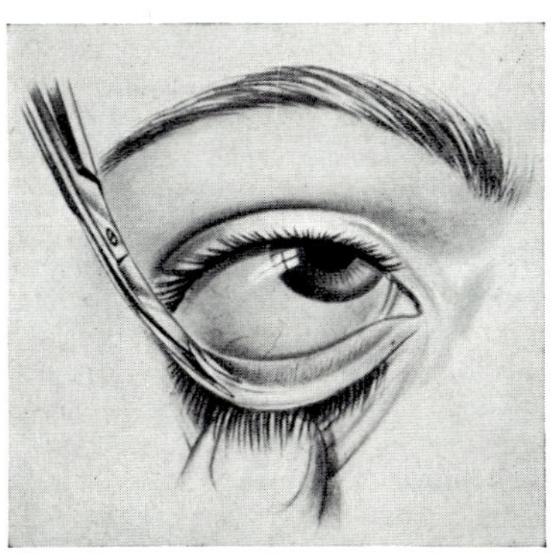

Fig. 461.—Tarsorrhaphy; the lower lid is everted and its posterior sharp edge is being cut off with scissors.

If the skin of the lids is sensitive, infiltrate them with lignocaine; if insensitive, no injection is needed. Evert the lower lid, and, with a pair of squint scissors curved on the flat, cut off the posterior sharp margin of the lid (*Fig.* 461) for the middle two-thirds of its extent. Evert the upper lid and treat it similarly. Unite the lids by three double-armed No. 1 silk sutures passed from their conjunctival surfaces forwards so as to co-apt the raw areas, and tie fairly firmly. A dressing is applied, which can be changed daily. The stitches are removed at the end of a week, by which time a firm adhesion will have formed. This is usually left for 3 months. At the end of this time, divide about 1 mm. of the adhesion on the nasal side, repeating the process each month until only a narrow band 2 mm wide is left uniting the lids on a line overlying the temporal margin of the cornea. If the eye regains sensation, this band may also be divided; if not, it is wise to leave it, or the keratitis will recur.

An alternative to tarsorrhaphy is the use of a contact lens, the fitting of which requires considerable skill and experience, while a second alternative is division of the cervical sympathetic on the affected side. This is said to prevent the distressing nasal symptoms which may accompany trigeminal anæsthesia, and to prevent keratitis.

Inflammation of the Lid Margins (Blepharitis) is primarily an infection of the lash follicles and of the sebaceous and sweat-glands leading into them. For effective local treatment it is essential to remove the crusts of exudate and epithelial debris which cover them. This is best done by swabbing the lid margins with an alkaline lotion (p. 615), picking off with forceps any specially adherent crusts. A variety of different agents may then be applied: among them are Liquor Tinctorium, which is painted on; Ung. Hyd. Ammon., 1 per cent; Ung. Hyd. Hydroxy Nit. Nig., 0·5 per cent; and Ung. Albucid, 5 per cent, which are rubbed in for at least 5 minutes. Loose lashes should be removed, and, if possible, the Meibomian glands expressed (p. 615). Errors of refraction, particularly of the hypermetropic variety, should be corrected with glasses and the patient's general health attended to, special attention being paid to securing an adequate intake of vitamins A and B complex. Local treatment is usually carried out three times a day and should be continued until at least a fortnight after apparent cure, or the condition will relapse.

Penicillin ointment, 1000 units of the calcium salt per gramme of oculentum B.P., applied to the lid margins three times daily with a wooden probe for 3 to 10 weeks has been advocated but some patients become hypersensitive to it. Obstinate cases will sometimes react favourably to steroid treatment (*see* p. 627).

Ectropion.—Blepharitis and chronic conjunctivitis are sometimes associated with eversion of the lower lid and cannot be cured until this displacement is overcome. Mild cases can be dealt with by daily painting of the exposed conjunctiva with 2 per cent silver nitrate. More severe ones often respond to applications of the cautery, especially if combined with the passage of Snellen's sutures (*Fig.* 462). The lid should be infiltrated with lignocaine, everted, and with the electric cautery a series of punctures made 3–4 mm. behind the lid margin, and 2 mm. from each other, using a horn spatula to protect the cornea from the heat of the cautery. The punctures should pass into the tarsal plate, but not through it. Snellen's sutures may then be passed as shown in *Fig.* 462. If this procedure fails, a plastic operation will be required.

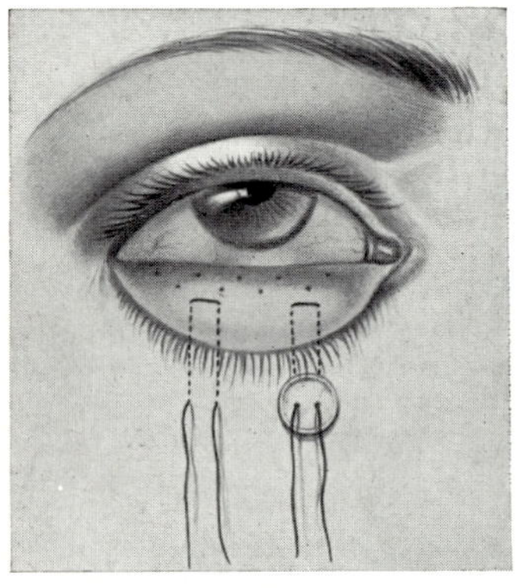

Fig. 462.—Snellen's sutures for the correction of ectropion. Two double-armed sutures are employed. They are passed through the most prominent part of the conjunctival swelling and brought out through the skin, being tied fairly tightly over pearl buttons, thereby pulling the lid back into position. The dots indicate the sites of application of the cautery.

2. LACRIMAL APPARATUS

The commonest task the house-surgeon will have to perform in this connexion
is to determine the patency, or otherwise, of the lacrimal passages. The first
thing to do is to press over the sac, situated on the side of the nose just below
the internal tarsal ligament, and see whether any mucus or pus regurgitates
through the lacrimal punctum. Should this occur, it is fairly conclusive evidence
of a block in the nasolacrimal duct. Absence of regurgitation does not, however,
prove patency of the duct, and in these cases, as also in those where pus is in
the sac, syringeing is required.

Syringeing is carried out as follows: instil two to three drops of 0·5 per cent
amethocaine at 5-minute intervals, evert the lower lid and rub a few crystals
of cocaine hydrochloride into the conjunctiva lining the inner surface of the
lid between the punctum and the inner canthus. Wait a further 3 minutes
and evert the lid again to expose the inferior punctum, inserting into it the

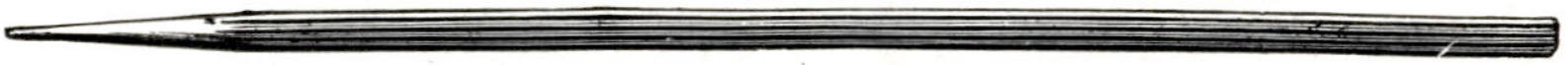

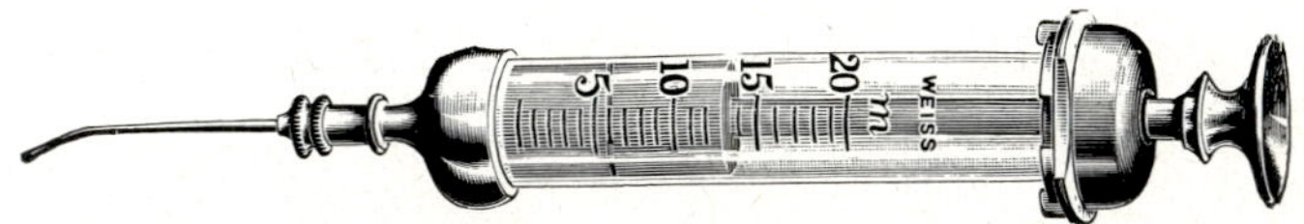

Fig. 463.—Nettleship's dilator for enlarging the lacrimal puncta.

point of a Nettleship's dilator (*Fig.* 463). If this is not at hand, or the point is
too blunt to enter the punctum, a sterilized safety-pin may be employed, but
it must be used carefully or a false passage will be made. The lacrimal cannula

Fig. 464.—Lacrimal cannula and syringe.

(*Fig.* 464) fitted to a 1-ml. syringe can then be passed into the inferior canaliculus
and the lacrimal passage syringed through with boracic lotion. Passage of
fluid into the throat can be avoided by making the patient bend his head forward,
when it will come out of the nose if the nasal canal is patent; if blocked, the
fluid will return by the upper punctum accompanied by mucus and pus, if
these have been present in the sac. Should the latter occur, the sac should
be washed clean with several syringefuls of boric acid lotion and then filled
with 2 per cent cocaine in 1–5000 adrenaline. After waiting for a few minutes,
fluid may pass into the nose, when syringeing is repeated. If it does not, the
question of probing will have to be considered. Before attempting this, it
is advisable to get the sac as clean as possible. This may be done by showing
the patient how to express the contents and instructing her to do so every hour
or so during the day. She should apply a little boric petroleum jelly to the
finger-tip each time to avoid excoriating the skin. A few days of this treatment
will usually suffice to convert the contents of the sac from mucopus to clear
mucus, and in elderly people may be enough to bring about relief of symptoms.

Probing.—To accomplish this painlessly, the eye should be anæsthetized as
for syringeing and the sac washed out with a little 4 per cent cocaine in adrenaline 1–10,000. The skin over the sac and nasolacrimal duct should be infiltrated

24

with 1 per cent lignocaine, some of the solution being injected deeply so as to pass if possible behind the sac and duct. A small-sized probe (No. 0 or 1, Bowman, *Fig.* 465) is passed through the dilated inferior punctum and along the canaliculus until it can be felt impinging on the lacrimal bone. The probe is raised into the vertical position so that it points towards the fold of the ala nasi,

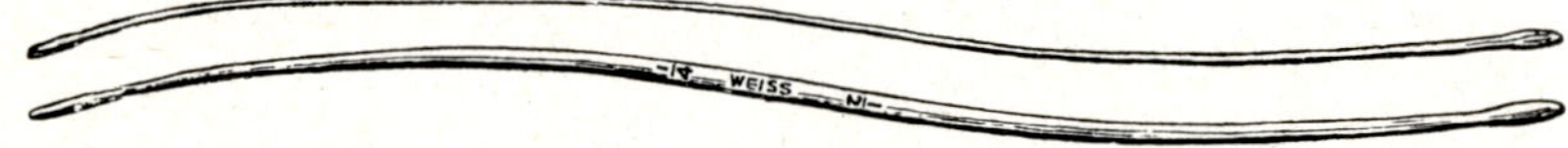

Fig. 465.—Bowman's probes.

and keeping its point a little backwards it will be felt to engage the opening of the nasolacrimal duct. A stricture will probably be encountered here, but with a little patience, this and others farther down the duct can usually be negotiated, and the probe passed into the inferior meatus of the nose. It is unwise to syringe immediately after, but local treatment for the eye and nose is indicated if the condition is not to relapse. The following régime has given satisfactory results; it is carried out three times daily and kept up for 3 to 4 weeks: glycerin of thymol, 1–8 as an eye lotion, and also for sniffing up the nostrils, drops of argyrol, 10 per cent, ephedrine, 1 per cent, for the eye and a decongestant spray for the nose.

Should this condition recur, probing may be repeated, but if this has to be done more than two or three times, excision of the sac or dacryo-cystorhinostomy should be performed.

Three-snip Operation.—This is a useful method of curing epiphora in elderly people, where, although the lacrimal passages are patent, troublesome watering of the eyes occurs. Inspection of such cases will show that the punctum is not in apposition with bulbar conjunctiva, either because of slight eversion of the lid from laxity of the orbicularis, or from atrophy of the lid tissues, leaving the punctum on the top of a tiny papilla where the tears cannot enter it. The eye is anæsthetized with a drop of 5 per cent cocaine and a little solid cocaine is

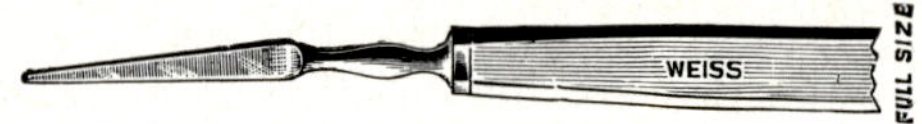

Fig. 466.—Stilling's knife for slitting up the lacrimal canaliculus.

rubbed into the conjunctiva of the lower lid from the punctum to its inner end. The punctum is dilated, the lid everted, and the canaliculus slit up by a Stilling's knife (*Fig.* 466) passed along it with its cutting edge directed towards the eyeball. Part of the posterior wall of the canaliculus is gripped in fine forceps and a small triangular portion removed by three snips with a pair of iris scissors (*Figs.* 467, 468).

Tonometry is used in cases of glaucoma to measure the intra-ocular pressure. The eye should be anæsthetized with two drops of 0·5 per cent amethocaine hyd. (B.P.) with a 5-minute interval (cocaine dilates the pupil, which might be dangerous; it also injures the corneal epithelium). The patient lies flat on a couch and is directed to hold his index finger of the same side above the eye, and look at it with both eyes open. The house-surgeon moves the patient's

Argyrol (Fassett & Johnson Ltd., Worsley Bridge Road, London, S.E.26).

hand until the eye to be examined is looking vertically upwards. The lids may have to be retracted; if so, it helps the patient to allow him to retract his lower lid with his unoccupied hand. The tonometer (*Fig.* 469) is applied vertically and

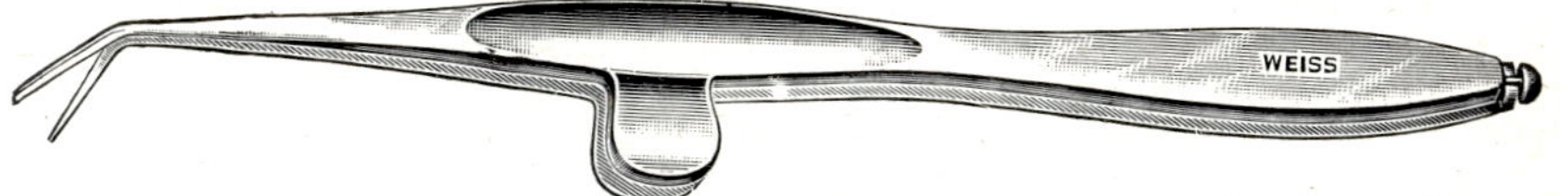

Fig. 467.—Iris scissors used for removal of posterior wall of lacrimal canaliculus. Also employed for iridectomy.

a reading is taken. The weight should be chosen so that the deflexion of the pointer is between 5° and 10°. The intra-ocular pressure is read off from the

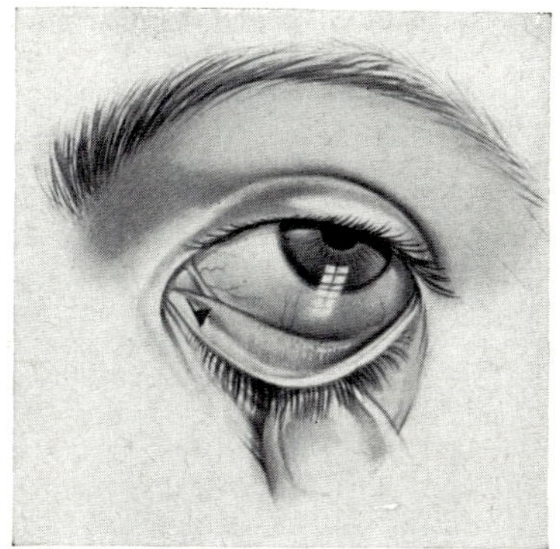

Fig. 468.—Three-snip operation completed, showing the triangle of tissue which has been removed to prevent healing of the slit canaliculus.

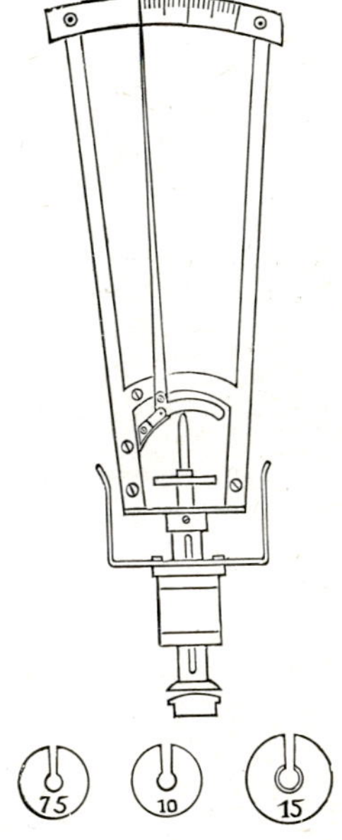

Fig. 469.—Tonometer.

table provided with the instrument. In recording the result, the deflexion and the weight used should be mentioned as well as the pressure, e.g., if it is a 7·5 weight with 6° deflexion, it would be recorded 6/7·5 = 23 mm. Hg. The normal pressure is from 15–25 mm. Hg, though figures up to 30 mm. may, in the absence of other symptoms, be taken as high normal. Tensions of 30–45 mm. are called + 1; 45–70 mm., + 2; and above 70 mm., + 3.

A source of error in this procedure is the variation which may be present in rigidity of the sclera. Patients with a high degree of scleral rigidity may appear to have modest hypertension for years without loss of field. Patients with low scleral rigidity may appear to have a normal or even subnormal tension and yet be losing field—the so-called low-tension glaucoma.

The applanation tonometer overcomes this difficulty by measuring the force required to flatten a small area of cornea, thus displacing much less aqueous than the Schiotz instrument. Should this not be available, an indication of abnormal scleral rigidity can be assumed if there is much difference in the estimated tension with the different weights.

3. AFFECTIONS OF THE CONJUNCTIVA

Trauma.—The removal of foreign bodies has already been described (p. 615, *see also* p. 625); burns from acids or alkalis demand immediate irrigation of the eye. The best immediate treatment is to immerse the face with eyes open in a basin of water. A drop of fluorescein is instilled after irrigation, to determine the extent of conjunctival damage, and the integrity or otherwise of the cornea. In the event of the latter being damaged, a drop of 1 per cent atropine should be used; if not, it can be omitted, but paraffin liq. (B.P.) should be instilled in both cases, the instillation being repeated 4-hourly, after gentle irrigation with normal saline. Later treatment should include the daily examination for adhesions between the conjunctiva lining the lids and that covering the eyeball (symblepharon), and the breaking down of them by a blunt probe or a glass rod. Should a large surface be involved, a mucous membrane graft will be required.

Particularly dangerous are the burns resulting from ammonia or lime. In the former, although the initial injury may appear slight, rapid necrosis of the cornea may ensue, and in the latter the cornea may also be seriously affected. In the case of lime burns, the patient's lids are often firmly closed and a useful preliminary procedure is to paralyse the orbicularis by an injection of 2 ml. of lignocaine adrenaline on to the ramus of the lower jaw a fingerbreadth below the condyle. All the particles should then be carefully picked out, the lids being separated by Desmarres' retractors, after instillation of a few drops of 0·5 per

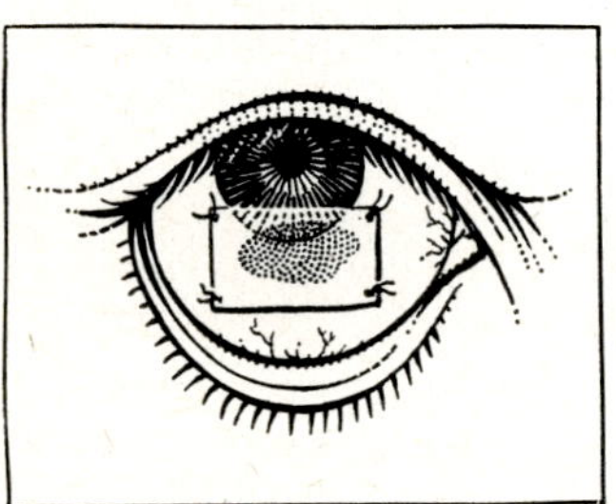

Fig. 470.—Graft held by four sutures. Dots indicate burnt area. Care should be taken not to cover too much of the corneal surface.

cent decicain or amethocaine. The conjunctival sac should be copiously irrigated with warm saline with the lids everted and this is followed by exploring the fornices with a small camel-hair brush moistened with liquid paraffin, care being taken to brush them clean. If the conjunctiva, and particularly the limbus, is affected, a subconjunctival injection of 5 mm. of saline should be made beneath the area and repeated daily to prevent formation of adhesions, after which hydrocortisone ointment 2·5 per cent can be applied, also daily, both being continued for a period of 2 weeks or so.

These measures have now almost ousted surgical procedures, but in severe cases the following is sometimes employed:—

1. Instil antibiotic drops every minute for 10 minutes.

2. Instil decicain or amethocaine 0·5 per cent.

3. Cover the burnt area of the eyeball with from 2 to 4 layers of human amniotic membrane (amnioplastin) cut to the correct size and fixed in position with stitches of 0 black silk at the corners.

4. Insert the stitches through the bulbar conjunctiva (*Fig.* 470).

5. Instil antibiotic.

Amnioplastin (London Hospital, London, E.11).

6. Bandage both eyes for 48 hours.

Conjunctivitis.—The treatment of this disease is a large subject, and only a few general points can be touched upon here.

1. If possible, identify the organism by taking a smear and culture from the conjunctival sac, using a diphtheria swab or a platinum loop and plating out on blood-agar. This should be done before treatment has started, but the latter should begin immediately the swab has been taken. If a culture is grown, the opportunity should be taken to test the sensitivity of the organism to various antibiotics.

2. Treat the less inflamed eye first.

3. Bathe the eye with sterile saline 1 per cent, instilling antibiotic drops, e.g., sulphacetamide 10 per cent, until the bacteriological report is available when if the infecting organism is sensitive to penicillin or some other antibiotic, dramatic results may be obtained by its use.

4. Apply a bland ointment, containing the chosen antibiotic, to the edges of the lids, especially at night to prevent the lashes sticking and so converting the conjunctival sac into a closed incubator. An alternative plan is to instil a drop of paroleine (sterile liquid paraffin) at night.

5. Avoid pads, bandages, cocaine because it injures the corneal epithelium, and adrenaline because it interferes with the natural processes of cure.

6. Do what is possible to encourage local and bodily resistance.

7. Prevent spread:

a. Keep all utensils, undines, trays, etc., scrupulously clean.

b. Use a separate swab for each eye and destroy after use.

c. In serious cases, the house-surgeon or nurse should wear gloves and goggles when treating the eye.

d. If only one eye is involved, especially if the conjunctivitis is severe, protect the fellow eye by a cone of X-ray film (*Fig.* 471) or a Buller's shield (*Fig.* 472).

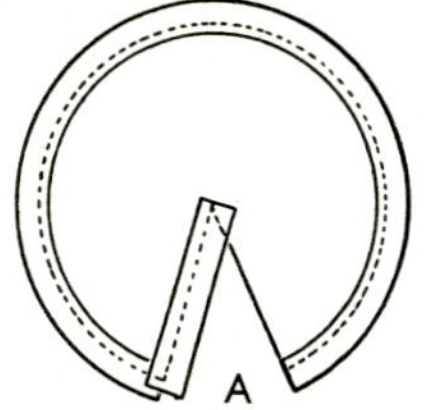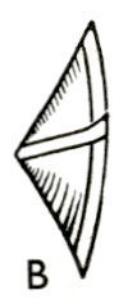

Fig. 471.—A, Disk of X-ray film (emulsion removed by hot water) sufficiently large to cover eye, segment removed and edges bound with strapping. B, Cone ready for application over eye.

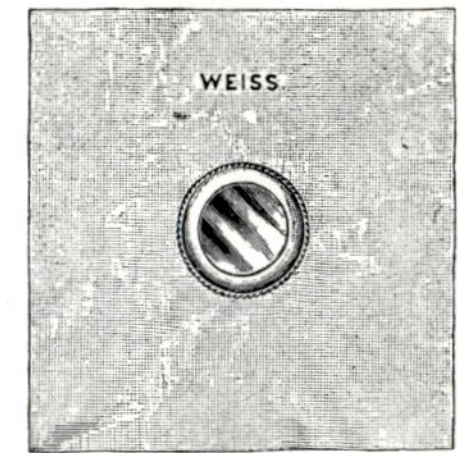

Fig. 472.—Buller's shield, consisting of a watch-glass surrounded by strapping.

8. In some cases stimulate local changes by painting the everted lids with silver nitrate, 1 per cent, every 24 hours, or, in milder cases, instil silver proteinate B.P.C., 10 per cent, night and morning. This treatment should not be continued for longer than 2 weeks, or permanent silver staining (argyrosis) of the conjunctiva ensues.

9. In cases of persistent uni-ocular conjunctivitis look for: (*a*) A foreign body, conjunctival concretion, or inturned lashes; (*b*) Lacrimal sac infection (*see* p. 619).

Paroleine (Burroughs, Wellcome & Co., Euston Road, London, N.W.1).

There are some twenty different types of conjunctivitis, with numerous sub-groups; one of particular importance in tropical countries is **trachoma**. It can be diagnosed by the presence of follicles up to 1 mm. in diameter on the upper fornix and tarsus and the presence of new vessels growing down into the cornea from its upper margin (pannus). Treatment varies, but one line is to give full doses of sulphathiazole for 10 days and to paint the conjunctivæ daily with 30 per cent sulphacetamide. It is not possible to deal here with the differential diagnosis of other forms of conjunctivitis though this is important from the therapeutic stand-point. Suffice it to say that the causative agent may be bacteria, a virus (e.g., trachoma), fungi, spirochætes, allergic hypersensitivity, mechanical (e.g., ectropion or entropion), or some unidentified agent, e.g., Parinaud's conjunc-tivitis, and that treatment has to be modified accordingly. In all cases, however, the above general principles hold good.

A few more points remain for comment. Inspection of the eyes is best carried out in diffuse daylight, and it is usually advisable to evert the lids (*see* p. 614). In adults this is simple, but in babies the following technique is advised: sit opposite the nurse, who holds the child's body with its hands down to its sides, the head being grasped in a towel between the house-surgeon's knees. Wash away all secretion and endeavour to separate the lids, being careful not to press upon the eyeball, when they will usually become everted. It is important to wear goggles while doing this, because the pus in the conjunctival sac may be under pressure and spurt up into the examiner's eyes when the lids are separated. It is usually necessary to examine the cornea in these cases, and if the lids do not open easily, small bent-wire retractors must be slipped under their edges and gently separated. By this means, pressure is not exerted on the eyeball and so the risk of causing an ulcer of the cornea to rupture is avoided. Should the eyeball roll upward in the effort to keep the eye closed, it usually suffices to wait a short time with the lids separated, and it will then roll down.

The employment of sulphonamides, penicillin or other antibiotics, particularly in ophthalmia neonatorum, has rendered frequent irrigations seldom necessary. The technique is to instil drops of penicillin, 2500 units per ml., every 5 minutes until the eye is free of discharge, which takes $\frac{1}{2}$ to 3 hours; then at longer intervals. One per cent saline, provided it is freshly made, is often used for irrigation, but a buffered solution of correct pH is really better, for example:—

℞	Boric Acid	0·40 G.
	Potassium Chloride (anhydrous)	0·25 G.
	Sodium Carbonate	50 mg.
	Aq. Dest.	ad 30 ml.

Alternatives are hyd. oxycyanide 1–6000, dettol 1–400, and glycerin of thymol 1–8.

4. AFFECTIONS OF THE CORNEA

Injuries.—*Abrasions* of the cornea are apt to be overlooked, since when fresh the transparency of the cornea is not interfered with. When any corneal injury has taken place, and an abrasion is suspected, a drop of fluorescein will stain the denuded area a bright green. The eye is bathed, a drop of atropine is instilled, and a pad and bandage are applied. Boracic bathing should be repeated every 4 hours. As a rule, the pad can be taken off in 24 hours. If the surface is not covered in that time, another drop of atropine should be put in and the pad or dark glasses replaced. If the patient finds the pressure of a pad intolerable, dark glasses with side pieces can be substituted for it.

Dettol (Reckitt & Coleman Ltd., Hull, Yorks).

Foreign bodies★ embedded in the cornea are mostly particles of steel or emery from the emery-wheel or grit from an engine. Careful examination with a loupe is often required for their detection, as they are frequently very small and difficult to find. A drop of fluorescein is of great assistance in doubtful cases, the staining area indicating the position of the foreign body. Another useful indication is a slight but definite contraction of the pupil on the affected side due to reflex irritation of the iris. This is often accompanied by some ciliary flush, occupying that part of the limbus which is adjacent to the foreign body. The removal must be done with as little injury to the corneal epithelium as possible. Occasionally, after dropping in a little 4 per cent cocaine, the foreign body may be so loosened that it can be removed by means of a little cotton-wool, soaked in boric acid, on the end of a glass rod. If this does not suffice, a corneal spud should be used (*Fig.* 473), and the removal must be complete.

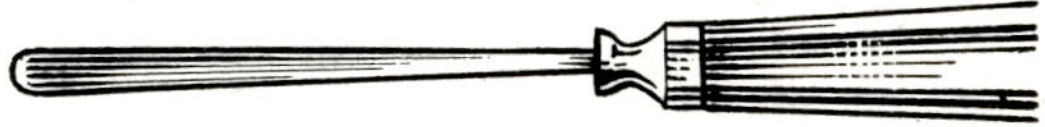

Fig. 473.—Corneal spud.

The eye is well cocainized, and a strong light focused on it by an assistant. The patient is told to look fixedly in whatever direction enables the operator to get the best view of the object to be removed. If the spud fails to remove it, recourse may be had to a discission needle (*Fig.* 474), but in digging out foreign bodies

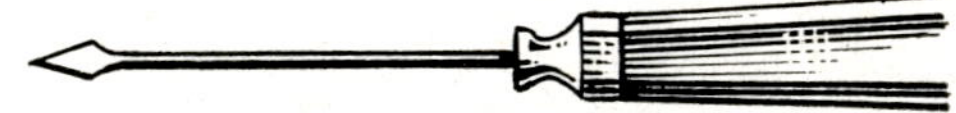

Fig. 474.—Discission needle.

with this, care must be exercised not to injure the cornea more deeply than is necessary. After removal, bathe carefully, put in a small piece of atropine ointment, and bandage the eye. If a discission needle is not available, a fine hypodermic needle attached to a 1-ml. syringe is a useful substitute; since the point is bevelled, it can be passed under the foreign body to loosen it and allow of its removal.

Perforating wounds of the cornea are apt to have serious consequences, and the house-surgeon should obtain the services of one who has had special training in ophthalmic surgery. *Fig.* 475 shows a small linear perforating wound of the cornea through which a globular portion of iris has prolapsed, bringing about a pear-shaped deformation of the pupil.

In all cases of perforating wounds, whether simple or complicated, the house-surgeon must be carefully on the watch for keratic precipitates. It is not the eye which passes into a condition of general suppuration which is most likely to set up *sympathetic ophthalmia*: such an eye is removed, and with its removal usually all danger is past; but the eye which remains inflamed and irritable, and in which there appear on the back of the cornea tiny round dots, is almost

---

★ A metallic foreign body sometimes stains the cornea, in which case at first sight it may appear to be still present when, in fact, it has been removed.

certain, if left, to cause a sympathetic inflammation in the other eye. Such an eye may have to be excised but can sometimes be saved by steroid treatment, e.g., prednisolone, 15 mg. daily for 3 weeks, then gradually reduced; to maintain electrolyte balance 450 mg. potassium chloride are given daily.

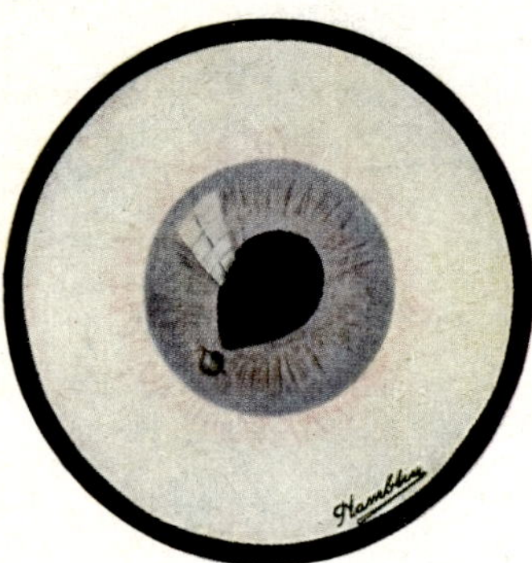

Fig. 475.—Small perforating wound of the cornea.

Corneal Ulcers.—Should the ulcer be secondary to purulent conjunctivitis or obviously infected, a smear should be made on a microscope slide and stained by the Gram method. If the organisms are Gram positive they should be sensitive to tetracycline B.P., bacitracin, or penicillin; if Gram negative to polymyxin. If the ulcer is of the dendritic type, it is almost certainly herpetic in origin and is best treated by carbolizing as described below. If not severe, ulcers will usually react favourably to very simple treatment. The first essential is to secure rest for the eye. For this purpose atropine drops (0·5 per cent) are put in, and the eye is covered with a pad lightly bandaged on. Only in cases in which the ulcer is complicated by conjunctivitis with a large amount of secretion is this latter abandoned. The atropine paralyses the action of the iris and ciliary muscles, and so acts as a physiological splint, while the pad keeps the eyelids at rest over the cornea. Frequently during the day the eye should receive an instillation of the chosen antibiotic or the insertion of an antibiotic ointment. It is advisable in all cases of corneal ulceration to inquire into the habits of the patient. In children especially, attention should be given to the condition of the alimentary tract. Small doses of compound rhubarb powder (0·75–1G.) may be prescribed, to be taken three times a day. In adults, a pill of calomel and colocynth at night, followed by a saline purge in the morning, is often of great service in initiating the treatment.

When the ulcer is of a more severe nature it becomes necessary to adopt other local measures. Of these the most generally useful is painting with pure carbolic acid

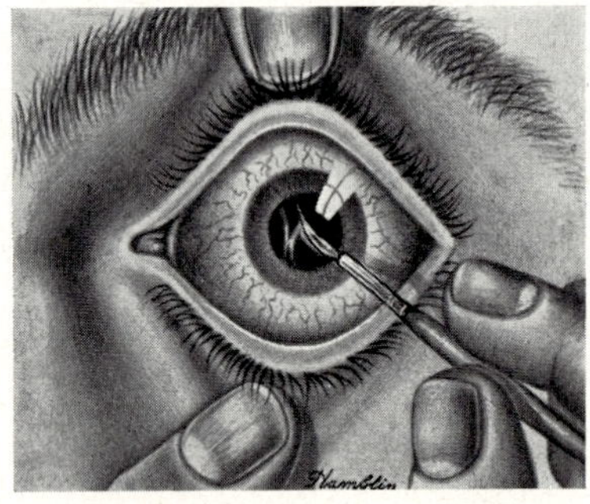

Fig. 476.—Application of pure carbolic to an ulcer of the cornea—for technique *see* text. The application is being made with a camel-hair brush, and the patient should be recumbent.

(*Fig.* 476). First put in two drops of cocaine, and then a drop of fluorescein (being careful to mop up any excess with a pad of absorbent wool). After a few seconds wash out the fluorescein with cocaine, and the ulcer will be found stained bright green. With two fingers of the left hand hold the lids gently apart; dry the surface of the ulcer with a small piece of sterilized blotting-paper, and touch the whole stained surface with a small camel-hair brush soaked in pure carbolic acid. Dry off any excess of this with blotting-paper and wash out the eye with saline or boric lotion before allowing the lids to close. The end of a wooden match carefully pointed and soaked in carbolic is an excellent substitute for the brush. If the ulcer is of the advancing type, most attention should be devoted to the advancing edge. The benefit of using pure carbolic is that it is itself an anæsthetic. After touching with phenol, continuous boric acid fomentations, with free hot bathings at each change, and atropine drops twice a day, should be ordered.

Pus forming in the anterior chamber (hypopyon) is not in these cases a sign of serious inflammatory involvement of the iris and ciliary body. The pus is usually sterile. It is probably most frequently seen in pneumococcal ulceration. It may form very rapidly, and with a healing ulcer it will become absorbed as rapidly as it forms. If it is necessary to perform paracentesis, the hypopyon should be washed out with normal saline.

When an ulcer is deep and there is a likelihood of perforation, no treatment is so valuable as lamellar keratoplasty. If an ulcer is allowed to perforate spontaneously, it is almost certain that the iris will prolapse in the rush of aqueous that takes place, and, lying in contact with the edges of the ulcer, will certainly become adherent if not removed. Should the ulcer become torpid, ionizing radiation, e.g., by Grenz rays, may stimulate it to heal.

5. SUBCONJUNCTIVAL INJECTIONS

These are being increasingly used in the treatment of inflammatory conditions of the eye, and are performed as follows: after instillation of decicain 0·5 per cent (or amethocaine)—3 drops at 3-minute intervals—a speculum is inserted, a fold of conjunctiva is picked up with fixation forceps, and the injection made by passing a fine hypodermic needle through the conjunctiva into the subconjunctival space. The usual site for injections is the lower outer quadrant of the eyeball, but other positions can be used. A solution used for hypopyon ulcers of the cornea is:—

℞	Crystalline Penicillin	1,000,000 units
	Mydricaine (a mydriatic)	0·30 ml.
	Adrenaline 1–1000	0·30 ml.
	Aq. Dest.	ad 1 ml.

Steroids.—Cortisone is also given by subconjunctival injections and is sometimes mixed with hyalase. Steroid treatment is contra-indicated if there is any possibility of a virus infection, e.g. dendritic ulcer.

Steroids have become increasingly used for self-limiting diseases such as uveitis and perivasculitis. Other indications are scleritis, pan-ophthalmitis, and temporal arteritis.

Contra-indications comprise peptic ulcer, pulmonary tuberculosis, diabetes, vascular hypertension, mental illness, congestive heart failure, and dendritic ulcer (*vide infra*).

Possible but rare complications during steroid treatment comprise Cushing's syndrome, defective glucose metabolism, increased protein metabolism, calcium absorption, osteoporosis, potassium depletion, restriction of growth in children, and posterior cortical cataract.

Mydricaine is a non-proprietary preparation containing atropine and a local anæsthetic (obtainable from Moorfields Eye Hospital, London).

For lesions limited to the anterior chamber, predsol may be used in the form of drops, instilled hourly or every half-hour, according to the severity of the case. Hydrocortisone ointment is placed inside the lower lid to maintain treatment during the night.

Systemic treatment is needed if the disease is farther back. In this case, give 15 mg. of prednisolone daily, doubling the dose in 3 days if there is no improvement.

In obstinate cases the dose may have to be increased further, up to as much as 60 mg. a day.

An alternative method, requiring in-patient treatment, is to start with 60 mg. of prednisolone daily. In both cases when improvement occurs, the dose should be reduced gradually, periodic blood examinations being carried out.

Recent work goes to show that some of the contra-indications quoted above are not so important. Thus, if diabetes should develop during treatment, it can be dealt with, and, if a tuberculous focus should light up, it can be controlled. The outlook therefore for steroid therapy would seem to have improved.

B. IN THE WARDS

1. CATARACT

Pre-operative Treatment for Cataract Cases.—The lids and conjunctiva should be carefully inspected for signs of conjunctivitis, and the patency or otherwise of the lacrimal passages determined by pressure over the sac (*see* p. 619), or in doubtful cases by syringeing. Conjunctival swabs and cultures were at one time taken in every case. This is done at least 48 hours before operation, because it takes this length of time for the culture to grow. *Staph. albus* and *B. xerosis* (a diphtheroid) are regarded as non-pathogenic, but the presence of *Staph. aureus*, pneumococcus, streptococcus, etc., demands postponement of operation, and local treatment with lotions and drops until a clean culture is obtained. It is important, when taking the second culture, to stop all treatment for the previous 24 hours. Some surgeons nowadays omit cultures, and, according to their writings, with no untoward effect, especially if penicillin drops, 2500 units per ml., are employed pre-operatively.

The patient should be admitted the night before operation, when a mild laxative is given, and the opportunity is taken of testing the urine, estimating the ocular tension, and measuring the blood-pressure. If the latter is raised, special precautions (e.g., blood-letting) may be required if intra-ocular hæmorrhage at operation is to be avoided. It is also usual to cut the lashes, using scissors which have been dipped in petroleum jelly, so that the hairs adhere to the blades instead of going into the conjunctival sac.

The administration of a pre-operative sedative is advisable, various drugs being used. It is important to choose one which will not cause vomiting. In the writer's experience, nembutal 0·1–0·2 G., according to the weight of the patient, an hour before operation, is satisfactory. If this is done, a further 0·2 G. about 12 hours later usually secures a good night's sleep. Only a light easily digested breakfast should be allowed.

If the operation is to be done with a dilated pupil, a drop of sterile watery homatropine and cocaine, 2 per cent, is instilled $1\frac{1}{2}$ hours before, and repeated in 5 minutes. The cocaine drops (5 per cent) are started 40 minutes before operation and repeated every 10 minutes for three further instillations, and then every 5 minutes. At the last instillation, a drop is put into the fellow eye too. The patient should be told to keep his eyes closed between instillations or the corneal epithelium may become hazy. It is inadvisable to cover the eye because it may open and sustain a corneal abrasion from the under-surface of the pad. A fair proportion of cataract extractions and glaucoma operations are performed nowadays under general anæsthesia, in which case pre-operative medication is under the control of the anæsthetist.

Post-operative Treatment.—In the absence of pain, both eyes are usually covered for 48 hours, and during this period the patient is kept as quiet as possible. If corneoscleral sutures have been employed, it usually suffices to cover only one eye. It is no longer considered necessary for him to lie flat, because doing so often produces severe pain in the lumbar region. The usual procedure is to nurse him in the semi-recumbent position, and for this purpose a Lawson Tait bed is admirable, particularly as the patient can be kept comfortable by altering his position a little now and again, without disturbing him.

He should be carefully watched during the first few days to prevent him rubbing the eye during sleep or on waking. Whenever possible, a special nurse should be employed day and night for this purpose, failing which the sleeves of the night attire should be pinned over the breast while the patient is unattended. Some form of protection to the eyes is advisable: Fuch's lattice shield can be employed if procurable, but this is rather heavy, and just as good or even better is a cartella eye shield (*Fig.* 477). A satisfactory dressing consists of a small square of tulle gras over the closed lids, surmounted by a pad small

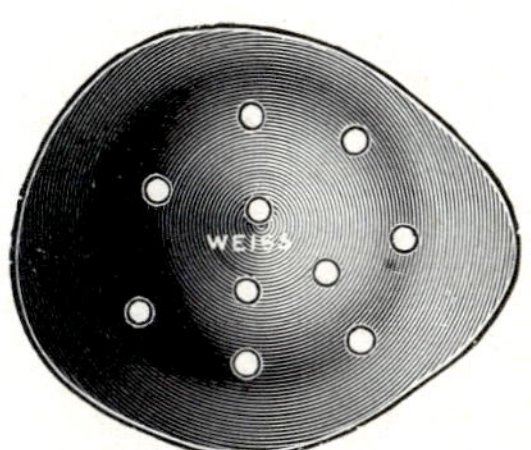

Fig. 477.—Cartella shield.

enough to be covered by the cartella and secured in place by a strip of zinc oxide strapping. Two strips of the same material are used to fix the shield and no bandage is required.

At the first dressing, the utmost gentleness should be employed. The pads are carefully soaked off by a few drops of sterile saline from a pipette. This is seldom necessary if a layer of tulle gras has been applied to the closed lids at the end of the operation. The edges of the lids are cleaned with pledgets of sterile cotton-wool wound around small sticks and soaked in sterile saline, being careful to exercise no direct pressure on the lids, but to employ the pledgets in the same way as a painter would a brush. If, as is usually the case, the upper lid of the operated eye is held down by a stitch, this should be left in situ, the plaster securing the lower end to the cheek being detached. The stitch can then be used to raise the upper lid, without exerting pressure on the lid itself. If all is well with the eye the stitch can be removed, but, if complications have occurred, it may be useful to re-attach it to the cheek. The unoperated eye should be opened first and the procedure carried out in a partly darkened room. To open the operated eye, the patient should be told to try first to open both for himself. If this is not possible, he should open the unaffected eye, while the house-surgeon gently draws down the lower lid of the operated eye, and, by means of the stitch, gently draws up the upper lid. Some form of inspection lamp should be at hand, with which focused light can be directed from the side on to the eye.

A quick glance should suffice to tell if:—

a. The pupil is round (i.e., the iris has not prolapsed through the wound).

b. The anterior chamber has re-formed (i.e., the wound has become sealed).

c. The anterior chamber is free of blood.

A drop of atropine is instilled and a pad applied. The other eye should have a cover over it which is secured above but not below, so that the patient can take an occasional look by raising the cover, but he should not be allowed to do much of this. After the lapse of a further 48 hours, the dressing is removed if all is well, and dark glasses with side-pieces are worn during the day, the protective cardboard shield being worn at night.

During the first 4 days the food should be soft enough not to require mastication, and if the bowels do not act naturally a mild aperient can be given on the evening of the third day. It is usual for the patient to get up for an hour or two on the fifth day, staying out of bed for gradually increasing periods each succeeding day. With modern technique—corneoscleral stitches and a sutured conjunctival flap—it is possible to allow the patient out of bed considerably earlier, sometimes on the day following the operation and to cover only the operated eye. In these cases, the corneoscleral stitch has to be removed, usually on the tenth day, unless some absorbable material has been used.

Removal of the stitch is an operation of some delicacy and in nervous subjects thiopentone anæsthesia may be required, though usually local measures will suffice. In these cases, 4 drops of cocaine 4 per cent or decicain 0·5 per cent are instilled at 3-minute intervals. The upper lid is then gently raised with a squint hook or silver wire retractor and a few crystals of solid cocaine applied to the region of the stitch, the recumbent patient being directed to look towards his feet. The eye is kept closed for a further 3 minutes, washed out with a few drops of penicillin, and the patient told to look down again, the upper lid being gently retracted if necessary. The knot of the suture is now grasped with fine forceps and pulled gently forwards so as to allow one blade of a fine pair of scissors to be passed under the silk, which is then cut through to allow the suture to be removed.

Conjunctival sutures, if of the interrupted type, frequently cut out, but if they have to be removed they should be dealt with before the corneoscleral suture in case the patient squeezes his eye.

Complications.—

1. *Hæmorrhage.*—It sometimes happens that a leakage of blood occurs from the wound into the anterior chamber (hyphæma) about the fourth or fifth day after operation, particularly if the incision has been scleral rather than at the limbus. Should this occur, the patient should be kept in bed, the eye covered with a pad (both, if the hæmorrhage is large) and some form of hæmostatic serum given. Hemostyl by the mouth for four or five mornings is usually satisfactory, particularly if it is combined with adequate doses of vitamins C (200 mg.), and K (20 mg.), three times daily.

2. *Iris Prolapse.*—This is shown by the iris protruding through the wound and by the pupil being oval. Treatment calls for a high degree of skill and should not be attempted by the inexperienced. If the prolapse is only slight or is threatening, instillation of eserine, 0·5 per cent, may suffice.

3. *Infection.*—This again calls for skilled handling, the administration of sulphonamides, antibiotics, and cortisone, and the application of short-wave diathermy being among the measures used. Its occurrence is shown by increased redness of the eye, exudate in the anterior chamber, and sometimes, but not always, by pain.

2. GLAUCOMA CASES

A. **Chronic.**—Pre-operative treatment is the same as on p. 628, except that it is important not to dilate the pupil. Cocaine does have this effect, therefore local

---

Hemostyl (Don S. Momand Ltd., London, N.W.1).

anæsthesia is procured by instillation of a drug such as decicain, 0·5 per cent, using the time schedule already given. It is usual nowadays, however, to perform the operation under general anæsthesia. If under local, a retrobulbar injection of 1·5 ml. of lignocaine and adrenaline is used. If the operation is to be an iris inclusion, miotics should be discontinued for 12 hours before; if a trephine, they need not be.

Post-operative treatment is much the same as for cataract cases, except that only one eye is covered if its fellow, the unoperated one, is also glaucomatous and is having miotic drops. If iris inclusion has been performed, instillation of pilocarpine, 2 per cent, is started at the first dressing and gentle massage is usually begun then, too. This is done by directing the patient to look upwards and exerting pressure with the finger through the lower lid on to the ball of the eye, making slight rotary movements. During the first week massage is done for half a minute, twice daily, a drop of 2 per cent pilocarpine being instilled

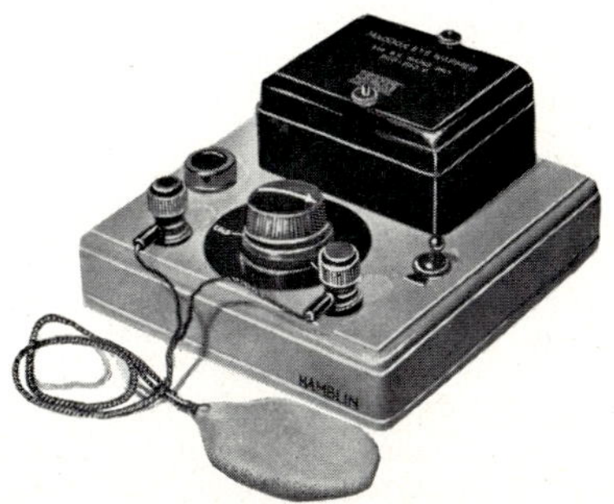

Fig. 478.—Electric heater.

5 minutes previously. At the end of the first week the period is increased to 1 minute, and, in a few more days, to 2 minutes. The patient is shown how to massage the eye himself and is advised to continue this and the pilocarpine for 6 months.

If the operation has been a trephine, atropine is generally used for the first fortnight or so and massage is not done. In both cases, stitches are removed under cocaine at the end of the first 10 days.

B. **Acute.**—Preliminary measures comprise the administration of a free purge, and the administration of diamox* 250 mg. 6-hourly for 24 hours, and then twice daily. Eserine, 1 per cent, in ol. ric. is instilled every 10 minutes for half an hour, then every half-hour until the tension falls or operation is decided upon. The first instillation should be into both eyes, because of the liability of the fellow eye to develop the same condition.

The application of an electric heater (*Fig.* 478), retro-ocular injection of lignocaine and adrenaline, or the use of short-wave diathermy is often helpful, if diamox fails to lower the tension.

---

* Diamox (Lederle Laboratories Ltd., London, W.C.2), a diuretic, diminishes the secretion of aqueous. It is given by mouth, 250 mg. 6-hourly for 24 hours, then twice daily, and may produce a marked lowering of intra-ocular pressure. During the time of its administration it is advisable to give Pot. Bicarb. 0·6 G. t.d.s. in the form of a mixture by mouth.

In the absence of nephritis or marked arterial degeneration, slow intravenous injection of a hypertonic solution may bring the tension of the eye down. Recommended solutions are sucrose, 25 per cent in 400 ml.; dextrose, 50 per cent in 100 ml.; or sodium chloride, 30 per cent in 50 ml. The first is given over a period of 45 to 60 minutes, the others can be given more quickly. Urea is sometimes used and the technique is to give 1 G. in 15 ml. of water three times daily for a week, then tail off gradually if the pressure comes down.

If the ocular tension can be brought down before operation, its performance is easier and the result more likely to be satisfactory. It can be carried out under general anæsthesia—thiopentone (*see* p. 123) is particularly useful—or after retro-ocular injection of lignocaine and adrenaline. The advantage of the latter is that it often softens the eye, especially if a 2 per cent solution is used. The simplest way of doing this is by inserting a long-fine hypodermic needle through the lower lid, along the junction of the floor and lateral wall of the orbit for 4 cm., turning the point medially towards the end of its travel, and injecting 1·5–2 ml. of 1 per cent lignocaine. It is usually advisable to wait 10 minutes before commencing the operation.

Post-operative treatment is on the lines already laid down for cataract.

3. DETACHED RETINA

While operating for this condition, it is essential to make periodic ophthalmo-scopic examinations; the cornea must, therefore, be clear, and anæsthetic drops are not used. The pupil, however, should be well dilated with atropine instilled three times daily for 2 days before operation, a final drop of phenyl epinepherine 10 per cent being put in 2 hours before the patient goes to the theatre. Whenever possible the operation is performed under general anæsthesia. Should this be impossible, however, local anæsthesia can be secured by lignocaine (1 per cent) injections: (1) Through the lower lid at the junction of the middle and outer thirds, the needle being passed along the bony floor of the orbit for 1·5 in. (3·75 cm.) before 1·5 ml. are injected; (2) From the outer canthus, infiltrating upper and lower lids.

After operation, the lids are closed and covered with a small piece of tulle gras. Over this on each side are placed pledgets of cotton-wool, carefully packed so as to support the eyes. The cotton-wool pads are secured by four strips of isinglass or zinc-oxide plaster. Over this is placed a binocular pad of cotton-wool held in place by a cataract bandage. A cardboard shield can be used as well if necessary.

The patient should be arranged in bed so that as far as possible the hole in the retina is in a dependent position. The first dressing is done in 3 days, and the second after another 3 days, at which time a rapid ophthalmoscopic exami-nation may be made. Subsequent dressings are done on alternate days and on each occasion a drop of atropine is instilled into the eye. The eyes are kept covered for 3 weeks, at the end of which time the patient dons detachment spectacles—dark glasses with side pieces, the lenses rendered opaque with black paper or vulcanite, except for a central hole about 2 mm. in diameter (*Fig.* 479). These are usually worn for a further 2–3 months, their object being to prevent the patient moving his eyes about and so re-detaching the retina before it has become firmly fixed.

Modifications in the operative treatment of retinal detachment have been introduced recently. By their use, a higher percentage of successes is obtained.

The underlying principle is to bring the sclera nearer the retina. There are various ways of doing this. The simplest is to pass a thread of supramid around the eyeball under the insertions of the extra-ocular muscles and tying it sufficiently tight to indent the sclera, but not to cause retinal arterial pulsation. Alternative methods comprise lamellar resection of a crescent of sclera, sewing the

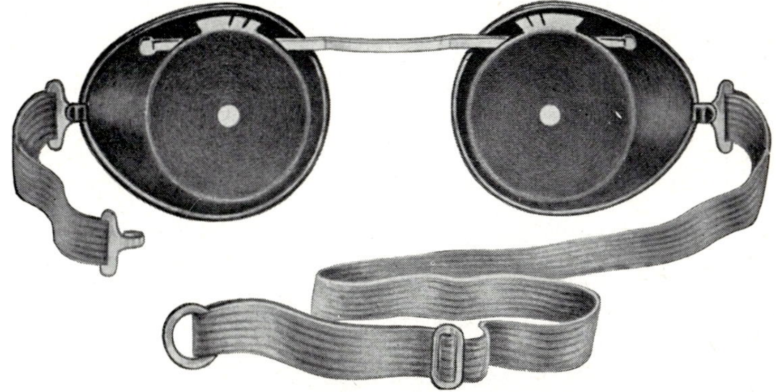

Fig. 479.—Detachment glasses.

edges together, or embedding some neutral substance such as silicone rubber before doing so.

After-treatment is usually simpler. Both eyes are covered at first, but after 3–4 days, if all is going well, only the operated eye is covered. The patient is allowed out of bed in a week and home in 12 days.

4. CORNEAL GRAFTS

Pre-operative treatment is the same as for other intra-ocular operations. The post-operative régime varies with different surgeons and techniques. A typical one is: First dressing 36–48 hours after operation when a culture is taken from the conjunctival sac and gutt. atropine 1 per cent and penicillin are instilled. Subsequently, the eye is dressed daily, the cornea being cocainized and cleaned of mucus adhering to it, after which, atropine 1 per cent and penicillin are instilled. Cortisone drops are begun on the tenth day and continued for several weeks, to prevent vascularization of the graft. The sutures are removed between the tenth and fourteenth days.

5. SQUINT

The angle of deviation should be estimated before operation, so that the latter can be regulated to meet the needs of the case. There are several methods of which Priestly-Smith's is the simplest. His tape is in two pieces joined by a ring; one is plain and the other is marked in degrees on a tangent scale, so that with the two tapes at right angles to each other, the angle between the plain tape and a point on the marked one is indicated by the marking (*Fig.* 480).

To use the tape, the patient puts a finger through the distal end of the plain tape, and holds it against her cheek. The house-surgeon holds the proximal ring against an electric ophthalmoscope, which he shines into the patient's eyes, directing her to look at the light, and notes the position of the corneal

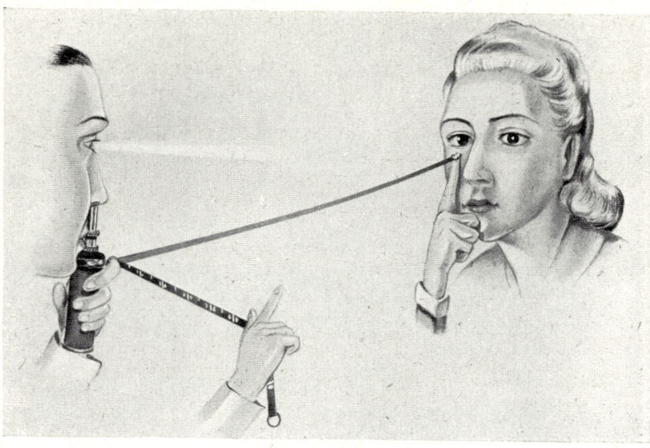

Fig. 480.—Examination for squint by Priestly-Smith tape. When looking straight, the patient has a convergent squint in the left eye. When fixing examiner's finger with her right eye, the left eye swings outwards and brings the corneal reflex into the centre of the pupil. The angle of squint is 45°, i.e., number opposite which examiner's finger is placed on tape when left eye appears to be straight.

reflection of it in the straight eye—it is usually a little to the inner side of the centre of the pupil. He now takes the marked tape between his fingers, asks the patient to watch them, and moves them along the tape until the corneal reflex in the squinting eye corresponds with the position it occupied in the previously straight eye. The number covered by his fingers on the marked tape will represent the angle of the squint.

The majority of squint operations are performed under general anæsthesia, and the patient should be adequately prepared for this. If local anæsthesia is used, deep injections into the orbit are needed, though some surgeons rely on cocaine drops aided perhaps by rubbing a little solid cocaine into the conjunctiva over the insertions of the muscles which are to be operated upon. The patient's face should be covered by a mask with a slit in it for the eye, and the surgeon and his assistants usually wear gloves.

Both eyes are covered after operation, and the first dressing is done 24–48 hours later. The pads are not usually discarded until 4–5 days later, when detachment spectacles can be worn for a further 10 days. The conjunctival stitches are removed under cocaine in a week, but if the child is nervous they can be left and will cut out in a few weeks. There is sometimes considerable swelling and redness of the conjunctiva after a squint operation, but if this is unaccompanied by rise of temperature or pulse it need occasion no anxiety. If there is reason to suspect infection, a culture should be taken, sulphonamides or antibiotics given, and hot bathing instituted.

6. ENUCLEATION

Enucleation of the eye is again usually performed under general anæsthesia, though local instillation of cocaine and retro-ocular injections as for detached retina will allow of its being done painlessly. The main point in post-operative treatment is to prevent hæmorrhage from the socket, which is achieved by packing it with petroleum jelly gauze before putting on the pad, or by incorporating a small ball of gamgee tissue in the pad and bandaging it firmly. If the optic nerve is divided by tightening a wire snare, instead of using a pair of scissors, there is little if any bleeding.

7. PTOSIS OPERATIONS

These require special after-treatment, because the eye cannot be closed and the cornea is therefore exposed. The simplest method is to apply a celluloid cone (*see* p. 623), fixing it all the way round with strapping so as to make it air-tight; the presence of drops of condensed moisture on the inside of the cone indicates that this has been achieved and that the eye can be left with its cornea exposed and no risk of ulceration. Another method is to cover the cornea by the lower lid, which is drawn up by means of a suture passed through it and attached to the forehead by strapping.

OPHTHALMOSCOPY

The electric ophthalmoscope provides a means for ready examination of the fundus oculi. Although interpretation of the findings requires considerable experience, it has been thought advisable to illustrate some of the more important surgical conditions which may be disclosed by the use of this instrument. These are depicted in *Figs*. 481–485.

Fig. 481 shows a normal fundus except for the greyish-white area underlying the upper temporal vessels. This is caused by the presence of a very early glioma of the retina (retinoblastoma), a highly malignant growth occurring in children at the age of about two years. It is not usually diagnosed until a more advanced stage, when it has filled the vitreous chamber and forms a white mass visible in the pupil.

Fig. 482 shows the appearances produced by a malignant melanoma of the choroid in the upper outer quadrant of the fundus. The retina is pushed forwards by the underlying growth, some of the vessels of which are visible. The retinal vessels appear darker over the affected area because of the lack of red reflex behind them.

Fig. 483 explains the appearances seen in *Fig*. 482. It is a vertical section of an eye containing a malignant melanoma of the choroid. Ophthalmoscopically the appearances would be similar to those in *Fig*. 482, except that the whole retina is detached, the portion not overlying the growth being separated from the back of the eye by an accumulation of fluid. This is a common complication in melanoma and makes ophthalmoscopic diagnosis from a simple detachment of the retina more difficult. The small brown area in the upper part of the iris represents a second melanotic growth.

Fig. 484 represents an advanced stage of papillœdema, i.e., œdema of the optic disk (or papilla) brought about by an increase in cerebrospinal fluid pressure.

Compare with the disk in *Fig*. 481, and note: (1) blurring of edges; (2) striate hæmorrhages; (3) turgescence of veins; (4) partial hiding of arteries; (5) wrinkles

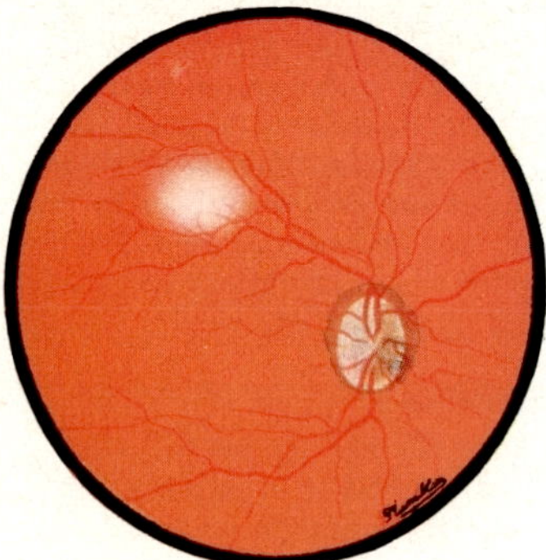

Fig. 481.—Early glioma of the retina (vel. retinoblastoma).

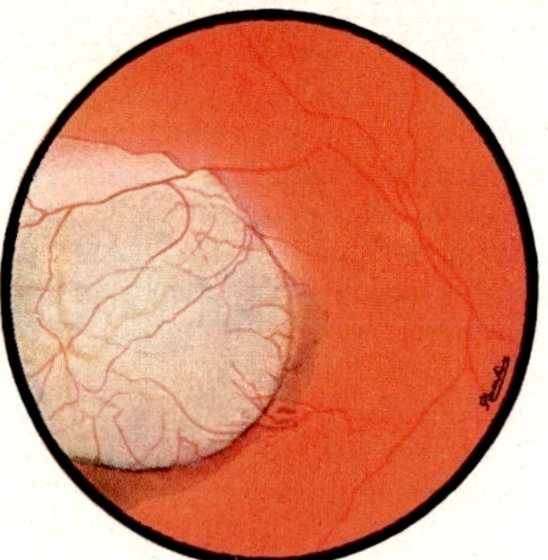

Fig. 482.—Melanoma of the choroid.

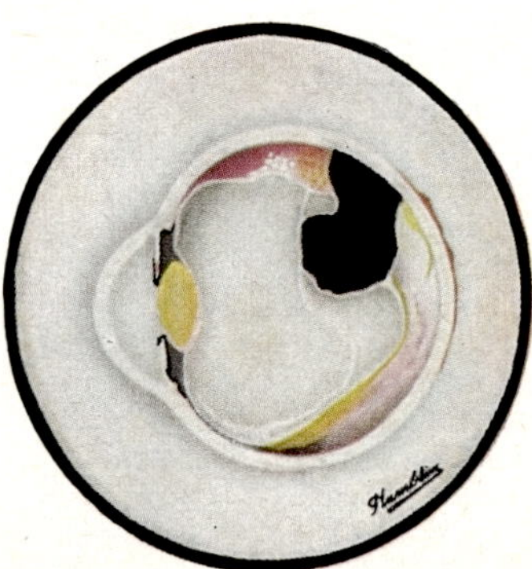

Fig. 483.—Vertical section of an eye containing a melanoma of the choroid.

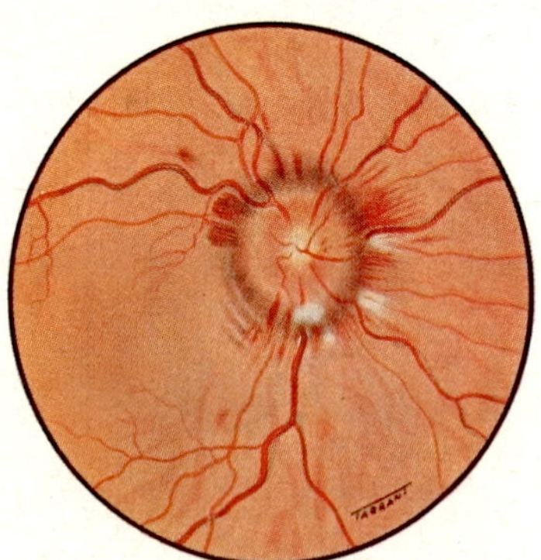

Fig. 484.—An advanced stage of papillœdema.

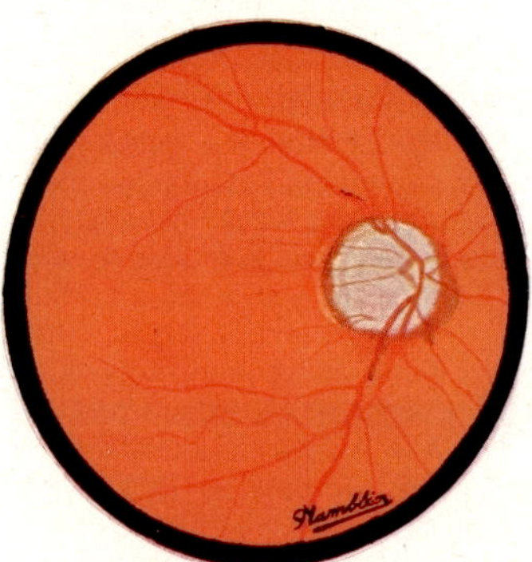

Fig. 485.—Optic atrophy.

in retina on temporal side of disk, concentric with its margin; (6) presence of a fan figure at the macula. This is not often seen, and its presence usually indicates that the rise in cerebrospinal fluid pressure has been rapid, e.g., in a subtentorial tumour; it is not shown in *Fig.* 484.

Fig. 485 shows the appearances in one of the forms of optic atrophy. The disk is greyish-white in colour and shows the stippling of the lamina cribrosa. The edges of the disk are clear and the calibre of the vessels unaffected. Such a condition is seen in tabes and in diseases (e.g., pituitary tumour) where optic atrophy is due to pressure on the nerve behind the point where the vessels leave it. In optic atrophy due to other causes (e.g., consequent on papilloedema) the vessels are usually reduced in calibre.

CHAPTER XLIII

EAR, NOSE, AND THROAT

By D. F. N. HARRISON

I. THE EAR

EXAMINATION OF THE EAR

THE house-surgeon must know how to examine the ear thoroughly, be able to recognize and treat the common and often very painful lesions of the external part of the auditory apparatus, and understand the principles of management of middle-ear infections.

It is obviously essential that any doctor who is prepared to diagnose and treat ear disease should be conversant with the normal appearances of those parts of

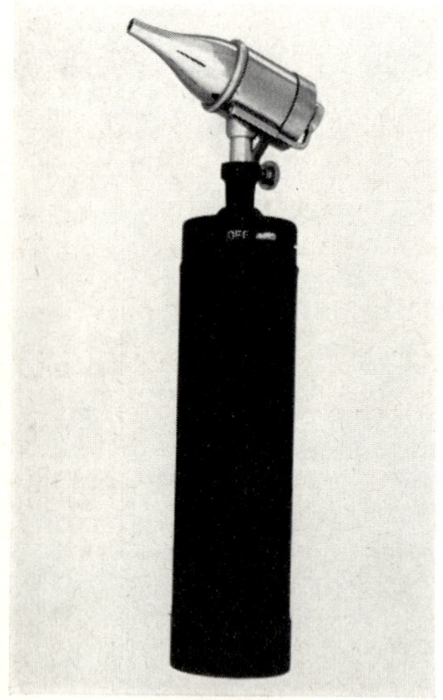

Fig. 486.—Battery-operated electric auroscope.

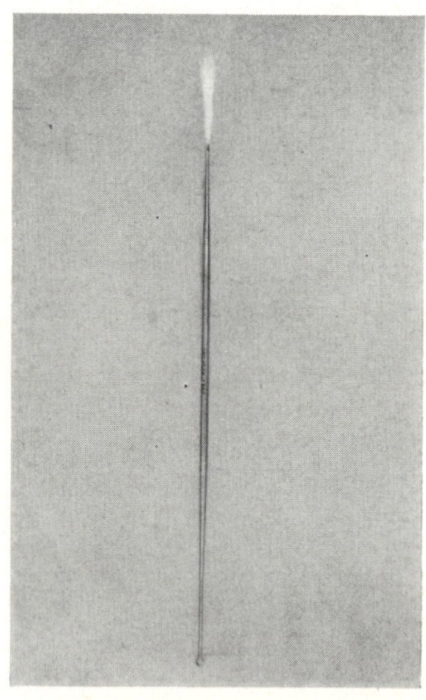

Fig. 487.—Jobson Horne wool carrier.

the auditory apparatus which can be readily inspected. These include the pinna and surrounding skin, external auditory meatus, and the tympanic membrane.

The pinna is readily available both for inspection and palpation, but a modern battery-operated electric auroscope (*Fig.* 486) is essential to examine the external

auditory meatus and tympanic membrane (or drumhead), although in skilled
hands the head mirror with appropriate light source has the advantage of
leaving both hands free for intrameatal manipulations.

Auroscopy.—In the adult the meatus runs a tortuous course and is straightened by lifting the pinna upwards and backwards, whilst gently pulling it outwards. However, in babies and young children the tympanic membrane is
almost horizontal and, since the bony meatus is undeveloped, the external canal
is virtually collapsed upon the drumhead. Exposure of the meatus and tympanic membrane is carried out by pulling the pinna downwards and backwards.
After selecting the appropriate aural speculum the instrument may be gently
introduced for a distance of about 0·5 in. (1·25 cm.). Soft wax and debris may
have to be removed to give an adequate view of these structures. Wooden ear
sticks are invariably too thick and provide poor adhesion for cotton-wool. It
is therefore advisable to use a proper wool carrier (*Fig.* 487), making certain
that the cotton-wool projects for a short distance beyond the end of the instrument to avoid damaging the drumhead.

The healthy tympanic membrane is greyish-white in colour and can be distinguished from the adjoining meatal skin by the handle of the malleus which lies
obliquely along its centre axis. From the tip of this ossicle a cone of light can
be seen passing downwards and forwards to the edge of the membrane (*Fig.*
488). This feature may be absent if the tympanic membrane is retracted, scarred,
or contains chalk patches, and
in such cases the short process
of the malleus may be unduly
prominent. In young children,
particularly when crying, it is
not uncommon for the drumhead to be pink in colour, but
this should not be confused with
early otitis media.

**Patency of the Eustachian
Tube.**—This may be tested by
observing movement of the cone
of light when the patient auto-
inflates. This test should not be
carried out if the patient has a cold or has pus in the nose or nasopharynx, for
fear of forcing infection into the middle ear.

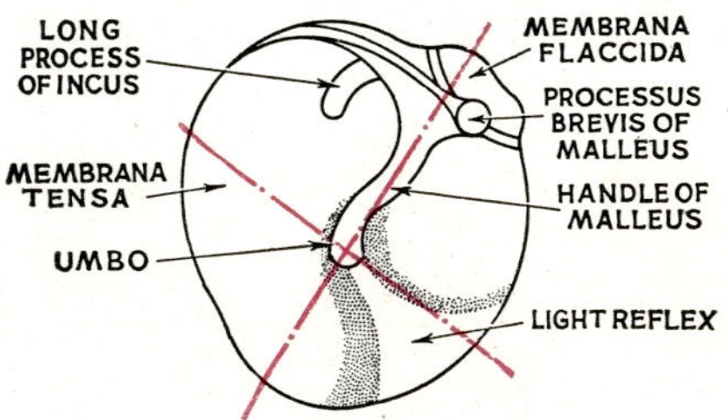

Fig. 488.—Diagram of the right tympanic membrane
as viewed through the electric auroscope.

Hearing Tests.—These should only be performed after ensuring that there is
no wax or discharge in the external ear. Both ears must be tested separately
with a conversation voice and then a soft whisper. In reasonably quiet surroundings a normal person will hear a whisper at 20 ft. (6 metres). The tuning
fork (usually of 256 double vibrations) is useful for differentiating between conductive and perceptive deafness. It should be activated by striking a prong against
the elbow—not a firm surface such as a table as overtones will be produced.
Normally an airborne sound is heard for about twice as long as when the fork is
placed on the bone of the mastoid process. The duration of bone conduction
is reduced in perceptive deafness, whilst in conditions which impair sound
conduction across the middle ear the sounded tuning fork will be heard better
by bone conduction than by air conduction.

In any examination carried out upon the auditory apparatus adequate illumination and the utmost gentleness are imperative.

HÆMATOMA OF THE PINNA

Trauma to the pinna may lead to bleeding between the cartilage and perichondrium. This condition is common in boxers and, if the hæmatoma is allowed to organize, the resulting fibrosis will lead to distortion of the pinna—the cauliflower ear.

Aspiration of the unclotted blood is effective if the patient is seen soon enough. This procedure must be carried out aseptically to prevent subsequent infection and perichondritis. Following removal of the blood, a pressure dressing must be applied to prevent reaccumulation. Cotton-wool pads are placed in front and behind the ear, and a crêpe bandage is then applied to bind the ear against the side of the skull. If the blood has clotted, surgical evacuation is desirable, the incision being placed along the margin of the helix.

REMOVAL OF WAX

Wax is usually removed by syringeing, but this method is inadvisable if there is a history of previous ear discharge. In such cases the wax may be removed under direct vision using a wax hook, a procedure which is both difficult and dangerous in a young child.

Normal saline, at a temperature of 38° C. (100° F.), is usually used as an irrigating fluid. Variations from this temperature may lead to labyrinthine

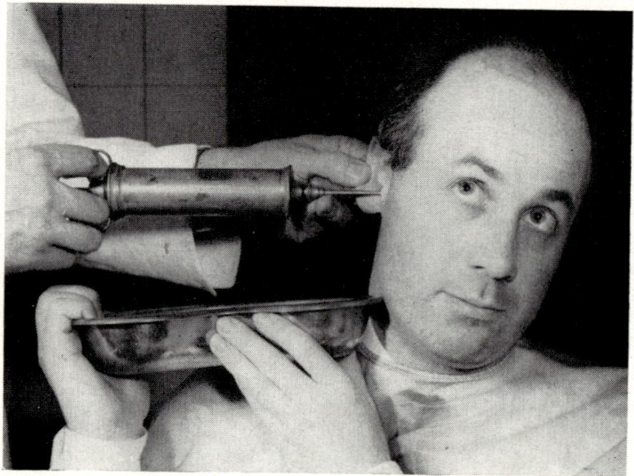

Fig. 489.—Syringeing the ear.

irritation and vertigo. A Higginson's syringe attached to a metal cannula is perhaps the safest instrument to use for irrigation, although metal syringes are in common use. Care must be taken with the latter to ensure that the nozzle is firmly attached to the body of the syringe. When using either instrument the metal cannula must be supported in the external ear to prevent sudden head movements forcing the metal end into the deep meatus or even perforating the tympanic membrane. It is extremely doubtful if excessive pressure of the irrigating fluid has ever perforated a normal tympanic membrane; the usual practice is to maintain a pressure consistent with the comfort of the patient (*Fig.* 489).

Before beginning the irrigation the meatus is straightened by pulling the pinna in the appropriate direction and the fluid is then directed along the meatal roof —never directly onto the wax plug. After syringeing and inspection to ensure that no wax remains, the meatus is gently mopped with cotton-wool.

If the wax is found to be extremely hard then it should be softened before any attempt at removal is made. Instillation of a few drops of olive oil twice a day for a week is invariably effective. Some proprietary preparations cause painful skin reactions and should be avoided.

FOREIGN BODIES IN THE EXTERNAL AUDITORY MEATUS

Most foreign bodies are deliberately introduced into the ear by the patient, although occasionally insects enter accidentally or a piece of cotton-wool is left behind after aural toilet. Consequently the majority of patients are either children or are mentally retarded.

Many metallic objects will cause meatal inflammation (otitis externa) and ill-advised attempts at removal invariably result in bleeding and swelling, which makes subsequent removal difficult if not impossible. These objects are best removed by syringeing, which is an effective method of removing most small objects. However, vegetable matter, if hydroscopic, may swell; it may best be removed with small forceps under direct vision. If the object is a close fit in the meatus syringeing will drive it deeper and the best method of removal is by passing a blunt hook beyond the obstruction and then drawing both out laterally. This method is the safest for the majority of foreign bodies, but requires gentleness and patient co-operation. Forceps must *never* be used for smooth, rounded bodies such as beads.

If an insect is alive it should be killed by instilling surgical spirit into the external ear.

A general anæsthetic is necessary for the removal of all foreign bodies in children and apprehensive adults.

Occasionally the object is tightly impacted in the deep meatus and removal necessitates opening the meatus via a post-auricular approach—a procedure requiring surgical experience but rarely requiring emergency action.

FURUNCULOSIS

A furuncle, or boil, is an infection of a hair follicle usually with *Staphylococcus pyogenes* and only occurs in the cartilaginous part of the external auditory meatus. It is frequently associated with otitis externa which causes irritation and scratching, but recurrent furunculosis is not uncommon in diabetics.

The inflammation causes tenderness in the external ear and is aggravated by moving the pinna or opening the jaw. Increased meatal swelling may result in complete occlusion of the lumen with deafness. Extension of infection outside the cartilaginous meatus produces post-auricular œdema and forward displacement of the pinna. Such patients may be diagnosed as suffering from acute mastoiditis if no view of the tympanic membrane is possible (*Table XVIII*).

Pain is severe but resolves rapidly when the furuncle bursts. In the early stages of the infection local heat is soothing and if the meatus is not occluded it may be packed with narrow ribbon gauze impregnated with magnesium sulphate paste. However, in severe cases, especially with post-auricular œdema, antibiotic therapy is indicated and systemic penicillin is the antibiotic of choice. Cloxacillin or fucidin may be needed for resistant staphylococci (*see* p. 75).

Table XVIII.—DIAGNOSTIC SIGNS OF FURUNCULOSIS AND ACUTE MASTOIDITIS

SIGN	FURUNCULOSIS	ACUTE MASTOIDITIS
Displacement of pinna	Forwards	Classically forwards and downwards
Post-auricular tenderness	Diffuse	Maximum tenderness over mastoid tip and antrum
Palpable lymph-nodes	Pre-auricular and infra-meatal	Absent
Movement of pinna	Pain	No pain
Deafness	Conductive	Conductive

OTITIS EXTERNA

The skin lining the external auditory meatus is normally resistant to infection. However, exposure to a hot humid environment together with local trauma from scratching reduces this resistance and may lead to infection with organisms such as *Bacillus pyocyaneus*, *B. proteus*, and *Staph. aureus*.

Secondary otitis externa may result from the constant bathing of the meatal lining with pus in patients with a chronic suppurative otitis media and the tympanic membrane must be examined in every patient with otitis externa at some stage of the disease.

In the acute stage the symptoms are similar to those of meatal furunculosis, with soreness and later pain in the ear accentuated by movements of the jaw or pinna. Examination of the meatal skin shows it to be red and swollen with pus in the external auditory meatus. After taking a swab for detection of the invading organism, the lumen should be cleared of all discharge and this must be carried out both gently and thoroughly. The meatus is then packed with $\frac{1}{2}$-in. ribbon gauze impregnated with glycerin and ichthyol or, if available, hydrocortisone cream. Topical antibiotics should be avoided since they frequently lead to skin sensitization and prolongation of symptoms.

In the chronic stage the main complaint is of recurrent irritation—often worse at night—and discharge. Reduction in the calibre of the meatus due to thickening of the skin makes aural toilet difficult, but thorough cleansing of all pus and debris is essential and may be aided by dipping the cotton-wool swabs in 1 per cent cetavlon. Daily packing with cortisone-impregnated ribbon gauze usually enlarges the meatus and will reduce irritation. Later this cream can be applied by the patient directly to the external meatus. Once again topical antibiotics should be avoided.

Fungal Infection.—Failure to respond to the above régime may be due to fungal infection. This condition appears to be increasing in frequency, probably as a result of ill-advised and over-enthusiastic use of local antibiotics. The fungi most commonly encountered are *Aspergillus niger* and *Candida albicans*, and both cause irritation in the ear and occasionally acute pain. Meticulous removal of all debris from the meatus is essential in the control of this condition and should be followed by the application of specific anti-fungal agents such as nystatin cream or amphotericin B lotion. In resistant cases the mercury preparation penotrane is valuable, but treatment must always be maintained, whatever the drug employed, for at least one week after the external auditory meatus has returned to normal. The patient should be warned to protect the ears from the ingress of water or shampoo by the use of petroleum jelly-impregnated cotton-wool plugs, for these conditions show a marked tendency to relapse.

Penotrane (Ward, Blenkinsop & Co Ltd., Wembley, Middlesex).

ACUTE OTITIS MEDIA

Acute infections of the middle-ear cleft are usually the sequel to upper respiratory tract infections or complicate the exanthemata. In young children the Eustachian tube is both wide and straight; consequently milk or vomit may readily enter the middle ear when the child is lying down, and result in infection.

The commonest organisms to cause middle-ear infection are the *Streptococcus pneumoniæ* and *Hæmophilus influenzæ*, and the symptoms of this condition will vary according to the organism, age of the patient, and degree of pneumatization of the mastoid air cells.

The presence of pathogenic organisms in the middle ear results in engorgement of the mucosa and pouring out of secretion into the cavity. This increase in pressure causes pain,

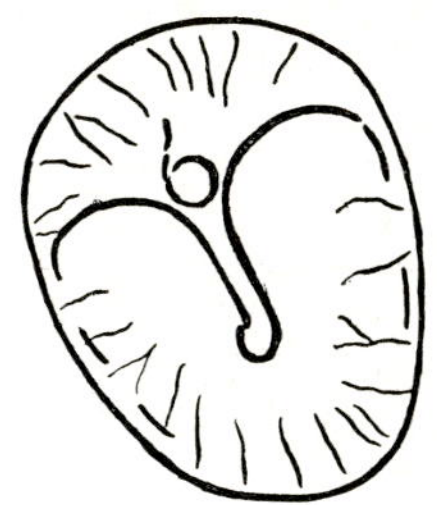

Fig. 490.—Early acute otitis media.

frequently in the mastoid process, and eventually rupture of the tympanic membrane secondary to interference with its blood-supply.

Early symptoms are therefore:—

1. Deafness—due to the mucosal swelling.
2. Pain—a result of increased intratympanic pressure.
3. Discharge—if the tympanic membrane ruptures.

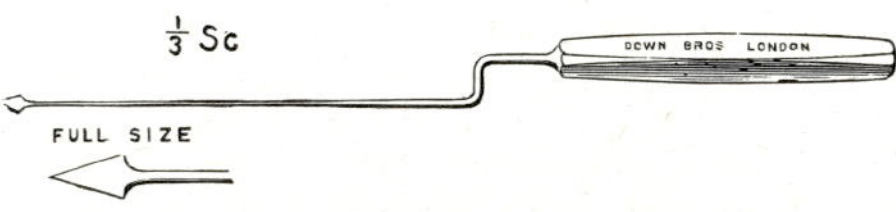

Fig. 491.—Fagge's myringotome.

The earliest change produced in the drumhead is a leash of vessels running down the handle of the malleus and multiple small vessels extending from the periphery of the drum towards the centre (*Fig.* 490). There may be spontaneous regression at this stage, but if the infection progresses to a suppurative otitis the entire membrane becomes red and increased pressure in the middle ear will cause bulging outwards into the meatus and eventually rupture.

Treatment.—In the earliest infections the use of inhalations of menthol or tinct. benz. co. twice daily together with vasoconstrictor nose drops—ephedrine 0·5 per cent in normal saline —will encourage drainage of the middle-ear secretions down the Eustachian tube. Warm olive-oil ear drops are soothing, but antibiotic drops are ineffective with an intact tympanic membrane.

Myringotomy.—If relief of symptoms does not occur within 12 hours, or the patient is

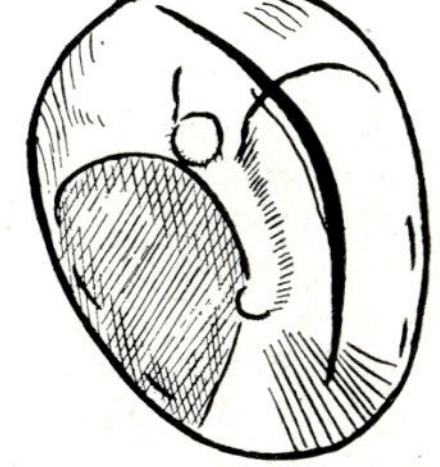

Fig. 492.—Incision for myringotomy.

first seen with a red bulging drum then myringotomy should be carried out under general anæsthesia. This can be performed through the speculum of an electric auroscope using a fine myringotomy knife (*Fig.* 491). The incision is made at the point of maximum convexity and from below upwards just behind the handle of the malleus (*Fig.* 492). Blood and pus may have to be gently sucked out. This procedure brings rapid relief from pain and after a full course of systemic antibiotics the incision should heal and hearing return to normal. In all probability the ear will begin to discharge following myringotomy and the pus must be removed by gentle swabbing followed by insufflation of 2 per cent iodine in boracic powder. In young children aural toilet may be impossible and syringeing with an all-rubber instrument will be safer and more effective. When possible the meatus should be dried afterwards and iodine-boracic powder inserted.

Management in Infants.—Acute otitis media is common in infants and, because the tympanic membrane is particularly tough at this age, otorrhœa is usually a late symptom. The patient cannot complain of pain in the ears or deafness and medical attention is usually sought because of restlessness, poor feeding, diarrhœa, and vomiting, or because the baby is generally unwell. Pulling or rubbing of the ears may draw attention to this region—or be explained as teething pains, the diagnosis only being established after examination of both tympanic membranes using an electric auroscope. The meatus and speculum are small and the drumhead difficult to see. Although the membrane may be red and bulging this is less common than a dull, lustreless, full appearance or even only a loss of the light reflex.

If pus is thought to be present then myringotomy under general anæsthesia is indicated. Alternatively, chemotherapy or antibiotic therapy may be started, although this will rapidly mask many of the acute symptoms and make evaluation of the final state of the treated ear difficult. It is therefore essential that adequate dosage of such drugs be both given and maintained for at least 48 hours after the return of the temperature to normal.

The *criteria of effective therapy* for all age-groups are return of the tympanic membrane to a normal appearance, cessation of discharge, and normal hearing.

ACUTE MASTOIDITIS

There will be inflammation of the mastoid air cells in most cases of acute otitis media, but these changes are usually reversible. If, however, bony caries occurs in the intercellular partitions then infection may continue, resulting in an increase in aural discharge, low-grade pyrexia, deafness, and pain. Most severe cases of acute otitis media are treated by antibiotic therapy and the dramatic clinical picture of primary acute mastoiditis—with the pinna pushed forwards and downwards by post-auricular œdema or a subperiosteal abscess—is rare.

The diagnosis of latent mastoiditis caused by inadequate or ineffective therapy is a difficult clinical problem and persistent low pyrexia, recurrence of pain, continuing deafness, or profuse creamy discharge must be considered as highly significant signs necessitating surgical intervention.

Treatment.—Simple cortical mastoidectomy (Schwartze) will effectively remove all infected air cells, but requires previous surgical experience. Intensive systemic antibiotic therapy (usually penicillin) extending over several weeks can cure some cases of acute mastoiditis, perhaps at the expense of hearing, but the presence of a subperiosteal abscess, profuse otorrhœa, or evidence of seriously raised pressure in the middle ear warrants urgent surgical decompression.

Intracranial extension of infection is uncommon in acute infections of the middle-ear cleft, but is indicated by severe headache, high fever, rigors, vertigo, or diplopia (the latter due to sixth-nerve involvement). Treatment is usually primarily with systemic penicillin and where possible oral sulphadiazine or sulphamezathine. It is essential that therapy is continued until the disease is cured or surgical intervention performed.

CHRONIC OTITIS MEDIA

Chronic middle-ear disease is progressively destructive and although the damage may be stopped it can never be reversed. The presenting symptom is invariably otorrhœa; this may be persistent or intermittent and secondary to either recurrent infections ascending the Eustachian tube or more serious descending infections from bony disease in the mastoid antrum.

Thorough cleansing of all discharge from the external auditory meatus will enable the tympanic membrane to be seen and the perforation identified (*Fig.* 493). In those cases where the discharge is primarily mucoid the perforation is

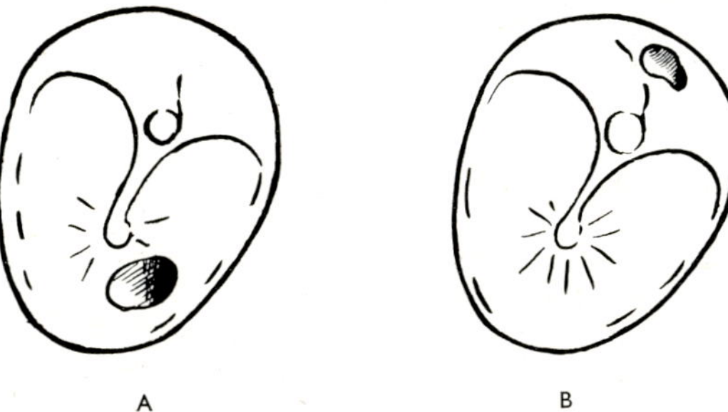

Fig. 493.—Defects in the tympanic membrane: A, central perforation; B, attic perforation.

usually central and in the antero-inferior quadrant of the tympanic membrane —hearing loss is minimal. This condition may follow an attack of scarlet fever or measles or previous acute middle-ear disease. Prognosis is good in that there is no risk to life, but deafness may increase and it may be impossible to dry the ear permanently.

Treatment.—Careful regular aural toilet is essential and if the discharge is profuse syringeing may be employed rather than mopping with cotton-wool swabs. The use of antibiotic drops or powders is rarely of value and systemic antibiotics should be reserved for acute exacerbations of infection. Spirit drops (SVR 25 per cent) will keep the ear clean and boracic iodine powder can be insufflated twice a week in the more persistent cases.

Reparative surgery (myringoplasty) is extremely successful in closing central perforations in those patients whose ears have remained dry for at least 6 months.

Attico-antral disease, where there is destruction of muco-endosteum and bone in the mastoid antrum and attic region of the middle ear, is invariably associated with an acellular mastoid process. Granulation tissue may grow from the surface of eroded bone and protrude into the deep meatus as a polyp. The disease is always progressive, although periods of remission are not uncommon.

The otorrhœa is purulent and offensive. Cholesteatoma (a grey shining mass of desquamated squamous epithelium) may be visible in the meatus or protruding through the tympanic perforation. The latter is usually in the upper and posterior part of the drumhead and is either in the pars flaccida or marginal (*see Fig.* 493).

Deafness is progressive and pain is not a feature of this condition unless there is an acute infection, invasion of dura, or neoplastic change.

Treatment is necessary to remove the danger to life from intracranial extension, to arrest deafness, and to stop otorrhœa. The patient is aware only of the deafness and discharge; many accept both as normal and seek attention late in the development of their disease.

Skilled attention is required in all cases and, although conservative therapy, such as polypectomy or aural toilet, may delay the progress of the disease, radical surgical intervention is invariably required.

REFERRED PAIN IN THE EAR

In the majority of patients pain in the ear is secondary to ear disease. However, because of the complexity of the sensory nerve-supply to this region, pain may be referred from remote areas whose sensory nerve-supply also sends branches to the ear.

The ear is supplied by sensory branches from the second and third cervical nerves and from branches of the fifth, ninth, and tenth cranial nerves.

Referred pain to the ear may therefore come from lesions of the upper cervical intervertebral disks, osteoarthritic changes affecting these vertebra, or fibrositis in the neck muscles.

Infections or neoplasms arising in the distribution of the fifth cranial nerve may cause referred otalgia. Particularly common are lesions affecting the lower jaw and teeth such as dental caries, impacted wisdom teeth, and arthritic changes in the temporomandibular joint.

The pharynx (with the exception of the nasopharynx) and posterior part of the tongue derive their sensory supply from the ninth and tenth cranial nerves, and infections (such as tonsillitis), ulceration (tuberculous), or neoplasms in this region frequently cause pain in the ears and may even present primarily with this symptom.

Whenever otalgia cannot be satisfactorily explained by local disease, search must be made in those areas where referred pain could be initiated.

II. THE NOSE AND ACCESSORY SINUSES

The primary functions of the nose are threefold:—
1. As part of the respiratory airway.
2. Heating, humidifying, and filtration of inspired air.
3. Olfaction.

Although external and intranasal examination gives some indication of the effectiveness of the nose as a pathway for respiration, it is not possible to determine by simple means the value of the nasal mucous membrane for air conditioning or defence against inspired bacteria.

EXAMINATION OF THE NOSE

A knowledge of the normal anatomical features as revealed by clinical examination is essential if those appearances consequent upon pathological changes are to be appreciated. Diffuse illumination is adequate for external examination of the nose, but bright, focused, reflected light using a head mirror is necessary for the proper examination of the nasal passages in all except the very young. In the latter patients an electric auroscope with a large speculum gives an adequate view and is particularly useful when searching for foreign bodies.

Inspection of the external nose will reveal displacements due to new or old traumatic injuries, swellings of varied aetiology and importance, and, perhaps most important of all, whether air is passing through both nostrils. This can be simply confirmed by the use of a wisp of cotton-wool held in front of each nares.

The true shape of the nostrils tends to vary with the ethnic origin of the patient. They are approximately pear-shaped and lined with skin. Adequate examination can often be carried out without the aid of a nasal speculum—particularly useful when a painful condition such as nasal furunculosis is present. However, the introduction of the appropriate size of nasal speculum (*Fig.* 494) does allow inspection of much of the nasal passages and septum. It

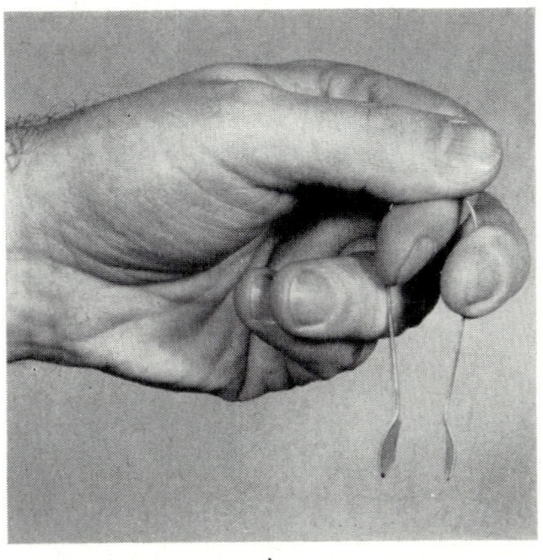
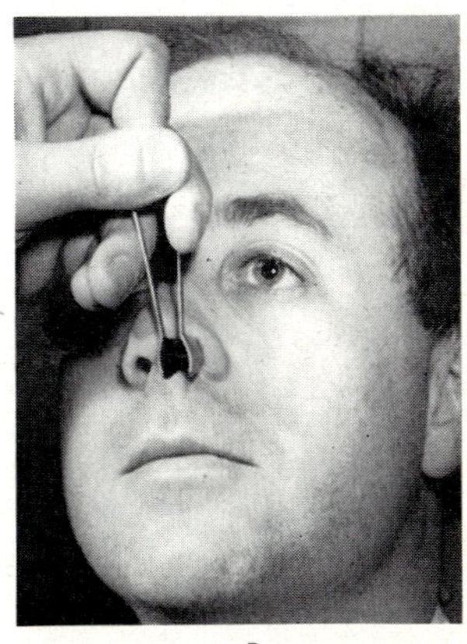

A   B

Fig. 494.—Use of Thudichum speculum: **A** method of holding and, **B**, insertion of speculum.

is never possible to adequately examine the whole of this region for invariably the nasal septum is deviated either in its cartilaginous or bony portions, and, since the adult nasal passage is 3 in. (7·5 cm.) long and appears as a long narrow slit, only the anterior halves of both inferior and middle turbinates are viewable without the prior use of local vasoconstrictors.

Normal, ciliated, columnar epithelium in the nose is pink, moist, and smooth. Variations from this appearance such as hypertrophy, polypi, or the presence of pus or excessive secretions must be noted. Swellings, particularly if ulcerated or friable with a tendency to bleed, are always pathological.

The paranasal sinuses, comprising maxillary antrum, frontal, and sphenoidal sinuses together with the ethmoidal labyrinth, are not available for direct inspection although abnormal secretions or growths usually present themselves in the nose. Valuable information concerning disease of these sinuses can be obtained by examination of the nose and from radiographic examination. Transillumination of the maxillary and frontal sinuses is of less help.

Radiographic Examination.—Both the taking and interpretation of standard views of the paranasal sinuses require experience. In the occipitomental position (*Fig.* 495) the petrous apices are projected below the floor of the maxillary antra.

A 25° tilt enables the frontal sinuses and ethmoidal labyrinth to be clearly shown (*Fig.* 496), although a lateral view is also helpful, whilst the submento-vertical projection shows the sphenoidal sinuses and base of skull.

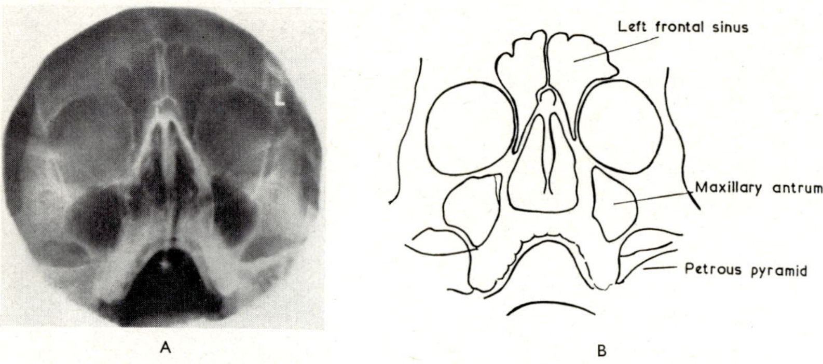

Fig. 495.—A, Standard occipitomenta position; B, Key line drawing.

Transillumination.—A specifically designed light carrier is introduced into the centre of the mouth and the patient then examined in a darkened room. It is essential to control the intensity of illumination and to have a small light

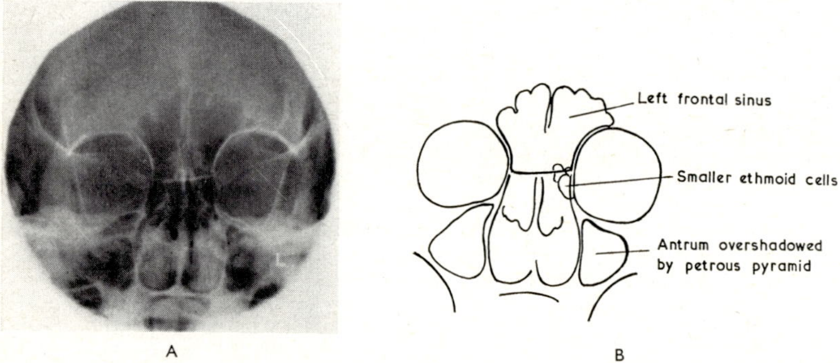

Fig. 496.—A, Standard 25° tilt; B, Key line drawing.

source. If the maxillary antra are both equal in size and normal then both will transmit the light to an equal extent as revealed by the infra-orbital crescent of light. Any condition interfering with the transmission of the light—such as mucopus, thickened antral lining—will produce a difference in intensity between the two sides. For illumination of the frontal sinuses the light source is applied to the bony floor above the medial canthus of the eye. Because of the frequency of variations in development of the frontal sinuses this test is unreliable and its value in detecting or confirming maxillary antral disease probably depends on the experience of the surgeon using this technique.

VASOCONSTRICTION OF THE NASAL MUCOSA

Occasionally it is necessary to shrink the nasal mucosa to allow adequate inspection of the air-passages. If limited intranasal manipulations, such as antral lavage, cauterization, or polypectomy, are required, it is useful to use a preparation which provides both local anæsthesia and vasoconstriction. Cocaine, in concentrations of 5, 10, and 20 per cent, remains the most commonly used preparation and is frequently diluted with equal parts of 1–1000 adrenaline. The solution may be sprayed into the nose or applied on ribbon gauze or cotton-wool pledgets. It must *never* be injected. Some people are unusually sensitive to cocaine and absorption of even small quantities will lead to increase of pulse-rate, rise in blood-pressure, and symptoms of intoxication. Pallor and sweating from stimulation of the vasomotor centre are early signs of toxicity and in such cases any swabs or packs must be immediately removed. Barbiturates may be needed in more severe cases and where there is respiratory failure artificial respiration.

Vasoconstrictor preparations containing naphthazoline (such as privine and fenox) are to be avoided for, although producing intense local vasoconstriction, they are liable to be followed by prolonged congestion of the mucosa.

FRACTURES OF THE NOSE

Most fractures of the nasal bones are compound, either the overlying skin or nasal mucous membrane being breached.

The commonest deformity encountered is displacement of the nasal skeleton away from the site of injury and the nasal bones are usually impacted. More

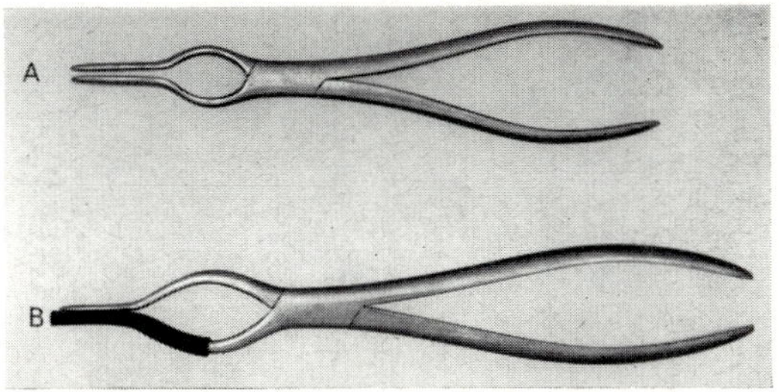

Fig. 497.—A, Ashe's forceps; B, Walsham's forceps.

uncommonly the whole nasal 'cap' may be displaced to one side, such as may occur after a glancing blow, or a heavy blow delivered from the front may push the whole nose inwards whilst at the same time splaying the nasal bones outwards.

A history of previous trauma, epistaxis, and later perhaps a black eye will confirm the diagnosis, but œdema rapidly develops and if reduction is not possible within a few hours of injury it is better to wait for 3–4 days.

Radiographic findings are of limited value and careful digital and intranasal examination, carried out either before or after the onset of reactionary œdema, is the most effective way of establishing the type of deformity.

Privine (Ciba Laboratories Ltd., Horsham, Sussex).
Fenox (Boots Pure Drug Co. Ltd., Nottingham).

Reduction should be carried out under general anæsthesia together with endotracheal intubation and pharyngeal packing, since bleeding is frequently brisk. Disimpaction is performed with Walsham's forceps and any septal deformity corrected with Ashe's septal forceps (*Fig.* 497). The mobilized and straightened nose is fixed in position with the aid of a plaster-of-Paris splint and in most cases no nasal packing is required or advisable. The splint may be removed after a week, but the nose should not be blown for a further week.

FRACTURE OF THE MALAR BONE

The malar forms the lateral buttress of the orbit and helps to protect the eye and maintain the normal facial contour. Fractures of this bone, resulting in displacement inwards and downwards, frequently involve the infra-orbital nerve, cause bleeding into the maxillary antrum, and always produce unevenness of the infra-orbital margin—a 'step down' is felt on palpation.

The disability is primarily cosmetic and the displacement should be reduced as soon as possible.

Treatment.—Under general anæsthesia an incision is made within the hairline on the side of the fracture and after exposure the temporal fascia is incised. This allows an elevator to be passed downwards under the arch and the displaced bone can be reduced by firmly lifting the fragment forwards and upwards. Reduction when complete shows no tendency to redisplacement (*Fig.* 498).

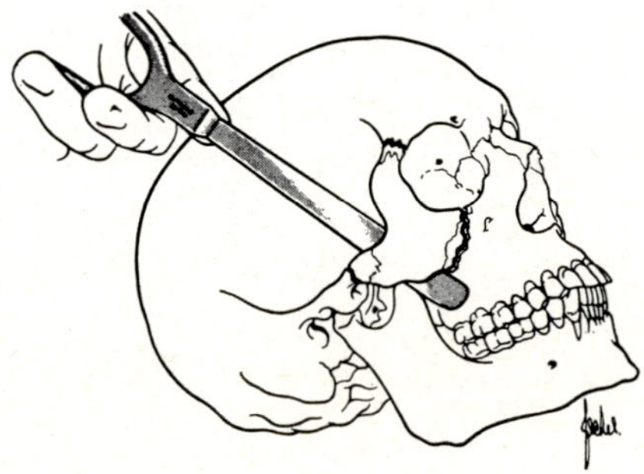

Fig. 498.—Elevation of a fractured malar bone. In reduction a Bristow's elevator is placed under the zygomatic arch.

Local fractures of the malar affecting only the zygomatic arch can be reduced using a similar technique.

SEPTAL HÆMATOMA

Collection of blood under the septal mucoperichondrium or mucoperiosteum commonly results from nasal trauma, either accidental or after surgical operations such as submucous resection (SMR).

A large bilateral hæmatoma will produce complete nasal obstruction and the dusky red swelling of the blood-filled sac is readily visible inside the nares.

If the blood, or more frequently blood-clot and serum, is not evacuated there is a considerable risk of infection and necrosis of cartilage. Evacuation should be carried out as aseptically as possible, usually by means of an incision into the most prominent part of the hæmatoma. The contents are aspirated and the wall then lightly packed against the underlying cartilage to obliterate the dead space. If evidence of infection or fresh bleeding is found a gauze wick may be left in the incision to maintain drainage.

Unless a septal abscess is present antibiotics are not usually required.

EPISTAXIS

The nasal mucous membrane is richly supplied with blood-vessels and bleeding from the nose is a frequent occurrence both in childhood and in adult life. Any condition which increases the vascularity of the mucous membrane, such as the common cold, may lead to mild bleeding, but the commonest cause in childhood is local irritation in the nose from deposition of dust on the anterior part of the septum. Scratching with the finger-nail leads to superficial ulceration, crusting, and intermittent bleeding.

Treatment.—Ung. Hydrarg. Oxid. Flav. placed nightly for a few weeks on both sides of the septum will effectively deal with this problem. Pinching the nostrils together for at least 10 minutes will invariably stop any epistaxis originating on the front of the septum, but occasionally recurrent bleeding is secondary to rupture of one or more prominent vessels on the septum and these should be

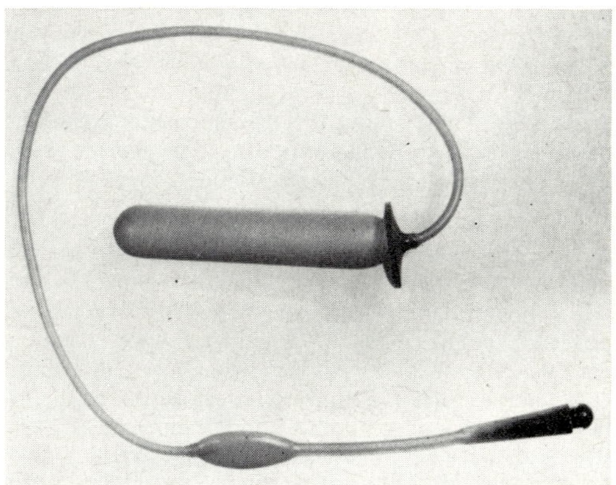

Fig. 499.—Simpson's balloon for the control of epistaxis.

coagulated either with the electro-cautery—a dangerous instrument in unskilled hands—or by the application of silver nitrate or a chromic acid bead.

In adult life similar aetiological factors exist, but the possibility of a neoplasm in the nasal passages must always be considered. Deviations of the nasal septum may result in alterations in the respiratory air currents and deposition of dust —treatment is correction of the obstruction.

Hypertensive epistaxis is both a dangerous and a frightening condition. In the elderly patient loss of vascular elasticity can hinder normal hæmostasis and lead to a torn vessel continuing to bleed. The cause of the epistaxis may be apparent on inspection and coagulation or packing the nose with ½-in. ribbon gauze impregnated with 5 per cent cocaine diluted with an equal volume of 1–1000 adrenaline will stop the bleeding. No nasal pack should be left in situ for longer than 24 hours unless systemic antibiotics have been given.

25

If these measures fail to control the hæmorrhage all packs should be removed and a well-lubricated rubber balloon attached to a small catheter passed along the floor of the nose (*Fig.* 499). The balloon is inflated with air until it completely fills the nasal airway and, since it conforms to all variations in the shape of the nose, bleeding is controlled.

When all other efforts have failed to control bleeding it may be necessary to ligate the external carotid, internal maxillary, or anterior ethmoidal arteries. These are ligated in continuity by external approaches.

Epistaxis can be both serious and fatal and there should be no hesitation in giving whole-blood transfusion whenever the patient's general condition gives cause for worry (*see* p. 43).

Adequate sedation is essential to assist in allaying anxiety and in reducing the unavoidable unpleasantness of thorough packing of the nose.

VESTIBULAR FURUNCULOSIS

The aetiology of boils in the nasal vestibule is the same as elsewhere in the body. However, the condition does present certain special features in the nose. Because of the adhesion of the skin to the underlying cartilage there is minimal room for expansion and consequently this is an acutely painful condition.

All furuncles in the nose are potentially dangerous because of the communication that exists between the facial (into which the nasal veins drain) and ophthalmic veins. Neither contain valves and infection in the nasal vestibule can travel directly by a process of thrombophlebitis to the cavernous sinus. Although the risk of this happening is small it is safer to treat all except the earliest nasal furuncle with systemic antibiotics. Squeezing or incision of the lesion imposes a risk of spreading the infection and must be avoided.

NASAL OBSTRUCTION

Most of the conditions responsible for partial or total nasal obstruction are acquired. Atresia of the posterior part of the nasal passages is, however, usually congenital and, if bilateral, the newborn baby will have serious feeding and breathing problems. Diagnosis may be confirmed by persistent nasal obstruction unrelieved by cleansing or ephedrine nose drops, and inability to pass a catheter through the nose into the pharynx. Perforation of the obstruction can be carried out and the opening maintained by the regular passage of a soft catheter. However, a general anæsthetic is necessary and previous experience by the surgeon of this procedure is advisable.

Foreign Body in the Nose.—Most foreign bodies found in the adult nose have been accidentally introduced, sometimes following surgical operations. They are, however, uncommon when compared with children, where for many reasons pieces of paper, buttons, and other handy objects are frequently pushed into their own or other children's noses. If undetected, symptoms of unilateral obstruction with purulent discharge usually develop. Examination of the anterior nares or nasal passages—and in very young children the electric auroscope is helpful— invariably reveals the object. If the foreign body has not been pushed in too far or is not impacted between the middle turbinate and septum, removal is possible without anæsthesia. Grasping forceps should not be used as a sudden jerk may force the object further backwards. The foreign body should be drawn forward by passing a right-angled probe behind it. Persistence of symptoms following removal could indicate further undetected objects in the nose. If examination under general anæsthesia is necessary care must be taken not to push the object into the nasopharynx where it might be inhaled.

Objects allowed to remain undisturbed in the nose for long periods become coated with magnesium and calcium salts forming a rhinolith. The resulting hard concretion may be too large for removal via the anterior nares and piecemeal destruction in situ may be required.

Nasal Allergy.—Paroxysmal swelling of the nasal mucous membrane with irritation, sneezing, and watery rhinorrhœa is usually associated with exposure to foreign antigens, such as occurs in hay fever. However, a more common and less specific condition termed 'perennial nasal allergy' or vasomotor rhinitis will produce similar symptoms. In addition to abnormal sensitivity to house dust and other common antigens, attacks may be provoked by changes in temperature and physical or psychological strain.

The nasal mucosa is pale blue and boggy, the inferior turbinates being so swollen as to completely occlude the nasal airway.

Avoidance of the appropriate antigen, if possible, and use of systemic antihistamines and topical corticosteroids will help to relieve symptoms, but persistent swelling of the inferior turbinates may require submucosal diathermization. The surface epithelium should never be destroyed by cauterization since this does not help the patient and may lead to the formation of adhesions.

Nasal Polypi.—These are pedunculated masses of œdematous nasal mucosa and are not to be considered as neoplasms. Invariably they originate from the middle turbinate or the middle meatus, and may enlarge to block the whole nasal airway or produce distension of the nasal framework. In most cases the aetiology is unknown, but may be a combination of allergy and chronic inflammation.

Removal can be carried out under general anæsthesia, but if local anæsthesia is desirable cotton-wool carriers dipped in a mixture of equal parts of 10 per cent cocaine and 1–1000 adrenaline should be packed around the polypi. After a period of 10 minutes an open wire snare (*Fig.* 500) is gently coaxed around

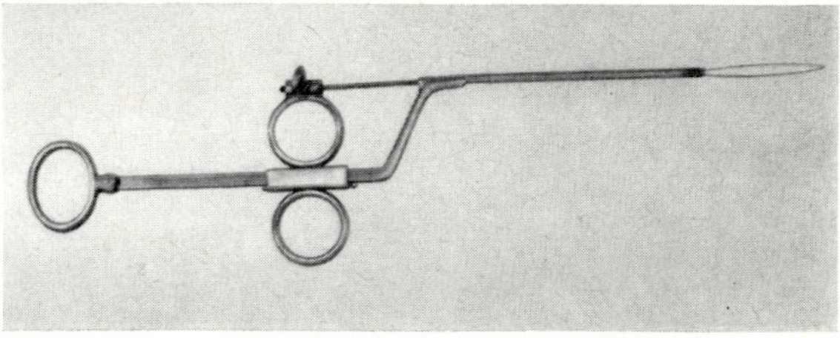

Fig. 500.—Glegg's nasal polypectomy snare.

the swelling and worked laterally towards the narrow pedicle. After tightening, the polyp can be avulsed and any small polypoidal remnants removed under direct vision with grasping forceps.

Any polypi showing unexpected toughness or friability, especially if associated with a tendency to bleed on touching, should be sent for histological examination.

ACUTE SINUSITIS

The most frequent cause of acute sinusitis is ascending infection during an acute rhinitis or common cold. Normally the nasal, ciliated columnar epithelium with its mucous blanket offers a protective barrier to infection, but poor general health, repeated exposure to upper respiratory tract infections, or mechanical obstruction from a deviated nasal septum or polypi may reduce the effectiveness of this defence mechanism. The regular use of cilia-paralysing nose drops such as cocaine or adrenaline will have a similar effect.

The pathological changes produced in the mucosal lining of the sinuses are those of acute inflammation and if the drainage openings (or ostia) of these sinuses are occluded then these secretions must accumulate within the cavities.

General symptoms of malaise, headache, and pyrexia are common together with dull pain located to the affected region. Characteristically the pain of maxillary sinusitis is made worse by coughing or stooping, and that of frontal sinusitis is worse in the morning. There may be reddening or œdema of the overlying skin and pain on pressure.

Examination of the nose will show a generalized erythema and after the use of vasoconstrictors pus may be visible in the middle meatus or on the posterior wall of the oropharynx.

Treatment.—Local measures designed to restore normal drainage using 1 per cent ephedrine in normal saline nose drops t.d.s., and steam inhalations with the

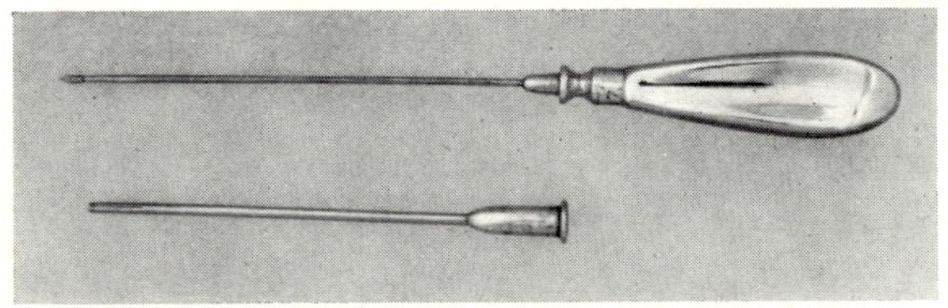

Fig. 501.—Lichtwitz trocar and cannula.

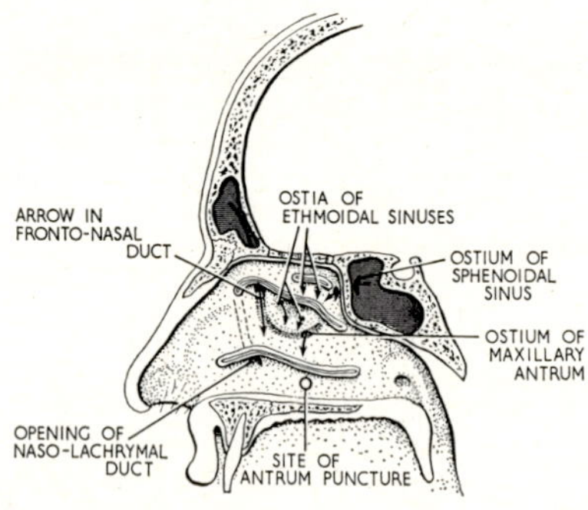

Fig. 502.—Diagram illustrating site of antral puncture.

addition of menthol or Friars' balsam (tinct. benz. co.) are useful and give considerable relief. In more severe cases systemic antibiotics are indicated, but should be preceded by nasal swabbing to determine the infecting organism and its sensitivity. Local antibiotics are useless.

Persistence of symptoms despite intensive medical therapy, together with radiological evidence of opacity in the antrum, is an indication for antral lavage.

Except in children or highly nervous adults, this minor procedure is carried out under local anæsthesia. The nose is sprayed with 10 per cent cocaine and after a few minutes a cotton-wool carrier soaked in a similar solution or impregnated with cocaine paste is gently introduced beneath the inferior turbinate coming to lie against the medial wall of the maxillary antrum. After removal of the wool carrier this bony wall is punctured with the straight Lichtwitz trocar and cannula (*Figs.* 501, 502), care being taken not to push the instrument into the cheek or orbit. The trocar is removed and a Higginson's syringe filled with normal saline at body temperature is connected to the cannula. Gentle irrigation causes the antral contents to flow through the maxillary ostium into the nose. If the ostium is blocked with œdematous mucosa, polypi, or inspissated mucopus, then pain will be produced on attempted irrigation and a second cannula may be introduced alongside the first to 'decompress' the antrum. Antral lavage should not be carried out during the acute stage of the infection.

Cannulation of the fronto-nasal duct to relieve an acute frontal sinusitis is no longer justifiable. If infection has not been relieved by medical means and there is radiological evidence of a fluid level, external drainage can be performed by perforation of the bony floor of the sinus above the medial end of the eyebrow. This is often the point of maximum tenderness in acute frontal sinusitis. After evacuation of the contents of the sinus a small plastic tube is introduced, this permitting irrigation of the cavity with an appropriate antibiotic solution or vasoconstrictor drops. Return of normal drainage into the nose usually occurs within 3–4 days and the tube should then be removed.

III. LARYNX

The interior of the larynx cannot be examined directly without the use of anæsthesia. However, indirect laryngoscopy is usually sufficient to establish a provisional diagnosis and is feasible in most adults. Children invariably require a general anæsthetic for any laryngoscopy.

INDIRECT LARYNGOSCOPY

Adequate illumination from an electric headlamp or head mirror is essential and a variety of laryngeal mirrors should be available together with tongue-holding cloths and some method of warming the mirrors (*Fig.* 503). The patient must be seated comfortably and fully relaxed if co-operation is to be expected, and dentures should be removed prior to examination. The tongue is extended and held in a gauze tongue square, care being taken not to pull too vigorously downwards on to the lower incisor teeth. A mirror warmed to body

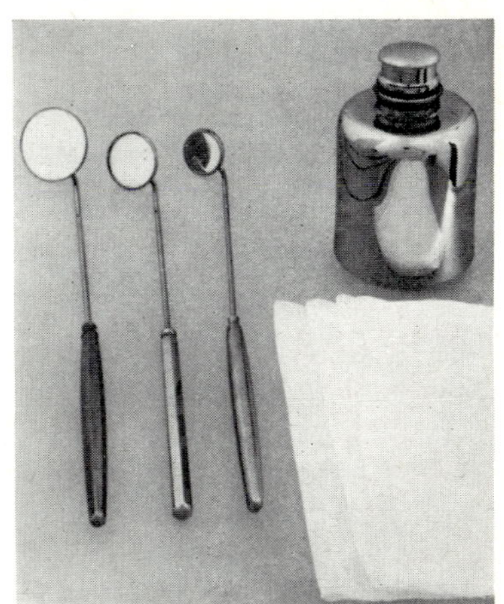

Fig. 503.—Instruments required for indirect laryngoscopy.

temperature is passed face downwards over the dorsum of the tongue and placed firmly against the soft palate. By tilting the mirror face the various structures in the valleculæ, larynx, and hypopharynx can be seen (*Fig.* 504).

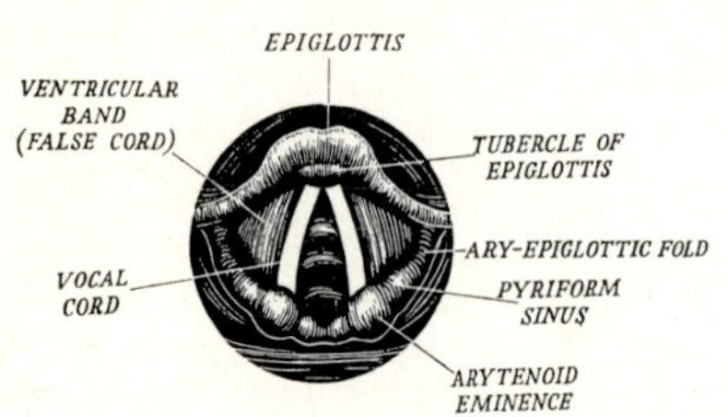

Fig. 504.—Larynx as seen on indirect laryngoscopy.

Even with care some patients are unable to tolerate the presence of any foreign object in their mouth. Preliminary spraying of the throat with 2·5 per cent cocaine or the sucking of an amethocaine lozenge abolishes sensation and usually enables the examination to be completed.

It is never possible to view all the structures in and around the larynx at any one time, and the laryngeal mirror must be gently tilted in various directions to enable complete inspection of this region.

Occasionally the epiglottis may overhang the larynx to such an extent that adequate visualization of the glottis is impossible; in such cases direct laryngoscopy is essential.

The mobility of the vocal cords can be tested by asking the patient to phonate 'e–e–e–e', and this will also bring the anterior commissure into view.

DIRECT LARYNGOSCOPY

The most effective method of viewing the interior of the larynx is by direct vision using one of the many laryngoscopes which are commercially available (*Fig.* 505). These differ primarily in their method of illumination and varying sizes and shapes are available for all requirements.

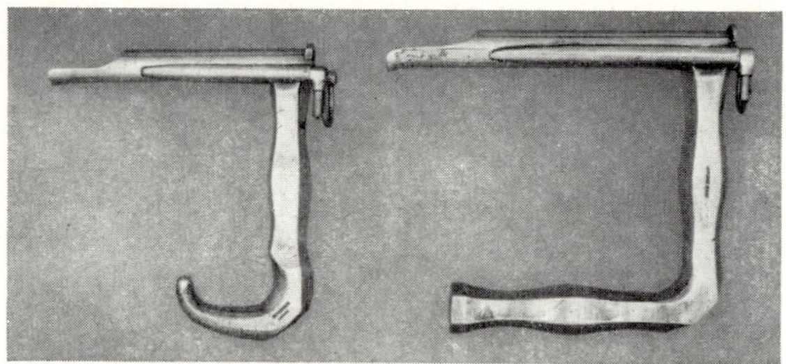

Fig. 505.—Adult and child laryngoscopes.

Although direct laryngoscopy can be carried out under general anæsthesia (and is preferable to children), most surgeons prefer to use local anæsthesia since this does not interfere with the movement or tension of the vocal cords and the view is not obstructed by the presence of an endotracheal tube.

Half an hour prior to spraying the throat with 4 per cent lignocaine, the patient is given one tablet of amethocaine (65 mg.) to suck and is instructed not to swallow his saliva to minimize toxic absorption. After thoroughly spraying the oral cavity, tongue, and pharynx with approximately 5 ml. of the solution, the lips and alveolar margin should be wiped with the lignocaine. Swabs wrung out in the same preparation are held in both pyriform fossæ for 10 minutes using Krause's carriers. This blocks the internal branches of the superior laryngeal nerves and anæsthetizes the laryngeal mucosa. Finally, the interior of the larynx and upper trachea can be sprayed under direct vision—this gives adequate anæsthesia for up to 1 hour, although this period may be reduced in heavy smokers or chronic bronchitics.

LARYNGEAL OBSTRUCTION

The gap between the vocal cords is the narrowest space that air must pass through on its way to the lungs. Consequently any condition which reduces this lumen may lead to inspiratory stridor and possibly asphyxia. In severe cases the inspiratory effort will suck in the soft tissues at the root of the neck and intercostal spaces. Cyanosis is a late and often terminal sign.

Acute Infections.—In the adult larynx, acute infections, though causing hoarseness, pain, and discomfort, are rarely dangerous. Similar infections in the child are, however, potentially serious, especially if diphtheritic, since the glottic space is relatively small and mucosal œdema readily causes obstruction to breathing. Most cases follow an upper respiratory tract infection, but the possibility of an inhaled foreign body must be considered and direct laryngoscopy may be necessary. Systemic antibiotics have reduced the seriousness of this condition and should be supplemented by measures designed to make the tenacious secretions less viscid—such as steam inhalations, steam tents, or aerosol inhalers (*Fig.* 506).

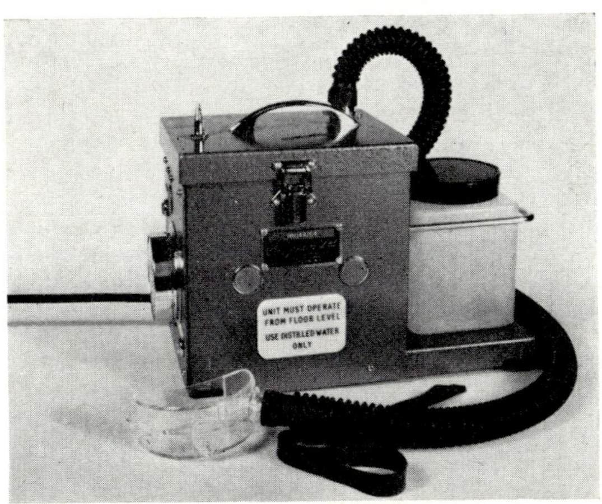

Fig. 506.—Electrically operated humidifier.

Acute laryngotracheobronchitis is always a serious condition usually affecting children under the age of 5 years. Because of the widespread mucosal involvement and tenacious nature of the secretions, the child may become exhausted in its efforts to cough and breathe. If intensive chemotherapy and nursing care

are not producing rapid relief then tracheostomy must be considered (*see* p. 16) to aid tracheobronchial toilet and oxygenation.

Œdema.—Although some œdema may accompany most acute infections of the larynx, non-infective causes are more dramatic and important. Angio-neurotic œdema, cardiac failure, trauma from ingestion of caustics, inhalation of irritant gases, or direct injury to the larynx, can all produce rapidly increasing stridor and dyspnœa.

Indirect laryngoscopy reveals gross swelling of the larynx and also the size of the residual glottic chink. Treatment will largely depend upon the severity of the condition, varying from medical therapy such as hypodermic adrenaline in acute allergy to urgent tracheostomy.

Paralysis of the Vocal Cords.—All the intrinsic muscles of the larynx, except the cricothyroid, are supplied by the recurrent laryngeal nerves. Paralysis of one nerve leads to the homolateral vocal cord becoming immobile and eventually coming to lie approximately in the midline of the glottic aperture (*Fig.* 507 A). Except for transient hoarseness this condition may be asymptomatic and un-suspected, especially if the opposite vocal cord crosses the midline to close the

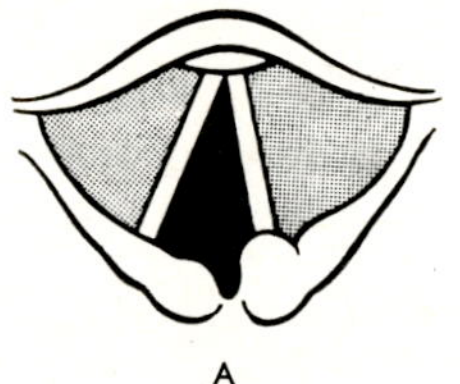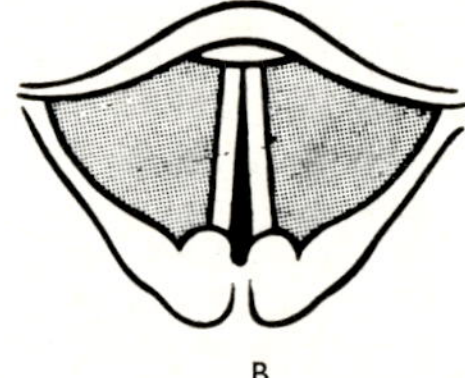

Fig. 507.—A, Unilateral vocal cord paresis; B, bilateral vocal cord paresis.

glottic chink. Prognosis depends upon the cause, but 30 per cent are idiopathic, and spontaneous recovery may occur in this group and in those secondary to thyroidectomy. Neoplasms of the thyroid, œsophagus, and bronchus obviously carry a bad prognosis.

Bilateral recurrent nerve paralysis is a far more serious condition but occurs rarely in comparison with unilateral paralysis. The commonest cause is thyroid-ectomy and, if both vocal cords take up a position of full adduction (*Fig.* 507 B), then dyspnœa and stridor will be acute and urgent tracheostomy required. Paralysis secondary to neoplastic disease generally occurs more slowly and allows time for compensation by the patient. Some patients with bilateral paralysis following thyroidectomy recover some function of their vocal cords. The remainder must decide between a permanent tracheostomy tube fitted with a speaking valve, and surgical correction of their disability. The latter, if successful, is invariably accompanied by an imperfect voice.

Laryngeal Growths.—An uncommon but important cause of persistent hoarse-ness with stridor and dyspnœa occurring in childhood is the development of multiple papillomata on the laryngeal mucosa. If not controlled, these may reach sufficient size to cause death and in advanced cases will need a tracheo-stomy. Removal may lead to rapid recurrence and a virus aetiology has been suggested.

Malignant tumours growing within the larynx produce progressive obstruc-tion of the airway. When involving the vocal cord hoarseness is an early symptom and this increases as the vocal cord becomes immobilized by deep infiltration or increasing tumour bulk. Discomfort in the throat is a common complaint, but pain is rare in the early stages.

IV. THROAT

Adequate examination of the mouth and oropharynx can best be carried out with the aid of good illumination and the appropriate-size metal tongue spatula. The nasopharynx can only be seen indirectly with a head mirror, reflected light, and a small warm postnasal mirror. This examination is difficult and requires experience. Nasopharyngoscopes are not suitable for routine use and are potentially harmful in unskilled hands.

ULCERS IN THE MOUTH

Aphthous Stomatitis.—This is the commonest form of ulceration in the oral cavity affecting all age-groups. Although it is occasionally associated with dyspepsia the condition is probably psychosomatic in origin. In response to anxiety or stress, or quite spontaneously, one or more vesicles appear on the buccal mucosa, favourite sites being the alveolar margins, orolingual folds, and cheek mucosa. The vesicles break to leave shallow painful ulcers surrounded by a narrow area of erythema. Within a few days most ulcers will have healed spontaneously, although single, large, deeper ulcers may persist for weeks. However, there is a strong tendency for recurrence of symptoms and an individual may never be free from at least one painful ulcer.

Painting the ulcer with 2 per cent silver nitrate or alum will reduce the pain. Corlan (hydrocortisone) pellets held beneath the tongue are invariably helpful, but adcortyl (triamcinolone) in orabase, when smeared over the ulcers, will give spectacular and prolonged relief.

Vincent's Angina.—The infection is due to a fusiform bacillus and a large spirillum, both normal inhabitants of the mouth, and ulceration is usually on the tonsil, although the soft palate and gums may be involved.

The ulcer is deep with considerable tissue destruction, slough, and general toxæmia. Upper deep cervical nodes are invariably palpable and tender—the throat is extremely sore and the breath foul-smelling.

Treatment is by systemic penicillin and hydrogen peroxide mouth-washes. Since the infection can be readily transmitted to others by the use of ineffectively washed crockery, the patient should be isolated if possible and full barrier precautions instituted for the first few days of the illness.

Recovery is usually followed at a later date by tonsillectomy.

Thrush.—This infection is from the fungus *Monilia albicans* and, although most frequently seen in debilitated and under-nourished children, it is not uncommon in adults receiving prolonged courses of systemic antibiotics or where penicillin pastilles have been sucked for long periods.

The whole of the oral mucous membrane may be covered with superficial white patches—the palate is invariably involved. Dysphagia may be slight and there is usually no systemic disturbances although, if the infection is uncontrolled, the patient's condition may become serious.

Mucosal lesions may be painted with 1 per cent aqueous solution of gentian violet; in severe cases nystatin suspension, 4 ml. q.d.s., may be administered.

Blood Diseases.—Acute leukæmia is a fulminating lethal disease which frequently presents as widespread ulceration in the mouth associated with bleeding from the gums and generalized lymphadenopathy. The patient is

Corlan (Glaxo Laboratories Ltd., Greenford, Middlesex).
Adcortyl-A in orabase (E. R. Squibb & Sons, Twickenham, Middlesex, and New Brunswick, New Jersey, U.S.A.).

usually young and the general condition poor. Although the total white count may not be raised in the early stages of this disease, examination of the blood-film will show large numbers of immature cells.

Agranulocytosis is most frequently secondary to administration of toxic drugs such as pyramidon, but most effective cytotoxic drugs in use against cancer are toxic to the bone-marrow and produce moderate to severe leucopenia.

Ulceration occurs throughout the whole oral mucosa, the ulcers at first being small with clean bases and no surrounding erythema. Progression of the condition will lead, however, to considerable tissue destruction.

The drug must be stopped immediately and systemic antibiotics given to protect the patient from infection. Pentnucleotide 40 ml. per day given intra-muscularly will stimulate the bone-marrow to produce new granulocytes; mean-while a fresh blood transfusion is of value.

PERITONSILLAR ABSCESS (QUINSY)

Most cases of acute tonsillitis, no matter how they are treated, recover completely. Occasionally, however, a tonsillar abscess previously localized to the intratonsillar cleft will burst through the tonsil capsule into the space between the tonsil and superior constrictor muscle. This condition, acute peritonsillitis, usually occurs about the fourth day of an acute tonsillitis and leads to an immediate increase in the severity of the patient's symptoms. Toxæmia is marked and intense trismus makes inspection of the tonsillar region difficult. Swallowing is extremely painful or impossible, and saliva dribbles from the corners of the mouth. Œdema of the soft palate is usual and later in the disease a yellow area of necrosis may be visible on the anterior pillar of the fauces—this is the point where the abscess will eventually discharge.

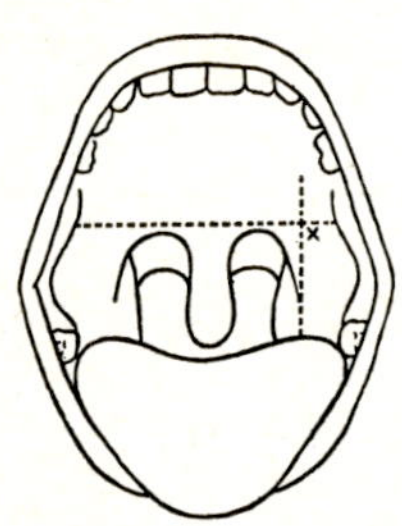

Fig. 508.—Semi-diagrammatic outline to indicate site for opening peritonsillar abscess.

Treatment.—If pus is thought to be present then it must be evacuated, but in the early stages of this infection the condition is primarily one of inflammatory œdema and a 10-day course of systemic penicillin (triplopen 1 ml. b.d.) will produce complete resolution.

Evacuation of a peritonsillar abscess should be performed either under local anæsthesia or, more usually, without anæsthesia to minimize the risk of inhalation of pus.

Unless the point of entry is already obvious the sinus forceps or guarded knife blade should be inserted into the classic site (*Fig.* 508) for a distance of at least 0·5 in. (1·25 cm.). The abscess is invariably deeper than expected and the pericapsular space may not be reached at the first attempt. A successful approach will be rewarded by a flow of pus and rapid relief of pain for the patient.

Tonsillectomy should be performed 4–6 weeks after an attack of acute peri-tonsillitis since recurrence of infection is common.

Parapharyngeal Abscess.—Infection of the parapharyngeal space may occur during acute tonsillitis or pharyngitis from retrograde thrombophlebitis. More commonly the infection follows trauma such as tonsillectomy or perforation of the pharyngeal wall by a foreign body.

Triplopen (Glaxo Laboratories Ltd., Greenford, Middlesex).

Swelling of the neck with medial displacement of the lateral pharyngeal wall occurs and later laryngopharyngeal œdema. Dysphagia, trismus, and toxæmia may lead to a mistaken diagnosis of peritonsillar abscess.

External drainage of the parapharyngeal space together with intensive systemic antibiotic therapy minimizes the risk of mediastinitis or carotid hæmorrhage.

Acute Retropharyngeal Abscess.—Up to the age of 5 years most children possess a number of small lymph-nodes situated in their retropharyngeal areolar tissue. Infection of these nodes, usually from a nasopharyngitis, may result in a suppurative lymphadenitis.

The child is usually under the age of 1 year and following an upper respiratory tract infection develops a mild pyrexia and dysphagia, and may hold its head stiffly to one side. More advanced infection will cause difficulty in breathing and stridor.

Examination is invariably difficult, but a red swelling may be seen on the posterior pharyngeal wall a little to one side of the midline. Accumulation of saliva or food debris may obscure the view.

Palpation must be extremely gentle to avoid rupturing the abscess, for spontaneous rupture is likely to be followed by inhalation of pus and death. Except in the earliest case when a systemic antibiotic is indicated, the abscess should be deliberately opened with the child on its back and the head slightly lowered. The mouth is held open with a gag and the evacuated pus removed by suction. Even mild dyspnœa may require a temporary tracheostomy.

Emergency incision can be carried out with the child's head hanging over the edge of a table. Once the pus is flowing the child can be turned on to its side with the head lower than the trunk—'the tonsil position'.

The organism is usually a staphylococcus and systemic antibiotic therapy must be continued for at least 48 hours after complete cessation of all symptoms.

COMPLICATIONS FOLLOWING TONSILLECTOMY AND ADENOIDECTOMY

Adenotonsillectomy is the commonest operation carried out under general anæsthesia and it is not surprising that there are a number of quite common post-operative complications. Many of these occur after the patient has left hospital, especially if the tonsils have been removed by the guillotine operation where the period of hospitalization may be only 24 hours.

Hæmorrhage.—Reactionary bleeding occurs during the first 48 hours after operation and examination of the tonsillar fossæ will show blood-clot on the affected side. This clot must be completely removed revealing the site of the oozing. A cotton-wool swab soaked in 1–1000 adrenaline and then squeezed almost dry is held in the fossa for at least 10 minutes. This procedure may need repeating, but if bleeding continues then ligation of the bleeding point must be carried out under general anæsthesia. With the decrease in popularity of the guillotine operation reactionary hæmorrhage is becoming less common.

Secondary hæmorrhage, however, occurs about the seventh post-operative day and is the result of sepsis. Some bright-red staining of the saliva may precede more vigorous bleeding and blood-clot is usually visible in the tonsil fossa. Systemic antibiotics should be given, blood-clot removed, and pressure applied. If ligation of a vessel is required this may be difficult since the tonsil bed is usually friable—a pack of gelfoam may have to be sewn in situ. Fortunately conservative measures invariably control the bleeding, but the patient should be kept in bed for several days until the temperature is normal.

Bleeding from the adenoid bed is the result of incomplete removal and re-examination of the nasopharynx under anæsthesia may be necessary. Post-nasal packs are unpleasant for the patient and not particularly effective. A transfusion of fresh whole blood may be needed to control bleeding in resistant cases.

Loss of blood in young children is always a serious matter and careful watch must be kept on the pulse-rate, blood-pressure, and general condition. All vomit must be kept for examination, for swallowing of blood may be undetected and true blood-loss be underestimated. There should be no hesitation in giving a blood transfusion when necessary.

Pulmonary Complications.—Even with care it is likely that over half of all the children undergoing tonsillectomy inhale some blood into their tracheo-bronchial tree. Fortunately, pulmonary complications are rare, but the development of dyspnœa, cough, and pyrexia following this operation would suggest an area of pulmonary atelectasis. Clinical and radiological examination of the chest will confirm the diagnosis and systemic penicillin therapy with vigorous physiotherapy invariably produces complete resolution. If this improvement does not occur, bronchoscopy with aspiration of the occluding plug are indicated.

Inhalation of a foreign body, such as a deciduous tooth or gauze swab, is fortunately unusual but would inevitably lead to the formation of a lung abscess.

Earache.—Referred pain from the tonsillar fossæ to the ears commonly occurs about the fifth post-operative day. The tympanic membranes should always be inspected since acute otitis media may be present. Only mild analgesia is necessary and the pain usually disappears within 48 hours.

SWALLOWED FOREIGN BODIES

Most of the foreign bodies, such as coins or meat bones, which are inadvertently or deliberately swallowed either stick in the œsophagus or pass freely into the stomach.

However, sharp spicules of bone sometimes lodge in the base of the tongue, tonsil, or pharyngeal wall. Dysphagia is acute, but the patient is usually able to localize the position of the foreign body with great accuracy. If the pharyngeal wall has been perforated there may be swelling of the neck, but usually no external abnormality is visible.

Examination of the mouth, tongue, and pharynx must be thorough and carried out with a headlight to leave both hands free. A fish bone may be seen sticking in the lower pole of the tonsil and can be grasped with suitable angled forceps. Frequently an area of bruising is seen and marks the site at which the mucosa has been scratched. It may, however, conceal the broken tip of a bony fragment and every patient must be observed for at least 48 hours. Persistence of symptoms indicates either infection or residual fragments, and examination under anæsthesia is essential.

Radiological examination of the neck can be helpful, but many common foreign bodies are not radio-opaque or opacities may be confused with areas of cartilaginous ossification. A negative radiograph must never be taken as conclusive evidence that a foreign body is not present.

CHAPTER XLIV

'MEDICAL OPERATIONS'

By F. DUDLEY HART

WHILE the procedures described in this chapter are usually performed in medical wards, the house-surgeon must be prepared to undertake them in the overall management of his patients. Medical diseases frequently co-exist with surgical lesions.

VENESECTION

The removal of blood from a patient was once a very popular form of treatment, and in some cases venesection is still a valuable measure. The condition that benefits most markedly is chronic congestive cardiac failure, where the patient, dyspnœic, distressed, and with distended veins in the neck, is much relieved by withdrawal of 250–500 ml. of blood. Other indications are hypertension with symptoms of severe headache and general distress, polycythæmia vera with like symptoms, acute congestive failure with pulmonary œdema, and some cases of status epilepticus and acute uræmic convulsions (where the benefit is largely due to relief of the heart). Over-enthusiastic blood transfusion or saline infusion may overload the heart. Severe anæmia is an absolute contra-indication to venesection.

Technique.—Place a sphygmomanometer band around the arm high up towards the shoulder and keep the pressure between 40 mm. and 70 mm. Hg. Feel the pulse to make certain the pressure is not so high as to cause obliteration of the arterial pulse. Infiltrate a small area with local anæsthetic over the most suitable vein—preferably the median cubital. Take a wide-bore, conical needle with a sharp point (e.g., French's needle) and attach to it a piece of sterile tubing. Fill the needle and tube with 3·8 per cent sodium citrate solution and clamp the bottom of the tubing. Slide the needle through the area anæsthetized, first through the skin, then obliquely through the wall of the vein. Hold a graduated receiver containing citrate solution below the tubing, unclamp, and collect the amount required—usually 250–500 ml. The whole process takes about 15–20 minutes. The blood may clot in the needle if an unsuitable needle of too small bore is used, or if it is not correctly in the vein.
Alternatively, the Fenwal's apparatus (p. 46) may be used.

TREATMENT OF ANASARCA

The practice of puncturing swollen areas to relieve the patient of œdema is much less popular than it was and has largely been replaced by mercurial and oral diuretics (*see* p. 664) and sodium-free diets. It is purely a palliative measure, and, though often attended by temporary relief, has seldom a lasting effect. The wounds in such swollen, waterlogged, and devitalized tissues tend to become infected, and the actual process may be very unpleasant to the patient.
A cardiac bed, with the foot low, is the best method of nursing such patients. A waterproof sheet is placed over the foot of the bed, tucked to form a gutter running into a suitable receptacle. The feet should be frequently dried and kept warm, otherwise they become cold and clammy with fluid.

Technique.—A length of fine perforated polythene tubing is threaded through a small nick in the skin some 2 in. (5·0 cm.) into the subcutaneous tissues. Alternatively, a trocar and cannula may be introduced through locally anæsthetized skin into the subcutaneous tissue. The trocar is withdrawn and perforated polythene tubing inserted through the cannula into the subcutaneous œdematous tissue; the cannula is then removed over the tubing, which is left in situ. Asepsis must be rigid. The tubes should be removed after 48–72 hours as they become much less effective after the first two days and increasingly liable to become infected. With each of these methods improved results can be obtained by the injection near the puncture sites of hyalase to facilitate flow of fluid through the tissues.

PARACENTESIS ABDOMINIS

In certain conditions the abdomen becomes distended with fluid: (1) as part of a generalized œdema; (2) due to tuberculous or malignant ascites; or (3) due to portal obstruction. Removal of fluid in such cases may give relief, and may be resorted to as a palliative measure when the patient is suffering discomfort from abdominal distension. Although the fluid is likely to return, it does not always do so, and after two or three aspirations no more may collect.

The fluid is under positive pressure, and as it is clear and watery no difficulty is experienced in its aspiration. A Southey's or other fine trocar and cannula is attached to a tube, which drains into a large receptacle at the side of the bed. The rate of drainage can be controlled by a bulldog clip.

The best site is either in one or other iliac fossa, or in the middle line 1–3 in. (2·5–7·5 cm.) below the umbilicus, care being taken first to empty the bladder. The intestine, even if touched, recedes before the cannula, and there is little chance of injuring it if reasonable care is taken. If nothing else is available, a hollow needle of medium bore may be used.

Technique.—At the site of election, 3–6 ml. of local anæsthetic are infiltrated into the abdominal wall including the parietal peritoneum, the skin is nicked with a scalpel, and the trocar and cannula inserted, usually with a rotary movement. With an abdominal binder, gradually tightened as the abdomen lessens in size, the fluid drains into the receptacle. As much fluid as required is drained, and tilting the patient to the side aspirated facilitates the drainage and lessens the negligible risk of bowel injury. Rapid emptying of the abdomen is not desirable as it may be followed by collapse of the patient.

MERCURIAL DIURETICS

The above-mentioned methods of withdrawing œdema fluid are only called for when other forms of diuresis are either contra-indicated or fail to work. Mercurial diuretics are very effective diuretics. Mersalyl (B.P.) contains approximately 39 per cent of mercury, and is still an excellent alternative to oral agents.

Indications.—Generalized œdema as in congestive cardiac failure or chronic nephrosis.

Contra-indications.—Renal insufficiency (as in acute and chronic nephritis), urinary obstruction (e.g., enlarged prostate), purpuric states. The patient should not be given the drug if he is unable to concentrate the urine above a specific gravity of 1020.

Technique.—The patient is at rest in bed with fluids charted on an intake-output chart. Salt intake is best restricted. One ml. of the drug is injected intramuscularly, not intravenously, as a test dose, followed in a few hours by a further 1 ml. if no adverse effects are noted. Injections are best given in the morning so that the action is largely over by nightfall. If satisfactory diuresis is obtained 2 ml. are given intramuscularly 2–4 days later, the injection being repeated every 2–7 days as desired. A satisfactory response is anything from 1 to 4 litres' increase in output over intake a day.

Undesirable effects may be vomiting, nausea, stomatitis, diarrhœa, fever, abdominal pain or discomfort, headache, hæmaturia, or (rarely) circulatory collapse. An acute attack of gout may be precipitated by the drug in a gouty subject and in such cases tab. colchicine 0·5 mg. is given twice or thrice daily over the period of mersalyl administration.

ORAL DIURETICS

Tablets and Dose.—Chlorothiazide, 500-mg.; hydrochlorothiazide, 50-mg.; hydroflumethiazide, 50-mg.; frusemide in 40-mg. tablets. Two tablets of one of these substances are taken by mouth each morning or two or three times a week. Alternatively, ethacrynic acid, 50 mg. daily, raising the dose if necessary. They are potent diuretics in themselves and can be used in conjunction with mersalyl in resistant cases of œdema. They are relatively non-toxic, the only likely unwanted effect being hypokalæmia from loss of potassium in the urine. Because of this effect a potassium supplement is commonly given in the evenings between administration of the diuretic. Frusemide is very expensive.

SPLENIC PUNCTURE

Splenic puncture as a diagnostic measure is—with reasonable care—a safe procedure, and may be required in splenic enlargement where Gaucher's disease is suspected. It is also used to measure pressure in portal hypertension and in the study of certain hæmatological conditions associated with splenomegaly. In kala-azar it is apt to be dangerous, and, though still often used, has largely given place to marrow-blood culture and venous-blood culture in special media.

It is important to check bleeding, clotting, and prothrombin times before any percutaneous biopsy procedure is carried out.

Technique.—Fix the enlarged spleen firmly against the lower border of the ribs. The organ is now felt quite superficially under the palpating fingers. Insert a large-bore needle with syringe attached, push in until the point is well into the spleen, and aspirate a portion of tissue into the needle. Keep up the negative pressure while withdrawing the needle. Apply firm pressure on the needle wound for 2 minutes with a swab.

The same technique may be used when the usual biopsy is impossible in soft tissues elsewhere. Aspirate the tissue—e.g., malignant glands of the neck—and, with negative pressure maintained in the syringe, give the needle a lateral jerk before withdrawal. This detaches the tissue aspirated, and prevents it being left behind on withdrawing the needle.

LIVER BIOPSY

While liver biopsy can be performed under direct vision using a peritoneoscope, needle biopsy is not infrequently required to assist in diagnosis when laparotomy is contra-indicated. Needle biopsy should only be performed upon patients able to co-operate intelligently with the operator. The usual site is in the seventh intercostal space in the anterior axilla or through the anterior abdominal wall when the liver is enlarged anteriorly below the costal margin; the former site is to be preferred. The true position of the liver should always be verified by percussion before biopsy.

Technique.—Local anæsthetic is injected into the skin, diaphragm, and hepatic capsule, and a small incision made with a scalpel into the skin at the site of election. If, after 5 minutes, oozing of blood continues it is best to abandon the procedure as the prothrombin time is probably unduly prolonged. Before performing biopsy it is wise to test the prothrombin time and, if prolonged, to give vitamin K_1 30–50 mg. by mouth or intravenously until the prothrombin time becomes normal. It is probably wise in most doubtful cases to give 30 mg. of vitamin K_1 daily for 3 days prior to the biopsy and, as an additional precaution, to have 1 pint of blood (550 ml.) cross-matched ready for use should it be required. The patient must remain in bed for 24 hours after the investigation, on a 15-minute pulse chart for the first 6 hours of this period. It is dangerous to perform biopsy in the face of prolongation of prothrombin or clotting time, and generally speaking cases of definite obstructive jaundice should not be submitted to liver biopsy. A Menghini needle is inserted through the incision down to the liver capsule; steady suction is then applied to the piston of the syringe as the needle is passed into the liver to the required depth. It is necessary to thrust and aspirate at the same time to get a suitable specimen, and the patients must hold their breath in expiration while this is done.

Alternatively, after infiltration of local anæsthetic from skin to hepatic capsule in the 9th intercostal space in the mid-axillary line, a trocar and cannula may be inserted to a point where they are just in contact with the liver capsule. The trocar is then withdrawn and a Vim-Silverman needle (p. 428) inserted into the liver through the cannula whilst the patient holds his breath in full expiration. The trocar is then drawn over the divided points of the needle to cut a neat small core of tissue out of the liver. The needle and cannula are then rapidly withdrawn. The same pre- and post-operative measures are instituted as outlined above.

It should be emphasized that liver biopsy carries definite risks—hæmorrhage, biliary peritonitis, pneumothorax, penetration of abdominal viscera, and dissemination of pyogenic infection. Nevertheless, it frequently gives very useful information.

BONE-MARROW BIOPSY

In many blood diseases it is of great advantage to ascertain what changes have taken place in the blood-forming tissues. The sternum is the most suitable bone, for it is superficial and accessible, and the marrow changes are there early and well marked. Some cases of leukæmia and multiple myelomatosis can only be diagnosed with certainty by sternal biopsy. In certain infections the causative organisms may be seen in marrow smears, e.g., malaria, kala-azar, filariasis, and trypanosomiasis, and culture from marrow blood occasionally gives positive results in enteric fever and pyogenic infections when venous blood-cultures have been negative. If biopsy is being done for the four tropical diseases mentioned above the needle and aspirating syringe must be completely dry. Malignant cells are sometimes seen in cases of secondary bony deposits. Large amounts of marrow are sometimes aspirated, stored, and re-infused later into patients with advanced malignant disease being treated by whole-body irradiation or perfusion with cytotoxic drugs. About 400 ml. may have to be aspirated (using a three-way syringe and closed system) from multiple puncture sites over the iliac crests and sternum.

Technique.—The marrow may be aspirated through a medium-bore needle quite easily, but in some cases (e.g., aplastic anæmia and myelosclerosis) it is desirable to examine the histological structure of the blood-forming tissue. In such cases local anæsthetic is injected over the site of election near the centre of the body of the sternum, using a fine needle with short bevel, the skin, subcutaneous tissues, and periosteum being infiltrated. An incision is then made and the periosteum cut and retracted. With a small trephine an area of bone 1 cm. in diameter is removed, together with a small spoonful of marrow. The latter is transferred to a sterile test-tube containing Wintrobe's mixture, the bone space is packed with bone wax, and the periosteum and skin are sutured. For Wintrobe's dry oxalate mixture place 0·1 ml. of a solution of 0·2 per cent potassium oxalate and 0·3 per cent ammonium oxalate into the test-tube for each 0·25 ml. of fluid to be aspirated and dry in the incubator. The marrow fluid clots very rapidly, so thorough mixing with the oxalate solution should not be delayed. Direct smears may be made if the fluid is not to be immediately examined.

Alternative Technique.—If simple aspiration of marrow tissue is all that is required this may be done as follows:—

Use a sternal puncture trocar and cannula similar to that illustrated in *Fig*. 509. An area near the centre of the body of the sternum opposite the third rib is infiltrated with local anæsthetic down to and including periosteum, and the needle is thrust through the area anæsthetized until the point touches bone. The guard is now adjusted so that it is some 3 mm. from the skin surface, and with a few sharp taps with a small hammer or a sharp thrust the needle is driven through the outer table into the marrow. Aspiration is effected as above, 0·24 ml. being added to the oxalate mixture. If the point of the needle is in marrow, aspiration is as easy as from a vein.

Sternal puncture may be performed at any age, but in childhood the aspiration should be from the centre of the manubrium sterni and the needle should be gently pushed through by hand, not driven by a hammer. Premedication is desirable. Both in adult and child the procedure is free from complications and is painless but for a drawing sensation in the sternum during the actual aspiration.

INDUCTION OF ARTIFICIAL PNEUMOTHORAX

Induction of an artificial pneumothorax is the procedure by which air is introduced into the pleural cavity, so separating the surfaces of visceral and parietal pleuræ, lowering the negative pressure in the pleural sac, lessening the normal tension of the lung, thereby allowing relaxation and partial rest of that organ. It is a passive partial collapse, and in no sense an active collapse by compression. The circulation through such a collapsed lung is decreased.

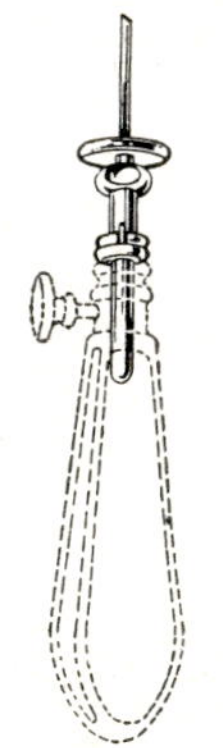

Fig. 509. — Needle suitable for marrow aspiration or intravenous venography.

Indications.—The usual indication for induction of an artificial pneumothorax is pulmonary tuberculosis with cavitation. It is also performed: (*a*) for

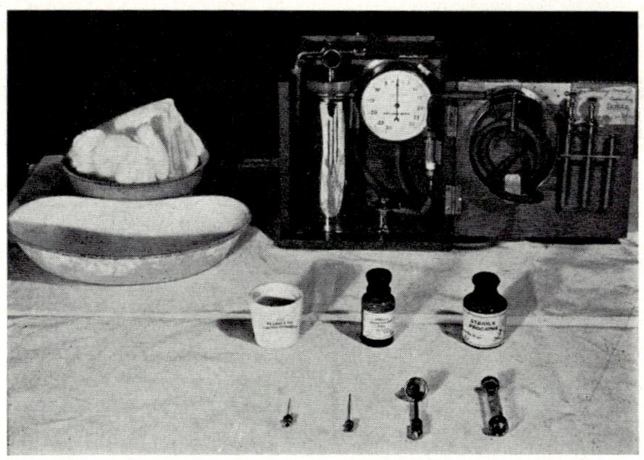

Fig. 510.—The Maxwell artificial pneumothorax apparatus with induction and refill needles in the rack. Local anæsthetic (2 per cent lignocaine) and adrenaline in case of pleural shock.

diagnostic purposes to decide whether a tumour is in the lung or chest wall; (*b*) prior to thoracoscopy; (*c*) for certain other conditions mentioned in this chapter.

26

Apparatus.—Many types of apparatus are on the market, of which that of James Maxwell (*Fig.* 510) is perhaps the most compact. That most commonly used in hospitals is the Lillingston-Pearson apparatus, as it is simple and easily kept in running order. *Fig.* 511 shows the apparatus ready for use. Coloured water is present in the two bottles. For an induction the fluid levels in both bottles are equal when ready for use; for a refill Bottle I is full and Bottle II has fluid up to the zero mark. If an air lock prevents the flow of fluid from I to II the mouth is applied to the open glass tube in Bottle I and a few millilitres of fluid are blown from one bottle to the other to start the flow. The coloured water in the manometer should be level with the zero mark before starting.

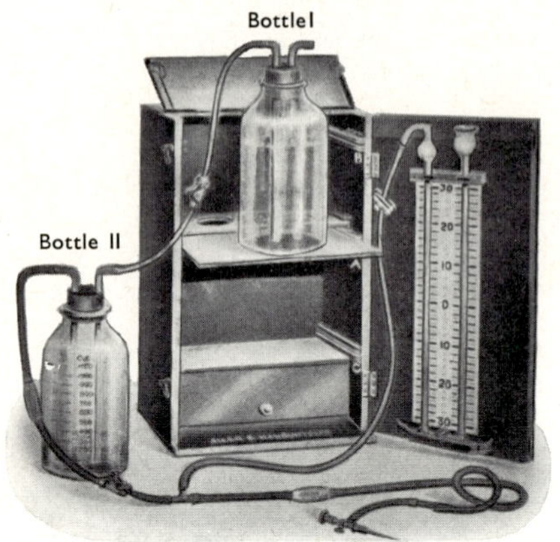

Fig. 511.—The Lillingston-Pearson artificial pneumothorax apparatus.

The principle is simple: when fluid flows from Bottle I to Bottle II the air in the latter is forced along the rubber tubing through two cotton-wool filters and so through the needle into the pleural sac. To start the flow the tap on the needle is opened, and the clips on each side of Bottle II are opened. The amount of air introduced is read on Bottle II—i.e., if the fluid level has risen from zero to 600, 600 ml. of air have been introduced. Readings are taken from the left of the manometer, a negative reading being shown by a rise above zero, a positive by a fall. Care should be taken to pinch the tube if the patient coughs, for the high positive pressure so caused may blow the fluid out of the manometer. For an induction an induction needle such as Rivière's (*Fig.* 512) or Küss's (*Fig.* 513) is used. On withdrawing the trocar care should be taken that the cap does not leave the end of the needle, for if this occurs the pleural sac is thrown open to the room air. This will not happen if it is first seen that the cap is firmly screwed on. Refills are done with refill needles such as Saugmann's (*Fig.* 514). As soon as the point is in the pleural space the stylet is withdrawn,

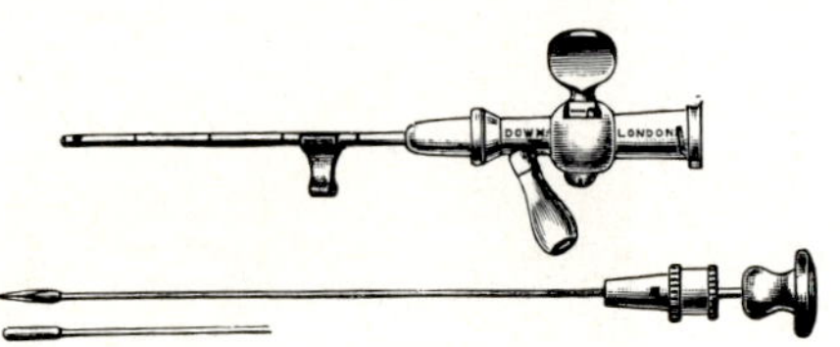

Fig. 512.—Rivière's needle.

the tap turned on, and the air introduced. Alternatively, a Morland's needle may be used for refills. This requires no stylet, the tube being attached to the end of the needle.

Technique of Induction of an Artificial Pneumothorax.—The apparatus is placed on a table or trolley alongside the bed with all taps closed and the fluids at equal levels in the two bottles. The patient lies comfortably flat on the bed on his unaffected side with only one pillow to support his head. His arm is thrown upwards in front of his face to expose the axilla on the affected side. After cleaning the skin an area over the site of election—usually the 4th–6th space in the mid- or anterior axillary line—is infiltrated with 5–8 ml. of local anæsthetic, care being taken to raise a small bleb in the skin, to avoid the ribs, and to infiltrate right down to the parietal pleura. The induction needle is then attached to the apparatus, and with a rotary movement the needle is passed through the skin and down between the ribs. When the pleura is reached the trocar is withdrawn and the cannula passed through the parietal pleura into the pleural sac. The needle tap is turned on, and a negative excursion on the manometer shows that the cannula is in the pleural sac. Any excursion on the manometer of less than 3 cm. is discounted. A common reading is −16

−11, an excursion of 5 cm., but anything from −30 −36 to −6 −2 may be seen. A reading of −1 +1 means that the end of the cannula is in the lung, and it should be gradually withdrawn until a suitable reading is obtained. A gradually rising

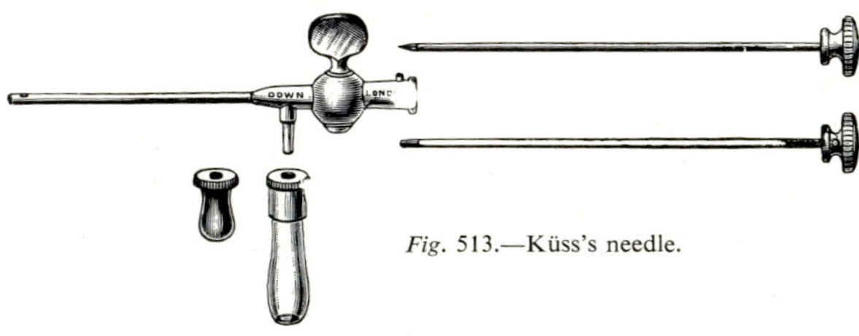

Fig. 513.—Küss's needle.

positive pressure indicates that the cannula is in a blood-vessel, and it should be withdrawn before blood flows through the rubber tubing into the apparatus. If no reading at all is obtained, either the cannula is in the chest wall or a pleural effusion, or the needle or tube is blocked. The trocar should be passed into the cannula and the tubing pinched several times to make certain this is not so. If still no reading is obtained it is likely that the lung is adherent in this area, and the process should be repeated in a fresh place—preferably in the 7th or 8th space posteriorly. The third and last site to be tried is high in the axilla or in the 2nd to 4th spaces anteriorly, care being taken to avoid the heart and great vessels.

When a suitable reading is obtained the taps are turned on, allowing the air to be *sucked* into the chest by the negative pressure

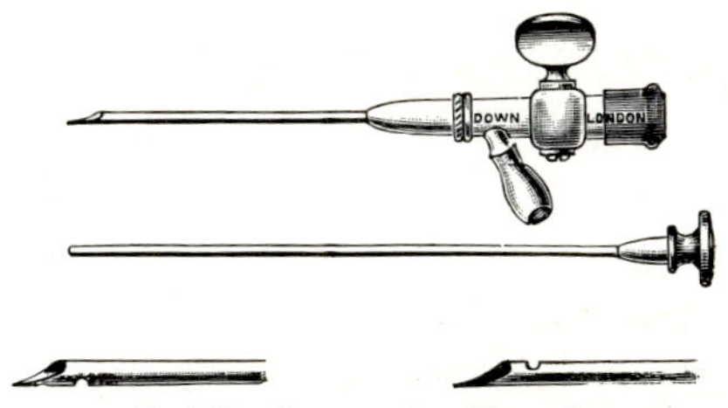

Fig. 514.—Saugmann's refill needle.

in the pleural sac. As the fluid level falls in Bottle I it may be raised so that the fluid levels remain equal in the two bottles. Any amount of air from 100 ml. to 500 ml. is introduced.

The final pressure should be a negative one, and the tap should be closed periodically to take a reading. A slight excursion throughout the induction is seen on the manometer which indicates that the cannula is still in the pleural space. A common reading obtained is −16 −12: 250 ml.: −13 −9. On no account should the pressure be left positive. A reading such as −12 −6: 100 ml.: −2 +2 means that adhesions are present between visceral and parietal pleuræ and only a small pocket of pleural sac has been filled with air. The final reading should not be lower than −4 −0. The needle is then withdrawn, the puncture wound covered with cotton-wool and collodion, and the patient ordered absolute rest for the subsequent twenty-four hours, lying on the side most comfortable to him—preferably the side induced. He is asked not to cough, and is given linctus codeinæ if a troublesome cough is present.

A possible danger must be emphasized. An intractable cough arising during induction may be due to puncture of the lung. This usually occurs when anæsthetizing the deeper structures; moreover, the sudden inspiratory movement may break off the needle in the chest wall.

Complications.—

1. *Bleeding from the puncture wound.* This is easily controlled by a pad and firm pressure for ten minutes.

2. *Pleural shock.* At any time during the induction the patient may become shocked. His pulse becomes weak and rapid, his blood-pressure drops, and his skin becomes cold, pale, and clammy. The induction is immediately stopped, and the patient is treated for shock. The cause of this complication is unknown.

3. *Tightness or discomfort in the chest.* In mild degree this is of no significance, but if severe the patient should be examined to ascertain if the breath-sounds are

absent, the percussion note hyper-resonant, or the heart displaced. Any of these signs may indicate a superadded spontaneous pneumothorax caused by the tearing of a pleural adhesion or laceration of the lung. A refill needle is inserted and a reading taken. If a positive pressure is present, air should be gradually withdrawn until the patient is eased. This is done by reversing the flow in the two bottles, so that the fluid runs from Bottle II to Bottle I (*Fig.* 515).

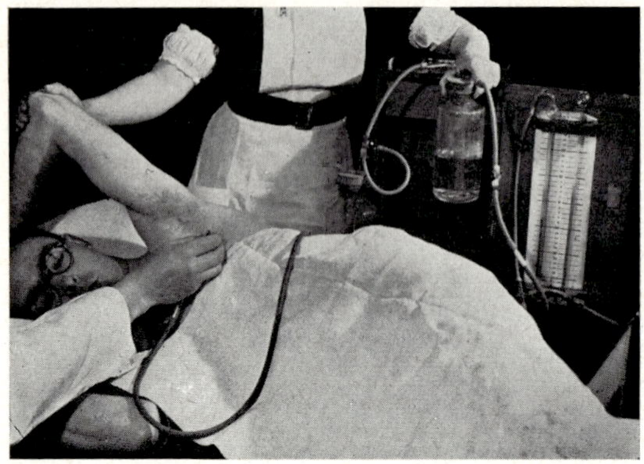

Fig. 515.—Artificial pneumothorax. If too much air has been introduced into the chest, elevation of Bottle II of the artificial pneumothorax apparatus sucks some air back. Note the positive pressure on the left limb of the water manometer (+ 7).

4. *Subcutaneous emphysema.* A mild degree of this is commonly present after induction and is of no significance.

5. *Hæmoptysis.* This probably means that the lung has been injured by the trocar during induction. It is never severe. The patient is reassured and told that slight staining of the sputum may persist for some hours but is of no significance.

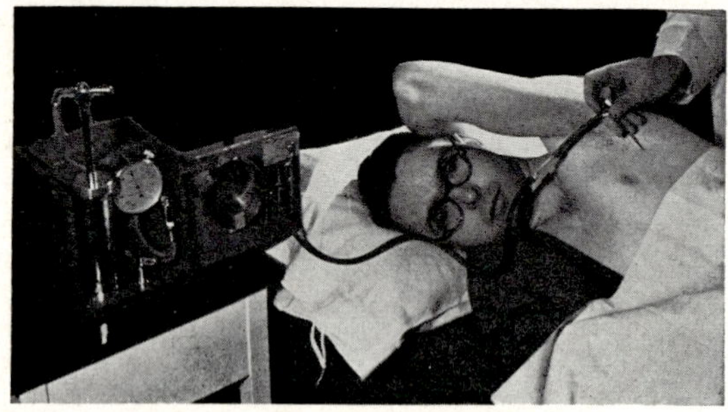

Fig. 516.—A refill of an artificial pneumothorax in progress. Note negative pressure on manometer.

6. *Air embolism.* This is the most dangerous of all complications and, though rare, is not infrequently fatal. The usual history is that, with no definite swing on the manometer, the impatient operator has run in 20 ml. or more air. If the point of the needle is in close relation to a vessel, often in a vascular adhesion, air may enter the pulmonary circulation and rapidly pass to the brain, causing convulsions,

coma, paresis of arm, leg, and/or face, and possibly death. Often the patient has peculiar sensations at the commencement of the embolism and knows something is going radically wrong. The needle must be withdrawn immediately if there is the slightest suspicion of air embolism. For treatment of air embolism *see* p. 8.

Refills.—After the induction of an artificial pneumothorax a refill should be performed after twenty-four hours, and subsequently (if desired) after 2, 4, and 8 days, maintaining the collapse at weekly intervals as found necessary. Treatment is controlled by radiographs and screening. Satisfactory collapse is usually not achieved until the fourth or fifth refill. Refills (*Fig.* 516) are performed with a suitable refill needle, using the same technique as for an induction. The fluid is run from Bottle I to Bottle II, the latter starting with the fluid level at zero. The amount of air introduced is read, and varies from 200 to 700 ml. The first three refills should not exceed 500 ml. The final pressure should never be positive, i.e., should not exceed $-2 +2$.

The only physical sign after the induction of an artificial pneumothorax is lessening of the breath-sounds on that side. After two or three fills the breath-sounds may disappear completely, but the percussion note remains normal. A mediastinal shift may or may not occur, and is of little or no significance after the third refill unless extreme and/or causing symptoms.

ARTIFICIAL PNEUMOPERITONEUM

Artificial pneumoperitoneum is used as a form of therapy in selected cases of pulmonary tuberculosis, usually in conjunction with phrenic paresis, the air under the diaphragm effecting a much greater elevation of that muscle than can be obtained by phrenic paresis alone. With few exceptions pneumoperitoneum is performed only when a satisfactory artificial pneumothorax cannot be obtained. It may also be used as a diagnostic investigation to locate the site of an intra-abdominal mass or as a preliminary to peritoneoscopy.

Technique.—With the patient lying flat over pillows placed in the small of the back to throw the lumbar spine into slight lordosis, the skin and abdominal wall are infiltrated with local anæsthetic at a point between the umbilicus and the left costal margin. A convenient spot is some 2–2½ in. (5–6 cm.) above and to the left of the umbilicus, preferably just lateral to the rectus abdominis muscle. The initial injection of air is made through an artificial pneumothorax induction needle (*see above*) or a suitable long wide-bore needle. The needle is thrust slowly through the abdominal wall to avoid perforation of the intestine, a very rare complication. When it is thought that the peritoneal cavity has been reached a small quantity of air is introduced; if the needle point is still in the abdominal wall a sharp rise occurs in the manometric pressure. Pressure readings from the peritoneal cavity are variable and unreliable and often none can be obtained, so if no sharp rise in pressure occurs on the manometer air is slowly run in, 500–800 ml. Subsequent refills are given much as with an artificial pneumothorax, the amount of air given depending on radiological and clinical control. When established, an artificial pneumoperitoneum usually needs some 1000 ml. of air weekly or fortnightly to maintain satisfactory elevation of the paralysed diaphragm. Pressure readings, even with refills, are unsatisfactory and may be anything from $+ 0$ to $+ 12$ cm. of water. The presence of air in the abdomen is therefore verified when performing a refill by aspirating a little air into the local anæsthetic after infiltration of the abdominal wall.

Complications.—
1. Shoulder-tip pain on the side of the unparalysed diaphragm. Mild analgesics or elevation of the foot of the bed are all that is necessary.
2. Perforation of the bowel.
3. Air embolism.
4. Mediastinal emphysema.
5. Peritoneal effusion.
The last four are rare.

AIR REPLACEMENT OF A PLEURAL EFFUSION

The patient sits on a couch with his head and shoulders upright. For comfort it is better to have his back supported, as the replacement, if difficult, may take time. He puts the arm on the affected side well forwards to expose his axilla, and leans slightly to the opposite side.

Two areas are infiltrated with local anæsthesia, one high in the axilla between the 3rd and 4th or the 4th and 5th ribs, the other lower in the 7th interspace in the posterior axillary line, in the 6th space in the mid-axillary line, or posteriorly in the

7th–8th space below the angle of the scapula. Two such areas are anæsthetized, and a small portion of fluid from both areas withdrawn into the syringe, to make certain fluid is present at both sites.

Into the lower area an aspirating needle is inserted and connected with the aspirator. Commonly used types are Dieulafoy's and Potain's. The latter has certain disadvantages, but is the model to be found in most hospitals. Its chief drawback lies in the irregularity of its suction, but for general purposes it is a very useful apparatus. Dieulafoy's aspirator is a large syringe with a two-way cock.

Through the upper area an artificial pneumothorax refill or induction needle is inserted and connected up with the artificial pneumothorax apparatus. If fluid extends above the site of the upper needle—as shown by aspiration of a few drops into the local anæsthetic syringe—a refill needle is used; if not, an induction needle, and readings are taken from the start.

Aspiration is commenced, and the upper needle kept closed if in fluid. After some 280 ml. have been withdrawn, insert air via the upper needle from the artificial pneumothorax apparatus (*Fig.* 517). Continue the aspiration, never allowing air to enter from above faster than fluid is escaping below. As the fluid level sinks below the

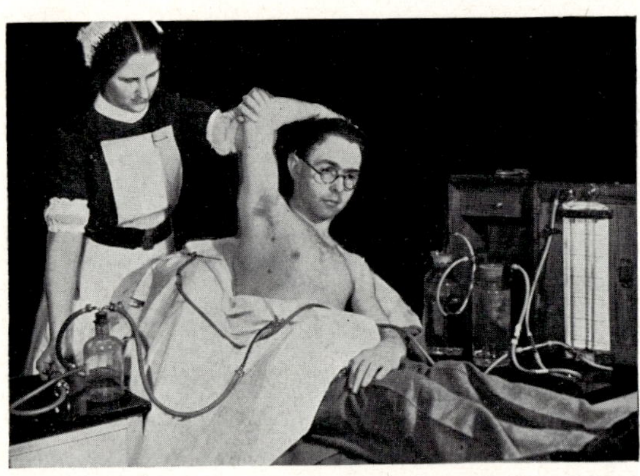

Fig. 517.—Air replacement of a pleural effusion. Potain's aspirator is on the left of the picture, the needle to be inserted into the chest at the lower mark. The Lillingston-Pearson artificial pneumothorax apparatus is on the right, the needle to be inserted at the upper mark on the chest wall.

upper needle a swing in the manometer of the artificial pneumothorax apparatus becomes apparent. The intrapleural pressure is kept slightly negative—a swing of −6 −2 is suitable. A high negative, such as −12 −8, means that too little air has been introduced and too much fluid removed. When the flow becomes less steady through the aspirator and interrupted by air-bubbles, let the patient lean over to the affected side. In this way all the fluid may be aspirated.

The final reading is then taken, and should be slightly on the negative side. Both needles are removed, the puncture wounds covered with cotton-wool and collodion, or cotton-wool alone, and the aspirated fluid and introduced air measured.

HÆMOPTYSIS

Hæmoptysis, if copious, may cause sudden death. The cause is almost always bleeding from a ruptured artery in a cavity; such a cavity is usually of tuberculous origin. Hæmorrhage may also occur from bronchiectasis, neoplasms, and other lesions. The patient may become drowned in his own blood, which is partly coughed out and partly inhaled into all parts of the lung.

Treatment.—The immediate treatment is to lower the head over the side of the bed if the patient is choking, and allow the blood to flow from the lung bases towards the bifurcation of the trachea, whence it will be coughed up. Usually the bleeding is too slight to warrant this procedure. Morphine always does more good than harm, as such a patient is anxious and terrified at the sight of his own blood, and imagines death to be imminent. Nothing seems to soothe as much as morphine. Only 10 mg. should be given, for tuberculous subjects seem to respond more readily than others to the injection. The patient is ordered absolute rest. If bleeding is copious and continues, and the signs of cavitation, clinical and/or radiological, are present on one side, an artificial pneumothorax may be induced on that side. Complete collapse of the cavity for hæmoptysis necessitates introduction of much more air than is permissible in any other condition at one fill. Anything up to 1200 ml. may be introduced, but at the first sign of distress the procedure should be stopped. Usually only 400–600 ml. are necessary. Shift of the heart and mediastinum does not matter if no distress is caused. The fill should be repeated if bleeding continues.

SPONTANEOUS PNEUMOTHORAX

The usual causes are rupture of an emphysematous bulla or pulmonary tuberculosis. A patient with an artificial pneumothorax may rupture an adhesion containing lung tissue and develop a spontaneous pneumothorax in addition. Symptoms may be absent or slight, or there may be severe pain in the side, palpitations, or shock. The onset is acute. Diagnosis is made on the signs of a displaced heart and absence of breath-sounds on one side. The percussion note is usually hyper-resonant, but not always so.

Treatment.—Take a radiograph to verify the diagnosis unless the condition is urgent. Insert an artificial pneumothorax needle into the affected side, connect with the artificial pneumothorax apparatus, and take a reading; but if the patient is not distressed it is best to leave him alone without taking pleural pressures. Instead of the normal negative pressure (about $-14 -8$) the swing shows $-2 +2$ or a positive reading such as $+2 +6$. If not distressed the patient is left severely alone; if short of breath and in pain, remove sufficient air to give him relief, but no more than 700 ml. at one time. The air is withdrawn by reversing the flow in the bottles of the artificial pneumothorax apparatus. If acutely urgent and the physical signs are such as to warrant the diagnosis, and if no artificial pneumothorax apparatus is to hand, thrust into the chest any wide-bore needle. The best site is in the 7th space in the axilla, but almost anywhere between 2nd and 9th ribs will do. The air will be heard to rush out if under great pressure. This often occurs where a valvular leak is present, allowing air to enter the pleura, but none to leave.

If the dyspnœa is increasing, a valvular pneumothorax is almost certainly present. In such a case leave the needle in and attach to it tubing and an under-water seal drainage bottle (p. 309). When the patient coughs bubbles will appear through the tube only if the fistula has persisted. A rubber catheter or polythene tube can be introduced anteriorly via a cannula into the pleural space and left retained to the chest wall with a stitch. This is infinitely preferable to an indwelling needle, which may puncture or tear the expanding lung.

If fluid appears in the pleural space the condition is probably tuberculous; if not, probably non-tuberculous though spontaneous hæmothorax may occur, albeit rarely. The emphysema cases are common, and almost all get well on rest alone, no removal of air being necessary. If the lung in such a case is slow in re-expanding, removal of air occasionally may accelerate the process.

LUMBAR PUNCTURE

Rigid asepsis must always be maintained in performing this procedure, preparation being as for a surgical operation.

Contra-indications.—It must be stressed at the outset that lumbar puncture is contra-indicated in situations where a great rise in cerebrospinal fluid pressure is liable to be encountered from space-occupying lesions within the skull. Clinically, these must be suspected from the triad of headaches, vomiting, and papillœdema, with the presence of the latter finding necessitating seeking expert neurological advice before proceeding with the investigation.

A fine-bore needle (*Fig.* 518) is preferable to a larger one, as it may be less likely to cause headaches as outflow of cerebrospinal fluid is slower. This, however, remains controversial.

Position of the Patient.—This is all-important, for the spine must not be rotated. One of two positions may be used:—

1. The lateral position, with the patient lying on a flat surface, back flexed as much as possible with lumbar vertebræ in line with the edge of the bed. A bed-board under the mattress is often necessary to give an absolutely flat surface;

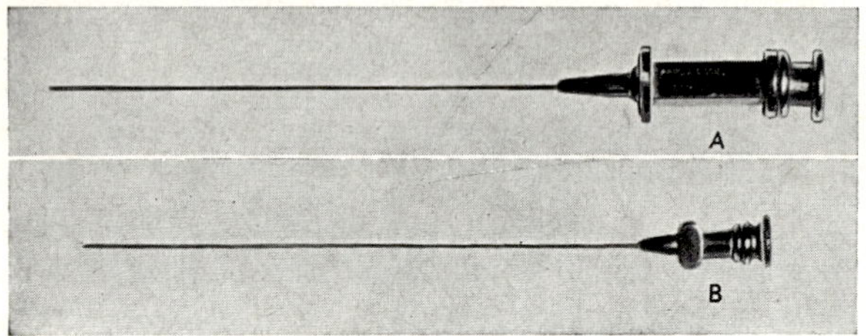

Fig. 518.—A, Barker's needle; B, A smaller lumbar puncture needle
for routine use.

in the case of a child a table-top may be used. The nurse should face the patient with one arm under the flexed knees and one on the neck to maintain full spinal flexion and prevent sudden movements which might break the needle while in situ (*Fig.* 519). A roller towel passed around neck and knees may be used in flexing and immobilizing difficult semi-conscious patients.

2. The upright position, with the patient sitting on a bed or chair with legs down and back bent forwards, a nurse standing by to support the patient, who for this position must be fully conscious and co-operative.

Position 1 is much to be preferred in almost all cases. The whole procedure is explained beforehand to the patient, who must be warned not to strain or cough during the puncture. For puncture in children, *see* p. 570.

Site of Puncture.—The site of election is between L.3–4 vertebræ; this space lies on a line joining the uppermost points of the iliac crests (*Fig.* 520). A line dropped perpendicularly from the uppermost iliac crest to the vertebral column will be accurate enough if spinal posture is as it should be. The skin is sterilized and isolated with sterile towels, and local anæsthetic is injected into the skin between the two adjacent spinous processes to raise a small bleb, local anæsthetic being then injected deeper down towards the theca. The usual preparation of the skin is with surgical spirit and iodine, so that contamination by either bacteria or spores may be avoided. Cetrimide (cetavlon) is irritant to the theca and is best avoided for this procedure. The lumbar puncture needle is then inserted through the anæsthetized area perpendicular to the skin and then inclined very slightly towards the patient's head. When the ligamentum flavum is penetrated, a slight 'give' is felt. Sometimes a second 'give' is felt just beyond, as the dura mater is punctured. The stylet is then withdrawn and spinal fluid should drip evenly into the sterile tube. Usually, however, pressures have to be taken first, unless it is only a simple examination of the fluid that is required.

Measuring Cerebrospinal Fluid Pressure.—The pressure should in most cases be measured with a manometer such as is shown in *Figs.* 521 and 522, particularly when pressures are low and a block is suspected. With the needle inserted through the interspinous ligament, the stylet is withdrawn and the manometer fitted. The dura is then entered and cerebrospinal fluid enters the manometer

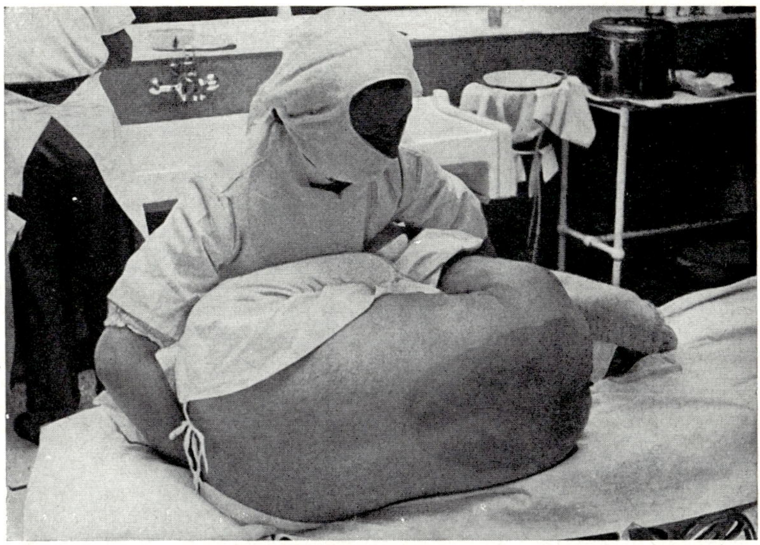

Fig. 519.—An assistant places one arm under the knees and the other around the back of the neck in order to flex the spine as fully as possible.

and pressures are taken. After warning the patient what is about to happen, Queckenstedt's test is performed, i.e., the nurse assisting presses gently but

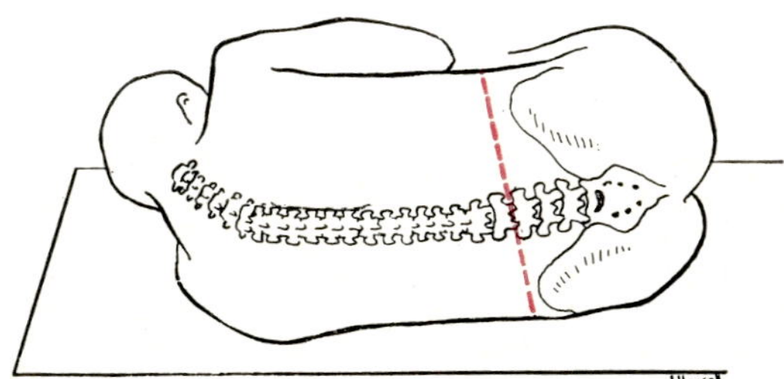

Fig. 520.—Method of defining the interspace between the 3rd and 4th lumbar vertebræ.

firmly on the internal jugular vein or veins and the rise in fluid pressure is noted, also the speed of rise after jugular pressure and of fall after release. It is essential for the patient to be completely relaxed and breathing naturally and evenly during the manœuvre, as any straining or holding of breath elevates the fluid pressure. Normal pressures vary between 100 and 200 mm., sitting pressures being higher than lying. Pressures above 200 mm. in a relaxed patient are abnormal. A slow or absent rise and fall with Queckenstedt's test may indicate a spinal (intrathecal) blockage.

Dry Tap.—To insert a needle and obtain nothing is a humbling experience which happens to every graduate occasionally, however efficient he may be. The usual excuses are osteo-arthritis or spinal adhesions, but the truth is almost

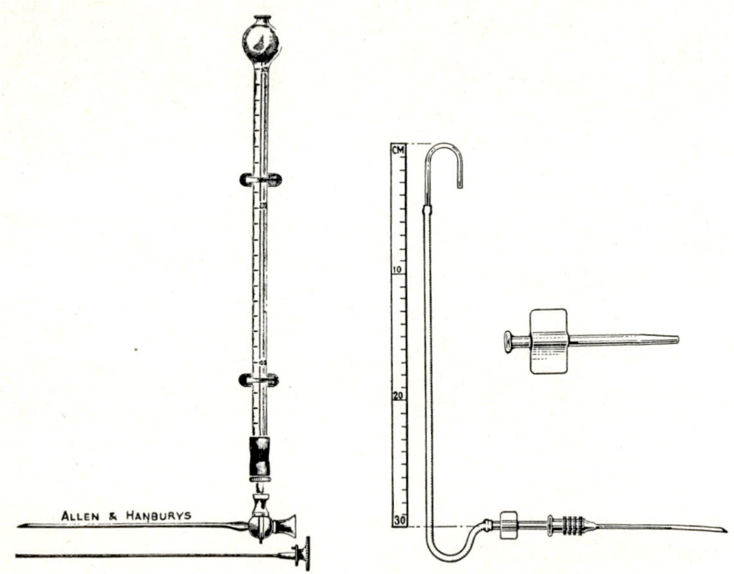

Fig. 521.—Greenfield's spinal manometer.   *Fig.* 522.—Northfield's apparatus for measuring the cerebrospinal fluid pressure. (*Inset*, the adaptor.)

always faulty position of the patient and inaccurate siting of the needle. A twisted curved spine due to a sagging mattress is a far more common cause of failure than osteo-arthritis. In severe ankylosing spondylitis, however, it may be impossible to obtain a specimen, for, both in this and other conditions, spinal flexion may be impossible. It is amazing how far from the desired spot the point of the needle may be in some cases: if the patient complains of pain radiating down the leg, the needle may have struck one of the roots of the cauda equina.

Cerebrospinal Fluid Specimens.—The essence of a satisfactory lumbar puncture is to take off as little fluid as will satisfy the pathologist as slowly as possible through a suitable fairly fine strong needle. Headaches subsequently often mean 'too much fluid off too quickly'. The fluid is dripped into two sterile bottles, which are marked (1) and (2). The first may contain blood-cells if a blood-vessel has been struck and only the second one may be truly representative of the spinal fluid. When pressures are taken with a manometer, the fluid from the manometer is run into sterile bottles for examination.

Complications.—Headache is the only common complication. Prevention is better than cure and a slow non-traumatic tap is the best way to avoid this side-effect, which can be very distressing. It is wise after lumbar puncture on a hospital in-patient to rest the patient in bed with feet slightly elevated for the rest of the day, but in an out-patient, as in the venereal disease clinic, only an hour or less may be possible. The headache is probably due in many cases to lowered pressures in the theca, and simple analgesics, rest with feet elevated, and abundant fluids by mouth are usually all that are indicated. Infections of the theca or extra-thecal tissues are, happily, rare. The patient should not be told to expect a headache: this is a certain way of increasing the prevalence of this complication in the suggestible. If headache is troublesome and persistent it may sometimes be relieved by giving fludrocortisone 0·5–1 mg. by mouth, repeating 0·5 mg. once if necessary after 8–10 hours.

VACCINATION AGAINST SMALL-POX (VARIOLA)

Small-pox is no longer endemic in Britain, but the rapidity and ease of air travel makes reinfection of an unvaccinated community a very real and ever-present danger. The community can be persuaded, but not ordered, to be vaccinated (for compulsory vaccination was given up in 1946). Those unfortunates not vaccinated in infancy may later in adult life, in the face of infection or before travel to foreign countries, have to be vaccinated, and often suffer much greater reactions and more complications.

Vaccination in Infancy.—It is best, therefore, to perform primary vaccination between the second and twelfth months, a good time being about the fourth month, though recent figures strongly suggest that the safest period is between 1 and 2 years. Except in the face of an epidemic it is wise to avoid vaccination in the first few weeks of life.

Mass vaccinations of a whole community on the appearance of a case of small-pox is not now advocated, but contacts of such a case and their household contacts should be vaccinated or revaccinated without delay as a matter of urgency. Unless actual signs of small-pox are present, vaccination may give some measure of protection even if carried out in the early incubation period. Those who have seen an outbreak of small-pox and what it can do to an individual or to a community have no doubts as to the wisdom of vaccination, preferably under 2 years of age. Variola major has an overall mortality-rate of around 25 per cent, and the hæmorrhagic forms are almost invariably fatal.

Vaccination produces an active immunity to small-pox by introducing a small quantity of lymph containing the living vaccine virus into the deeper layers of the epidermis. This lymph is supplied in sealed capillary tubes, and should be stored in a cool dark place such as a domestic refrigerator. Maximal immunity occurs after 2 to 3 weeks, though some immunity usually lasts some 3 to 4 or more years. International regulations demand revaccination for travellers into endemic areas every 3 years.

Indications for vaccination are: (1) where the individual is proceeding into an area where small-pox is endemic, (2) exposure to a known or suspected case of small-pox, or (3) where the individual's occupation carries particular risks of infection (e.g., medical attendants, nurses in fever hospitals, ambulance drivers).

Technique.—The site of choice is the lower part of the posterior border of the deltoid muscle: scarring here is not unduly apparent. If the leg is preferred in infants the site should be 1 in. (2·5 cm.) above the external malleolus, and in children or adults, the thigh. If it is necessary to clean the skin, simple soap and water is all that is required. Antiseptics should not be used as they may destroy the virus. The vaccine lymph is ejected from the capillary tube on to the cleaned area and a handy method is to blow the lymph out with a teat from an infant's bottle, the unbroken tube of lymph being passed through the small opening in the teat, then both ends broken off. The tube is then pulled down into the teat and the lymph blown out, as in *Fig.* 523. The multiple-pressure method is effective, relatively painless, and non-traumatic, is not likely to be associated with secondary infection, and shows a higher success rate in revaccination than does the scratch technique. A straight sterilized needle, flat-sided or triangular in section, is moved rapidly up and down through the drop of lymph and pressed repeatedly downwards (*Fig.* 524) gently but

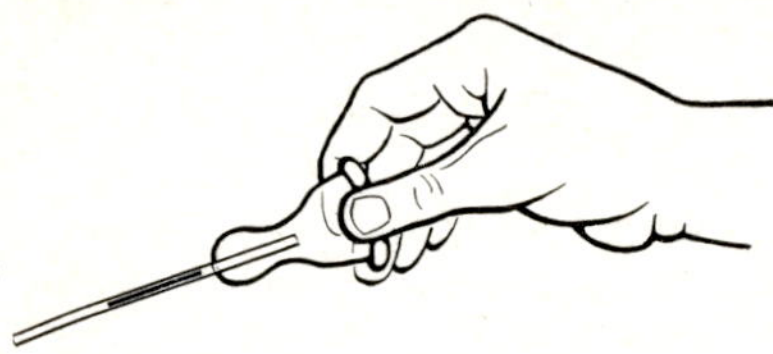

Fig. 523.—Method of transferring lymph from the capillary tube, using a teat from a feeding bottle.

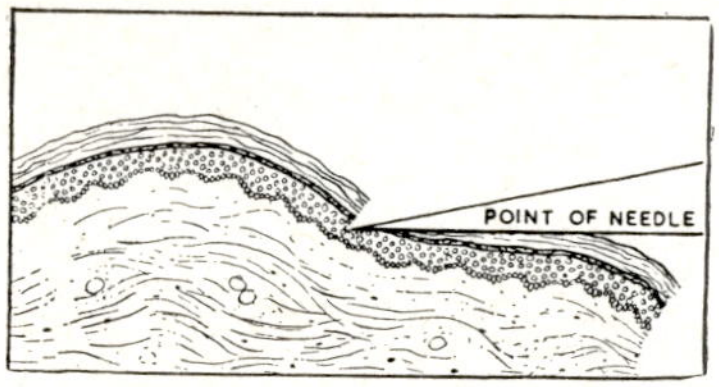

Fig. 524.—Multiple-pressure method of vaccination. A rapid up-and-down motion of the side of the needle, the point of which enters the drop of the vaccine.

firmly on the skin. Some thirty pressures are rapidly applied with an up-and-down movement perpendicular to the skin. Excess lymph is removed with sterile cotton-wool. No immediate dressing is essential, but some prefer to apply a light sterile, *non-antiseptic* dressing for the first few days to reduce the risk of accidental self- or cross-vaccination.

Course of Events after Vaccination.—

Primary Vaccination.—After 4 days a small red slightly itching papule appears, becoming vesicular the next day, and an area of inflammation appears around it (*Fig.* 525). After about a week the inflammation subsides and a scab forms, which separates 10 to 14 days later. Some systemic features may appear a week after vaccination in both adults and infants.

Revaccination.—If there is no skin response within a week of vaccination, the procedure should be repeated, and again a third time if persistently negative. If after three attempts no positive reaction is obtained, it is assumed, unless the quality of the lymph is in question, that the immunity level is still high from previous vaccination, and it is recorded as 'no local reaction to revaccination (repeated)'. The reaction may appear early and run a short course, the 'accelerated' reaction, indicating that some immunity remains from previous vaccination. Local irritation without vesiculation may occur after 2–3 days. This may or may not indicate immunity, and is recorded as 'maximal local reaction (non-vesicular) 2nd/3rd day'. Occasionally a previously vaccinated individual reacts as in primary vaccination, indicating that all previous immunity has disappeared. This is recorded as 'typical (primary) vaccinia'.

The antibody response to revaccination is more rapid and reaches a higher level than can be obtained by primary vaccination, hence the importance of immediate vaccination of contacts of a known case. Routine revaccination should be performed, in any case, in children between 8 and 12 years of age, and those dealing with cases of small-pox, such as doctors, nurses, and ambulance personnel, should be revaccinated annually.

Complications.—After successful primary vaccination there may be a mild fever for 4–8 days, but this is not strictly speaking a complication but a part

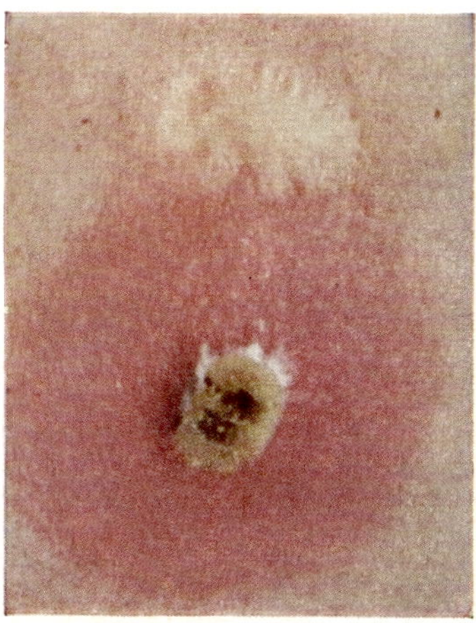

Fig. 525.—Successful vaccination. Appearance on the eighth day.

of the normal march of events. Similarly axillary adenitis is usually present to some degree on the affected side. Inflammatory changes subside in a few days, or up to 3 weeks. True complications have been classified as follows:—

Local Complications.—Necrosis and ulceration of the vaccination site are more common in adults after primary vaccination. Satellite vesicles may occur. Keloid and hypertrophic scars are not uncommon and do not always follow severe local reactions. Bacterial infection (impetigo and erysipelas) is very rarely seen.

Distant Complications.—

1. *Non-specific Vascular Reactions.*—Erythema multiforme or toxic erythema may both occur some 13 days after primary vaccination, starting near the site of vaccination. Allergic purpura and urticaria may also occur.

2. *Eruptions of vaccinial vesicles* may develop at a distance from the vaccination site as a result of skin contamination (accidental inoculation vaccinia) or blood-borne spread (generalized vaccinia). Vesicles of accidental inoculation appear about a week after primary vaccination, often on skin previously broken by previous infection, as in acne, or eyelids, conjunctivæ, lips, or vulva may be affected.

Generalized (*blood-borne*) *vaccinia* may be: (1) mild and sparsely spread, occurring some 10 days after vaccination. The lesions may sometimes be confused with modified small-pox. A much more serious though rare complication is (2) progressive vaccinia (vaccinia gangrenosa), where the vaccination site fails to heal normally and the lesion extends and ulcerates, the ulcer enlarging and deepening, sometimes developing satellite lesions. It is usually associated with disorders of immune response such as hypoglobulinæmia and chronic leukæmia, or in patients receiving corticosteroids or antimetabolic agents. It is usually fatal. (3) Eczema vaccination is a generalized vaccinia occurring in an eczematous patient, the pustular eruption being worse in the eczematous areas. It carries a mortality of about 6 per cent, being particularly dangerous to children under 5 years of age. Administration of antivaccinial hyperimmune gamma-globin has reduced this mortality considerably and apparently restricted the spread of skin reactions. (4) Aseptic meningitis, osteitis, and encephalitis are rare.

Vaccination of pregnant women in the first 3 months has not been followed by an increase of abnormalities in the offspring, but cases have been reported of premature macerated infants with skin and viscera covered with vaccinia pocks, whose mothers received primary vaccination in the second trimester. In general it is wise not to vaccinate patients at any time during pregnancy.

Contra-indications.—Vaccination should be postponed if there is eczema or dermatitis, gastro-enteritis, acute infections, sepsis, or marked debility, or if there has been recent exposure to infectious disorders such as measles or pertussis. Premature infants should only be vaccinated when they are thriving and only where there is special risk of infection with small-pox. Hypogammaglobulinæmic, corticosteroid-treated, and other patients particularly at risk should be given antivaccinial hyperimmune gamma-globulin in the other arm at the time of vaccination if exposed to a case of small-pox. In general it is wise to avoid vaccination in pregnancy unless there is a very real risk of variola.

CHAPTER XLV

TREATMENT OF SNAKE-BITE

By Bruce C. Paton

THE world contains about 2700 different species of snake of which the majority are harmless. The poisonous snakes are, however, widely distributed throughout the world and are found in every type of terrain except subarctic and arctic areas, at high altitudes, and in some zoologically isolated areas such as New Zealand. Since the Garden of Eden enmity has existed between snakes and man, but most of the aggression has been man's. With the exception of the king cobra, the mambas, and a few South American species, the poisonous snakes do not generally attack man spontaneously, and bite only in defence or because they have been disturbed or trodden upon.

The mortality-rate from snake-bite is not generally as high as imagined although in some areas, such as India, 20,000 to 30,000 people die annually from snake-bite. Burma has probably the highest incidence of death from snake-bite, 15 per 100,000. But in the same geographic area, Thailand, infested by snakes and with a largely rural population of 27 million, only records about 250 deaths from snake-bite per year. In the United States there were 138 deaths between 1950 and 1959 (compared with approximately 350,000 deaths from automobile accidents in the same period).

The likelihood of dying from snake-bite depends upon:—

1. The size and type of snake.
2. The depth and effectiveness of envenomation.
3. The treatment administered.

The doctor cannot influence the first two factors but is obviously of prime importance in the third.

PRECAUTIONS IN SNAKE-INFESTED COUNTRY

Do's.—

1. Know what types of poisonous snakes may be encountered.
2. Provide appropriate specific antivenom.
3. Wear suitable clothing: ankle-length boots, long trousers.

Don'ts.—

1. Place your hands on ledges, down holes, or under rocks where an unseen snake may be hiding.
2. Walk around barefoot or with sandals, especially at night.
3. Walk around at night without a light: most poisonous snakes are more active at night than by day.
4. Camp in heavily wooded or brush areas without clearing the ground.
5. Disturb snakes: *never* pick them up unless you are *certain* they are harmless.
6. Examine the mouth and fangs of freshly killed snakes except with a stick: reflex action in a dead snake has been known to cause a severe bite.
7. Be unduly afraid. Most snakes will go quietly away if given a chance: therefore, when faced by a snake keep still and do not provoke the snake to attack—it can move much quicker than you.

Killing a Snake.—Most snakes are easily killed by a blow with a stick on or behind the head. The back can also be easily broken, but a blow near the tail will not disable the snake. There is no guarantee that just because a snake has inflicted one bite that it does not have enough venom left to inflict another that is potentially serious. Therefore, although an attempt should be made to kill the snake, take care. Most snakes can only strike for a distance of about one-third to one-half of their length. The smaller the snake, the closer you can get without danger.

TYPES OF POISONOUS SNAKES

The zoological classification of poisonous snakes is quite complex, but for medical purposes most poisonous snakes fall into one of three categories:—

1. Elapidæ: cobras, kraits, mambas, coral snakes, Australian tiger snake, taipan.

2. Crotalidæ: rattlesnakes, moccasins, copperhead, Russell's viper, Malayan pit viper, puff adder.

3. Hydrophidæ: sea snakes.

The recognition and identification of a poisonous snake are sometimes very simple (e.g., if there is a rattle on the tail) and occasionally difficult. There are no certain features by which a poisonous snake can be differentiated from a non-poisonous except for the presence of fangs.

The Elapidæ all have short fixed fangs at the front of the upper jaw. A few, like the South African boomslang, have posteriorly placed fangs and, because of this, are rarely able to bite a man effectively. The Crotalidæ have larger, retractable grooved fangs also at the front of the upper jaw which project when the snake's mouth is opened.

The most important poisonous snakes found in various geographical areas are outlined below.

1. BRITAIN AND EUROPE

Vipers.—About eight species of viper occur in Europe, but only one occurs in Britain. They are found on mountains, moors, and fields. Some of the European species are occasionally quite aggressive. Death from snake-bite is rare in Britain and only 2 deaths were recorded in England and Wales in 19 years; in France and Italy combined there are about 20 deaths per year.

2. NORTH AMERICA

a. **Rattlesnakes.**—These are widely distributed and found in all types of terrain, but mostly open, sandy, rock country. The largest diamondbacks are extremely dangerous, but the smaller types (prairie, massasauga) seldom cause fatalities, and are usually not aggressive; they cause 70–80 per cent of bites in the U.S.A. The venom is cytotoxic.

b. **Water Moccasins.**—These are always in or near water, are good swimmers, and adopt a threatening attitude with the mouth wide open. The venom is cytotoxic.

c. **Copperheads.**—These are found both in dry country and deep forest. Bites are rare because these are timid, non-aggressive snakes. The venom is cytotoxic.

d. **Coral Snakes.**—These are found only in certain southern areas. They are not aggressive and bites are rare, but the venom is very toxic. This is the only elapid snake in the U.S.A. The venom is neurotoxic.

3. SOUTH AMERICA

a. **Rattlesnakes.**—There are five species and they are widely distributed. The tropical rattlesnake is the commonest and most dangerous. The venoms are cytotoxic and neurotoxic.

b. **Bushmasters.**—These are large, aggressive forest snakes. They are not usually found near habitations. The venom is cytotoxic and neurotoxic.

c. **Fer-de-lances.**—There are several species, some being large and dangerous. The venom is cytotoxic.

d. **Coral Snakes.**—These live mostly underground and are not aggressive. The venom is neurotoxic.

4. AFRICA

a. **Mambas.**—These are black or green, and are widely distributed in deep forest, woodland, and bush, up to 5000 feet. They are aggressive, especially during breeding, and are extremely swift. The venom is neurotoxic.

b. **Cobras.**—

i. *'Spitting' Cobras.*—These are black-necked or ringhals. They spit a fine spray of venom in self-defence, usually directed towards the eyes causing severe pain and conjunctivitis, and can also bite in the usual manner.

ii. *Eight Other Species.*—These are distributed in hot, dry country and forests, and are rare above 5000 feet. They are often found near houses, especially if rats are plentiful. They are not usually aggressive. The venom is neurotoxic.

c. **Vipers.**—

i. *Puff Adders.*—These are very widely distributed, in dry forest and bush. They are sluggish till roused and are very venomous.

ii. *Night Adders.*—These are nocturnal and are often found near water. The widest distribution is in south and tropical Africa.

iii. *Horned Adders.*—These are small and bury themselves in sand.

iv. *Berg Adders.*—These are found on high South African mountains.

v. *Gaboon Vipers.*—These are large and extremely venomous, but are rare.

vi. *Sand Vipers.*—These are found in the deserts of North Africa.

All these vipers have mainly cytotoxic venoms.

5. INDIA AND SOUTH-EAST ASIA

a. **Cobras.**—

i. *Common Cobras.*—These are widely distributed poisonous snakes. Their colour and pattern are variable. They are usually dark bluish black, with some white marks on the throat. They characteristically spread their spectacled hood when alarmed or angered and coil, with head erect, for striking position. They cause most of the deaths. They are found often in or near houses and eat rats. They are not usually aggressive. The venom is neurotoxic.

ii. *King Cobras.*—These are found in deep jungle, are very aggressive especially when breeding, and grow to 18 ft. They eat other snakes. Bites are rare because of habitat; recovery from bite is probably infrequent. The venom is neurotoxic.

b. **Kraits.**—There are several varieties, and are mostly banded yellow or white and black. They are nocturnal, not aggressive, but very venomous. The venom is neurotoxic.

c. **Vipers.**—

i. *Russell's Vipers.*—They are found in open sunny country and are not vicious. The venom contains a powerful coagulant.

ii. *Malayan Pit Vipers.*—These are the commonest cause of bites in Malaya. They are distributed in North Malaya only.

27

d. **Sea Snakes.**—These are common off the shores of India, Burma, and the Malaysian Peninsula; they are usually found in coastal waters and are liable to be caught in fishing nets. A sea snake seldom bites unless it is handled. The toxic effects are not often severe.

6. AUSTRALIA

All are **Elapid snakes** with mainly neurotoxic venoms.

a. **Tiger Snakes.**—These are widely distributed, aggressive, and the commonest cause of fatal bites.

b. **Taipans.**—These are found mostly on Cape York Peninsula. They are large, being up to 9 ft. long. They are very vicious and venomous, and recovery is most unlikely unless antivenom is given immediately.

c. **Death Adders.**—These are common in sandy areas and are easily trodden upon. They are not aggressive but are very poisonous.

d. **Brown Snakes.**—There are many species, and they have a wide distribution. They are not aggressive.

e. **Copperheads.**—These are found in southern Australia in swampy areas, and are not usually aggressive.

f. **Red-bellied Black Snakes.**—These are king brown snakes. They are found in marshy areas and streams, and are dangerous to swimmers and bathers. Their bites are not usually lethal.

7. FAR EAST

Most varieties resemble those found in South-east Asia.

In Japan.—The mamushi and habu—the two commonest *vipers*—cause 80 to 90 deaths per year.

In Taiwan.—There are several local species of *cobras* and *vipers*, and they cause 100 to 200 deaths per year.

HAS THE PATIENT BEEN BITTEN?

A frightened patient at whom a snake has struck will naturally assume that he has been seriously bitten. This may or may not be true and the evaluation of the severity of envenomation should be based on objective clinical evidence, not on the history.

Snake venoms contain several toxic proteins with enzymatic actions. The proportions of these toxins vary in the poisons of different snakes, and the resultant symptoms differ accordingly.

Toxins.—The main toxins are:—

1. Proteases (thrombase, hæmorrhagin, anticoagulin) causing local cellular necrosis, disruption of capillaries, and alterations in coagulation.

2. Phosphatidases, causing hæmolysis.

3. Neurotoxins, resulting in paralysis of respiratory centre, 9th, 10th, 11th, and 12th cranial nerves; curare-like action at motor-nerve end-plates.

4. Cardiotoxins.

5. Hyaluronidase, assists in spreading of other toxins.

6. Cholinesterase.

There are two main categories of snake venom: (1) cytotoxic and hæmotoxic, and (2) neurotoxic.

1. Cytotoxic and Hæmotoxic Venoms.—The rattlesnakes, vipers, and adders have mainly cytotoxic venoms which give a marked local reaction with severe pain, swelling, and ecchymosis. There may, in addition, be systemic symptoms of nausea, vomiting, hæmolysis, hæmorrhage into respiratory, gastro-intestinal, and urinary tracts, headache, and shock.

2. Neurotoxic Venoms.—The cobras, kraits, mambas, and coral snakes have neurotoxic venoms, which cause deep local pain without severe local reaction but with cranial nerve and respiratory symptoms preceding shock—diplopia, hearing difficulties, vertigo, incoherence, locomotor disturbances, muscle spasms, severe headache.

EXAMINATION OF THE PATIENT

In examining the patient, note:—

1. Marks of Bites.—Characteristically the double fang mark with or without additional teeth marks points to the bite of a venomous snake. The bite of a non-poisonous snake is usually a U-shaped impression of small teeth marks (*Fig.* 526). The South African boomslang has back fangs and sea-snake bites are often overlooked because of the small fangs and teeth.

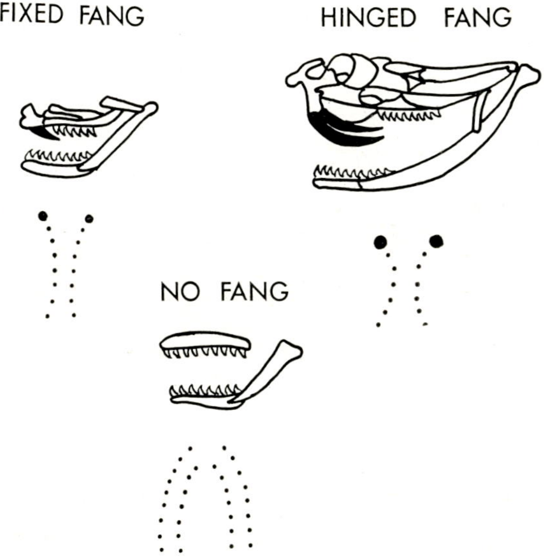

Fig. 526.—Cutaneous impressions of snake-bites. *Top left*: fixed fang, cobra; *top right*: hinged fang, rattlesnake; *bottom*: no fangs, non-poisonous snakes.

2. Local Reaction.—A severe reaction within an hour is a reliable indication of a viper bite. The more rapid and severe the reaction the greater the degree of envenomation.

3. Local Pain.—In the presence of fang marks, local pain, with or without swelling, usually means that the snake was poisonous. A serious bite by some species (e.g., coral snake) may sometimes occur with very little local reaction, but be followed after several hours by systemic symptoms. If fang marks are present, but neither local nor general symptoms develop, either the snake was not poisonous or envenomation did not occur.

4. Systemic Symptoms.—These are cranial nerve disturbances, hæmorrhage, shock, nausea and vomiting, and respiratory difficulty. Hysterical reactions with diplopia, swallowing difficulties, sensory loss of the 'stocking and glove' type, hyperventilation, and perioral tingling may be deceptive, but should not delay the institution of treatment.

TREATMENT

Considerable controversy still exists over the best management of snake-bites. This is probably because most bites are not fatal and the low mortality may mistakenly be ascribed to the treatment. If envenomation is minimal the chances of serious consequences are slight and, therefore, the most energetic therapeutic measures are unnecessary and should be withheld until the magnitude of the poisoning becomes evident.

SELF-ADMINISTERED FIRST-AID

1. If possible, kill the snake for identification.

2. If the snake is known to be poisonous, or if uncertain, lie or sit down, put a tourniquet 2–4 in. (5–10 cm.) above the bite, tight enough to occlude venous return only. Suck on wound if accessible.

3. Send for help if possible. Do not run. Activity increases rate of absorption.

4. The main aim of treatment is to get to specific antivenom as quickly as possible. If the antivenom can be brought to the patient, this is better than the patient walking to the antivenom. With a serious bite, the patient should, if possible, be carried. If carrying the patient is impossible, the relative dangers of awaiting help or walking for aid depend upon individual circumstances of time, distances, terrain, and type and severity of bite.

PRIMARY TREATMENT

The therapeutic measures in order of importance are: (1) specific antivenom, (2) immobilization, (3) use of a tourniquet, and (4) incision and suction.

1. Specific Antivenom.—Specific antivenom is available for most species of poisonous snake throughout the world (*Table XIX*). Nearly all the antivenoms are made from horse serum and, therefore, their use carries a significant risk of allergic reactions. The principles in the use of antivenom are:—

a. Do not use horse serum antivenom unless *significant symptoms of envenomation,* local or systemic, exist.

b. Always *test for sensitivity* to horse serum by conjunctival (or intradermal) test. Place one drop of undiluted horse serum or antivenom into the conjunctival sac: a positive result is indicated by lacrimation, burning, or itching within 5 to 30 minutes. For intradermal testing, inject 0·05–0·1 ml. of antivenom 1–10 dilution intradermally. Urticaria, erythema, and swelling in 5 to 30 minutes indicate a positive test. The more rapid the response, the more positive the result.

c. Use *specific antivenom* whenever possible. There is no point in using anti-neurotoxins if the venom is a cytotoxin. But polyvalent serum is available in many parts of the world.

d. Site of administration. Antivenom can be injected around the bite, intramuscularly or intravenously. The most effective route is intravenous, but this carries the greatest risk of allergic reactions. Have adrenaline, antihistamines, or hydrocortisone I.V. at hand if the antivenom is given intravenously. Dilute the dose in 250 ml. normal saline for intravenous use.

e. The dosage depends upon the type of antivenom and instructions accompanying the serum should be followed. Because the antivenom counteracts the concentration of venom, larger doses of antivenom must be used in children than in adults because the volume of distribution of the venom is smaller in a child and the concentration, therefore, higher.

Table XIX.—INSTITUTES FROM WHICH ANTIVENOM CAN BE OBTAINED. IN COUNTRIES IN THE MIDDLE EAST SUPPLIES ARE AVAILABLE FROM LOCAL PASTEUR INSTITUTES

GEOGRAPHIC AREA	SNAKE	SOURCE OF ANTIVENOM	
		Country	Producer
Britain	Common European viper	Britain	Allen & Hanbury's Ltd., 7 Vere Street, London, W.1
Europe	All European adders	Germany	Behringwerke, Aktiensgesellschaft, Marburg-Lahn
		France	Institut Pasteur, Service de Sérothérapie, 36 Rue du Doctor-Roux, Paris
		Italy	Instituto Sieroterapico, Milan
Iran	Cobras and vipers. Polyvalent serum	Iran	Razi Institute, P.O. Box 656, Teheran, Iran
India	Cobra, krait, viper	India	Haffkine Institute, Bombay Central Research Institute, Kasauli
Pakistan	Polyvalent serum for all venomous snakes	Pakistan	Razi Institute, P.O. Box 656, Teheran, Iran
South Africa	All important types	Union of South Africa	S.A. Institute for Medical Research, Johannesburg FitzSimon's Snake Park Laboratory, Durban
Burma	Cobras and vipers	Burma	Burma Pharmaceutical Industries, Rangoon
S.E. Asia	King cobra, cobra, Russell's viper, Malayan pit viper, banded krait	Thailand	Queen Saovabha Memorial Institute, Bangkok
	Sea snake	Australia	Commonwealth Serum Laboratory, Melbourne
Australia	Tiger snake, death adder, taipan, brown snake, king snake, blacksnake, copperhead	Australia	Commonwealth Serum Laboratory, Melbourne
N. America	Rattlesnake, moccasin, copperhead	U.S.A.	Wyeth Laboratories, Philadelphia, Pennsylvania
	Coral snake	Brazil	Instituto Butantan, Caixa Postal 65, São Paulo
S. America	Bushmaster, fer-de-lance, rattlesnake, coral snake	Brazil	Instituto Pinheiros, Ruo Teodoro, Sampaio, 1860, São Paulo Instituto Butantan, Caixa Postal 65, São Paulo

f. If the patient is sensitive to horse serum, make dilutions of antivenom of 1–10 and 1–100. Inject 0·1 ml., 0·2 ml., 0·5 ml. of 1–100 dilution at 15-minute intervals and repeat with 1–10 dilution. If there is no reaction, give undiluted antivenom.

g. If the bite is obviously *serious* and the patient is *sensitive* to horse serum, (i) give a suitable dose of antihistamine and 100 mg. hydrocortisone I.V.,

(ii) inject 0·3–0·5 ml. of 1–1000 adrenaline subcutaneously, and (iii) inject the antivenom very slowly intravenously, being prepared to stop antivenom and give additional doses of adrenaline if necessary.

h. The possibility of *serum sickness* developing 1 to 3 weeks after the treatment should always be considered. The incidence of serum sickness is directly related to the size of the dose initially used.

2. Immobilization.—Venoms are absorbed by the lymphatics and lymphatic drainage is greatly accelerated by movement. Total immobilization is advisable if possible. At all costs, stop excited, hysterical reactions.

3. Use of a Tourniquet.—The application of a tourniquet is probably only of value if carried out within 2 to 10 minutes of the bite. It should be tightened enough to occlude lymphatic and venous drainage and should be released for 30 seconds every 20 minutes and not continued for longer than 2 hours. Release the tourniquet slowly after giving antivenom.

Many authorities no longer regard the tourniquet as effective treatment, and limbs have been lost unnecessarily because of too tight a tourniquet maintained for too long.

4. Incision and Suction.—The depth at which a snake injects its venom depends upon the length of the fangs and the adequacy of the bite. It would be rare for venom to be injected more than ¾ in. (2 cm.) beneath the skin, but, because the fangs are curved, the site of injection is not immediately deep to the puncture marks. Too shallow an incision is inadequate and too deep an incision may be dangerous. Also, after a few minutes, the cytotoxins become fixed to the tissues and are difficult to extract. Inexpert incision is often dangerous or inadequate and a source of secondary infection.

Most authorities are now against incision as an effective therapeutic measure.

Suction is only likely to be effective in the very earliest stage after the bite and the value of this measure is also in doubt. Excessive massaging of the bitten area in an attempt to suck out poison may actually aid in its spread. Snake venoms are innocuous if taken orally, therefore sucking on a wound with the mouth is safe provided there are no cracks on the lips or mouth.

Fasciotomy.—If a limb becomes extremely tense and swollen, some hours after a bite, fasciotomy with release of the tension in the muscular compartments may be vital in saving the limb. Under local anæsthesia a small (1½–2 in., 3·8–5 cm.) vertical incision is made over the mid-portion of the three muscular compartments. A small vertical nick is made with the scalpel in the fascia, and slightly opened scissors are pushed upwards and downwards to split the fascia extensively. The tense œdematous muscles immediately bulge into the incision.

ADDITIONAL MEASURES

1. Antibiotics.—The mouths of all snakes are infested with bacteria and a wide-spectrum antibiotic should always be given as part of the treatment.

2. Antitetanus.—A booster dose of toxoid or antitetanus serum must be given with suitable precautions (*see* p. 67).

3. Steroids.—Some authorities, especially in India, have claimed that adrenal steroids are very valuable in the treatment of cobra bites and are specific antidotes to neurotoxins. The evidence for this is not conclusive, but in cases of severe elapid envenomation steroids may be given, but not as an alternative to antivenom. Give 100 mg. hydrocortisone I.V. in severe cases. Steroids may also be valuable for the treatment of allergic manifestations appearing later due to serum sickness.

4. Blood and I.V. Fluids.—Some toxins produce severe hæmolysis resulting in a rapid fall in hæmatocrit, anæmia, and even renal shutdown. Blood should be cross-matched and available for all cases of severe crotalid bite and should be used according to the standard indications for blood replacement. Intravenous fluids are a useful vehicle for giving antivenom intravenously and an I.V. drip should be started on severe cases. The usual indications should be used for the use of intravenous fluids for replacing fluids lost by vomiting or diarrhœa.

5. Cold.—The use of local cold has been advocated especially for the treatment of rattlesnake bites. The bitten limb is immersed in iced water to diminish pain, reduce local reaction, and slow down absorption and enzymatic action of the venom. This form of treatment has not been widely accepted and should only be used with the knowledge that immersion of a foot in iced water for more than 30 minutes may cause cold injury as severe in its effects as the bite.

6. Respiratory Assistance.—The usual cause of death from neurotoxic venom is respiratory paralysis. The widespread availability of anæsthesia equipment and ventilators should enable prolonged respiratory assistance to be given. An endotracheal tube can be inserted, and a self-inflating bag attached to an anæsthetic machine or a ventilator used to maintain ventilation for as long as necessary. The endotracheal tube can safely be used for 24 hours until the necessity for a tracheostomy is apparent. In the field, mouth-to-mouth respiration must be attempted and could conceivably be continued for a long time.

7. Sedation.—Narcotics and analgesics may be essential for the relief of pain. The injection of a local anæsthetic around the bite may sometimes be helpful. Morphine in doses likely to depress respiration should never be given if the venom is neurotoxic unless methods for controlling and assisting respiration are available.

SUMMARY

Most snake-bites are preventable with suitable care and precautions in snake-infested country.

Snake-bites are not usually fatal and if the patient arrives alive at the hospital he should live.

The mainstay of all treatments is the administration of adequate quantities of specific antivenom.

CHAPTER XLVI

THE HOUSE-SURGEON AND THE PATHOLOGY DEPARTMENT

By B. Joan Haram

The house-surgeon is the liaison officer between the pathological and surgical departments. In hospitals without a resident pathologist, he may be responsible for certain investigations during the night or when the regular laboratory staff is not on duty.

I. THE COLLECTION OF SPECIMENS FOR PATHOLOGICAL INVESTIGATION

A. GENERAL

1. It is most important that all specimens be labelled clearly with the patient's name, unit number, age, ward, the nature of the specimen, and the date (and sometimes the hour) of collection.

2. Each specimen should be accompanied by a request form giving a few clinical notes concerning the patient, including the length of his illness (an essential point in the case of blood sent for the Widal reaction, for example), drugs given, and stating the nature of the investigation required.

3. All specimens should reach the laboratory as soon as possible after collection.

B. PROCEDURE FOR CERTAIN SPECIAL INVESTIGATIONS

1. Tissues for Histological Examination.—These should be put into a suitable container and covered immediately with 10 per cent formol–saline. Soft tissues such as the brain should be placed on a layer of cotton-wool. The amount of fixative must be sufficient to cover the specimen.

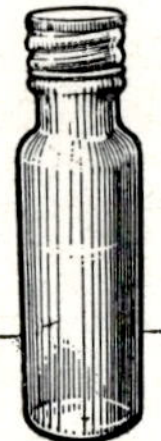

Fig. 527.—Screw-capped bottle for pathological specimens.

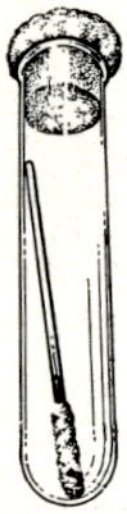

Fig. 528.—A swab stick. This pattern enables the surgeon in the operating theatre to handle the stick without contaminating his sterile gloves.

Material from diagnostic biopsies, such as endometrial or bronchial epithelium, must be handled particularly carefully.

2. Smears for Exfoliative Cytology.—It is essential that smears for cytological examination should be fixed *wet*, immediately they have been made. A satisfactory method is to drop the slide into a Coplin jar filled with 95 per cent ethyl alcohol. Fixation will be complete in 15 minutes, but if necessary the slides may remain in this fixative for several days. Staining by Papanicolaou's method, or with hæmatoxylin and eosin, may then be carried out.

3. Specimens for Culture.—

a. Pleural, ascitic, or cerebrospinal fluid, samples of pus, and catheter or midstream specimens of urine should be sent in sterile screw-capped bottles (*Fig.* 527). In the case of pleural fluids, part should be collected into a dry container and part into a bottle holding a few crystals of potassium oxalate to prevent coagulation.

b. Throat, nasal, cervical, and other swabs should be sent to the laboratory before the infected material has had time to dry. Sterile swab sticks in sterile test-tubes are supplied for use in the wards and operating theatres (*Fig.* 528).

c. Vaginal swabs to be investigated for *Trichomonas vaginalis* should be rotated in a tube containing about 2 ml. of *warm* saline and examined immediately. The trichomonad has a pear-shaped body, a single nucleus, and three to five flagella. It is 14–16 μ in size (*see Fig.* 540, p. 699).

d. Sputum and stools are preferably collected into disposable cartons.

Fig. 529.—Bottles containing media. A, Sloped medium (nutrient agar), for culture of various swabs; B, Fluid medium (serum broth), for culture of various swabs; C, Cooked meat medium, for anaerobes.

4. Culturing Techniques.—

In the absence of the pathologist it is advisable to culture specimens in some routine medium (*Fig.* 529).

a. Fluids and pus should be inoculated on to blood-agar plates and in cooked meat medium.

b. Urines should be inoculated on to McConkey plates.

c. Swabs may be cultured on agar slopes, blood-agar plates, or into serum broth. If diphtheria is suspected, Lœffler's medium should be used.

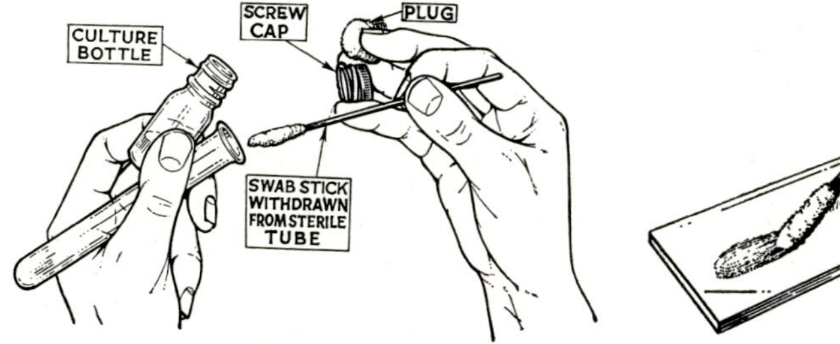

Fig. 530.—The technique of inoculating culture medium.

Fig. 531.—Method of making a smear on a microscope slide.

The technique, which requires some practice, is shown in *Fig.* 530. It is advisable to loosen the screw cap of the bottle before commencing the procedure. After completing the culture the swab should be smeared over the centre of a microscope slide (*Fig.* 531). The smear can then be stained and examined if required. To culture a swab on a blood-agar plate in order to identify a hæmolytic organism, the following method is recommended. The swab should be rubbed on one corner of the plate and the inoculum spread by means of a platinum loop in horizontal and vertical lines across the surface (*Fig.* 532). The incubator should be kept at a temperature of 37° C., and most of the cultures may be read after 18–24 hours' incubation. Certain organisms such as the *Neisseria* have a slower rate of growth and cultures of these should not be reported as negative until after at least 48 hours' incubation. In the absence of a pathologist or technician, specimens of urine and fæces not requiring immediate attention should be kept in the refrigerator, thus preventing the multiplication of any organisms present.

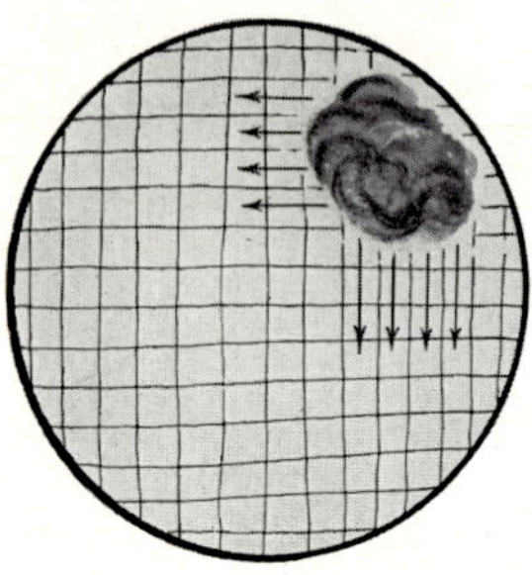

Fig. 532.—Method of inoculating a plate.

d. Sputa should be inoculated on to blood-agar and McConkey plates.

e. Stools should be inoculated into selenite broth and subcultured on the following day on to desoxycholate and McConkey plates. Stools to be examined for parasites, ova, and worms should be kept warm and examined as soon as possible after collection.

5. Collection of Blood.—Certain investigations are carried out on serum, others on plasma, whole blood, or cells. As laboratories differ in the methods they employ, it is advisable to find out, whenever possible, the type of sample and quantity of blood required. As a general guide, clotted blood should be supplied for grouping, cross-matching, Coombs' test, Wassermann reaction, and most routine chemical analyses. Whole blood, *not* clotted, is required for cell-counts, hæmoglobin estimation, and sedimentation rate.

To obtain Serum.—From 5 ml. to 10 ml. of blood are withdrawn by venepuncture, using a sterile dry syringe free from alcohol or other spirit. If a tourniquet is used, this should be released as soon as the needle is in the vein. The blood is transferred to a dry sterile test-tube, centrifuge tube, or screw-capped bottle, and allowed to clot. The amount of serum obtained is approximately half the volume of the blood withdrawn.

For chemical analyses a fasting specimen is preferable, and the serum should be separated as soon as possible after clotting has taken place. If not used immediately, serum may be stored in the refrigerator at between 0° and 4° C.

To obtain Whole Blood or Plasma.—Blood is withdrawn as in the case of serum, but placed in a tube containing several crystals of potassium oxalate or sequestrene, and shaken to prevent clotting.

Exceptions:—
a. For blood-sugar estimations, sodium fluoride is used as the anticoagulant. This prevents glycolysis.
b. For the sedimentation rate estimated by Westergren's method, 3·8 per cent sodium citrate is used as the anticoagulant, 1·6 ml. of blood being added to 0·4 ml. of citrate.
c. For the estimation of prothrombin time, 0·2 ml. of blood is added to 1·8 ml. of 3·8 per cent sodium citrate. The contents of the tube are mixed by inversion and centrifuged at 1500 r.p.m. for 5 minutes. The supernatant plasma is removed and may be kept in the refrigerator at 4° C. for a few hours if the test cannot be carried out immediately.
d. For blood-culture, the skin in the antecubital fossa is cleaned especially thoroughly with spirit and ether, and 5–10 ml. of blood removed with a sterile, dry syringe.

Varying amounts of blood are then added to three or four culture tubes containing different fluid media such as broth, glucose, bile-salt broth, or serum broth, and cooked meat medium.

e. Estimation of bicarbonate should be carried out on plasma. Blood should be collected under paraffin into a bottle containing heparin. The contents are mixed by gentle rotation, centrifuged, and the plasma carefully withdrawn.

A convenient tube for the collection of blood is sold by Bayer Products Ltd., and is called a Behring venule (*Fig.* 533). Plain tubes and tubes containing oxalate, fluoride, broth, etc., are supplied. The needle is encased in a glass

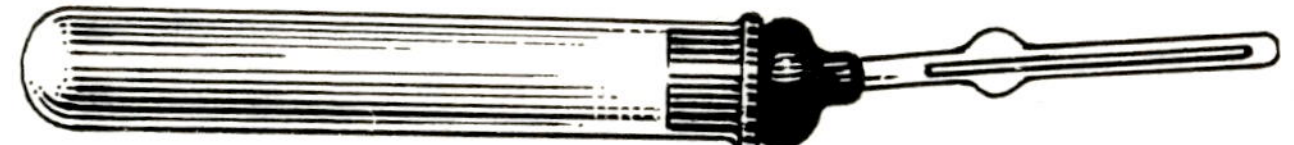

Fig. 533.—The Behring venule.

sheath. A 'vacuum' in the tube draws up the blood from the vein. These tubes are particularly convenient when specimens of blood have to be sent through the post.

II. THE TECHNIQUE OF CERTAIN EXAMINATIONS
EXAMINATION OF THE BLOOD

The following are among the most important of the investigations which the house-surgeon may be called upon to carry out himself.

1. Blood Grouping and Compatibility Tests

Now that stored blood is readily available to most hospitals through the Blood Transfusion Service, transfusion has become increasingly used for a wide variety of conditions.

Warning: (1) It is emphasized by the highest authorities that, of all pathological tests, blood grouping carries the greatest responsibility, and should never be carried out by anyone who has not received special instruction in modern techniques. A house-surgeon responsible for these tests in the absence of the pathologist should make himself familiar with every detail of the routine procedure to be used.

(2) No patient, except in grave emergency, should be given a transfusion unless the ABO and Rhesus group of patient and donor have been verified, and a compatibility test carried out. Rarely is blood transfusion so urgently required as to justify the use of Group O Rhesus-negative blood for an ungrouped patient. It should be understood clearly by all concerned that grouping and compatibility tests require 2–3 hours for full incubation, and that more rapid methods are not reliable. If the avoidance of delay is essential, the patient should be given a preliminary infusion of plasma or dextran while the compatibility tests are being completed.

A full description of the methods of grouping and direct matching will be found in *Practical Hæmatology* by J. V. Dacie and similar textbooks. Only a short summary will be included here.

a. ABO Grouping.—One drop of an approximately 2 per cent saline suspension of the patient's red cells is placed in each of two small glass rimless test-tubes, 7×50 mm. in size. (The suspension is prepared by adding a large drop of blood from ear or finger to 50 drops of physiological saline in a small agglutination tube.) An equal volume of anti-A serum is added to one, and of anti-B serum to the other. The tubes are capped, left at room temperature for one hour, and then examined microscopically (*Fig.* 534).

RESULTS

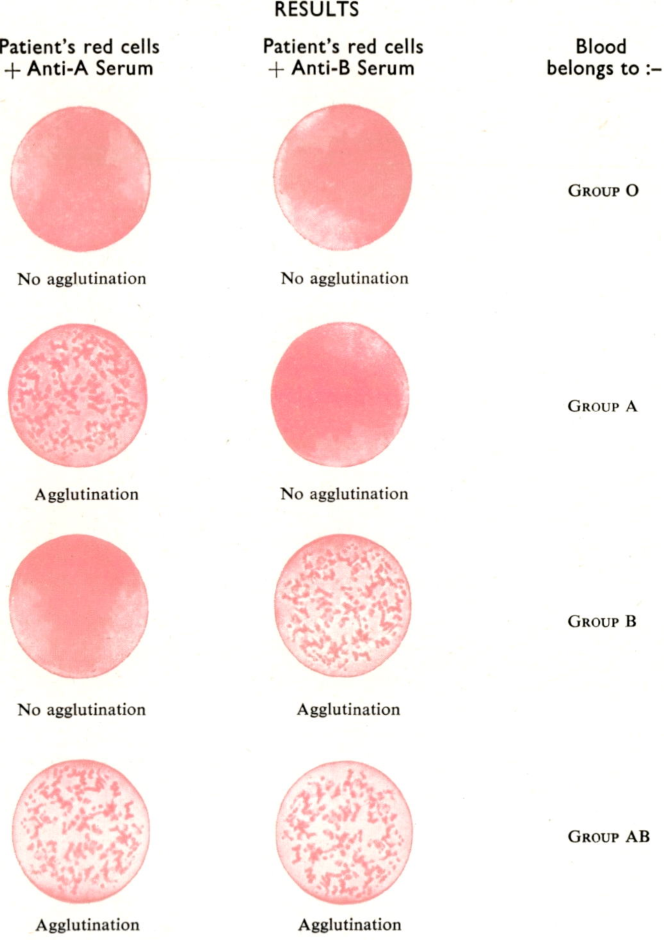

Fig. 534.—Chart showing method of identifying the different blood groups.

It is desirable to give a recipient blood of his own group, although in an emergency Group O blood can be given without great danger.

b. Rhesus Grouping.—The easiest method is to use serum containing saline agglutinins. One volume of a saline cell suspension is mixed in a small test-tube with one volume of Rh anti-D serum. The tube is capped and incubated at 37° C. (98·6° F.) for 2 hours. The deposited cells are drawn up with a Pasteur pipette, spread on a slide, and examined under the microscope. If the cells have agglutinated the patient is Rhesus positive; if no agglutination has occurred, the patient is Rhesus negative.

Owing to the scarcity of sera containing saline agglutinins, anti-D serum containing albumin agglutinins is often supplied. The tube is set up as before, and incubated for 1½ hours. The supernatant fluid is pipetted off the button of red cells, and replaced by one drop of 20 per cent albumin, without disturbing the cells. After incubation for a further half-hour the test is read as before. Known D-negative and D-positive cells should be set up as controls. All pregnant women should be tested for Rh as well as ABO, and no woman of child-bearing age or young girl should be given a transfusion without first determining her Rhesus group.

c. Direct Matching.—It is advisable for every patient to have his or her blood group determined before a major operation. Should it be thought probable that blood transfusion will be needed, sufficient blood should be taken for the compatibility test. The serum, when separated, should be stored in the refrigerator and will then be readily available when required. A fresh specimen of serum must be obtained before each subsequent transfusion.

The best direct matching procedure involves carrying out two tests, one in saline at room temperature, to detect ABO incompatibility, and an indirect Coombs' test to detect antibodies of the albumin-agglutinating type. The latter *must* be carried out if the history of the patient suggests any possibility of previous immunization, for example, from the transfusion of Rhesus-positive blood to a Rhesus-negative recipient, or from a Rhesus-positive infant having sensitized a Rhesus-negative mother. The technique for the test is beyond the scope of this book. The minimum routine for all transfusions should be a saline and an albumin test, both carried out at 37° C. (98·6° F.). For the saline test, a drop of the recipient's serum is added to a drop of a 2 per cent saline suspension of donor's cells, and incubated for 2 hours. For the albumin

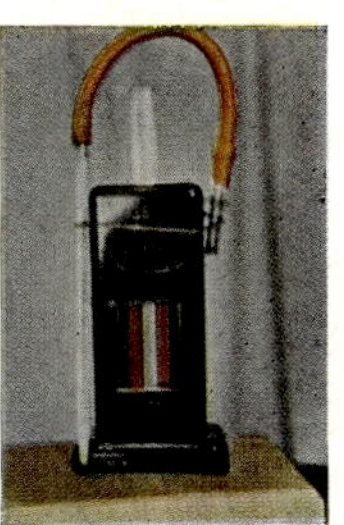

Fig. 535.—Sahli's hæmoglobinometer.

test, a drop of the saline suspension of donor's cells is centrifuged, the supernatant removed, and the cells re-suspended in 20 per cent albumin. This tube also is incubated for 2 hours. After incubation, the cells are transferred to a slide and examined under the microscope. If the donor's red cells are compatible with the recipient's serum, no agglutination of the red cells will have occurred.

2. Estimation of Hæmoglobin

The house-surgeon will probably find it most useful to be familiar with the Sahli method as this can be used by daylight or by artificial light, and most laboratories are equipped with the apparatus (*Fig.* 535).

a. The Sahli Method.—The graduated tube is filled to the mark 10 with *N*/10 hydrochloric acid. The patient's ear or finger is pricked, and after wiping away the first two drops, 20 c.mm. of blood are collected in the marked pipette. The tip is wiped and the blood blown out to the bottom of the acid, the pipette being rinsed by drawing acid in and out a few times. The hæmoglobin is converted into acid hæmatin, and the apparatus is allowed to stand until conversion is complete. This may take 5 to 30 minutes according to the graduation of the instrument. The fluid is then diluted with distilled water until it matches the standard.

As different instruments have standards which represent different amounts of hæmoglobin per 100 ml. of blood, it is essential that the observed reading be adjusted so that 100 per cent is equivalent to 14·8 G. of hæmoglobin per 100 ml. of blood.

b. The Oxyhæmoglobin Method, using the M.R.C. grey-wedge photometer.— Many laboratories now use this apparatus; 0·02 ml. blood is washed into 4 ml. $N/150$ NH$_4$OH. After mixing, the solution is matched in the photometer against a rotating grey wedge, using a green filter.

c. The E.E.L. portable colorimeter is now readily available and very simple to use.

3. Leucocyte Count

A leucocyte count is often required urgently. The ear or finger is pricked as before and blood drawn up to the mark 0·5 on the white-cell pipette (*Fig.* 536).

Diluting fluid consisting of 1 per cent acetic acid, coloured with crystal or gentian violet, is then sucked up until the level of the fluid reaches the 11 mark, care being taken to avoid the introduction of air. The ends of the pipette are

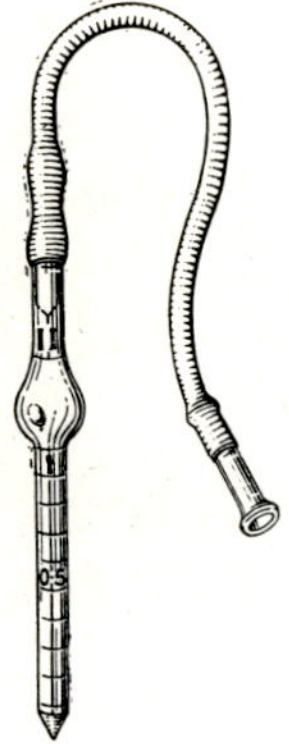

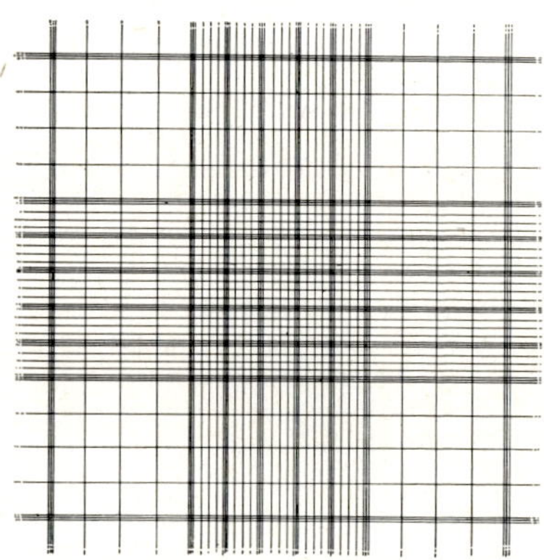

Fig. 536.—Pipette for counting leucocytes. Note the markings 0·5, 1, and 11, and the white bead.

Fig. 537.—Improved Neubauer counting chamber.

covered by the thumb and middle finger respectively, and the pipette is shaken in order to mix the diluent with the blood. The count must be made within an hour of collecting the blood. After a further mixing of the contents of the pipette, about a third is blown out, and a drop is then run in under the cover-slip of the counting chamber, which must be scrupulously clean. Air bubbles must be avoided and the drop must not be allowed to flow over the edge of the counting chamber. The cells are allowed to settle for five minutes. Using a Neubauer counting chamber (*Fig.* 537), all the leucocytes in the four large ruled squares at the corners of the chamber are counted and an average for one square obtained.

An alternative method for taking a leucocyte count is to add 0·05 ml. of blood (using a 50 c.mm. pipette) to 0·95 ml. of the diluting fluid in a small tube. The tube is corked and the contents mixed thoroughly. A drop is then run under the coverslip of the counting chamber as before.

Calculation: The area of each large corner square is 1 sq. mm. Since the depth of the chamber is one-tenth of a mm., the number of cells counted in 1 sq. mm. is that contained in 0·1 c.mm. of diluted blood. The blood has been diluted 20 times. The total number of white cells per c.mm. is, therefore, the number counted in one corner square multiplied by 200.

4. Differential Cell-count

When collecting blood for hæmoglobin estimation or cell-count, blood-films should invariably be made. The appearance of the film will establish the presence of any degree of anæmia, leucocytosis, or leucopenia; in fact, a well-spread and carefully stained preparation may be a more reliable guide to diagnosis than a cell-count carried out by a tyro.

The film must be made on a clean grease-free slide. A small drop of blood is placed at one end, and the end of another slide is placed over the drop and moved along to make the film (*Fig.* 538). The more acute the angle formed by the spreading slide to the smeared slide, the thinner will be the blood-film which results. When dry, the film may be stained with Leishman's stain.

Leishman's Stain.—The slide is covered with the stain for two minutes to fix it. About the same amount of distilled water or a buffer solution of pH 6·8 is added and well mixed, a metallic sheen on the surface of the stain denoting that the correct pro-

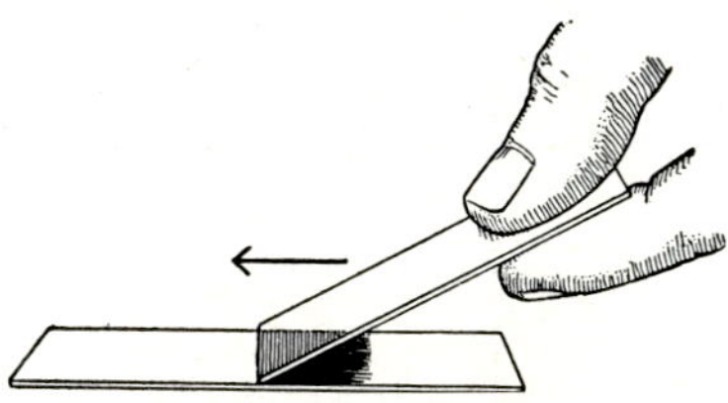

Fig. 538.—Making a blood-film.

portions have been attained. After at least five minutes the film is washed with distilled water or buffer, leaving the water on the slide until the film has a mauvish-pink appearance. It is then left to dry.

Before making the differential count the whole of the film should be examined with a low-power objective in order to acquire a general impression of the blood-picture and to see whether the smear has been evenly spread. Polymorphonuclear leucocytes tend to congregate at the edges of a film, so that to obtain a truly representative count the cells should be counted over a wide area, including those in the centre as well as those at the edge. At least 200 cells should be counted.

Malarial Films.—Blood-films for malarial parasites should be taken several times a day during an attack. Both thick and thin preparations should be made and stained by the usual methods.

5. Sedimentation Rate

The blood is collected into citrate as described on p. 692 and, after thorough mixing, drawn up into a Westergren tube which is graduated in mm. from 0 to 200. The tube is placed vertically in a special stand, the red cells gradually sediment, and the clear column of plasma is measured after one hour. The answer is expressed as follows: Erythrocyte Sedimentation Rate, x mm. in one hour.

6. Estimation of Fibrinogen

A rapid slide test, for hypofibrinogenæmia is now available as 'Fi-test'.

Fi-test (Hyland Laboratories, Los Angeles, U.S.A., and Baxter Laboratories Ltd., High Wycombe, Bucks).

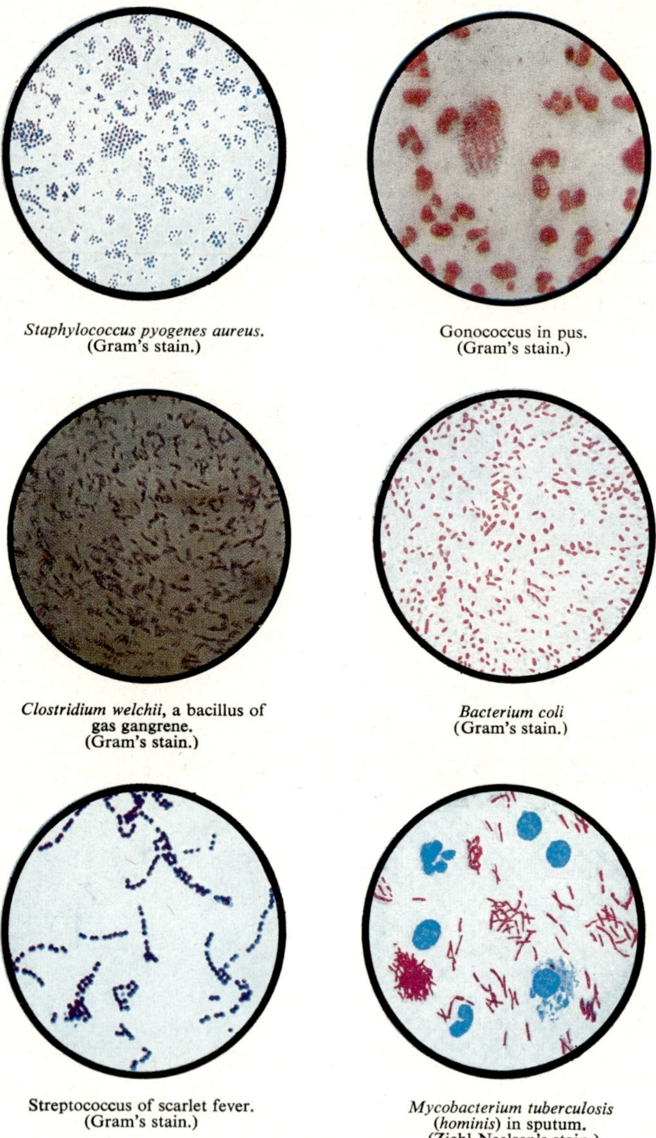

Fig. 539.—Illustrations of micro-organisms.

EXAMINATION OF PUS
(*Figs.* 539, 540)

The colour, consistency, and smell should be noted, also the presence or absence of gas bubbles, or the 'sulphur' granules which occur in actinomycosis.

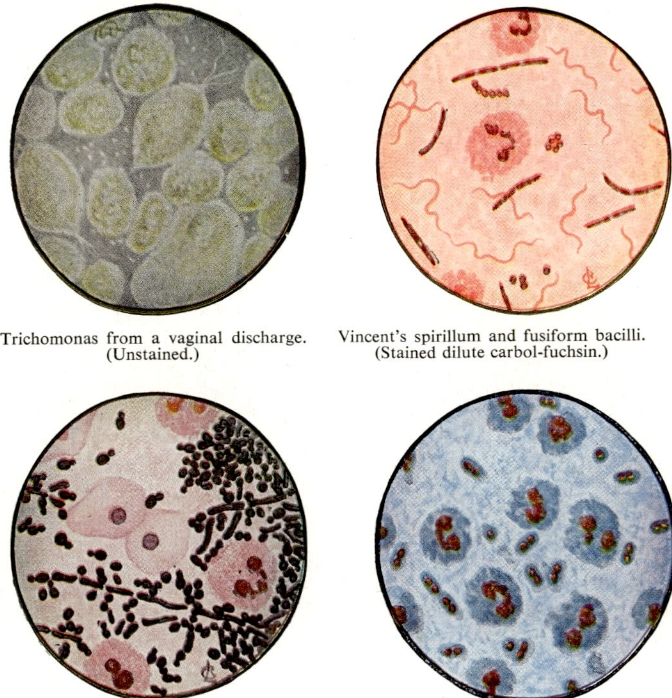

Trichomonas from a vaginal discharge.
(Unstained.)

Vincent's spirillum and fusiform bacilli.
(Stained dilute carbol-fuchsin.)

Thrush.
(Gram's stain.)

Pneumococci.
(Muir's stain.)

Fig. 540.—Four preparations of important diagnostic significance.

A 'wet' preparation should be made by placing a drop of pus on a slide, covering with a cover-slip, and examining with a one-sixth objective. Polymorphs, epithelial cells, and crystals should be identified.

Smears for Staining.—To find out what organisms are present, a loopful of pus is spread thinly on a slide and stained.

a. Gram's Method.—The smear is fixed by passing the slide quickly through the flame of a Bunsen burner. Debris is removed by washing with a 2 per cent solution of acetic acid. The slide is then covered with crystal or methyl violet, which is almost immediately washed off with Gram's or Lugol's iodine. After one and a half to two minutes, the iodine is washed off with absolute alcohol or industrial spirit until no more violet stain comes away. The film is then counterstained with neutral red or dilute carbol-fuchsin and, after ten or twenty seconds, washed with water, blotted, and dried.

The slide is examined with the one-twelfth objective, and it should be possible to recognize, or at least suspect, the presence of staphylococci, streptococci, pneumococci, actinomycotic filaments, gonococci, and some of the Gram-positive bacilli such as *Cl. welchii* and *B. anthracis*.

b. Ziehl-Neelsen's Method.—This is used for the identification of tubercle bacilli. The smear is fixed as before and covered with strong carbol-fuchsin stain. The slide is heated until steam rises, and kept gently warmed for about ten minutes, care being taken to prevent the stain from drying. The slide is washed in water and then covered with alcohol. After five minutes the alcohol is washed off and the slide immersed in a small bath or jar containing 25 per cent sulphuric acid. After decolorizing for at least fifteen minutes it is removed, washed in water, and counterstained with methylene blue for about thirty seconds. The excess is washed off, and the slide is blotted, dried, and examined with the one-twelfth objective.

c. Weak Carbol-fuchsin.—If Vincent's stomatitis (*Fig.* 540) is suspected the smear made from the ulcer is stained for a minute with 5 per cent carbol-fuchsin and then washed with water. The typical fusiform bacilli and spirochætes show up clearly by this method.

The same stain can be used to reveal the presence of monilia found in thrush and also frequently present in vaginal discharges. These yeasts are oval bodies rather larger than a red blood-corpuscle. Branching hyphæ may also be detected.

d. 'Negative' Capsule Stain.—Pneumococci may be identified by using the indian ink wet film method. A small portion of a colony is added to a loopful of undiluted indian ink on a slide. A cover-slip is placed on top and pressed down under a pad of blotting paper. The capsule appears as a clear light zone between the cell outline and the dark background.

EXAMINATION OF CEREBROSPINAL FLUID

A full examination of the cerebrospinal fluid is somewhat outside the scope of the house-surgeon, but a cell-count, using a Fuchs-Rosenthal counting chamber, can be easily performed.

About 1 ml. of the fluid is pipetted into a test-tube and stained for a few minutes with a loopful of crystal violet. A drop of the fluid is then run in under the cover-slip on the counting chamber. All the cells in the cross-ruled area of the chamber are counted, and the number obtained is divided by three. This gives the number of cells in 1 c.mm. of fluid, since the ruled area holds about 3 c.mm. of fluid. If the cells are too numerous to be counted by this method, a Neubauer chamber is used instead and the necessary calculation made.

A purulent fluid from a case of meningitis should be centrifuged and the deposit stained by Gram's method. This will often reveal the causative organism such as the meningococcus, pneumococcus, or *Hæmophilus influenzæ*.

A simple test for detecting a decrease in the dextrose content of the fluid may be carried out as follows: 0·25 ml. of Fehling's solution is boiled with 1 ml. of cerebrospinal fluid. Normally a heavy red precipitate will form, the supernatant fluid still retaining its blue colour. If the sugar content is diminished, the precipitate will be decreased or absent and the supernatant fluid pale or colourless.

PROSTATIC AND VESICULAR MASSAGE

In cases of suspected acute or chronic vesiculitis, diagnosis can often be established by examination of the secretion obtained from prostatic and vesicular massage per rectum.

A drop collects at the external meatus and is placed on a microscope slide. This is immediately covered with a cover-slip and excess fluid absorbed by means of blotting-paper, the cover being lightly compressed during the process. The bladder should always be emptied before massage. The slide is then examined microscopically with a one-sixth objective (*Fig.* 541).

A pathological fluid is more viscid than the normal secretion. On microscopical examination pus cells and bacteria (*Fig.* 542) are often plentiful.

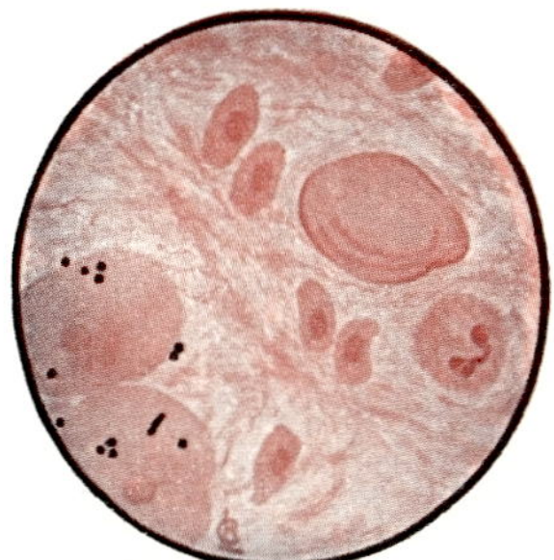

Fig. 541.—Film of fluid expressed by prostatic massage in a normal man. Stained Gram + basic fuchsin, it shows: prostatic cells, corpus amylaceum, polymorphonuclear leucocyte, urethral epithelial cells, with a few cocci and a diphtheroid. (Oil immersion × 1000.)

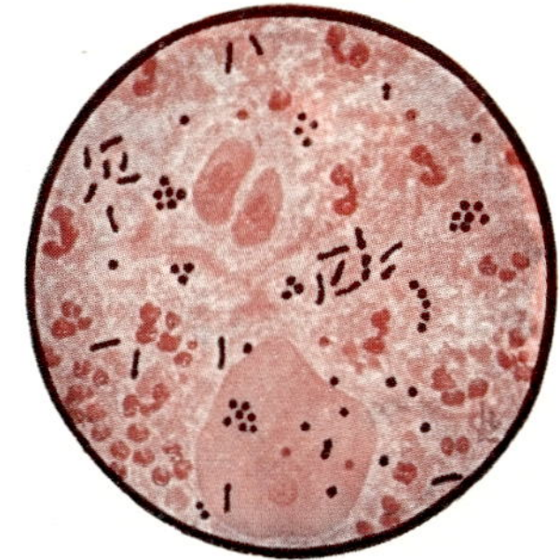

Fig. 542.—Film of prostatic fluid in a case of chronic prostatitis. Stained as in *Fig.* 541, it shows: prostatic cells, urethral epithelial cell, numerous pus cells (very degenerated), staphylococci, streptococci, diphtheroid bacilli.

EXAMINATION OF URINE

This is dealt with in Chapter XXXI.

RENAL FUNCTION TESTS

The techniques for these are described in Chapter XXXI.

PENTAGASTRIN AND AUGMENTED HISTAMINE TEST

This procedure is described in Chapter XXVI.

EXAMINATION OF FÆCES FOR OCCULT BLOOD

The only qualitative test commonly performed on fæces is for the detection of hæmoglobin and its derivatives, derived from bleeding into the alimentary tract. Since a normal diet contains hæmoglobin and myoglobin (in meat) and since minor degrees of bleeding (e.g., from the gums) are almost universal, it is obviously a matter of difficulty to assess the significance of weakly positive tests for blood pigments. With definite negative results there is no difficulty; strongly positive tests are likewise easy to interpret; between these extremes, one can only record the strength of the reaction on a tough scale as +, + +, + + +, etc., and repeat the test after withdrawing meat from the diet for a day or two.

1. The Orthotolidine Test.—

Reagents.—4 per cent orthotolidine in glacial acetic acid.

   3 per cent hydrogen peroxide (10 vols.).

Equal parts of the above reagents are prepared freshly before each test.

Method.—Make a suspension of a small quantity of fæces in distilled water. Use clean glassware. Boil the suspension for a few minutes, and cool.

On a clean filter-paper, place a few drops of the fæcal suspension, and also a few drops of the working solution. Allow the fluids to run together.

A definite blue colour at the junction of the liquids indicates a positive test.

A blank should be run with each test, i.e., distilled water only, boiled, cooled, and placed on filter paper with orthotolidine solution. Any blue colour resulting from a blank test will indicate exhaustion of stock orthotolidine solution.

The orthotolidine best has been largely replaced by:—

2. Hæmatest Tablets.—

These are similar in composition to 'Occultest' tablets, but adjusted to a lower level of sensitivity for use with faeces rather than urine.

Hæmatest (Ames Co., Stoke Poges, Bucks).

Make a *thin* smear of fæces on the filter-paper square, using a glass rod or spatula. (Do not use an emulsion or suspension.) Place one tablet at the edge of the smear, and put one drop of water on the tablet. After 10 seconds, put a second drop on the tablet so that it flows down on to the paper. *Exactly two minutes later*, note any blue colour on the *paper*. Ignore any colour on the tablet or the smear.

III. TABLE OF LABORATORY NORMALS

It must be appreciated that techniques in different laboratories vary, and that with regard to many investigations authorities vary in their evaluation of the normal range. Always ascertain the values accepted as normal by your own laboratory. For most of the blood chemistry investigations (except sugar) send at least 5 ml. clotted blood to the laboratory.

DISTRIBUTION OF BLOOD GROUPS IN EUROPEANS.—

Group O, 46 per cent.   Group B, 9 per cent.
Group A, 42 per cent.   Group AB, 3 per cent.
                 Rhesus positive, 85 per cent.

HÆMOGLOBIN.—
90–110 per cent or 13·3–16·3 G. per 100 ml.

RED BLOOD-CORPUSCLES.—
Men, 4·5–6·5 millions per c.mm. Women, 3·9–5·6 millions per c.mm.

WHITE BLOOD-CORPUSCLES.—
Total: 4000–10,000 per c.mm.
Differential:—

Polymorphs { Neutrophil, 40–75 per cent. Basophil, 0–1 per cent.
           { Eosinophil, 1–6 per cent.
Monocytes, 2–10 per cent.
Lymphocytes, 20–50 per cent.

ERYTHROCYTE SEDIMENTATION RATE (Westergren's Method).—
3–5 mm. in one hour (men). 4–7 mm. in one hour (women and children).

BLOOD CHEMISTRY.—
Amylase, 50–180 units per 100 ml.
Bicarbonate, 24–32 mEq. per litre.
Bilirubin, total 0·1–0·5 mg. per 100 ml.
Calcium, 4·2–5·2 mEq. per litre; 9–11 mg. per 100 ml.
Chlorides, 96–106 mEq. per litre or 560–620 mg. per 100 ml. (as NaCl),
    (plasma or serum).
Cholesterol, 140–270 mg. per 100 ml. (plasma or serum).
Magnesium, 1·5–1·85 mEq. per litre.
Phosphatase (acid), 1–3 units (King and Armstrong).
            (alkaline), 3–13 units (King and Armstrong).
Phosphorus (inorganic), 1·7–2·6 mEq. per litre or 2–4 mg. per 100 ml.
Potassium, 4·5–5 mEq. per litre or 15–20 mg. per 100 ml. (plasma or
    serum; abnormally high if blood hæmolysed).
Proteins (total), 5·8–8·6 G. per 100 ml.
Sodium, 137–148 mEq. per litre or 316–340 mg. per 100 ml. (plasma or
    serum).
Sugar, 80–120 mg. per 100 ml. (use oxalate + fluoride tube).
Transaminases, SGOT, 4–20 i.u. per litre; SGPT 2–15 i.u. per litre.
Urea, 20–40 mg. per 100 ml.
Uric acid, 1–4 mg. per 100 ml. (whole blood).

CHAPTER XLVII

THE HOUSE-SURGEON AND THE DEPARTMENT OF RADIODIAGNOSIS

By Lewis A. Gillanders

It is customary for the departmental staff of large X-ray units to perform all the techniques which require the attention of a doctor, and in these circumstances the house-surgeon is rarely called upon to give practical assistance. In smaller departments, however, he may well find himself incorporated into the medical team. It is all-important that the house-surgeon should have a clear understanding of the practical procedures which are being carried out on his patients whether he is involved in their performance or not, since he is inevitably concerned both with their preparation for radiology and in their after-care.

Space does not permit description of all the numerous radiological procedures which are employed nowadays. The more common ones will be described in detail; examinations relating particularly to the special departments, e.g., obstetrics, neurosurgery, and cardiology, will be omitted here.

THE USE OF THE X-RAY DEPARTMENT

The Department of Radiodiagnosis provides a comprehensive ancillary medical service. Close co-operation between the users of the department and its staff is essential if the quality of this service is to be of a high standard. It should always be remembered that radiology *supplements* physical examination of the patient, and that there should be clear clinical indications before any patient is X-rayed. Should a number of radiological investigations be contemplated, much time and trouble will be saved if consideration is given to the order in which these investigations are to be performed; for example, if a barium meal is carried out, several days may require to elapse before the abdomen is clear enough of barium to allow the performance of an intravenous pyelogram or an examination of the lumbar spine.

PROTECTION FROM IONIZING RADIATION

Large doses of radiation are potentially dangerous and involve somatic and genetic hazards to man. The radiation hazard is particularly important in the case of children, young adults, and pregnant women where the number of radiological examinations should be kept to a minimum. The staff of the X-ray department will give helpful advice on this subject. Under no circumstances should a repeat examination be carried out for convenience, e.g., when previous X-ray films are temporarily mislaid.

While in the X-ray department, the house-surgeon is subject to the advice of the Radiation Safety Officer regarding his personal protection. Protective measures include the wearing of a lead-rubber apron when working within range of the X-ray beam, and sheltering within a protective cubicle during radiographic exposures.

REQUESTS FOR RADIOLOGICAL EXAMINATION

Requests for radiological examinations should be compiled with care. The following information should be provided on the request form:—

1. *Name.*—The surname and Christian names are essential for the correct filing of patients' record cards in the department; also hospital unit number, if any.

2. *Age and sex* are important as they have a bearing on certain X-ray appearances.

3. *Address.*—Many patients have the same Christian name and surname.

4. *Occupation.*—In certain conditions the patient's occupation has a direct bearing on the pathological process.

5. *Ward or department.*—This is essential for the delivery of films and reports.

6. *Under the care of.*—The name of the consultant in charge of the case should be quoted.

7. *Previous X-ray examination.*—The date of the most recent X-ray report should be quoted.

8. *Clinical abstract.*—This should be brief but relevant. In the investigation of the alimentary tract, concise details of any previous abdominal operations should be included.

9. *Investigation required.*—This should be stated clearly without any technical instructions from the point of view of radiology.

10. *Date and signature of the doctor.*—This is essential as responsibility for the request must be known.

RADIOGRAPHY OF THE ACUTE ABDOMEN

In cases of this kind invaluable help may be obtained from plain films. It is usual for two radiographs to be taken, preferably in the X-ray department.

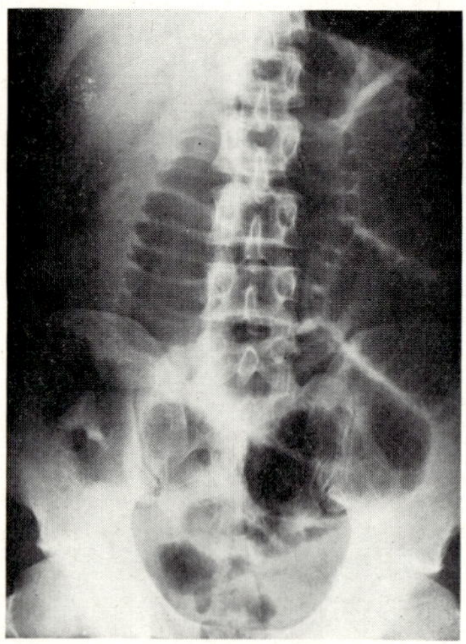

Fig. 543.—Supine film of abdomen. Small bowel obstruction. Grossly distended loops of small bowel located centrally in the abdomen. Absence of gas in cæcum and colon.

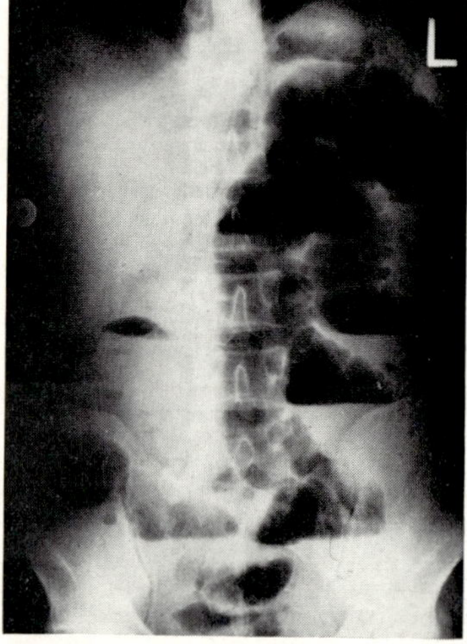

Fig. 544.—Same patient: erect film of abdomen. Numerous fluid levels are demonstrated in the small bowel.

One film will be taken supine and the second erect (*Figs.* 543, 544). Should the patient be unable to stand, the film is taken with the patient lying on one side, the X-ray beam being directed in the horizontal projection. The supine film shows the soft-tissue shadows of the various organs, normal and abnormal calcifications, and demonstrates the distribution and appearance of bowel gas to the best advantage. The erect film, which must include the diaphragmatic region, is used to show the presence of pneumoperitoneum due to perforation of a hollow viscus (*Fig.* 545). The presence of fluid levels in the small or large bowel is an important finding, e.g., in cases of intestinal obstruction or paralytic ileus. Fluid levels will show only when the X-ray beam has been projected horizontally, i.e., with the patient erect or in the lateral decubitus position.

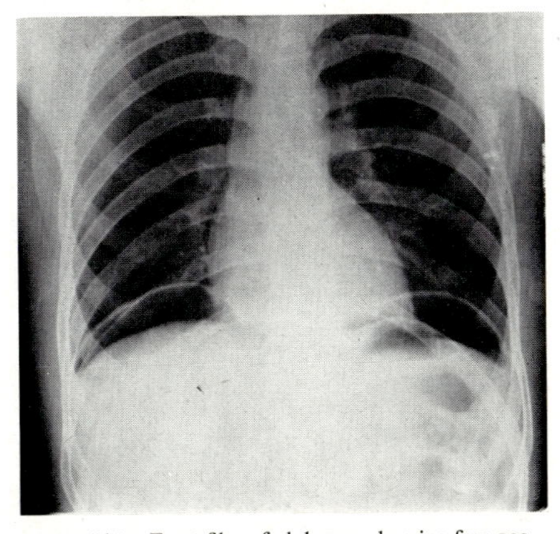

Fig. 545.—Erect film of abdomen showing free gas below the diaphragm.

Contrast media may be given orally to elucidate a lesion in the alimentary tract. In cases of hæmatemesis, oral administration of a water-soluble organic iodine preparation such as gastrografin may be preferred. This medium gives a gastric mucosal pattern similar to barium; it is unsatisfactory for anatomical study of the small-bowel mucosa but gives good colonic definition. Functional assessment of the alimentary tract can be obtained by this medium which is well tolerated should it enter the peritoneal cavity. On occasion it may be helpful to produce opacification of the biliary or renal tracts as an emergency procedure.

POST-OPERATIVE PYREXIA

Radiography of the chest is routine for the patient who develops a pyrexia following an abdominal operation. It is sometimes necessary to direct attention to the possibility of a subphrenic abscess. It cannot be stressed too strongly that portable radiography of the chest is a most unsatisfactory examination in such a case. Almost without exception it should be possible to bring the patient to the

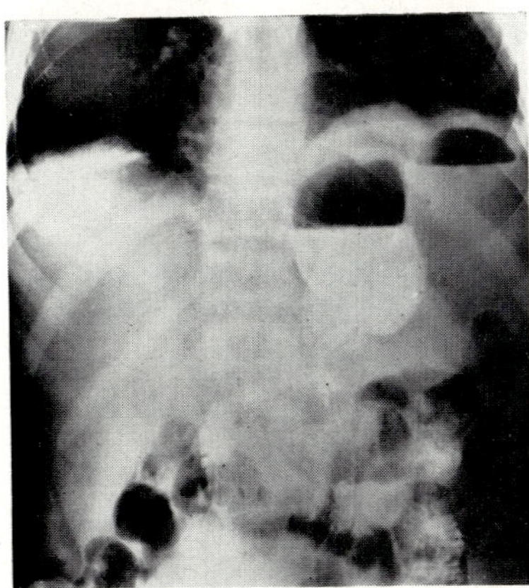

Fig. 546.—Erect film of diaphragmatic region. There is a left-sided subphrenic abscess containing a fluid level on the lateral aspect of the stomach, the latter being outlined by contrast medium.

X-ray department in order that screening and films of the diaphragm and upper abdomen can be carried out. Oral administration of contrast medium can be very useful to separate the various gas shadows in the upper abdomen and demonstrate displacement of normal structures by the mass of the abscess itself (*Fig.* 546).

TRAUMATIC CASES

The radiologist may not always be available to give immediate advice in accident cases. It is particularly important here that the radiographer should

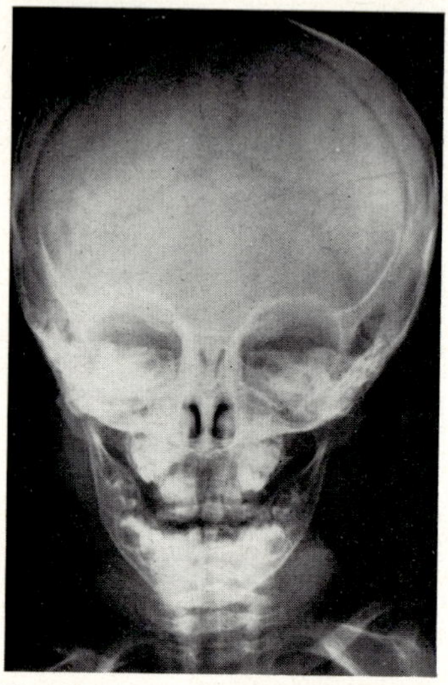

Fig. 547.—Postero-anterior view of a normal skull in a child.

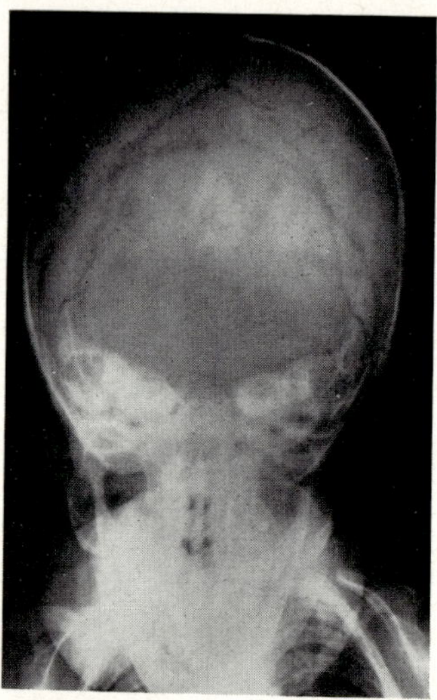

Fig. 548.—Towne's (half axial antero-posterior) view of skull.

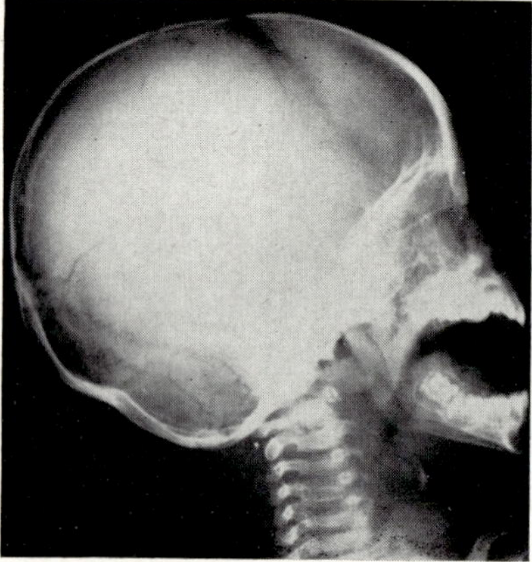

Fig. 549.—Lateral view of skull.

be informed of the precise region to be examined. Standard radiographic projections have been carefully designed to show a particular bone to the best advantage and the advice of the radiologist or the radiographer should always be adhered to in this connexion. Some modifications of the usual techniques may occasionally be required, but it is unwise to invent new projections which may cause confusion in diagnosis. Two views of a fracture at right-angles to one another should be taken whenever possible. A few remarks pertaining to injuries to some specific parts of the skeleton may be useful.

In **head injuries,** the standard projections are: (1) postero-anterior, (2) Towne's view, (3) both lateral views. In these particular films the frontal, occipital, and parietal bones respectively are adjacent to the film and show in sharp relief (*Figs.* 547, 548, 549). Fractures of the vault of the skull are demonstrated with a high degree of accuracy. Radiographic demonstration of fractures of the base of the

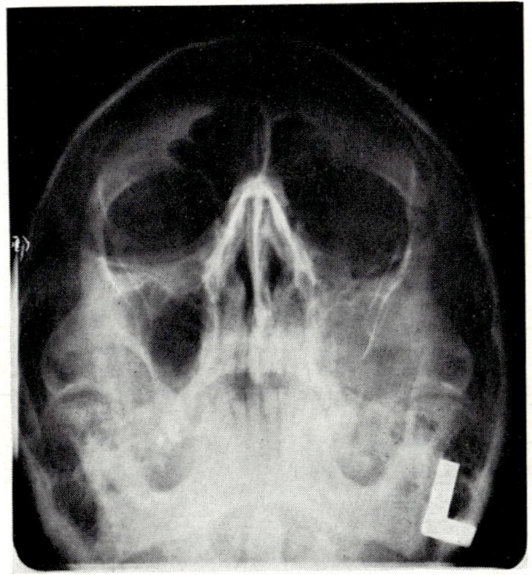

Fig. 550.—Occipitomental view of skull showing a depressed fracture of the left malar bone. There is fracturing of the infra-orbital ridge and lateral wall of antrum and separation of the fronto-malar suture.

skull is unsatisfactory but may be inferred by obvious extension of a fracture of the cranial vault coupled with the clinical signs. Fissure fractures have to be distinguished from suture lines and the normal vascular grooves. Supplementary view of sinuses or mastoid bones may be required where leakage of cerebrospinal fluid is apparent. A depressed fracture of the skull is indicated by the double density of overlapping bone fragments. Tangential views of the affected region may be useful.

A depressed fracture of the **malar bone** may be obscured by soft-tissue swelling of the cheek and will seldom be seen on the standard views of the skull. Special views have been designed for this region to show the degree of depression of the fracture and any associated damage to the maxilla and zygomatic process (*Fig.* 550).

Displacement of the odontoid process of the axis will be seen easily (if looked for) in the lateral view of the **cervical spine** (*Fig.* 551), but may be missed in the anteroposterior unless a special view is taken through the open mouth (*Fig.* 552). Lateral radiography of the upper dorsal spine is made difficult by the bulk of

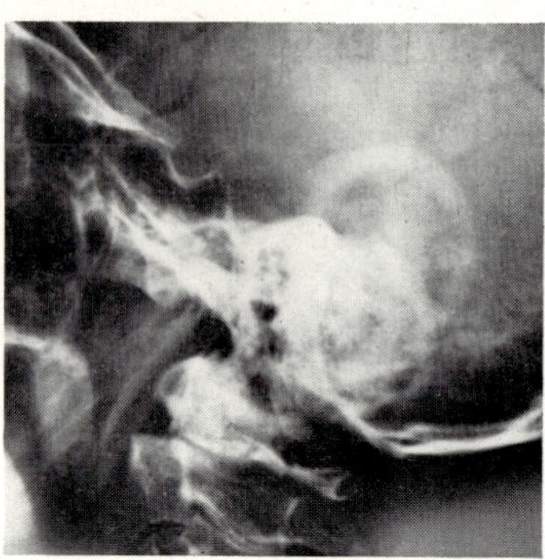

Fig. 551.—Lateral view of base of skull and upper cervical region. The base of the odontoid process is fractured transversely and displaced posteriorly in relation to the body of the axis.

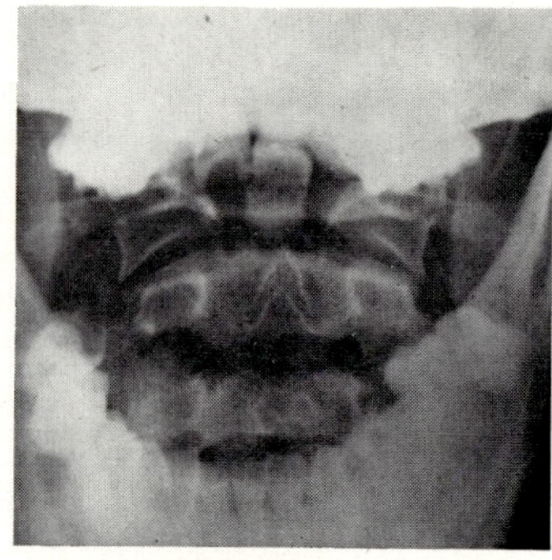

Fig. 552.—Same case. Antero-posterior view through the open mouth showing the fracture of the odontoid process.

the shoulder-girdle and it is usual for slightly oblique views of this region to be substituted. Good lateral views of the lumbar spine in an immobilized patient are difficult to obtain by portable apparatus. Radiographs in varying degrees of obliquity are necessary for the complete demonstration of the apophyseal joints, intervertebral foramina, pedicles, and laminæ.

Injuries to **the elbow** region, particularly in children, should be analysed with care. Comparable views of the opposite joint are helpful. Following reduction of a posterior dislocation of the elbow-joint, persistent displacement of the epiphysis or the medial humeral epicondyle into the elbow-joint may be overlooked. In wrist injuries, special views are required to show the scaphoid bone to the best advantage.

Chest radiography may show evidence of lung trauma, e.g., surgical emphysema, pneumothorax, or pleural effusion. A normal X-ray film of the chest has sufficient penetration to show the middle and upper ribs only, the lower ribs being obscured by the density of the trunk and abdominal viscera. Where there is any possibility of a rupture of **the spleen**, it is wise to ask for a radiograph of the abdomen; the lower ribs will be clearly shown and the splenic shadow itself can be examined. Evidence of hæmoperitoneum may be seen. An intravenous pyelogram is an essential examination in cases of hæmaturia following abdominal trauma.

SPECIAL INVESTIGATIONS

The contrast media used in these special investigations are listed at the end of the chapter (p. 729).

ALIMENTARY TRACT

Sialography.—In cases of swelling of the glands due to calculous disease, sialectasis, or tumour, radiographic demonstration of the salivary glands and ducts is obtained by the retrograde injection of contrast medium (*see* p. 729). The procedure is contra-indicated in acute sialitis.

Technique.—The orifice of the parotid salivary gland lies opposite the second upper molar tooth, and that of the submandibular salivary duct in the sublingual papilla near the midline. The appropriate area is dried by a gauze swab and the duct located by massaging the gland and observing the discharge of saliva. Salivation can be augmented by giving the patient a slice of lemon to suck. Preliminary dilatation of the duct orifice by means of a lacrimal dilator may be required. (*Fig.* 553.) A thin metal olivary-tipped cannula or a

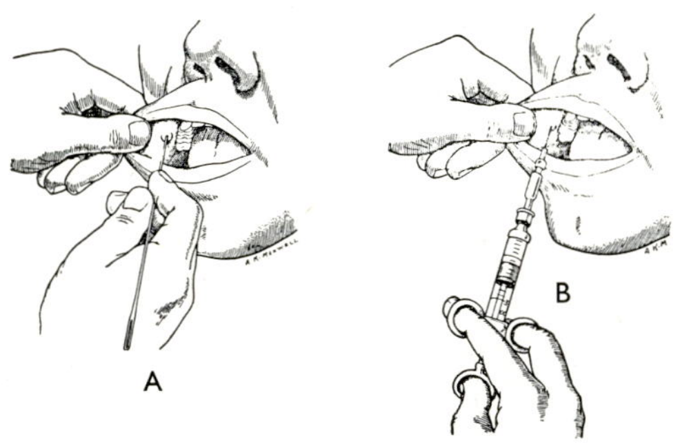

Fig. 553.—Technique of parotid sialography. **A,** The duct orifice is located, and dilated if necessary by a probe. **B,** The opaque medium is injected.

fine polythene catheter is used for the introduction of the contrast medium. The cannula or catheter should be connected to the syringe and the entire system filled with contrast medium at the beginning. About 0·5 ml. of contrast medium is generally sufficient and the injection should be stopped when the patient complains of pain. The instrument should remain in the duct during radiography in order to prevent the escape of contrast medium.

BARIUM STUDIES

These examinations are normally carried out in the X-ray department by the radiologist. The patient is examined under the fluorescent screen, radiographs being taken at appropriate stages during the examination. (Contrast media, *see* p. 729).

1. Barium Swallow.—This is generally understood to refer to the investigation of a morphological process of the pharynx or œsophagus only; it is also used, however, in suspected cases of mediastinal lymphadenopathy and in the assessment of cardiac chamber enlargement or abnormalities of the great vessels near the base of the heart.

2. Barium Meal.—This comprises an examination of the œsophagus, stomach, and duodenum. The patient is examined first in the erect and then in the horizontal position, when a routine search is made for gastro-œsophageal reflux.

3. Barium Series (or 'Meal and Follow-through' Examination).—This means a full barium meal, followed by regular filming of the small bowel and at least the proximal half of the colon (*Fig.* 554). Excess mucus in the small bowel may cause clumping or fragmentation of ordinary barium to occur and a preparation specially resistant to flocculation is therefore employed. The radiologist will not be prepared to give an opinion on a pathological process in the colon during a follow-through examination since filling of the large bowel is often patchy due to fluid absorption; in addition, it is impossible to assess the distensibility of the bowel wall by this method. For these reasons, a barium enema is the method of choice in the investigation of the colon and ileocæcal region. Barium by mouth may have to be used, however, in cases of incontinence.

4. Barium Enema.—It is inadvisable to perform this examination immediately following sigmoidoscopy, despite the fact that one may be tempted to do so in order to save further bowel preparation. The reason for this advice is that a complete or incomplete perforation of the bowel is occasionally produced if a rectal biopsy has been performed during the endoscopic procedure.

The conventional method is to administer a suspension of barium sulphate into the rectum by gravitational feed. The flow of contrast medium is usually continued until the terminal ileum is reached. The radiologist observes colonic filling on the fluorescent screen and takes radiographs as

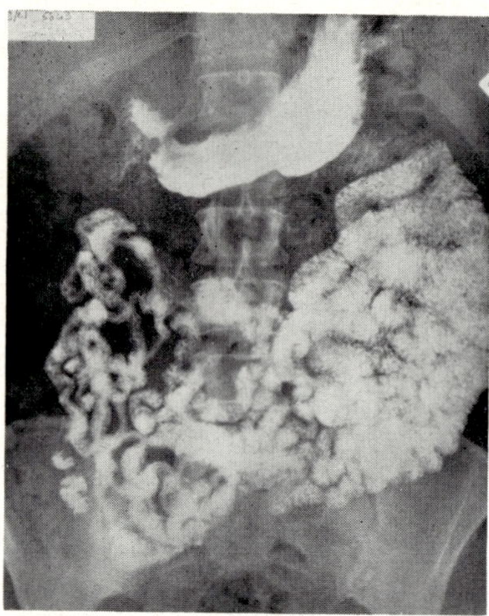

Fig. 554.—Prone film of abdomen one hour after administration of 250 ml. of barium sulphate. About half of the barium remains in the stomach, while the 'head' of the meal has reached the lower ileum. The feathery pattern of the normal small intestine is shown.

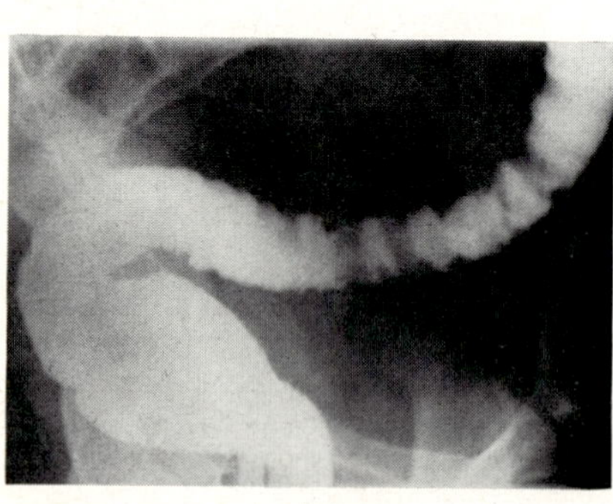

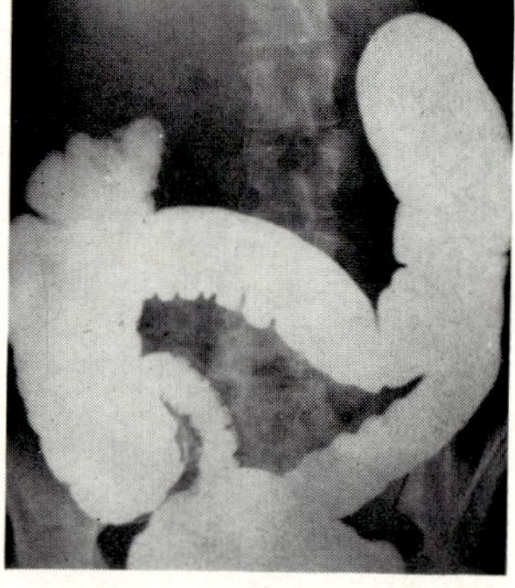

A   B

Fig. 555.—A, Barium enema. Oblique view of the pelvis to show rectosigmoid junction. B, Barium enema. Postero-anterior view. There is complete filling of the large bowel and terminal ileum.

required (*Fig.* 555), including at least one film following evacuation when the mucosal pattern is seen to advantage (*Fig.* 556). Relief pictures to enhance the demonstration of small polypi are obtained by a double-contrast technique which consists of pumping air into the colon by a Higginson's syringe after the barium has been evacuated (*Fig.* 557). Extremely thorough preparation of the bowel is vital for the barium-enema technique to be successful. Repeat examination is mostly required in the investigation of colonic polypi, where 'air contrast' barium enemas are not performed routinely.

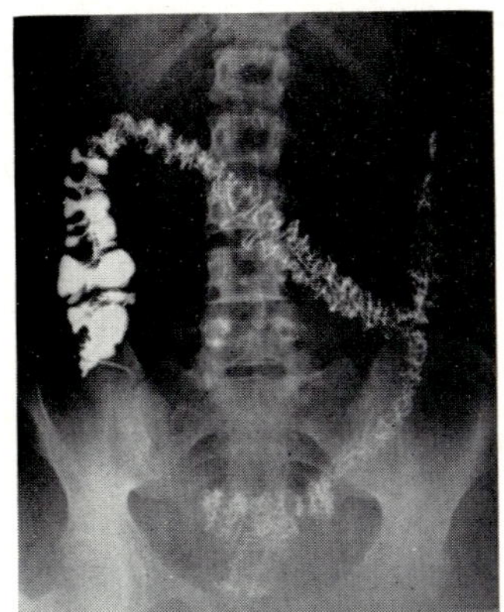

Fig. 556.—Barium enema. Post-evacuation film. The mucosal pattern of the collapsed colon is clearly demonstrated.

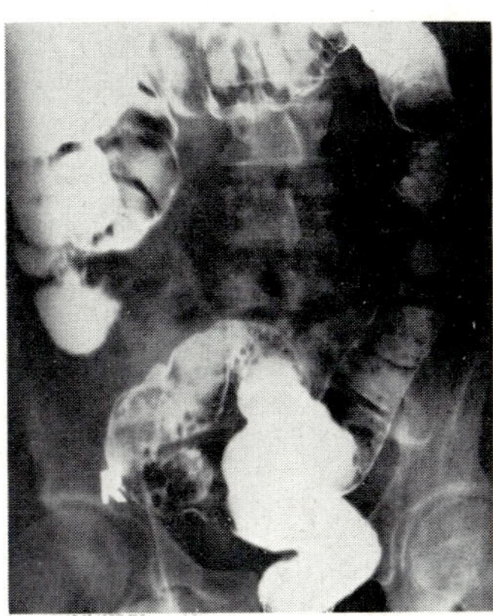

Fig. 557.—Barium enema with air contrast. Supine film. The colon is distended with air while barium continues to provide a mucosal coating. Numerous small rounded filling defects are seen which represent colonic polypi.

BILIARY TRACT

A plain radiograph of the gall-bladder region is taken in all cases, as it is possible for faintly calcified gall-stones to be obscured by a dense contrast medium during cholecystography. Any form of cholecystography will be unsuccessful where the serum bilirubin is greater than 3 mg. per cent—when clinical jaundice will be present.

Oral Cholecystography.—This procedure is designed to show the function of the gall-bladder and the presence or absence of gall-stones; demonstration of the bile-ducts is uncertain by this method. The technique depends both on the capability of the gall-bladder mucosa to concentrate, and on the patency of the cystic duct. It is of no value when the gall-bladder has been removed. Contrast medium—*see* p. 729.

The contrast medium is given at 7 p.m. and radiographs are taken at 9 a.m. the following day, in order to allow time for absorption of the contrast medium to occur from the alimentary tract and concentration to take place in the gall-bladder. Films of the gall-bladder are taken in both prone (*Fig.* 558) and erect positions; the latter projection is used since small stones may be best seen floating in the gall-bladder (*Fig.* 559). Further films are commonly taken half an hour following a fatty meal to show the contractibility of the gall-bladder and possibly demonstrate the duct system.

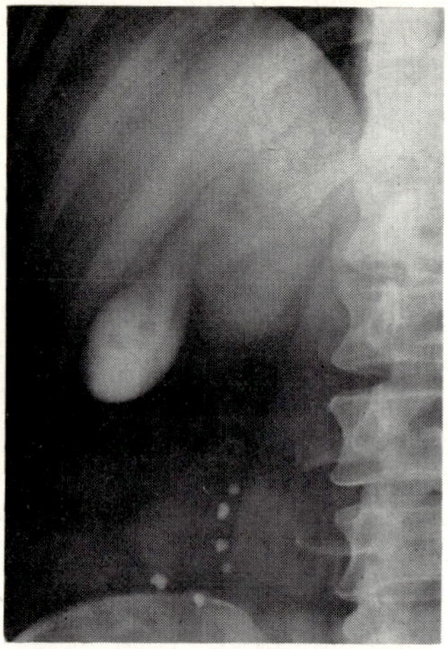

Fig. 558.—Cholecystogram. Prone film. Normally concentrating gall-bladder containing radiolucent calculi.

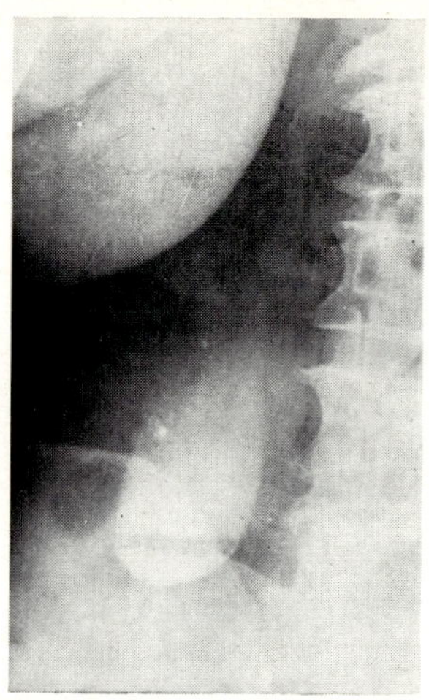

Fig. 559.—Cholecystogram. Erect film. A layer of tiny non-opaque calculi is seen floating within the contrast medium in the gall-bladder.

If there is non-opacification of the gall-bladder in a patient with a normal liver, it is wellnigh certain that the gall-bladder is diseased. Non-opacification, however, is due occasionally to failure to take the telepaque tablets, to failure of absorption of the contrast medium, e.g., in cases of pyloric stenosis, or to severe vomiting or diarrhœa caused by reaction to the contrast medium. It is customary in many departments to repeat the examination for confirmation. When the gall-bladder fails to fill, more precise information as to the state of the biliary tract can be obtained by the intravenous method of cholecystography.

Intravenous Cholecystangiography.—Twenty ml. of biligrafin forte (p. 729) are given slowly intravenously. The shadow of the bile-ducts begins to appear about 15 minutes later. Providing the cystic duct is patent, the gall-bladder fills and is seen to the best advantage in about 2 hours after injection (*Fig.* 560). It is important to remember that the concentrating power of the gall-bladder cannot be assessed by this method. The examination will occasionally fail owing to the contrast medium being excreted entirely by the kidneys.

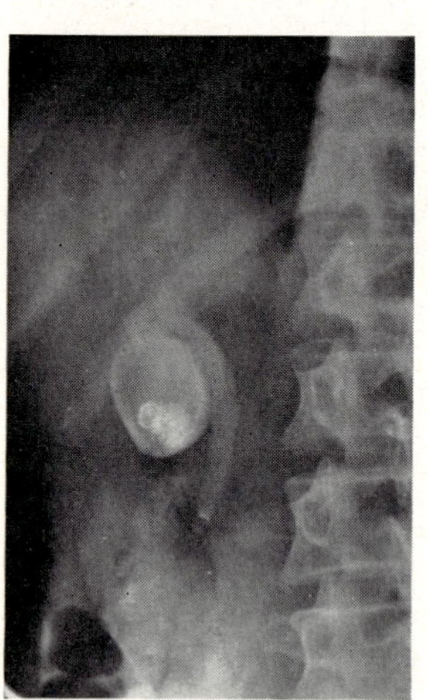

Fig. 560.—Intravenous cholecyst-angiogram. The common bile-duct is outlined; there is a small opaque calculus at the lower end. The gall-bladder has filled and is seen to contain multiple opaque calculi.

The intravenous cholangiogram, which is the only satisfactory procedure when the gall-bladder has been removed, has proved invaluable in the investigation of the 'post-cholecystectomy syndrome'. The examination is unreliable in cases of internal biliary fistula, and a barium meal is probably the best method of investigation here.

Operative Cholangiography.—The technique is designed to demonstrate the hepatic and common bile-ducts during operation. (Contrast medium—hypaque 25–45 per cent, p. 729.) The patient lies on a specially designed cassette tunnel incorporated into the operating table-top, which allows a number of X-ray films to be taken. The cystic duct is exposed. It is catheterized with a fine polythene catheter connected to a 20-ml. syringe, the entire system being filled with saline from the outset. Bile is aspirated to check that the air seal is secure. The syringe is then changed for one containing contrast medium and the plunger again withdrawn to ensure removal of air bubbles. Radiographs of the common bile-duct are taken with the operating table tilted 10–15° to the right. It is customary to take three films as quickly as possible following the injection of 3–4 ml., 7–8 ml., and 10–12 ml. of contrast medium (*Fig.* 561).

Operative Film with T-tube in Position.—At this stage radiography is less rewarding due to the leakage of contrast medium and the fact that the sphincter of Oddi is often in spasm and prevents adequate demonstration of the lower end of the common bile-duct.

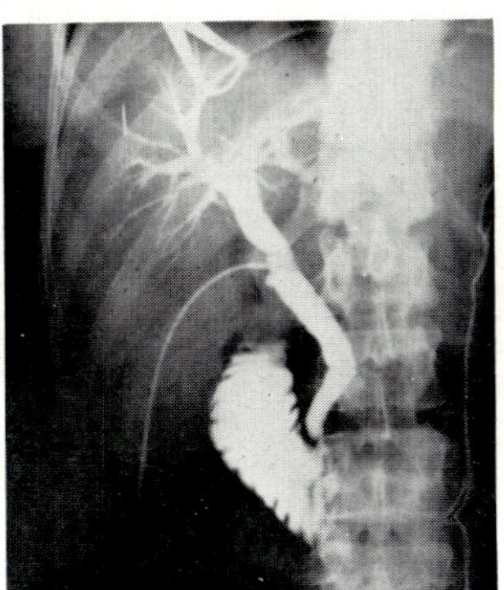

Fig. 561.—Operative cholangiogram via a catheter inserted into the cystic duct. Antero-posterior view. There is good filling of the intrahepatic, common hepatic, and common bile-ducts with free flow of contrast medium into the duodenum.

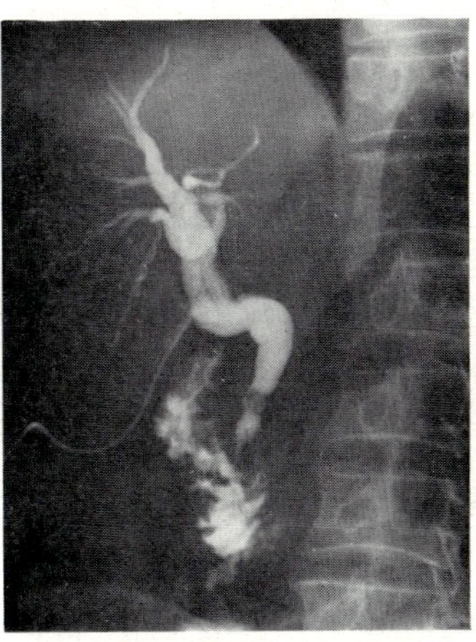

Fig. 562.—T-tube cholangiogram. Antero-posterior film. Despite good flow into the duodenum there is a large faceted non-opaque calculus near the lower end of the common bile-duct.

The introduction of air-bubbles may be prevented by placing the T-tube in position while it is being continuously irrigated with saline. Two or three films are exposed using slightly larger amounts of contrast medium than in the earlier procedure.

T-tube Cholangiography.—This is normally carried out in the X-ray department about 10 days after operation. It is normally done under fluorescent screen control. (Contrast medium—*see* p. 729.) A 20-ml. syringe containing contrast medium is connected directly to the end of the tubing. Bile is aspirated together with any air-bubbles which are present. The syringe is then held vertically and the contrast medium allowed to flow in by gravity. The rate of flow is controlled by varying the height of the syringe from the table-top and by stopping the flow completely during radiography. Two or three fractionated quantities are injected in order to demonstrate the hepatic and the common bile-ducts and the passage of contrast medium into the duodenum (*Fig.* 562).

URINARY TRACT

The intravenous injection of contrast medium is the most frequently employed method of demonstrating the urinary tract. It may be supplemented by retrograde technique when excretion is poor or when the lower urinary tract is being investigated.

Intravenous Pyelography.—This examination demonstrates both the function and anatomy of the kidneys in addition to providing delineation of the ureters and bladder. Plain radiographs of kidneys, ureters, and bladder are taken routinely prior to the intravenous injection of at least 40 ml. of contrast medium. (Contrast medium—*see* p. 729.) If the examination is carried out carefully in patients who are well prepared, the necessity for retrograde pyelography is markedly reduced. Films of the kidneys are generally taken at 5 minutes, 10 minutes, and 30 minutes after injection (*Fig.* 563); the number of radiographs

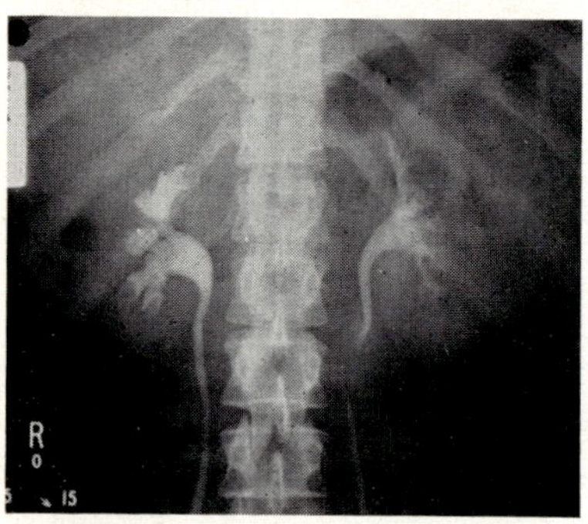

Fig. 563.—Intravenous pyelogram. Ten-minute film. Normal function and appearance of both kidneys.

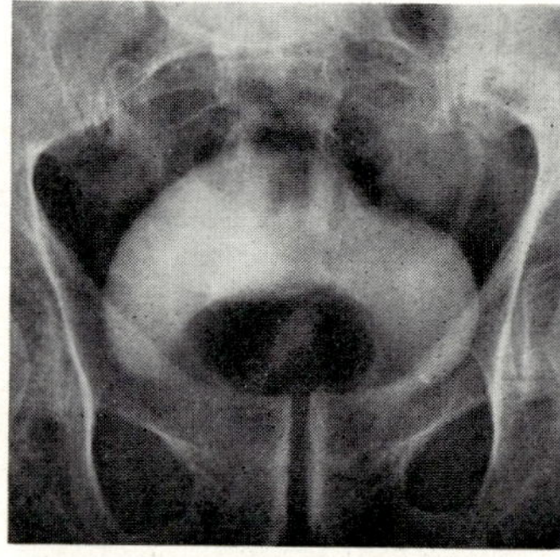

Fig. 564.—Intravenous pyelogram. Film of bladder area. The large, smooth, rounded filling defect in the base of the bladder is due to prostatic hypertrophy.

may require modification depending on the disease process under investigation. Radiographs of the bladder before and after micturition are helpful in the determination of residual urine (*Fig.* 564).

The level of blood-urea should be estimated if it is thought likely to be elevated. A double dose of contrast medium should be given if the blood-urea is in the region of 75 mg. per cent. With higher levels of blood-urea, drip infusion pyelography (*see* p. 715) may be helpful. Infants and children tolerate relatively large amounts of contrast medium (1·5 ml. per kg. body-weight). At least 5 ml. may thus be given to infants, and 10 ml. to small children. In infants, the feed prior to the examination should be omitted and a sedative given. A drink of lemonade or similar beverage at the end of the injection will distend the stomach and show the kidneys to advantage.

Where intravenous injection proves impossible in infants, the contrast medium can be given subcutaneously. Strict aseptic precautions are necessary. Ten ml. of contrast medium are given to infants and children up to the age of 5 years. This quantity should be diluted to 30 ml. with sterile distilled water containing 1000 units of hyaluronidase. It is important that the hyaluronidase solution be prepared freshly. The injection is made subcutaneously in two divided doses over the scapulæ; absorption is aided by massaging the site of injection. The first radiograph is usually taken at about 30 minutes.

Drip Infusion Pyelography.—This technique gives pyelograms of improved quality and a more complete demonstration of ureters and bladder. Pyelograms may also be obtained in cases of renal failure with blood-urea levels as high as 150 mg. per cent. The technique is contra-indicated in oliguria. (Contrast medium—*see* p. 729.)

Technique: The method depends on the intravenous infusion of relatively large amounts of contrast medium of the order of 0·5–1 ml. per kg. of body-weight without fluid restriction. The salts contained in the contrast medium normally produce an adequate diuresis. The latter can be augmented by giving an equal quantity of 5 per cent dextrose in water. A convenient technique is to use a 1-litre infusion bottle of dextrose solution, discarding the unwanted amount and adding the contrast medium to the remainder. An infusion pack containing 250 ml. of dilute contrast medium is now available commercially. The infusion is given through the standard giving set over a period of about 5 minutes. Films are required in about 10 minutes' time; in cases of delayed excretion due to ureteric obstruction or renal failure, late films up to 24 hours may be helpful.

Reactions to Contrast Media of the Organic Iodine Type.—Intravenous pyelography should not be performed in a patient known or suspected to have myelomatosis, since renal failure may be precipitated. Care should be exercised in patients with a strong history of allergy; an antihistamine such as piriton 10 mg. may be given beforehand, either intramuscularly or intravenously. The contrast medium can be varied where reaction has occurred previously. It is generally agreed that test doses of contrast media are unreliable. The customary practice is to inject 1–2 ml., and wait for 1 minute before giving the whole amount. The main injection of urografin or hypaque can be given rapidly but it is recommended that biligrafin should be given more slowly, preferably taking up to 10 minutes.

Minor reactions, such as a general feeling of body warmth, coughing, dizziness, or nausea and vomiting, usually disappear spontaneously within a few minutes. Symptoms such as rhinorrhœa or pruritus will be relieved by antihistamines. Severe reactions, which are rare, take the form of urticaria or angioneurotic œdema, respiratory difficulty, or circulatory collapse. The most useful drug for immediate use is adrenaline 1–1000 solution, in a dose of 0·5 ml. subcutaneously. The action of adrenaline can be reinforced by hydrocortisone 100 mg. intravenously if necessary.

Retrograde Introduction of Contrast Medium into the Urinary Tract.—Strict asepsis is essential in the following procedures:—

Retrograde Pyelography.—This examination should not be performed prior to intravenous pyelography unless renal failure exists. Where this examination is carried out under X-ray screen control, accuracy of filling is ensured and ureteric function is demonstrable. When a 'blind' radiographic procedure is used the routine is as follows:—

Piriton (Allen & Hanburys Ltd., Bethnal Green, London, E.2).

28

A plain film with the ureteric catheter in position is obligatory in order to obviate injection into the renal substance via a mal-positioned catheter. The catheter should be withdrawn until it is in the renal pelvis and aspirated prior to injection. The syringe containing contrast medium is connected to the catheter by a small hypodermic needle or by a special adaptor which clamps tightly over the outer wall of the catheter. It is important to ensure that the injecting system is free of air. An organic contrast medium (*see* p. 729) is used; under no circumstances should sodium iodide be employed. About 4–8 ml. of contrast

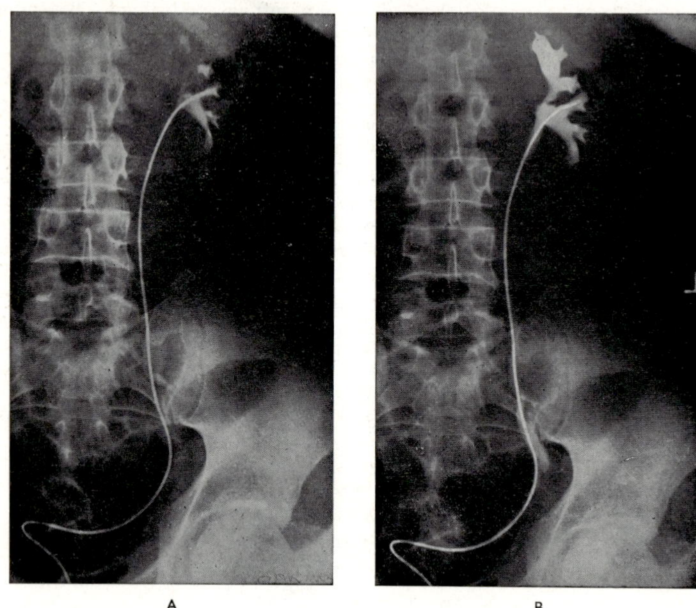

A   B

Fig. 565.—A, Retrograde pyelogram showing pelvis incompletely filled; B, More solution has been introduced and pelvis is now completely filled.

medium are normally required to fill the collecting system. The conscious patient will complain of pain when the pelvi-caliceal system is full, but this is an unsatisfactory guide and it is better to introduce a small amount of contrast medium initially and give an augmented injection in order to obtain complete filling (*Fig.* 565). Overfilling may result in pyelotubular, pyelolymphatic, or pyelovenous backflow (*Fig.* 566). These complications do not appear to be serious, although the pictorial result is spoiled.

Cystography.—Radiographic demonstration of the urinary bladder is obtained following catheterization by the introduction of warmed urografin, 15–60 per cent strength, the higher concentrations being required for the demonstration of the urethra. About 350 ml. of contrast medium are used in an adult with normal bladder capacity. Antero-posterior and both oblique films are taken and a further film after emptying the bladder. The examination is usually performed to show bladder diverticula. Standard cystography is not particularly useful in bladder tumours as the tumour mass is obscured by the contrast medium.

Micturating Cystography. — This examination is designed to show the bladder neck and urethra and to determine the presence or absence of ureteric reflux. General anæsthesia is

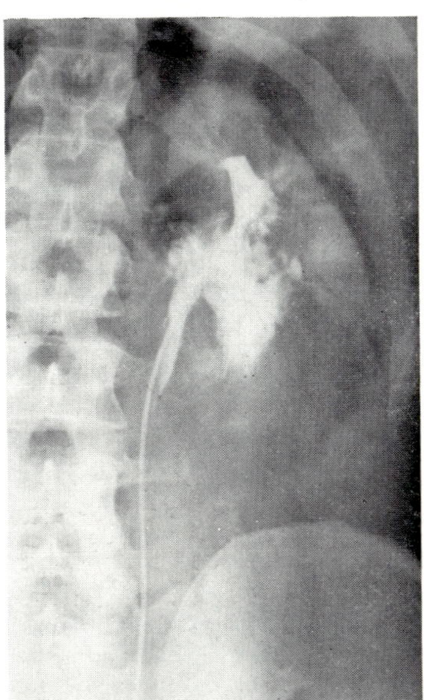

Fig. 566.—Left retrograde pyelogram. Over-filling of the pelvis has caused pyelotubular and pyelolymphatic backflow of contrast medium.

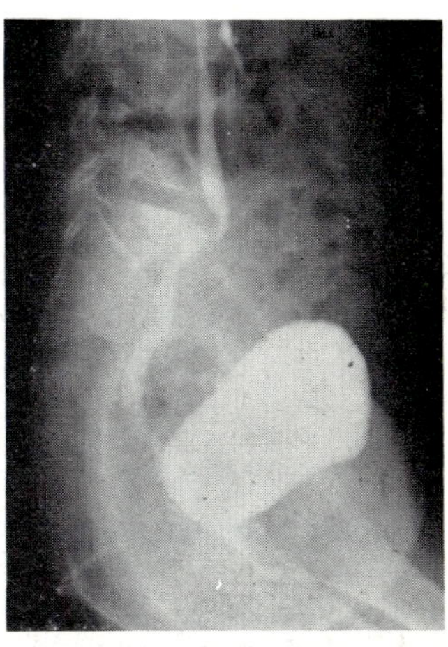

Fig. 567.—Micturating cystogram. Female patient. Lateral film taken during micturition. The bladder neck and urethra are demonstrated. Ureteric reflux is occurring.

not used as the essence of the examination is to have a voluntary micturition. It is rare for a child of over 6 years to be uncooperative. In children it has been found helpful for the bladder catheterization to be performed under familiar surroundings at ward level. The bladder should first be allowed to drain through the catheter; it is then filled with contrast medium using a 20-ml. or 50-ml. syringe. The amount of contrast medium given is appropriate to the age and build of the patient. For a child of 7 years about 120 ml. are required. A film is taken of the filled bladder. The patient is instructed to micturate voluntarily, further radiographs being exposed in both antero-posterior and lateral projections during the act (*Fig.* 567).

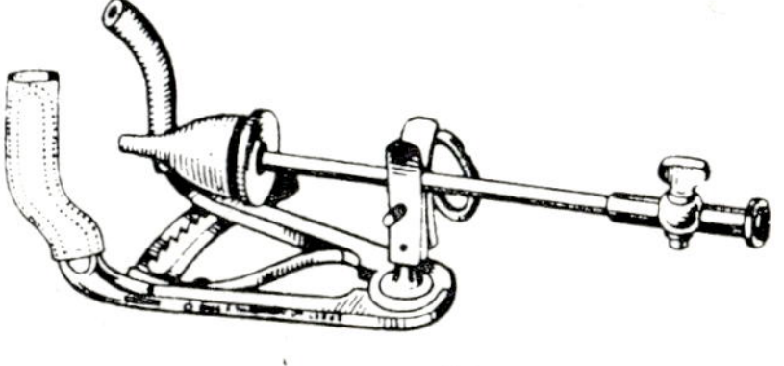

Fig. 568.—Knutsson's penile clamp.

Urethrocystography.—This technique consists of retrograde injection of contrast medium into the male urethra to show congenital, traumatic, or inflammatory lesions of the urethra and bladder neck. (Contrast medium—*see* p. 729.) The patient empties his bladder and lies on the X-ray table. The prepuce is retracted and the glans and external meatus are cleaned with antiseptic. The penis is gripped behind the glans by the blades of a special penile clamp (*Fig.* 568). The rubber acorn at the end of the cannula is introduced into the external meatus as far as possible and fixed in position by means of a clamping screw. The

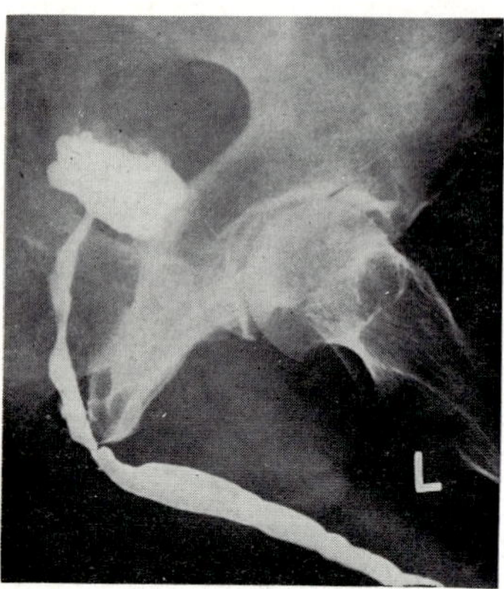

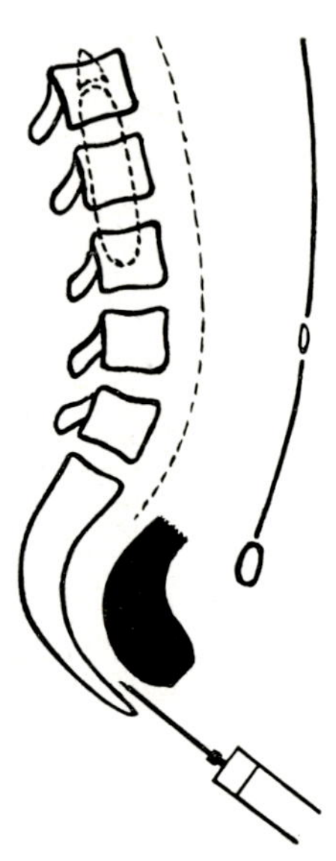

Fig. 569.—Male urethrogram. A stricture is present in the bulbous urethra.

patient is then placed in the oblique position and the injection commenced using a 50-ml. syringe. Several films are taken during the examination. At the stage of filling, a burning sensation will be experienced by the patient. A feeling of resistance will be felt by the operator when the contrast medium reaches the external sphincter; this will pass off when the sphincter relaxes. The injection is continued until the bladder base is outlined; this may require up to 40 ml. of contrast medium (*Fig.* 569).

Fig. 570.—Presacral air insufflation. Diagram of method. The needle is introduced into the perineum between the anus and the tip of the coccyx. The long dotted line represents the posterior parietal peritoneum in the midline.

Complications: Reflux may occur into the veins of the corpus callosum and is particularly liable to occur where there is urethral stricture. No ill-effects occur from this. The patient should be warned that hæmaturia may be found following the procedure.

Presacral Gas Insufflation.—This technique is used in the investigation of adrenal gland enlargement (particularly tumour) but is sometimes of value in determining the exact renal contours. (Contrast medium—air or oxygen is generally employed. Carbon dioxide obviates the possibility of air embolus but its rapid diffusion into the tissues means that radiography must be carried out with speed; repeat injections of this gas are required.) Premedication in adults is advisable, e.g., omnopon 20 mg. About 1000 ml. of gas are sufficient for the average patient. In cases of phæochromocytoma the blood-pressure should be monitored frequently and an injection of phentolamine should be available.

Technique: The patient is placed in the knee–elbow position. The assistant draws the buttocks apart and the skin of the natal cleft is cleaned with antiseptic. A needle about 12·5 cm. long of about 18 gauge with a stylet is introduced through the skin about half-way between the coccyx and the anus, and directed backwards in the direction of the curvature of the sacrum (*Fig.* 570). The position of the needle tip in the presacral space is checked by a gloved finger in the rectum. The stylet is removed and the needle aspirated to ensure that the tip does not lie in a blood-vessel. Gas is introduced either by a syringe or a Maxwell pneumothorax box. With the latter the air will normally percolate

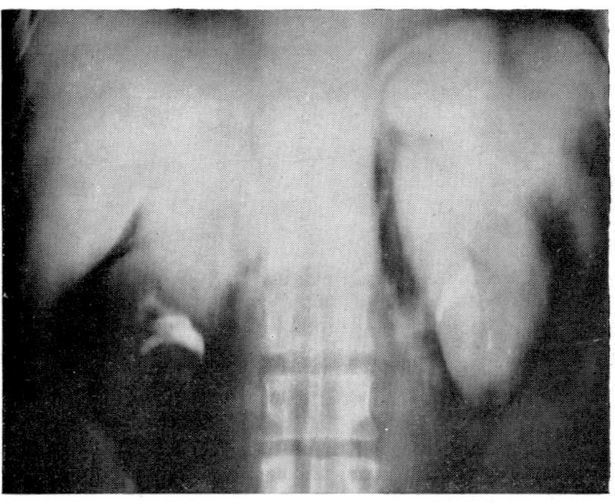

Fig. 571.—Presacral air insufflation (with intravenous pyelogram). Antero-posterior tomogram demonstrates a large right adrenal tumour. The large round opacity above the left kidney is caused by fluid in the gastric fundus.

at the rate of 50–100 ml. per minute. (Some authors recommend an initial injection of local anæsthetic and then 20 ml. of saline into the presacral space prior to the injection of gas.) If no flow of gas occurs, slight adjustment of the needle tip is usually all that is required. The patient complains of pain in the back during and following the injection of gas. He should then sit erect for about 10 minutes following the injection. A plain radiograph of the abdomen is taken supine. An asymmetrical distribution of gas can be corrected by lying the patient on the side which is well filled for 10–15 minutes. Tomography is usually employed (*Fig.* 571).

VASCULAR INVESTIGATIONS

One of the major developments in radiology in recent years has been the direct demonstration of the vascular system by arteriography. This has resulted from the development of contrast media of low toxicity and the numerous techniques which have emerged following the ingenious method of percutaneous arterial catheterization, devised by Seldinger of Sweden. (Contrast medium— hypaque or urografin, p. 729.)

In the investigation of the aorta and its main branches, the catheter is introduced into a convenient peripheral artery. The femoral or axillary arteries are most commonly used; alternatively, the brachial or carotid arteries may be employed. For demonstration of the aorta the contrast medium must be delivered rapidly in order to produce sufficient concentration. Hand injection is generally sufficient to allow demonstration of branch vessels. Examination of the thoracic aorta is obtained by guiding a radio-opaque catheter into the ascending part of the arch under X-ray screen control (*Fig.* 572). A non-opaque

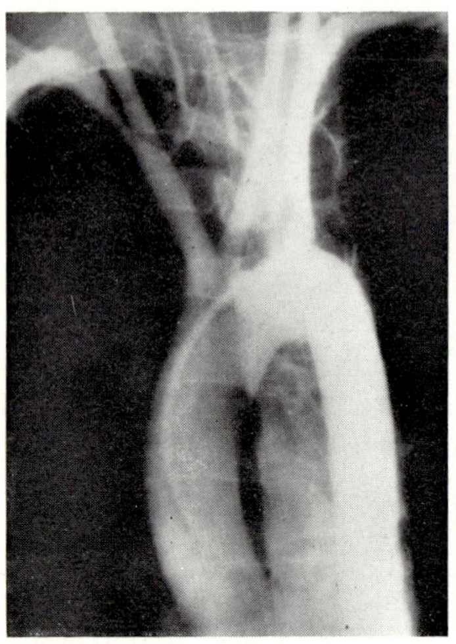

Fig. 572.—Arch aortogram. The tip of the catheter lies in the ascending arch of the aorta.

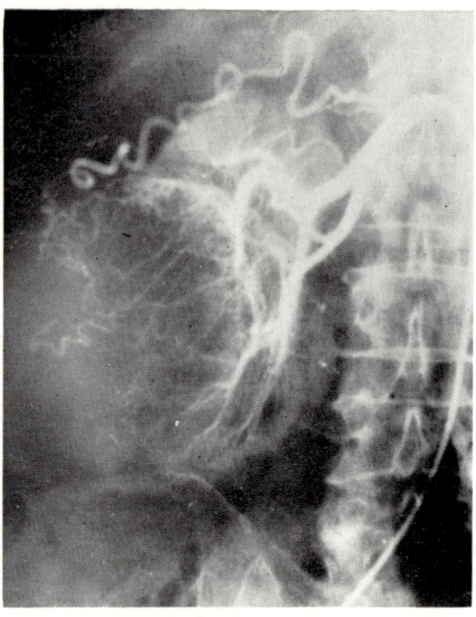

Fig. 573.—Selective right renal arteriogram. The tip of the catheter lies in the main renal artery. There is a large highly vascular carcinoma extending from the lower two-thirds of the kidney.

catheter is commonly used for standard abdominal aortography, while for selective arteriography a radio-opaque catheter is introduced into the desired branch of the aorta (*Fig.* 573).

Complications are few when arteriography is undertaken by experienced workers. The commonest minor complication is bleeding from the puncture site. Aortic dissection due to the introduction of the catheter tip beneath an atheromatous plaque has been recorded.

Translumbar Aortography.—This technique is still preferred by some workers and is the only satisfactory alternative method when tortuous iliac arteries do not allow retrograde passage of a femoral catheter and where catheterization of other branches of the aorta is inadvisable. The contrast medium is introduced into the abdominal aorta by direct needle puncture (*Fig.* 574). In order to minimize complications, this procedure should be done only by persons who are adequately experienced in the technique.

The examination is carried out under general anæsthesia with the patient lying prone. The needle is introduced into the lumbar region on the left side about 7·5 cm. lateral to the midline and is directed slightly medially to pass immediately adjacent to the bodies of the lumbar vertebræ. Once the aorta has been punctured, a test injection is given to ensure that the needle is positioned correctly before proceeding to the main injection.

Complications: Retroperitoneal bleeding occurs commonly, either from the aortic puncture or due to tearing of lumbar arteries. This hæmatoma may prove embarrassing during nephrectomy or sympathectomy. An incorrect position of the needle tip may lead to dissection of the aorta; if this involves the origins of major branches, the organs supplied may be subjected to acute ischæmia. Most cases of paraplegia which have been recorded were caused by contrast media which were particularly neurotoxic.

Peripheral Arteriography.— The demonstration of limb arteries is most commonly performed by direct needle puncture of femoral, subclavian, or brachial arteries. The subject of carotid angiography will not be dealt with in this chapter.

Percutaneous Splenoportal Venography.—Demonstration of the portal venous circulation is used in cases of portal hypertension due to extrahepatic or intrahepatic portal vein obstruction, or splenic vein thrombosis. The

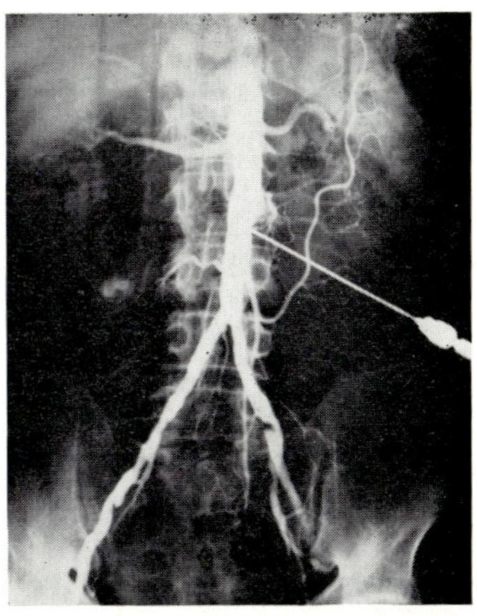

Fig. 574. — Aortogram. Translumbar method. There is marked atheromatous irregularity of the iliac arteries. The right renal, the splenic, and inferior mesenteric arteries have also filled.

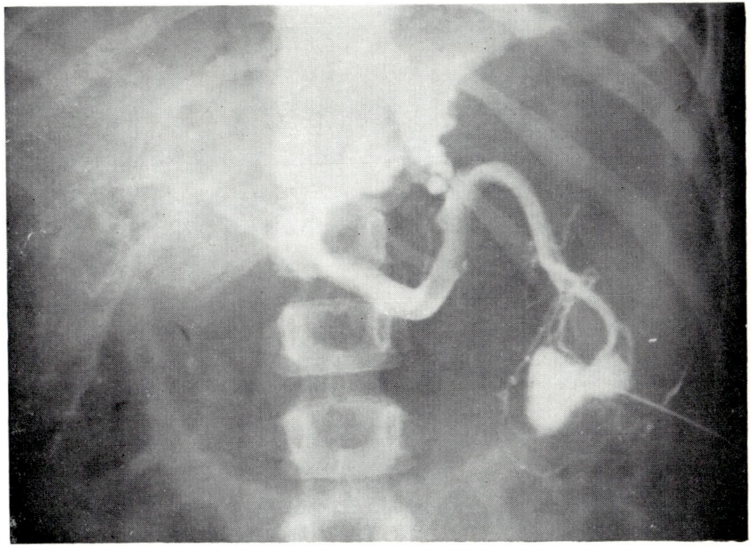

Fig. 575.—Percutaneous splenoportal venogram. The splenic and portal veins are patent. Large gastric and œsophageal varices are demonstrated. The stomach is outlined by gas.

contra-indications are: deep jaundice even with a normal prothrombin level, a prothrombin level within twice the normal range for the particular laboratory, or a platelet count less than 100,000 per c.mm. Ascitic fluid is removed prior to puncture of the spleen. (Contrast medium and post-operative care—*see* pp. 729, 730.)

The examination is carried out with aseptic precautions under local anæsthesia in adults and under general anæsthesia in children. In adult patients a premedication of 100 mg. of pethidine is given. An 18-gauge needle, about 10 cm. in length and containing a stylet, is inserted into the eighth or ninth intercostal space in the mid-axillary line. Satisfactory placement within the splenic pulp is checked by X-ray screening and the injection of a small test dose of contrast medium. At least ten films of the upper abdomen are taken during the main injection of 40 ml. of contrast medium (*Fig.* 575). In a small portion of cases bleeding from the spleen may complicate the procedure.

RADIOGRAPHY IN INFANTS AND CHILDREN

In the first few hours of life radiography may be called for in cases of respiratory or circulatory difficulty due to *diaphragmatic hernia* (*Fig.* 576).

The diagnosis of *œsophageal atresia* is suspected on the basis of excessive amounts of mucus in the mouth and pharynx and attacks of choking and cyanosis when feeding is attempted. The blind upper pouch may be seen on

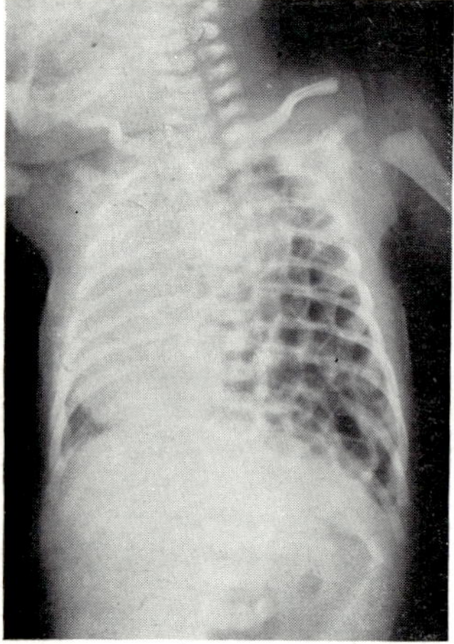

Fig. 576.—Erect film of chest in a new-born infant with diaphragmatic hernia. Loops of bowel containing gas are seen in the left hemithorax. There is considerable displacement of the mediastinum to the right.

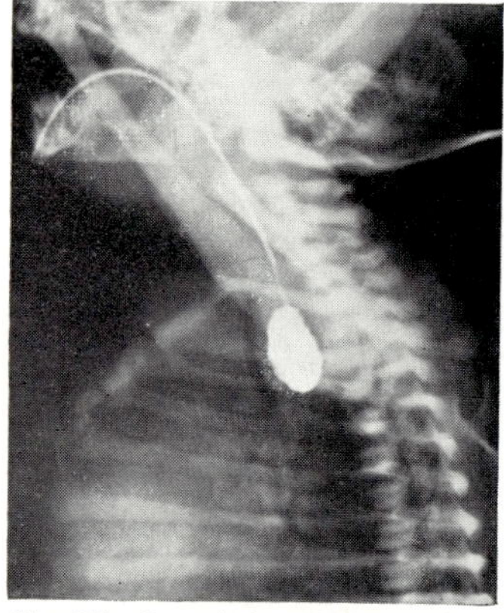

Fig. 577.—Lateral view of the thorax in a new-born infant with œsophageal atresia. A soft catheter has been introduced into the pharynx; the catheter has been arrested in the blind upper œsophageal pouch which is outlined by a small quantity of contrast medium.

plain films of the chest, but contrast examination is generally required for confirmation. The examination is performed under screen control. A soft rubber catheter is passed into the pharynx where it becomes arrested at the level of the carina. A very small amount of neohydriol is introduced into the tube—just sufficient to show the pouch. Spot radiographs are taken (*Fig.* 577), the contrast medium being aspirated immediately thereafter.

In suspected cases of *intestinal obstruction,* the usual supine and erect films of the abdomen are employed. Gas is normally present throughout the small and large bowel within 12 hours of birth but onward passage of air into the colon may be delayed by some hours in prematurity. Radiological differentiation between small and large bowel may prove difficult and barium enema is sometimes required to show the state of the colon. The bowel proximal to a complete obstruction will be gas-distended while that distally is collapsed and devoid of gas (*Fig.* 578). In cases of stenosis, air will be present distally but may be reduced in amount. Contrast medium is often required, particularly for the examination of the duodenum, where stenosis is commoner than atresia.

Pyloric Stenosis. — Radiological investigation is usually asked for only in atypical cases. Plain films are seldom helpful as they are usually normal, but characteristic appearances are shown in the majority of cases using contrast medium. The infant is examined just before a normal feed time and barium is administered by a feeding bottle under screen control. There is usually some delay in initial gastric emptying. Demonstration of the pattern of the prepyloric region is extremely important. It may be

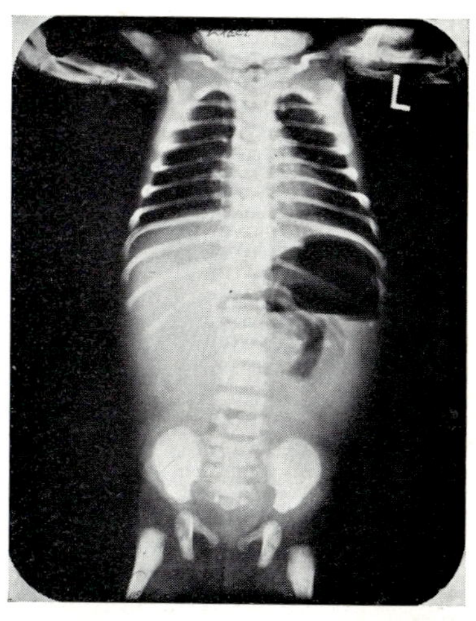

Fig. 578.—Erect film of abdomen in a new-born infant. Case of ileal atresia. Fluid levels are seen in stomach and jejunum. There is a complete absence of gas in the ileum.

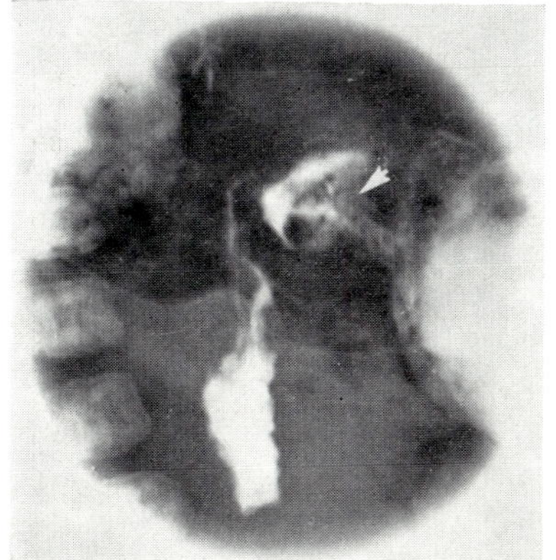

Fig. 579.—Barium meal. Congenital hypertrophic pyloric stenosis. There is marked elongation and narrowing of the pyloric antrum (arrow).

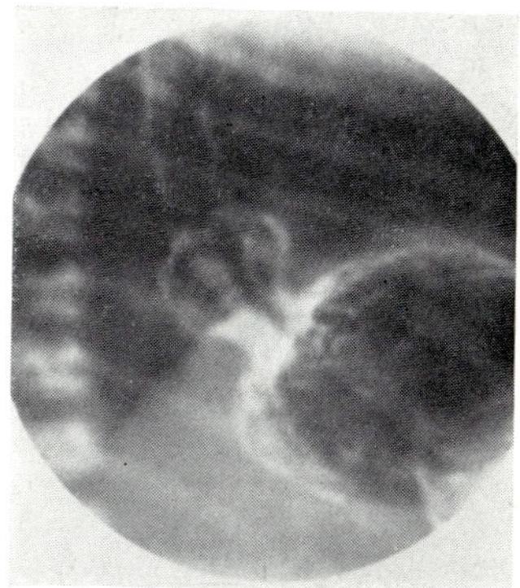

Fig. 580.—Barium meal. Oblique view of diaphragm in an infant. A sliding type of hiatus hernia of the stomach is outlined above the diaphragm.

necessary to keep the child in the X-ray department for an hour before this can be obtained (*Fig.* 579).

Hiatus Hernia.—Excessive regurgitation and/or vomiting after meals, sometimes accompanied by the presence of fresh or altered blood in the vomit, may

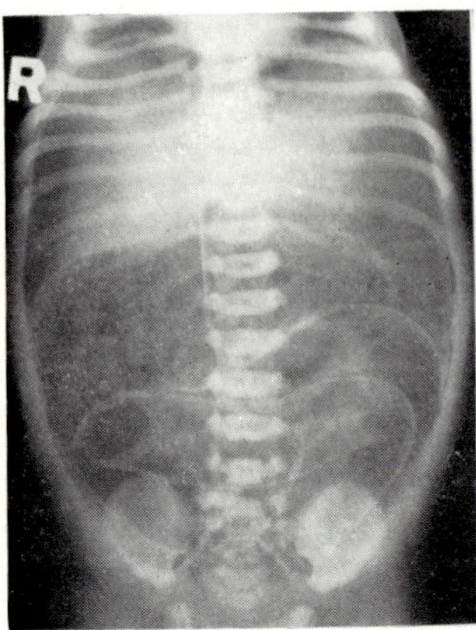

Fig. 581.—Supine film of abdomen. Meconium ileus. Note typical mottled appearance of gas mixed with gelatinous meconium in dilated small bowel loops. Perforation of distended small intestine has produced pneumoperitoneum.

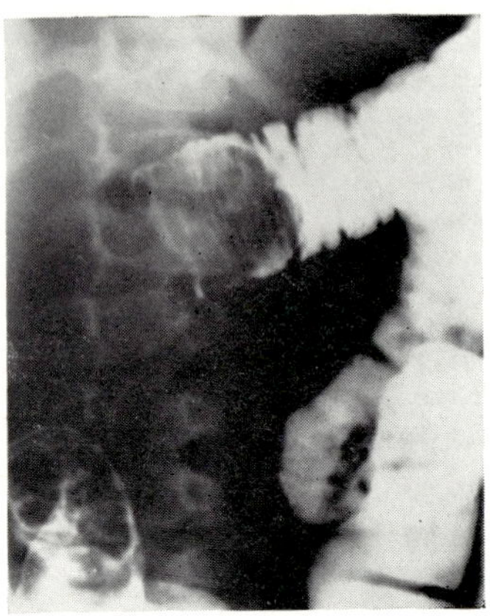

Fig. 582.—Barium enema. Intussusception. The intussusceptum is shown projecting into the barium column in the transverse colon.

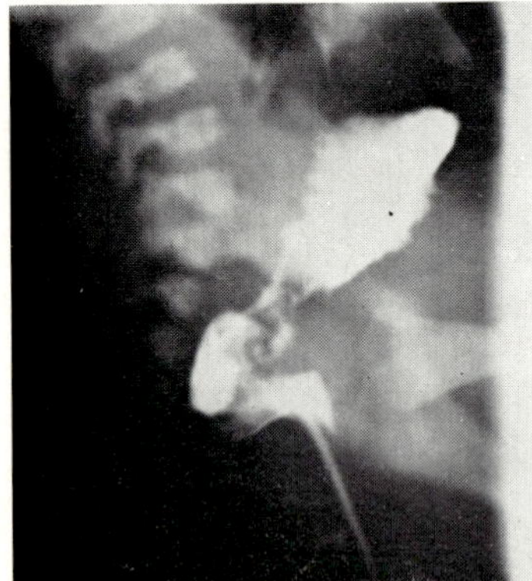

Fig. 583.—Barium enema. Lateral film. Hirschsprung's disease. The narrowed aganglionic segment is demonstrated (arrow).

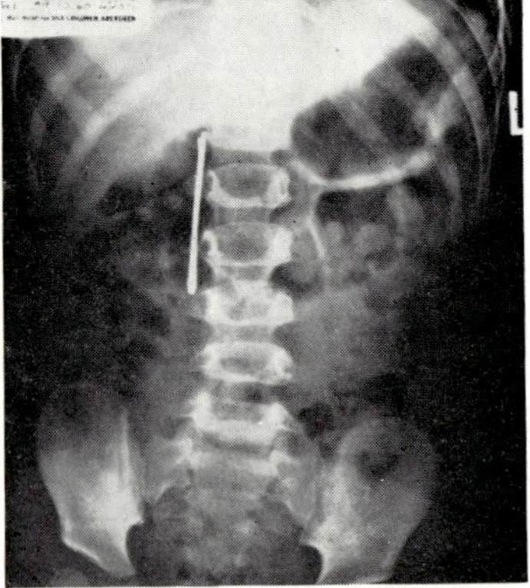

Fig. 584.—Supine film of abdomen. Kirbygrip impacted in second part of duodenum.

prompt a radiological examination for a sliding type of hiatus hernia (*Fig.* 580).

Meconium Ileus.—In this condition, symptoms of intestinal obstruction may appear, i.e., vomiting, abdominal distension, and failure to pass meconium.

Plaques of intra-abdominal calcification may be seen on plain radiography if perforation of distended bowel has occurred in utero. The presence of gas within the distended small-bowel contents produces a characteristic mottled appearance (*Fig.* 581).

Obstruction of the large bowel is rare. In cases of *imperforate anus*, a lateral film following inversion of the child for several minutes may be of value to show the distance between the distal rectum and the anus. An opaque marker is placed at the customary position of the latter.

Intussusception.—Signs of intestinal obstruction may be seen on plain X-ray films. Barium enema may be requested in cases of doubt, but this is of value only where the intussusception has extended into the large bowel (*Fig.* 582).

Barium enema is used in the differential diagnosis of *megacolon* and *Hirschsprung's disease*. It may be required in the latter condition when it presents in the form of an 'acute abdomen'. In megacolon, dilatation of the bowel will commence at the rectum, whereas in Hirschsprung's disease the colon is dilated only above the area devoid of ganglia. Usually the aganglionic segment is short (*Fig.* 583). Complete filling of the colon is not attempted in these cases in view of the danger of water intoxication.

Foreign Bodies.—It is important that the pharynx and œsophagus as well as the entire abdomen is included in the radiographic examination. When a foreign body lodges in the œsophagus, the most common site is the cervical part. The majority of foreign bodies which reach the stomach will be discharged in the fæces, and examination of the latter should be the 'test of cure' rather than repeated radiography. Relatively long thin metal objects such as kirby-grips may become impacted in the second part of the duodenum (*Fig.* 584). In this case, several days should be allowed to lapse before radiography is repeated. Should the object remain in a constant position in the duodenum, operation is likely to be required. It is important that a check film should be taken immediately prior to the operative procedure. Occasionally contrast media are required in the search for a non-opaque foreign body. It is wise to include a radiograph of the chest in all cases since inhalation of foreign material may sometimes pass unrecognized in young children.

RESPIRATORY TRACT

Bronchography.—Delineation of the bronchial tree is obtained by the introduction of contrast medium such as dionosil into the trachea. Coating of the bronchi is obtained by suitable positioning of the patient. In cases of bronchiectasis, postural drainage should be performed for a few days prior to the examination. In view of the fact that the larynx is anæsthetized, patients should be warned not to take anything by mouth for 3 hours following the procedure. (Contrast media—*see* p. 729; dionosil oily is less irritant than its aqueous counterpart.)

Trans-glottic Method.—This simple method consists of dripping the contrast medium into the larynx. Topical anæsthesia is begun by giving the patient a lozenge of local anæsthetic 20 minutes before the examination. The larynx is then sprayed with 4 per cent lignocaine, while the patient is encouraged to take deep breaths. A 20-ml. syringe coupled to a 10-cm. length of rubber or plastic tubing is used for the injection. The tongue is gripped and drawn forward, the tip of the tubing is placed over the back of the tongue and the contrast medium is slowly expressed; the patient is instructed to breathe easily and refrain from swallowing. The contrast injection is made in three divided amounts and positioning is carried out following each separate injection. Radiography is then performed as quickly as possible.

Trans-nasal Route.—This entails the introduction of a curved rubber or gum elastic catheter (size 7 or 8 English) into the trachea via the nostril. The pharynx and larynx are first sprayed with 4 per cent lignocaine. The nostril is then anæsthetized by a cotton-wool pledget on the end of a wooden stick. The tongue is drawn forward and the catheter passed down the nose through the glottis.

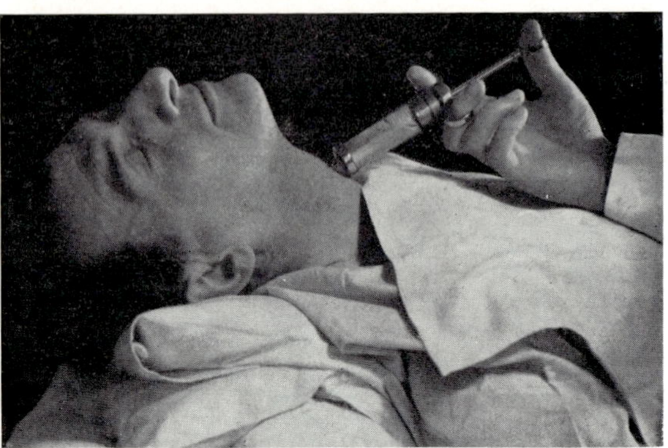

Fig. 585.—Bronchography. Cricothyroid method.

Its entry into the trachea is confirmed by closing the mouth and opposite nostril when air will be heard to pass through the catheter. Local anæsthetic (0·5 ml.) is then introduced into the catheter; this frequently provokes a short bout of coughing. The contrast medium is then introduced as above.

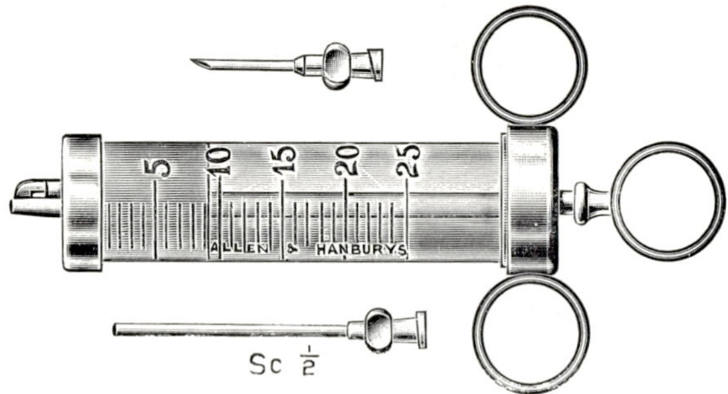

Fig. 586.—Syringe, filler, and needle, for cricothyroid method of bronchography.

Cricothyroid Route.—The patient lies supine with the head extended. The skin is treated with local antiseptic solution. The cricothyroid membrane is identified and local anæsthetic introduced into the skin and deeper tissues. An intra-muscular needle attached to a small syringe is now introduced into the trachea through the cricothyroid membrane (*Fig.* 585). Puncture of the tracheal lumen is confirmed by withdrawing the plunger of the needle when air will bubble back into the syringe. About 1 ml. of local anæsthetic is then injected rapidly. The syringe and needle should be removed immediately following this since coughing is provoked. The contrast medium is introduced by a special short, bevelled needle (*Fig.* 586). Three separate injections of contrast medium are made, the position of the needle being checked on each occasion by withdrawing air from the trachea. The needle is removed before the patient occupies the third position. Local bleeding at the injection site is quickly controlled by local pressure. The patient should be warned to press on the puncture site should he cough at the end of the examination.

Positioning in Bronchography.—It is most essential that positioning of the patient is performed correctly if filling of all the bronchial segments is to be obtained. Demonstration of one side only should be performed at one sitting. The patient remains inclined to this side during the examination. The positions are as follows:—

1. Leaning backwards 20°.
2. Leaning forward to within 15° of the horizontal.
3. Lying on one side with the long axis of the body slightly below the horizontal, the patient being rotated backwards and forwards for a few moments.

Amount of Contrast Medium.—This varies according to the size of the patient and the pathological process under suspicion. An adult normally requires about

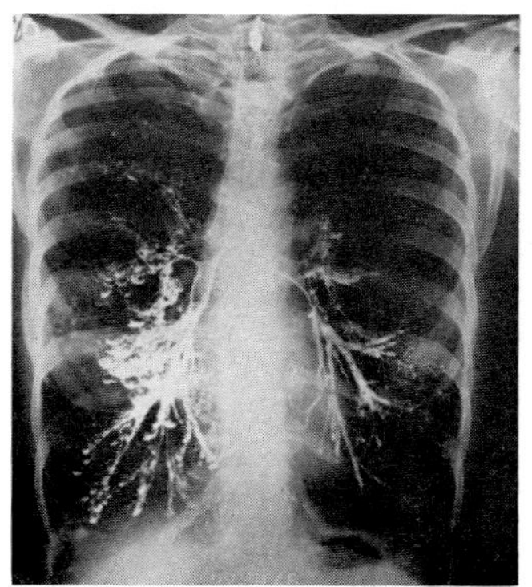

Fig. 587.—Bronchogram. Postero-anterior view. Saccular bronchiectasis of the right middle lobe.

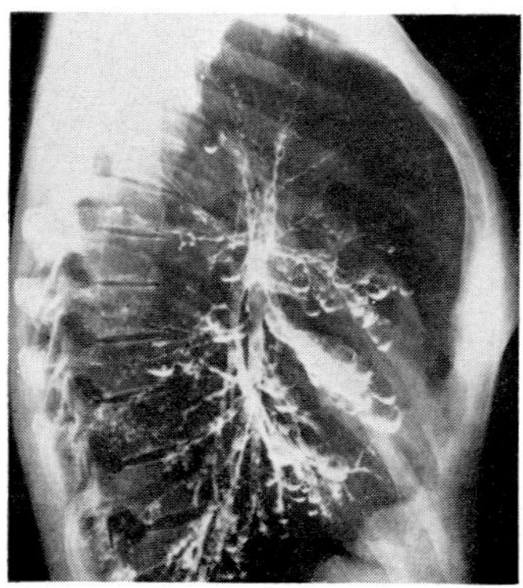

Fig. 588.—Bronchogram. Right lateral view. The contracted and bronchiectatic right middle lobe is demonstrated. There is also bronchiectasis involving the anterior segment of the right lower lobe.

12–15 ml. of contrast medium for each side. More may be required in a case of bronchiectasis. For children, proportionately less can be given, e.g., for a child of 7 or 8 years about 6 ml. will suffice.

Bronchography in Children.—In children under 10 years of age general anæsthesia is necessary. The contrast medium is introduced through a polythene catheter which is inserted down the endotracheal tube. The catheter should be measured beforehand and marked to ensure that the tip does not pass beyond the endotracheal tube. It is also important that the endotracheal tube itself is not so long that it will extend beyond the carina. Following induction of anæsthesia and intubation of the trachea, the child is first held in the sitting position and leaning towards the side to be examined. The child can continue to breathe quietly and it is not necessary to produce respiratory paralysis. The cap of the endotracheal tube is removed and the polythene catheter inserted. Three separate amounts of contrast medium are given, positioning being carried out at the end of each injection, following which the polythene tube is removed. The child lies first on the side to be examined and then supine, the anæsthetist controlling respiration momentarily while postero-anterior, lateral, and oblique films are taken (*Figs.* 587, 588, 589). The bronchi are cleared by suction at the end of the examination.

SINOGRAPHY

This is the radiological demonstration of the source and ramifications of fistulæ and abscess cavities by a contrast medium. (Type of contrast medium—endografin, urografin, or neohydriol, p. 729). The oily medium neohydriol has a

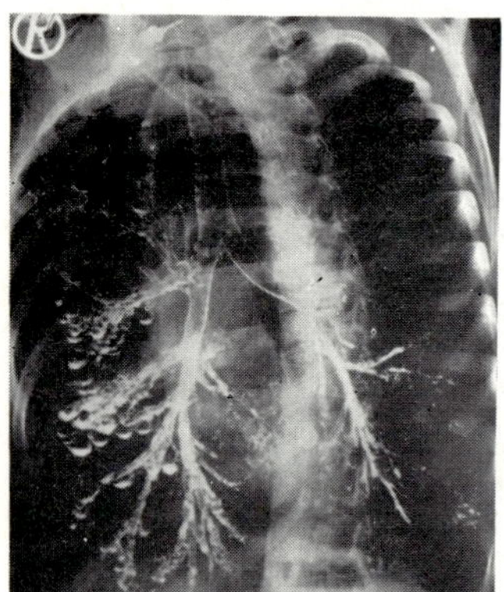

Fig. 589.—Bronchogram. Left anterior oblique views (same patient as in *Figs.* 587, 588).

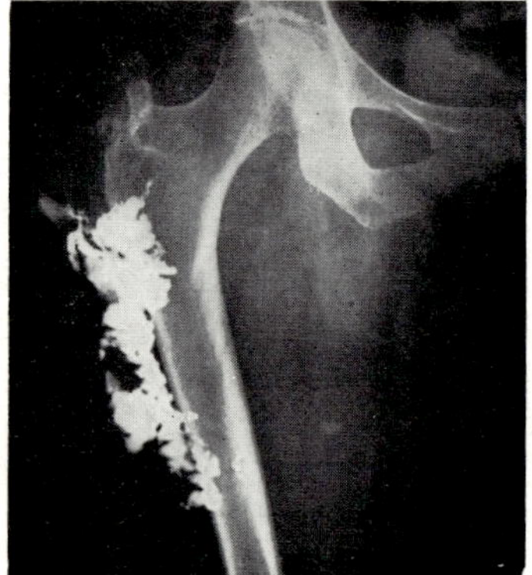

Fig. 590.—Sinogram. Case of chronic osteomyelitis with fistula. The wide extent of the fistulous tract is demonstrated.

high radiographic density and is preferable when the track is fine and of small capacity.

Technique.—Initial gentle probing of the sinus will give a guide as to its direction. If the track extends deeply, filling is best obtained by using a polythene catheter of suitable diameter. A rubber acorn applied to the end of the syringe or tubing will prevent leakage if compressed against the sinus mouth during introduction of the medium; the operator's hands must be removed from the area to be irradiated immediately prior to radiography (*Fig.* 590). It is important to record the position of the sinus mouth relative to the body surface with a small radio-opaque marker. The sinus opening should be uppermost during the injection in order to avoid leakage and the injection should continue until resistance is felt or leakage is apparent.

A. SUGGESTED LIST OF CONTRAST MEDIA

EXAMINATION	CONTRAST MEDIUM	STRENGTH	SUPPLIER
Sialography	Neohydriol fluid	40 per cent	May & Baker Ltd., Dagenham, Essex, England
Barium meal	Micropaque		Damancy & Co. Ltd., Ware, Herts, England
Barium series	Raybar, BAS 16		Damancy & Co. Ltd.
Barium enema	Micropaque		Damancy & Co. Ltd.
'Gastrografin' meal	Gastrografin	76 per cent	Schering A.G., Berlin
Oral cholecystogram	Telepaque	6 × 0·5 G. tablets	Bayer Products Ltd., Division of Winthrop Group Ltd., Surbiton-on-Thames, England
Intravenous cholecystogram	Biligrafin (Forte)	50 per cent	Schering A.G., Berlin
Cholangiography (operative and post-operative)	Hypaque	25–45 per cent	Bayer Products Ltd.
Intravenous pyelography	Hypaque	45 per cent	Bayer Products Ltd.
	Urografin	60 per cent	Schering A.G., Berlin
Retrograde pyelography	Hypaque	25 per cent	Bayer Products Ltd.
Cystography Micturating cystography	Urografin	15–60 per cent	Schering A.G., Berlin
Cysto-urethrography	Hypaque	45 per cent	Bayer Products Ltd.
	Umbradil Viscous U	35 per cent	Astrapharm Ltd., Surbiton, Surrey, England
Hysterosalpingography	Endografin	50 per cent	Schering A.G., Berlin
	Diaginol viscous	40 per cent	May & Baker Ltd.
Aortography (thoracic)	Conray '480'		May & Baker Ltd.
Aortography (abdominal)	Hypaque	65 per cent	Bayer Products Ltd.
Peripheral arteriography	Hypaque	45 per cent	Bayer Products Ltd.
Selective aortic branch arteriography	Urografin	60 per cent	Schering A.G., Berlin
Spleno-portal venography	Hypaque	85 or 65 per cent	Bayer Products Ltd.
Bronchography	Dionosil (oily or aqueous)		Glaxo Laboratories, Greenford, Middlesex, England
	Neohydriol viscous	40 per cent	May & Baker Ltd.
Sinography	Urografin	60 per cent	Schering A.G., Berlin
	Neohydriol fluid	40 per cent	May & Baker Ltd.
Colonic actuator	Veripaque		Bayer Products Ltd.

B. PREPARATION OF PATIENTS FOR X-RAY EXAMINATION

It is recommended that the patient be allowed up out of bed if permissible from the clinical point of view, since this helps to minimize the amount of gas in the bowel.

Barium Meal, Barium Swallow, Barium Series.—
1. Aperient*—two nights before examination.
2. Low-residue diet—day before examination.
3. Nothing to eat or drink from the night before examination.

Barium Enema.—
1. Aperient—two nights before the examination.
2. Low-residue diet—day before examination.
3. Veripaque enema†—one hour prior to examination.
4. Tea and toast breakfast on morning of examination.

Straight Film of Gall-bladder, Kidneys, Ureters, and Bladder. Retrograde Pyelogram, and Intravenous Cholecystangiography.—
1. Aperient—two nights before the examination.
2. Low-residue diet—day before examination.

Emergency Erect and Supine Films of Abdomen.—No preparation is advised.

---

* Aperient—Dulcolax is generally preferred, in a dose of 1–2 tablets.

† Veripaque enema—1 vial Veripaque powder (3 G.) to 2 litres of water. The patient should retain the enema for as long as possible before evacuation.

Dulcolax (Boehringer Ingelheim Ltd., Isleworth, Middlesex).

Cholecystogram (Oral).—
1. Fat-free meal at 7 p.m. on the day before X-ray examination.
2. Contrast medium taken orally half an hour after this meal.
3. No further food, but fat-free fluids may be taken as desired.
4. Cholecystogram from 9 a.m. on the day following administration of the contrast medium.
Intravenous Pyelogram.—
1. Aperient—two nights before examination.
2. Low-residue diet and restricted fluid intake—day before examination.
3. No fluid of any sort for 8 hours prior to examination.
Percutaneous Splenoportal Venography.—
1. Aperient—two nights before examination.
2. Low-residue diet—day before examination.
3. Test dose of contrast medium to be given the day before examination.
4. Tea and toast only, 4 hours before examination.
5. Parenteral sedative 45 minutes before the examination.
N.B.—Half-hourly pulse chart to be kept for 12 hours following examination.
Aortography (Translumbar and Retrograde).—
1. Aperient—two nights before the examination.
2. Low-residue diet the day before examination.
3. Premedication if general anæsthetic to be given.
4. In all cases other than translumbar aortography, groins to be prepared.
N.B.—Before any form of angiography will be carried out, a signed permission form for anæsthetic and operation should be received by the X-ray department.

CHAPTER XLVIII

MANAGEMENT OF ADVANCED CARCINOMA
AND CARE OF THE DYING

By A. P. M. Forrest

More than 100,000 people die from cancer in England and Wales each year. The terminal stages of malignant disease may be prolonged and the alleviation of pain and misery is an essential part of medical care. Effective palliation may vary with the type of tumour. Some have properties which allow the use of relatively specific measures. Carcinomas of the breast, prostate, or thyroid can be influenced beneficially by alteration in the endocrine environment, carcinoma of the adrenal by the administration of the specific adrenal cytotoxin $o'p'$DDD and carcinoma of the thyroid by radioactive iodine. However, in the majority of cancers one has to depend on non-specific methods of treatment, either with the aim of inhibiting the growth of the tumour itself or of alleviating the symptoms which are produced.

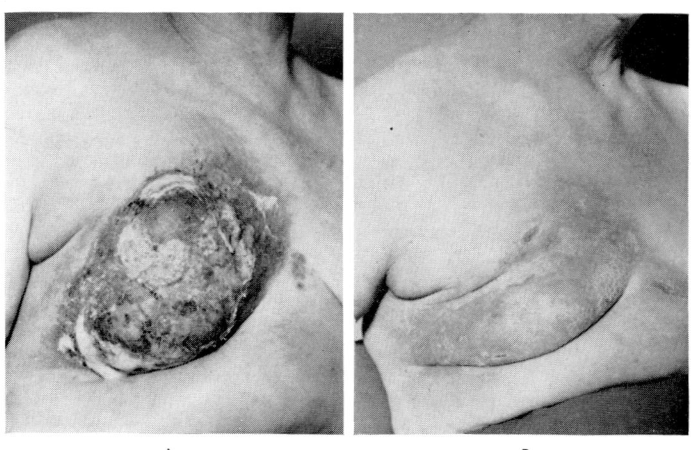

A   B

Fig. 591.—Palliation of advanced local cancer by radiotherapy: A, Before treatment; B, After treatment.

LOCAL PALLIATION

Surgery.—Surgical excision of tumour masses has little application in the later stages of malignant disease unless in an attempt to relieve severe alteration in function, for example, intestinal obstruction caused by abdominal metastases, or paraplegia resulting from deposits in the spinal canal. In such cases the house-surgeon must make it clear to the relatives that operation is not being undertaken with the prospect of cure, but to relieve a complication which, if left alone, would only cause additional suffering.

Radiotherapy.—The development of apparatus capable of delivering ionizing radiations of high energy has widened the scope of radiotherapy in cancer. Deep-seated large tumour masses may now be treated with minimal disturbance to nearby normal tissue. Most frequently radiotherapy is used in advanced disease to heal ulceration from a superficial tumour or to relieve the pain of bone metastases (*Fig.* 591).

Treatment with radioactive isotopes may also prove worthwhile, particularly in cancer of the thyroid. Metastatic deposits can be encouraged to take up radioactive iodine if the remaining function in the thyroid is first ablated by surgery or by a large dose of the isotope. Isotopes of gold (^{198}Au) and yttrium (^{90}Y) have also been used for the control of malignant effusions and micro-aggregates of colloidal gold or yttrium can be injected intra-arterially to irradiate, internally, a tumour mass. These methods of treatment are highly specialized.

When the surgeon has decided that radiotherapy is to be the main or an adjuvant line of therapy, the house-surgeon should contact the radiotherapy department at an early stage; when the radiotherapist sees the patient, he should ensure that all necessary records, X-rays, and pathology reports are available. Finally, the house-surgeon should ascertain details about out-patient attendances and follow-up, and inform the surgeon and family doctor about the proposed arrangements.

CANCER CHEMOTHERAPY

Two main groups of drugs are used to inhibit the growth of tumours: (1) alkylating agents, (2) antimetabolites. As they act by interfering with the capacity of cells to divide, they affect all rapidly growing and dividing cells. As the capacity for growth of certain normal cells in the body equals or exceeds that of a tumour, the dose of these drugs is limited by their effect on normal tissues. Particularly susceptible are the bone-marrow, the intestinal epithelium, and the germinal epithelium of the gonads.

A miscellaneous series of compounds—steroids, vitamin B_{12}, certain antibiotics, urethane, and colchicine—are also used to inhibit tumour growth.

Chemotherapeutic agents are mainly used systemically for the treatment of Hodgkin's disease, leukæmia, malignant lymphoma, adenocarcinoma of the ovary, and chorion carcinoma. Their value in other tumours is less well defined, but they have a place in the treatment of mammary cancers, myelomatosis, and embryonal sarcomas. Their local administration can give useful palliation in solid tumours, particularly when these are confined to a limb or organ.

I. ALKYLATING AGENTS

Alkylation is the substitution of an alkyl group (CH_3; C_2H_5; C_3H_6; etc.) in a compound. Being electrophilic, these alkyl groups are attracted to a variety of sites on a molecule, particularly inorganic or organic ions and amino or sulphide groups. Biological alkylation implies the substitution of alkyl groups for hydrogen in the molecule of deoxyribonucleic acid (DNA) which is the main protein of the cell nucleus. As this occurs predominantly in the primary phosphate groups, phosphate esters are formed (*Fig.* 592).

Most biological alkylating agents are polyfunctional and contain two or more active alkyl groups. Their attachment to different sites on the DNA molecule thus forms 'cross-linkage' or 'bridging' between two groups on one molecule or between two molecules, and results in molecular distortion and

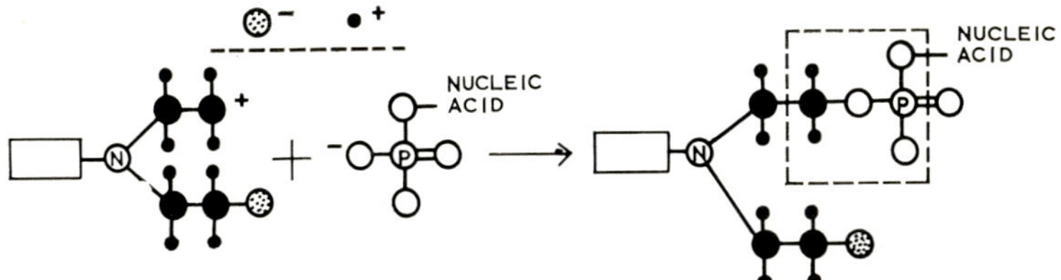

Fig. 592.—Biological alkylation. Esterification of primary phosphate groups of DNA — intramolecular and intermolecular cross-linkage.

fragmentation and clumping of chromosomes (*Fig.* 593). Mitosis is thus suppressed. Alkylation of the cytoplasmic protein, ribonucleic acid (RNA), also occurs but is relatively unimportant.

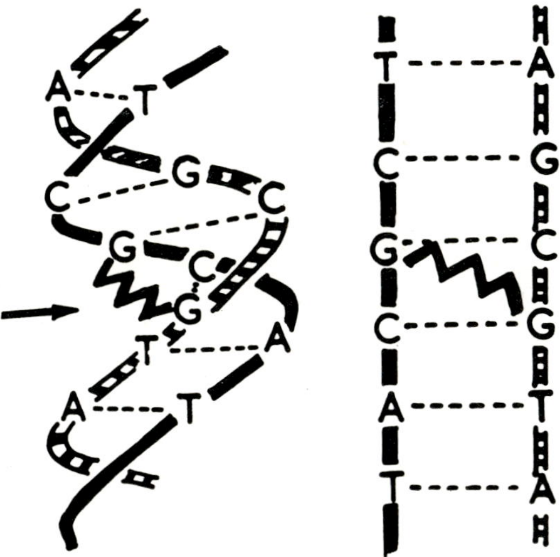

Fig. 593.—Diagrammatic representation of the reaction of a bifunctional alkylating agent with DNA. The order of bases along the DNA molecular chain is indicated by their initial letters (adenine, thymine, guanine, cytosine), and the alkyl chain by the zigzag line. The diagram on the right is a simplified version of the double helix (left).

Alkylating agents used for cancer chemotherapy are grouped as follows:—

1. Mustards.—Derivatives of mustard gas (sulphur mustard), which was used for chemical warfare in Flanders in 1917, these compounds all contain two or more chloro-ethyl groups (CH_2CH_2Cl) which are responsible for their alkylating properties. The first compound used therapeutically was *nitrogen mustard*, a solid, in which two chloro-ethyl groups are attached to nitrogen. A wide range of alkylating mustards have since been synthesized by the attachment of chloro-ethyl groups to various organic and inorganic nuclei (*Table XX*).

Table XX.—The Mustards used as Cytotoxic Agents

Prosthetic Group		Cytotoxic Agent
Ions:	Sulphur	Mustard gas
	Nitrogen	Nitrogen mustard (mustine)
Organic acids:	Phenylalanine	Melphalan
	Phenylbutyric	Chlorambucil
Sugars:	Mannitol	Mannomustine
Antimalarial drugs:	Quinacrine	Quinacrine mustard
	Choloroquine	Chloroquine mustard
Phosphoric acid ester:		Cyclophosphamide
Pyrimidine base:	Uracil	Uracil mustard

It was believed initially that these various compounds might show a degree of specificity of action. For instance, *phenylalanine mustard (melphalan)* was synthesized in the hope that it might be taken up selectively by malignant melanoma, which utilizes phenylalanine to form tyrosine and melanin. Similarly *cyclophosphamide*—in which the alkylating groups are inactive until split off by tissue phosphatases—was developed in the belief that activation might take place selectively in malignant tissue, which is known to have a rich supply of these enzymes. These assumptions have not proved valid. At the same time, different tumours vary in their sensitivity to different agents and *in vitro* methods of assessing this are under trial.

2. Ethyleneimines.—These compounds depend for their alkylating properties on ethylene groups attached to tyrosine (*triethylene melamine, TEM*), phosphoramide (*triethylmelamine phosphoramide, TEPA*), and *triethylmelamine thiophosphoramide, thio-TEPA*), or a synthetic resin (*triethylene glycol diglycidyl ether, ethoglucid*). Being more stable than the majority of mustards they can be administered orally.

3. Alkyl-sulphonates.—The most important member of this group of esters of alkane sulphonic acid is *myleran*. It has virtually no pharmacological action other than suppression of the white-cell series and is used predominantly in the treatment of leukæmia.

II. ANTIMETABOLITES

Unlike the alkylating agents, these chemotherapeutic agents owe their action to their chemical similarity to the natural substrates used in the enzymatic synthesis of nucleic acids. As a result they are incorporated in the synthetic pathways and block the uptake of the natural metabolites which are essential for the synthesis of cell protein. In the absence of normal synthesis of DNA, cell division is suppressed. These drugs are classified according to their site of action (*Fig.* 594).

1. Folic-acid Antagonists.—Folic acid is essential for the formation of tetrahydrofolic acid which is concerned with the metabolic transfer of single carbon units. The folic-acid antagonists—derivates of 4-aminopterin (e.g.,

Mustine (Boots Pure Drug Co. Ltd., Nottingham).
Thiotepa (Lederle Laboratories Ltd., Bush House, Aldwych, London, W.C.2).
Uracil mustard (Upjohn Ltd., Crawley, Sussex).

amethopterin—methotrexate)—act by competitive inhibition of folate reductase which converts folate to di- and tetrahydrofolates. This action can be circumvented by supplying tetrahydrofolate in the form of *citrovorum factor* (*folinic acid*) which, if given within 4 hours, will prevent cell destruction. Folic-acid antagonists are particularly useful in the treatment of chorion carcinoma.

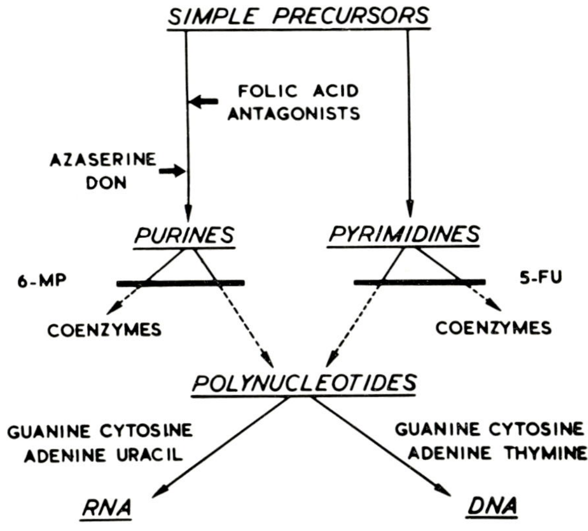

Fig. 594.—Sites of actions of antimetabolites.

2. Pyrimidine Antagonists.—Thymine (5-methyluracil) is the unique basic component of DNA. The substitution of fluorine for the methyl group forms a stable compound *5-fluorouracil* (*5-FU*) which competes for thymine in the thymidylate synthetase enzyme system and inhibits DNA synthesis.

3. Purine Antagonists.—The sulphur analogue of hypoxanthine, *6-mercaptopurine* (*6-MP*) blocks the incorporation of purines into the nitronucleotides and prevents the formation of a wide range of co-enzymes. It is mainly used in the treatment of leukæmia. *Azothioprine* (*imuran*), a derivative of 6-MP, also is used for immunosuppression in homotransplantation.

III. MISCELLANEOUS PRODUCTS

The natural *vinca* alkaloids found in the periwinkle (*vinblastine*), certain antibiotics (*actinomycin* D), and the synthetic compound ethyl carbamate (*urethane*) have cytotoxic properties which are useful for the treatment of leukæmias. A derivative of the insecticide DDT, *o'p'*DDD, is selectively toxic against adrenocortical cells and can inhibit adrenal tumours. They will not be considered further here.

ADMINISTRATION

Systemic therapy, initially by the intravenous route, is commonly used. If the problem is one of control of a localized, inoperable tumour intra-arterial

Methotrexate (Lederle Laboratories Ltd., Aldwych, London, W.C.2).

infusion or perfusion allows a higher concentration of the drug to reach the site of the disease.

Intravenous Therapy.—*Nitrogen mustard* is still one of the most useful compounds for initial therapy, particularly in the advanced case. To counteract nausea and vomiting it is best given as a single large dose (0·4 mg. per kg.) in a 1–1000 solution (1 mg. per ml.). An intravenous drip of dextrose 6 per cent or saline 0·9 per cent is commenced in the evening and a sedative (400 mg. pentobarbitone) and an anti-emetic (10 mg. prochlorperazine) given. Once the patient is asleep the dose of mustard is injected into the drip tubing. No further dose is required for 6 weeks and then only if the leucocytes have returned to normal levels.

Alternatively, one can use one of the other alkylating agents either as a single large dose or as daily administration of a smaller dose. *Chlorambucil*, 0·2 mg. per kg. (5–10 mg.) orally per day for 3–6 weeks, or *cyclophosphamide* up to 4·8 mg. per kg. (200–300 mg.) intravenously three times a week for 2–3 weeks are convenient for use.

Blood-counts are done before each dose. Reduction in white cells or platelets indicates postponement of further treatment until recovery occurs.

Oral Administration.—If the disease has been controlled by initial intravenous administration, maintenance therapy will be required. This is started 1 month

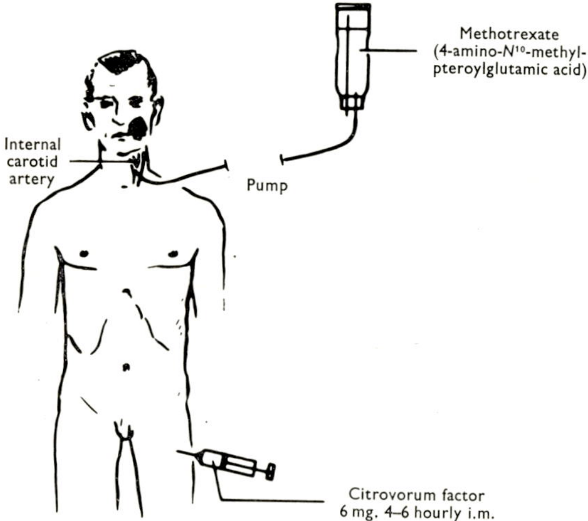

Fig. 595.—Antimetabolite-metabolite combination. Course of treatment 5–10 days.

after the intravenous course and can be given most conveniently by the oral route. The dose is dependent upon maintaining a white-cell count of 2000–5000, and will be in the order of 0·15–0·2 mg. per kg. for chlorambucil or 1·3 mg. per kg. daily for cyclophosphamide.

Intracavitary Injection.—Nitrogen mustard or thio-TEPA is the drug of choice. A needle is inserted into the pleural or abdominal cavity, as much fluid as possible is withdrawn, and the cytotoxic agent (0·2–0·6 mg. per kg. nitrogen mustard or

10–50 mg. thio-TEPA) in 0·9 per cent saline is injected. The amount of diluent may vary—20 ml. for the chest and 50–100 mg. for the abdominal cavity are suitable. Following the injetion the patient is turned to lie on his back and his front and on either side, each for 10 minutes, to allow maximum contact of the drug.

Intra-arterial Infusion.—The main artery supplying the tumour is cannulated either by open operation or by a percutaneous technique. If several arteries are supplying the tumour those not used for cannulation may be ligated. The tumour then derives its remaining blood-supply largely from the vessel through which infusion is to take place. The drug to be infused is dissolved in 500 ml. of 0·9 per cent saline which is connected to the cannula and administered either by gravity (in which case the bottle must be suspended at a height great enough to overcome the patient's arterial pressure) or by an infusion pump.

A variety of agents can be added to the infusion fluid, e.g., ethoglucid, 5-fluorouracil, or methotrexate. Suitable doses are given in *Table XXI*. In this country, amethopterin (methotrexate), 50 mg. daily, has been used most frequently. To minimize systemic effects citrovorum factor, 6 mg. q.i.d., is administered intramuscularly (*Fig.* 595).

Table XXI.—Normal Doses of Cytotoxic Agents

Chemotherapeutic Agent	Total Dose of Initial Course	Administration
Alkylating Agents Nitrogen mustard	0·4 mg. per kg.	I.v.—single injection or divided doses over 4–5 days
Melphalan	1–2 mg. per kg.	I.v.—as nitrogen mustard Oral—5–10 mg. daily for 2–3 weeks (maintenance: 1–3 mg. daily after rest of 1 month)
Chlorambuci	4 mg. per kg.	Oral—0·2 mg. per kg. per day (5–10 mg.) for 2–3 weeks (maintenance: 2–4 mg. daily)
Thio-TEPA	0·8–1·2 mg. per kg.	I.v. or i.a.—0·2 mg. per kg. daily for 5 days (maintenance: 0·2 mg. per kg. per week)
Cyclophosphamide	40 mg. per kg.	I.v.—2–4 mg. per kg. daily for 6–8 days and then twice weekly Oral—maintenance: 50–200 mg. daily
Ethoglucid	250 mg. per kg.	I.v.—200–250 mg. per kg. each 3–5 weeks, then 100 mg. per kg. per week I.a.—50 mg. per kg. per day
Antimetabolites Methotrexate	100–200 mg.	Oral—5–10 mg. three times a week for 6–8 weeks I.v.—Divided dose over 2–5 days I.a.—50 mg. per day for 6–10 days with citrovorum factor
5–FU	50 mg. per kg.	I.v. or i.a.—15 mg. per kg. per day for 5 days, then 7·5 mg. per kg. on seventh and ninth day, or 10 mg. per kg. per day for 2 weeks
5–FUDR	100 mg. per kg.	I.v. or i.a.—double dose of 5–FU

It should be noted that the doses recommended are approximate only, as the dose administered is largely based on the extent of hæmatological depression.

Confirmation that the cannula is correctly placed in the feeding vessel is essential before the infusion is started. This is done by injecting either fluorescein (2–3 ml. of 5 per cent solution) and observing the distribution of fluorescence in ultra-violet light, or sulphan blue (disulphine blue), 0·25–0·5 ml. per kg., 6·2 per cent solution, the distribution of which is visible in daylight.

Recent technical developments include the construction of small portable clockwork pumps into which the patient can inject his daily dose of anti-tumour drug. A plastic cannula can be left in an artery for long periods of time and, when not in use, it is heat sealed.

Regional Perfusion.—The tumour-bearing part of the body, usually a limb, is isolated from the general circulation and perfused through an artery and vein by a pump oxygenator (*Fig.* 596). The cytotoxic agent (nitrogen mustard,

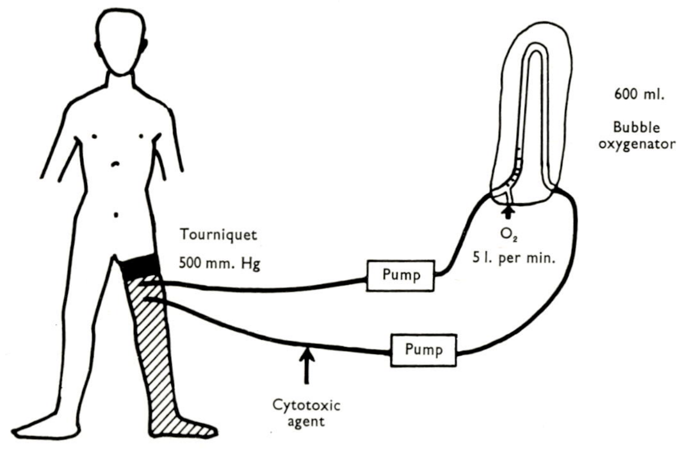

Fig. 596.—Perfusion of leg with cytotoxic agent by means of a bubble oxygenator–pump circuit.

0·8 mg. per kg.; phenylalanine mustard, 1·5 mg. per kg.) is then injected into the extracorporeal circuit. If the limb or organ is suitably isolated, the amount which reaches the marrow and gastro-intestinal tract is small; consequently high concentrations, up to fifteen to twenty times those normally used, can be achieved at the tumour site.

Satisfactory isolation of the perfused part from the general circulation is not easy; in the case of a limb, this is usually done by a pneumatic tourniquet. Leakage into the general circulation can be assessed by injecting ^{131}I-albumen or ^{51}Cr-labelled cells into the extracorporeal circuit and counting the radioactivity over the heart (*Fig.* 597).

Following the injection of the cytotoxic drug, perfusion is maintained for 45 minutes in the case of nitrogen mustard or 90 minutes in the case of phenylalanine mustard so as to allow complete metabolism of the drug. Before reconnecting the circulation, an exchange transfusion of the extracorporeal circuit is performed to flush out any unmetabolized drug.

Disulphine blue (I.C.I. Ltd., Pharmaceuticals Division, Macclesfield, Cheshire).

Perfusion with cytotoxic agents has been used to treat tumours in limbs, pelvis, brain, head and neck, lungs, abdominal viscera, and liver. The technique is complex and not without danger and its use has been confined to a few specialized centres.

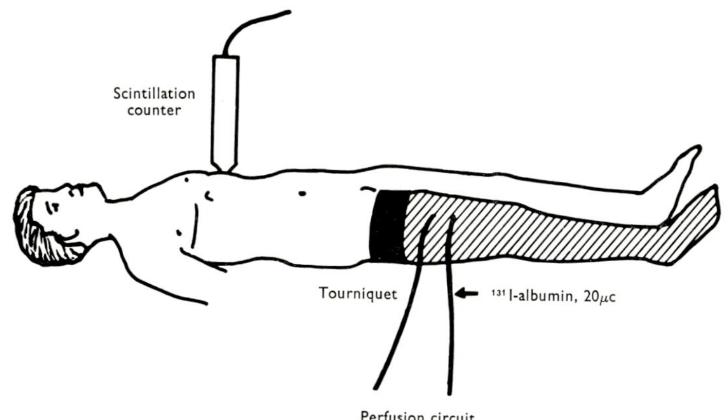

Fig. 597.—Method of assessing leakage in perfusion.

ENDOCRINE TREATMENT

Alteration of the endocrine status has greatest application in cancer of the breast and of the prostate.

I. BREAST CANCER

Like the normal breast, the behaviour of mammary cancer is influenced by its endocrine environment (*Fig.* 598). This, in turn, is dependent upon the hormones of the ovaries, adrenals, and pituitary gland. Alteration of their secretory activity, by pharmacological or surgical means, may effect a temporary remission of the cancer and thus relieve the symptoms of advanced disease.

Oophorectomy and Radiation Castration.—Suppression of ovarian function by surgery or radiotherapy is indicated in the premenopausal patient with advanced cancer of the breast and benefit will follow in approximately one-third of patients. If oophorectomy fails to control the disease, further endocrine ablation—by adrenalectomy or hypophysectomy—is unlikely to be useful. Œstrogens must not be given to counteract the hot flushes which may follow castration, as these may reverse a beneficial effect.

Administration of Hormones.—Three main groups of sex hormones have been used in the treatment of advanced cancer of the breast: œstrogens, androgens, and progestogens. In general, they should be reserved for postmenopausal or castrated premenopausal women, in whom an initial course of hormone therapy should precede adrenalectomy or hypophysectomy.

Œstrogens.—Diethylstilbœstrol, 5 mg. t.i.d. by mouth, is the simplest preparation to use. Stilbœstrol is superior to androgens in healing soft-tissue and visceral lesions and probably of equal value in bone metastases. In the dose recommended it has few side-effects other than nausea. In patients with bone metastases hypercalcæmia may occur, and the serum calcium level should occasionally be checked. Sometimes in older women vaginal bleeding may be produced; patients should be warned beforehand of this possibility.

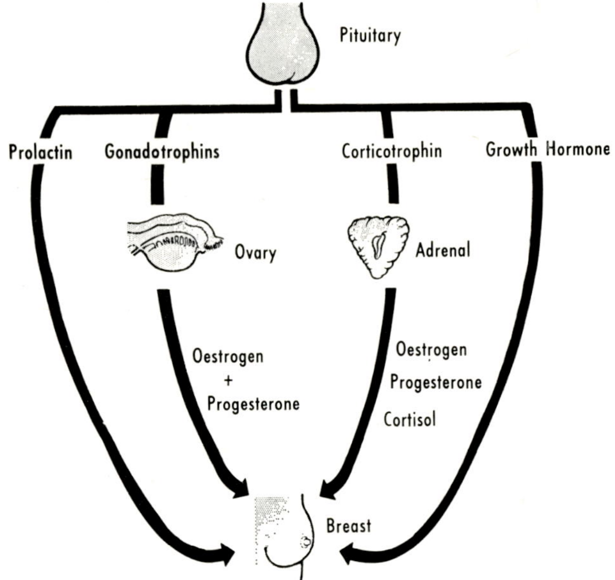

Fig. 598.—Endocrine control of the breast.

Androgens.—Testosterone propionate, 100 mg. three times a week, or the phenyl-propionate ester of 19-nortestosterone (durabolin), 25 mg. a week intramuscularly, are the usual preparations used in Britain. Oral therapy with methyl testosterone, 5 mg. t.i.d., can also be given. Masculinization with hirsutism, acne, deepening of the voice, and enlargement of the clitoris can be disturbing. Hypercalcæmia and liver damage are possible dangers.

Progestogens.—Various derivatives of 19-nortestosterone, administered intramuscularly or orally, have been used in the palliative treatment of cancer of the breast. Some lesions apparently are resistant. Norethisterone, 15–60 mg. per day by mouth, gestonorone, 200 mg. per week intramuscularly, and 17-hydroxyprogesterone, 250 mg. a week intramuscularly, are suitable compounds.

Appropriate hormone therapy will produce a response within 4–6 weeks. If this does not occur in that time administration of the drug should be stopped and one of another group tried.

Adrenalectomy and Oophorectomy.—Surgical removal of the adrenals and ovaries is indicated in postmenopausal patients who have failed to respond to hormone therapy or in whom an initial remission has run its course. Premenopausal women who have initially responded to castration may have further benefit if the adrenals are removed when relapse occurs.

Durabolin (Organon Laboratories Ltd., Morden, Surrey).

The operation can be performed in one or two stages. If the one-stage operation is used, it is important to cover this with adequate steroid replacement. If a two-stage procedure is preferred, steroid cover is usually required for the second side only.

Table XXII.—RÉGIME FOR STEROID COVER FOR PATIENTS UNDERGOING ADRENALECTOMY OR FOR ADRENALECTOMIZED PATIENTS UNDERGOING FURTHER SURGICAL PROCEDURES, USED IN THE SURGICAL UNIT, CARDIFF

DAY	ORAL	INTRAMUSCULAR	INTRAVENOUS	TOTAL
−2	—	50 mg., 10 p.m. and 4 a.m.	—	100 mg.
−1	—	50 mg. 6-hourly (10 a.m., 4 p.m., 10 p.m., and 4 a.m.)	—	200 mg.
Day of operation	—	50 mg. 6-hourly	200–500 mg.	400–900 mg.
+1	—	50 mg. 6-hourly	100–200 mg.	300–500 mg.
+2	—	50 mg. 6-hourly	—	200 mg.
+3	50 mg., 10 a.m. and 4 p.m.	50 mg., 10 p.m. and 4 a.m.	—	200 mg.
+4 +5	50 mg., 8 a.m. and 4 p.m.	50 mg. at midnight	—	150 mg. .... 150 mg.
+6 +7	25 mg., 8 a.m. and 4 p.m., and 50 mg. at midnight	—	—	100 mg. .... 100 mg.
+8 +9	25 mg. 8-hourly (8 a.m., 4 p.m., and midnight)	—	—	75 mg. .... 75 mg.
+10	25 mg. b.d. (10 a.m. and 10 p.m.)	—	—	50 mg.

It should be noted that, in this régime, a 'day' refers to a 24-hour period from 8 a.m.

Replacement Dosage.—Depot injections of cortisone acetate, 50 mg. intramuscularly 6-hourly, are started 36 hours before operation (total pre-operative dose 150 mg.). An intravenous drip is set up pre-operatively and hydrocortisone sodium succinate, 100 mg. per 500 ml., infused slowly during the operation. Intramuscular cortisone is continued post-operatively in the above dose, the needs for intravenous hydrocortisone being determined by the systolic blood-pressure, which is recorded each 30 minutes in the first 48 hours. The drip is usually discontinued on the second or third post-operative morning, and the dose of intramuscular cortisone reduced according to the ability of the patient to take cortisone by mouth.

As cortisone insufficiency is most likely to be missed during the night it is a good policy to give the evening dose of cortisone by injection for the first 5 or 6 post-operative days.

The total daily dose of cortisone is gradually reduced until by the time the patient is due to leave hospital the oral dose of cortisone is 25 mg. in the morning and 25 or 12·5 mg. in the evening. Fludrocortisone acetate, 0·1 mg.

daily, is started on leaving hospital. Its potent mineral-corticoid action avoids the need for supplements of salt. A typical régime is shown in *Table XXII*.

Tests of adequacy of maintenance therapy are physical well-being, serum electrolytes, and the maintenance of systolic arterial pressure on assuming the upright posture.

Medical Adrenalectomy.—Large-dose steroid therapy (prednisone, 5–10 mg. t.i.d.) can be used to suppress pituitary and adrenal function in advanced breast cancer. It is not as effective as surgical removal of the adrenals, and side-effects, of which obesity is the most troublesome, are common. Because of this some surgeons use a smaller dose (5 mg. prednisone twice a day).

This method of suppressing adrenal function is preferable to surgery in the seriously ill patient and is particularly of value in patients with cerebral metastases (in whom its anti-inflammatory effects reduce œdema) and with hypercalcæmia from bone metastases.

Hypophysectomy.—This operation can now be performed by the trans-ethmoidal, transphenoidal route, or by the implantation, through the nose or ethnoids, of radioactive yttrium (*Fig.* 599). Both these methods of pituitary

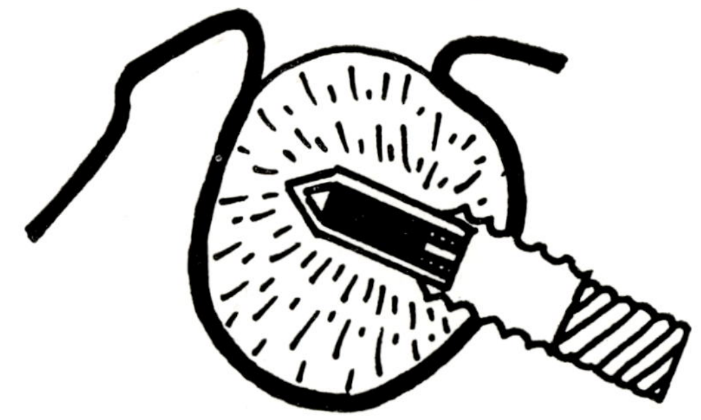

Fig. 599.—Implantation of the pituitary with yttrium-90 rods introduced through a screw-tipped trocar. Characteristics of yttrium 90: β 2·24meV. Max. penetration 11 mm. Half-life 64 hr.

ablation cause less disturbance to the patient than transcranial hypophysectomy or adrenalectomy. Adequate steroid cover for the transethmoidal operation is provided by giving the patient 100 mg. cortisone acetate intramuscularly pre-operatively, and then 50 mg. 6-hourly intramuscularly, started on return to the ward. This dose is continued for 2–3 days and then oral medication, at pro-gressively reduced dosage, is given.

Yttrium implantation can be performed safely without cortisone cover and *maintenance therapy* with oral cortisone 37·5 mg. daily is started 3–4 days post-operatively. Following hypophysectomy, adequate steroid balance can be maintained by cortisone acetate, 37·5 mg. by mouth daily (25 mg. in the morning and 12·5 mg. in the evening). As aldosterone secretion continues in the absence of the pituitary, fludrocortisone is not required.

Diabetes insipidus may be a problem after hypophysectomy but can be controlled by pitressin, given as the tannate in oil (5 units each 48 hours). Care must be taken to warm and shake the ampoule until the small yellow sediment of active peptide is dissolved. It may also be administered as pitressin snuff

(40-mg. capsule) or as a nasal spray (synthetic lysine vasopressin, 50 units per ml.). These the patient should use each time she empties her bladder.

A hypophysectomized patient also requires *thyroid maintenance therapy* to compensate for the suppression of thyrotrophin (TSH) secretion. Secondary myxœdema can be prevented by *l*-thyroxine, 0·1 mg. once or twice daily. This is usually started 4–6 weeks after operation, and after tests of thyroid function have been performed.

Dangers of Adrenal/Pituitary Ablation.—

1. *Adrenal Crises.*—Following adrenalectomy, and, less commonly, hypophysectomy, patients may be admitted to hospital in acute adrenal insufficiency, owing to insufficient maintenance cortisone. Symptoms are loss of appetite, floppiness, headache, and muscle pains, leading to hypotension and collapse. Pyrexia may be a feature.

Treatment is by intravenous cortisol hemisuccinate, 100 mg. intravenously, followed by 200 mg. per 500 ml. 0·9 per cent saline infused over 2–3 hours, the rate depending on the clinical response. A régime of cortisone therapy similar to that after adrenalectomy can then be instituted. Blood should be taken before treatment is started for electrolyte estimations and a sample of plasma refrigerated for later estimation of cortisol. If the serum sodium and chlorides are low, aldosterone, 0·5 mg. 4-hourly, should also be given by the intramuscular or intravenous route. A suitable preparation for intravenous use is aldocorten.

2. *Acute Hypothyroidism.*—Occasionally a hypophysectomized patient may be admitted in hypothyroid coma, which should be suspected if they appear myxœdematous and if the body temperature is low. Thyroid replacement of tri-iodothyronine (liothyronine sodium B.P., 100 μg. intravenously or intramuscularly, followed by 20 μg. 6-hourly) must be given carefully and combined with intravenous cortisol therapy. Otherwise adrenal insufficiency may follow restoration of normal metabolism.

Cytotoxic Agents.—These may also be used in advanced cancer of the breast but are best reserved for those tumours which do not respond to endocrine therapy.

Carcinoma of the Male Breast.—Male patients with advanced cancer of the breast, irrespective of their age, should be treated initially by orchidectomy. Other forms of endocrine treatment should be reserved for those who fail to respond.

II. PROSTATIC CANCER

The symptoms of cancer of the prostate—retention of urine and pain from osteosclerotic bone metastases—can be relieved by œstrogen therapy (stilbœstrol, 5 mg. t.i.d.). If symptoms are severe, initial control should be attempted using systemic therapy: either œstradiol benzoate (5 mg. intramuscularly daily) or stilbœstrol diphosphate (500 mg. on first day, then 1 G. intravenously daily for 6 days) is given. It was believed that this latter compound would be activated selectively by the prostatic phosphatases, but this is not the case and it has no advantage apart from its availability for intravenous use. Œstrogen therapy leads to the enlargement of the male breast after a few weeks of treatment.

If œstrogen therapy fails to control the disease, orchidectomy may be performed or steroids (prednisolone, 5 mg. t.i.d.) given. Hypophysectomy also has been used to control unresponsive cases. Serial estimations of serum acid phosphatase are of value as an objective index of progress.

III. THYROID CANCER

Papillary carcinoma of the thyroid may be temporarily improved by inhibition of the secretion of pituitary thyrotrophin (TSH) by the administration of tri-iodothyronine (liothyronine sodium B.P., 100 μg.) or *l*-thyroxine (thyroxine sodium B.P., 0·4 mg. daily).

CARE OF THE DYING

In the management of malignant disease the time comes when the doctor must cease in his attempts to prolong life—'the good doctor is aware of the distinction between prolonging life and prolonging the act of dying' (Lord Horder). When this point is reached the doctor should prepare the patient and his relatives for the inevitable end. Relatives most commonly prefer that patients spend their few remaining weeks or months in familiar surroundings and this aspect of care falls most frequently on the family doctor. However, they may be admitted to hospital for 'terminal care', particularly if symptoms are severe.

It is not within our terms of reference as doctors to hasten death. Nevertheless, when in advanced malignant disease death is clearly in sight, it is not justifiable to employ artificial methods of supporting or replacing vital body systems when the patient's comfort does not call for such measures—

> Thou shalt not kill, but need'st not strive
> Officiously to keep alive.

The latest antibiotics are not needed for a terminal bronchopneumonia. In his dying hours, the paramount consideration is the patient's comfort. Consequently it is the doctor's responsibility to relieve physical and mental distress and to prepare the patient for the end. It is shirking this responsibility to leave the care of the dying patient to others. The tact and patience of a considerate doctor can do much to allay the patient's fears and comfort the relatives.

RELIEF OF PAIN

Pain in malignant disease tends to be constant, and constant control is required. This implies the prescription of a regular schedule of pain-relieving drugs which should be designed to anticipate rather than to treat pain. Under no circumstances should a patient ever be in the position of 'watching the clock' for his next dose of analgesic; nor should he feel the need to justify it by first experiencing pain.

The drugs available for the relief of pain are the analgesics and the narcotics. These can be potentiated by the phenothiazines, which also will control nausea and vomiting, or by sedatives, which will ensure adequate sleep.

Mild Pain.—Aspirin (600 mg.), codeine phosphate (30–60 mg.), dihydro-codeine bitartrate (50 mg.), methadone (10 mg.), and paracetamol (1 G.), are all useful analgesics for the control of mild pain and can be given 4- or 6-hourly (*Table XXIII*). If aspirin is used, it should be in soluble (calcium aspirin) buffered (without acid) form. Aspirin, phenacetin, and codeine are combined as Tab. Cod. Co., and although the dose of codeine is only 8 mg. per tablet, there appears to be an additive effect. In Tabs. A.P.C. caffeine is substituted for codeine; these should not be given at night. Paracetamol (panadol), the active metabolite of phenacetin, is used increasingly.

It is normal to give, as an adjuvant to these mild pain-relievers, promazine (sparine) or chlorpromazine (largactil), 25–75 mg. 6-hourly, and barbiturates or chloral hydrate.

Panadol (Bayer Products Co., Surbiton-on-Thames, Surrey).

Moderate and Severe Pain.—When pain is more severe, the narcotics morphine or diamorphine (heroin) are unquestionably the best drugs available. Oral medication should be started with four daily doses of 1–2 ml. nepenthe to which is added aspirin (600 mg.) or codeine phosphate (30 mg.).

The Brompton mixture (morphine hydrochloride, 15 mg.; cocaine hydrochloride, 10 mg.; gin, 4 ml.; honey, 4 ml.; aq. chlorof. ad 15 ml.) is a useful preparation, and initially a mixture containing a smaller dose of morphine (e.g., 5 mg.) may be sufficient. The strength can be increased gradually.

Methadone, dihydrocodeine, and pethidine also can be used to control moderate pain but in patients with advanced malignancy they take second place to the natural opiates. Recommended doses are given in *Table XXIII*.

Table XXIII.—The Commonly Used Narcotics

	Equivalent Subcutaneous Dose to 10 mg. Morphine in Terms of Pain Relief (mg.)	Range of Doses Employed (mg.)
Natural alkaloids:		
Morphine	10	10–60
Diamorphine	3	5–10
Semisynthetics:		
Codeine	120	30–60
Dihydrocodeine (DF 118)	60	30–60
Synthetics:		
Pethidine	1000	25–100
Methadone (physeptone)	10	5–10
Levorphanol (dromoran)	3	2–4

Nausea can be controlled by syrup of prochlorperazine maleate, 5–10 mg., and additional sedation by syrup of chlorpromazine, 25–50 mg.

Once pain is severe parenteral therapy will be required. It is usual to start with 10 mg. morphine sulphate or 5 mg. diamorphine hydrochloride subcutaneously 4- or 6-hourly and to increase the dose as necessary. Doses in excess of 60 mg. morphine or 10 mg. diamorphine are not normally required. When prescribing narcotics in dosages above those normally employed, it is advisable for the house-surgeon to have the order countersigned by a more senior colleague.

Side Effects of Morphine.—Morphine and its derivatives may cause nausea, vomiting, drowsiness, respiratory depression, depression of the cough reflex, and constipation. Diamorphine has the advantage that it does not cause vomiting or constipation. Nausea can be prevented by promazine (sparine), cyclizine (marzine), or dimenhydrinate (dramamine), 25–50 mg.; drowsiness by amphetamine (benzedrine) or dexamphetamine sulphate (dexedrine), 5–10 mg.; and respiratory depression by nalorphine hydrobromide (lethidrone) or levallorphan tartrate (lorfan), 10 mg. intravenously.

DF 118 (Duncan, Flockhart, & Evans Ltd., Birkbeck Street, London, E.2).
Dromoran (Roche Products Ltd., 15 Manchester Square, London, W.1).
Physeptone (Burroughs, Wellcome & Co., Euston Road, London, N.W.1).
Pethidine is known in N. America as demerol (Winthrop Laboratories Inc., New York 18). The official title in the U.S.P. is meperidine hydrochloride.
Sparine (John Wyeth & Brother Ltd., Maidenhead, Berks).
Largactil (May & Baker Ltd., Dagenham, Essex).
Marzine, Lethidrone (Burroughs, Wellcome & Co., Euston Road, London, N.W.1).
Dramamine (G. D. Searle & Co. Ltd., Lane End Road, High Wycombe, Bucks).
Benzedrine, Dexedrine (Smith, Kline, & French Laboratories Ltd., Welwyn Garden City, Herts).
Lorfan (Roche Products Ltd., 15 Manchester Square, London, W.1).

Alcohol itself may prove a useful adjuvant, and there is much to be said for a bottle of whisky or brandy at the bedside.

Interruption of Pain Pathways.—If severe pain of nerve-root or spinal origin is present, a neurosurgeon should be consulted about cordotomy. Recently methods of interrupting pain pathways in the medulla by the percutaneous insertion of electrocoagulating electrodes have been under trial and may prove more applicable in patients with malignant disease.

Alternatively, the posterior nerve-roots corresponding to the segmental distribution of the pain can be blocked by the intrathecal injection of phenol in glycerin or phenol in iophendylate (myodil) in a dilution of 1 G. in 20 ml. It is advised that the site of injection is one segment above the involved nerves and that the patient is positioned in such a way that the neurotoxic solution bathes the involved roots. An anæsthetist should be consulted.

OTHER SYMPTOMS OF ADVANCED CANCER

Pain is not the only symptom of advanced malignancy, and vomiting, dysphagia, cough, dyspnœa, ulceration, or fungation may cause distress. The following are brief guides to management:—

Vomiting.—If not caused by mechanical obstruction, suspect drug toxicity. The vomiting may be psychological and reassurance, careful diet, iced water, sedatives, and anti-emetics may help.

Dysphagia.—If mechanical obstruction is present, consider giving relief by insertion of Moussin–Barbin or similar tube. Inability to swallow saliva is distressing and frequent mouthwashes may help. Gastrostomy and jejunostomy may only prolong suffering and are now seldom used.

Mouth Cancer.—Advanced cancer in the mouth may be very painful but frequent antiseptic washes and local anæsthetic sprays can help. Salivation may be a problem and it is difficult to control dribbling. Conversely, a dry mouth leads to cracked tongue and lips and episodes of fungous infection—lip ointments, boiled sweets, and fungicides (nystatin) may help. A painful red tongue may respond to tablets of nicotinamide.

Cough is best controlled by linctus codeine or diamorphine.

Dyspnœa can be very distressing but bronchial relaxants (ephedrine, amino-phylline, and atropine) and sedatives (amylobarbitone, 30 mg., or chlor-diazepoxide, 5–10 mg. t.i.d.) can help. An open window may give great relief.

Fungating Growth.—Frequent dressings with liquid paraffin, eusol in paraffin, or proflavine emulsion may control discomfort and odour. Fortunately, the patients themselves are rarely troubled by the unpleasant smell, but isolation with aerosols or 'smoke bombs' may be required for the sake of relatives and nursing staff.

GENERAL CARE

Fæcal impaction is best prevented by twice-weekly enemas or suppositories. Aperients should be used only in small doses, particularly if the patient is bedridden. As narcotics constipate, the patient should be assured that lack of a daily bowel movement is not harmful.

Incontinence of urine and fæces may be troublesome: the former indicates the insertion of an indwelling catheter of Gibbon type. A urinary antiseptic should be given (*see* p. 72).

Bed-sores.—Frequent attention to the skin or the provision of a sheepskin rug or ripple mattress helps to prevent bed-sores in the bedridden patient (p. 477).

Myodil (Glaxo Laboratories Ltd., Greenford, Middlesex).

Sleep.—Adequate restful sleep should be achieved by sedation, preferably with chloral hydrate (1–1·5 G.) or dichloralphenazone (welldorm) (50–1300 mg.). Barbiturates tend to cause a 'hangover' but may be required. An initial dose of 100 mg. increasing to 150 or 200 mg. until an effect is observed is advised.

THE DYING

Death from malignant disease is usually a gradual process of withdrawal and thus the sympathetic doctor can do much to help the patient and his relatives. The patient should be encouraged to talk and his questions answered frankly and simply. While it is not our duty to tell a patient he is about to die, it is equally not in his interests to deny him the truth should he choose to know it. All humans have responsibilities and worries and many will die happier if they first have the opportunity to leave their affairs in good order. For this reason frank discussion should not be avoided until the patient is moribund, by which time it is frequently too late.

Dying patients require constant encouragement and must never be passed by on the ward round. The hospital chaplain should be informed about a dying patient as soon as possible so that he can establish a relationship of trust and help the patient overcome his fears. Religious faith can help a man bear his trials with strength and expectation, and a doctor, whatever his own beliefs, must never say anything to destroy hope for a new and better life.

Relatives also require encouragement and help. Frequently they are reluctant to accept the truth and the house-surgeon may have to repeat, many times, the reasons for the patient's condition if misunderstanding is later to be avoided. Above all, he must do his utmost to allay the inevitable sense of guilt which relatives feel by his assurance that everything possible has been done. Under no circumstances must he indicate that something more might have been done or that the patient or his relatives were at fault in not seeking medical care at an earlier date. Relatives should be told not to discuss the patient's condition when with him and not to whisper at the foot of his bedside. Acuity of hearing is often preserved until the end. They should be encouraged to help to show their love for the patient by performing little tasks for his comfort.

As death approaches it should be remembered that the peripheral circulation will fail and subcutaneous injections of narcotics may cease to be effective. Drinks of iced water, cool sponging, and an electric fan help to keep the patient cool. There is no need for the patient to spend his last hours on his back and by turning him on his side choking can be prevented. The 'death rattle' is due to retained bronchial secretions and may be reduced by a timely injection of atropine.

HAS DEATH OCCURRED?

It is not always easy to be certain that a patient is dead. This is particularly true when the patient has had brain metastases, has been artificially cooled down, or is being maintained on a ventilator. The embarrassment of the young doctor is increased when there are relatives present, anxiously awaiting his verdict.

With advanced malignant disease there is no place for resuscitative measures and a little time can be taken to make certain that death has occurred. But when confronted by a sudden, unexpected death in an otherwise fit patient, cardio-respiratory resuscitation must be started *immediately* by external cardiac massage and inflation of the lungs and the hospital 'crash team' summoned (*see* p. 1).

The usual method of determining the presence of death is by auscultation with a stethoscope over the apex of the heart for sounds of circulatory activity

Welldorm (Smith & Nephew Pharmaceuticals Ltd., Welwyn Garden City, Herts).

and over the trachea and bronchi for any respiratory sounds. Silence in the room or ward is essential as the sounds may be very feeble. At least 2 minutes (by the clock) must be spent on auscultation. If there is any doubt it is advisable to come back in 5 minutes' time and again listen; in the meantime the relatives are told that life is not yet extinct.

Fragmentation of the blood columns in the retinal vessels as seen through the ophthalmoscope is another test of death that is sometimes employed. The most rapid and certain confirmation is that provided by a monitoring electrocardiograph, the complexes flickering to a steady line on the screen of the oscilloscope.

In a patient who is being maintained on a ventilator, fixed dilated pupils are a sign of irreversible cerebral damage which can be confirmed by the finding of flat electro-encephalography tracings. In the presence of these signs it is justifiable to disconnect the ventilator and observe whether spontaneous respiration returns within 1 minute. If so, the patient is not dead and the ventilator should be reconnected.

Death and Transplantation.—When there is any possibility of the organs of a dying patient being used for transplantation, then the attending doctor must make the decision that the patient is dead and that his vital body systems are no longer capable of independent activity—it must never be made by a member of the transplantation team.

CHAPTER XLIX

THE ADMINISTRATIVE DUTIES OF THE HOUSE-SURGEON

By the late W. D. LOVELOCK-JONES

THE hospital exists for the sake of the patients. The very word 'hospital' (Latin, *hospitium*) means a place where guests are received. Being a house of hospitality all patients within the walls of a hospital should therefore be treated as guests; this is a basic and changeless concept that has prevailed for centuries. In common with other members of the medical and nursing staff, the house-surgeon must never display the arrogance of office. On the other hand, he should preserve a certain dignity; jokes and levity are out of place, for they are liable to be mistaken by outsiders. Bad language must never be used; evidence of haste and of indecision should be avoided. Another axiom is never to make remarks in front of a patient or his relatives that might impugn the treatment given by the outside doctor, such as 'This patient should have been sent to hospital much earlier'. Such indiscretions cause endless trouble. Smoking should be avoided in any place where the doctor may be seen by patients or the public.

The house-surgeon throughout his stay in hospital should not assume responsibilities which he is not sufficiently experienced or qualified to shoulder. If in any real doubt or difficulty he must consult his seniors.

Contacts with the Patient's Doctor.—When he telephones requesting the admission of a patient, a general practitioner should not be subjected to a 'third degree' interrogation—as if he were subintelligent. House-surgeons and other resident hospital doctors must remember that as a rule general practitioners are very busy and conscientious persons, and that most of them have held a hospital appointment similar to that which gives the present holder the authority to admit patients. The house-surgeon should ascertain the main facts of the case, previous admissions, etc., and in particular what drugs have been given. If asked to readmit a known chronic case, the matter should be referred to the consultant surgeon.

Should the general practitioner telephone subsequently concerning the diagnosis or the findings at operation of his patient, the house-surgeon must studiously avoid adopting a patronizing attitude, especially if the diagnosis after admission differs from that made by the practitioner. It should be recalled that the facilities of the hospital can, and in most instances do, render diagnosis much easier. In spite of this (perhaps because too much reliance was placed on laboratory reports, etc.) all those with considerable experience can recall occasions where the diagnosis made by the patient's doctor was after all the correct one, and had it been acted upon the results might have been happier.

Admission of Patients.—When he receives a message that a patient—whether written for or sent to the hospital urgently—has arrived, the house-surgeon should go to the receiving room *at once*. In the event of another duty on which he is engaged being so impelling as to delay this course, the house-surgeon should send a message to the sister or nurse-in-charge of the receiving room, asking her to arrange for another member of the resident staff to see the patient on his behalf. Nothing damages the reputation of a hospital more than publicity concerning an ill patient kept waiting unnecessarily.

First on Call.—During the whole of the term that he is first on duty call ('taking in' as it is known colloquially) the switch-board operator must be kept informed of the house-surgeon's whereabouts. Only by so doing can the switch-board operator carry out his responsible duties efficiently and avoid keeping an outside doctor (who is, perhaps, telephoning from a call-box on a cold night) waiting while he (the switch-board operator) rings all round the hospital in an endeavour to locate the house-surgeon on duty.

Most large hospitals have a location signalling system, either by means of coloured lights (stationary or flashing) or, better still, one whereby the house-surgeon on duty wears a receiver in his breast pocket which buzzes when he is wanted on the telephone.

Examination of New Patient.—*A patient whose urgent admission has been arranged by telephone should be sent straight to the ward*, where he must be examined by the house-surgeon as soon as the nursing staff have had time to put the patient to bed, unless obviously the presence of a doctor is required before the patient is moved from the stretcher. The house-surgeon will find that 'putting the patient to bed' includes entering the name, age, address, religion, the date and time of admission, as well as the name and address of the patient's nearest relative, on the case-sheet, and taking and charting the temperature and the pulse-rate. Realizing that all this is saving him trouble, on entering the ward the house-surgeon should inquire if the patient is ready to be seen, and if not, instead of exhibiting signs of impatience, he can employ his time profitably by reviewing some particular point concerning another patient until he is notified that the new patient is ready to be seen.

The admitting house-surgeon must be able to recognize a really ill patient at once—and immediately notify his senior—either registrar or consultant, who will then be responsible. In the recognition of a seriously ill patient, the newly appointed house-surgeon should not be too proud to receive the help of experienced sisters, who so often give this most valuable aid unobtrusively.

Drunk or Dying?—This is a well-recognized perplexity. That the patient's breath smells of alcohol is no criterion. If, after due consideration, the casualty officer comes to the conclusion that the patient is inebriated on no account should he just write on the record 'C_2H_5OH' and feel satisfied that that will meet the diagnostic requirements expected of him. On the contrary, he must record the signs that led him to this conclusion in sufficient detail to warrant the diagnosis, remembering that to be biased because the patient is drunk is at variance with medical ethics. Should, as is frequently the case, there have been an accident and the patient is brought to hospital because of an injury, a consultation with the ward house-surgeon is imperative even if the injury appears trivial. It must be remembered that Court proceedings may follow, in which event one (or both) of the hospital residents who examined the patient will be called as a medical witness. Careful notes of the findings will then be of untold value. To read the actual notes made at the time the patient was brought to hospital will not only assist the Court but will place the medical witness in an unassailable position. A house-surgeon should *not* take blood or breath alcohol samples from motorists for the police; this is the duty of the police doctor.

Refusal to Admit.—The house-surgeon who refuses to admit a patient frequently assumes heavy responsibilities. The usual excuse for the refusal is shortage of beds. It is difficult to believe that the admitting staff (nursing as well as surgical) of any hospital worthy of the name cannot arrange for an extra bed to be made up so that a perforated peptic ulcer or patient with a ruptured spleen has not to be sent elsewhere. Transfer of patients requiring urgent treatment can seldom be justified. When there is no other general hospital in the area, the patient *must* be admitted. In a city, if it appears likely that the patient cannot be admitted, it is much better to send him on at once, after conducting an examination in the ambulance, rather than to keep him waiting in the Casualty Department. Now that British hospitals are nationalized and regarded as public property criticisms for refusal to admit are much more common.

Ward Work.—The house-surgeon should make morning and evening visits to the wards and go at all times when sent for urgently. His morning rounds should be timed to suit the convenience of the sister—for instance, he should not arrive just as she is about to supervise the serving of the patients' midday meal. The new house-surgeon is strongly advised to make inquiries as to when the patients' main meals are served, when bed-making is undertaken, and the days and times set as visiting hours for the patients' relatives and friends. It is best to enter these times in the front of his notebook, for should his routine visits coincide with any of these busy times he is bound to be received by the nursing staff with at least a degree of coldness, which is quite understandable.

Case Notes.—In the careful writing up of case notes the house-surgeon learns much—indeed it is the main source of his tuition. When there is a possibility of litigation, e.g., after an accident, careful detailed records are essential. Should the hospital's board of management seek recognition for its house posts to be suitable for the F.R.C.S. or other higher examinations, when the representatives of the Examining Board in question visit, particular attention is paid to the case notes. Follow-up work, research, statistics, etc., will all be vitiated unless accurate records are kept. As well as the case history and investigations a provisional diagnosis should be written down, and thereafter daily progress notes. At the time of discharge, the final diagnosis is entered along with any recommendations to the outside doctor and any follow-up dates.

Investigations.—It is the *results* of investigations that are of value. See that the results are available when the surgeon goes round, telephoning the laboratory if need be (and in emergencies).

Referring Patients to Other Departments.—When patients are referred to special departments for investigation or treatment (e.g., Radiodiagnosis, Radiotherapy, Physiotherapy, Biochemistry, Electrocardiography) the appropriate forms should be completed in each case with full details of what is required. Heads of departments frequently complain that the form that has been drawn up by the department in question is incompletely or inaccurately filled in, and this often leads to delay in investigation and treatment of the patient.

Requests for Further Opinion.—If a specialist's opinion is required by the surgeon, a 'Request to see' form should be completed and passed to the house-physician or house-surgeon attached to the consultant concerned, having first ascertained that the latter is available. An urgent request merits a personal interview or telephone call rather than a form.

Seeking the Help of the Medical Social Worker.—The recovery of patients is often impeded if they are worried over personal or family matters. The notice of the medical social worker (almoner) should be called to such patients and much help can be given. She can arrange financial help, can contact employers about keeping the patient's job for him, arrange convalescence, and can help in other ways.

Visiting by the Patient's Relatives and Friends.—The house-surgeon is advised to refer this matter to the sister-in-charge. In the case of a patient who is dangerously ill the relatives must be allowed to come whenever they wish, but the time they actually remain with the patient must be regulated by the sister-in-charge, often after consultation with the house-surgeon. The house-surgeon should be available at least twice per week to interview relatives and answer their questions.

'Is it Cancer, Doctor?'—To this question the house-surgeon swiftly should reply, 'Investigations are not yet completed; in any case that is a question you must put to the surgeon-in-charge, not to me.'

Consent for a Surgical Operation.—No operation should be performed without the consent of:—

The patient, if he or she be 21 years of age or over, or

The patient's guardian, should the patient be under 21 years of age.

A brief, non-technical explanation of the proposed operation and why it has been recommended should be given before requesting the patient or the patient's guardian to sign the consent form. The form recommended by the Medical Defence Societies is a particularly good one, and it will therefore be reproduced here.

OPERATION CONSENT (*Patient*)

SURNAMES (Block Letters)	FIRST NAMES (Block Letters)	UNIT NUMBER

I, the undersigned, hereby agree to the Hospital Authorities carrying out whatever treatment and operations they may consider necessary in my interests and I also agree to the administration of local or general anæsthesia as may be considered necessary.

Signature ....
Address ....
....
Date........... ....

No promise should be given as to who will perform the operation.

In a case of dire emergency, if consent cannot be obtained immediately the consultant surgeon is unlikely to wait for it, the life-saving nature of the operation being sufficient justification for its performance.

In the case of certain gynæcological operations that might cause sterility or interfere with marital relations, if the patient is a married woman the consent of her husband must be obtained in addition.

Qualified Consent.—It should be noticed that the above consent form stipulates 'Whatever treatment and operations they may consider necessary . . .' That is, in effect, what is known as *unqualified* consent. By *qualified* consent is meant that the patient (or, in the case of a child, the parents) specifies for what operation or what procedure consent is given or, as is more usual, for what operation or procedure consent is *not* given. Perhaps the most common of these qualified consent problems met with in Europe, the U.S.A., and Australia concerns Jehovah's Witnesses who, by reason of a clause in their faith, are forbidden to receive another's blood into their veins. In the case of a child whose parents, in giving consent for their child to undergo an operation, stipulated that no blood transfusion should be given, the situation was dealt with in the following way: The parents were told that should a blood transfusion be deemed necessary to preserve the child's life they would be notified. If within one hour they did not come to the hospital bearing a magistrate's order restraining the surgeon from performing a blood transfusion, the transfusion would be given. It is highly improbable that the parents *and* the magistrate would take it upon themselves to restrain the surgeon in these circumstances.

From time to time other problems of this kind present—almost always they can be circumvented by patient, constructive argument, but on no account must the house-surgeon or his chief belittle or attempt to prove that the patient's religious beliefs are ill-founded. That is the very way to get consent withheld adamantly.

Pre-operative Preparations.—Every patient going to have an operation should have his name, unit number, and diagnosis written on a plastic bracelet which is attached to his wrist. Similar details should appear on the operation list and be used for sending for the next patient for theatre. The house-surgeon or registrar must mark with indelible ink which side is to be operated on. Digits should be named so that there is no possibility of error.

Dangerous Drugs.—These must not be ordered over the telephone. The correct dose must be entered legibly and signed—*initials are not sufficient.* It should be noted especially that sedative or narcotic drugs should be ordered only for the benefit of the patient; they should never be ordered for administrative or nursing convenience.

On Notification of Infectious Diseases.—The inadvertent admission into a general ward of a patient, especially a child, suffering from an infectious or contagious disease may have serious consequences. If such a patient is seen in the admitting room, he or she should be screened off and consultation held as to the best means of transferring the patient and disinfecting the room or ward into which the patient was received.

A list of notifiable diseases and other information concerning notification and quarantine, etc., will be found on the inside back cover.

On Notification of Industrial Diseases.—All cases of disease that may have arisen as a result of working with chemicals, carcinogenic agents, and the like, must be notified to the Chief Inspector of Factories. Further information upon this subject will be found on the inside back cover.

On Divulging Information concerning Patients.—The relationship between a doctor and his patient is essentially private and confidential. On this basis a patient answers questions and gives information which he or she might not wish others to know, therefore information so obtained must not be divulged without the patient's consent. Should information be required for governmental or legal purposes, e.g., reports to Ministries, insurance companies, or solicitors, the consent of the patient or his legal adviser should be obtained in writing. Inquiries concerning the patient's condition from outsiders—especially the patient's employer—require careful consideration and only such information as the patient gives consent for must be imparted. Even to relatives, information should not be given without thought. A simple inquiry from a husband about his wife may be made with a divorce in view.

On Signing Certificates.—Every certificate should be read carefully, to ensure that the statements contained therein are within one's knowledge and true. It is illegal to ante-date or post-date a certificate—a certificate is true only for the time at which it is signed. Never certify today something you expect will be true tomorrow.

On Discharging Patients from Hospital.—When, as is usually the case, there is pressure on the hospital beds it is imperative that no patient remains in hospital longer than is necessary. Consequently the house-surgeon should make regular rounds for the express purpose of selecting and writing up patients fit for discharge or for transfer to a convalescent home, if such be affiliated to the hospital. Every reasonable precaution must be taken to ensure that a patient is not discharged until he or she is fit (*a*) to make the journey without undue fatigue, and (*b*) to fend for himself sufficiently in the surroundings in which he will find himself. If there is any doubt about the patient's home conditions it is a wise precaution to inquire about them. Often the patient's doctor will be able to help in this direction, and in necessary cases he will arrange for a district nurse to visit the patient. It is essential that the patient be examined by the house-surgeon on the morning of the day of discharge to ensure that there is no reason for cancelling the arrangement. Omission of this step has resulted in public censure and damage to the reputation of the hospital, as well as claims for damages.

A short note for his own doctor should be sent with each patient at the time of his discharge; in it are briefly summarized the investigations, diagnosis, and recommended treatment. It may be many days before the outside doctor receives a detailed discharge letter from the surgical registrar or consultant. Faulty communications are a frequent cause of misunderstanding between hospital staff and family doctors.

Patients taking their own Discharge.—The patient must be permitted to take his discharge whenever he wishes to do so. Should he select an inconvenient time to leave the hospital an effort to persuade him to stay is permissible, but he cannot be compelled to give reasonable notice of his intention to depart. If he is medically unfit to go, he should be asked to sign an acknowledgement that he is leaving against medical advice, but again it must be remembered that he cannot be compelled to sign such an acknowledgement. If he refuses to sign, it is a good practice to have a witness that he has been advised, but refuses, to stay in hospital.

Maternity Department.—All births, both live and still, must be notified to the Medical Officer of Health. Legally the child is said to be born alive if it breathes or shows other signs of life, after separation from its mother. If a period of gestation of less than 28 weeks results in a dead fœtus, the case is one of abortion or miscarriage. The words 'abortion' and 'miscarriage' mean the same thing, and the distinction formerly made between them has been abandoned.

If a feeble newborn child dies before it is seen by a doctor, it is always wise to notify the Coroner, who will take such action as he thinks fit in the circumstances.

Each hospital has its own routine procedure to prevent the grave occurrence of mistaken identity of newborn babies. Before the child is removed from the labour ward a strip of adhesive strapping bearing the name should be attached to its skin. As soon as convenient, this is replaced by two labels in the form of tapes. On each is written in marking ink, name, religion, and date of birth. If there are two mothers in the ward with the same surname—sufficient additional detail for unmistakable identification should be added. One tape is placed around the ankle and the other around the wrist. It is important to have two labels in case one should become detached. When the tape labels are fixed, the temporary strapping is removed, and the identity checked by a second nurse.

Abortions.—There is little doubt that many abortions are induced by criminal action. If the patient herself is at fault, it is no part of the doctor's duty to report the matter to the police, although the Coroner must be informed should she die. If the abortion is known to be the work of a professional abortionist, the doctor who hides the fact carries a heavy responsibility, for other lives are at stake. He should try to persuade the patient to allow information to be given to the police. However, the patient should not be requested to make a dying declaration, which commences 'I, so and so, believe myself to be at the point of death'. If questioned why no attempt was made to obtain a dying declaration the house-surgeon must explain to the authorities that such phraseology is prejudicial to the possible recovery of the patient, and that it is his (the house-surgeon's) duty to fan the embers of life.

Therapeutic Abortion.—In Britain, under the 1967 Abortion Act, a pregnancy may be terminated when: (1) its continuance would endanger the life of the pregnant woman, or (2) cause injury to her physical or mental health greater than if the pregnancy were terminated, or (3) cause similar risk of injury of her existing children, or (4) where there is substantial risk that the child, if born, would suffer from serious physical or mental abnormalities. Two doctors must sign a certificate indicating on which of these grounds the termination is justified, and the surgeon who performs the operation should retain the certificate for 3 years. The operation may only be performed in hospitals or nursing homes specifically approved. A doctor may on grounds of conscience refuse to participate in arrangements for an abortion, but he should refer the patient to another practitioner.

The patient's consent to the necessary operation should be obtained in writing. In the case of a married woman, the husband's approval should be obtained if possible. In the case of a girl over the age of 16, while desirable, the consent of her parents is not strictly necessary. An abortion must not be performed at the parents' insistence when the girl is unwilling.

The doctor performing the termination must notify the chief medical officer on a statutory form within 7 days of every abortion he performs and provide some additional information.

Deaths.—Some hospitals insist that a house-physician or house-surgeon must be summoned to verify that death has taken place; this may not always be necessary. In the case of a patient whose death is expected, to call the house-surgeon from his bed at 3 a.m. to verify that the patient is clinically dead seems to be a work of supererogation. The sister will make a note on the case-sheet stating the date and the time of death—and this entry must be signed. If the relatives are not present at death they should be informed immediately by messenger or telegram. They should also be informed when to come for the death certificate and then told about the office hours of the Registrar of Births and Deaths. Every consideration and sympathy must be shown to the relatives. Sometimes they wish to see the body; a nurse should always accompany them to the mortuary—and care should be taken to ensure that the body is in the Chapel of Repose before the relatives are admitted.

Certification of Death.—*See* Chapter LI.

Reporting to the Coroner.—*See* Chapter LI.

Post-mortem Examinations.—Routine post-mortem examinations are most desirable in everyone's interest, for it is to the benefit of all concerned that everything possible should be learnt about fatal cases. No necropsy should be carried out without the permission of the nearest relative, or, if the death is within the province of the Coroner, without his authorization. Relatives who are reluctant can usually be persuaded to give consent if good reasons are put to them with sincerity and clarity and they can be convinced that information likely to benefit others will be obtained and that there will be no discernible disfigurement.

Reporting to the Police.—The police are most helpful to hospitals and their courtesies should always be reciprocated. Information should be given to the police in the following:—

a. Accident cases. Progress of injured patients, etc.

b. Criminal abortion (*see above*).

c. In regard to patients who have been guilty of some criminal offence and who have been apprehended by the police.

d. Attempted suicide. Attempted suicide is a crime in England and the facts must be reported to the police, and to the hospital's Administrative Officer at the earliest possible moment. As a rule, if it can be avoided, the police are reluctant to take action. Full notes must be made of all circumstances of the attempted suicide, including the method of obtaining the drug or weapon.

The hospital may be at fault in allowing access to poisonous drugs. In many instances the action of the patient can be attributed to a disordered mind and a consultation with a psychiatrist should be sought as soon as the patient is well enough. Very often the patient is transferred to a mental hospital. (Scottish Law is different in regard to attempted suicide.)

ON BEING PREPARED FOR POSSIBLE LITIGATION

On qualification every registered medical practitioner, no matter where he is working, should join one of the Medical Defence Societies. Since British hospitals became State supported and the members of the medical profession enrolled in a National Health Service, the general public regard the hospitals as their property and medical men as their servants, and as a consequence there has been a remarkable increase in the number of claims for damages against doctors—many of them frivolous. Another strong incentive to bring such actions is that it is now possible for the plaintiff without sufficient means to obtain free legal aid, so if unsuccessful he has nothing to lose. The house-surgeon therefore should take all reasonable care in his dealings with patients and in the keeping of accurate case-histories, which undoubtedly are bound to stand him in good stead if the evil day of litigation falls upon him—this advice holds good in all parts of the world.

CHAPTER L

MEDICO-LEGAL REPORTS

By the late DONALD C. NORRIS

IN recent years there has been a considerable increase in the number of cases in which a patient claims money payments in respect of injury or illness. Such claims may be made under various statutes, or at common law, and the doctor may be asked to assist by giving a medical report, to be used as evidence in such proceedings, and, if necessary, by attendance as a witness at the hearing of the case in Court.

Importance of Proper Hospital Records.—Since any such report must be based upon observations made in the course of treatment, it is most important that these observations should be recorded carefully at the time they are made, or as soon afterwards as is practicable, and that they should be complete, legible, and free from ambiguities and omissions. It may be months or even years after the event before a medico-legal report is called for, and nothing can be more embarrassing than to search through a mass of vague, badly written notes in an attempt to compile a clear, connected account of what injuries were sustained, what abnormalities were found on examination, what treatment was given, and what progress made. Care should be taken that "Right" and "Left" are inserted when describing the site of any bodily condition noted, and that fingers are described by their *names* (index, middle, ring, or little) and not by numbers in order that no doubt exists as to the identity of the finger concerned. Abbreviations, if used, should be unmistakable and the results of special investigations given so that they can be found *readily*. (Too often, one finds a note "For X-ray" —and only by searching the file can one find the result of this investigation.) Operation findings should be explicit and complete, and information given as to previous injuries and illnesses. Range of movement should be given in degrees, and figures given for temperature, pulse-rate, blood-pressure, and other observations capable of being expressed in figures. The situation of wounds, scars, etc., should be stated, with diagrams where appropriate.

Consent.—The patient's consent should be obtained, except as stated below, before any information about his case is given to third parties. Some hospitals have a printed form which the patient is asked to sign, giving his consent to such disclosure. The patient must understand clearly the purpose of the disclosure, and to whom it is to be made. If he is unable, owing to mental or physical disability, to give such consent, it should be obtained from his nearest relative or other properly authorized agent.

The doctor may, in a few instances, be under a statutory obligation to give information about a patient, regardless of his consent: thus, he may be required to notify the proper authorities that the patient is suffering from infectious disease, or from some scheduled industrial disease: he is also bound to answer questions in Court, if so directed by the Judge, as to his findings in examining a patient. This is so even if the witness is bound by statute to treat such information as confidential.

Thus, in the case of *Garner* v. *Garner* it was held by the Court that a doctor was bound to give evidence that a woman patient was suffering from venereal disease.

although she was under treatment by him in a clinic set up under the provisions of the Public Health (Venereal Diseases) Regulations, 1916, which expressly forbid the disclosure of such information to third parties. On the other hand, in a case reported in *The Lancet* (1934, **2**, 835) a doctor was asked in Court to give evidence about a patient attending a tuberculosis dispensary, and he successfully pleaded that he was forbidden to do so, by the Public Health (Tuberculosis) Regulations, 1930, breach of which carried a penalty of £100.

Claims for money payments in respect of disability may be made under various statutes or at common law; the more important of these statutes are as follows:—

1. *Fatal Accidents Acts*, 1846–1908.—If the breadwinner of a family is killed in an accident in circumstances which entitle him to damages, these Acts give a right to his dependants to sue for the financial loss brought about by his death. The doctor may then be asked to estimate the expectation of life of the dependants —if this is below average, they are not entitled to receive as much as they would had their lives been first-class.

2. *The Law Reform* (*Miscellaneous Provisions*) *Act*, 1934.—This extended the list of dependants who might be entitled to sue under the Fatal Accidents Acts, and provided that when one or other of the parties in an action for negligence dies after the right arose, the action may be continued by or against the estate of the deceased litigant. Damages in such a case may include an item in respect of "Loss of expectation of life" of a deceased plaintiff. In the case of *Benham* v. *Gambling*, 1941, the House of Lords decided that the Court should assess the value of the deceased's prospects of a "Happy life"—so that, presumably, the sum to be awarded would be reduced if the life, had it continued, would not have been a happy one, e.g., on account of a permanent disability.

3. *The Employers' Liability Act*, 1880.—This Act gave a right to a workman in certain specified industries to bring an action against his employer if the workman was injured by reason of defects in the "ways, works, plant or machinery" provided by the employer. As long ago as 1904 this Act was pronounced to have been "a failure" in a report by a Government committee, and it is now seldom invoked.

4. *The Workmen's Compensation Acts*, 1897–1945.—These Acts set out to provide money payments ("Compensation" for loss of earnings) during disability for workmen injured by an accident "Arising out of and in the course of" their employment. These Acts provided for a simple procedure by which some 98 per cent of claims were settled without litigation. However, many such claims gave rise to disputes in which medical evidence was called for to determine, amongst other things, whether disability was present, and if so in what degree, and whether it was due to or aggravated by an accident. These Acts also applied in cases in which a workman contracted a disease due to his employment, and certain diseases common in particular industries were scheduled, e.g., nystagmus and "beat hand" in miners, and cataract in glass workers.

These Acts were repealed by the National Insurance (Industrial Injuries) Act, 1946, except as regards cases which arose before that date—these have now become very uncommon.

5. *The Disabled Persons* (*Employment*) *Act*, 1944.—This Act marked the dawn of a more enlightened attitude towards disabled persons, and the obligations of society towards them. It sets out "To make further and better provision for enabling persons handicapped by disablement to secure employment, or work on their own account." It provides for a register of disabled persons, to be maintained at Employment Exchanges throughout the country; enrolment is

voluntary, and certain classes of person, including those in receipt of disability pensions from the Services, are entitled to be registered without further inquiry. In most cases, however, medical evidence is called for in support of the application for registration under this Act. For this purpose it is not necessary to state the cause of disability, since this is irrelevant—the only thing which matters is to establish that there is some substantial handicap to obtaining or keeping employment, and to give such particulars of this handicap as will best assist the official dealing with the case (the Disablement Resettlement Officer or D.R.O.) to advise the applicants as to suitable employment. Generally speaking, this official wants to know, not what faculties the applicant has lost, but what faculties remain and what limitations there are to his working capacity. This information is sought by the issue of an eight-page leaflet, "Form D.P. 1", which the applicant is asked to have completed by his medical attendant. These forms may be obtained at any Employment Exchange, and it is recommended that the Hospital resident should make himself familiar with the form, so as to be able to complete it without delay when required.

It is very desirable that, in any case which appears likely to entail a substantial impairment of earning capacity for six months or more (this being the period contemplated in this Act as justifying registration), the patient should be informed as soon as practicable about the benefits to which this Act entitles him; and it is often a good plan to ask the D.R.O. to attend at the hospital to discuss with the patient and his doctor the steps which should be taken to secure rehabilitation. The D.R.O. is usually well informed about the facilities in his district for placing disabled persons in employment, and he will always be glad to have any guidance which the doctor may be able to give him as to any special hazards imposed by the patient's physical condition. Thus, certain chest complaints may make it undesirable that the work should entail exposure to extremes of temperature or to dust; while cardiac cases may require work on the level, or sedentary work; loss of the sense of smell may make a man unfit for employment in a gas works; while liability to attacks of giddiness may incapacitate him from working on scaffolds or ladders.

6. *The National Insurance Industrial Act*, 1965; *The National Insurance Act* 1965–66; and *The National Health Service Act*, 1946.—These three Acts might well be considered together, since they marked the establishment of a new system by which the Welfare State took over the administration, to a large extent, of services to provide for treatment of disabled persons, including payment of financial benefits during periods of sickness or disablement from injury. These Acts and subsequent amendments are administered largely by Government agencies, particularly the Departments responsible for health and the social services, employment and productivity.

Officials of these Ministries are empowered to deal with claims for sickness and injury benefits, and patients are examined, where necessary, by Medical Boards set up by the Ministry, at which the degree of disability is assessed according to a percentage rating, and payments made according to a schedule on a statutory scale. These Medical Boards often call for hospital records to assist them in arriving at a suitable assessment, and they may ask for a medical report if these records are not sufficiently clear. Regulations under these Acts provide for a wide discretion of the authorities to increase the scale of benefit to meet special needs—including costs of attendance, the maintenance of dependants, provision of surgical or nursing appliances, etc. The aim is to see that everything possible is done to provide for the needs of the handicapped person and to facilitate his recovery and resettlement as an independent worker so far as may be practicable.

In a number of centres special committees have been set up at which members of the medical and surgical staff of a hospital meet regularly for consultation with representatives of the Ministries concerned, with local employers, trade union officials, the Disablement Resettlement Officer, physiotherapists, occupational therapy workers, and others, and difficult problems of treatment, training, and placement in employment are discussed. Such an arrangement can be of the greatest value to the disabled persons concerned, and serves to avoid the waste and disappointment and distress which can arise so easily after the acute stage of an illness or injury has passed and return to gainful employment has become the main object of treatment.

Claims at Common Law.—Speaking generally, statutory remedies are limited to particular classes of persons, or to special types of loss, they are often limited in amount, and subject to special procedure. At common law, however, the injured party may claim not only "Special damages", including all his out-of-pocket expenses—loss of earnings, damage to clothing, costs of treatment, etc.—but also "General damages", viz., a sum in respect of pain and suffering, loss of capacity for social and recreational activities, and for loss of expectation of life.

In such a case it is therefore desirable that the doctor should deal in his report not only with technical details, but should give some information about the patient's family and social setting, recreations, etc., where these may have been affected by the accident. The effects of the injuries on his working capacity should be mentioned, and also on his ability to feed and dress himself, to travel, and to manage his affairs. In short, the report should state two things—what sort of injuries the patient has sustained, and what sort of patient has sustained these injuries.

Before starting to write his report, the doctor should be careful to *read his instructions*, which will often explain exactly what information is required, and may give details of special points on which inquiry should be made.

Arrangement of Reports.—Insurance companies sometimes send a printed form, with a request that the doctor will complete this by entering answers to a series of questions. This form of report is particularly useful in life assurance examinations, and other cases in which presumably healthy persons are to be examined; but in cases of injury or illness it is usually better for the doctor to construct his own report, in which irrelevant material can be omitted, and the salient features of the case given their proper emphasis. It makes for clarity if the matter is arranged under cross-headings, such as History of Accident, Previous Medical History, Present Complaints, Condition on Examination, and Opinion. *Diagrams are often useful, to illustrate loss of amputated parts, restriction of movement in joints, size and position of scars, and outline of fragments in cases of fracture.* If separate documents are to be sent—e.g., prints of radiographs, copies of pathological reports, etc.—it is advisable to give a list of these in a covering letter, in case they should become mislaid. *Original documents, e.g., X-ray negatives, reports signed by the pathologist, etc., should not be sent out of the hospital; care should, however, be taken that copies are accurate and legible, and include the full name of the patient and the date of examination.*

Doubtful Cases.—

The house-surgeon may be in doubt as to some important aspect of the case, e.g., whether the condition found is due to the accident, or as to the diagnosis. Such doubts should, if possible, be resolved before a report is sent, but in no case should they find expression in a vague or ambiguous report. If the difficulty is such as could be resolved by some further tests or observations, then these should be undertaken if possible, or at least should be indicated in the report. Thus, it is unsatisfactory to say, "He is making a good recovery, although the fracture has not yet healed soundly"; the doctor should suggest a further examination at such a time as would probably enable him to give a final opinion as to whether bony repair has been secured or not. It is useless to report that a patient is "either a malingerer or a neurotic"—a definite opinion should be expressed, giving the grounds on which this is formed, or some further tests suggested which would resolve such a doubt. If information is then provided that the patient has been seen to engage in a strenuous game, it would be justifiable to report: "In view of the information furnished by you, and of my own examination of this case, I am of the opinion that A.B. is fit to resume his ordinary work."

The Doctor in the Witness Box.—Many medical men regard attendance at Court as an ordeal which they would avoid gladly; they fear that Counsel will seek to extort admissions and turn them to the advantage of his client, with little regard for the truth, and will seek to damage the character of the medical witness. Actual experience of cases before the courts will soon dispel any such apprehensions. Provided that he has given a careful and accurate report, based on properly kept records, and that he is prepared fully to substantiate in evidence everything which appears in the report, and to explain clearly how he arrives at his opinion, his appearance in the witness box should prove to be an interesting and valuable experience, and he may gain the satisfaction of knowing that his evidence has been of real assistance to the Court and to the parties concerned.

The doctor should remember that legal procedure, however tedious and unreasonable it may appear, has been built up over the centuries as being the best way to secure a decision on matters in dispute, and to do justice between the parties; he should count it a privilege to be able to take part in this useful work, remembering that it is usually in the best interests of the patient that such a decision should be made, taking into account all the relevant circumstances. This is particularly so in cases in which the patient's recovery is being retarded by anxiety about a claim.

Notice that his attendance is required in Court may be given informally by letter or telephone; if he cannot attend, or feels that his evidence would be of little value, he should say so at once, giving his reasons, so that alternative arrangements can be made.

The Subpœna, and the matter of *Fees for attendance at Court*.—The doctor may be handed a document called a 'subpœna', which is a summons issued by the Court, directing him to attend there at a stated time and remain there until he is released. Once such a document has been put in his hands he is bound to obey it, under risk of penalty of fine or even imprisonment for 'contempt of court'. If he cannot attend at the stated time he should at once inform the Court, and give his reasons, and ask for further directions. Service of a subpœna should be accompanied by 'conduct money' (usually one guinea) which is meant to cover costs of travel to Court. Having arrived there, he is bound to give evidence of fact if called upon, but he need not give 'expert evidence' (i.e., opinion) unless his fees have been paid or guaranteed. If nothing has been arranged about his fees, he is entitled to ask the party calling him to undertake to pay these; if no agreement can be reached as to fees the witness may appeal to the Judge—this should be done before he takes the oath. The best plan about fees is to agree these with the party calling him, before he goes to Court. If it is left until after the case is over, the doctor may find his account unsettled, and the solicitor concerned may merely refer him to the client, who may have lost the case, and have no funds. It would be improper to make a bargain that the fees will be paid only if the claimant wins his case, but there is no objection to an arrangement that payment of an agreed account will be deferred until the conclusion of the hearing in Court.

Although the witness swears to tell "the truth, the whole truth, and nothing but the truth", this phrase has a narrow, technical meaning. Actually, he will seldom be allowed to tell all he knows, but only to answer questions briefly—usually by saying "Yes" or "No" to the questions set by Counsel. These questions are often very skilfully devised, so that while the doctor is led to reply to each question quite correctly, the general inference which Counsel seeks to draw from the whole series of answers may be very different from the true opinion of the witness. If a doctor thinks he is being unfairly treated, or that a wrong construction is being put on his evidence, he should say so to the Counsel calling him, or in the last resort he may make a protest to the Judge. It is a bad mistake to lose one's temper in the witness box; this is likely to lead to one's evidence being discredited.

The rules of evidence exclude not only everything which is irrelevant, but also all that is 'inadmissible', such as hearsay; thus a doctor will not be allowed to quote the observations of an eminent consultant with whom he saw a case, although such an opinion might be most important, and quite clearly relevant; the proper way to bring in such evidence is to call the consultant himself as a witness.

When he attends Court, the doctor should remember that he is at the service of justice, and should place himself unreservedly in the hands of Counsel, and should do to the best of his ability what is required of him. He should not be offended if the case turns out to be such that medical evidence is of little or no value, so that he may spend a good deal of time at Court without being called upon at all to give evidence; he should console himself with the reflection that he is entitled to his fees whether he is put into the witness box or not, so long as he actually attends Court when summoned to do so.

A useful booklet has been published by the Medical Defence Union dealing with the matter of fees in medico-legal cases, with other information relating to the duties and responsibilities of the doctor who may become involved in such cases.

Another publication in this field which is strongly recommended is *A Doctor's Guide to Court*, 2nd ed. (1967), by Professor Keith Simpson. (London: Lewis, 45s.)

CHAPTER LI

CERTIFICATION OF DEATH AND REPORTING TO THE CORONER

By J. Burton

In the past 900 years a system of reporting deaths has evolved in England and Wales through the old Common Law requirements that all deaths must be reported to the coroner where there might be some financial benefit to the Crown and, more recently, through the statutory requirements that a register must be kept of all deaths and that information must be supplied by the doctor in attendance on the deceased.

As a result of this concurrent evolution there is considerable overlapping of the duties of all those concerned in investigating and recording the causes of death. Any doctor who has attended the deceased is bound by a double duty, first, to report to the coroner any death that is violent or unnatural or of which the cause is unknown, and, secondly, to give a certificate to the registrar stating the cause of death to the best of his knowledge and belief, if he is able to do so.

The performance of one of these duties does not, in law, absolve him from the other, but this causes little difficulty in practice as a short telephone conversation with the coroner's officer usually resolves any difficulties and then either the doctor certifies the death or the coroner assumes all further responsibility.

The majority of deaths are due to natural causes and are dealt with by the doctor's certificate and registration by the registrar. The Births and Deaths Registration Act, 1953, states that, when the deceased person has been attended during his last illness by a registered medical practitioner, that practitioner shall sign a certificate in the form provided, stating to the best of his knowledge and belief the cause of death, and shall forthwith deliver that certificate to the registrar. Notice must also be given to the person qualified to register the death, usually the next relation, that the certificate has been signed. It is a common practice to deliver the certificate to a relation to be handed over at the time of registration, thus avoiding the delay caused by posting the certificate.

Completing a Death Certificate.—The certificates are supplied in book form and the book contains instructions as to the manner in which the certificate should be completed. These instructions should be read carefully before the certificate is filled in, as an improperly completed certificate will be returned by the registrar, causing delay in registration and possibly interfering with any proposed arrangements for the funeral. This causes unnecessary inconvenience and distress to the relations of the deceased.

The certificate requires the *cause of death* to be stated, not the manner of dying. This should be given as accurately and concisely as possible.

The wording should be checked against the list of undesirable terms or terms requiring further information that is given on pp. 4–6 of the certificate book.

The site of any cancerous growth should be accurately recorded when it is known, even if it has been surgically removed before death, as this information is needed for classification.

In some cases, particularly in old people or patients with a chronic disease, the condition directly causing the death would not have killed an otherwise healthy person. The contribution made by age or a second condition is recorded as a 'significant condition contributing towards death but not related to the disease causing it' under clause II of the cause of death on the certificate. Examples of entries of direct and contributory causes of death are given on p. 7 of the book of certificates. It is not necessary to record co-existing diseases or injuries if they played no part in causing the patient's death. If a doctor has any doubts about the form of the certificate he may always ask the coroner for advice. This is not the same thing as reporting the case to the coroner—although he may advise that the case should be reported. It may be necessary to explain the situation to a relative who might otherwise believe that some apparently significant injury has been concealed.

There is no fee payable for issuing a death certificate and there is an obligation on the doctor attending in the last illness to give a certificate if he can state the cause of death, on pain of a penalty. This duty applies even where the death is violent or unnatural.

Inability to Complete a Death Certificate.—In certain cases it is not possible for the doctor attending the patient in his last illness to give a cause of death and so complete a death certificate. Refusal to give a cause should not be due to insufficient information as to the *complete* nature of the patient's illness. Death from carcinomatosis or from chronic cardiac failure is a natural cause of death, even though the exact site of the primary growth or the nature of the valvular lesion of the heart is not certain.

In any case of doubt the case should be reported to the coroner who may well say that he is satisfied that the case does not come within his jurisdiction.

POST-MORTEM EXAMINATION

A doctor should never refuse to give a certificate when he can supply a cause of death simply in order to force the relations to consent to a post-mortem examination when they are unwilling to give that consent. If an autopsy is necessary to establish the cause of death then the coroner should have been informed.

There is no objection to a private post-mortem examination being made when the cause of death is known and is a result of natural causes. The examination should be performed, with the consent of the relations of the deceased, before the death certificate is completed, as the autopsy may reveal some material condition which was hitherto unsuspected.

A space is provided on the back of the death certificate to be initialed if further information, as, for example, a histological or bacteriological report, is likely to become available in the future.

During the post-mortem examination is may become apparent that the death should have been reported to the coroner, as where signs of poisoning or unsuspected trauma are revealed on internal examination. In such cases the autopsy should be suspended and the coroner informed as quickly as possible.

HUMAN TISSUE ACT, 1961

The provisions of this Act apply:—

1. When a person has requested, either in writing or orally in the presence of two witnesses, that his body be used for therapeutic purposes or for medical education or research, or

2. When the person in possession of the body is satisfied that the deceased expressed no objection and the next of kin do not object to use of tissues from the deceased.

The Act allows a fully registered doctor, who is satisfied that life is extinct, to remove the required part of the body. If there is any reason to believe that an inquest or coroner's post-mortem examination may be required, the coroner must authorize any interference with the body.

When organs, such as kidneys, are to be transplanted, it is essential to remove them as soon as possible after death. In order to do this and to arrange for the recipients to be prepared, the coroner must be approached before the patient dies. It is unfortunate that the patient with a head injury and irreversible cerebral damage is the ideal donor and also the most likely subject for a forensic inquiry.

The coroner gives his consent whenever possible, but the removal of a substantial part of the body can make the subsequent interpretation of the pattern of injuries very difficult. It is not likely that consent would be given when a charge of homicide was pending.

The doctor must have had the consent of the patient or of the relatives in addition to that of the coroner before he removes any tissue.

REFERENCE TO THE CORONER

When a doctor has certified the cause of death the registrar is under a duty to refer any of the following cases to the coroner:—

1. Where it appears from the certificate that the doctor signing it had not attended the deceased within 14 days of death or examined the body after death.

2. Where the cause of death, as certified, was due to violence or neglect, abortion, or in suspicious or unnatural circumstances.

3. Where the death occurred during an operation or before recovery from the anæsthetic.

4. When the death was due to any industrial disease or industrial poisoning.

This list will be seen to include all cases of poisoning by drugs, whether due to overdosage, toxic side-effects or allergy, and to poisoning by alcohol, acute or chronic. Deaths due to cirrhosis of the liver, unless certified as non-alcoholic, will be reported. The lapse of a period of time, however long, between an event which requires to be reported and the death of the patient does not make it unnecessary to report the case to the coroner.

Note.—It will be seen that there may be some days' delay before the registrar can notify the coroner of the circumstances of any death, particularly when the certificate is handed to a relation who has 5 days in which to register the death. To overcome this delay the doctor should notify the coroner's officer directly of any death that he does not believe to be due to natural disease or in which he thinks the coroner may have jurisdiction. There is a space on the back of the certificate for the doctor to initial if he has informed the coroner.

CREMATION

In cases where the death is due to apparently natural causes and the relations wish to have the deceased cremated, the doctor signing the death certificate gives, in addition, a Form B for the purposes of cremation. There must also be a confirmatory certificate from a second registered medical practitioner, who must be of at least 5 years' standing and who is not a relation of the deceased or the certifying doctor, nor a partner of the certifying doctor. These certificates, which require to be completed in considerable detail, are sent to the crematorium referee who may require a post-mortem examination or further inquiries to be made before furnishing the certificate for disposal.

A fee of 2 guineas is recommended for completion of these certificates, but the first certificate must be supplied by a hospital doctor without charge under the terms of his service.

Where a case is referred to the coroner these certificates are not required. The coroner issues his own certificate for cremation. Under the Cremation Regulations, 1965, it is now permissible to cremate a person who had left instructions to the contrary, and to cremate bodies that have undergone anatomical dissection and also unidentified remains.

STILLBIRTH

The law with regard to certification and registration of stillbirths is in a somewhat unsatisfactory state. A stillborn child is one which has issued forth from its mother after the 28th week of pregnancy and which did not at any time after being completely expelled from its mother breathe or show other signs of life. A certificate must be signed by the doctor or midwife, if one was present, that the child was not born alive. The birth, not the death, is registered within 6 weeks. If no doctor or midwife was present the mother may still register the birth within 6 weeks and make a declaration that the baby was born dead and no medical assistance was at hand. By this time it is difficult to prove otherwise. If the registrar has any reason to believe that the child was born alive he must inform the coroner.

THE CORONER

The coroner is a duly appointed barrister, solicitor, or medical practitioner, of at least 5 years' standing in his profession, whose duty it is to hold an inquiry on any dead body within his jurisdiction that is believed to have died a violent or unnatural death, a sudden death of which the cause is unknown, or in prison or in such place or under such circumstances as to require an inquest.

The coroner is not put upon inquiry until the death is reported to him and the advisability of doctors reporting certain cases directly to the coroner has already been considered. In Northern Ireland, under the Coroners' Act (Northern Ireland), 1959, a statutory duty is imposed upon every medical practitioner, registrar of deaths, funeral undertaker, occupier of a dwelling or person in charge of any premises where a deceased person was residing, who has reason to believe that the deceased person died:—

1. Either directly or indirectly as a result of violence or misadventure or unfair means, or

2. As a result of negligence or misconduct or malpractice on the part of others, or

3. From any cause *other than* natural illness or disease for which he had been seen and treated by a registered medical practitioner within 28 days prior to his death, or

4. In such circumstances as may require investigation (including death as a result of the administration of an anæsthetic).

The aforementioned person shall immediately notify the coroner within whose district the body of such deceased person is of the facts and circumstances relating to the death.

There is no such statutory duty in England and Wales, but this recent Act may serve as in indication of the types of case that should be reported to the coroner, although the period of 28 days mentioned is too long. If the doctor has not seen the deceased within 14 days of his death or examined the body afterwards, the registrar will report the death to the coroner.

In short, in any case where a certificate of death cannot be completed giving a natural cause of death, unconnected with any previous accident or notifiable disease, however long before, or where the last attendance on the deceased was not within 14 days of death, the coroner should be informed. There will then be no delay in completing any investigation and no risk of criticism by the coroner if the delay has hampered his inquiries.

The mere reporting of a case to the coroner, through his officer, does not mean that there will have to be an inquest. When a case is reported to the coroner, the coroner's officer, who is usually a policeman, makes some inquiries regarding the circumstances of the death and interviews the deceased's relations; the coroner sees the death certificate, if there is one, and may ask for further information from the certifying doctor. Some coroners have a form to be filled in giving details of deaths in hospital following an operation.

INQUIRY

As a result of this preliminary investigation the coroner will embark on one of three courses:—

1. He may issue a Form A stating that he is satisfied that the cause of death is as certified and that no further inquiry is necessary.

2. He may order a post-mortem examination by a suitable pathologist. A fee of 5 guineas is paid for this and a total of 8 guineas if the pathologist has to give evidence at an inquest. Additional fees are paid for special examinations such as barbiturate analysis. In the case of a death in hospital, a hospital pathologist should not perform the examination if he does not wish to do so or the conduct of another member of the staff might be called into question or any relative of the deceased has objected to his performing the examination. If the autopsy reveals that the death was due to natural causes—and this can include a properly performed operation necessitated by a natural condition—a Form B is issued by the coroner, the death registered, and no inquest held. The coroner should inform the relatives of the deceased, the doctors treating him, interested government departments, and, if necessary, the police of the time and place of the post-mortem. They may then be represented by a doctor at the autopsy if they wish, but the coroner need not delay the autopsy on this account. A doctor who wishes to be present at an autopsy should keep in touch with the coroner's officer, particularly when the body is removed to a public mortuary, and should ask for any particular specimen to be saved for his inspection if he is not certain that he can be present at the time of the autopsy.

3. He may hold an inquest. This is an inquiry held in public with evidence taken on oath from witnesses. Interested parties at an inquest may be represented by a lawyer and any person whose conduct might be called into question must be summoned or given notice of the hearing.

VERDICT

If any person is charged or is to be charged before the magistrates with murder, manslaughter, or infanticide, or causing death by dangerous driving, the inquest is adjourned for the trial to proceed. In all other cases the inquest proceeds before the coroner alone or sitting with a jury. A jury is always summoned when there is any chance that the verdict may result in a named person's committal to the assizes and where any Act requires a jury to be summoned, as in road traffic deaths.

After hearing the evidence the coroner or jury bring in a verdict stating who the deceased was, and when, where, and by what means he came to his death. The jury, but not the coroner alone, can bring in a verdict of murder, manslaughter, or infanticide by a named person. In this case the accused person is committed to the assizes for trial on the inquisition.

The verdict of the jury must not be framed in such a way as to appear to determine any question of civil liability. Despite this, the coroner's inquest is a valuable source of information for the legal representatives of any person who might sue or be sued as a result of the death in question. Any doctor whose actions might be questioned or criticized by the relations of the deceased is well advised to be legally represented and put his case forward at an early stage, even when there is no suggestion that there may be a verdict of manslaughter against him.

Finally, the coroner or jury makes any recommendation which is likely to prevent recurrences of fatalities similar to that in respect of which the inquest is being held. If there is any possibility that a system of work is likely to come under criticism, as in performing major surgical operations at a place remote from a blood bank, the persons responsible would be well advised to inform the court that the system has been or is being altered, before the rider is recorded and adverse publicity follows it.

CHAPTER LII

DEATH CERTIFICATION IN SCOTLAND

By Gilbert Forbes

CERTIFICATION of death is a duty imposed on members of the medical profession, which must be performed without fee, and failure to certify renders the doctor liable to a penalty. It is therefore necessary for practitioners to understand their obligations fully regarding certification.

It is illegal to dispose of a dead body without a registrar's certificate or a procurator fiscal's order.

In Scotland the statutes bearing on the subject are the Births, Deaths, and Marriages (Scotland) Acts, 1854–1960, and the Registration of Stillbirths (Scotland) Act, 1938. Under the former Acts the practitioner who has been in attendance on the deceased during his last illness must supply the registrar with a certificate of the cause of death to the best of his knowledge and belief. This certificate must be provided within 7 days. Should he fail to do so, the registrar must send him a certificate form partly filled in, with the request that the completed form be returned to him within 3 days after receipt, under a penalty not exceeding 40 shillings in case of failure. Although it is the responsibility of the doctor to transmit the certificate to the registrar, he usually employs the nearest relative as a messenger and hands the certificate to him. The registrar on receipt of an acceptable certificate will register the death and issue a certificate of registration, on which disposal of the body can be carried out. Before a doctor can usefully sign a death certificate without reference to the procurator fiscal, he must have been in attendance during the last illness, he must know the cause of death, and he must regard the death as due to natural causes.

The death certificate in Scotland does not contain, as in England, a notice to the informant. The certificate proper is directed to the registrar of the appropriate district and it certifies that the doctor attended the deceased, giving the date and place of death. In the body of the certificate should appear entries as to the disease or condition directly leading to death (and this does not mean the mode of dying, such as syncope, asphyxia, or coma), followed by the morbid conditions, if any, leading to the primary cause of death, and, last, any other significant condition not related to the disease or condition causing it, but contributing to a significant degree to the cause of death. There are spaces in which the duration of the fatal conditions are to be entered. The doctor should also indicate whether the certified cause takes account of post-mortem information, whether information from a post-mortem may be available later, or whether a post-mortem is not proposed. In certifying death, general terms, such as heart disease, must not be employed and the nature of the disease must be specifically stated. Each certificate of death must be on the appropriate form and books of certificate forms can be obtained by registered medical practitioners from the Registrar of Births, Deaths, and Marriages. There is no legal obligation on a practitioner to view the body after death to verify the fact of death, but he is well advised to do so. *Under no circumstances* should a practitioner be tempted to sign blank certificates or to sign a certificate of death of a person while he is still alive, though critically ill. This may expose the practitioner to a charge of false certification and his action might be deemed 'infamous conduct in a professional respect' by the General Medical Council, and might result in erasure of the practitioner's name from the Medical Register.

When not to issue a Certificate.—There are certain circumstances under which a Scottish practitioner should decline to issue a death certificate and should report the death to the procurator fiscal. The following general rules will act as a guide:—

1. If called to a sudden death and you have not seen the patient before, then you cannot issue a certificate and should report the death to the procurator fiscal.

2. If you have been attending a patient for some illness and he dies suddenly and unexpectedly, and you do not know the cause of death, then you should notify the procurator fiscal.

3. If you have been attending a patient for an illness which you expect to end fatally at any time and you have seen the patient recently (say within 14 days), you may issue a certificate, but you should view the body.

4. If you have not attended a patient recently but you knew that he was suffering from some condition likely to end fatally, then you may issue a certificate if you examine the body after death. In such cases you are advised to consult the procurator fiscal, who will advise you whether to certify or not.

5. If the deceased died as a direct or indirect result of an accident, notify the procurator fiscal.

6. Notify deaths in prison.

7. If an operation or an anæsthetic has contributed or may have contributed to the cause of death, notify the procurator fiscal.

STILLBIRTHS

The Registration of Stillbirths (Scotland) Act, 1938, requires that all stillbirths in Scotland be registered. For the purposes of the Registration Acts every birth will fall into one of three categories:—

1. A child who, whatever the duration of the pregnancy, breathes or shows any other sign of life after complete extrusion from the mother is a live birth and the birth must be recorded in the Register of Births. If the child dies, no matter how soon after birth, both the birth and the death should be registered.

2. The birth of a child before the end of the 28th week of pregnancy which shows no sign of life is not required to be registered. It is an abortion.

3. The birth of a child after the 28th week which does not show any sign of life is a stillbirth and must be registered as such in the Register of Stillbirths.

The informant in the case of a stillbirth must deliver to the registrar a stillbirth certificate signed by the doctor or midwife. The certificate, addressed to the registrar, certifies that the doctor or midwife was present at the stillbirth or has examined the body and that the child was not born alive. The doctor or midwife is further expected to state the probable cause of death of the child (Population (Statistics) Act, 1960). If no doctor or midwife was in attendance at the birth or examined the body, or if for any other reason his or her certificate cannot be obtained, then the informant must make a declaration to this effect and that the child was not born alive. It is unlawful to have the body of a stillborn child buried without a certificate from the procurator fiscal or the registrar.

A live birth must be notified to the Medical Officer of Health by the doctor or the father within 36 hours, and the birth must be registered with the Registrar of Births, Deaths, and Marriages within 21 days in Scotland.

CREMATION

Very closely linked with the subject of death certification is that of cremation, and the patient's relatives are entitled to expect that their doctor will be conversant with the regulations. The Cremation Acts of 1902 and 1952, and the regulations made thereunder, are applicable to Scotland as well as to England and Wales. The legal provisions with regard to cremation are contained in the Cremation (Scotland) Regulations made under these Acts, the most important being those of 1935. The death of the deceased must have been registered in the ordinary way and the registrar's certificate of registration must be produced. If the death has occurred in Northern Ireland an equivalent certificate of registration must be shown. When death has taken place in England or Wales, an acknowledgement by a coroner that notice of the intention to remove the body out of England or Wales has been received by him, together with an intimation that he does not intend to hold an inquest, or a certificate following an inquest is issued by the coroner. No cremation can take place if the deceased has specifically stated in writing to this effect, as, for example, in a Will. There are a number of documents other than the death certificate and the registrar's certificate of registration which must be completed before cremation can be authorized by the medical referee to the cremation authority:—

Form A.—This is an application to be made out by the executor or nearest surviving relative of the deceased, and this must have its contents verified by being countersigned by certain specialized categories of persons (member of parliament, barrister, solicitor, justice of the peace, medical practitioner, bank manager, etc.).

Form B.—This is an initial medical certificate to be completed by the usual medical attendant of the deceased, who certifies that he has attended the deceased before death and seen and identified the body after death.

Form C.—This is a confirmatory medical certificate which must be completed by a medical practitioner of at least 5 years' standing in his profession, who is neither a relative of the deceased nor a relative nor partner of the doctor completing Form B and who has consulted with the doctor signing Form B. He should have made an external examination of the body and have made some further inquiry, e.g., a post-mortem dissection or consultation with a relative or someone who has nursed the deceased.

Form F.—Normally these three documents, with the registrar's certificate of registration, are all submitted to the medical referee of the cremation authority. The cremation authority must appoint a medical referee and a deputy, and the appointments must be notified to the Secretary of State and the Scottish Home and Health Department. The medical referee considers the documents and, if he is satisfied with the cause of death, and is satisfied that it has been established that all the regulations have been fully complied with and that there is no occasion for further inquiry, he will complete Form F authorizing the cremation. On the other hand, in the event of any suspicious circumstances coming to his knowledge, whether revealed in the application, or the certificates, or otherwise, and in particular if the cause of death assigned on the medical certificates be such as might be due to poisoning, violence, illegal operation, privation, or neglect, or if there is any reason to suspect that death occurred while the deceased was under an anæsthetic, the medical referee must report the matter immediately to the procurator fiscal for investigation.

Form D.—If a post-mortem examination is carried out by or at the direction of the medical referee, or privately, because Forms B and C cannot be obtained, then the pathologist completes Form D which supersedes Forms B and C.

Form E.—Form E is completed by the procurator fiscal following the investigation of a case on his behalf. This supersedes Forms B, C, and D.

POST-MORTEM EXAMINATIONS

The Human Tissue Act, 1961, makes it lawful to conduct post-mortem examinations in hospitals, or rather removes any doubt as to their legality. It also gives authority for the removal after death of parts of the body which may be required for therapeutic purposes, for medical education, or for research. It should be pointed out that no post-mortem examination or other interference with a body ought to be made if the case is one calculated to put the procurator fiscal on inquiry.

THE INVESTIGATION OF SUDDEN AND UNNATURAL DEATHS

In Scotland there are no coroners and no inquests. The procurator fiscal performs the duties of the coroner, but while the coroner holds public inquests on a variety of cases other than deaths from natural causes, which are dealt with under Section 21 of the Coroners' Amendment Act, 1925, the procurator fiscal usually holds his inquiries in private. Under the Fatal Accidents and Sudden Death Inquiry (Scotland) Act, 1906, provision is made for public inquiries in the case of fatal accidents or in other cases where the Lord Advocate considers that the circumstances warrant a public inquiry. In these circumstances the procurator fiscal petitions the sheriff to hold a fatal accident inquiry and the sheriff gives his authority to cite witnesses and sits with a jury of seven. The evidence is led by the procurator fiscal and interested parties may be legally represented. Medical evidence is nearly always called at fatal accident inquiries.

INDEX

A disease caused by a chemical or any physical agent with which the patient comes in contact during the course of his employment must be notified to the Chief Inspector of Factories,* Baynards House, 1–13, Chepstow Place, Westbourne Grove, London, W.2. It should be understood that notification does not bind the doctor to his opinion that the disease is due to this or that agent; it merely puts the onus on the authorities to investigate the cause of the disease in that particular patient.

The importance of a good occupational history cannot be overstressed in all suspected cases of industrial disease.

Notifiable Industrial Diseases

Aniline Poisoning

Anthrax

Arsenical Poisoning

Carbon Bisulphide Poisoning

Chrome Ulceration, i.e., due to chromic acid of bichromate of potassium, sodium, or ammonium, or any preparation of these substances

Chronic Benzene Poisoning. Benzene used as an industrial solvent is perhaps the greatest cause of occupational leukæmia at the present time

Compressed-air Illness

Epitheliomatous Ulceration due to tar, pitch, bitumen, mineral oil or paraffin, or any compound, product or residue of any of these substances. It may not be obvious that the worker handles any of these materials when he describes the nature of his employment. For instance a brush-maker can use one of these derivatives to fix the bristles; a lens-grinder embeds the glass in pitch before grinding. The doctor should therefore ask specifically if any of these carcinogens are or were used in the trade which the patient follows or followed in the distant past. Of oils and paraffin, shale oil is the most potent

Lead Poisoning—this may be present as acute abdominal pain

Manganese Poisoning

Mercurial Poisoning

Phosphorus Poisoning

Toxic Anæmia

Toxic Jaundice, i.e., jaundice due to tetrachlorethane or nitro or amino derivatives of benzene or other poisonous substances

The notification should state the name, address, and occupation of the patient; the disease; the name and address of the factory (in the case of a painter, the premises on which he was working); the notifying doctor's name and address and the date of notification.

Forms for the purpose may be obtained from the Chief Inspector's Office, but a letter giving the above details will be accepted as a notification.

NEW AND OLD NOMENCLATURE FOR BACTERIA

New Nomenclature	Old Nomenclature
Escherichia coli	B. coli
Neisseria gonorrhœæ	Gonococcus
Pseudomonas aeruginosa	B. pyocyaneus
Mycobacterium tuberculosis	Tubercle bacillus
Clostridium welchii	B. Welchii
Salmonella typhi	Typhoid bacillus

---

* In Northern Ireland notification should be made to the Chief Inspector, Ministry of Health and Social Services, Dundonald House, Upper Newtownards Road, Belfast BT4 3SF.